D0757868

# High-Risk Pregnancy

## A Team Approach

**Second Edition**

Robert A. Knuppel, MD, MPH

Professor and Chairman
Department of Obstetrics & Gynecology
University of Medicine & Dentistry of New Jersey
Robert Wood Johnson Medical School
New Brunswick, New Jersey


Joan E. Drukker, RNC, MS

Adjunct Professor, School of Nursing
University of Pittsburgh
Director of Nursing, OB Services
Magee-Womens Hospital
Pittsburgh, Pennsylvania

**W.B. SAUNDERS COMPANY**
*A Division of Harcourt Brace & Company*
Philadelphia • London • Toronto • Montreal • Sydney • Tokyo

**W.B. SAUNDERS COMPANY**
*A Division of*
*Harcourt Brace & Company*

The Curtis Center
Independence Square West
Philadelphia, Pennsylvania 19106

RG
x . 571
.H45
1993

| | |
|---|---|
| **Library of Congress Cataloging-in-Publication Data** | |

High-risk pregnancy : a team approach / [edited by] Robert A. Knuppel,
   Joan E. Drukker.—2nd ed.
      p.  cm.
   Includes bibliographical references and index.
   ISBN 0-7216-3455-9
    1. Pregnancy, Complications of.  2. Labor, Complicated.
  I. Knuppel, Robert A.  II. Dauphinee, Joan E. Drukker.
   [DNLM: 1. Labor Complications.  2. Pregnancy Complications.
  WQ 240 H6375]
  RG571.H45  1993
  618.3—dc20
  DNLM/DLC

                                       91-43072

High Risk Pregnancy, A Team Approach, 2nd ed. ISBN 0-7216-3455-9

Printed in United States of America

Last digit is the print number:     9     8     7     6     5     4     3

*To*
*Herman and Marion Knuppel,*
*my father and mother.*

**Robert A. Knuppel**


*Eric Dauphinee, my husband,*
*for his support and patience.*

**Joan Drukker Dauphinee**

# Contributors

SHERRY ALLISON-COOKE, MA
Senior Research Associate, National
Perinatal Information Center,
Providence, RI
*Adaptations to Perinatal Regionalization*

MEICHELLE ARNTZ, RNC, BSN,
ACCE
Seminar Instructor, Weber State College;
Brigham Young University; Utah
Technical College UT; Unit Coordinator,
Fetal Assessment Center; Nursing
Coordinator, Perinatal Outreach,
Humana Hospital, Las Vegas, NV
*Preterm Labor*

GRETCHEN M.-E. AUMANN, BSN,
PhD
Assistant Professor Ob/Gyn, University
of Pittsburgh School of Medicine; Magee
Women's Hospital; Consortium Ethicist,
Consortium Ethics Program, University
of Pittsburgh Center for Medical Ethics,
Pittsburgh, PA
*Risk Assessment for Pregnant Women*

MARGARET M. BAIRD, LTC (P),
MSN, BSN
Head Nurse, Antepartum Service,
Walter Reed Army Medical Center,
Washington, DC
*Risk Assessment for Pregnant Women*

ABBE BENDELL, RN, MBA
Assistant Director of Nursing, Women's
Hospital Center, University of Miami;
Jackson Memorial Medical Center,
Miami, FL
*Cesarean Birth*

PAMELA G. BLAKE, RN, MSN
Clinical Nurse Specialist, Department of
Obstetrics and Gynecology, University of
Mississippi Medical Center, Jackson, MS
*Disseminated Intravascular Coagulation,
Autoimmune Thrombocytopenic Purpura,
and Hemoglobinopathies*

WINSTON A. CAMPELL, MD
Associate Professor, Obstetrics and
Gynecology; Associate Director,
Maternal-Fetal Medicine; Director,
Maternal-Fetal Intensive Care Unit;
John Dempsey Hospital, University of
Connecticut Health Center, Farmington,
CT
*Prolonged Pregnancy*

MARIA S. CASTILLO, RN, BSN
Department of Obstetrics and
Gynecology, Bexar County Hospital
District, Brady Green Community Clinic,
San Antonio, TX
*Bleeding in Pregnancy*

ROBERT C. CEFALO, MD, PhD
Professor of Obstetrics and Gynecology;
Director, Division of Maternal-Fetal
Medicine; Assistant Dean, Head of the
Office of Graduate Medicine Education,
University of North Carolina School of
Medicine, Chapel Hill, NC
*Nutrition in Pregnancy*

IRA J. CHASNOFF, MD
Associate Professor, Pediatrics,
Northwestern University Medical School;
President, National Association for
Perinatal Addiction Research and
Education, Chicago, IL
*Substance Abuse in Pregnancy*

BONNIE FLOOD CHEZ, RNC, MSN
Director, Women's Center, University
Community Hospital, Tampa, FL
*Fetal Assessment*

VICKI G. COLBURN, RN, BSN, MEd
Clinical Educator, Labor and Delivery,
Women's Hospital Center, University of
Miami, Jackson Memorial Medical
Center, Miami, FL
*Cesarean Birth*

DONALD R. COUSTAN, MD
Professor and Chairman, Obstetrics and
Gynecology, Brown University School of
Medicine; Obstetrician,
Gynecologist-in-Chief, Women and
Infants Hospital of Rhode Island,
Providence, RI
*Diabetes Mellitus in Pregnancy*

M. DOUGLAS CUNNINGHAM, MD
Professor of Clinical Pediatrics and
Neonatology, Division of
Neonatal/Perinatal Medicine,
Department of Pediatrics, California
College of Medicine, University of
California, Irvine; Medical Director,
Neonatology, Saddleback Women's
Hospital, Laguna Hills, CA
*Newborn Care in the Delivery Room*

MARINA DEVINEY, RT, RDMS
Senior Sonographer, University Hospital,
MacDonald Hospital for Women,
Cleveland, OH
*Ultrasound in Pregnancy*

JANICE M. DODDS, EdD, RD
Associate Professor in Nutrition, School
of Public Health, University of North
Carolina at Chapel Hill, Chapel Hill, NC
*Nutrition in Pregnancy*

JOAN E. DRUKKER, RNC, MS
Adjunct Professor, School of Nursing,
University of Pittsburgh; Director of
Nursing, OB Services, Magee-Womens
Hospital, Pittsburgh, PA
*Developing the Perinatal Team
Approach; Hypertension in Pregnancy;
Twins and Other Multiple Gestations*

ELIZABETH L. FABBRI, BSN, RDMS
Perinatal Nurse Specialist, Obstetrical
Ultrasound Department, Crawford Long
Hospital of Emory University,
Atlanta, GA
*Antepartum Assessment of the Fetus*

SEBASTIAN FARO, MD, PhD
Professor and Chairman, Department of
Gynecology and Obstetrics, Division of
Infectious Diseases, University of Kansas
School of Medicine, Kansas University
Medical Center, Kansas City, Kansas
*Perinatal Infections*

DAVID E. GAGNON
Clinical Assistant Professor, Brown
University Medical School; Executive
Director, National Perinatal Information
Center, Providence, RI
*Adaptations to Perinatal Regionalization*

STUART Z. GROSSMAN, JD
Grossman & Roth, Grand Bay Plaza,
Miami, FL
*The Nature of Lawsuits Related to
Obstetric Care*

EDWIN R. GUZMAN, MD
Assistant Professor, Maternal-Fetal
Medicine Division, Robert Wood
Johnson Medical School, University of
Medicine and Dentistry of New Jersey;
Specialist, St. Peter's Medical Center,
Robert Wood Johnson University
Hospital, New Brunswick, NJ
*Premature Rupture of the Membranes*

HUNTER A. HAMMILL, MD
Assistant Professor, Section of Infectious
Disease, Department of Obstetrics and
Gynecology, Baylor College of Medicine,
Texas Medical Center, Houston, TX
*AIDS in Pregnancy*

GARY D. V. HANKINS, MD
Professor of Obstetrics and Gynecology,
Uniformed Services University of the
Health Sciences; Chair, Department of
Obstetrics and Gynecology, Wilford Hall
US Air Force Medical Center, San
Antonio, TX
*Critical Care of the Pregnant Patient*

REGINA HANSON, RDMS
Sonographer, Advanced Technology Lab,
Bothell, WA
*Ultrasound in Pregnancy*

CAROL J. HARVEY, RNC, MS
Project Director, The Center for High
Risk and Critical Care Obstetrics,
Department of Obstetrics and
Gynecology, University of Texas Medical
Branch at Galveston, Galveston, TX
*Critical Care of the Pregnant Patient*

MILDRED G. HARVEY, RNC, MSN
Affiliate Faculty, University of
Tennessee, College of Nursing;
Obstetrical Clinical Nurse Specialist,
Baptist Memorial Hospital East,
Memphis, TN
*Maternal Adaptations to Pregnancy*

ROBERT H. HAYASHI, MD
J. Robert Willson Professor of Obstetrics,
Director of Maternal-Fetal Medicine,
Department of Obstetrics and
Gynecology, University of Michigan
Medical School, Ann Arbor, MI
*Bleeding in Pregnancy*

WILLIAM N. P. HERBERT, PhD, MD
Professor, Department of Gynecology and
Obstetrics; Associate Director,
Maternal-Fetal Medicine, University of
North Carolina, School of Medicine,
Chapel Hill, NC
*Nutrition in Pregnancy*

JOHN F. HUDDLESTON, MD
Professor and Director, Division of
Maternal-Fetal Medicine, Department of
Obstetrics and Gynecology, University of
Alabama at Birmingham,
Birmingham, AL
*Antepartum Assessment of the Fetus*

CHARLES J. INGARDIA, MD
Assistant Professor of Obstetrics and
Gynecology, University of Connecticut;
Director, Maternal-Fetal Medicine,
Hartford Hospital, Hartford, CT
*Additional Medical Complications in
Pregnancy*

KENNETH A. KAPPY, MD
Director of Obstetrics and Gynecology,
Newark Beth Israel Medical Center,
Newark, NJ
*Premature Rupture of the Membranes*

MARSHA E. KAYE, RN, MSN
Pediatric Nurse Practitioner, National
Association for Perinatal Addiction
Research and Education, Chicago, IL
*Substance Abuse in Pregnancy*

KENNETH R. KELLNER, MD, PhD
Associate Professor, College of Medicine,
Shands Hospital, University of Florida,
Gainesville, FL
*Grief Counseling*

JOHN H. KENNELL, MD
Professor of Pediatrics, Case Western
Reserve University, School of Medicine;
Attending Pediatrician, Chief, Division of
Child Development, Rainbow Babies'
and Children's Hospital, Cleveland, OH
*Parent Counseling*

MARSHALL H. KLAUS, MD
Adjunct Professor of Pediatrics,
University of California School of
Medicine; Director of Academic Affairs,
Children's Hospital, Oakland, CA
*Parent Counseling*

ROBERT A. KNUPPEL, MD, MPH
Professor and Chairman, Department of
Obstetrics and Gynecology, Robert Wood
Johnson Medical School, University of
Medicine and Dentistry of New Jersey,
New Brunswick, NJ
*Developing the Perinatal Team
Approach; Hypertension in Pregnancy;
Twins and Other Multiple Gestations*

MARIAN F. LAKE, RNC, MPH
Instructor, Department of Obstetrics and
Gynecology, Robert Wood Johnson
Medical School, University of Medicine
and Dentistry of New Jersey, New
Brunswick, NJ
*Grief Counseling*

JEFFREY LIPSHITZ, MB, ChB, MRCOG, FACOG
Professor of Obstetrics, University of Las Vegas Medical Center; Director, Perinatal Center Las Vegas, Las Vegas, NV
*Preterm Labor*

DEITRA L. LOWDERMILK, RNC, PhD
Clinical Associate Professor, School of Nursing, University of North Carolina, Chapel Hill, NC
*Sexual Intimacy During Pregnancy*

TREVOR MACPHERSON, MB, ChB, FRCOG
Associate Professor of Pathology, University of Pittsburgh School of Medicine; Chief of Pathology and Director of Research, Magee-Womens Hospital, Pittsburgh, PA
*Placental Pathology*

JAMES N. MARTIN, Jr, MD
Professor, Director Division of Maternal-Fetal Medicine, Department of Obstetrics and Gynecology, University of Mississippi Medical Center, Jackson, MS
*Disseminated Intravascular Coagulation, Autoimmune Thrombocytopenic Purpura, and Hemoglobinopathies*

ANNE L. MATTHEWS RN, PhD
Assistant Professor, Departments of Pediatrics and Nursing, University of Colorado; Associate Director, Genetic Counseling Program, University of Colorado Health Sciences Center and Genetic Services, The Children's Hospital, Denver, CO
*Genetic Counseling*

JOHN S. McDONALD, MD
Professor and Chairman, Department of Anesthesiology, Ohio State University Hospitals, Columbus, OH
*Anesthesia Principles for Labor and Delivery*

MARY McTIGUE, RNC, BSN
Associate Director of Nursing, Elizabeth General Medical Center, Elizabeth, NJ
*Premature Rupture of the Membranes*

SISTER JEANNE MEURER, CNM, MS
Associate Professor, Department of Community and Family Health, College of Public Health, University of South Florida, Tampa, FL; Board of Directors, SSM Health Care System, St. Louis, MO
*Prevention and Public Health in Obstetrics*

FRANK C. MILLER, MD
Professor and Chairman, Department of Obstetrics and Gynecology, University Hospital, University of Kentucky, Lexington, KY
*Fetal Assessment*

MICHAEL L. MORETTI, MD, FACOG
Director of Antepartum Testing and Ultrasound, Department of Obstetrics and Gynecology, St. Vincent's Medical Center of Richmond, Staten Island, NY
*Maternal Adaptations to Pregnancy*

JANE M. MURPHY, MPA
Director of Social Services, Medical Social Worker, Humana Women's Hospital of Tampa, Tampa, FL
*Psychosocial Implications of High-Risk Pregnancy*

C. A. MURTAGH, PA-C
Clinical Instructor, Baylor College of Medicine; HIV Clinical Obstetrical Coordinator for the Baylor Pediatric AIDS Clinical Trial Unit at Texas Children's Hospital and St. Luke's Episcopal Hospital; Special Mother's Coordinator for Pregnant Women with Substance Abuse Problems at The Shoulder and Ben Taub General Hospital, Houston, TX
*AIDS in Pregnancy*

DAVID J. NOCHIMSON, MD
Professor and Vice Chairman, Obstetrics and Gynecology, Associate Dean, School of Medicine, John Dempsey Hospital, University of Connecticut Health Center, Farmington, CT
*Prolonged Pregnancy*

JOSEPH G. PASTOREK II, MD
Professor and Chief, Section of Infectious
Disease, Member Section of
Maternal-Fetal Medicine, Department of
Obstetrics and Gynecology, Louisiana
State University School of Medicine,
New Orleans, LA
*Perinatal Infections*

KENNETH G. PERRY, Jr, MD
Assistant Professor, Department of
Obstetrics and Gynecology, Division of
Maternal-Fetal Medicine, University of
Mississippi Medical Center, Jackson, MS
*Disseminated Intravascular Coagulation,*
*Autoimmune Thrombocytopenic Purpura,*
*and Hemoglobinopathies*

ROY H. PETRIE, MD, ScD
Professor of Obstetrics and Gynecology,
Division of Maternal-Fetal Medicine,
Washington University, St. Louis, MO
*Labor; Induction of Labor*

JEFFREY P. PHELAN, MD, JD
Director, Maternal-Fetal Medicine,
Pomona Valley Hospital Medical Center;
San Antonio Community Hospital,
Pasadena, CA
*Cesarean Birth*

PATRICIA M. PIERCE, MD
Clinical Assistant Professor, Department
of Obstetrics and Gynecology, University
of Nevada (Reno); CA Humana Hospital
Sunrise, University Medical Center,
Women's Hospital, Las Vegas, NV
*Preterm Labor*

ELIZABETH FRANCES PITCHER, RN
Perinatal Clinical Nurse Specialist,
Hartford Hospital, Hartford, CT
*Additional Medical Complications in*
*Pregnancy*

WILLIAM F. RAYBURN, MD
Professor and Director, Division of
Maternal-Fetal Medicine, Department of
Obstetrics and Gynecology; Professor,
Department of Pharmacology, University
of Nebraska Medical Center,
Omaha, NE
*Medications in Pregnancy*

DEBORAH ROBBINS, RN, BSN, MPA
Senior Perinatal Consultant, Hill-Rom,
Boston, MA
*Psychosocial Implications of High-Risk*
*Pregnancy*

LEE ROTONDO, RN, MEd
Diabetes Nurse Specialist, Women and
Infants Hospital, Providence, RI
*Diabetes Mellitus in Pregnancy*

BARBARA C. RYNERSON, MS, RNC
Staff, School of Nursing, University of
North Carolina, Chapel Hill, NC
*Sexual Intimacy During Pregnancy*

ANN C. M. SMITH, MA
Consultant, Genetic Counselor,
Department of Obstetrics and
Gynecology, Georgetown University,
Washington, DC
*Genetic Counseling*

DOUGLAS L. TAREN, PhD
Asssistant Professor, Department of
Community and Family Health, College
of Public Health, University of South
Florida, Tampa, FL
*Prevention and Public Health in*
*Obstetrics*

KATHRYN E. TePAS, MSN, NNP
Instructor, Maternal-Child Nursing,
Eastern Kentucky University; Unit
Director, Special Care Nursery, Mount
Carmel Medical Center; Advisory Board
and Faculty for Central Ohio Regional
NNP Program, Columbus, OH
*Newborn Care in the Delivery Room*

JEAN CLAUDE VEILLE, MD
Associate Professor, Director of
Obstetrics, Special Studies, Director of
Maternal-Fetal Medicine, Fellowship
Program, North Carolina Baptist
Hospital; Forsyth Memorial Hospital,
Winston-Salem, NC
*Ultrasound in Pregnancy*

ANTHONY M. VINTZILEOS, MD
Professor, Obstetrics and Gynecology and
Pediatrics, PHS Professor and Endowed
Chair in Maternal-Fetal Medicine;
Director, Maternal-Fetal Medicine and
Obstetrics, John Dempsey Hospital,
University of Connecticut Health Center,
Farmington, CT
*Prolonged Pregnancy*

JULIE WEST, RNC, BSN
Perinatal Nurse, Arkansas High Risk
Pregnancy Program, Department of
Obstetrics and Gynecology, University of
Arkansas for Medical Sciences, Little
Rock, AR
*Fetal Assessment*

ATHANASIA M. WILLIAMS, RN, BSN
Staff, Department of Obstetrics and
Gynecology, Columbia Presbyterian
Medical Center, New York, NY
*Labor; Induction of Labor*

GAIL S. WILLIAMS, BSN
Perinatal Nurse Specialist, Division of
Maternal-Fetal Medicine, University of
Alabama, School of Medicine,
Birmingham, AL
*Antepartum Assessment of the Fetus*

# Preface

The response to the first edition of *High Risk Pregnancy: A Team Approach* has encouraged the publisher and coeditors to develop this second edition. The second edition continues to offer the perinatal team health care provider a comprehensive digest of the information necessary for modern health care of women with complicated pregnancies.

In addition to the most up-to-date, clinically relevant information available, this edition provides an incisive look at areas of rapid changes in women's health care. It is desired by the coeditors and authors that this text, while unique in being coauthored by physicians and nurses, will address many of the issues that unfortunately become isolated within medical or nursing arenas.

The genesis of this second edition is complementary to that of the first. While it builds on new information, its primary theme is to enhance communication between nursing and medical services. All too often, unnecessary schisms between the two approaches develop as a result of backgrounds and guidelines. The spirit of this textbook emanates from the need to continue to bridge these gaps and coordinate our services to better help our patients. Furthermore, it appears unreasonable to us to have individuals who work so closely together receive education and information that may be disparate and not developed in a symbiotic environment.

This textbook continues to represent the collective efforts of leading experts in obstetrics and gynecology. The editors would like to thank these busy and productive individuals for their time and effort in preparing this new edition.

The second edition contains several new chapters on "Prevention and Public Health in Obstetrics," "AIDS in Pregnancy," "Substance Abuse in Pregnancy," "Placental Physiology," and "Critical Care of the Pregnant Patient." This edition also emphasizes greater consumer sensitivity. The authors have recognized the patient as a person and emphasized communication and counseling techniques, as well as physical care.

We hope this edition meets the goals and expectations of our readers. We look forward to hearing your comments and suggestions regarding the contents of the entire textbook.

ROBERT A. KNUPPEL, M.D., M.P.H.
JOAN E. DRUKKER DAUPHINEE, R.N.C., M.S.

# Contents

# List of Patient Care Summaries

**PART I**

General
Considerations and
Assessment

# CHAPTER 1

# Developing the Perinatal Team Approach

Robert A. Knuppel and Joan Drukker Dauphinee

The team approach involves cooperation, collaboration, and communication. In obstetrics, this is a multispeciality approach focusing on total care management for the patients, their fetuses, and their families. The concept and development of the team are not unique to medicine. Examples of successful and unsuccessful teams are witnessed daily in politics, industry, and athletics. Although the products and outcomes in perinatal care are of higher cultural value, the management of the team is essentially the same.

A part of the team approach has been discussed in the literature as case management or managed care. The goals of a team approach system are not only quality care but also cost effectiveness. Bigelow and Young (1991) studied the effect of case management and found that case-managed clients received more services and experienced an improved quality of life as well as a reduction in hospital admissions. Although case management is designed to fit its specific institution, each system shares a common thread: a single health care professional who oversees, manages, and is accountable for the total health care management for the patient. This professional is usually a nurse, physician, or social worker who coordinates the day-to-day activities of the patient. The case manager assesses the need for resources to support and sustain health care management goals and monitors the patient regimen. Appropriate discharge planning and home health care are also coordinated by the case manager.

Case management describes critical paths and patient care time lines to outline the management a patient receives. These critical paths are also used by the perinatal team to manage patient care. Critical paths are specific and delineate when the patient should achieve certain care goals. When these goals are not met, the team discusses changes in the patient's care to get care back on track. Moving the patient along her particular critical path will help with timely discharges within diagnosis related groups (DRG), define appropriate length of stay, or may allow earlier discharge. If discharge should occur sooner than outlined by the critical path, then the management should be examined to determine if the length of stay could be shortened for other patients. The critical paths help to sequence interventions to avoid last minute oversights that might delay discharge planning.

An example of how critical paths can assist the team with care of the diabetic patient follows. At the Thursday high-risk clinic, the nurse and physician assess diabetic patients. If the patients need further education or increased insulin control, they are admitted on Friday. Although some tasks can be accomplished on Friday, many services are not available until Monday. Therefore, the patients are spending 3 unnecessary days in the hospital. If admissions are changed to Monday, the average length of stay for the patient is decreased, in most cases, from 4 to 5 days to 2 days. This is obviously more cost effective as well as more palatable for the patient and, therefore, increases patient compliance.

Because routine care is established for patients through critical paths, they serve as valuable orientation tools for nurses, residents, and other health care professionals. They can also be used to educate referring hospitals in the region, thus expanding the team approach to the referring hospitals in conjunction with the tertiary center.

Another advantage to team management is that as home health care for antepartum and postpartum patients continues to increase, resources can be redistributed. Nurses who work in the hospital can make home visits to these patients in addition to providing care within the hospital, thereby providing continuity of care.

## Leadership

The team must first develop a structure and hierarchy of command. The resources available are the key to the growth of the team. The constituents of the team are dictated by institutional goals, geography, competition, and myriad sociopolitical factors. Each team is designed based on these constraints; to ignore these would set up unrealistic goals that initiate frustration and discontent. On the other hand, some of these obstacles, such as restrictions on education and academic pursuits, can be overcome by educating the resistant forces.

The "Chief Executive Officer" of the medical and perinatal hierarchy is generally a physician. The same person is usually the director of obstetrics. The maternal and child nurse director is parallel to the physician. Just as the medical director coordinates the physicians, the nursing director directs the nurses. The nurse hierarchy is more structured and should adapt well to a team approach. The leadership qualities necessary to effectively lead the team are extensive and difficult to enumerate. There is no question, however, that the structure of the entire system comes from the top. The hiring, firing, purchasing, cost containment, and direction are guided through the physicians, who are comparable to CEOs of the health care team. These team leaders should fit comfortably into the framework of the institution and pick the right people to whom the leaders can delegate responsibility and authority.

The complexity of the team depends on the resources the organization wishes to provide. Table 1–1 provides an extensive list of team

**Table 1–1**
CONSTITUENTS OF THE OBSTETRIC TEAM

Perinatal nurse
Neonatologist
Obstetric anesthesiologist
Sonographer
Geneticist
Maternal fetal medicine specialist
Medical physician with special interest in pregnancy
Biostatistician epidemiologist
Maternal dietician and lactation consultant
Social worker
Ethicist
Risk manager
Respiratory therapist
Occupational therapist
Physical therapist
Dietician

members located in an institution who provide a majority of services in a perinatal system. As the chapter on regionalization (see Chapter 4) strengthens the concept that resources are more important than levels of care, the services the team provides are more important than the designation of levels of care.

The patient and her family are an integral part of the perinatal team. Discussions of care and treatment, critical paths, progress, and outcomes contribute to successful patient care. When families play a role in health care decisions, their compliance is increased, and they are usually more satisfied with the patient's care (Giuliano, 1991).

Table 1–2 outlines several microsystems from which the individual can choose a subset for his or her perinatal unit. Obviously, these roles overlap. The strengths of one division should not weaken the other divisions, nor should the weaknesses of one drain the others. Rather, the structure of the system and the lines of authority should identify weaknesses and provide support and guidance for improvement. The structure allows

**Table 1–2**
PERINATAL TEAM MEMBERS

Director of Obstetrics/MCH Nursing Director
Directors who will collaborate with the Team Leaders:
Head Nurses/Nurse Managers
Director of Research
Director of Ultrasonography
Director of Ambulatory Care
Director of Outreach Education (CMEs and CEUs)
Director of Genetics
Director of Medical Complications and Critical Care

clear communication, rapid decision-making, and authority. Responsibility is thereby delineated and focused. The obstetric team should meet frequently enough to make sure the system is reasonably responsive to change. This may mean daily or weekly meetings in addition to daily rounds that are made by part or all of the team. Monthly morbidity, genetics, and even department meetings should be open to *all* members of the team.

The physician directors must align themselves with the nurses (Table 1–3) and complement the medical directive. Although it is recognized that nursing and medicine traditionally have separate authorities, it makes sense to have a nurse and physician share the direction of the team.

The nurse codirector interacts with the various perinatal team members outside of the medical field while the physician codirector orchestrates the medical personnel. Working together, they can coordinate the entire team. The nurse case manager is probably a clinical nurse specialist or nurse manager, who reports to a director or vice president. The case manager manages patient care issues and collaborates with the director or vice president on administrative issues. The nurse case manager is the most consistent member of the team, because changes occur in rotations of perinatologists, attending physicians, residents, and students.

Perinatal team members ideally view their work as a vocation rather than as employment. The work place then assumes an importance beyond being defined as a place where the job is performed. Pride becomes an intangible, important reward for the team members that should be attainable within the system.

The evolution of the perinatal team has been relatively slow, considering the explosion of perinatal technology. The number of disciplines and the amount of information required for effective communication has enlarged. Cognitive stimulation is essential to understanding and enjoyment in the work place.

## Education

The employer should consider ongoing education essential to the health care and stability of his or her economic unit. The education should be both intramural and extramural. Nurses are often the last to be subsidized for education, yet they are the frontline care providers the client will contact within an institution or even a private practice setting. In reality, the nurse is the representative of the office, hospital, and home care team; his or her education should be paramount. Furthermore, cross-fertilization of perinatal issues is integral to intellectual growth. One unit can respond to inevitable questions from patients only if each unit is knowledgeable about the other units' procedures and policies. This is true among services within the hospital as well as between hospitals.

The dietician requires particular specialization in maternity and medical complications. The social worker should understand the prognosis and extent of the complication to effectively communicate to the patient, referring agency, or third-party insurance carrier. All members need to recognize the positive value of quality assurance and risk management.

## An Example of a Team Development

An obstetrician and either a head nurse, clinical specialist, or case manager, with input from the maternal and child director of nursing, decide to develop the team concept. Meetings are established first with labor and delivery nurses to define their goals. Statistics are generated to directly influence shifting of resources, if necessary. Policies and procedures are reviewed and updated with both nursing and physician input.

As the labor and delivery unit becomes more directed, the leaders turn to the ante-

**Table 1–3**
NURSING SERVICES

Antepartum unit
Antepartum surveillance unit
Ambulatory and home care services
Labor and delivery unit
Postpartum unit
Critical care unit
Nurses to assist in invasive perinatal procedures
Liaison to neonatal intensive care unit (NICU),
    normal newborn, and home nursing

partum care within the institution. The antepartum area is considered a unit with ongoing education and consistent nursing specialization in antepartum surveillance. The nurses join with a maternal-fetal medicine (MFM) specialist, a social worker, and a dietician to make rounds daily. Patient care rounds are held each week to determine the needs of the patient. Representatives from ambulatory care, labor and delivery, occupational therapy (OT), and physical therapy (PT) are also in attendance for continuity. A computer-generated hard copy of the patient's name, gestational age, and complications is provided daily to all units involved in the longitudinal care of the patients.

Postpartum care should not be forgotten, even when normal outcomes occur. Continued support after this difficult time is important for parenting and follow-up for mothers and infants with complications. Therefore, neonatology and mother-baby nurses are an integral part of the team.

The extension of continuity of care is now turned toward the clinic and private office. Antepartum surveillance must be reported to the responsible physician daily. This could easily be achieved through telecommunication to the office or clinic the moment the procedure has been completed.

Other specialities are then included in the team as needs arise. Genetic evaluation is one of the newest team responsibilities. A geneticist, counselor, and sonographer are necessary to evaluate the fetal condition in women older than 35 years of age, women exposed to potential teratogens, and women who have a history of genetic disorders. This unit evaluates any fetus at risk from genetic or environmental exposure and is very important to the advancement of research and education. The development of a multidisciplinary fetal evaluation panel will enable regions to develop strength and expertise in molecular genetics, embryology, fetal syndromes, and techniques for early fetal assessment. Although 98 percent of the perinatal genetic procedures result in a normal outcome, it is vital that team members remember that the possibility of undergoing invasive procedures and receiving information that the fetus may be at risk is as stressful as one can imagine for the pregnant women. Team members should place themselves in the position of the mother who is normal but over 35 years of age. What does

the patient envision when she is aware that a 7-centimeter needle will be placed through her abdomen into the sac of fluid or into the baby's placenta, and that in 1 in 350 pregnancies, the fetus may be found to be abnormal? Strong psychologic support and a continuance of sensitivity to the difficulties faced by these mothers will help health care professionals to extend more humanistic care.

Unlike a decade ago, the need for establishment of fetal imaging 7 days a week along with chorionic villus cultures and molecular genetics place a demand of the highest priority on institutions that wish to provide genetic services. Obviously, ethics is intimately involved. Each institution considers the negative and positive aspects of handling these very difficult cases. Often, physicians and referring institutions take these procedures less seriously until they have had an abnormal outcome. It is then that the backup of a well-educated, up-to-date team, including social worker, genetic counselor, medical geneticists, and advanced sonographers, becomes paramount. This is a very costly system, and serious thought must be given to whether it can be effectively developed within a particular unit.

The newness of this genetics program emphasizes the ongoing growing pains of the perinatal team. It is, therefore, incumbent on us to maintain ongoing education in case discussion. Ignorance within the unit leads to lack of understanding, fear, hostility, and insensitivity to many of the patients' complaints.

Finally, the team has now developed into a well-honed, large unit that communicates, cooperates, and pursues new challenges to provide quality patient care. It requires constant change on a microsystem level over the next several years (Table 1–4).

**Table 1–4**
AREAS TO EMPHASIZE IN DEVELOPING A TEAM

Communication
Cooperation
Exchange of information
Education of team members
Telecommunications
Pride

## Summary

The development of quality care requires commitment, resources, and leadership. It is wise to visit other centers to evaluate their successes and failures. No two programs are identical; however, new ideas on administration, construction, resource management, and patient care can be brought home and molded to your system. The codirectors and hospital administrators should visit these sites to encourage a better understanding of what can be developed. Community outreach is essential to delineate the needs of the community. Response to community care will be misdirected unless time is spent with community leaders to discuss the regional care needs. Furthermore, biostatisticians and epidemiologists help the unit to keep the needs of the community in focus.

It takes caring, educated, self-starting individuals to make the team successful; time must be allowed for the team to grow and mature. As described here, the perinatal team can be in various stages of development and have various corresponding needs. The young, newly developed team benefits greatly from leadership that provides structure and direction while simultaneously allowing freedom for growth. A team that has been functioning for several years may need to review its priorities, and at the same time, take pride in its accomplishments. The established team, although continuing to meet regularly and provide patient care, may be experiencing benign neglect. Review and revitalization of protocols with the possible addition of new members may energize this team.

Regardless of how long the unit has been in existence, leaders must be aware that the lack of personal chemistry destroys the most efficient unit over a prolonged period of time. Leaders must be actively involved in team function and must continuously evaluate the team's effectiveness. Data collection and analysis helps provide objective evidence of success and the need for new direction.

## References

Bigelow DA, Young DJ: Effectiveness of a cast management program. Community Ment Health J 27(2):56–60, 1991.

Dunston J: How managed care can work for you. Nursing 90, pp. 115–123, October 1990.

Giuliano KK, Poirier CE: Nursing care management: critical pathways to desirable outcomes. Nurse Management, 22(3):52–55, 1991.

Rogers M, Swindle D: Community-based nursing care pays off. Nursing Management, 22(3):30–34, 1991.

Wolfe K: Using information to optimize case management. AAOHN-J, 38(10):504–6, 1990.

# CHAPTER 2

. . . . . . . . . . . . . . . . . . . . . . . . . . . . . . . . . . . . . .

# Risk Assessment for Pregnant Women

Gretchen M.-E. Aumann and Margaret M. Baird

Fifty years ago it was not uncommon to know or at least to know of someone who died in childbirth. At that time every young woman about to become a mother was realistically concerned about her safety. A healthy baby was considered an extra dividend. From the obstetric viewpoint, maternal survival was of primary importance and in some instances even living fetuses were sacrificed for the mother's safety (Burchell and Gunn, 1980).

The focus of obstetric care has changed during the past years. There has been a significant reduction in maternal mortality and morbidity as a result of advances in the management of disorders that have an adverse effect on the pregnant woman. However, there has been a less significant reduction in perinatal mortality and morbidity. In many ways, morbidity exerts a more profound economic effect than mortality (Wallace, 1971).

"The perinatal death rate is . . . like an iceberg, for we see only a portion of ill results, the deaths. But we must not forget the submerged and large fraction, the near deaths and the harm which they may cause. The correlation is suggestive because some causes of death—premature delivery, asphyxia during labor, rhesus incompatibility—are known to be associated with the occurrence of mental or physical defects in some of the survivors. With a reduction in perinatal mortality there will also follow *pari passu* a diminution in perinatal morbidity." (Mixon and Hickson, 1952).

---

The views of the authors do not purport to reflect the position of the Department of the Army or the Department of Defense.

Childbirth itself is described as part of the continuum of human development, affected by physical, biologic, psychologic, and social factors (Chez et al, 1977). The ideal time for assessment of this event is well before the antenatal period, because the majority of factors affecting perinatal outcome are present prior to conception (Hobel, 1976). Additionally, most pregnant patients have already passed the period of fetal development most greatly affected by adverse factors by the time they first seek prenatal care. Consequently, to promote perinatal safety, it is necessary to identify those who are at risk and then to provide the specific care required to prevent death or damage.

Because the fetus in any given pregnancy is now at greater risk than the mother, the concept of "at risk" is applied to both maternal and fetal outcome. A "high-risk" pregnancy is defined as one in which the mother or the fetus has a significantly increased chance of death or disability, when compared with a "low-risk" pregnancy in which an optimal outcome is expected for both (Chez et al, 1977). The perinatal period, as a stage on the continuum, is unique in that outcome is frequently reliant upon the early recognition and management of problems. Assessment of the existence of risks, together with appropriate and timely intervention, can help prevent disabling conditions both during the neonatal period and in future stages along this linear continuum.

The aim of obstetric care is to concentrate resources on improving perinatal outcome. A multidisciplinary approach—an expensive form of health care requiring highly skilled manpower, equipment, and specialized facilities—is necessary to achieve this aim. The concept of regionalization of perinatal care implies the concentration of personnel and equipment in designated medical centers, where care is provided for all high-risk pregnancies in a defined geographic area. This approach to care of the obstetric patient is cost-effective and makes better use of highly skilled personnel, contributing to improved perinatal outcome.

This chapter discusses the philosophy and history of screening for the high-risk pregnancy. Standards of normal prenatal care are presented. Definitions and classifications of high-risk pregnancy are discussed, including socioeconomic, demographic, maternal, medical, and fetal factors contributing toward increased risk in pregnancy. Recommendations for prevention of perinatal morbidity are presented, along with a summary of goals for improvement in outcome.

## History and Philosophy of Risk Assessment in Obstetric Care

The idea that certain events that occur during the antenatal and intrapartum periods can have an adverse effect on the infant in later life is not a new one. As early as 1862, the association between abnormal labor and premature birth, and the child's subsequent mental and physical status was noted by London physician W. J. Little. It was not until the 1950s, nearly 100 years later, that significant work was done on even one specific abnormal neonatal outcome, that of cerebral palsy. In 1951, a retrospective study by Lilienfeld and Passamanick showed that five factors—prematurity, multiple birth, previous stillbirths, toxemia, and placental abnormalities—were associated with later development of cerebral palsy in the infant (Hobel, 1976).

These investigators also found that prematurity or other neonatal conditions alone were associated with an increased incidence of epilepsy. Additionally, they noted that the combination of a neonatal condition with maternal complications was associated with a twofold increase in the incidence of epilepsy. By 1955, it was clear that the five factors were related to perinatal morbidity and mortality.

In 1957 and 1958, Donnelley and associates and Wells and associates, respectively, identified socioeconomic status, maternal age, and birth interval to be significant factors in perinatal mortality, particularly in conjunction with the previously identified factors. These studies served to validate a later study by Prechtl (1967), whose data suggested that nonoptimal conditions occur in association with each other (Hobel, 1976).

Two major prospective studies published in the 1960s and 1970s furthered progress in identification of risk factors. These were the British Perinatal Mortality Survey (Butler and Bonham, 1963), which reviewed all births in Great Britain during a short period, and the Collaborative Perinatal Study, *The Women and Their Pregnancies* (Niswander and Gordon, 1972), which examined a small population for several years. These studies clearly implicated the interrelationship among perinatal factors and made an early attempt to identify factors responsible for later morbidity in children up to age 7 years. They also identified 13 additional factors adversely affecting perinatal outcome, including lack of prenatal care, length of labor, and smoking (Table 2–1).

In total, there are 21 factors identified in these studies as significantly contributing to increased perinatal mortality and morbidity. All of these factors are almost evenly divided between historical and pregnancy-related factors. These studies, therefore, provided the criteria necessary for the development of specific risk assessment techniques.

Risk assessment systems are used to provide a rational basis for identifying differential or prophylactic interventions that may be required in the course of pregnancy, labor, or delivery. Based on factors identified in early studies as well as subsequently recognized factors, formal risk-scoring systems attempt to improve pregnancy outcomes for mothers and babies by quantifying risk factors according to their relative contribution to adverse perinatal outcomes. Several risk-assessment tools have been developed, including the popular scoring system of Hobel and associates (1976). A summary of these systems can be seen in Table 2–2.

An example of a risk-assessment tool for preterm labor that used quantitatively weighted factors can be seen in Table 2–3. A trend has developed to remove numerical weights from the risk assessment process (Holbrook et al, 1989). Factors are either

**Table 2–1**
LITERATURE SURVEY OF DETERMINANTS OF
PERINATAL MORBIDITY AND MORTALITY

| Investigations | Factors |
| --- | --- |
| Lilienfeld and Parkhurst (1951) and Lilienfeld and Passamanick (1955) | 1. Prematurity<br>2. Multiple birth<br>3. Previous stillbirth or infant death<br>4. Toxemia<br>5. Placental abnormalities |
| Donnelly et al (1957) and Wells et al (1958) | 6. Socioeconomic status<br>7. Maternal age<br>8. Birth interval |
| Butler and Bonham (1969) and Butler and Alberman (1969) | 9. Parity<br>10. No prenatal care<br>11. Prolonged labor<br>12. Short labor<br>13. Breech birth<br>14. Smoking |
| Niswander and Gordon (1972) | 15. History of infertility<br>16. Organic heart disease<br>17. Diabetes<br>18. Urinary tract infection<br>19. History of vaginal bleeding<br>20. Incompetent cervix<br>21. Hydramnios |

Data from Hobel CJ, *In* Spellacy W (ed): Management of the High Risk Pregnancy. Baltimore, University Park Press, 1976.

present or absent. However, although no weights are used, identifying some variables as major factors, and others as minor factors, implies that a form of weighting has occurred.

Criteria for an effective scoring system include the following: first, the method should be comprehensive, well validated, objective, and reliable in scoring by multiple users; second, it must be relatively simple, cost effective, and readily accepted by both health care providers and patients; and finally, the system should be reasonably predictive, showing a correlation between increasing risk score and worsening perinatal outcome (Goodwin, 1969).

Given the complex and dynamic nature of pregnancy, the prospect of a single risk-assessment system fulfilling these criteria is not particularly bright. For instance, most obstetric researchers would agree that about one third of the problems that can arise during a pregnancy actually arise at the time of delivery and are not predictable by the systems presently in use (Forney and Whitehorne, 1982; Rayburn et al, 1987).

Wilson and Schifrin (1980) comment that the diagnosis of low-risk pregnancy is one to be made only in retrospect. Moreover, a tension exists between the general public's expectations of ideal outcome for mothers and infants sought through risk assessment and the realities of contemporary obstetric care and knowledge as quantified in risk assessment systems.

For example, when a risk assessment system works well there are few false-negative and false-positive results. The *sensitivity* of a risking system indicates its ability to identify correctly patients with a certain problem or condition. A high false-negative rate means that many women and infants who actually are at risk remain unidentified throughout the assessment periods. *Specificity* is an indication of the system's ability to identify those women without a problem. Therefore, a false-positive rate is a measure of the number of women inappropriately assessed as high risk.

Cutoff points or threshold values for high risk are essentially arbitrary, depend on the goals of the users, and reflect the societal values and resources available to provide obstetric care. Decreasing the number of false-negative assessments made would increase the proportion of pregnancies identified as high risk, and would concomitantly increase the number of patients requiring intensive services. In addition, increasing the sensitivity to lower the proportion of false-negative results would decrease the specificity of the system, thereby subjecting women inaccurately called high risk to expensive interventions they may not need or want.

At present, no one particular assessment tool has been identified as ideal. It is generally recognized, however, that a combination of preconception, prenatal, and intrapartum factors contribute to placing the mother/infant dyad at risk. These factors and their potential for risk are identified and discussed in light of present research.

## Standards of Prenatal Care

The prenatal period involves complex physiologic changes and emotional adjustments for the pregnant woman. These changes affect not only the woman and the fetus but also her family and the significant others in her social environment. Whatever

*Text continued on page 15*

**Table 2–2**

SUMMARY OF REPORTED OBSTETRIC RISK-SCORING SYSTEMS

| Author(s) | System | Year(s) Data Collected | Sample Size | Type of Study* | Purpose | When Used | Period Assessed | Definition of High Risk | Predictive Ability (High Risk Only)† | Outcomes Studied |
|---|---|---|---|---|---|---|---|---|---|---|
| Rogers | Risk register | 1959, 1964 | 13,020 | R | Detect handicapped children | Birth to 1 month | Antepartum Intrapartum Neonatal | 1 or more factors present | | Neonatal death |
| Donahue and Wan | Prematurity risk score | 1965, 1966 | 1716 | R | Predict premature births | | Antepartum Neonatal | Sum of (factor value × weighted variable) = 25th percentile | | |
| Prechtl | Obstetric complications score | 1967 | 1378 | R | Predict abnormalities | Day 2 to day 14 | Antepartum Intrapartum Neonatal | ≤ 7 factors present | | |
| Effer | Prognostic risk score | 1967 1968 | 211 350 | P | Identify high-risk prenatal patients | Onset of labor | Antepartum Intrapartum Neonatal | Correction factor × sum of factors 43 > 50 | | Perinatal mortality 1-min Apgar score |
| Nesbit and Aubry | Semi-objective grading system (Maternal-Child Health Care Index) | 1969 | 1001 | R | Identify patients with poor outcomes | Initial prenatal visit | Antepartum | Sum of factors 100 < 70 | *Preterm Delivery* / *Low-birth-weight:* Sens = .469 / .432; Spec = .713 / .728; +PV = 102 / .196 | Preterm delivery, low-birth-weight, labor complications, cesarean delivery, perinatal morbidity and mortality |
| Goodwin et al | Antepartum fetal risk score | 1969 | 936 | R | Predict fetal risk | Onset of labor | Antepartum | Sum of factors ≥ 6 | *Perinatal Mortality* / *5-min Apgar < 4:* Sens = .778 / .673; Spec = .971 / .979; +PV = .830 / .805 | Perinatal mortality 5-min Apgar score < 4 |
| Yeh et al | Antepartum fetal risk score | 1971, 1973 | 266 | P | Evaluate Goodwin's high-risk scoring system | Onset of labor | Antepartum | Sum of factors ≥ 4 | | 1- and 5-min Apgar < 7 Umbilical arterial blood pH at birth Fetal scalp blood pH Fetal heart rate patterns |
| Morrison and Olson | Antepartum fetal risk score (Goodwin et al) | 1977 | 16,733 | P | Test validity of Goodwin's scoring system | Antepartum | Antepartum | Sum of factors ≥ 3 | Sens = .679; Spec = .820; +PV = .070 | Perinatal mortality |
| Foy and Backes | Antepartum fetal risk | 1977 | 96 | P | Evaluate Goodwin's high-risk scoring system | Onset of labor | Antepartum | Sum of factors ≥ 4 | *Perinatal Morbidity* / *Perinatal Mortality:* Sens = .875 / 1.0; Spec = .925 / .80; +PV = .70 / .05 | Perinatal morbidity and mortality |

*Table continued on following page*

**Table 2–2**

SUMMARY OF REPORTED OBSTETRIC RISK-SCORING SYSTEMS *Continued*

| Author(s) | System | Year(s) Data Collected | Sample Size | Type of Study* | Purpose | When Used | Period Assessed | Definition of High Risk | Predictive Ability (High Risk Only)† | Outcomes Studied |
|---|---|---|---|---|---|---|---|---|---|---|
| Copeland et al | Antepartum fetal risk score (Goodwin et al) | 1977 | 5459 | R | Education | Ante- and intrapartum, neonatal periods | Antepartum Intrapartum Neonatal | None | Correlation of increasing risk with worse outcome | Apgar scores, birth weight, prematurity, neonatal intensive care, perinatal mortality |
| Akhtar and Sehgal | Prepartum and intrapartum risk-scoring method (modified from Copeland et al) | 1978 | 300<br>924 | R<br>P | Identify high-risk patients | Ante- and intrapartum periods | Antepartum Intrapartum Neonatal | Sum of factors >6 | **Sens** / **Spec** / **+PV**<br>.70 / — / —<br>.255 / .899 / .259<br>.251 / .900 / .279<br>.356 / .898 / .211 | Perinatal mortality, preterm birth, low-birth-weight, Apgar score < 7 |
| Edwards et al | | 1974–1977 | 2085 | P | Predict neonatal morbidity and mortality | Antepartum | Antepartum | Sum of factors ≥ 7 | Sens = .886<br>Spec = .545<br>+PV = .06 | Perinatal mortality |
| Haeri et al | Perinatal mortality risk score | 1969, 1970 | 7912 | P | Find statistically valid method that has good prediction and is easy to use | First visit | Antepartum | Sum of factors ≥ 4 | Sens = .329<br>Spec = .865<br>+PV = .057 | Perinatal deaths |
| Stembera et al | Identification of high-risk factors | 1969, 1972 | 3500 | P | Predict high-risk neonate and infant | Ante- and intrapartum, neonatal infancy | Antepartum Intrapartum Neonatal Infancy | Sum of factors ≥ 40 | | |
| Hobel et al | Screening to predict high-risk neonate | 1969, 1971 | 738 | P | Predict high-risk neonate | Ante- and intrapartum, neonatal periods | Antepartum Intrapartum Neonatal | Sum of factors ≥ 10 | **Antepartum**<br>Sens = .504<br>Spec = .685<br>+PV = .228<br>**Intrapartum**<br>.669<br>.701<br>.293 | Neonatal morbidity and mortality |
| Sokel et al | Hobel et al | 1976 | 1275 | P | Predict high-risk neonate | Ante- and intrapartum periods | Antepartum Intrapartum | Sum of factors ≥ 10 | **Antepartum**<br>Sens = .842<br>Spec = .521<br>+PV = .051<br>**Intrapartum**<br>.974<br>.550<br>.062 | Perinatal death and Apgar scores < 7 |
| Baruffi et al | Hobel et al | 1977, 1978 | 1600 | R | Predict high-risk neonate | Ante- and intrapartum periods | Antepartum Intrapartum | Sum of factors ≥ 10, ≥ 20 | **Antepartum Risk ≥ 10**<br>Sens = .379<br>Spec = .724<br>+PV = .259<br>**Intrapartum Risk ≥ 20**<br>.648<br>.552<br>.259 | Neonatal morbidity |
| Winters et al | Hobel et al | | 62 | R | Evaluate usefulness of Hobel's risk-assessment system | Postpartum | Antepartum Intrapartum | Sum of factors ≥ 10 | Sens = 1.0<br>Spec = .091<br>+PV = .058 | "Poor neonatal outcome" defined as sum of any of the following: |

*Table continued on following page*

| Author | Name of score | n | Year | R/P | Purpose | Period | Scoring method | Results | Outcome |
|---|---|---|---|---|---|---|---|---|---|
| Rey et al | | 665 | | R | Evaluate Hobel's risk-assessment system | Ante- and intrapartum, neonatal periods | Sum of factors ≥ 10 | Higher scores during ante- and intrapartum periods were significantly associated with more neonatal complications | 1. Apgar score ≤ 5 at 1 or 5 min<br>2. Low-birth-weight (< 2500 g)<br>3. Large for gestational age<br>4. Estimated gestational age < 37 weeks or > 42 weeks<br>5. Neonatal problems<br>6. Neonatal intensive care unit admission |
| Fedrick | | 793 | 1976 | R | Antenatal identification of women at risk of preterm delivery | Antepartum | Multiplication of factors ≥ 5 | **Primiparas** Sens = .094 Spec = .996 $^+$PV = .291    **Multiparas** Sens = .253 Spec = .992 $^+$PV = .347 | 1- and 5-min Apgar scores<br><br>Preterm birth |
| McCarthy et al | Antepartum fetal risk score | 230 585 | 1974 1976 1977 | R | Predict neonatal death | Antepartum | Sum of factors ≥ 76 | Sens = .006 Spec = .99 $^+$PV = .195 | Neonatal mortality |
| Jones et al | Prenatal risk of interhospital transfer leading to neonatal death | 1021 | 1974 to 1977 | P | Predict transfer of infants for neonatal intensive care | Antepartum | Sum of factors ≥ 7 | **Neonatal Death** Sens = .706 Spec = .983 $^+$PV = .041    **Transfer** Sens = .688 Spec = .749 $^+$PV = .150 | Neonatal death; interhospital transfer for perinatal care |
| Adelstein and Fedrick | | 490 | 1978 | R | Predict low-birth-weight infant at term | During third trimester | Multiplication of scores = composite relative risk | | Low-birth-weight |
| Kennedy | Women Infant Care obstetric risk score | 1328 | 1973, 1978 | R | Identify pregnant women at risk for poor neonatal outcome | Antepartum | Sum of factors ≥ 50 | Sens = .266 Spec = .833 $^+$PV = .129 | Low-birth-weight |
| Halliday et al | Prenatal risk score | 1268 | 1974, 1978 | R | Predict high-risk neonate | Postpartum Neonatal | Sum of factors ≥ 7 | Sens = .677 Spec = .750 $^+$PV = .064 | Perinatal mortality |
| Pavelka et al | Thalhammer's scoring system | 162 | 1977 to 1978 | P | Predict prematurity | First visit | Sum of factors < 30 | | Premature delivery (≤ 36 weeks) |
| Creasy et al | Modified from 1978 Papiernik-Berkhauer's | 1092 | 1978 | P | Predict spontaneous preterm delivery | Antepartum | Sum of factors | **Overall** Sens = .904 Spec = .644 $^+$PV = .304    **Primiparas** .926 .312 .208    **Multiparas** .899 .767 .327 | Preterm birth |

**Table 2–2**

SUMMARY OF REPORTED OBSTETRIC RISK-SCORING SYSTEMS *Continued*

| Author(s) | System | Year(s) Data Collected | Sample Size | Type of Study* | Purpose | When Used | Period Assessed | Definition of High Risk | Predictive Ability (High Risk Only)† | Outcomes Studied |
|---|---|---|---|---|---|---|---|---|---|---|
| Fortney and Whitehorne | Index of high-risk pregnancy | | | R | Test predictive validity of multiple discriminant analysis derived model | Ante- and intrapartum periods | Antepartum Intrapartum | Sum of factors ≥ 6, ≥ 7 | **Sum of factors ≥ 6** Sens = .689 Spec = .776 ⁺PV = .084 · **Sum of factors ≥ 7** .561 .888 .112 | Perinatal mortality, low-birth-weight (≤ 2500 g) |
| Wilson and Sill | High-risk pregnancy score | | 148 150 | P R | Identify high-risk patients for perinatal loss | Antepartum | Antepartum | Sum of factors 100 < 40 | Sens = 1.64 Spec = .938 ⁺PV = .375 | Cesarean delivery, perinatal deaths, preterm births |
| Sirivongs and Parisunyakul | Screening high-risk pregnancy | 1978, 1979 | 503 | P | Predict high-risk neonate | Ante and intrapartum periods | Antepartum Intrapartum | Sum of factors ≥ 7 | Correlation of increasing risk with worse outcome | Preterm delivery, assisted delivery, cesarean delivery, abnormal puerperium, Apgar score < 7, birth weight |
| Guzick et al | Multiple logistic model | 1980 | 2865 | P | Predict preterm delivery | Antepartum | Antepartum Intrapartum | Statistically significant factors correlated with preterm delivery | Max attributable risk = 6.26  **Probability of Preterm Delivery** / Sens / Spec / ⁺PV — .1 .622 .794 .227; .2 .433 .902 .301; .4 .106 .987 .443; .6 .043 .997 .550 | Preterm delivery |
| Smith et al | Antepartum scoring system | 1981 | 451 | R | Predict low-Apgar-scoring infants | Onset of labor | Antepartum Intrapartum | Sum of factors ≤ 10 | Sens = .68 Spec = .79 ⁺PV = .33 | 1-min Apgar ≤ 5 |
| Coburn et al | Antepartum fetal risk | 1982 | | R | Predict fetal risk | Last prenatal visit | Last prenatal visit | Sum of factors ≤ 4 score | **Perinatal Mortality** Sens = .23 Spec = .12 ⁺PV = .22 · **Low-birth-weight** Sens = .22 Spec = .12 ⁺PV = .13 | Perinatal mortality, low-birth-weight (≤ 2500 g) |

From Wall EM: A review of obstetric risk-scoring systems. J Fam Prac 27(2):153–163, 1988. Used with permission.
\* R = retrospective; P = prospective
† Sens = sensitivity; Spec = specificity; ⁺PV = positive predictive value

**Table 2–3**
RISK OF PRETERM DELIVERY

| Score | Socioeconomic Status | Past History | Daily Habits | Current Pregnancy |
|---|---|---|---|---|
| 1 | 2 children at home<br>Low socioeconomic status | 1 abortion<br>< 1 yr since last birth | Work outside home | Unusual fatigue |
| 2 | < 20 yr<br>> 40 yr<br>Single parent | 2 abortions | More than 10 cigarettes per day | Weight gain of 12 lb by 32 wk<br>Albuminuria<br>Hypertension<br>Bacteriuria |
| 3 | Very low socioeconomic status<br>< 5 ft<br>< 100 lb | 3 abortions | Heavy work<br>Long tiring trips | Breech at 32 wk<br>Weight loss of 5 lb<br>Head engaged<br>Febrile illness |
| 4 | < 18 yr | Pyelonephritis | | Metrorrhagia after 12 wk<br>Effacement<br>Dilatation<br>Uterine irritability |
| 5 | | Uterine anomaly<br>Second trimester abortion<br>DES exposure | | Placenta previa<br>Hydramnios<br>Uterine myoma |
| 10 | | Premature delivery<br>Repeated second trimester abortion | | Twins<br>Abdominal surgery |

EDB (estimated date of birth): _____
HIGH-RISK:     Yes     No

From Creasy RK, Herron MA: Prevention of preterm birth. Semin Perinatol 5:299, 1981.

happens to mother and fetus during the antepartum period is of critical importance to both. Adaptation is demanded of both in an ongoing sequence of events designed to prepare the fetus for life outside the uterus.

The growth of the fetus and the accompanying physical changes that occur during gestation are relatively unpredictable. However, the feelings and behaviors accompanying these changes may be more diverse, depending upon the unique characteristics and situation of the individual woman. Through early and continuous prenatal health care the pregnant woman and her family can be assisted in successfully adapting to these changes. Health care includes the ongoing assessment of the mother's physical and emotional health and assessment of fetal health and development. Pregnancy provides an optimal opportunity for preventive health care, maintenance, and education. Although the primary goal of antepartum care is to ensure a healthy mother and baby, a goal of equal importance is to promote an optimal physical and emotional experience for the family.

The physiologic process of pregnancy itself is normal. This process, however, imposes stresses to which both mother and fetus must adapt. Ideally, a woman is in an optimal state of health and free from exposure to harmful substances prior to conception. Because this is not always the situation, health care, if not already begun, should begin as soon as pregnancy is suspected. Prenatal care, therefore, becomes a screening process to differentiate those babies and mothers at jeopardy (high risk) from those in little danger (low risk). To be effective, such an assessment system must be based on a thorough and uncompromising search for those factors that may endanger the pregnancy. Obviously, the participation of the woman in prenatal care is essential in identifying and treating problems that may threaten her or her fetus.

With the advent of regionalization, perinatal care is now, in many cases, being provided by an interdisciplinary team that includes an obstetrician, a nurse, a nurse-midwife, a nutritionist, and a social worker. In some settings, pharmacists are added to this team. Each of these professionals has a distinct function and collectively can assist the patient and her family in achieving an optimal pregnancy experience. This team approach can also be more cost effective through better utilization of health care providers.

The primary health care provider for the pregnant woman is in an ideal position to assess not only the physiologic process but also (1) the way in which the patient is adapting to the pregnancy, (2) the supports and resources available to her, and (3) the lifestyle and personal belief system subscribed to by the woman and her family (Becker, 1982). Early, frequent, and continuing contact with the pregnant woman provides an ideal opportunity to assess for and identify existing and potential problems that may place the woman and/or her fetus at risk.

Becker (1982) has developed a prenatal assessment guide that can assist health care providers in gathering a more comprehensive data base from which care specific to the needs of the individual patient can be planned and implemented. This prenatal assessment guide consists of three parts (Table 2–4). The first deals with aspects of physical and psychologic adaptation to pregnancy. The second focuses on aspects of the woman's personal belief system and lifestyle that may affect her health and the health of the fetus. The third aims to identify the support systems and resources available to the patient that may influence the course and outcome of her pregnancy.

## DIAGNOSIS OF PREGNANCY

Of fundamental importance is establishment of the diagnosis of pregnancy. If this is confirmed by correlation of historical information, physical examination, and laboratory tests, the estimation of gestational age and estimated date of confinement at this early visit will minimize confusion as the pregnancy continues. Estimation of gestational age is most accurate in the early first trimester and becomes subject to increasing error as the pregnancy develops.

There are many presumptive signs of pregnancy. The most frequent is amenorrhea, which is often the first evidence to the patient of possible conception. Some patients may not be aware of pregnancy until other symptoms appear. These include nausea, vomiting, breast fullness, urinary frequency, constipation, fatigue, and enlarging abdomen.

Certain signs of pregnancy are highly suggestive of the diagnosis. These include uterine enlargement, softening of the uterine isthmus (Hegar's sign), and vaginal and cervical cyanosis (Chadwick's sign). Also, a positive laboratory test for human chorionic gonadotropin (hCG) is indicative of pregnancy (Brunel, 1980). Estimation of gestational age by uterine size is one of the most important elements of the first examination. The detection of fetal heart tones at about 10 to 12 weeks of gestation is possible with an ultrasonic Doppler, whereas the fetal heart rate cannot be heard until about 17 weeks with a DeLee stethoscope; in most pregnancies, fetal heart tones will be heard by at least 19 weeks' gestation (Pritchard and MacDonald, 1978). The estimated date of confinement can be calculated by Nägele's rule: Add 7 days to the first day of the last menstrual period and subtract 3 months. However, irregular or prolonged menstrual cycles, or a known single sexual exposure can cause variations from this calculation.

In decreasing rank of accuracy, the criteria for estimating date of birth are:

1. Basal body temperature chart with coital record;
2. Ultrasound between 7 and 10 weeks menstrual age, documenting crown-rump length;
3. Serum hCG;
4. Urine pregnancy testing, depending on type of test;
5. Two ultrasounds prior to 26 weeks' gestation;
6. Last menstrual period, in which cycle is normal and regular.

## INITIAL PRENATAL CARE

Once there is a confirmed diagnosis of pregnancy, an initial visit should be scheduled as soon as it is feasible. During the initial interview with the woman, careful attention to detail is necessary. This first visit is to assess risk and establish a plan of care, and should include:

1. A careful screening history.

**Table 2–4**
PRENATAL ASSESSMENT GUIDE*

## I. Aspects of Adaptation

Age
Initial response to this pregnancy
Planned or unplanned pregnancy
Feelings about this pregnancy
Desired family size
Perception of pregnancy affecting present activities and responsibilities
Perception of parenthood affecting future activities and plans
Current developmental tasks of pregnancy: how coping with pregnancy; fantasies about pregnancy; changes in mood and effect on others
Sexual functioning during pregnancy: changes in; feelings about and/or problems with
Nature of verbal interest expressed about self and fetus
Preparation for: prenatal classes (type, when completed series?); place of delivery; care for other children in mother's absence; care for new sibling
Menstrual history: problems with; last normal menstrual period; expected date of confinement
Height and prepregnancy weight
Obstetric status: course, abdominal assessment, quickening, fetal heart sound, blood pressure, urinalysis, weight and pattern of gain, signs of any major complications of pregnancy
Medical history: illness (date)—treatment, outcome, surgery: childhood diseases; current immunization status; allergies; venereal disease; emotional problems
Family medical history: illnesses, emotional problems, genetic defects (both sides of family)
Loss of significant other in past year
Food intolerance (lactose, nausea/vomiting); food cravings; pica
Iron, vitamin, and/or mineral dietary supplements used
Elimination patterns: changes/problems with remedies used
Pattern of rest, sleep: difficulties with; remedies used

## II. Aspects of Personal Belief System and Lifestyle

Date first sought prenatal care this pregnancy and in prior pregnancies
Reasons for seeking and receiving prenatal care
Beliefs about pregnancy and childbirth; cultural beliefs subscribed to with regard to childbearing (antepartum, intrapartum, postpartum)
Racial–ethnic group
Beliefs about role of father during pregnancy and labor, and role in child care
Perception of needs of fetus
Perception of needs of infant and proposed methods to meet those needs
Contraceptive history: methods used; failures and/or problems with; knowledge of alternate methods; willingness to use
Patterns of use of tobacco, alcohol, prescription and nonprescription drugs, illegal drugs; perception of effects of these substances on health of self and fetus
Patterns of nutrient intake: food dislikes; history of/method(s) of dieting
Planned method of infant feeding; why chosen
Occupation: Present, former, hours of duty per day, work requirements, hazards, amenities, plans regarding current occupation
Recreational activities: Plans to continue with; use of seat belt in car; pets in home
Community activities
Perception of health care personnel and agencies; prior experiences with
Date of last physical examination including breast exam, Pap smear, chest x-ray, and dental checkup
Breast self examination; done regularly?; if not, interested in learning about?

## III. Aspects of Support

Address: How long there, housing accommodations, phone, plans to move (if so, when where to, why?)
Level of education and future plans regarding education
Religious preference; nominal or active involvement?
Marital status; how long married
Father of baby: age, occupation, educational level, racial–ethnic group, religious preference
Family composition; household members
Communication patterns with significant others
Communication patterns with health personnel
Perception of support system (mate, family, friends, community agencies): how available? how willing to use?
Perception of meaning of this pregnancy to significant others; mate's response to news of pregnancy
Type of prenatal service receiving; perception of adequacy of available transportation to receive medical care
Social service/community agencies involved with: how long? name of contact person?
Self concept and perceived ability to cope with life situations
Body image: prepregnancy; currently; response to physiologic changes of pregnancy
Mate's response to body changes in pregnancy
Feelings about parenting that woman received as a child; history of separation from mother—what age?
Prior experiences with infants; knowledge of infant care
Feelings about previous pregnancies, labor, puerperium, and mothering skills
Knowledge of reproduction, labor and delivery, and puerperium

* From Becker CH: Comprehensive assessment of the healthy gravida. JOGN Nurs 11:375, 1982.

2. A general to specific physical examination designed to exclude risk factors.

3. Routine laboratory screening (Table 2–5).

4. Individually indicated maternal laboratory evaluation (Table 2–6).

5. Careful fetal assessment.

6. Specialized studies to ascertain fetal well-being and/or fetal maturity as individually indicated.

Patient biographic data—age, race, religion, marital status, and social and economic factors—must be carefully considered at this time. Historical data should include obstetric history (gravidity, parity, and details of previous pregnancies), menstrual history, and contraceptive history. A complete medical history must be obtained to screen for medical problems that may cause compli-cations or be aggravated by the pregnancy. These include diabetes mellitus, hypertension, thyroid disorders, cardiac disease, and seizure disorders. The initial history must also note hospitalization, prior surgery, medications taken, allergies, smoking, alcohol, and drug usage. A conventional review of all organ systems should be performed. Items of significance from the family history are multiple gestation, diabetes mellitus, hypertension, preeclampsia and eclampsia, bleeding disorders, and hereditary illnesses (e.g., hemophilia, Down's syndrome, and Tay-Sachs disease) (see Chapter 32). During the physical examination, attention should be directed to specific organ systems as a positive history is elicited. A general examination should especially evaluate the blood pressure, weight, height, optic fundi, thyroid, lungs, heart, abdomen, and extremities.

**Table 2–5**
GENERAL LABORATORY EXAMINATIONS

| Tests | Initial Visit | 26–30 Weeks | 36 Weeks | Findings that Signal Further Assessment |
|---|---|---|---|---|
| **Blood Tests** | | | | |
| 1. Complete Blood Count (CBC) | | | | |
| (a) Hemoglobin (Hgb)* or | X | X | X | Hgb $<10$ g/dl[d] |
| (b) Hematocrit (Hct)* | | | | Hct 32 percent or less |
| (c) White blood cell count (WBC) | X | | | 15,000 mm or more |
| (d) Differential smear (Diff) | X | | | Cellular abnormalities and/or decreased platelets |
| 2. Blood Group | X | | | |
| 3. Rh Factor | X | | | Mother: Rh-negative Mate: Rh-positive or unknown |
| 4. Antibody Screen | X | | | A titer defined by the laboratory |
| 5. Serology for Syphilis | X | | Repeat† | Positive |
| 6. Rubella Screen (titer) | X | | | A titer of 1:8 or less, or a significant rise in titer |
| 7. Two-Hour Postprandial Blood Sugar | Obtain‡ | X | X | 145 mg/dl§ or more |
| 8. Hepatitis B | X | | Repeat‖ | Positive |
| **Urine Tests** | | | | |
| 1. Urine Bacteria Screen | X | X | | Positive |
| 2. Urine Glucose and Protein | AT EACH VISIT | | | Protein 1+ or more Glucose 1+ or more |
| **Cervical Tests** | | | | |
| 1. Papanicolaou smear (Pap smear) | X | | | Positive |
| 2. Culture for gonorrhea | X | | Repeat† | Positive |

\* Usually one or the other is needed, not both.
† Repeat test if woman is at risk for reinfection.
‡ Obtain specimen if high-risk pregnancy or if history is inadequate.
§ Note that in current literature mg/dl may be used instead of the more traditional mg/100 ml; 1 deciliter (dl) = 100 ml. Norms may be different depending on laboratory variability.
‖ Repeat test if woman is in high-risk group or was exposed to Hepatitis B at any time during pregnancy.

**Table 2–6**
SPECIFIC LABORATORY EXAMINATIONS

| Tests | Initial Visit | 24–28 Weeks | 36 Weeks | Findings that Signal Further Assessment |
|---|---|---|---|---|
| Blood Tests<br>Antibody screen<br>(Rh-negative woman) | X | X | X | Significant, as defined by the local laboratory* |
| Oral glucose tolerance test<br>(OGTT) | | 24–28 wks<br>X | | plasma threshold 140 mg/dl |
| Human Immunovirus<br>(HIV) | offer screening to at-risk women at initial visit | | | Positive |
| Maternal serum-Alpha<br>Fetal Protein | initial visit counsel; offer test to be done at 15–20 weeks | | | ≥2.0 MoMs |
| Sickle Cell Screen | X | | | Positive for trait or anemia* |
| Tay-Sachs Screen | X | | | Carrier* |
| Cervical Test<br>Herpesvirus hominis,<br>Type 2 | When physical findings indicate at any prenatal visit | | X | Positive |
| Skin Test<br>Tuberculosis | X | | | Positive |

\* Test the woman's male partner.

## LABORATORY DATA

Pregnancy induces dramatic changes in maternal body systems. Laboratory findings must be evaluated in terms of pregnancy norms rather than nonpregnancy norms. *Individual laboratories determine their own pregnancy norms, and normal values vary with the technique used.* Also, considerations such as climate and altitude may influence the norm for that population (Schneider, 1978).

Table 2–5 identifies tests for the low-risk pregnancy woman. Abnormalities in these routine tests or positive findings in the history and physical examination may indicate the need for further specific tests (see Table 2–6).

## SUBSEQUENT PRENATAL CARE

The recommended frequency of prenatal visits is monthly, starting at the first indication of pregnancy, until 28 to 30 weeks; a visit every 2 weeks until 36 weeks; and weekly from 37 weeks until delivery. It is beneficial to see the patient weekly starting at the 18th week to gather information about fetal heart tones, uterine size, and quickening, in order to more firmly establish the correct gestational age. Once fetal heart tones are heard and quickening occurs, the patient can again be seen monthly until 30 weeks' gestation.

## SUBSEQUENT HISTORY

Information regarding changes in the woman's physical, emotional, and social status should be reviewed and noted at each visit. Problems and concerns identified previously should be followed up. Information regarding prenatal education classes, child care classes, Lamaze classes, breastfeeding classes; and other helpful programs should be provided, along with encouragement for the woman to utilize these resources. Ongoing assessment, counseling, and education in several areas are necessary (Table 2–7).

## SUBSEQUENT PHYSICAL ASSESSMENT

At each subsequent prenatal visit the following physical parameters should be assessed:

**Table 2–7**
Prenatal Assessment/Teaching Guide*

| | |
|---|---|
| 1Δ | Medical care during pregnancy<br>Body changes<br>Fetal development<br>Drugs, alcohol, smoking effects<br>Safety<br>Communicable diseases<br>Danger signs<br>Nutrition and weight gain<br>Minor discomforts; how relieved<br>Sexual activity<br>Hygiene<br>Exercise and rest<br>Emotional adjustments |
| 2Δ | Traveling<br>Infant feeding plans<br>Preparation for childbirth<br>Signs/symptoms of labor<br>Hospitalization<br>Home preparation<br>Sibling/family preparation |
| 3Δ | Family planning |

* 1Δ = 1st trimester; 2Δ = 2nd trimester; 3Δ = 3rd trimester.

### Maternal

1. Weight
2. Blood pressure
3. Urinalysis
4. Edema
5. Uterine growth
6. Laboratory tests as indicated (see Table 2–5)

### Fetal

1. Gestational age
2. Quickening and presence of daily fetal movements
3. Fetal heart tones
4. Fundal height
5. Specific assessments as indicated:
   A. Ultrasound (biophysical profile)
   B. Amniocentesis
   C. Electronic fetal heart rate (FHR); non-stress test (NST)/contraction stress test (CST)

## PARENTING ASSESSMENT

Allen and Mantz (1981) report that being "normal," that is, medically and obstetrically healthy, may carry an underestimated risk factor. Being labeled as normal may cause health care providers to overlook this group of patients who may not be coping well with childbearing, but whose clues are often too subtle and thus overlooked until an acute emotional or social crisis occurs.

Over the course of 2 years, 180 families were studied in a project designed to provide appropriate nursing care to patients potentially at risk, although designated as normal. These criteria were as follows:

1. Significant ambivalent or negative feelings toward pregnancy after 20 weeks' gestation.
2. Insecure or negative feelings about mothering skills.
3. Inappropriate positive feelings about pregnancy or mothering.
4. Inadequate nuclear family support.
5. Inadequate extended support system.
6. Current or historically significant psychiatric problems (Allen and Mantz, 1981).

Therefore, in addition to the ongoing physical assessment, counseling, and education, parenting assessment must also be a continuing process. An important concern of health care providers who are committed to the promotion of healthy parenting is the prevention of child abuse and neglect. Early identification and treatment during pregnancy of those parents who are at high risk for becoming neglectful or abusive toward their children is the responsibility of all members of the health care delivery team (Field et al, 1985).

Josten (1981) has devised a "prenatal assessment of parenting" guide, offering health care providers a framework for the prenatal identification of women who need assistance with their parenting skills and attitudes. On the subject of identifying parents at risk, Josten states: "It would be unethical to evaluate women prenatally on their parenting ability unless the intention was to offer them assistance. Those women identified at high risk need help so that child abuse and neglect can be prevented. I suggest using an intervention approach that focuses initially on the woman's difficulties with the developmental task of pregnancy and then the problems present in her life situation."

## CONTINUING ASSESSMENT OF RISK

As pregnancy progresses, the woman should have all risk factors reassessed. At times, patients initially identified as being "low risk" develop problems later in gestation (Table 2–8). In fact, it has been suggested that the current concept and definition of the term "low risk" needs to be reexamined: As Wilson and Schifrin (1980) have noted, "In labeling a small group of patients 'high risk' we may paradoxically be creating an elite class of obstetric patients destined to receive the best care the specialty has to offer. The emphasis on 'high risk' may convince both physicians and lay individuals alike that a patient not considered 'high risk' is 'low risk.' 'Low risk' in turn may be interpreted to mean negligible risk—an unfortunate conclusion."

# Identification of a High-Risk Pregnancy

A high-risk pregnancy is one in which the mother or fetus has a significantly increased chance of death or disability (Hobel, 1979). In order to achieve optimal perinatal outcome, all factors contributing to mortality and morbidity in a particular pregnancy must be identified and acted upon early. This section identifies and categorizes high-risk pregnancy factors and outlines the reasons for each factor's designation. The factors may be divided into the categories of socio-

**Table 2–8**
RISK FACTORS IN EARLY AND LATE STAGES OF PREGNANCY

| Stage | High-Risk Factors | Moderate-Risk Factors |
|-------|-------------------|-----------------------|
| *Early Pregnancy* | Failure of uterine growth or disproportionate uterine growth | Unresponsive urinary tract infection |
| | Exposure to teratogens (radiation, infection, chemicals) | Suspected ectopic pregnancy |
| | Pregnancy complicated by isoimmunization | Suspected missed abortion |
| | Need for antenatal genetic diagnosis | Severe hyperemesis gravidarum |
| | Severe anemia (9 g or less hemoglobin) | Positive VDRL test |
| | Substance abuse | Positive gonorrhea screening |
| | | Anemia not responsive to iron treatment |
| | | Viral illness |
| | | Vaginal bleeding |
| | | Mild anemia (9–10.9 g hemoglobin) |
| *Late Pregnancy* | Failure of uterine growth or disproportionate uterine growth | Hypertensive states of pregnancy (mild) |
| | Severe anemia (less than 9 g hemoglobin) | Breech, if cesarean section is planned |
| | More than 42 1/2 weeks' gestation | Uncertain presentations |
| | Severe preeclampsia | Need for fetal maturity studies |
| | Eclampsia | |
| | Breech, if vaginal delivery is planned | Postdate pregnancy (41–42 1/2 weeks' gestation) |
| | Moderate to severe isoimmunization (necessitating intrauterine transfusion or neonatal exchange transfusion) | |
| | Placenta previa | |
| | Hydramnios or oligohydramnios | Induction of labor |
| | Antepartum fetal death | Suspected fetopelvic disproportion at term |
| | Thromboembolic disease | |
| | Premature labor (less than 37 weeks' gestation) | Floating presentations 2 weeks or less from the EDC |
| | Premature rupture of membranes (less than 38 weeks' gestation) | |
| | Tumor or other obstruction of birth canal | |
| | Abruptio placentae | |
| | Chronic or acute pyelonephritis | |
| | Multiple gestation | |
| | Abnormal oxytocin challenge test | |
| | Falling urinary estriols | |
| | Prolonged rupture of membranes | |
| | Diabetes | |

Adapted from Babson SG, Pernoll ML, Benda GI (with the assistance of Simpson K): Diagnosis and Management of the Fetus and Neonate at Risk, 4th ed. St. Louis, CV Mosby, 1980.

economic, demographic, and medical (Table 2–9). There is considerable overlap of the various categories, and it will become apparent that the first category, socioeconomic, achieves more importance as control or improvement occurs within the purely medical category (Chez et al, 1977).

## SOCIOECONOMIC FACTORS

**Socioeconomic Status.** The many social factors that place a fetus at greater risk are interrelated. Such conditions as overcrowding, poor standards of housing and hygiene, and poor nutrition are closely associated with high rates of infant and child morbidity and mortality. Poverty and low educational status are at the root of these problems, and in countries where social and economic improvement has occurred, there has also been a decrease in perinatal mortality (Chez et al, 1977).

**Parental Occupation.** Occupation of the father, as a reflection of socioeconomic status, is related to profound differences in the incidence of prematurity and infant mortality. Kessner and colleagues (1973) have reported that the lowest incidence of perinatal loss occurs in cases in which the father is in a professional or managerial position, whereas the highest rates of loss are seen in situations in which the father is absent altogether. Between these two extremes, the incidence of loss gets higher as one goes down the socioeconomic spectrum, with the rate increasing through the ranks of sales/clerical workers and skilled craftsmen, until it has doubled in families in which the father is in a semi-skilled or manual labor occupation.

It has further been demonstrated that a correlation exists between the occupation of the mother's father and the incidence of perinatal loss; that is, women from a higher socioeconomic background have a lower incidence of perinatal loss than those from a less affluent one (Kessner et al, 1973).

**Social Environment.** The effects of maternal social environment on the outcome of pregnancy are recognized to be both multiple and profound. "Social environment" itself is described as the summation of numerous factors, including the family's standards of health and hygiene, housing and financial status, emotional and social support, and so on. The effects may be direct or indirect and

may be difficult to separate within the context of socioeconomic status. It is the interrelationship of these factors, rather than any single factor, that works to affect the outcome of pregnancy.

A pilot study in 1966 from a health care unit in South Philadelphia (Fed Res Grant IR 18-H 50 1135-01) provided some interesting observations: The majority of the families came from a deprived family background and low socioeconomic group. If the pregnant patient was married, there frequently was marital disharmony and disruption, wife and child abuse, and little help or support from relatives. The environment itself was grossly unhygienic. Recurrent infections and "poor health" were frequently noted within the family. Educational needs were, for the most part, unmet and ignored. Single-parent families were commonplace and accepted. Financial support was, at best, inadequate, with the pregnant patient frequently being the main wage earner. The adverse influences of this history of social, emotional, nutritional and financial deprivation on reproductive outcome were numerous. Reproductive histories obtained from female relatives of the pregnant patient included a high rate of reproductive loss, significant evidence of premature labor, low-birth-weight infants, and a high proportion of children with mental retardation or learning disabilities. These types of outcomes were traced through one or more generations and could be repeated in the next.

**Marital Status.** The frequency of cases of low-birth-weight infants and the perinatal mortality rates of infants born to unmarried mothers are double those of the children of married women. Marital status alone is not necessarily an indicator of potential risk for mother and fetus so much as it is an indicator of an unwanted/unplanned pregnancy. These pregnant women, especially if unwed or teenagers, tend to have limited access to health care and may leave advice unheeded. Statistically, pregnancy complications occur more frequently in unmarried than in married women (Brown, 1988).

**Psychologic High-Risk Factors.** When a woman becomes pregnant the entire family prepares for change. The support and guidance that the family receives during this preparation period will influence the family's ability to cope with the stress of this pregnancy and with its changes in family structure, as well as with other life stresses

**Table 2–9**
CATEGORIZATION OF HIGH RISK PREGNANCY FACTORS

**Socioeconomic factors**
1. Inadequate finances
2. Poor housing
3. Severe social problems
4. Unwed, especially adolescent
5. Minority status
6. Nutritional deprivation
7. Parental occupation

**Demographic Factors**
1. Maternal age under 16 or over 35 years
2. Overweight or underweight prior to pregnancy
3. Height less than 5 feet
4. Maternal education less than 11 years
5. Family history of severe inherited disorders

**Medical Factors**
**A. Obstetric History**
1. History of infertility
2. Previous ectopic pregnancy or spontaneous abortion
3. Grandmultiparity
4. Previous stillborn or neonatal death
5. Uterine/cervical abnormality
6. Previous multiple gestation
7. Previous premature labor/delivery
8. Previous prolonged labor
9. Previous cesarean section
10. Previous low-birth-weight infant
11. Previous macrosomic infant
12. Previous midforceps delivery
13. Previous baby with neurologic deficit, birth injury, or malformation
14. Previous hydatidiform mole or choriocarcinoma

**B. Maternal Medical History/Status**
1. Maternal cardiac disease
2. Maternal pulmonary disease
3. Maternal metabolic disease—particularly diabetes mellitus, thyroid disease
4. Chronic renal disease, repeated urinary tract infections, repeated bacteriuria
5. Maternal gastrointestinal disease
6. Maternal endocrine disorders (pituitary, adrenal)
7. Chronic hypertension
8. Maternal hemoglobinopathies
9. Seizure disorder
10. Venereal and other infectious diseases
11. Weight loss greater than 5 pounds
12. Malignancy
13. Surgery during pregnancy
14. Major congenital anomalies of the reproductive tract
15. Maternal mental retardation, major emotional disorders

**C. Current OB Status**
1. Late or no prenatal care
2. Rh sensitization
3. Fetus inappropriately large or small for gestation
4. Premature labor
5. Pregnancy-induced hypertension
6. Multiple gestation
7. Polyhydramnios
8. Premature rupture of the membranes
9. Antepartum bleeding
   a. Placenta previa
   b. Abruptio placentae
10. Abnormal presentation
11. Postdatism
12. Abnormality in tests for fetal well-being
13. Maternal anemia

**D. Habits/Habituation**
1. Smoking during pregnancy
2. Regular alcohol intake
3. Drug use/abuse

in the future. Therefore, it is important to identify psychologic maladaptation to pregnancy. Maladaptations may increase anxiety, and it has been suggested that increased anxiety can cause physical complications during pregnancy, including preterm labor (Crandon, 1979; Creasy, 1981). It is also recognized that child battering, mental illness, and many psychosomatic illnesses result from unhealthy mother-infant-family relationships.

## DEMOGRAPHIC FACTORS

**Maternal Age.** The relationship between maternal age and pregnancy outcome has long been recognized. Studies have shown that the optimal age for childbearing is between 20 and 30 years, with a steadily increasing risk of perinatal mortality when the woman is over 30 years of age. Children of mothers 19 years and younger and the firstborn of mothers 35 years of age and older are at an increased risk for prematurity and other pregnancy complications such as pregnancy-induced hypertension (PIH) and congenital anomalies (Niswander and Gordon, 1972). Additionally, babies born to women over 35 years of age have an increased risk of genetic defects such as Down's syndrome and other genetic abnormalities (Crandall et al, 1986).

**Maternal Education.** Correlations have been indicated between the number of years of schooling completed by a pregnant woman and perinatal death rate, birth weight, and the rate of neurologic abnormalities seen in the child at 1 year of age. As the length of the mother's education increases, perinatal morbidity and mortality rates drop significantly. It is thought that this association occurs not because education in itself decreases problems in pregnancy but that length of education is a useful index of general socioeconomic status.

**Maternal Height.** Short stature of the mother (less than 5 ft) has been associated with increased perinatal morbidity and mortality in several studies. The primary reason suspected for this association is that short maternal stature may be a reflection of adverse environmental conditions and poor nutrition as a child. Because stature relates to pelvic dimensions, short women have a higher incidence of operative delivery, including cesarean section because of cephalopelvic disproportion.

**Maternal Weight and Weight Gain.** Women who are underweight or overweight for height and age at the beginning of pregnancy are at risk for poor perinatal outcome (Abrams and Laros, 1986). Both of these parameters reflect previous nutritional status of the mother. Women who are underweight and/or fail to gain the recommended 28 to 40 lb during pregnancy are at risk for having low-birth-weight infants. Women who are overweight and/or gain more than 35 lb during pregnancy are at risk for developing preeclampsia and having large-for-gestational-age babies. Fetuses weighing more than 4000 g (9 lb) are frequently associated with an increased likelihood of dystocia during labor, fetal distress, maternal and infant birth trauma, and consequently, an increased incidence of perinatal morbidity and mortality.

## PREVIOUS OBSTETRIC PROBLEMS

In women who have had an obstetric complication or a perinatal loss, there is a tendency for the problem to "repeat" in a subsequent pregnancy (Shapiro et al, 1968). This is true for all of the factors listed in the high-risk pregnancy classification (see Table 2–9).

**History of Infertility.** Conceptions following medical or surgical treatment of infertility carry a considerable high-risk factor. There is a high prevalence of multiple gestation and associated preterm labor in women treated for infertility, and, therefore, an increase in the perinatal morbidity and mortality rates.

**Previous Ectopic Pregnancy and Spontaneous Abortion.** For women of any parity who have had an ectopic pregnancy, there is a significantly higher perinatal mortality rate in subsequent pregnancies. The incidence of infertility in patients who have had an ectopic pregnancy is high, as is the chance of a repeat ectopic conception (Kadar and Romero, 1990). In women who have had two or more spontaneous abortions, the risk of a repeat abortion is significantly increased. However, should the pregnancy proceed beyond the second trimester, a history of previous abortion does not predispose the woman to premature labor (Cavanagh and Talisman, 1969; Kadar and Romero, 1990).

**Previous Stillbirth or Neonatal Death.**
A history of a previous perinatal death, especially if the cause is unknown, is an indication of high-risk status. The perinatal mortality rate in these women is even higher than in those who have had a previous spontaneous abortion or a premature live birth (Butler and Bonham, 1969; Goldsmith, 1990).

**Uterine/Cervical Abnormality.** Abnormalities of the uterus/cervix such as a bicornuate uterus, uterine septum, and incompetent cervix are frequently associated with repeated spontaneous abortions and premature labor. A large number of abnormalities of the genital tract remain undetected unless a complication of pregnancy or delivery alerts the health care provider to the need for a thorough investigation. Congenital uterine malformation should be suspected if there is a history of repeated spontaneous abortions, malpresentations, and malpositions during labor.

**Previous Preterm Labor/Delivery.**
Preterm labor is one of the most challenging problems facing perinatal health care providers (McCormick, 1985). Despite recent clinical advances, preterm birth is still associated with up to 85 percent of nonanomalous neonatal deaths and is the cause of handicaps in the survivors at rates reported as high as 40 to 85 percent (Creasy, 1990; Dweck, 1977; Marriage and Davies, 1976). A woman who has had a previous premature labor and/or delivery has a significantly higher chance of delivering prematurely with a subsequent pregnancy. Depending on the etiology of the preterm birth, the history of one previous preterm birth is associated with a risk of recurrence of 25 to 50 percent, and the risk increases with each subsequent preterm birth (Creasy, 1990). There is also an increased chance that the patient will have a stillbirth or neonatal death (Cavanagh and Talisman, 1969; Creasy, 1990).

The etiology of preterm labor remains incompletely understood, although certain risk factors have been identified (Creasy, 1990). Because prediction of preterm labor is the first step toward prevention, several authors have attempted to develop risk assessment systems, with varying success. A summary of several of these systems can be seen in Table 2–10. Most recently, a risk prediction system for preterm labor was outlined by Holbrook and associates (1989) (Table 2–11). This system reinforces the importance of both past reproductive history and current pregnancy conditions in the prediction and prevention of premature labor.

**Previous Macrosomic Infant.** A macrosomic infant is one who, at term, weighs more than 4000 g or is large for his or her gestational age. A woman who has previously had, or is suspected of carrying, a large infant is at risk for having or developing diabetes during pregnancy, with all its concomitant problems. The infants themselves are at increased risk for morbidity (including low newborn blood sugars) and mortality as a result of unstable maternal metabolic condition, placental insufficiency, and even if the mother is not diabetic, birth trauma due to difficult delivery, shoulder dystocia, and other complications.

**Grandmultiparity.** Increasing parity increases the risk of pregnancy wastage both in terms of higher mortality rates and an increased risk of neurologic and congenital anomaly. In general, the lowest perinatal mortality rate and incidence of obstetric complication occurs in second and third pregnancies, and the highest in fifth and subsequent pregnancies. The frequency of anemia, hypertensive disease of pregnancy, antepartum and postpartum hemorrhage, as well as the number of cesarean sections, almost doubles for each of these complications in women of increasing parity (> para 4) compared with women of lower parity.

**Maternal Medical History/Status.** Certain maternal disease states diagnosed prior to pregnancy, at the time of initial physical examination or at any time during the pregnancy, may have a significant influence on the outcome of the pregnancy for both fetus and mother (see Table 2–9). These states are discussed in the following paragraphs.

*Maternal Cardiac Disease.* The diagnosis of organic heart disease includes rheumatic heart disease, hypertensive heart disease, and congenital heart disease. Fetal death rates are substantially increased in women with any of these diagnoses; in fact, the stillbirth rate is doubled compared with that in women without organic heart disease. The presence of organic heart disease also significantly increases the risk of delivery of a low-birth-weight infant (<2500 g).

*Maternal Pulmonary Disease.* Bronchial asthma is a rather common respiratory disease; pregnancy does not seem to have any consistent effect on it. The effect of pregnancy on asthma generally follows the rule

**Table 2–10**
SUMMARY OF REPORTED OBSTETRIC RISK-SCORING SYSTEMS BASED ON
LOW-BIRTH-WEIGHT OR PRETERM BIRTH

| Authors | Year Published | System | Definition of High Risk | Definition of Preterm Birth and Low-Birth-Weight | Predictive Ability | |
|---|---|---|---|---|---|---|
| Kaminski et al | 1973 | Risk of preterm delivery | Score ≥ 8.5 | Preterm ≤ 36 weeks<br>Low-birth-weight ≤ 2500 g<br>Term— low-birth-weight | *Preterm birth*<br>Sens = .30<br>Spec = .68<br>⁺PV = .17 | *Low-birth-weight*<br>Sens = .39<br>Spec = .63<br>⁺PV = .10 |
| Herron et al | 1982 | Risk of preterm delivery | Score ≥ 10 | Preterm birth ≤ 37 weeks | *Preterm birth*<br>Sens = .43<br>Spec = .85<br>⁺PV = .07 | |
| Main and Gabbe | 1985 | Risk of preterm delivery | Score ≥ 10 | Preterm birth ≤ 37 weeks | *Preterm birth*<br>Sens = .48<br>Spec = .68<br>⁺PV = .23 | |
| Main et al | 1987 | Risk of preterm delivery | Score ≥ 10 | Preterm birth ≤ 37 weeks | *Preterm birth*<br>Sens = .26<br>Spec = .80<br>⁺PV = NS. | |
| Holbrook et al | 1989 | Risk of preterm delivery | Score ≥ 10 | Preterm birth ≤ 37 weeks | *Preterm birth*<br>Sens = .40<br>Spec = .86<br>⁺PV = .13 | |

**Table 2–11**
MAJOR AND MINOR RISK FACTORS IN
PREDICTION OF SPONTANEOUS
PRETERM LABOR*

**Major**

| | |
|---|---|
| Multiple gestation | Previous preterm delivery |
| DES exposure | Previous preterm labor/ term delivery |
| Hydramnios | Abdominal surgery during pregnancy |
| Uterine anomaly | History of cone biopsy |
| Cervix dilated > 1 cm at 32 weeks | Cervical shortening < 1 cm at 32 weeks |
| Second-trimester abortion × 2 | Uterine irritability |

**Minor**

| | |
|---|---|
| Febrile illness | Cigarettes—more than 10/day |
| Bleeding after 12 weeks | Second-trimester abortion × 1 |
| History of pyelonephritis | More than 2 first-trimester abortions |

* Presence of one or more major factors, two or more minor factors, or both, places patient in high-risk group.

From Holbrook RH Jr, Laros RK Jr, Creasy RK. Evaluation of a risk-scoring system from prediction of preterm labor. Am J Perinatol 1988, 6:62. Reprinted by permission of Appleton & Lange, Inc.

of thirds: one third of patients improve during pregnancy, one third remain unchanged, and one third deteriorate. Women who have deterioration of asthma during one pregnancy will often experience a similar occurrence in a subsequent pregnancy (Weinstein and Dubin, 1979). The fetuses may be at increased risk for intrauterine growth retardation, preterm labor-delivery, stillbirth, or neonatal death (Benedetti, 1990).

***Diabetes Mellitus.*** Diabetes is deleterious to pregnancy in a number of ways. The adverse maternal effects that are likely to be encountered are as follows:

1. The likelihood of preeclampsia/eclampsia is increased fourfold.

2. Infection occurs more often and is likely to be more severe.

3. The fetus frequently is macrosomic, and its size may lead to difficult delivery with injury to the infant and the birth canal.

4. The tendency for fetal condition to substantially deteriorate prior to the onset of labor, as well as the possibility of dystocia,

increases the frequency of cesarean section with its incumbent maternal risk.

5. Postpartum hemorrhage is more common.
6. Polyhydramnios is common.

Maternal diabetes also affects the fetus/neonate in a variety of ways:

1. Perinatal death rate is considerably higher.
2. Morbidity as a result of birth trauma or respiratory distress syndrome is common.
3. Congenital anomalies, including sacral agenesis or caudal dysplasia, anencephaly, open spina bifida, and cardiac anomalies, are more frequent.
4. The infant is more likely to inherit diabetes.
5. Persistent maternal hyperglycemia probably contributes to the increased risk of intrauterine death, respiratory distress syndrome, hypoglycemia, and other morbidity (Gabbe, 1991).

***Maternal Thyroid Dysfunction.*** Thyroid disease appears to have an adverse effect on pregnancy outcome. Hypothyroidism results primarily in an increase in the stillbirth rate. Hyperthyroidism shows a slight association with increased neonatal mortality rate, a significant increase in the frequency of delivery of low-birth-weight infants, and an overall drop in the mean birth weight. Once the diagnosis of thyroid disease is made in pregnancy, therapy may be complicated by the presence of the fetus. Drugs that may be beneficial to the mother can be harmful to the fetus, and this must be taken into account when a therapeutic decision is made (Burrow and Ferris, 1982).

***Gastrointestinal/Hepatic System Diseases.*** With the exception of hepatitis and appendicitis, maternal gastrointestinal disease does not generally cause any increased risk in pregnancy. Hepatitis appears to be associated with an increase in low-birth-weight infants and an increased incidence of infection of the infant. Appendicitis appears to increase the rate of premature labor, fetal death, and low-birth-weight infants, most probably as a result of infection, regardless of whether surgery is performed.

***Chronic Hypertension.*** In most cases of chronic hypertension, high blood pressure is the only demonstrable finding. A few patients, however, show secondary alterations that are often grave, not only in relation to pregnancy but also with regard to maternal

life expectancy. These include hypertensive cardiac disease, arteriosclerotic renal disease, and retinal hemorrhages and exudate. Frequently, the babies of mothers with chronic hypertension show evidence of intrauterine growth retardation. The incidence of abruptio placentae and PIH also has been noted to be increased.

***Renal Disease/Urinary Tract Disease.*** Renal diseases such as glomerulonephritis, nephrotic syndrome, polycystic disease of the kidney, and previous nephrectomy/renal transplant vary in their effect on pregnancy outcome, depending on the severity of the disease. Most commonly, they are associated with increased risk for premature labor, intrauterine growth retardation, and placental insufficiency leading to antepartum fetal distress.

Acute urinary tract infection, if undiagnosed or untreated, may lead to premature labor (Prithcard et al, 1985).

**Current Obstetric Status.** Ideally, if a woman participates in prenatal care, identification and treatment of problems that may threaten her or her fetus will be accomplished. Prenatal care, therefore, is a screening process that incorporates the historical and social factors mentioned previously with constant surveillance of the mother and fetus as the pregnancy continues. Some of the factors contributing to poor perinatal outcome in relation to the current pregnancy are discussed later (see also Table 2–9).

***Late or No Prenatal Care.*** Prenatal care that is inadequate, late, or nonexistent is the single greatest predictor of poor perinatal outcome, particularly in regard to low-birth-weight infants (Sachs et al, 1987). In two groups of women matched for age, parity, and risk assessment, studies at the University of Tennessee (Ryan et al, 1980) demonstrated that perinatal outcome was substantially altered by amount of prenatal care. Analysis of outcomes revealed marked differences in pregnancy outcome between the group of women who had less than four prenatal visits and those who had four or more visits. Other studies have corroborated data showing that women with late or no prenatal care had a significantly higher rate of premature labor, premature delivery, low-birth-weight infants, and stillborns (Nesbitt, 1990).

***Antepartum Bleeding.*** Antepartum bleeding is defined as bleeding from the vagina after the 28th week of gestation and prior to the onset of labor. The etiology includes (1) placenta previa, (2) abruptio placentae, (3) local causes such as cervical polyps or erosions, and (4) unknown etiology in which a specific cause cannot be found.

Placenta previa, and consequent bleeding from a placenta partly or wholly attached to the lower uterine segment, is a complication frequently associated with multiparity and older gravidas. Women who have had a placenta previa tend to repeat this complication in subsequent pregnancies. Overall incidence of placenta previa is 1 in 200 pregnancies at term. Incidence increases significantly with maternal age, parity, previous placenta previa, and most importantly, previous uterine surgery (Bender, 1987).

Maternal mortality associated with placenta previa has been reduced to less than 1 percent, but maternal morbidity from this complication is still as high as 20 percent (Atrash et al, 1990; Cavanagh et al, 1982).

Prematurity is the prevalent cause of perinatal mortality associated with placenta previa. Despite the availability of neonatal intensive care, the perinatal mortality rate remains as high as 20 percent, with intrauterine hypoxia and developmental anomalies also complicating the situation.

Abruptio placentae is described as the premature separation of a normally implanted placenta from the uterine implantation site with ensuing retroplacental bleeding, which may or may not cause vaginal bleeding. Abruption of the placenta is most commonly associated with hypertension of any origin, including preeclampsia. Hypertension is 5 times more common in women with severe abruption. High parity and a history of previous abruption have also been implicated. In a study by Pritchard and coworkers (1970), 47 percent of women with abruptions severe enough to cause fetal death were hypertensive. Women having their 7th child were 6 times more likely to have an abruption than were primiparous women. Other factors implicated as possible causes of abruption are trauma, sudden uterine decompression (particularly with polyhydramnios), short umbilical cord, and uterine leiomyomas and anomalies. Recurrence rates of placental abruption range from 1 in 6 to 1 in 18 pregnancies (Patterson, 1979).

Maternal mortality in abruptio placentae ranges from 2 to 10 percent in severe cases with associated fetal death. Perinatal mortality approaches 35 percent, the major determinants being length of gestation and fetal condition at the time of presentation (Clark, 1990).

In general, antepartum bleeding is associated with significantly increased risks for premature labor and delivery, intrauterine growth retardation, fetal and maternal anemia, and perinatal death (Clark, 1990).

***Multiple Gestation.*** Perinatal mortality in twins is 2 to 3 times higher than in single births. The predominant cause of perinatal death is prematurity. Other major complications include placenta previa, intrauterine growth retardation, twin-to-twin transfusion, prolapsed cord, premature separation of the second placenta, and malformations. Women with a multiple gestation have an increased incidence of preeclampsia, anemia, polyhydramnios, and postpartum hemorrhage.

***Pregnancy-Induced Hypertension (PIH).*** PIH is one of the hypertensive disorders of pregnancy, and a major contributor to maternal, fetal, and neonatal morbidity and mortality. Complications of PIH are the second most common cause of maternal deaths (Atrash, 1990). PIH is divided into three categories: 1) hypertension alone, 2) preeclampsia, and 3) eclampsia. Diagnosis of preeclampsia is based on increased blood pressure plus proteinuria or generalized edema. Eclampsia is characterized by the symptoms cited plus convulsions (Gant and Pritchard, 1990).

The incidence of PIH in the United States is approximately 6 to 8 percent. PIH seems to be higher in blacks for each age and parity group, and it runs in families. The incidence is also higher in young, primiparous women and in multiparous women over 35. It is frequent in women with twins, diabetes, chronic hypertension, polyhydramnios, and hydatidiform mole. Approximately one third of women who have had PIH previously will develop it in subsequent pregnancies (Burrow and Ferris, 1982).

Maternal effects of PIH range from relatively transient to serious morbidity, such as renal damage or cerebral vascular accident, to death of the mother or fetus, or both. Fetal problems include increased incidence of intrauterine growth retardation, abruptio placentae, preterm birth, stillbirth, and mental retardation in surviving offspring.

PIH is a major cause of perinatal mortality and is the second leading cause of maternal death in the United States (Cavanagh et al, 1982).

At present, it is not possible to prevent PIH. It is possible, however, to identify patients who are especially prone to develop the disease. Conditions that predispose a woman to develop PIH include:

1. First pregnancy
2. Multiple pregnancy
3. Chronic hypertension
4. Hydatidiform mole
5. Chronic renal disease
6. Malnutrition
7. Diabetes
8. Hydrops fetalis
9. History of PIH in family or in previous pregnancy
10. Age less than 20 or greater than 30
11. Patient's developing polyhydramnios

***Premature Rupture of the Membranes.*** Premature rupture of the membranes, that is, rupture prior to the onset of labor, is a major perinatal complication and is responsible for at least 30 percent of preterm deliveries (Garite, 1990; Kaltreider, 1980). The incidence of premature rupture of the membranes is reported to be 8 to 10 percent of all pregnancies that extend beyond 20 weeks' gestation (Garite, 1990; Gunn et al, 1970). It is associated with a high perinatal mortality rate, attributable primarily to delivery of premature, low-birth-weight infants. Depending on management, premature rupture of the membranes can also be associated with significant perinatal morbidity, including premature delivery, maternal and/or fetal infection, and fetal respiratory distress syndrome. Other problems, such as breech presentation, prolapsed cord, transverse lie, aplastic lungs, and positional limb deformities of the fetus due to the lack of "cushioning" normally provided by amniotic fluid, have also been reported. It is felt by several authors that preexisting infection may contribute significantly to premature rupture of the membranes.

***Intrauterine Growth Retardation.*** Intrauterine growth retardation (IUGR) complicates approximately 3 to 7 percent of all pregnancies. Babies born at or below the 10th percentile of mean weight for gestation are at greater risk of antepartum death, perinatal asphyxia, neonatal morbidity, and later developmental problems. Babies with IUGR have a perinatal mortality rate that is 8 times that of normal infants (Butler and Alberman, 1969).

Two types of fetal growth retardation—asymmetric and symmetric—have been described. In asymmetric IUGR, there is increasing disproportion in head-to-body ratios. This type of IUGR is the more common and is known as "brain sparing," because the last organ to be deprived of essential nutrients is the brain. Asymmetric IUGR is most commonly caused by adverse effects applied during the latter part of pregnancy. A common example is placental insufficiency resulting from such conditions as PIH, chronic hypertension, multiple gestation, chronic abruption, smoking, and alcoholism. Symmetric IUGR is non–brain sparing, occurs less commonly, and can be the result of an acute maternal infection, chromosomal abnormalities in the fetus, maternal drug addiction, or maternal malnutrition.

Whatever the cause and type of IUGR, affected babies are at increased risk for death or damage during both the antepartum and intrapartum period. Prompt identification and continued follow-up of the fetuses during pregnancy can mean the difference between life and death for these babies, as well as affecting the quality of life in those that survive.

At present, diagnostic accuracy of IUGR is less than optimal. Diagnostic screening for IUGR infants includes meticulous use of McDonald measurements between 20 and 34 weeks, accurate assessment of gestational age, and serial ultrasonography as appropriate, along with a review of the patient's history to look for factors predisposing her baby to IUGR (Table 2–12).

***Rh Isoimmunization.*** In the early 1960s, Rh hemolytic disease of the newborn was responsible for 5000 to 6000 perinatal deaths annually. Medical science, in the space of one generation, has elucidated the pathogenesis of the disease, outlined a plan for prenatal diagnosis and intrauterine and neonatal treatment, and developed a method for prevention of the disease that has resulted in total prevention of the severe form now being within reach. With optimal management at a tertiary level perinatal center, perinatal mortality from Rh erythroblastosis has been reduced from 14.3 to 1.5 percent (Bowman, 1978).

The simple step of determining a woman's Rh status should be done at the initial examination for all pregnant women. Every Rh-

**Table 2–12**
FACTORS CAUSING FETAL
GROWTH RETARDATION

**Maternal Factors Causing**
**Fetal Growth Retardation**
    Chronic lung disease
    Cyanotic heart disease
    Severe anemias
    Malnutrition
    Low calorie consumption
    Malabsorption conditions
    Surgical bypass procedures
    Smoking
    Drug addiction
**Placental Factors Causing**
**Fetal Growth Retardation**
    Small placenta in hypertensive women
    Circumvallate placenta
    Abnormal implantation site
    Placental infarcts
    Abruptio placentae
**Fetal Factors Causing**
**Fetal Growth Retardation**
    Congenital anomalies
    Trisomies
    Intrauterine infections
        AIDS*
        TORCH†

From Spellacy WN: Intrauterine growth retardation. *In*
Eden R, Boehm F: Assessment and Care of the Fetus.
Norwalk, CT, Appleton & Lange, 1990, p 644. Reprinted by
permission of Appleton & Lange, Inc.
* AIDS = Acquired immunodeficiency syndrome.
† TORCH = *T*oxoplasmosis, *R*ubella, *C*ytomegalovirus
(CMV), and *H*erpes simplex virus (HSV).

negative woman carrying a child fathered by an Rh-positive man should be tested for antibodies in every pregnancy, starting with the first prenatal visit. Past history should be elicited from the woman and should include the following:

1. History of transfusion of incompatible blood
2. Outcome of previous pregnancies
   a. Rh factors of infants
   b. Severity of hemolytic disease
   c. Gestational age at intrauterine death, if any
   d. Questionable autopsy confirmation of erythroblastosis
3. Existing conditions implicated in predisposition to Rh isoimmunization
   a. PIH
   b. External version
   c. Abruptio placentae

Once this information is obtained, appropriate measures—including amniocentesis, cordocentesis, intrauterine fetal transfusion, and planning for possible early delivery—can be instituted.

Prevention is the key to eradicating this disease. With assiduous attention to detail in caring for all Rh-negative women (regardless of outcome of pregnancy) and appropriate use of Rh immunoglobulin, this goal may be possible (Bowman, 1990).

***Prolonged Pregnancy.*** Prolonged pregnancy is a common obstetric problem with potentially profound consequences. Three definitions are important at the outset:

1. *Postdatism*—the pregnancy has gone beyond the expected date of birth.
2. *Prolonged pregnancy*—the length of gestation has exceeded 42 weeks.
3. *Postmaturity*—a pediatric diagnosis based on neonatal examination.

The incidence of prolonged pregnancy ranges from 7 to 12 percent, with an average of approximately 10 percent. The diagnosis of prolonged pregnancy starts at the first prenatal visit with an accurate and meticulous estimation of gestational age, taking into account the last menstrual period, last normal period, dates of negative and positive pregnancy tests, history of oral contraceptive use, history of menstrual irregularity, and pelvic examinations. Later important determinations are based on hearing fetal heart tones with a fetoscope at 20 weeks, fundal height measurements, and ultrasonography when appropriate. All of these are necessary in order to "date" the pregnancy and to later differentiate between postdatism and prolonged pregnancy should the need arise.

The perinatal impact of prolonged pregnancy may be severe: Perinatal mortality for these infants is increased 2 to 3 times relative to term infants and, in small-for-gestational-age infants, 7 times. Morbidity includes birth trauma, meconium aspiration, and hypoglycemia. Developmental defects in surviving infants have been identified.

The vast majority of prolonged pregnancies are idiopathic; however, anencephaly, trisomy 18, and placental sulfatase deficiency have all been implicated in the etiology of this syndrome.

### Habits/Habituation

***Smoking during Pregnancy.*** Cigarette smoking during pregnancy has been demonstrated to be detrimental to the fetus. The mechanism of the effect of smoking on the outcome of pregnancy is still obscure, but it is believed to be related to decreased placental perfusion of the smoker. Studies have shown that among pregnant women who smoke, particularly those who smoke more than 20 cigarettes per day, the incidence of premature labor and delivery is significantly increased. There is also a strong correlation between smoking and low birth weight, premature infants, and stillbirths. Evidence has also been presented that smoking during pregnancy increases the incidence of bleeding, abruptio placentae, placenta previa, and premature and prolonged rupture of the membranes (Kleinman et al, 1988). In addition, infants of smoking mothers tend to continue to be smaller at 1 year of age when compared with offspring of nonsmoking mothers. Women who cannot stop smoking should be urged to at least reduce the number of cigarettes smoked to 10 or fewer per day (Smith, 1979).

*Alcohol.* Infants born to mothers who drink alcohol on a regular basis are at risk for fetal alcohol syndrome, a combination of fetal alcohol syndrome facies, mental retardation, intrauterine growth retardation, and developmental failure. The world rate for fetal alcohol syndrome has been estimated at approximately 1.9/1000 live births. In the United States, where 60 to 80 percent of all fetuses are exposed to some alcohol during the prenatal period, fetal alcohol syndrome is estimated to be the leading cause of mental retardation.

In addition to full fetal alcohol syndrome, there is a range of adverse outcomes that have been related to prenatal alcohol exposure. Risk of spontaneous abortion is doubled, and risk for stillbirth is significantly increased. The most consistent effect of alcohol exposure is a twofold increase in the rate of intrauterine growth retardation over the pregnant population in general. Interventive efforts toward ceasing or significantly reducing the amount of alcohol consumed have resulted in improved outcomes, depending on when cessation or reduction occurred (Brown, 1988).

*Medications and Substance Abuse.* Although some animal studies have suggested that certain drugs cause teratogenic effects, these studies cannot always be applied to humans, and some drugs have not been tested at all. The best recommendation is that no medication be taken during pregnancy unless absolutely necessary (Drukker, 1983). See Chapter 9 for a more detailed discussion.

The increasing use of the street drug crack cocaine has brought a precipitous increase in the rates of preterm labor and delivery, fetal congenital anomalies, abruption, and IUGR. Intravenous drug abusers are at risk for all of these complications, as well as a greatly increased risk for maternal and/or neonatal AIDS. The outlook for pregnant women who abuse drugs is further complicated by maternal medical disorders associated with drug abuse. These include hepatitis, multiple abscesses, thrombophlebitis, pulmonary embolus, anemia, nephrotic syndrome, and sexually transmitted diseases. (See Chapter 10 for a more detailed discussion.)

*"If we are interested in quality then let us know what can assure it; likewise let us understand those events which are responsible for developmental delay" (Hobel, 1977).*

At conception, every fetus receives his or her own genetic potential through his or her parents. This genetic potential for intelligence, development, and quality of life is subjected to numerous environmental, physical, social, and psychologic obstacles along the continuum of pregnancy. How or if the fetus survives depends a great deal on the health care provided the mother.

To be born too soon, too small, unwanted, or uncared for has dire consequences for the child not only in terms of physical problems but also in terms of mental and emotional development. Problems during pregnancy, labor, and delivery have too often affected the fetus in ways that may make the achievement of his or her genetic potential impossible.

Therefore, we see two major goals. The first is to ensure accessibility to the appropriate health care system for all women.

Our second goal is to reduce the number of low-birth-weight infants born. Although this group represents only 1 percent of all liveborn infants, it contributes to over half of the neonatal mortality in parts of the United States.

"Low-risk" pregnancy is a diagnosis made only in retrospect. Continuous and thorough assessment of and intervention for mother and fetus prenatally, during the intrapartum period, and neonatally is a means of contributing toward the quality of life for them as individuals and for all of us.

# References

Abrams BF, Laros RK: Prepregnancy weight, weight gain and birthweight. Am J Obstet Gynecol 154:503–509, 1986.

Adelstein P, Fedrick J: Antenatal identification of women at increased risk of being delivered of a low birth weight infant at term. Br J Obstet Gynaecol 85:8, 1978.

Akhtar J, Sehgal N: Prognostic value of a prepartum and intrapartum risk-scoring method. Southern Medical Journal (Birmingham AL) 73(4):412–414, 1980.

Allen E, Mantz ML: Are normal patients at risk during pregnancy? JOGN Nurs 10:348, 1981.

Arsenault PS: Maternal and antenatal factors in the risk of sudden infant death syndrome. Am J Epidemiol 111:279, 1981.

Atrash HK, Koonin LM, Lawson HW, et al: Maternal Mortality in the United States, 1979–1986. Obstet Gynecol 76(6):1055–61, 1990.

Babson C, Benson R: Management of the High Risk Pregnancy and Intensive Care of the Neonate. St. Louis, CV Mosby Co 1975, pp 1–21, 276–281.

Baruffi G, Strobino DM, Dellinger WS Jr: Definitions of high risk in pregnancy and evaluation of their predictive ability. Am J Obstet Gynecol 148:781, 1984.

Becker CH: Comprehensive assessment of the healthy gravida. JOGN Nurs 11:375, 1982.

Bender S: Placenta previa and previous lower uterine segment cesearean section. Surg Gynecol Obstet 98:625, 1990.

Benedetti T: Cardiopulmonary disorders. In Eden R, and Boehm, F (eds): Assessment and Care of the Fetus. Norwalk, CT, Appleton & Lange, 1990.

Berg CJ, Druschel CM, McCarthy BJ, et al: Neonatal mortality in normal birth weight babies: does the level of hospital care make a difference? Am J Obstet Gynecol 161(1):86, 1989.

Bowman JM: Maternal blood group immunization. In Eden R, and Boehm F (eds): Assessment and Care of the Fetus. Norwalk, CT, Appleton & Lange, 1990, pp 749–766.

Bowman JM: The management of Rh-isoimmunization. Obstet Gynecol 52:1, 1978.

Brewer DW, Aubry, RH: Physiology of pregnancy, clinical pathologic correlations. Postgrad Med 52:110, 1972.

Brewer DW, Aubry RH: Physiology of pregnancy, clinical pathologic correlations. Postgrad Med 53:221, 1973.

Brown SS (ed): Prenatal Care: reaching mothers, reaching infants. Washington, DC, National Academy Press, 1988.

Brunel LE: Prenatal care. In Niswander KR (ed): Manual of Obstetrics: Diagnosis and Management. Boston, Little, Brown & Co 1979, pp 27–35.

Burrow GN, Ferris TF: Medical Complications During Pregnancy, 2nd ed. Philadelphia, WB Saunders Co, 1982.

Burchell RC, Gunn J: The new birth experience. JOGN Nurs 9:250, 1980.

Butler NR, Bonham DG: Perinatal Mortality: The First Report of the 1958 British Perinatal Survey. Edinburgh and London, E & S Livingstone, Ltd, 1969.

Butler NR, Alberman ED: Perinatal Problems: The Second Report of the 1958 British Perinatal Mortality Survey. Edinburgh and London, E & S Livingstone, Ltd, 1969.

Cammu H, Verlaenen H, Derde MP: Premature Rupture of Membranes at Term in Nulliparous Women: a hazard? Obstet Gynecol 76(4):671–74, 1990.

Canadian Task Force on the Periodic Health Examination: The periodic health examination. Can Med Assoc J 121:1193, 1979.

Catalano PM, Capeless EL: Fetomaternal Bleeding as a Cause of Recurrent Fetal Morbidity and Mortality. Obstet Gynecol 76(5, part 2):972, 1990.

Cavanagh D, O'Connor TCF, Knuppel RAK: Obstetric Emergencies. Philadelphia, JB Lippincott Co, 1982, Chapters 1,2,6,9,11.

Cavanagh D, Talisman FR: Interval between pregnancies. In Cavanagh D (ed): Prematurity and the Obstetrician. New York, Appleton-Century-Crofts, 1969.

Cetrulo CL, Freeman R: Bioelectric evaluation in intrauterine growth retardation. Clin Obstet Gynecol 20:137, 1977.

Chez RA: A clinical approach to the therapy of premature labor. In Gluck L (ed): Intrauterine Asphyxia and the Developing Fetal Brain. Chicago, Year Book MediCal, 1977, pp 139–148.

Clark S: Third trimester hemorrhage. In Eden R, Boehm F (eds): Assessment and Care of the Fetus: physiological, clinical and medicolegal principles, Norwalk, CT, Appleton & Lange, 1990, p 631.

Coopland AT, Peddle LJ, Baskett TF, et al: A simplified antepartum high-risk scoring system form: statistical analysis of 5459 cases. Can Med Assoc J 116(9):999, 1977.

Crandall BF, Lebherz TB, Tabash K: Maternal age and amniocentesis: should this be lowered to 30 years? Prenat Diagn 6(4):237–42, 1986.

Crandon AJ: Maternal anxiety and obstetric complications. J Psychosom Res 23:109–111, 1979.

Creasy RK: Preterm labor. In Eden R, Boehm F (eds): Assessment and Care of the Fetus. Norwalk, CT: Appleton & Lange, 1990, pp 617–630.

Creasy RK, Herron MA: Prevention of preterm birth. Semin Perinatol, 5:295, 1981.

Creasy RK, Gummer BA, Liggins GC: System for predicting spontaneous preterm birth Obstet Gynecol 55:692, 1980.

Dauphinee JD: Risk assessment. In Mandeville LK and Troiano NH (ed): High-Risk Intrapartum Nursing. Philadelphia, JB Lippincott Co, 1992.

Davidson EC Jr: A Strategy to Reduce Infant Mortality. Obstet Gynecol 77 (No. 1):1–6, 1991.

Donahue CL Jr, Wan TT: Measuring obstetric risks of prematurity: a preliminary analysis of neonatal death. Am J Obstet Gynecol 116:911, 1973.

Degeorge FV, Nesbitt RL, Aubry RH: High risk obstetrics. VI. An evaluation of the effects of intensified care on pregnancy outcome. Am J Obstet Gynecol 111:650, 1971.

Donnelly FJ, Flowers CE, Creadice RN, et al: Parental, fetal, and environmental factors in perinatal mortality. Am J Obstet Gynecol 74:1245, 1957.

Douglas CP: Prenatal risks: an obstetrician's point of view. In Aladjem S (ed): Risks in the Practice of Modern Obstetrics, 2nd ed. St. Louis, CV Mosby Co, 1975.

Drukker J: Antenatal Assessment. Part I. Maternal profile. NAACOG Update Series, Continuing Professional Education Center, Inc, Princeton, NJ, 1983.

Dweck HS: The tiny baby: past, present, and future. Clin Perinatol 4:425, 1977.

Easterling TR, Benedetti TJ, Schmucker BC, et al: Maternal Hemodynamics in Normal and Preeclamptic Pregnancies: a longitudinal study. Obstet Gynecol 76(6):1061–70, 1990.

Edwards LE, Barrada MI, Tatreau, et al: A simplified antepartum risk-scoring system. Obstet Gynecol 54(2):237, 1979.

Effer SB: Management of high-risk pregnancy: report of a combined obstetrical and neonatal care unit. Canad Med Assoc J 101(389):55, 1969.

Eisner V, Pratt MW, Hexter A, et al: Improvement in infant and perinatal mortality in the United States, 1965–1973. I. Priorities for intervention. Am J Public Health 68:359, 1978.

Fedrick J: Antenatal identification of women at high risk of spontaneous pre-term birth. Br J Obstet Gynaecol 83:351, 1976.

Field T, Sandberg D, Garcia R, Rosario M: Prenatal problems, postpartum depression and early mother-infant interactions. Dev Psychol 12:1152–1156, 1985.

Fortney JA, Whitehorne EW: The development of an index of high-risk pregnancy. Am J Obstet Gynecol 143:501, 1982.

Foy JE, Backes CR: A study of the relationship between Goodwin's high-risk scoring system and fetal outcome. J Am Osteopath Assoc 78:113, 1978.

Gabbe SG, Niebyl JR, Simpson JL: Obstetrics: Normal and Problem Pregnancies, 2nd ed. New York, Churchill Livingstone, 1991.

Gant N, Pritchard J: Pregnancy induced hypertension. In Eden R, Boehm F (eds): Assessment and Care of the Fetus. Norwalk, CT, Appleton & Lange, 1990.

Garite TJ: Premature rupture of the membranes. In Eden R, Boehm F (eds): Assessment and Care of the Fetus: Physiological, Clinical, and Medicolegal Principles, Norwalk, CT, Appleton & Lange, 1990, p 631.

Gillogley KM, Evans AT, Hanson RL, et al: The perinatal impact of cocaine, amphetamine, and opiate use detected by universal intrapartum screening. Am J Obstet Gynecol 163(5):1535, 1990.

Goldsmith J: Neonatal morbidity. In: Eden R, Boehm F (eds): Assessment and Care of the Fetus. Norwalk, CT, Appleton & Lange, 1990.

Goodwin JW, Dunne JT, Thomas BW: Antepartum identification of the fetus at risk. Canad Med Assoc J 101(458):57, 1969.

Gunn GC; Mishell DR, Morton DG: Premature rupture of the fetal membranes: a review. Amer J Obstet Gynecol 106:469, 1970.

Guzick DS, Daikoku NH, Kaltreider DF: Predictability of pregnancy outcome in preterm delivery. Obstet Gynecol 63:645, 1984.

Haeri AD, South J, Naldrett J: A scoring system for identifying pregnant patients with a high risk of perinatal mortality. J Obstet Gynaecol Brit Commonw 81:535, 1974.

Halliday HL, Jones PK, Jones SL, et al: Method of screening obstetrics patients to prevent reproductive wastage. Obstet Gynecol 55:656, 1980.

Harper RG, Sokal MM, Sokal S, et al: The high risk perinatal registry. A systematic approach for reducing perinatal mortality. Obstet Gynecol 50(3):264, 1977.

Hein HA, Brumeister LF, Papke KR: The Relationship of Unwed Status to Infant Mortality. Obstet Gynecol 76(5, Part 1):763, 1990.

Heron MA, Katz M, Creasy RK: Evaluation of a preterm birth prevention program: preliminary report. Obstet Gyneocol 59:452–456, 1982.

Higgins AC, Moxley JE, Pencharz PB, et al: Impact of the Higgins nutrition intervention program on birth weight: a within mother analysis. J Amer Dietetic Assoc 89:1097, 1989.

Hobel CJ: Recognition of the high risk pregnant woman. In Spellacy W (ed): Management of the High Risk Pregnancy. Baltimore, University Park Press, 1976, pp 1–28.

Hobel CJ: Identification of the patient at risk. In Bolognese RJ (ed): Perinatal Medicine: Clinical Management of the High Risk Fetus and Neonate. Baltimore, Williams & Wilkins, 1977, pp 1–25.

Hobel CJ, Youkeles L, Forsythe A: Prenatal and intrapartum high risk screening II: risk factors reassessed. Am J Obstet Gynecol 136:1051–1056, 1979.

Hobel CJ, Hyvarinen MA, Okada DM, et al: Prenatal and intrapartum high-risk screening. 1. Prediction of the high-risk neonate. Am J Obstet Gynecol 117:1, 1973.

Holbrook RA Jr, Laros RK Jr, Creasy RK: Evaluation of a risk-scoring system for prediction of preterm labor. Am J Perinat 6:62, 1989.

Jellinek MS, Murphy JM, Bishop S, et al: Protecting severely abused and neglected children—An unkept promise. N Engl J Med 323(No. 23): 1628–30, 1990.

Jones PK, Halliday HL, Jones SL: Prediction of neonatal death or need for interhospital transfer by prenatal risk characteristics. Med Care 17:796, 1979.

Josten L: Prenatal assessment guide for illuminating possible problems with parenting. MCN 6:113, 1981.

Kadar N, Romero R: Ectopic pregnancy. In Eden R, Boehm F (eds): Assessment and Care of the Fetus. Norwalk, CT, Appleton & Lange, 1990.

Kaltreider DF, Kohl S: Epidemiology of preterm delivery. Clin Obstet Gynecol 23:17, 1980.

Kamiaski M, Goujard, Rumeau-Rouquette C: Prediction of low-birth-weight and prematurity by a multiple regression analysis with maternal characteristics known since the beginning of pregnancy. Int J Epidemiol 2:195–204, 1973.

Kappy KA, Cetrulo CL, Knuppel RA, et al: Premature rupture of the membranes: a conservative approach. Am J Obstet Gynecol 134:655, 1979.

Kennedy ET: A prenatal screening system for use in a community-based setting. J Am Diet Assoc 86:1372, 1986.

Kessner DM, Singer J, Kalk CE, et al: A selected review of the epidemiology of infant mortality. In Contrasts on Health Status, Vol. 1: Infant Death: An Analysis by Maternal Risk and Health Care. Washington, D.C., Institute of Medicine, National Academy of Sciences, 1973, pp 110–113.

Kleinman JC, Pierre MB Jr, Madans JH, et al: The effects of maternal smoking on fetal and infant mortality. Am J Epidem 127:274–282, 1988.

Kopp CB, Kaler SR: Risk in infancy: origins and implications. Amer Psychol, Feb 1989, p 224.

Kugler JP, Connell FA, Henley CE: An evaluation of prenatal care utilization in a military health care setting. Milit Med 155:33, 1990.

Laifer SA, Darby MJ, Scantlebury VP, et al: Pregnancy and liver transplantation. Obstet Gynecol 76(6):1083, 1990.

Larks SD, Larks GG: Factors associated with birth conditions. Biol Neonate 20:134, 1972.

Lilienfeld AM, Parkhurst E: A study of the association of factors of pregnancy and parturition with the development of cerebral palsy. A preliminary report. Am J Hyg 53:262, 1951.

Lilienfeld AM, Passamanick B: The association of maternal and fetal factors with the development of cerebral palsy and epilepsy. Am J Obstet Gynecol 70:93, 1955.

Little WJ: On the influence of abnormal parturition, difficult labours, premature birth and asphyxia neonatorum, on the mental and physical condition of the child, especially in relation to deformities. Trans Obstet Soc London 3:293, 1862.

Main DM, Gabbe SG: Risk scoring for preterm labor: where do we go from here? Am J Obstet Gynecol 157:789–93, 1987.

Main DM, Richardson D, Gabbe SG, et al: Prospective evaluation of a risk scoring system for predicating preterm delivery in black inner-city women. Obstet Gynecol 69:61–66, 1987.

Marriage KJ, Davies PA: Neurological sequelae in children surviving mechanical ventilation in the neonatal period. Arch Dis Child 52:176, 1977.

Martin JN Jr, Blake PG, Lowry SL, et al: Pregnancy complicated by preeclampsia-eclampsia with the syndrome of hemolysis, elevated liver enzymes, and low platelet count: how rapid is postpartum recovery? Obstet Gynecol 76(5, Part 1):737–742, 1990.

McCarthy BJ, Schultz KF, Terry JS: Identifying neonatal risk factors and predicting neonatal deaths in Georgia. Am J Obstet Gynecol 142:557, 1982.

McCormick MC: The contribution of low birthweight to infant mortality and childhood morbidity. N Engl J Med 312:82–90, 1985.

Minkoff HL, Henderson C, Mendez, et al: Pregnancy outcomes among mothers infected with human immunodeficiency virus and uninfected controls. Am J Obstet Gynecol 163:1598, 1990.

Mixon WCW, Hickson EB: A Guide to Obstetrics in General Practice. Staples Press, London, 1952.

Mold JW, Stein HF: Sounding board: the cascade effect in the clinical care of patients. N Engl J Med 314(8):512–514, 1986.

Molfese VJ, Thomas BK, Bennett AG: Perinatal outcome: similarity and predictive value of antepartum and intrapartum assessment scales. J Reprod Med 30:30, 1985.

Moos MK, Cefalo RC: Preconceptional health promotion: A focus for obstetrical care. Am J Perinat 4:63–67, 1987.

Morrison I, Olsen J: Perinatal mortality and antepartum risk scoring. Obstet Gynecol 53:362, 1979.

Naeye RL, Blank WA: Influences of pregnancy risk factors on fetal and newborn disorders. Clin Perinatol 1:187, 1974.

Nesbitt REL, Aubry RH: High-risk obstetrics. II. Value of semiobjective system in identifying the vulnerable group. Am J Obstet Gynecol 103(7):972, 1969.

Nesbitt TS, Connell FA, Hart LG, et al: Access to obstetric care in rural areas: effect on birth outcomes. Am J Public Health 80(7):814–818; 1990.

Niswander K, Henson G, Elbourne D, et al: Adverse outcome of pregnancy and the quality of obstetric care. Lancet 2(8407):827–31, 1984.

Niswander KR, Gordon M: The Women and Their Pregnancies. Philadelphia, WB Saunders Co, 1972.

O'Brien WF, Knuppel RA, Torres C, Sternlicht D: Potential prenatal predictions of Down syndrome: a statistical analysis. Am J Obstet Gynecol 163:179, 1990.

Odendaal HJ, Pattinson RC, Bam R, et al: Aggressive or expectant management for patients with severe preeclampsia between 28–34 weeks' gestation: a randomized controlled trial. Obstet Gynecol 76(6):1070–1076, 1990.

Orleans M, Haverkamp AD: Are there health risks in using risking systems? The case of perinatal risk assessment. Health Policy 7:297–307, 1987.

Owen J, Goldenberg RL, Davis RO, et al: Evaluation of a risk scoring system as a predictor of preterm birth in an indigent population. Am J Obstet Gynecol 163(3):873–79, 1990.

Patterson MEL: The aetiology and outcome of abruptio placentae. Acta Obstet Gynecol Scand Suppl 58:31, 1979.

Paul RH, Hon EH: Clinical fetal monitoring. V. Effect on perinatal outcome. Am J Obstet Gynecol 114:529, 1974.

Pavelka R, Riss P, Parschalk O, et al: Practical experience in the prevention of prematurity using Thalhammer's score. J Perinat Med 8:100, 1980.

Peabody FW: The care of the patient. J Am Med Assoc 88:877, 1927.

Pearse WH: Quality of care-A primer. Obstet Gynecol 77(1):145, 1991.

Prechtl HFR: Neurological sequelae of prenatal and perinatal complications. Br Med J 34:763, 1967.

Pritchard JA, MacDonald PC: Hypertensive disorders in pregnancy. In Williams Obstetrics, 15th ed. New York, Appleton-Century-Crofts, 1978, p 552.

Pritchard JA, MacDonald PC, Gant WF: Preterm and postterm pregnancy and fetal growth retardation. In Williams Obstetrics, 17th ed. Norwalk, CT, Appleton-Century-Crofts, 1985.

Rayburn WF, Johnson MZ, Hoffman KL, et al: Intrapartum fetal heart rate patterns and neonatal intraventricular hemorrhage. Am J Perinatal 4(2):98–101, 1987.

Rey HR, James LS, Wiele RV: Interrelationship between risk factors of pregnancy, perinatal events and outcome. Soc Gynecol Invest 8:70, 1977.

Rogers MGH: The risk register—A critical assessment. Med Officer Nov 17, 1967:253.

Ryan GM, Sweeney P, Solola A: Prenatal care and pregnancy outcome. Am J Obstet Gynecol 129:876, 1980.

Sachs BP, Brown DA, Driscoll SG, et al: Maternal mortality in New England: trends and prevention. N Engl J Med 316:667–672, 1987.

Scott DE, Pritchard JA: Anemia in pregnancy. In Milunsky, A (ed): Clinics in Perinatology. Philadelphia, WB Saunders Co, 1974.

Schneider KD: Primary care of the pregnant woman: laboratory tests. A Staff Development Program in Perinatal Nursing Care. White Plains, NY, National Foundation–March of Dimes, 1978.

Seidman DS, Ever-Hadani P, Gale R: Effect of maternal smoking and age on congenital anomalies. Obstet Gynecol 76(6):1046–1051, 1990.

Sirivongs B, Parisunyakui S: Risk pregnancy screening: a simple method for non-physicians to screen the high-risk pregnancy. J Med Assoc Thai 67(suppl 2):15, 1984.

Shapiro S, Schlesinger ER, Nesbitt REL: Infant, Perinatal, Maternal, and Childhood Mortality in the United States. Cambridge, MA, Harvard University Press, 1968.

Smith M, Stratton WC, Roi L: Labor risk assessment in a rural community hospital. Am J Obstet Gynecol 151:569, 1985.

Smith D: Mothering Your Unborn Baby. Philadelphia, WB Saunders Co, 1979.

Sokol RJ, Rosen MG, Stojkov J, et al: Clinical application of high-risk scoring on an obstetric service. Am J Obstet Gynecol 128:652, 1977.

Sylvain JPE: Regionalization of perinatal services and the use of high-risk scoring systems. Can Med Assoc J 130:1269, 1984.

Trotter CW, Chang PN, Thompson T, et al: Perinatal factors and the developmental outcome of preterm infants. JOGN Nurs, 11:83, 1982.

Wall EM: Assessing obstetric risk: a review of obstetric risk-scoring systems. J Fam Prac 27(2):153, 1988.

Wall EM, Sinclair AE, Nelson J, et al: The relationship between assessed obstetric risk and maternal-perinatal outcome. J Fam Pract 28(1):35, 1989.

Wallace HM: Factors associated with perinatal mortality and morbidity. Clin Obstet Gynecol 13:38, 1971.

Weinstein AM, Dubin BD, Podleski WK, et al: Asthma and pregnancy. JAMA; 241:1161, 1979.

Wells HB, Greenberg BG, Donnelly JF: North Carolina fetal and neonatal death study. I. Study design and some preliminary results. Am J Publ Health 48:1583, 1958.

Wilson EW, Sill HK: Identification of the high risk pregnancy by a scoring system. N Z Med J 78:437, 1973.

Wilson RW, Schifrin BS: Is any pregnancy low risk? Obstet Gynecol 55:653, 1980.

Winters S, Itzkowitz S, Johnson K: Prenatal risk assessment: an evaluation of the Hobel record in a Mount Sinai clinic population. The Mount Sinai Journal of Medicine 46:424, 1979.

Yeh SY, Forsythe A, Lowensohn RI, et al: A study of the relationship between Goodwin's high-risk score and fetal outcome. Am J Obstet Gynecol 127:50, 1977.

# CHAPTER 3

· · · · · · · · · · · · · · · · · · · · · · · · · · · · · · · · · · ·

# Prevention and Public Health in Obstetrics

Sister Jeanne Meurer and Douglas L. Taren

The type and quality of obstetric care have recently been reviewed in the United States Public Health Service Expert Panel report, *Caring for Our Future: The Content of Prenatal Care* (US PHS, 1989). The newly defined objectives of prenatal care in this report are based on the premise that the preconceptual period, the 9 months of pregnancy, and the postpartum period are the ideal times to ensure a healthy pregnancy outcome for the family. Thus, family planning, pediatric care, and parenting skills are also a part of this holistic model of prenatal care. To fulfill these objectives, attention must be given to the health of the woman, her social development, her family dynamics, and the availability of resources and services in the community. The basic components of prenatal care can be accomplished by (1) health promotion, (2) early and continuing risk assessment, (3) medical and psychosocial interventions, and (4) follow-up care (US PHS, 1989).

The focus of prenatal care is to improve perinatal outcomes by decreasing maternal and infant morbidity and mortality. The Institute of Medicine (1985) concluded from a comprehensive review of the literature that prenatal care has reduced the incidence of low birth weight. This reduction in low birth weight has been a major factor in lowering the infant mortality rate in this country over the past century. However, during the past decade there has been a stagnation in the downward trend for low birth weight and the infant mortality rate in the United

States compared with other developed countries. These findings are also corroborated by other recent comprehensive studies on perinatal care (National Commission to Prevent Infant Mortality, 1988; Sing et al, 1990).

The prevention and public health activities for improving perinatal outcomes need to address a broad range of issues to effect long-term changes. In order to facilitate these types of changes, public health policies need also to consider social problems such as dysfunctional families, poverty, hunger, homelessness, substance abuse, sexually transmitted diseases, AIDS, and the stresses of daily living in their plans of action. Clinical aspects of prenatal care cannot solve these problems alone, but act as a conduit to channel women into needed services that assist in the improvement of the physical and mental health of women, infants, and the family. To do this, prenatal care has to be available, accessible, affordable, and acceptable to those who need it.

## Obstacles to Prenatal Care

In 1987, the majority of pregnant women (76 percent) in the United States received prenatal care in the first trimester (NCHS, 1989). Disturbingly, 18 percent delayed their care to the second trimester, and 6.1 percent of the pregnant population either received care only in the third trimester or received none at all (NCHS, 1989). Concerted efforts by the perinatal team to enroll women into care must be increased if the infant mortality rate is to decrease in the near future. In this respect, the 1990 objective published by the Department of Health and Human Services (1980) was to have at least 90 percent of pregnant women start prenatal care in their first trimester of pregnancy. Unfortunately, this objective was not met, and the authors expect that this same objective for the year 2000 (Department of Health and Human Services, 1990) will not be accomplished.

A major reason why this objective is presently difficult to achieve is the presence of numerous obstacles that exist to prenatal care (Institute of Medicine, 1988; National Commission to Prevent Infant Mortality, 1990). These obstacles include the financing of prenatal care, inadequate systems capacity, poor organization practices and clinic atmosphere, and cultural and personal biases. These obstacles are most difficult to overcome by women who are poor, young, and unmarried and who are of African American, Hispanic, or Native American descent and have completed less than 12 years of education (NCHS, 1989). A careful review of 15 studies indicated that poverty and a low value placed on prenatal services were the most consistent factors associated with insufficient prenatal care (Institute of Medicine, 1988); similar findings from a survey of physicians were presented by the American College of Obstetricians and Gynecologists (ACOG, 1987). It is now necessary to remove these obstacles in order to plan programs that will increase the number of women enrolling early into prenatal care and lower the infant mortality rate in this country.

## FINANCING PRENATAL CARE

Women with private health insurance are more likely than uninsured women or Medicaid-enrolled women to receive early and adequate prenatal care (Cooney, 1985; Fisher et al, 1985). In 1985, approximately 14.6 million women of childbearing age (26 percent) either had no health insurance or had insurance that did not cover maternity care. More disturbingly, about half of the women in their childbearing years without insurance are either employed or have spouses who are employed (The Allen Guttmacher Institute, 1987).

For women below the poverty level, decreasing the financial obstacles to prenatal care has been accomplished by providing local assistance in completing applications for Medicaid eligibility (Contis et al, 1990). Nationally, the OMNIBUS Reconciliation Act of 1989 (US GAO, 1989) increased the income criteria for Medicaid to 185 percent of the poverty level. The increase to 185 percent of the poverty level was attained in some states by using state dollars to match federal dollars, thus enabling more pregnant women to seek health care. Providing universal access to health care has also been addressed through state and federal legislation. New York, Massachusetts, and Hawaii have introduced plans for state health insurance programs. Using single-payer systems and competitive models, these initiatives may also help constrain health care costs (Beauchamp et al, 1990).

## INADEQUATE SYSTEMS CAPACITY

Not having enough providers is a major obstacle to having an adequate system capacity for prenatal care. Long waiting times for appointments at private offices, local public health departments, and federal community health centers are a reflection of inadequate systems capacity (Institute of Medicine, 1988). These problems occur because of the increasing number of women with no health insurance or inadequate insurance, and the decreasing number of private providers accepting Medicaid insurance. Another major problem limiting capacity is the decreasing number of obstetricians, nurse-midwives, and public health nurses because of inadequate Medicaid reimbursement rates and increases in malpractice insurance premiums.

Many states have attempted to increase the system capacity by increasing Medicaid reimbursement rates, thereby encouraging provider participation. The National Public Health Service Corps is also being considered again as a mechanism to increase the number of providers in underserved areas (Brown et al, 1990). Finally, as presented earlier, creating state and federal legislation that will ensure universal access will increase the system capacity by providing the necessary funds and personnel.

## ORGANIZATION, PRACTICES, AND ENVIRONMENT

The acceptance and use of public health services are adversely affected by poorly organized systems, insensitive practices, and hostile atmospheres (Okada et al, 1980). Inadequate coordination between health departments, private physicians, community and tertiary hospitals, and other community agencies creates a confusing system for families, resulting in duplication of services or no services at all (National Commission to Prevent Infant Mortality, 1990). The practice of having multiple sites for various services has led to access problems because of inadequate transportation systems, a lack of child care facilities, and schedules that do not necessarily accommodate working parents, adolescents, and school-aged children.

Providing comprehensive care in single locations, "one-stop shopping" for women and families to obtain all their services, is one plan that has been promoted to decrease the burden on clients receiving care. This one-stop shopping will allow women and their families to make fewer trips to receive care, have more care provided at each visit, and improve the coordination among services for monitoring individual care and community changes. Under this plan, less child care is required, and personal schedules, especially for those who work, are less disrupted.

## CULTURAL AND PERSONAL OBSTACLES

A woman's attitude toward her pregnancy and toward prenatal care is influenced by her cultural values and beliefs. Poland and associates (1987) identified 6 cultural and personal factors affecting the amount of prenatal care a woman received. These factors were (1) the amount of insurance, (2) attitudes toward health professionals, (3) delays in suspecting pregnancy, (4) delays in telling others about the pregnancy, (5) perception of the importance of prenatal care, and (6) the woman's initial attitude about being pregnant. All of these factors imply that the social support that a women receives and her knowledge and understanding of prenatal care impact the decision to seek and continue care (Joyce et al, 1983). These researchers recommended that this information be used

to better market the public health system and identify women and families who are at greatest need for the support services that are an integral part of prenatal care.

# Identifying Risk Factors

The quantitative identification of prenatal risks for poor obstetric outcomes intensified during the 1970s (Bakketeig et al, 1981; Bragioner et al, 1984; Creasy et al, 1980; Kaminski et al, 1973, 1974; Newcombe et al, 1977; Papiernik, 1969). This intensification was brought about by basic statistical research on factors associated with premature and low-birth-weight infants with the advent of greater access to computers by medical investigators. The quantitative identification of risk factors has remained an important part of obstetric research because of its potential to assist the development of clinical care and public health policies (see Chapter 2). The risk categories that have received the most attention include past obstetric history, current pregnancy events, socioeconomic factors, psychosocial factors, and lifestyle patterns. Within the public prenatal care system, the identification of these risk factors needs to guide intervention policies and practices.

When identifying risk factors, one of the most important elements to consider is the dynamic process of the occurrence and disappearance of both clinical and nonclinical risks. Thus, the assessment of risk factors continually needs to be updated during prenatal care for the development of individualized care plans. For example, the employment status of women during pregnancy may be temporary in many families being served by public prenatal services, and continual updating of this information will inform clinicians about the availability of appropriate resources to these women. Similarly, several studies have suggested that food shortages have a monthly cycle, with the greatest food deficit the last week of the month, after resources from federal and state assistance programs have been depleted, and thus, dietary questionnaires may be answered differently depending on the week of the month they are given (Thompson et al, 1988; Taren et al, 1990). Further, the assessment of psychosocial stress of women may change from visit to visit. Finally, the dynamic process of all risk factors, both clinical (e.g., hemoglobin values, effacement and dilatation) and nonclinical, is in a constant state of change that modifies plans of action throughout the prenatal period.

## PSYCHOSOCIAL RISK FACTORS

Psychosocial stress before and during pregnancy has been reported to increase the risk of perinatal complications (Beck et al, 1980; McDonald et al, 1964; Newton et al, 1979). Psychosocial risk factors are measured by studying life changes within the year preceding pregnancy and during pregnancy, levels of social support, family relationships, and anxiety scores (Institute of Medicine, 1988; Poland et al, 1990). Further, a greater proportion of women who receive prenatal care through the public health system are also more likely to have psychosocial factors that put their pregnancies at risk because many of them are younger and less educated. Women with these characteristics have been reported to have an increased amount of psychosocial stress about their pregnancies and childbirth (Standley et al, 1979). This increased stress may also be compounded by a lack of informal social support networks and, therefore, should be targeted by programs that introduce support through nonmedical resources such as resource mothers (Heins et al, 1987; Moore et al, 1986; Oakley, 1985; Rook et al, 1985).

Obstetric complications, including prolonged labor, precipitate labor, preeclampsia, and clinical fetal distress and lower APGAR scores (Crandon, 1979), have been reported to be highly associated with increased anxiety as measured by the IPAT Anxiety Self-Analysis Form. Further, Norbeck and Tilden (1983) suggest that women who have a high level of stress, little social support, and anxiety may be identified early during pregnancy and thus benefit from appropriate intervention.

Our society is currently experiencing a change in the factors that produce stress in families, such as homelessness, drug dependency, increasing family and neighborhood violence, and isolation. Prevention and public health programs need to know the prevalence and impact of these problems on perinatal outcomes. Therefore, new instruments are needed for the identification of these modern day factors as a part of prevention and public health in obstetrics.

## ASSESSING PERINATAL RISKS IN PUBLIC HEALTH

Providing a composite score from a group of risk factors and diagnoses to identify women with low, medium, and high risk for adverse perinatal outcomes has been instituted in many clinics, hospitals, and regional programs (Creasy et al, 1980; Papiernik, 1984; Thalhammer et al, 1976). These scores provide a weight to factors that have been identified as predictors of poor pregnancy outcomes. Scoring systems have been developed for determining "poor outcomes," perinatal mortality, low birth weight, low birth weight at term, premature deliveries, low APGAR scores, and sudden infant death syndrome (Alexander et al, 1989). There are many similarities among the components of these scoring systems, such as young maternal age, previous preterm labor, smoking, repeated second trimester abortions, and twins, that place women at high risk. The advantage of these risk scores is that they provide an important systematic guide to the clinician as to which women have risk factors, the number of risk factors, and their association with poor pregnancy outcomes. Currently, the use of prenatal risk scores may be limited by the broadly defined psychosocial factors that are associated with preterm labor, and these scores need to be updated for current issues, as discussed in the previous section. Furthermore, care needs to be taken with these scoring systems to (1) limit the stress they may give women who are labeled high risk, (2) limit the burden on clinicians to decrease the risks or consequences of high scores, and (3) decrease false conclusions that changes (or no changes) in perinatal outcomes are due to the scoring system and not to other factors within the prenatal care environment (Alexander et al, 1989).

The sensitivity and specificity of a single risk score may also be different according to the population that the score is being judged against. In Florida, the sensitivity of a risk score appeared to be slightly better for African Americans and multigravidas (Taren et al, 1991a). The greater diagnostic value for multigravidas suggests that information gathered from previous pregnancy histories is extremely beneficial and is congruent with the emphasis put on these factors in the scoring systems. Differences in the sensitivity and specificity reported in the literature among populations are partially accounted for by the variation in the gestational age when the scores are conducted. However, decisions regarding what proportion of women are considered high risk depend on resources that are directed to these women.

# Public Health Interventions

The complexities and stressors in today's society that affect perinatal outcomes call on more resources than the traditional health care team can provide and the family can support. This is particularly true for those members of society who are most disenfranchised and most in need of comprehensive care. Future prevention and public health programs in obstetrics will need to emphasize the psychosocial components and interventions as well as the medical interventions. In fact, without this multidisciplinary focus, medical interventions most likely will not be carried out by the client and therefore will not help to solve societal issues.

The success of detailed public health policies and identification of risk factors in assisting women to have a positive and special pregnancy can be accomplished only when there exists a set of paths of care that coordinate individualized interventions. These paths of care consist of (1) informal and formal social and economic support systems; (2) access to nutritionists; (3) a standardized plan of office visits that is flexible to meet individual needs; and (4) access to the full spectrum of health care providers, including social services, nurse-midwifery services, and labor and delivery services.

Because current scoring systems are not predictive, the Florida Department of Health and Rehabilitative Services has developed a new system to identify appropriate paths of care that is based not on the quantitative risk score of a woman for a poor pregnancy outcome but on three categories of risk factors. Women are classified as having medical risks, risks for premature labor, or psychosocial risks. Depending on the risk category,

women receive individualized care; those who have medical risks see clinicians more often; those who have risks for premature labor receive cervical examinations more often; and women who have psychosocial risks receive appropriate professional services from social workers, nutritionists, and others. Although this method is currently being evaluated, the concept of individualizing paths of care is an important step in using current knowledge about risk factors associated with poor pregnancy outcomes.

## SUPPORT SYSTEMS

Support systems can be created through the use of professional and peer home visiting programs. A recently published US GAO study (1990) reports the following findings on home visiting by nurses:

1. Home visiting can help at-risk families become healthier and more self-sufficient.
2. Families that face obstacles to needed care and have difficulty accessing services (e.g., adolescent mothers, low income families, and families living in rural areas) benefit most from a structured home visiting program.
3. Home visits improved birth outcomes and child health and development, compared with children from families who did not receive these services.
4. Home visiting is most effective because it involves family participation.

Furthermore, the benefits to the families persisted over time, resulting in improved family functioning, better school performances, and better outcomes after high school (US GAO, 1990).

Few cost analysis studies have been performed in these programs, but those that have been completed demonstrate that delivery of preventative services (home visiting) can reduce serious and costly programs in the future. The US GAO report (1990) concluded that home visiting can be an effective intervention, and when combined with center-based and other community services, shows lasting positive effects.

## OFFICE VISITS

The Kessner Index and the guidelines set by the ACOG established the principles for determining the minimal number of prenatal visits for the general population of women. Both of these guidelines have recommended that a women be seen monthly until the end of the second trimester, every 2 to 3 weeks until the last month of pregnancy, and weekly thereafter. These guidelines represent the normal number of visits that the average woman may need during pregnancy. However, because these recommendations are being made for the general population, many women may warrant a different schedule of visits.

Further, the number of prenatal visits is not an indicator of quality of prenatal care. Obviously, the number of visits depends on when a woman starts prenatal care and the length of gestation. Kotelchuck and colleagues (1987) report that, after controlling for the gestational age at the first prenatal visit and the gestational age at birth, women in the national natality survey had an appropriate number of prenatal visits until the last month of pregnancy. Decreases from the recommended number of visits occurred toward the end of pregnancy, when clinic appointments become more frequent. This decrease was greater for African American women, who, the report assumed, were poorer and had more difficulty obtaining transportation. These modifications of the ACOG guidelines and Kessner index to account for appropriate durations of prenatal care have helped identify the behavior of patients in regard to their clinic visits, which should help in planning appropriate strategies to increase access to prenatal care.

## NUTRITIONAL CARE

The components of nutritional services in prenatal care need to include the provision of a nutritional assessment, nutrition education and counseling, and when appropriate, nutrient and food supplements. The basic elements of a nutritional assessment need to include dietary information, continual monitoring of weight gain, and hematologic data regarding anemia. Women who are having an abnormal weight gain pattern, who are anemic, and who have metabolic disorders (e.g., diabetes) need additional nutritional interventions.

The basic element of a dietary assessment needs to include information about a woman's usual dietary pattern. Recently, the Institute of Medicine (1990) stated that "dietary assessment serves as the foundation for appropriate nutrition counseling and intervention." Further, this report stated that "A pregnant woman's risk of dietary inadequacy may be assessed more efficiently and practically by a food frequency or diet history questionnaire." However, special attention must also be given to short-term food shortages, the daily distribution of calories for diabetic pregnant women, and the identification of eating disorder behaviors.

Assessing weight gain is also an essential role when monitoring the progress of pregnancy. For this reason, weight needs to be obtained accurately and with standardized procedures. Weight gain charts need to be used at each visit, completed accurately, and shown to pregnant women for education and counseling. Furthermore, liberal weight gain patterns need to be given to women in order to be consistent with the 25- to 35-pound weight gain recommendation for women with normal pre-pregnancy weights and single births (Institute of Medicine, 1990). Women with twins who go to term are recommended to gain between 35 and 45 pounds for having the greatest chance of a favorable outcome (Institute of Medicine, 1990).

Nutrient and food supplements need to be provided along with education and counseling. In the United States, referrals should automatically be given to women for the Special Supplemental Feeding Program for Women, Infants and Children (WIC). There are also numerous other food programs that pregnant women from low income families can use, including food stamps, special food cooperatives, public service programs such as SHARE USA, and the Expanded Food and Nutrition Education Program (EFNEP) from the Cooperative Extension Office of each state. However, no matter what program pregnant women use, the nutritional resources need to be tailored because of cultural values and religious beliefs that influence individual tastes and preferences. Different physiologic responses to pregnancy, such as morning sickness, pica, and food cravings also must be considered when conducting a dietary assessment and when implementing dietary interventions. Women also need to be instructed to have a sufficient food intake, good food selection, and a good distribution of food intake throughout the day (King, 1983).

## EDUCATION AND COUNSELING

The medical interventions that are necessary for the successful outcome of any pregnancy must be integrated with education and health promotion activities. Traditionally, prenatal education has been provided in both formal and informal settings. Office visits focused on individual medical complications and discomforts of pregnancy, whereas structured classes outside of the office visit focused on preparation for childbirth and parenting.

New areas for the perinatal team to incorporate into its education programs include nutrition counseling, exercise, stress reduction, work-related activities, appropriate use of medications, and ways to reduce or eliminate unhealthy habits such as smoking, alcohol consumption, and drug abuse during the preconceptual period and pregnancy.

Numerous studies have shown that successful implementation of prenatal education depends on efforts to change the behavior of all pregnant women and not only women who are considered to be at high risk for poor pregnancy outcomes (Christopherson, 1985; Papiernik, 1987). The importance in this approach is that group change fosters individual change. For example, the effect of prenatal education on early signs and symptoms of preterm labor has been shown to significantly decrease low-birth-weight infants when directed to all women and not just to women who are at high risk for preterm labor (Taren and Graven, 1991b). Childbirth education has also been reported to significantly reduce the use of anesthesia during labor compared with women who spent the same amount of time in classes but did not receive education on relaxation and breathing (Christopherson, 1985). Secondary effects of education may also exist, because the time spent by health care providers with pregnant women provides additional support to the women that can decrease their level of stress, build confidence for labor and delivery, and provide clues to the nonmedical factors influencing their pregnancies.

## REDUCING RISK BEHAVIORS

Areas for intense education and counseling are smoking cessation, alcohol avoidance, and abstinence from illicit drugs. Ideally the preconceptual period is the time to initiate this counseling and education.

**Smoking.** There is clear evidence that there is an association between maternal smoking during pregnancy and low birth weight (Department of Health and Human Services, 1980; Picone et al, 1982; Shiono et al, 1986). Women who enter their pregnancy as smokers can benefit from smoking cessation counseling. Mullen (1990) analyzed 13 studies on smoking intervention programs and found enough evidence to suggest that programs of smoking cessation can be effective in improving birth weights for infants of pregnant smokers. Health care providers need to incorporate into their practices a plan for smoking history status at the first visit as well as a plan for quitting smoking. Subsequent visits are to include reinforcement, written materials, and referrals to programs that specifically deal with smoking during pregnancy. The primary care provider needs to take the lead in counseling and education of the woman, and the entire team should reinforce this at each visit.

**Alcohol.** Alcohol use among women poses a serious risk factor for both maternal and fetal well-being. There is enough epidemiologic evidence to support an association between heavy drinking during pregnancy and congenital anomalies, including fetal alcohol syndrome, spontaneous abortions, and intrauterine growth retardation (Mullen et al, 1990). Important aspects of care for this perinatal problem are screening, diagnosis, and intervention. The personal history is the most practical way of identifying those who abuse alcohol. In order to improve accuracy in responses, a personal history should be specific and nonjudgmental. Sokol and associates (1989) have reported a new screening procedure, T-ACE, to identify pregnant women who consume the equivalent of 1 or more ounces of absolute alcohol a day. The T-ACE questionnaire may prove to be the ideal tool that a busy practitioner can employ to identify women who drink a significant amount of alcohol during pregnancy.

Education and counseling of pregnant women who abuse alcohol need to begin with the first visit, and ideally, at a preconceptual visit. Information must be provided about the effects of alcohol on the fetus, along with ongoing supportive counseling in a nonjudgmental manner. Counseling needs to focus

**Table 3–1**

## HEALTH PROMOTION ACTIVITIES DURING PRENATAL CARE

| | Prenatal Visit Schedule | | | | | | | | |
|---|---|---|---|---|---|---|---|---|---|
| | 1st visit | 2nd visit | 3rd visit | 4th visit | 5th visit | 6th visit | 7th visit | 8th visit | 9th visit |
| *Counseling to Promote and Support Healthful Behavior* | | | | | | | | | |
| Smoking cessation | * | * | * | * | * | * | * | * | * |
| Alcohol avoidance | * | * | * | * | * | * | * | * | * |
| Illicit drug abstinence | * | * | * | * | * | * | * | * | * |
| Teratogen avoidance | * | * | * | * | * | * | * | * | * |
| Nutrition | * | * | * | * | * | * | * | * | * |
| Maternal seat belt use | | * | | | | | | | |
| Work patterns | | * | | | | | | | |
| Safer sex | * | | | | | * | * | * | * |
| *General Knowledge of Pregnancy and Parenting* | | | | | | | | | |
| Physiological changes | * | * | * | * | * | * | * | * | * |
| Emotional changes | * | * | * | * | * | * | * | * | * |
| Sexuality | * | | * | * | * | * | * | * | * |
| Self-help for discomforts | * | * | * | * | * | * | * | * | * |
| General health habits | * | * | * | * | * | * | * | * | * |
| Early pregnancy classes | * | * | | | | | | | |
| Fetal growth & development | | | * | * | * | * | * | * | * |
| Breastfeeding promotion | | | | * | * | | * | * | * |
| Childbirth classes | | | | * | * | | | | |
| Perineal exercises | | | | * | * | | | | |
| Infant car seat use | | | | * | | * | * | * | * |
| Family roles | | | | * | | | * | * | * |
| Parenting classes | | | | | | * | | | |
| Signs and symptoms of labor | | | | | | * | * | * | * |
| Postpartum activity | | | | | | | * | * | * |
| Family planning | | | | | | | * | * | * |
| Newborn care | | | | | | | * | * | * |
| *Information on Proposed Care* | | | | | | | | | |
| Early prenatal care | * | | | | | | | | |
| Screening and diagnostic tests | * | * | * | * | | | | | |
| Content and timing of visits | * | * | * | * | * | * | * | * | * |
| Reporting danger signs | * | * | * | * | * | * | * | * | * |
| Signs and symptoms of labor | | | * | * | * | * | * | * | * |
| Preparation for labor and birth | | | | | | * | * | * | * |
| Review birth plan | | | | | | * | * | * | * |
| When to call | | | | | | * | * | * | * |
| Where to go in labor | | | | | | * | * | * | * |
| Preparation for post-term tests | | | | | | | | * | |

Adapted from Caring for Our Future: The Content of Prenatal Care. A Report of the Public Health Service Expert Panel on the Content of Prenatal Care. Department of Health and Human Services, Washington, DC, 1989.

on reducing alcohol consumption and coping strategies to deal with the psychodynamics of pregnancy and the challenges of sobriety. For women who cannot respond to the supportive counseling offered by the perinatal team during prenatal care visits, referrals and follow-up need to be made to an appropriate alcohol treatment program that deals with the medical aspects of pregnancy.

**Illicit Drug Use.** There was a significant increase in illicit drug use among pregnant women, especially those in urban areas, during the 1980s. This increase in drug use is also related to the greater prevalence of perinatal AIDS. Recent surveys suggest that more than 15 percent of women of childbearing age use cocaine; at least 10 percent of infants born in urban hospitals test positive for cocaine in the nursery (Frank et al, 1988; US GAO, 1990a). Intravenous drug use has been identified as the vehicle of infection for 52 percent of the women with AIDS (Scott, 1989). Further, the percentage of AIDS patients who are women increased by 33 percent between 1984 (6 percent) and 1989 (8 percent) (US Centers for Disease Control 1989). Results from several studies have demonstrated that maternal drug use causes an increased risk for preterm labor, produces addicted infants, and delays fetal and infant development (Chasnoff, 1985; 1987). Given the large prevalence of illicit drug use during pregnancy and the severity of problems that it causes, maternal drug abuse is a national problem requiring a joint effort from the public and private spheres for identifying and implementing solutions. Programs need to be established that focus on early identification during pregnancy, case management to ensure that these women have proper treatment, and follow-up.

Jones and Lopez (1990) identified three entry points at which drug-abusing and drug-dependent women may enter the health care system for some type of service: (1) drug rehabilitation programs that do not know that their patients are pregnant, (2) prenatal programs that fail to identify drug-using women, and (3) sexually transmitted disease clinics. These entry points into the health care system provide opportunities for health care providers to effectively identify this population. In addition to these entry points, health care professionals need to find other mechanisms to bring pregnant women into the prenatal care system. In developing these outreach programs, the punitive treatment of women (e.g., arrest, incarceration) has to be recognized as an important reason why women do not seek care. Greater success may be achieved with more positive programs that focus on case management, which includes family support and professional counseling.

## HEALTH PROMOTION ACTIVITIES

The timing of health promotion during pregnancy begins, ideally, during the preconceptual period. A team approach is necessary because no one health care provider has either the time or expertise in all these areas. Providing women and their partners with knowledge about healthy behaviors and the physical and emotional changes that occur during pregnancy gives them a sense of well-being and self-esteem. These activities will allow a woman and her family to assume more responsibility for this pregnancy and the health of the family. In Table 3–1, a summary of education and health promotion activities recommended by the US Public Health Service (1989) is presented. These are important guidelines that can be used to remind practitioners what types of information should be discussed with women during their prenatal visits.

As the United States continues to lead the world in technologic advances in perinatology and in the early identification and management of maternal-fetal abnormalities, it is now time to focus public policy on guaranteeing prevention and public health obstetric programs for all women. This will require the collective resources of the public and private sectors. Emphasis will need to be given to providing appropriate levels of care to those women who can most benefit from these services. This may mean that women with the highest socioeconomic risk need more comprehensive and personalized care, as addressed in this chapter.

## References

ACOG, Unpublished data, 1987.

Alexander S, Keirse MJNC: Formal risk scoring during pregnancy. *In* Chalmers I, Enkin M, Keirse MJNC (eds): Effective Care in Pregnancy and Childbirth. Oxford, Oxford University Press, 1989, pp 346–365.

Bakketeig LS, Hoffman HJ: Epidemiology of preterm

birth: results from a longitudinal study of births in Norway. *In* Elder MG, Hendricks CH (eds): Preterm Labor. London, Butterworths, 1981, pp 17–56.

Beauchamp DA, Rouse RL: Universal New York health care. A single-payer strategy linking cost control and universal access. N Engl J Med 323:640–644, 1990.

Beck NC, Siegel LJ, Davidson NP, et al: The prediction of pregnancy outcome: maternal preparation, anxiety, and attitudinal sets. J Psychosom Res 24:343–351, 1980.

Bragonier RJ, Cushner I, Hobel C: Social and personal factors in the etiology of preterm birth. *In* Fuchs F, Stubblefield P (eds): Preterm Births: Causes, Prevention and Management. New York, Macmillan Publishing Co, 1984, pp 64–97.

Brown J, Stone V, Sidel VW: Decline in NHSC physicians threatens patient care. Am J Public Health 80:1395–1396, 1990.

Chasnoff IJ: Cocaine use in pregnancy: prenatal morbidity and mortality. Neurotoxicology 9:291–293, 1987.

Chasnoff IJ, Burns WJ, Schnoll S, et al: Cocaine use in pregnancy. New Engl J Med 313:666–669, 1985.

Christopherson ER: Enhancing the effectiveness of health education strategies. Clin Perinatol 12:381–389, 1985.

Constantine JC, Taren DL, Keel J, et al: Increasing Medicaid client approval rates: The Hillsborough Medicaid Compliance Demonstration Project. American Public Health Association, October 3, 1990.

Cooney JP: What determines the start of prenatal care? Prenatal care, insurance and education. Medical Care 23(8):986–997, 1985.

Crandon AJ: Maternal anxiety and neonatal well being. J Psychosom Res 23:113–115, 1979.

Creasy RK, Gummer GA, Liggins GC: System for predicting spontaneous preterm birth. Obstet Gynecol 55:692–695, 1980.

Department of Health and Human Services: The Health Consequences of Smoking for Women: A Report of the Surgeon General. Washington, DC, 1980.

Department of Health and Human Services: Promoting Health/Preventing Disease: Year 2000 Objectives for the Nation. Washington, DC, 1990.

Fiori MC, Novotny TE, Pierce JP, et al: Methods used to quit smoking in the United States: do cessation programs help? JAMA 263:2760–2765, 1990.

Fisher ES, LoGerfo JP, Daling JR: Prenatal care and pregnancy outcomes during the recession: The Washington State experience. Am J Public Health 75:866–869, 1985.

Frank DA, Zuckerman BS, Amaro H, et al: Cocaine use during pregnancy: prevalence and correlates. Pediatrics 82:888–895, 1988.

Heins HC, Nuance NW, Ferguson JE: Improving prenatal outcome: the resource mothers program. Obstet Gyncol 70:263–266, 1987.

Institute of Medicine: Preventing Low Birthweight. National Academy Press, Washington, DC, 1985.

Institute of Medicine: Prenatal Care Reaching Mothers, Reaching Infants. National Academy Press, Washington, DC, 1988.

Institute of Medicine: Nutrition During Pregnancy. National Academy Press, Washington, DC, 1990.

Jones CL, Lopez RE: Drug abuse and pregnancy. *In* Merkatz IR, Thompson JE (eds): New Perspectives on Prenatal Care. New York, Elsevier, 1990, pp 273–318.

Kaminski M, Goujard J, Rumeau-Rouguette C: Prediction of low birth weight and prematurity by multiple regression analysis with maternal characteristics

known since the beginning of pregnancy. Int J Epidemiol 2:195–204, 1973.

Kaminski M, Papiernik E: Multifactorial study of the risk of prematurity at 32 weeks of gestation. J Perinatal Medicine (Berlin) 2:37–44, 1974.

King JC: Dietary risk patterns during pregnancy. *In* Weininger J, Briggs CM (eds): Nutrition Update, Vol 1. New York, John Wiley and Sons, 1983, pp 205–226.

Kotelchuck M, Costello C, Wise PB: Race differences in utilization of prenatal care services in the United States. Presented at the American Public Health Association, New Orleans, 1987.

McDonald RL, Parham KJ: Relation of emotional changes during pregnancy to obstetric complications in unmarried primigravidas. Am J Obstet Gynecol 90:195–201, 1964.

Moore ML, Meis PJ, Ernest JM, et al: A regional program to reduce the incidence of preterm birth. J Perinatol 6:216–220, 1986.

Mullen PD: Smoking cessation counseling in prenatal care. *In* Merkatz IR, Thompson JE (eds): New Perspectives on Prenatal Care. New York, Elsevier, 1990, pp 161–176.

Mullen PD, Glenday MA: Alcohol avoidance counseling in prenatal care. *In* Merkatz IR, Thompson JE (eds): New Perspectives on Prenatal Care. New York, Elsevier, 1990, pp 177–192.

National Center for Health Statistics (NCHS): Advance Report of Final Natality Statistics 1987. Monthly Vital Statistics Report Vol 38(3), June 29, 1989.

National Commission to Prevent Infant Mortality: Death Before Life: The Tragedy of Infant Mortality. Chiles L (Chairman), US Senate, Washington, DC, August 1988.

National Commission to Prevent Infant Mortality: Troubling Trends: The Health of America's Next Generation. Chiles L (Chairman), US Senate, Washington, DC, February 1990.

Newcombe R, Fedrick J, Chalmers I: Antenatal identification of patients "at risk" of pre-term labour. Proceedings of the 5th Study Group of the Royal College of Obstetricians and Gynaecologists, 5th & 6th October, 17–28, 1977.

Newton RW, Webster PA, Binu PS, et al: Psychological stress in pregnancy and its relation to the onset of premature labor. Br Med J 2:411–413, 1979.

Norbeck JS, Tilden VP: Life stress, social support, and emotional disequilibrium in complications of pregnancy: a prospective, multivariate study. J Health Soc Behav 24:30–46, 1983.

Oakley A: Social support in pregnancy: the "soft" way to increase birthweight? Soc Sci Med 21:1259–1268, 1985.

Okada LM, Wan TTH: Impact of community health centers and Medicaid on the use of health services. Public Health Rep 95:520, 1980.

Papiernik E: Community wide approaches to preventing preterm birth. *In* Chamberlin RW (ed): Beyond Individual Risk Assessment: Community Wide Approaches to Promoting the Health and Development of Families and Children. Washington, DC, National Center for Education in Maternal and Child Health. 1987, pp 145–175.

Papiernik E: Prediction of the preterm baby. Clin Obstet Gynecol 11:315–336, 1984.

Papiernik E: Coefficient du risque d'accouchement prématuré (CRAP). Presse Med 77:793–794, 1969.

Papiernik E: Prediction of the preterm baby. Clinics Obstet Gynecol 11:315–336, 1984.

Picone TA, Allen AH, Olsen PN, et al: Pregnancy outcome in North American women. II. Effects of diet, cigarette smoking, stress, and weight gain on placentas and neonatal physical and behavioral characteristics. Am J Clin Nutr 36:1214–1224, 1982.

Poland ML, Ager JW, Olson KL: Barriers to receiving adequate prenatal care. Am J Obstet Gynecol 157:297–303, 1987.

Poland ML, Ager JW, Olson KL, et al: Quality of prenatal care; selected social, behavioral and biomedical factors; and birth weight. Obstet Gynecol 75:607–612, 1990.

Rook KS, Dooley D: Applying social support research: theoretical problems and future directions. J Social Issues 41:5–28, 1985.

Scott G: Perinatal HIV-1 infection: diagnosis and management. Clin Obstet Gynecol 32:477–484, 1989.

Shiono PH, Klebbanoff MA, Rhoads GG: Smoking and drinking during pregnancy. Their effect on preterm births. JAMA 255:82–84, 1986.

Sing S, Forrest JD, Torres A: Prenatal Care in the United States: A State and County Inventory. The Alan Guttmacher Institute, Washington, DC, 1989.

Sokol RJ, Martier SS, Ager JW: The T-ACE questions: practical prenatal of risk drinking. Am J Obstet Gynecol 160:863–868, 1989.

Standley K, Soulle B, Copons SA: Dimensions of prenatal anxiety and their influence on pregnancy outcome. Am J Obstet Gynecol 135:22–26, 1979.

Taren DL, Graven SN: The sensitivity and specificity of a preterm risk score for various patient populations. J Perinatol 11:130–136, 1991a.

Taren DL, Graven SN: Nutritional and educational components of prenatal care and their association with low birth weight infants. Public Health Rep 106:426–436, 1991b.

Taren DL, Clark W, Chernesky M, et al: Weekly food servings and participation in social programs among low income families. Am J Public Health 80:1376–1378, 1990.

Thalhammer O, Coradello H, Pollak A, et al: Prospective and retrospective examination of an easily applicable score to predict the probability of premature birth defined by weight. J Perinat Med 4:38–44, 1976.

The Allan Guttmacher Institute: Blessed Events and the Bottom Line: Financing Maternity Care in the United States. New York, 1987.

Thompson FE, Taren D, Andersen E, et al: Within month variability in use of soup kitchens in New York State. Am J Public Health 78:1298–1301, 1988.

US Centers for Disease Control: HIV/AIDS Surveillance Report, AIDS Program, May 12, 1989.

US GAO (Government Accounting Office): Home Visiting. A Promising Early Intervention Strategy for At-Risk Families. GAO/HRD-90-83, Washington, DC, July 1990.

US GAO (Government Accounting Office): Drug-Exposed Infants. A Generation at Risk. GAO/HRD-90-138, June 1990a.

US GAO (Government Accounting Office) Medicaid: States Expand Coverage For Pregnant Women, Infants, and Children. Washington, DC, 1989.

US PHS (US Public Health Service): Caring for Our Future: the Content of Prenatal Care. A Report of the Public Health Service Expert Panel on the Content of Prenatal Care. Washington, DC, 1989.

# CHAPTER 4

# Adaptations to Perinatal Regionalization

David E. Gagnon and Sherry Allison-Cooke

## Background

Beginning in the 1970s, regionalization of perinatal and neonatal care has been instrumental in improving patient outcomes, especially neonatal survival rates. It has been 15 years since the publication of "Toward Improving the Outcome of Pregnancy" (Committee on Perinatal Health, 1976). This seminal document defined the regional concept for organizing perinatal services and issued recommendations for developing regional networks, including a delineation of the responsibilities and service offerings appropriate to community hospitals with level I nurseries, secondary care facilities with special care or Level II nurseries, and tertiary referral centers with level III neonatal intensive care units (NICUs).

Level I hospitals were identified as hospitals that would provide care for "uncomplicated maternity and newborn cases." Practitioners in these hospitals were urged to assess patient risk as early as possible and seek referral or consultation as appropriate for high-risk patients. In contrast, practitioners in level II hospitals would provide care for both uncomplicated and moderately complicated obstetric and newborn cases. These hospitals would be located in urban or suburban settings with a sufficiently large birth cohort to support more sophisticated care. Finally, level III hospitals would be regional centers responsible for 8000 to 12,000 births in the region. These referral centers would provide leadership in education and research and act as coordinators of care for high-risk patients in the region (Committee on Perinatal Health, 1976).

The approach outlined in "Toward Improving the Outcome of Pregnancy" was hierarchical in nature and it was assumed that a coherent structure would evolve in geographic regions across the country. Soon after the publication of these guidelines, there was indeed a very active movement to incorporate the structural elements of the report into perinatal care programs in many areas of the country.

## Status of Regional Programs

The original document, "Toward Improving the Outcome of Pregnancy," was based on several assumptions that may be no longer operable. For example:

*Regionalization implies the development, within a geographic area, of a coordinated, cooperative system of maternal and perinatal health in which, by mutual agreements between hospitals and physicians and based upon population needs the degree of complexity of maternal and perinatal care each hospital is capable of providing is identified. (Committee on Perinatal Health, 1976).*

This statement assumes that geography, not reimbursement, is the key component of the regional program. In a health care environment that witnesses large groups of people contracting for care with a given set of providers, the geographic organization of care has become the exception. There is also a need to recognize that, for better or worse, the American health system is committed to competition, not cooperation, to attain cost effectiveness in the delivery of care. Underlining this phenomenon is the rapid development of case law based on the principles of the Sherman Antitrust Act, which attacks mutual agreements among competing providers as collusion in the marketplace. Finally, the statement avoids the issue of who identifies the capability of a specific hospital to provide an acceptable level of care. In response to this last directive, some states have passed laws and administrative regulations to define the regional program. Unfortunately, as with any political process, lawsuits, exceptions, and unpunished violations have weakened these efforts. In general, the public sector is committed to reduce health care costs through competition and thereby benefit public employees and Medicaid recipients directly and the business community indirectly.

## The Successes of Regional Programs

It should not be taken as a negative that the Committee on Perinatal Health could not foresee the changes in health care that would occur at the end of the century. Its major contribution remains delineation of the crucial elements of a regional system to make appropriate care for high-risk patients available and accessible to mothers and their infants.

The objectives of the regional programs remain

- Delivery of quality care to all pregnant women and newborns.
- Maximal use of highly trained perinatal personnel and intensive care facilities.
- Assurance of reasonable cost effectiveness.

The committee was also clairvoyant in its description of the essential components of

the system:

*All physicians and hospitals in the regionalized system of maternal and perinatal health would be linked by a communication network which provides readily available expert telephonic and ambulatory consultation, basic continuing education for physicians, nurses, and allied health personnel in perinatal health care and, under certain circumstances, efficient and safe transferral of selected maternity cases with complications and selected sick newborns to another hospital possessing more comprehensive specialized maternal and perinatal services (Committee on Perinatal Health, 1976).*

The system's components—specialized clinical care, education, communication, referral and consultation, transport, and research—remain as critical today as they were in the early 1970s. These same components were the building blocks of perinatal programs across the country, and they remain essential to the success of these programs.

With encouragement from pilot programs funded by The Robert Wood Johnson Foundation and from programs supported by the states, perinatal regional care prospered during the 1970s. For the most part, the success of these programs corresponded with the successful leadership and the financial support of tertiary referral centers. The ability to gain support from community physicians and the primary hospitals they staffed was a difficult task and stands as one of the great successes of regionalization. Over the course of the decade, the regionalization of neonatal intensive care was highly successful; the regionalization of maternal and fetal care has lagged somewhat behind and remains a problem in many areas of the country (Allison-Cook et al, 1988; Gagnon et al, 1988). Nonetheless, there is general agreement that the regionalized approach to organizing perinatal services, even with its faults, has been a successful measure of improving perinatal outcomes (Gagnon et al, 1988).

In an evaluation study reported by McCormick and associates (1985) on the eight prototype sites funded by The Robert Wood Johnson Foundation, the authors identified a shift of deliveries from Level I to Level III hospitals between 1970 and 1979, indicating antepartum identification of high-risk pregnancies and sharp declines in neonatal mortality rates. These declines were not accompanied by increases in morbidity rates. In essence, the creation of systems of care based on the components of a regional program had a positive impact on improving pregnancy outcomes (McCormick et al, 1985).

The success of the regional programs is witnessed in a variety of settings. Urban areas as diverse as New York, Seattle, and Cleveland show improved outcomes as a result of regionalization (McCormick et al, 1985). The same holds true in rural areas such as Iowa (Hein, 1980). In general, the premise posed by the Committee on Perinatal Health in the early 1970s has worked, yet, widespread disappointment in regionalization persists.

In his editorial on regionalization, Kanto (1987), attributes the perceived decline in regionalization to "turf guarding, that is, the guarding of one's area of practice." He cites the inflexibility of government-designated levels of care as a form of Cvivsregio, eius religio (as the ruler, so the religion). As he declares, "The strictness and inflexibility of this method [of designation] have fostered the development of empires where political influences rather than the needs and welfare of the patient determined care" (Kanto, 1987).

Although Kanto's criticism may be strong, the fear of deregionalization is real. There is a lack of recognition of the changes in the health care environment, documented later in this chapter, in the adaptation of regional and perinatal systems to current demands. There is a fear that the gains acquired over the past 25 years with better-organized perinatal care will be lost.

Some of these fears should be seen in the context of the original intent of the Committee on Perinatal Health. In the early 1970s, there were a limited number of perinatal centers and trained professionals to staff these centers. In response to the need for specialists in neonatal and maternal and fetal medicine, the respective professional organizations encouraged training programs to develop these specialists. Institution of fellowships in neonatal medicine generated a relative plethora of specialists by the 1980s. Merenstein and associates (1986) identified

more than 1500 neonatologists in the United States in 1983. The National Perinatal Information Center (NPIC) in 1984 identified over 1600 such specialists (Muri and Schwartz, 1988). Both studies agree that there is an oversupply of these physicians. The growth in the maternal and fetal specialty has been much slower, with only half as many perinatologists as neonatologists.

As might be expected, the increased subspecialty capacity is mirrored by an increase in neonatal bed capacity. There is certainly a synergy between increases in the population of the profession and growth of NICUs or NICU beds; the result has been a dramatic expansion of NICUs in the nation. Between 1984 and 1988, there was a 46.9 percent increase in hospitals reporting NICUs. In addition, there was a 38.6 percent increase in NICU beds; this growth appears to continue at a rate of 5 to 7 percent per year (Lynch, 1991). Increasingly, the distribution of these services is spreading to less sophisticated community hospitals, and newly graduated neonatal fellows are accepting positions in new neonatal units. As pointed out in an article by Rachel Schwartz,

*The increasing pressure on Level II facilities to care for lower gram weight infants is clear. As the number of neonatologists available grows, the only barrier to providing more sophisticated services will be the availability of patients, since technology tends to proliferate along with the staff who require it. However, the number of high risk infants is not rising. In fact, the stability of the percentage of high risk infants at 6–7% of births overall has been documented, and much of the current focus in prenatal medicine is on the prevention of prematurity. In addition, the birth rate is not rising dramatically, and total births have also been fairly stable. The question becomes can the expanding infrastructure that is developing to care for high risk infants be supported from a quality standpoint by a stable population of high risk neonates?* (Schwartz, 1991).

To some degree, the story of the growth of perinatal regionalization is also a study of improved pregnancy outcomes. The once scarce resources are now available to all; the technology that was arcane a few years ago is now routine in all NICUs.

As in any market economy, the growth of service is a response to the laws of supply and demand. As the supply of neonatologists grew, there was increasing competition to become a staff member of a perinatal service unit in a tertiary hospital. Because the turnover of these services is consistently low, new graduates became available as an inducement to other units. In turn, these units have now become competitive with the regional perinatal centers.

In a recent survey by the NPIC, 26 states indicated they had regional plans and guidelines and had generated regulations to ensure the creation of such a system (NPIC, 1990).

## Decade of Change

During the 1980s, the American health care community was subjected to dramatic changes that have limited the ability to maintain regionally organized systems of care. These have been hallmarked by such developments as:

- New prospective payment schemes like the Diagnostic Related Groups (DRG) system replacing traditional retrospective fee-for-service reimbursement for hospital care.
- New managed care delivery arrangements such as Health Maintenance Organizations (HMOs) and Preferred Provider Organizations (PPOs) capturing significant market shares from traditional indemnity insurance plans.
- New patterns of medical practice, such as the shift to outpatient surgery and shorter inpatient stays, resulting in overbedded hospital markets, where facilities compete against each other for increasingly scarce inpatient days.
- New dimensions to the issue of medical malpractice liability, which has led physicians to alter traditional medical practices and to question the financial viability of certain medical subspecialties.

Each of these factors has contributed to the alteration of traditional perinatal regionalization. Regionalization of services is based on two critical goals, both of which can be considered somewhat fragile under the current health care environment. For regionalization to be achieved and maintained, hospitals must (1) accept a differentiation in roles, responsibilities, and services based on population distributions and patient needs in the surrounding areas; and (2) establish agreements among themselves on the referral and transport of mothers and babies according to the level of services required by specific patients. These goals are based on cooperation among facilities in order to maximize medical efficiency, quality of patient care, and cost effectiveness in a large geographic area. The changing health care environment may be making such cooperation antiquated (Gagnon, 1991).

As the perinatal community began to voice alarm during the 1980s about deregionalization, the NPIC recognized the need to assess the scope of this phenomenon and initiated a study of regionalization toward the end of the decade with funding by The Robert Wood Johnson Foundation (NPIC, 1989).

A key ingredient for successful regional functioning is an atmosphere of cooperation and mutual respect among the institutions and individuals encompassed by the perinatal system; otherwise, any semblance of regionalized delivery of services would be impossible. Unfortunately, competition is the antithesis of cooperation. Recognizing this potential threat to regional structures, the NPIC investigated the question of what has happened in the 1980s to the regional perinatal structures created during the 1970s. To this end, NPIC completed case studies in six cities across the country, conducting personal interviews with 226 individuals in 35 hospitals. Interview subjects included top level administrators, chief financial officers, medical chiefs of staff for perinatology and neonatology, and head nurses for labor and delivery, normal newborn nurseries, and NICUs (Allison-Cooke et al, 1988).

### STUDY PURPOSE

The purpose of these interviews was to glean from key decision-makers and clinicians their perceptions of the forces impacting on perinatal care today. Of particular interest are the subjects' perceptions of the relative importance and roles of state reimbursement, hospital competition, HMOs and PPOs, and medical malpractice liability in mediating potential changes in the face and forum of perinatal care.

During the site visits, NPIC staff frequently encountered friction in the perinatal community. Usually, the disagreement assumed the guise of tensions between university-based physicians and the community's physicians. These tensions were further exacerbated by the closed-door policies of many tertiary centers, the use of residents or nonclinicians in key communication positions, and the general lack of interaction between the academic and local medical communities.

Nonacademic tertiary centers seem to avoid many of these problems. They often stress an open-door policy for obstetricians that allows them to follow high-risk patients throughout their pregnancies, including delivery at the perinatal center or, if the patient has been maintained to term, in the obstetricians' usual admitting hospital. This helps to minimize the obstetricians' complaints of losing contact with patients and of feeling boxed out of the regional system of care.

A somewhat related issue involves the degree of competition that exists between level II and level III facilities in some locations. Viewed from the tertiary perspective, level II upgrades are often seen as profit-motivated, which frequently result in a compromised quality of care for certain high-risk infants. Viewed from the community hospital perspective, perinatal centers are often characterized as clinging to antiquated and unrealistic visions of regionalization, which place these centers at the zenith and relegate community hospitals forever to a level I status. This is considered unacceptable by urban hospitals, given the competitive and litigious pressures present in the health care environment of the 1990s. Competition is also mounting among tertiary centers, and this impacts on relations between their perinatal programs. New level III facilities tend to be viewed with even greater skepticism than upgraded level II facilities. The advent of these new services raises legitimate questions concerning resource allocations and cost efficiency and the volume of patients necessary to establish and maintain the skill levels required to adequately care for high-risk infants.

# Issues in Perinatal Regional Programs

The NPIC site visit team identified operating principles on which some regional programs had built more productive relations. The best provider relations, which produced more successful perinatal regions, were characterized in a few very basic ways:

- Defined and commonly accepted roles for levels I, II, and III.
- Some provision for exchange and cohesion between academic and community medicine.
- Minimal competition for patients either within or across level of care designations but particularly among NICUs or between Levels II and III.
- A general spirit of cooperation and mutual respect.

Achieving this mix of characteristics appears to be largely determined by the perinatal center and stems partly from policy (e.g., the role of residents and open versus closed admitting privileges) and partly from attitude. Academic institutions, particularly, need to develop and maintain sensitivity to both the pressures and prejudices present within their local medical communities if they are to remain in control of the more important aspects of perinatal regionalization, such as transfer decisions.

## INFANT TRANSFERS

Competitive pressures to maximize hospital occupancy rates have a negative influence on the appropriate transfer of high-risk infants. As level II facilities secure either in-house or contracted neonatologist coverage and upgrade their level of nursing care, they expand boundaries for retaining premature or low-birth-weight infants. Formerly, the criteria for transfer were less than or equal to 35 weeks' gestational age or less than or equal to 1500 g or requiring ventilatory support, but Level II facilities now frequently retain infants unless they are less than or equal to 30 to 32 weeks' gestational age or less than or equal to 1000 to 1250 g or need ventilatory support for periods longer than 2 to 24 hours. Cardiac, neurologic, and surgical cases are all transferred out from level II facilities. In fact, many Level III facilities transfer these cases to a children's hospital NICU, if one is available.

Staff in level II facilities are comfortable with the care being delivered in their special care nurseries. In fact, some neonatologists practicing in Level II facilities argue that although extremely high-risk infants benefit from the sophisticated technology available in NICUs, these settings constitute fairly stressful environments, and intermediate-risk babies may actually be better served by the less technical, more personal care provided by a level II facility.

Notwithstanding this argument, tertiary centers are apprehensive. Their chief concerns include the inability of level II hospitals to provide 24-hour in-house neonatologist coverage, lack of a sufficient array of support services, and less experienced nursing staffs. Although few tertiary centers actually maintain neonatologists in-house 24 hours per day, they usually have access to a greater number of full-time equivalents than do level IIs so that the NICU can be covered as necessary. Also, tertiary facilities generally have 24-hour coverage provided by pediatric and neonatal residents, which is not always the case in level II hospitals. Few level II hospitals have the equivalent depth of pediatric support services available in tertiary centers to help bolster their high-risk infant care. It is also more difficult for level II nurses to maintain specialty skill levels, since they generally treat fewer high-risk infants in their special care nurseries than do perinatal center NICU nurses. Finally, level II facilities seldom have a maternal fetal specialist on staff, or even on a consultant basis, to care for the high-risk mother (Allison-Cooke et al, 1988). The presence of this level of obstetric care is a prerequisite for a tertiary center.

It is unclear precisely where the lines of demarcation regarding transfer criteria should be drawn. A major problem is that the level II designation has evolved to cover such a broad spectrum of neonatal service capabilities that no single set of guidelines is appropriate to all intermediate care units.

## BACK TRANSFERS

The use of a level II nursery as a step-down unit for the perinatal center to reverse the transfer of infants no longer in need of ventilatory support emerged in the NPIC study as one technique that helps a perinatal network to function as a cooperative, interdependent unit. In contrast, paucity of back transfers can exacerbate resentments among physicians who lose contact with their patients after referral. This practice varies considerably among perinatal networks.

## TRANSPORT SYSTEMS

There were few serious criticisms about the arrangements for patient transport existing in the various NPIC study sites. Maternal transport is often achieved by nonspecialized modes such as regular emergency ambulance teams. This is sometimes considered to be less than optimal, especially in less populated areas.

In contrast, transport teams for high-risk infants are highly specialized, although their precise composition varies among perinatal networks. One comment heard repeatedly from doctors and nurses in community hospitals was a preference for the transport vehicle to be staffed by neonatal nurse practitioners rather than by residents, who were viewed as less experienced, less skilled and sometimes less political in their remarks. Some interview subjects noted a preference for the transport team to deploy while the mother is still in active labor rather than waiting until after the birth, as is the policy of some perinatal centers.

Although the specific components of neonatal transport systems vary from site to site, the general satisfaction rate is high. Unnecessary duplication of transport systems occurs in some areas. In many locations, however, multiple NICUs rely on the same transport service, which is sometimes jointly staffed by the various units, especially under consortium arrangements (Allison-Cooke et al, 1988).

## OUTREACH EDUCATION

Infant transport and outreach education have always been the cornerstone on which a successful perinatal network is built. Perinatal centers no longer enjoy the monopoly over outreach education that they once could claim, however, and lower level hospitals are becoming more discriminating in identifying their needs. In many instances, private neonatologists or newer level III hospitals have used this traditional strength of academic centers, that is, outreach, to establish their own networks in direct competition with the perinatal center.

To some degree, outreach always was a marketing tool. The original perinatal centers used it not only to improve quality of care in outlying hospitals but also to cement a relationship with those hospitals and practitioners that would include transfer agreements for sending high-risk infants to the perinatal center. Presently, outreach is an important tool for attracting larger market shares in areas where level III hospitals engage in open competition.

The role of outreach sometimes differs between more urban and rural sites. As urban level II hospitals become more sophisticated, they look to outreach as a means of upgrading their level of care, and they are increasingly interested in morbidity and mortality reviews. Physicians have become more accepting of morbidity and mortality reviews to help them avoid malpractice situations. In less populated states, outreach efforts link rural providers to urban specialists and allow rural obstetricians and family practitioners to continue to treat pregnant women in isolated areas despite rising malpractice fears (Allison-Cooke et al, 1988).

## IMPACT OF MEDICAID

State Medicaid reimbursement policies emerged from our NPIC interviews as much less important than the other factors under study. This is, in part, attributable to the fact that Medicaid covers a relatively small percentage of all inpatient care.

Widespread adoption of the latest Medicaid provisions, which offer states the option of greatly expanding their range of eligible mothers and babies, has increased the proportion of Medicaid-sponsored hospital care and enhanced the concomitant importance of Medicaid as a hospital payor. At present, the much greater issue is physician reimbursement and the resulting barriers to ambulatory-based obstetric care that are created when obstetricians close their doors to Medicaid patients. Hospitals can afford to accept Medicaid patients at reduced cost to occupy otherwise empty beds; however individual practitioners are far less able or willing to do this.

Although interview subjects judged Medicaid to have a mixed-to-negative overall impact, most would agree that Medicaid reimbursement rates are better than nothing, and in fact, Medicaid reimbursement for hospital care was generally believed to be reasonably adequate in four of the six case study sites.

Most of the key respondents to the NPIC interviews stated that Medicaid reimbursement policies had little to do with their hospitals' decision regarding perinatal and neonatal service offerings. In a similar vein, DRG reimbursement methodologies were seen as neutral in their influence on perinatal practice patterns (Allison-Cooke et al, 1988).

## IMPACT OF COMPETITION

Although competition among hospitals for patients was clearly rated the most important factor in the NPIC study (1988), opinions as to whether the competitive model of health care has a positive or negative impact on perinatal care and perinatal regionalization vary widely by level of care and professional affiliation as well as by geographic location. Competition is depicted by some as destroying regionalization, whereas others see it as a force of revitalization and progress. Administrators tend to look at the big picture for their hospital or for the total health care system, as opposed to only the perinatal care component, and believe that competition is much healthier than regulation. Obstetric and newborn nurses at community hospitals look at improvements in physical plant, equipment, program options, physician specialty coverage, and nursing education in their facilities and conclude that competition has been healthy for patients and clinicians alike. Many respondents point to the greatly expanded range of consumer choice in obstetric care as a direct benefit of hospitals competing for patient business.

Tertiary facility clinicians, on the other hand, are fairly unanimous in their assessment of health care competition as extremely injurious to perinatal regionalization. They express the concern that pressures for hospitals to diversify and be all things to all customers will spread some services, such as neonatal nursing, too thin and dilute skill levels among specialities that require minimum volumes of patients to maintain their adeptness.

At the heart of the competition in neonatal services is manpower acquisition and technologic proliferation, both of which are necessary for hospitals to upgrade their services and offer a higher level of care. As larger numbers of neonatologists become available, more level II hospitals will continue to hire them, buy new equipment, and establish special care nurseries in direct competition for a portion of the high-risk market formerly reserved for perinatal centers. Some tertiary facilities worry about their ability to compete successfully against these less expensive, sometimes more efficient level II hospitals. They also question whether or not these newer services are able to offer truly comparable levels of care and whether or not the total volume of high-risk infants is sufficient to support such a proliferation of units; this is often referred to as the level II problem.

Representing an opposing viewpoint, the community hospitals with significant obstetric services are proud of the progress they have made in upgrading to level II status; believe their enhanced ability to stabilize infants and receive back transfers improves the quality and efficiency of perinatal care; and feel that any expectation that they should remain as level I facilities is unrealistic in today's health care environment, in which local hospitals must offer a broader range of services to attract patients and HMO contracts and to cover themselves against malpractice suits. In contrast, birth hospitals in some cities have already achieved level II status, and this phenomenon seems to be viewed as less threatening in these environments. These level II hospitals seldom have maternal-fetal programs; they usually rely on maternal-fetal specialists in tertiary centers for this support. These different views reflect the complicated mix of direct and indirect costs and benefits attributable to competition in health care.

Administrators often view competitive pressure as a positive influence because it serves as a catalyst to running the hospital more like a business. This includes improving the physical plant in order to make the hospital more appealing to prospective patients as well as purchasing more sophisticated equipment and making other changes to attract more admitting physicians. This influence also compels hospitals to become more patient centered and to develop a broader range of program offerings in order to meet consumer demand for alternative birth arrangements. It clearly means learning to run the hospital in a more cost-efficient manner. On the other hand, competition erodes cooperation among hospitals, and cooperation is a mainstay of regionalization (Allison-Cooke et al, 1988).

## IMPACT OF HMOs

NPIC interview subjects were mixed in their evaluations of the importance of alternative delivery systems in their regions. In those areas where alternative delivery systems are a significant force, the perinatal professionals interviewed perceived their impact as largely negative. Clinicians, in particular, questioned whether cost considerations under alternative delivery models might not dominate medical considerations to the possible detriment of quality of care. Virtually the only positive ratings were from administrative or financial officers in hospitals where HMO contractual arrangements may secure more patient admissions.

Criticism of HMOs encompass a broad range of quality of care issues, including:

- Insufficient identification of high-risk mothers.
- Reluctance to use specialty consultants or tertiary care facilities.
- Services that are generally below par.
- Truncated lengths of stay, which impede maternal education and infant testing.

Some of these points relate to HMO generic policies and others to the discretionary power of general practice "gatekeepers," who screen cases and make referral for consultation and who bear the brunt of the financial risk and who feel the most direct pressure to avoid expensive specialty referrals or tertiary admissions.

Medicaid patients present special problems in accessing services under an HMO-style arrangement. Limits by HMOs on hospital length of stay place undue burden on young uneducated mothers with limited understanding of childbearing.

Medicaid HMO hospital networks may cut across traditional perinatal networks, disrupting regional relationships of referral and transfer. However, a much greater problem is the occasional need to subject babies to multiple transports because they were initially transferred to a hospital without an HMO contract. Medicaid HMO patients often identify themselves merely as welfare recipients so their high-risk infants are transported to the hospital's usual perinatal center. This necessitates a later, additional transport, which interrupts the continuity of care (Allison-Cooke et al, 1988).

## IMPACT OF MALPRACTICE

Malpractice issues were judged to be of moderate-to-low importance in all six NPIC sites. Administrators and financial officers tend to judge this issue as relatively benign, but clinicians believe that the issue is a serious problem. Reactions to its effects on quality of care in general and perinatal care were extremely varied. Many clinicians believe that the art of medicine is being lost in the overreliance on test results and defensible medical practices. Others believe that clearer standards of practice have emerged and that there is greater compliance with these standards. However, perinatal center representatives were fairly uniform in agreeing that malpractice worries have had virtually no impact on patient care practices at tertiary facilities.

The consequences of the current situation are seen more often as negative than positive, especially by community practitioners. The most glaring negative by-product of escalating litigation rates is the creation of access obstacles to ambulatory care, especially for uninsured, Medicaid insured, and rural mothers. Urban obstetricians are closing their practices to indigent and Medicaid patients who are prone to have high-risk babies and for whom any reimbursement received is unlikely to even cover the physician's malpractice premiums. Many experienced obstetricians and gynecologists are beginning to specialize in gynecology in order to minimize the risk of obstetric lawsuits. Family practitioners in isolated areas are dropping obstetrics altogether because of escalating insurance rates.

In addition to obstacles to access, malpractice is seen as a problem for hospitals in general terms of escalating premiums and as a negative factor in inducing unnecessary testing and cesarean sections. This combination results in greatly increased health care costs.

How these alterations in practice patterns apply to the quality of services rendered is much less clear and much more controversial. Some perinatologists and most obstetricians link the escalating cesarean section rate to fear of malpractice suits; many find this trend highly objectionable. There is an opinion, however, that fear of problem deliveries is influencing some providers to institute better referral and transfer practices, thus enhancing overall perinatal regionalization. Not surprisingly, the malpractice crisis is commonly cited as having improved documentation of care in the medical records.

Fear of malpractice emerges as a significant source of stress, especially for private practitioners. There is a common perception, true or not, that the instigation and outcome of lawsuits bear little relationship to quality of care, that is, that equity does not exist.

Concerns over malpractice liability are also affecting interprofessional relationships. Obstetricians and pediatricians, physicians and nurses debate the responsibilities of patient care and of documenting that care, such as interpreting and recording cord gases, APGARS, and incidence reports (Allison-Cooke et al, 1988).

## RELATIVE IMPACT OF ENVIRONMENTAL FACTORS

NPIC interview subjects registered extremely mixed opinions as to whether competition among hospitals has a positive or a negative impact on the delivery of perinatal services. Respondents from level II hospitals are more likely to hold extremely favorable views of competition as providing a catalyst to the acquisition of more sophisticated manpower and technology, whereas perinatal centers perceive hospital competition as extremely injurious to regionalized care.

HMOs, malpractice, and Medicaid are all viewed as exerting mixed-to-negative pressures on the organization and delivery of perinatal care, but this opinion varies substantially by geographic area. State Medicaid programs were more likely than the other two factors to receive clearly negative rather than mixed assessments, but this is largely attributable to Medicaid's ambulatory payment practices, which tend to be well below current market rates for obstetric services. In contrast, Medicaid reimbursement for inpatient care is believed to be relatively adequate.

Perceptions of the impact of alternative delivery systems on the organization and delivery of perinatal care vary according to market penetration and type of plan in place in the region. HMOs are capable of both creating and destroying perinatal networks as they shift large blocks of patient admissions and transfers. Whether this is perceived to be a positive or negative factor seems to be largely a function of the provider's success in competing for contracts within this system. Some observers are critical of the quality of care delivered by specific plans.

The current malpractice environment is producing a mixed impact in nearly all geographic areas. Consistent variations in opinion regarding the effect of escalating malpractice litigation emerge by physician affiliation and the level of care they provide. Community providers, especially obstetricians, feel the negative side effects of litigation far more strongly than do tertiary providers, who are often insulated from this problem by legislative or institutional safeguards. Tertiary physicians hold ambiguous opinions on the effect the fear of malpractice litigation may have on their professional peers in the community. Some physicians believe that escalating cesarean section rates, unnecessary testing, and obstetricians dropping or restricting their practices is the negative result of malpractice litigation, whereas others believe that a more litigious environment has forced improvements in the standard of practice.

The conclusions of the study were varied. The factor of competition was identified in this NPIC study to be of paramount importance to hospitals today in their ability to organize and maintain regionalized structures of perinatal care. This competition is manifested through community hospital acquisition of the manpower and technology necessary to upgrade to higher levels of care in order to compete for higher-risk patients, (i.e., the level II hospital problem). Highly controversial questions were raised concerning the appropriateness of altered service offerings and transfer patterns by level II hospitals vis-à-vis perinatal centers and how these changes have an impact on patient outcomes (Allison-Cooke et al, 1988).

# The Future of Regional Programs: The Perinatal Partnership

Recognizing that identified environmental factors affect perinatal regionalization, there is a need to articulate the establishment of a new alternative: perinatal networks based on equal partnerships rather than the traditional centralized strategy. Hospital requirements would be based on the needs of the hospitals' patients, not on system definitions such as levels of care. There would be no constraints on hospital service offerings, provided that they meet specified patient volume and quality of care standards.

All obstetric hospitals would be required to determine what types of patients they wished to treat, and these patient categories would then be matched to a set of manpower and technology resource requirements based on patient needs. Under this approach, referred to here as the Perinatal Partnership, patient care needs not provided by a particular hospital must be available through arrangements with other institutions, (e.g., transport or medical education agreements). This concept was established by a national committee that reviewed the findings of the NPIC study of regionalization. The consensus for a Perinatal Partnership seemed to many participants to be a way out of the conundrum of a disintegrating regional structure (NPIC, 1989).

The implementation of this type of approach requires that the community of perinatal professionals generate two sets of definitions:

1. Patient groups as a grouping algorithm for patients would need to be specified, based on characteristics such as birthweight and comorbidities.
2. Patient group resource requirements include manpower, training, technology, and patient volume requirements associated with each patient group.

Hospitals wishing to treat particular patient groups would be required to provide the levels of manpower, training, equipment, ancillaries and other resources specified by the patient group resource requirements needed for those patients. This approach would include safeguards to help ensure quality and cost effectiveness. For example, minimum volume requirements would be specified to maintain clinical skills and encourage economies of scale. All hospitals would participate in an area-wide quality assurance program, including morbidity and mortality reviews, to ensure against substandard care.

The Perinatal Partnership would retain many aspects of the study "Toward Improving the Outcome of Pregnancy," particularly, the incentives to participate in a network of perinatal hospitals. In order to meet the needs of all patients, hospitals must provide for:

• Maternal and neonatal transport
• Patient follow-up
• Data sharing
• Continuing education
• Multi-hospital monitoring and quality assurance
• Teaching and research
• Communication and consultation

Few hospitals can supply all these functions in isolation. A network of sharing institutions is needed (Fig. 4–1). This is consistent with the current trend toward multi-hospital systems and cooperative agreements (NPIC, 1989).

There are two major differences between the Perinatal Partnership approach and the original articulation of regionalization in the document *Toward Improving the Outcome of Pregnancy.* First, the new system would be built on the characteristics of patients to whom hospitals wish to provide services rather than around hospital characteristics.

The second major difference would be that regional care would not necessarily revolve around one central facility, although this would certainly be an acceptable organizational model. The major goal of a perinatal system is to provide for all the needs of all patients, either directly or through agreements among hospitals. In a traditional regional model, this goal is achieved by systemwide risk identification plus centralization of high-risk services in one tertiary level facility, which serves as a focal point for less sophisticated units. A Perinatal Partnership could also function in this manner, or it could involve more coequal, cooperative relationships with more facilities able to offer higher levels of care as long as they maintain

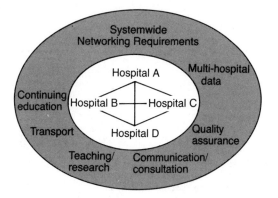

**Figure 4–1.** The Perinatal Partnership. An approach to organizing perinatal care in the 1990s. (From National Perinatal Information Center Perinatal Partnership, 1989.)

sufficient economics of scale and an appropriate level of quality of care is achieved and systemwide needs such as patient transport and provider education are met (NPIC, 1988).

## PERINATAL SERVICE REQUIREMENTS

In order for this approach to work, certain requirements must be met by hospitals, perinatal departments, and systemwide networks. These would include department, hospital, and system levels of application (Table 4–1). Departmental and support service criteria would correlate to the severity level of the patient-case mix that a given hospital chooses to serve. These criteria would constitute the perinatal group resource requirements for that institution. One of these guidelines would set a minimum of patients per month for optimal quality care. Other requirements would address specific staffing ratios, training levels, coverage guidelines, ventilation, and other treatment needs as well as quality of care outcome expectations.

The choice to provide services to patients at highest risk would rest with the institution and its clinical department. Implied in this approach, however, is that hospitals must meet all the perinatal group resource requirements for that patient group, including the minimum volume requirements. This approach would serve two purposes:

**Table 4–1**
THE PERINATAL PARTNERSHIP. AN OUTLINE
FOR FUTURE SPECIFICATION

| Perinatal System Requirements | Patient Groups |
|---|---|
| • Networking | • Birthweight |
| • Transport | • Ventilation |
| • Multi-hospital data | • Other conditions |
| • Quality assurance | • Other procedures |
| • Communication | • Other—to be specified |
| • Consultation | |
| • Continuing education | |
| • Teaching and research | |
| • Other—to be specified | |

**Patient Group Resource Requirements**

| *Hospital Requirements* | *Perinatal Department Requirements* |
|---|---|
| • Adequate revenue generation | • Neonatologist/patient ratios |
| • Networking | • Perinatologist/OB requirements |
| • Credentialing | • RN/patient ratios |
| • Adequate liability insurance | • RN training levels |
| • Quality assurance | • Pediatric coverage |
| • Other—to be specified | • Nighttime coverage |
| | • Ventilation services |
| | • Other treatments |
| | • Support services |
| | • Transport provisions |
| | • Follow-up |
| | • Continuing education |
| | • Quality assurance |
| | • Networking |
| | • Other—to be specified |

From National Perinatal Information Center. Perinatal Partnership, 1989.

first, it would enhance quality, and second, it would promote systemwide efficiency through economics of scale with sufficient numbers of patients to maintain an adequate standard of practice.

## HOSPITAL REQUIREMENTS

From the viewpoint of financial viability, all hospitals need to generate revenue sufficient to support the level of services they choose to deliver. They also must maintain adequate liability insurance, internal quality assurance credibility in their community, and a network of relationships with other institutions.

Economics stresses the relation of volume to efficiency in this instance. A larger volume of patients in specific patient groups is more efficient than smaller numbers,

thereby allowing the per case costs to drop. Although third party payors are increasingly interested in the price of care, clinicians and other observers worry whether or not cost containment may jeopardize quality services. When the guidelines explicitly delineate staffing, support services, and volume, however, a certain standard of quality becomes the only type of care available, and competition for patients can be based on cost without a trade-off against quality (NPIC, 1989).

## SYSTEM REQUIREMENTS

Although some hospitals will be able to operate perinatal services alone, without the cooperation of other hospitals, the majority will need to participate in a system level perinatal network, if for no other reason than to ensure that the volume of patients is maintained. These system components are essential support mechanisms that allow patients to receive quality care in appropriate settings. They include patient support; education, consultation, and communication arrangements; a shared information base; and areawide quality assurance programs (see Table 4–1 and Fig. 4–1).

Certain public sector obligations are also implied. Primarily, government needs to ensure that adequate financing is available to allow providers to deliver services to all patients, regardless of the pay source. In addition, an oversight function is needed to ensure that hospitals meet specified volume and patient outcome standards (NPIC, 1989).

## THE RESPONSE

The Perinatal Partnership approach does not eliminate competition. It does, however, confront the quality versus cost dilemma directly, by identifying that any hospital can provide high-risk services if it can meet both the patient volume and quality of care standards. This approach attempts to maintain the most valuable elements of "Toward Improving the Outcome of Pregnancy" while confronting the realities of hospital competition and the complexities of today's health care environment.

## QUALITY

The Perinatal Partnership approach is one in which quality of care is the primary goal. To guarantee quality, it is not sufficient to rely on structural variables such as adequate staffing ratios and equipment alone. These are components of quality but do not guarantee it. There must be an understanding of both what good care is and whether or not it is being provided.

Institutional and comparative quality assurance systems based on criteria, norms, and standards derived from a uniform data system with input from an expert panel are key. Both morbidity and mortality reviews are important but should emphasize morbidity indicators because these are primary patient outcome measures. An adequate area-wide quality improvement program would include at least four components:

- An information and data base support system
- A review system
- Standards and criteria for assessing structure, process, and outcome
- Corrective action measures such as feedback, education, regulations, and sanctions.

Funding for quality improvement needs to be systemwide and, if possible, independent of funding for the delivery of services. This activity must be recognized as a necessary function, because it would be the tool employed to ensure against abuses of the flexibility available to all institutions under the partnership approach (NPIC, 1989).

## DATA AND INFORMATION

There is also a need for national, or at least regional, information systems to support the planning, organization, delivery, and assessment of systems of perinatal care. The goal would be a functional data retrieval system with uniform information available for a variety of uses and users. To the greatest extent possible, the system should encompass the continuum of perinatal care outlined earlier. This need for data exists equally for current and future systems of care.

# Networking

One of the most positive aspects of regionalization and the one most threatened by competition is the establishment of cooperative relationships among institutions. Hospitals and perinatal teams should be responsible for establishing meaningful perinatal networks that encompass all or most of the resources necessary to meet the requirements of all patient categories.

All hospitals and perinatal personnel would participate in perinatal network functions to ensure that their patients are not placed in jeopardy because of self-serving attitudes or practices. Review of network agreements and participation should be within the purview of local, state, or federal agencies.

The principle of networking would continue the very positive example established by the regional systems in the 1970s. At the same time, by shifting the emphasis away from an attempt to impose a set structure on an elusive health care system to an approach that focuses on patient needs, the Perinatal Partnership would provide flexibility to respond to local situations.

# Organization and Structure

In the past, perinatal care has focused on the hospital setting. There is now an increasing awareness of health care professionals of the need to emphasize prevention and to establish a continuum of services from gynecologic and prenatal care through postpartum and neonatal and infant care. The need to specify timing, criteria, and content of care, especially prenatal care, also is recognized, as is the need to place more emphasis on the counseling and education functions of ambulatory providers.

The goals of any system of care should be guaranteed access, high-quality care, and cost efficiency. If these goals are achieved, structure and process are seen only as intermediate objectives that would not be the focal point of the Perinatal Partnership (NPIC, 1989).

# Access and Financing

It has become increasingly evident that levels and methods of financing health care services determine many characteristics of the delivery system. This fact would be equally true for the Perinatal Partnership approach as it is for the regional concept of care. All providers should be paid a fair rate for all patients, thus eliminating problems of access, indigent health care, dumping (poor patients sent to a public hospital), dual health care systems, and double standards of quality.

Inadequate or inequitable financing constitutes the most significant limitation to patient access; the greatest and most obvious problems lie in the area of indigent health care and overcoming access obstacles. Medicaid and other payors must recognize that reimbursement levels directly affect accessibility of services for their clients. Currently, a disproportionate share of Medicaid and indigent patients can place physicians and hospitals in financially precarious positions.

In the Perinatal Partnership approach, there is a link between reimbursement and quality through linking rates to patient care requirements. Specifically, hospitals electing to treat high-risk patients would be eligible only for payment for such services if they can meet the patient group resource requirements for those patients. Also, reimbursement systems should include incentives for better patient outcomes. There is a need for positive incentives to encourage early prenatal care, ensure high-risk screening and referral, and avoid unnecessary cesarean sections.

The Perinatal Partnership approach would mitigate many of the undermining characteristics of HMOs and managed health care systems. These systems could incorporate the resource and quality of care standards (patient group resource requirements) appropriate to their patient populations. One of the challenges before the perinatal community is to ensure that these evolving managed care systems make provisions for joining or developing adequate perinatal programs and that they meet the same guidelines as other providers (NPIC, 1989).

The continued emphasis on a regionalized structure based on the currently delineated levels of care is no longer effective in coping with the complexity of today's health care environment. There is a recognized need to restructure the approach to regionalized perinatal care. This approach must be more patient centered than facility centered. It should include a more active outreach to patients with access obstacles to both primary and referral care. The patient-centered approach to care places greater emphasis on the capability of practitioners and hospitals to care for specific high-risk patients. There should then be greater flexibility in the composition of hospital services. The perinatal services provided by hospitals should be defined by degree of sophistication rather than by level; in turn, the application of these services to patients must be measured by the outcome they produce rather than by their presence in a hospital.

The Perinatal Partnership concept encourages a more coequal status among providers as an alternative to hierarchical referral structure. Greater emphasis is placed on the primary physician following his or her patient with appropriate consultation. Greater use is made of back transport to ensure that patients are treated in their community by practitioners with whom they will relate on a permanent basis. Finally, attempts should be made to ensure quality and systemwide efficiencies by establishing standards for the outcome of care. It is understood that there is a relationship of economies of scale to support appropriate care standards.

Further study is needed to determine appropriate patient groups and patient group resource requirements. Further study is also required on manpower, staffing, and organizational structure to assure the successful implementation of such a partnership.

If the perinatal community wishes to maintain those elements of perinatal regionalization most worthy of preservation, it must adapt to these changes. The approach suggested in the Perinatal Partnership concept is one way to meet effectively the dramatic changes in the health care environment that have had an impact on both provider and patient. If perinatal regionalization is to prosper into the next century, it must adapt and change.

## References

Allison-Cooke S, Schwartz RM, Gagnon DE: A study of the impact of recent developments in the health care environment on perinatal regionalization. National Perinatal Information Center, 1988.

Gagnon DE: Managing the future: an examination of the neonatal intensive care unit. J Perinatol 11:2, 1991.

Gagnon DE, Allison-Cooke S, Schwartz RM: Perinatal care: the threat of deregionalization. Pediatr Ann 17:7, 1988.

Hein HA: Evaluation of a rural perinatal care system. Pediatrics. 6:6, 1980.

Kanto WP: Regionalization revisited. Am J Dis Child 141(4):403–404, 1987.

Lynch NK: Growth in neonatal intermediate care services. Perinatal Press. 13:16, 1991.

March of Dimes, The National Foundation: Committee on perinatal health: toward improving the outcome of pregnancy. Recommendations for the regional development of maternal and perinatal health services, 1988.

March of Dimes, The National Foundation: Committee on perinatal health: toward improving the outcome of pregnancy. Recommendations for the regional development of maternal and perinatal health services, 1976.

McCormick MC, Shapiro S, Stanfield BH: The regionalization of perinatal services. JAMA 253:6, 1985.

Merenstein G, Rhodes P, Little G: Personnel in neonatal pediatrics. Assessment of numbers and distribution. Pediatrics 78:3, 1986.

Muri JH, Schwartz RM: Neonatal special care services: questions of supply and demand. Perinatal Press 11:5, 1988.

National Perinatal Information Center (NPIC): Perinatal partnership: an approach to organizing care in the 1990s, 1989.

National Perinatal Information Center (NPIC): Survey of MCH directors in the 50 states. Unpublished, 1990.

Schwartz RM: Regionalization in an environment of competition and technology proliferation. Perinatal Press 11:1, 1988.

US Congress: Office of Technology Assessment: Neonatal intensive care for low birthweight infants: cost effectiveness. OTA-HCS-39. Washington DC, US Government Priority Office, 1987.

# CHAPTER 5

· · · · · · · · · · · · · · · · · · · · · · · · · · · · · · · · · · · · · · · · · ·

# Antepartum Assessment of the Fetus

John F. Huddleston, Gail S. Williams, and Elizabeth L. Fabbri

Although there has been steady and respectable improvement in perinatal outcome during recent years, a small percentage of pregnancies continue to terminate in either fetal mortality or serious morbidity. Although not all potentially disastrous outcomes can be predicted, a majority of pregnancies with such potential can be identified through screening methods (e.g., the history, the physical examination, and laboratory tests) and thus be labeled as high risk (Aubry and Pennington, 1973; Goodwin et al, 1969; Hoebel et al, 1973). Over the last two decades, several surveillance methods have been developed and used in managing these high-risk pregnancies—pregnancies that because of factors justifying the high-risk label would be expected, without effective surveillance methods and selective intervention, to produce the majority of cases of perinatal morbidity and mortality.

Pregnancies can be designated as high risk for any of several undesirable outcomes. For instance, the woman who has lost several babies because of recurrent preterm labor in the midtrimester presents a management problem different from the woman with long-standing diabetes mellitus who has had several stillbirths near term. Another pregnancy in the diabetic woman would be at risk for the inadequate provision of nutrients and of oxygen—that is, uteroplacental insufficiency.

Pregnancies considered to be at risk for uteroplacental insufficiency carry a serious threat for fetal growth retardation, intrauterine fetal demise, intrapartum fetal distress, and various types of neonatal morbidity. Factors such as insulin-requiring diabetes and hypertensive disorders can interfere with uterine blood flow, intervillous space perfusion, and placental exchange, and thus, may interfere with fetal nutrition and oxygenation (Parer, 1976). The potential for perinatal morbidity or mortality is thereby increased. Of the general types of surveillance methods that have been developed, those using electronic monitoring of the fetal heart rate and real-time ultrasonography have become the most widely used and accepted for fetal assessment in the management of those pregnancies at risk for uteroplacental insufficiency (Resnik et al, 1982). Through assessment of the at-risk fetus with antepartum electronic heart rate monitoring and sonography and, at times, biochemical monitoring, those pregnancies with normal uteroplacental exchange, as evidenced by repetitively normal tests, can confidently be managed with a hands-off policy. Of this large majority with normal tests, most can be carefully followed and be allowed to undergo spontaneous labor and delivery. For those few babies whose tests are abnormal—and thus suggest decreased uteroplacental function—corrective efforts can be effected, either to improve uterine blood flow or to remove the fetus from its unfavorable environment.

## Indications for Testing
(Table 5–1)

Maternal factors that place a pregnancy at risk for uteroplacental insufficiency include chronic and pregnancy-induced hypertension, chronic renal disease, insulin-requiring

**Table 5–1**
SUGGESTED INDICATIONS FOR ANTEPARTUM
FETAL ASSESSMENT

Chronic hypertension/pregnancy-induced
  hypertension
Chronic renal disease
Diabetes mellitus (insulin-requiring)
Cyanotic congenital heart disease
Rhesus (or other) isoimmunization
Homozygous hemoglobinopathies
Maternal abuse of cigarettes/alcohol/drugs
Previous unexplained stillbirth
Fetal growth retardation
Postdatism
Hydramnios/oligohydramnios
Decreased fetal movement
Multiple gestation
Premature rupture of membranes (PROM)
Third trimester bleeding
Arrhythmias
Sickle cell anemia
Maternal collagen vascular disease

diabetes mellitus, cyanotic congenital heart disease, isoimmunization, sickle cell diseases, cigarette and other substance abuse, and history of a previous pregnancy that terminated with an unexplained stillbirth. Other obstetric problems that place a pregnancy at such risk include fetal growth retardation, prolonged pregnancy (42 or more gestational weeks), hydramnios, and oligohydramnios. Testing should also be considered when there are maternal sensations of decreased fetal movement and in cases of multiple gestation.

Primary emphasis in this chapter is given to biophysical testing, because it is used more extensively. For the sake of completeness, biochemical testing methods will be outlined.

# Biophysical Testing Methods

Any fetus at risk for uteroplacental insufficiency is a candidate, as early as the 25th to 26th week of gestation, for biophysical fetal evaluation. The time chosen to begin testing depends on the circumstances surrounding the individual pregnancy and the neonatal survival data for tiny babies at a particular hospital or referral center. Generally, for at-risk pregnancies that are progressing well by clinical criteria, testing is started at about 32 to 34 weeks of gestation. The lower gestational age limit to begin testing is defined as

that at which, after consultation with the patient and her husband, one would do a cesarean delivery for fetal indications. In tertiary referral centers, this lower limit currently is about 25 to 26 weeks.

Two types of biophysical evaluation using fetal heart rate testing have achieved widespread acceptance for antepartum surveillance. The first described was the contraction stress test (CST), which relies for its interpretation on the fetal heart rate response to uterine contractions (Pose et al, 1969; Ray et al, 1972). Because even normal uterine contractions exert some hypoxic stresses to the fetus through impairment of uterine blood flow (Poseiro et al, 1969), uteroplacental function can be assessed through performance of the CST. If function (and thus fetal oxygenation) has been normal, these temporary interruptions of uterine blood flow do not disturb fetal oxygenation sufficiently to affect the heart rate (Parer, 1976). However, contractions may cause repetitive late decelerations if fetal basal oxygenation is low, a finding that implies impairment in uteroplacental exchange (Martin, 1978; Myers et al, 1973; Pose et al, 1969). A finding of a negative CST (no late decelerations with a contraction frequency of 3 in 10 minutes) has been found highly predictive of intrauterine survival for 7 subsequent days (Freeman et al, 1982; Huddleston and Freeman, 1982). Gabbe and associates (1978) have found CST results to be reliable even early in the third trimester.

The second of these biophysical tests is the nonstress test (NST), which relies for its interpretation on fetal heart rate reactivity, defined as accelerations of the heart rate found in response to fetal movements (Evertson et al, 1979; Rochard et al, 1976). As with the negative CST, a reactive NST is also highly predictive of intrauterine survival for 7 subsequent days (Freeman et al, 1982; Martin and Schifrin, 1977). However, a finding of a nonreactive pattern may imply that the fetus is acidotic, as a result of prolonged suboptimal oxygenation. In the evolution of fetal deterioration due to hypoxia, we consider that the appearance of late decelerations in response to contractions (positive CST) will precede loss of heart rate reactivity (nonreactive NST) (Huddleston and Freeman, 1982; Huddleston et al, 1984) (Fig. 5–1). Data obtained from experiments on rhesus monkey fetuses supported this clinical impression (Murata et al, 1982). On the

| | Metabolically Normal Fetus $\rightleftarrows$ | Critical Hypoxia During Contractions $\rightleftarrows$ | Fetus With Asphyxia |
|---|---|---|---|
| Basal Oxygenation | Normal | Subnormal | Subnormal |
| Contraction Stress Test | Negative | Positive | Positive |
| Acid-Base Status | Normal | Normal | Acidotic |
| Nonstress Test | Reactive | Reactive | Nonreactive |

Figure 5–1. Evolution of fetal deterioration due to hypoxia. Loss of reactivity, when due to hypoxia, is usually preceded by late decelerations, if the uterus is contracting. If this is the correct sequence of events, then the CST is a better indicator of fetal reserve, whereas the NST better defines acute fetal condition.

other hand, because a nonreactive pattern frequently exists for other reasons, a follow-up CST is generally performed to explain a nonreactive pattern. A positive CST suggests that this pattern is due to protracted fetal hypoxia; a negative CST suggests that the nonreactivity exists because of some other factor, such as fetal sleep or maternal ingestion of narcotic or sedative drugs (Martin and Schifrin, 1977).

Of these two biophysical tests used for fetal surveillance, the NST has become the primary test in many institutions, because it is simpler, requires less time, and is less costly than the CST (Resnik et al, 1982). In the authors' opinion, there remain, however, definite indications for the CST. Not only is it used to define fetal status when a nonreactive NST is found, but some institutions rely on the CST for primary testing of their pregnancies at highest risk. (At the authors' institutions, four conditions qualify: severe chronic hypertension, insulin-requiring diabetes, fetal growth retardation substantiated by ultrasound, and oligohydramnios) (Huddleston and Freeman, 1982). Moreover, data now available from the CST/NST Collaborative Study suggest that the CST may be a better predictor of fetal reserve, because its use for primary fetal surveillance seems to be associated with fewer stillbirths when compared with primary use of the NST (Freeman et al, 1982). Moreover, recent methods employing maternal nipple stimulation to produce uterine contractions may encourage more widespread use of the CST, because this test now compares favorably with the NST with regard to simplicity and, therefore, low cost (Freeman, 1982; Huddleston et al, 1984).

## THE CONTRACTION STRESS TEST

### CST Methodology

The gravida is placed in the left-lateral or semi-Fowler's position, in an attempt to prevent aortocaval compression (Scott and Kerr, 1963); such compression can reduce uterine blood flow and result in temporary fetal hypoxemia and an abnormal test, independent of the reason for which the pregnancy is being tested. External fetal monitoring equipment is then applied. Blood pressure is measured initially and at 10- to 15-minute intervals throughout testing. Any hypotension is noted and corrected by a change in maternal position. Baseline fetal heart rate and spontaneous uterine contractions are assessed for 15 to 20 minutes after application of the external fetal heart rate transducer and the tocotransducer. Care must be taken in positioning and tightly securing the tocotransducer to ensure that uterine activity and, if desired, fetal movements are recorded on the monitor strip. After the baseline recording has been obtained, uterine activity is assessed for adequacy and, if spontaneous activity is inadequate (arbitrarily defined as less than three palpable 40- to 60-second contractions in a 10-minute period), either oxytocin delivery is begun with an intravenous infusion pump, or contractions are initiated by intermittent nipple stimulation.

Some relative contraindications should be considered when administering the CST. These include placenta previa, previous uterine rupture, previous vertical cesarean section, preterm labor, incompetent cervix, and premature rupture of the membranes.

**Oxytocin Delivery via Intravenous Infusion Pump.** If spontaneous uterine activity is deemed inadequate following the 15- to 20-minute baseline period, a low-dose, slow intravenous infusion is begun (generally with either normal saline or Ringer's lactate solution). A controlled-rate infusion pump is used to regulate the oxytocin infusion, which is administered in a piggybacked fashion into the intravenous line. Oxytocin, diluted in normal saline, is begun initially at a rate of 0.5 to 1.0 milliunits/min and then increased (per protocol described in the oxytocin product literature) approximately every 30 minutes until an adequate contraction frequency is achieved. The typical rate of oxytocin delivery required to elicit adequate uterine activity is 4 to 5 milliunits/min; rarely will a gravida require more than 8 milliunits/min to achieve this activity (Huddleston et al, 1979; Huddleston and Freeman, 1982). The average duration of a CST employing this method of oxytocin delivery is reported to be 80 to 90 minutes (Schifrin, 1977).

**Oxytocin Release via Intermittent Nipple Stimulation.** As a result of impulses transmitted via thoracic sensory nerve roots, breast stimulation in the lactating woman causes the posterior pituitary to release oxytocin (Cobo, 1974). It has been suggested that nipple stimulation in the gravida is an alternative for achieving uterine contractions for CSTs, in lieu of intravenous oxytocin delivery (Freeman, 1982; Huddleston et al, 1984). However, the mechanism by which nipple stimulation causes contractions is not clear. Women wearing light clothing are instructed to rub one nipple, through their clothes with the palmar surfaces of their fingertips, for 2 minutes, and then to stop nipple stimulation for 5 minutes. If a woman has several layers of clothing on, she is instructed to stimulate one nipple through the brassiere. Stimulation is stopped immediately if a contraction commences during the 2 minutes of stimulation, because we found uterine hyperstimulation occasionally to occur with prolonged stimulation of the nipple (Huddleston et al, 1984). A gravida may alternate nipples during stimulation, in order to decrease the chances of producing nipple tenderness. A 7-minute cycle is composed of the 2 minutes of stimulation plus the 5 minutes of rest. On average, only 2 or 3 nipple-stimulation cycles are required to elicit adequate uterine activity, with the average

length of a CST using intermittent nipple stimulation being 40 to 45 minutes (including the 15- to 20-minute observation period) (Huddleston et al, 1984). Because of the simplicity and speed of this method, oxytocin is rarely used now to achieve a CST.

### CST Interpretations

**Negative.** CST results are interpreted in the classic manner (ACOG, 1987; Freeman, 1975). The CST is defined as negative when there are *no* late decelerations present on the tracing and uterine contractions have been adequate to sufficiently stress the fetus (three 40- to 60-second palpable contractions in a 10-minute period or a tetanic contraction lasting ≥90 seconds). Usually, fetal heart rate reactivity is seen (Figs. 5–2 and 5–3). The CST, when negative, generally is repeated every 7 days until delivery, unless severe clinical decompensation occurs (e.g., diabetic ketoacidosis or exacerbation of hypertensive disease). However, some researchers are advocating testing patients with insulin-requiring diabetes, gestational diabetes with a previous stillborn, postdate pregnancy, or intrauterine fetal growth retardation (IUGR) twice a week. With this strict, classic interpretation for the negative test, the authors and others have found a false-negative CST (fetal death occurring within 7 days of a negative test) rate of only 1 to 2 per 1000 cases (Freeman et al, 1982; Huddleston and Freeman, 1982). Thus, the authors have not seen reason to shorten the time interval between tests. About 80 to 85 percent of tests are negative.

**Positive.** In the absence of uterine hyperstimulation or supine hypotension, the presence of late decelerations with 50 percent or more of the contractions during a period of adequate uterine activity constitutes a positive CST (Huddleston and Freeman, 1982). However, it is unnecessary and actually undesirable to continue efforts to achieve three contractions in a 10-minute period if recurrent late decelerations are evident with contractions occurring less frequently. Reactivity may be present (Figs. 5–4 and 5–5).

From 3 to 5 percent of CSTs are classified as positive. The fetus with a positive CST is probably suboptimally oxygenated, at least at the time of testing (Freeman et al, 1976). Therefore, management of the positive CST fetus generally includes prompt interven-

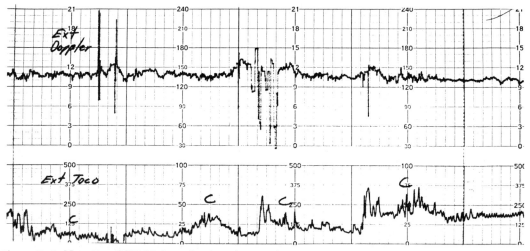

**Figure 5–2.** Negative CST. No late decelerations with a contraction frequency of at least 3 in 10 min.

tion. The fetus at term or post-term most frequently is delivered. The route of delivery is predicated on the presence of concurrent heart rate reactivity and on obstetric factors, such as cervical preparedness (assessed by the Bishop score [Bishop, 1964]) and fetal lie. It has been found that, if such conditions are favorable and the fetus is treated prophylactically for fetal distress (i.e., mother placed in the left-lateral position, hydrated intravenously, and given oxygen by mask), about half of these fetuses can safely endure the induction of labor with oxytocin (Braly and Freeman, 1977; Huddleston et al, 1979). However, if the positive CST is also nonreactive, the fetal condition is generally such that labor cannot be tolerated; cesarean delivery is generally employed in a pre-emptive manner for these patients. However, some institutions do give these patients a trial of labor. If fetal maturity is in doubt *and* if heart rate reactivity* is present on the positive CST tracing, an amniocentesis typically is performed for studies of pulmonary maturity. If such studies suggest that the fetus is immature *and* if the frequently assessed heart rate reactivity (or biophysical profile) remains reassuring, such a patient temporarily may be managed by having the gravida remain at bedrest with encouragement of the lateral position (Huddleston and Freeman, 1982). Some physi-

cians consider the use of glucocorticoids in an attempt to hasten fetal pulmonary maturity (Liggins and Howie, 1972). The management of such an immature fetus includes *daily* assessments for reactivity (NST) or biophysical profile. (A discussion of this test appears later in this chapter.) However, if these evaluations are not persistently reassuring, the fetus generally is transferred from its hostile intrauterine environment to a neonatal intensive care unit.

**Equivocal.** About 15 to 20 percent of CSTs are not interpretable as either negative or positive. These tests are designated as equivocal and impart little useful information concerning fetal well-being. They should be repeated within 24 hours, in an attempt to achieve a definitive result concerning fetal well-being. Equivocal tests may be further categorized as suspicious, hyperstimulated, and unsatisfactory (Huddleston and Freeman, 1982).

A CST is considered suspicious when late decelerations only intermittently are present with an adequate but not excessive contraction frequency (e.g., present with fewer than half of contractions). Usually, but not always, heart rate reactivity is present. Because only about one fifth of these suspicious tests become positive on repeat testing, and because a delay of 24 hours to repeat a suspicious test almost never results in fetal loss, such repeat testing is almost always employed unless the pregnancy is at term or beyond (Bruce et al, 1978; Huddleston et al,

---

* Heart rate reactivity is defined as 2 accelerations in a 20-minute period increasing 15 beats above the baseline and persisting for 15 seconds (reactive NST).

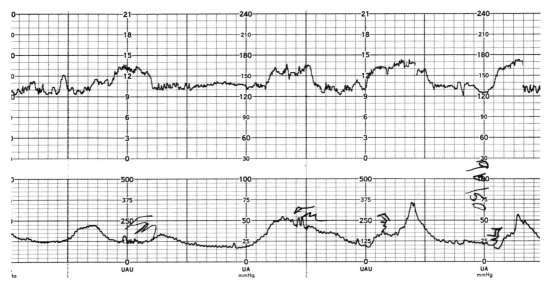

**Figure 5–3.** Negative CST. Reactivity associated with fetal movements (FM) is so pronounced as to perhaps cause confusion in interpretation. However, the baseline heart rate is 130 to 140 beats/min, and the return of the heart rate to baseline following the accelerations does not represent late deceleration.

1979). If reactivity is not present, a biophysical profile may provide additional information regarding fetal well-being.

In the presence of excessive uterine activity (contractions occurring more often than every 2 minutes and/or lasting more than 90 seconds) with associated late deceleration(s), a CST is labeled hyperstimulation. Because uterine sensitivity to oxytocin varies with each gravida, extreme care must be taken when introducing intravenous oxytocin or

when beginning intermittent nipple stimulation. Excessive uterine activity may even occur in the gravida who is contracting spontaneously. Allow the uterus to relax and restart the oxytocin at a lower dose or use less frequent nipple stimulation.

Occasionally, the quality of a tracing is such that an interpretation of the CST cannot be made confidently; such tests are termed unsatisfactory. Factors that may increase the chances for an unsatisfactory CST

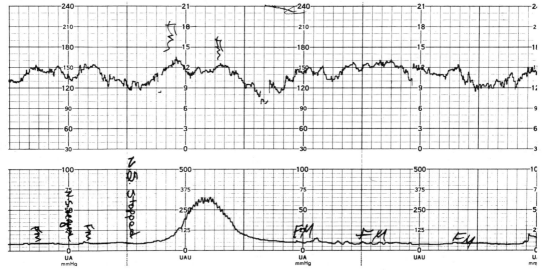

**Figure 5–4.** Positive, reactive CST. Only one contraction, with one late deceleration, is seen in this particular frame, which was chosen to display the obvious reactivity in response to fetal movements (FM).

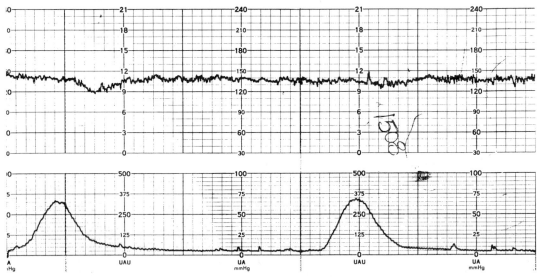

**Figure 5–5.** Positive, nonreactive CST. Recurrent late decelerations with no reactivity. This fetus has a high likelihood of intrapartum distress and an increased possibility of neonatal morbidity.

include extreme obesity, hydramnios, and a very active fetus. The effect of these factors can be reduced if the examiner remains with the patient and monitors the tracing. Uncommonly, an adequate contraction frequency may not be obtainable, and such a CST is also classified as unsatisfactory. This latter type of unsatisfactory result seems limited to those tests stimulated by exogenous oxytocin; our experience to date with the CST by intermittent nipple stimulation is that adequate uterine activity can be achieved in nearly all cases (Huddleston et al, 1984), the rare exceptions being those women with previous reductive mammoplasties that resulted in insensate nipples. Most gravidas with equivocal CSTs will, on follow-up testing within 24 hours, readily achieve an adequate frequency of contractions.

## THE NONSTRESS TEST

### NST Methodology

The NST is conducted much the same as the CST, except that there is no need for a means to elicit uterine contractions. The gravida is placed in the left-lateral or semi-Fowler's position, and the external fetal monitoring equipment is applied. Blood pressure is measured initially and at 10- to 15-minute intervals during testing, and any maternal hypotension is noted and corrected by changing the maternal position. Observation is made of the baseline fetal heart rate, of any spontaneous contractions occurring, and of any decelerations (most commonly of the variable type) evident on the monitor strip. Not infrequently, the gravida undergoing an NST is spontaneously contracting at a frequency sufficient to give a bonus: the added reassurance of a negative CST. Fetal movements are annotated on the monitor strip, either through a marker pressed by the patient or by writing "FM" on the strip. Fetal movements usually are manifested as a spike on the tocotransducer tracing and are generally audible over the monitor's speaker. Some gravidas in late pregnancy are unaware of any but the strongest fetal movement. However, it is not necessary for test interpretation to define these movements.

Because sleep and rest cycles are considered to occur at 20-minute intervals (Evertson et al, 1979), the sleeping fetus may be encountered during an NST. Usually, gentle manipulation of the fetus by the mother or the nurse or an external stimulus such as loud noise (Read and Miller, 1977) awakens the healthy but sleeping fetus and elicits fetal movements with reactivity. Such fetal stimulation generally serves to differentiate between a sleeping fetus and a fetus that is hypoactive because of reduced uteroplacental exchange.

Some institutions are using vibratory

acoustic stimulation to awaken the baby in utero. This response is similar to the startle reflex, which is seen in the newborn (Divon, 1985; Gagnon, 1986). Smith (1988) demonstrated that not only was the test shorter, but that there were fewer false nonreactive tests.

To use the acoustic stimulator, place the stimulator over the fetal vertex and evoke a sound pulse for 1 second. If there is no response after 1 minute, the 1-second sound pulse with a 1-minute interval can be repeated twice. Care should be taken not to overstimulate the fetus by pulsing too often. The reflex will stop even in a healthy baby. This is called habituation.

## NST Interpretations

Disturbances of autonomic influences on the fetal heart rate—and thus fetal metabolic health—can be evaluated through heart rate patterns of beat-to-beat variability and accelerations associated with fetal movements. With chronic suboptimal oxygenation, both a reduction of heart rate reactivity and a flattening of normal beat-to-beat variability are exhibited. The latter assessment is generally valid only during the intrapartum period, when the fetal heart rate is derived from a scalp electrode. Evaluation of apparent beat-to-beat variability is often misleading with external Doppler transducers. Therefore, interpretation of the

antepartum NST is based on the grosser changes of heart rate reactivity, which are of sufficient magnitude and duration so as not to be confused with the smaller heart rate changes (beat-to-beat variability), which may be spurious. This reactivity implies that, at the time of testing, the fetus (from an acid-base perspective) is metabolically normal (Parer, 1976; Resnik et al, 1982).

**Reactive.** The NST is defined as reactive when there are accelerations of the fetal heart rate of at least 15 beats/min and lasting at least 15 seconds at that rate (Fig. 5–6). Much has been published concerning the number of heart rate accelerations within a certain time frame required to justify a designation of reactive (Evertson et al, 1979; Mendenhall et al, 1980; Resnik et al, 1982). We have considered that two accelerations meeting the above-mentioned criteria within a 20-minute period suffice as a reactive test (ACOG, 1987; Resnik et al, 1982). Fetal movements may occur (a) spontaneously, (b) following abdominal palpation, (c) in response to spontaneous contractions, or (d) as a result of sonic stimulation (Read and Miller, 1977) or ingestion of fruit juice. A reactive NST, without variable decelerations, using whatever criteria one elects for the required number of accelerations, is a good predictor of fetal well-being for 1 week (unless severe clinical decompensation occurs) (Resnik et al, 1982). Some researchers are advocating testing twice a week for insulin-dependent dia-

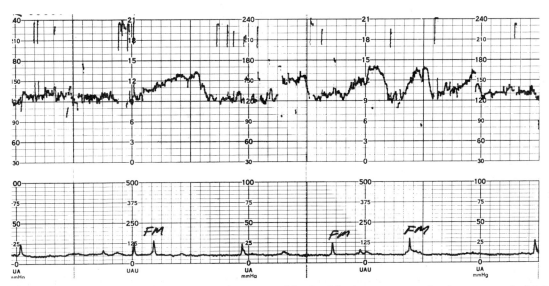

**Figure 5–6.** Reactive NST. Impressive accelerations of the fetal heart rate, occurring in response to fetal movements (FM).

betics, gestational diabetics with a previous stillborn, cases of postdatism, or IUGR. However, if variable decelerations are present (Fig. 5–7), one should suspect oligohydramnios, and further evaluation (generally ultrasound and a CST) should be pursued (Freeman et al, 1983).

**Nonreactive.** If the criteria for reactivity are not met, the NST is termed nonreactive. It must be ascertained, however, whether fetal sleep or a sedative drug (including ones that may have been obtained illicitly) may have been responsible for the nonreactivity. In such cases, prolonging the NST for an additional 20 minutes may provide a reactive test (Evertson et al, 1979; Resnik et al, 1982). Because a nonreactive NST in and of itself provides little or no useful information as to fetal well-being, a CST (or biophysical profile) should then be performed to provide a definitive answer. At the time of the CST, achieved either by intravenous oxytocin or through intermittent nipple stimulation, the fetus may begin to stir and the tracing may become reactive. In these cases, it is not necessary to continue with oxytocin delivery or nipple stimulation, unless there is some other clinical indication for the CST besides the transiently nonreactive NST.

Keegan and coworkers (1980) found that if the nonreactive NST was repeated later in the day, 98 percent of those tests became reactive. Therefore, some hospitals are now repeating the NST the same day before proceeding with further testing.

**Sinusoidal.** Sinusoidal patterns (Fig. 5–8) are seen as baseline oscillations at a frequency of 2 to 5 per minute, varying from 5 to 15 beats per minute, with an absence of heart rate reactivity (Rochard et al, 1976). Thus, the sinusoidal pattern is a variant of the nonreactive test, and the presence of good reactivity on any adjacent part of the tracing should preclude serious consideration of its being truly sinusoidal. The truly sinusoidal pattern is found usually in Rhesus-sensitized fetuses or in fetuses with severe fetomaternal bleeding; this pattern is rare, and it is an ominous sign (Modanlou et al, 1977; Rochard et al, 1976).

## PATIENT EDUCATION AND CONSIDERATIONS FOR THE NST/CST

Prior to initiating NST/CST testing, the procedure is fully explained to the patient and the support person by a member of the high-risk team. In some hospitals a consent form, which covers a single test or a series of tests, is signed before testing (Table 5–2). A thorough explanation of the reasons for and methods of testing is essential and helps

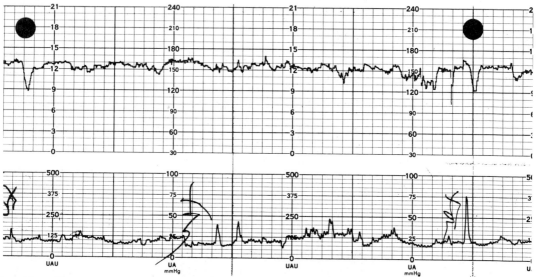

**Figure 5–7.** Nonreactive NST with variable decelerations. The fetus is moving (FM), but no accelerations meeting the criterion of 15 beats/min for 15 sec are seen. Several variable decelerations (dots) suggest vulnerability of the umbilical cord, most commonly due to oligohydramnios.

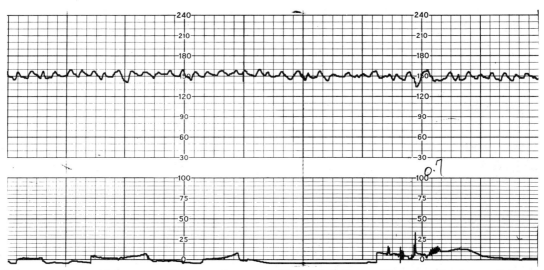

**Figure 5–8.** Sinusoidal pattern. Narrow, sine-wave–like undulations with no heart rate reactivity. An ominous tracing, most likely indicative of severe fetal anemia.

prevent most anxieties otherwise common in these patients. Testing on a weekly basis (or more often if required) is necessary for most women until delivery. These rare exceptions, for which testing is not repeated, include gravidas whose complaint is decreased fetal movement and whose initial test is normal (as long as fetal movements continue), and those few patients who no longer have an indication for testing. The majority of these are patients who on initial testing were considered to have exhibited signs of fetal growth retardation but for whom subsequent, careful ultrasonic assessment has shown no evidence of this problem.

The anticipated time requirement for testing should be explained and, when feasible, testing should be scheduled on the same day as the patient's medical appointment. When the test precedes the office visit, the practitioner can have the available results when the patient is examined. This coordination helps alleviate problems such as transportation and is especially appreciated by those women who might be working or who have small children at home. Some fetuses seem to be active at particular times of the day. If the mother notes that the fetus is active in the morning, it would be best to schedule her appointment for that time, in order to facilitate testing. Patients are encouraged to eat prior to testing, because this promotes greater activity by the fetus (Miller et al, 1978).

A well-informed patient is a more cooperative and willing patient for testing. Decreasing maternal anxiety by emphasizing that testing is not painful and that very few tests are abnormal is useful and will also help alleviate the problem of "no-shows" or cancellations. It is also possible that allaying fears might even reduce chances for a positive test result. Patients should be encouraged to participate in the testing by pushing the button to mark fetal movement, or verbally indicating when fetal movement has occurred. Because all of these mothers have been labeled high risk, most are relieved when the test indicates fetal well-being. Involving the mother in the testing also helps decrease the number of missed appointments. Patients may resume their previous level of activity immediately following testing.

Testing of multiple gestations can be accomplished by performing separate testing on each fetus, making certain that different heart rate baselines are distinguishable. With some multiple gestations, two recordings can be detected at the same time, which can shorten the duration of the test. However, the two ultrasound signals may interfere with each other, making the test difficult. Newer monitors now have external capabilities that do not interfere with each other, so that the test can be done with one monitor.

Because antepartum fetal heart rate testing usually takes a minimum of 10 to 15 minutes and may take as long as an hour or

**Table 5–2**
INFORMED CONSENT FOR NST AND CST

Because my pregnancy is complicated, it has been recommended that I have periodic evaluations of my baby's heartbeat (NST and/or CST) during the rest of my pregnancy. I understand that this will be done by placing small, painless, and (as far as is known) harmless devices on my abdomen to pick up the heartbeat and any of my baby's body movements (NST), as well as to pick up any contractions. I also understand that, because of my particular complication or because the NST may not be able to give a definite answer, I may be asked to rub one of my nipples, which will cause me to have a few contractions (CST). This has not been found to cause premature labor. I further understand that the response of the heartbeat, either to the baby's movements or to contractions, will determine whether the test is normal: (1) if normal (which most are), this is reassuring, but the test must be repeated every 7 days; (2) if slightly abnormal, the test will have to be repeated in a day or so; (3) if quite abnormal (which very few tests are), this will indicate that my baby may be in serious trouble and that I may need to be hospitalized for further tests or delivery.

It has been explained to me that these procedures have been performed thousands of times, both here and at other hospitals, and no ill effects on the baby have been related to the procedures.

I understand the above statements; I have been given the opportunity to ask questions, and the answers to my questions (if any) have been satisfactory. By signing this permit, I hereby agree to have these tests (NST and/or CST) performed for the remainder of my pregnancy.

Witness _____
Date _____

Signature _____
Date _____

so, it is an excellent time to educate the patient about what to expect during the prenatal period, labor and delivery, and the postpartum period. Not only is education easily accomplished during the testing period, but the rapport it develops offers an excellent opportunity for counseling. Therefore, the nurses performing the NST/CST testing are an integral part of the team, because they can provide much education, patient information, and counseling.

Inpatient testing is performed in the same manner as outpatient testing. However, although the NST has been performed in the office setting, most CST tests have been performed in the hospital setting or in offices adjacent to the hospital owing to the administration of intravenous oxytocin.

The cost of NST/CST testing probably varies from facility to facility, with the CST cost being slightly higher, especially if oxytocin is used. Factors included in determining cost are the expenses of intravenous supplies (this is not needed for the NST and is the reason for its lower cost), the time required for testing, and the time of a nurse specialist and his or her medical backup. In addition, equivocal tests need to be repeated until a definitive test result can be obtained. Most insurance carriers defray at least part of the expense involved in NSTs/CSTs.

## Biophysical Profile*

The biophysical profile is another test developed to help discriminate between fetuses that are well and those that are in distress (Manning et al, 1980). This test considers variables that reflect immediate fetal condition (heart rate reactivity, body movements, breathing, and tone) and a variable that reflects fetal condition over a longer time span (qualitative amniotic fluid volume). Prospective studies have suggested that observing a combination of biophysical variables may improve predictive accuracy over any one single variable (Baskett et al, 1987; Vintzileos and Campbell, 1989).

The biophysical profile is based on five observations. The first is the presence of reactivity by the NST, as has been described. The other four, which are diagnosed by ultrasound, are the presence of gross body movements (three discrete body/limb movements in 30 minutes); the presence of fetal breathing movements (at least one episode of 30 seconds of continual breathing in 30 minutes); the observation of good fetal tone (one extension/flexion cycle of a fetal limb with rapid return to the flexed posture in 30 minutes); and the presence of a normal amount of amniotic fluid (the presence of a pocket of fluid that is greater than 2 cm in two perpendicular planes).

Each parameter receives 2 points if normal and 0 points if abnormal; the maximal best score is 10, and the worst score is 0. Scores of 8 to 10 are considered reassuring, and testing can be repeated in a week unless fetal or maternal circumstances change. A score of 6

_____

* See also Chapter 6.

is considered equivocal and requires that testing be repeated within 24 hours. Scores of 2 or 4 are abnormal and indicate immediate evaluation for delivery. A score of 0 is considered a grave perinatal emergency, and delivery is recommended, provided there is some expectation for extrauterine survival (Manning et al, 1987). A 0 value for amniotic fluid volume generally heightens concern, regardless of other findings, provided the membranes are intact.

Of the major biophysical profile studies reported, the corrected perinatal mortality rate (exclusive of anomalous fetuses) has ranged from 1.9/1000 (Manning et al, 1985) to 26.6/1000 (Vintzileos and Campbell, 1987). In combining the studies of Baskett and colleagues (1987) and Manning and colleagues (1987), 16 stillbirths of structurally normal fetuses were observed among 23,396 patients when the last score prior to delivery was normal. This represents a false-negative rate of 0.68 per 1000, which compares favorably with that of the CST (Freeman et al, 1982).

The biophysical profile appears to offer the advantage of grading various degrees of fetal compromise. However, a theoretical concern with this profile is that it might not be as predictive of uteroplacental reserve as a test requiring a fetal stress, as does the CST. A study comparing the relative efficacies of the biophysical profile and the CST has not been reported.

A major advantage of the biophysical profile (apart from the actual biophysical assessment) is that, during real-time ultrasound examination, additional information may be gathered (e.g., fetal morphometrics and fetal anomaly screening).

## PATIENT EDUCATION AND CONSIDERATIONS

Most of the ultrasound components of the biophysical profile can be completed within 30 minutes. It is important to make the mother comfortable during that part of the examination. Education of the mother and her support person regarding the test is important. Educational materials should be presented to the couple prior to the test to prepare them for it. Photographs of other ultrasonic scans may help with the explanation. An explanation that the procedure is not painful is also helpful.

# Biochemical Fetal Evaluation

Biochemical assays of estriol and human placental lactogen (hPL) are now rarely used in assessing fetal well-being and placental function. The most common situation for current use of these tests is when the fetal monitoring test results are nonreassuring and the pregnancy is preterm. Even for those physicians occasionally ordering estriol or hPL assays, fetal monitoring tests are generally performed concurrently. The serum or plasma concentrations of both hormones increase as pregnancy progresses, and sharp or progressive decreases in concentration may indicate fetal jeopardy. Serial sampling, therefore, is essential for determining sequential changes and assessing fetal well-being. Estriol values correlate with fetal weight in the third trimester, and increasing hPL values parallel increasing placental mass.

## MATERNAL ESTRIOL MEASUREMENT

Production of the steroid hormone estriol by the placenta is dependent on proper functioning of the fetal adrenal gland and liver, and the amount produced is influenced by several factors. Length of gestation, multiple gestation, fetal and placental size, certain drugs (particularly glucocorticoids), maternal activity, maternal renal function, and glycosuria may affect either urinary or serum estriol levels and must be considered when interpreting values. In addition, maternal disease may affect test results. Low values from assays in a diabetic gravida are generally more ominous than low values in a hypertensive patient. A single assay is essentially worthless in terms of determining fetal condition, unless the value is so low as to indicate that fetal demise is imminent. Either urinary or plasma radioimmunoassays should be performed 2 to 3 times weekly, so that any impending fetal disaster may be determined and delivery affected if indicated. Any sharp (50 to 60 percent less than preceding value) or progressive decrease in serial values is suggestive of fetal jeopardy. The normal range of daily estriol excretion at term is from 10 to 30 mg, and the range for plasma estriol is 9 to 22 $\mu$g/dl. Results of 24-hour urinary estriol excretion are generally available in about 12 hours, and measurement of blood estriol levels may be returned within approximately 1 hour (Green and Touchstone, 1963; Kochenour, 1982).

## HUMAN PLACENTAL LACTOGEN LEVELS

A single-chain protein hormone, hPL, is released by the cytotrophoblast into the maternal circulation, where it can be detected as early as 20 to 40 days after implantation. Production slowly increases until 37 weeks' gestation, after which it remains the same or decreases slightly. By 42 weeks' gestation, an impressive decrease is seen (Zlatnik et al, 1979). As a result of associated increases in placental volume, higher hPL values are seen in multiple gestation, erythroblastosis, and poorly controlled diabetes. With these conditions, prediction of fetal well-being by hPL seems to be particularly inaccurate (Varner and Hauser, 1982). Conversely, lower values have been reported by some in pregnancies complicated both by fetal growth retardation and maternal hypertension. Radioimmunoassays for hPL generally are performed weekly, and the range for normal maternal serum values near term is 5.4 to 7.0 $\mu g/ml$. Values lower than 4 $\mu g/ml$ may represent fetal compromise after 30 weeks' gestation, and consistently low values may be as ominous as decreasing values (Spellacy, 1973). It has been suggested that hPL radioimmunoassays be performed serially on specific high-risk pregnancies as an adjunct to other fetal surveillance methods.

## INDICATIONS FOR ESTRIOL AND hPL RADIOIMMUNOASSAYS

Some fetuses at risk for uteroplacental insufficiency may be candidates for estriol and/or hPL radioimmunoassays. Both estriol and hPL assays have been claimed to be helpful in identifying possible postmaturity in postdate pregnancies if values are low, and both may be of some benefit in the management of hypertensive disorders of pregnancy. However, doubt has been cast over the value of hPL in predicting postmaturity (Berkowitz and Hobbins, 1977). Estriol assays may be beneficial for fetal surveillance when

maternal diabetes is present; hPL assays, however, have been reported to be of limited value in the management of this disorder (Spellacy, 1973). The diagnosis of fetal growth retardation may be suspected from hPL determinations but probably not as readily from serum assays for estriol. Moreover, neither assay has been shown to be of great benefit in the management of Rh isoimmunization. *Although these fetal surveillance methods are still practiced in a very few obstetric centers, there has been a progressive decrease in their clinical use over the last decade.*

## PATIENT EDUCATION AND CONSIDERATIONS

Because serial estriol assays must be performed 2 to 3 times weekly for reasonable surveillance of fetal well-being, a patient must be sufficiently motivated and concerned with her pregnancy to undertake the 24-hour urine collections and/or blood samplings that are required several times weekly (Kochenour, 1982). Patients who have transportation problems, who are working, or who do not have the money to cover the cost of serial assays will probably be unwilling or find it impossible to comply with this testing. Furthermore, outpatient management might be difficult for even the most compliant patient. Other factors that might affect the accuracy of results are the collection of an accurate 24-hour urine specimen, variations in fluid intake, the amount of bed rest, concurrent drug administration, and renal function. Although serial plasma assays would certainly be less time consuming for the gravida, blood sampling must still be done 2 to 3 times weekly (daily for diabetics) (Goebelsmann et al, 1973) for any impending disastrous changes to be appreciated and intervention effected. However, hPL measurements may require only weekly blood sampling but may not be as helpful.

Inpatient management results in more accurate outcomes for the 24-hour urine collections for estriol excretion assays and provides more control over factors such as fluid intake and bed rest. Problems with transportation to and from the clinic or office and working schedules are eliminated when the gravida is treated as an inpatient. Cost, however, is increased and, unless a patient's insurance coverage is excellent, could prove a financial burden for the patient and her family. Also, child care expenses and loss of wages, if the mother works, would further increase the burden. Therefore, management should be accomplished in the outpatient setting if at all possible. Motivation and reliability of the patient can effect accurate and therefore beneficial test results. Also, thorough patient education on collection of a 24-hour urine sample is essential. If, however, adequate teaching fails, or if the patient is unreliable or noncompliant, another means for assessing fetal well-being should be considered, rather than resorting to hospitalization. Even noncompliant and unreliable patients might be most willing to have weekly or even twice-weekly NSTs or CSTs for fetal surveillance, especially if these tests are performed on the same day as their medical appointment.

Approximately 15 percent of pregnancies in a referral center have indications that place them at risk for uteroplacental insufficiency, and antepartum fetal surveillance methods play an important role in the obstetric management of these women. Biophysical testing of the fetal heart rate is the most common method used, and the use of the biophysical profile is gaining acceptance. Biochemical fetal evaluations, when performed serially, may be of benefit in differentiating between the fetuses tolerating their environments well or poorly. However, biochemical testing has been virtually abandoned.

Biophysical fetal evaluations, especially of the fetal heart rate, have achieved the most widespread acceptance for antepartum fetal surveillance. These tests of the fetal heart rate can identify accurately, within these high-risk pregnancies, those fetuses (with negative CSTs and/or reactive NSTs) tolerating their intrauterine environments acceptably, and these normal tests usually need be repeated only weekly. Biophysical profile testing is used adjunctively in most centers. These reassuring tests are of great comfort to both the patient and the clinician, and test results are available immediately. Those few fetuses whose test results are abnormal and who are in possible jeopardy can be identified immediately, and corrective measures can be undertaken. Moreover, a policy of nonintervention can be followed in approximately 95 percent of these high-risk pregnancies undergoing fetal heart rate test-

ing, as only a small percentage (those with positive CSTs or low biophysical profile scores) will be at serious risk for impending disaster (Huddleston and Freeman, 1982).

## References and Recommended Reading

ACOG Technical Bulletin #107: Antepartum fetal surveillance. Washington, DC, American College of Obstetricians and Gynecologists, 1987.

Aubry RA, Pennington JC: Identification and evaluation of high-risk pregnancy: the perinatal concept. Clin Obstet Gynecol 16:3, 1973.

Baskett TF, Allen AC, Gray JH, et al: Fetal biophysical profile score in perinatal death. Obstet Gynecol 70:357, 1987.

Berkowitz RL, Hobbins JC: A reevaluation of the value of hCS determination in the management of prolonged pregnancy. Obstet Gynecol 49:156, 1977.

Bishop EH: Pelvic scoring for elective induction. Obstet Gynecol 24:266, 1964.

Braly P, Freeman RK: The significance of fetal heart rate reactivity with a positive oxytocin challenge test. Obstet Gynecol 50:689, 1977.

Braly PS, Freeman RK, Garite T, et al: Incidence of premature delivery following the oxytocin challenge test. Am J Obstet Gynecol 141:5, 1981.

Bruce SL, Petrie RH, Yeh SY: The suspicious contraction stress test. Obstet Gynecol 51:415, 1978.

Clark SL, Gimovsky ML, Miller FC: The scalp stimulation test: a clinical alternative to fetal scalp blood sampling. Am J Obstet Gynecol 148(3):274, 1984.

Clark SL, Gimovsky ML, Miller FC: Fetal heart rate response to scalp blood sampling. Am J Obstet Gynecol 15; 144(6):706, 1982.

Clark SL, Paul RH: Intrapartum fetal surveillance: the role of fetal scalp blood sampling. Am J Obstet Gynecol 1; 153(7):717, 1985.

Cobo E: Neuroendocrine control of milk injection in women. In Josimovich JF, Reynolds M, Cobo E (eds): Lactogenic Hormones, Fetal Nutrition, and Lactation. New York, John Wiley & Sons, 1974, p 433.

Dauphinee JD: Antepartum Testing: A challenge for nursing. J Perinatal Neonatal Nurs 1(1):29–48, 1987.

Divon MY, Platt LD, Cantrell CJ, et al: Evoked fetal startle response: a possible intrauterine neurological examination. Am J Obstet Gynecol 153(4):454, 1985.

Evertson LR, Gauthier RJ, Schifrin BS, et al: Antepartum fetal heart rate testing. I. Evolution of the nonstress test. Am J Obstet Gynecol 133:29, 1979.

Freeman RK: The use of the oxytocin challenge test for antepartum clinical evaluation of uteroplacental respiratory function. Am J Obstet Gynecol 121:481, 1975.

Freeman RK: Contraction stress testing for primary fetal surveillance in patients at high risk for uteroplacental insufficiency. Clin Perinatol 9:265, 1982.

Freeman RK, Anderson G, Dorchester W: A prospective multi-institutional study of antepartum fetal heart rate monitoring. I. Risk of perinatal mortality and morbidity according to antepartum fetal heart rate test results. Am J Obstet Gynecol 143:771, 1982.

Freeman RK, Anderson G, Dorchester W: A prospective multi-institutional study of antepartum fetal heart rate monitoring. II. Contraction stress test versus nonstress test for primary surveillance. Am J Obstet Gynecol 143:778, 1982.

Freeman RK, Goebelsmann U, Nochimson D, et al: An evaluation of the significance of a positive oxytocin challenge test. Obstet Gynecol 47:8, 1976.

Freeman RK, Huddleston JF, Petrie RH, et al: Ensuring optimum outcome for postdate pregnancy. Contemp Ob/Gyn 22(6):187, 1983.

Gabbe SG, Freeman RK, Goebelsmann U: Evaluation of the contraction stress test before 33 weeks' gestation. Obstet Gynecol 52:649, 1978.

Gagnon R, Hunse C, Carmichael L, et al: External vibratory acoustic stimulation near term: fetal heart rate and heart rate variability responses. Am J Obstet Gynecol 156(2):323, 1987.

Gagnon R, Patrick J, Foreman J, West R: Stimulation of human fetuses with sound and vibration. Am J Obstet Gynecol 155(4):848, 1986.

Goebelsmann U, Freeman RK, Mestman H, et al: Estriol in pregnancy. II. Daily urinary estriol assays in the management of the pregnant diabetic woman. Am J Obstet Gynecol 115:795, 1973.

Goodwin JW, Dunne JT, and Thomas BW: Antepartum identification of the fetus at risk. Can Med Assoc J 101:458, 1969.

Green JW, Jr, Touchstone JC: Urinary estriol as an index of placental function. Am J Obstet Gynecol 85:1, 1963.

Harvey CJ: Fetal scalp stimulation: enhancing the interpretation of fetal monitoring tracings. Perinatal Neonatal Nursing 1(1):13, 1987.

Hoebel CH, Hyvarinen MA, Okada DM, et al: Prenatal and intrapartum high-risk screening. I. Prediction of the high-risk neonate. Am J Obstet Gynecol 117:1, 1973.

Huddleston JF, Sutliff G, Carney FE, Jr, et al: Oxytocin challenge test for antepartum fetal assessment: report of a clinical experience. Am J Obstet Gynecol 135:609, 1979.

Huddleston JF, Freeman RK: Assessment of fetal well-being by antepartum fetal heart rate testing. In Bolognese RJ, Schwarz RH, Schneider J (eds): Perinatal Medicine: Management of the High Risk Fetus and Neonate, 2nd ed. Baltimore, Williams & Wilkins, 1982, p 129.

Huddleston JF, Sutliff G, Robinson D: Contraction stress test by intermittent nipple stimulation. Obstet Gynecol 63:669, 1984.

Ingemarsson I, Arulkumaran S, Paul RH, et al: Fetal acoustic stimulation in early labor in patients screened with the admission test. Am J Obstet Gynecol 158(1):70, 1988.

Keegan KA, Paul RH, Broussard PM, et al: Antepartum fetal heart rate testing. V. The nonstress test—An outpatient approach. Am J Obstet Gynecol 136:81, 1980.

Kochenour NK: Estrogen assay during pregnancy. Clin Obstet Gynecol 25:659, 1982.

Liggins GC, Howie RN: A controlled trial of antepartum glucocorticoid treatment for prevention of the respiratory distress syndrome in premature infants. Pediatrics 50:515, 1972.

Manning FA, Harmon CR, Morrison I, et al: Fetal assessment based on fetal biophysical profile scoring. III. Positive predictive accuracy of the very abnormal test (biophysical profile score = 0). Am J Obstet Gynecol 162:398, 1990.

Manning FA, Morrison I, Harman CR, et al: Fetal assessment by fetal biophysical profile scoring: experience in 19,221 referred high-risk pregnancies. II. The false-negative rate by frequency and etiology. Am J Obstet Gynecol 157:880, 1987.

Manning FA, Morrison I, Lange I, et al: Fetal assessment based upon fetal biophysical profile scoring; experience in 12,620 high-risk pregnancies. I. Perinatal mortality by frequency and etiology. Am J Obstet Gynecol 151:343, 1985.

Manning FA, Platt LD, Sipos L: Antepartum fetal evaluation: development of a fetal biophysical profile. Am J Obstet Gynecol 136:787, 1980.

Martin CB Jr: Regulation of the fetal heart rate and genesis of FHR patterns. Semin Perinatol 2:131, 1978.

Martin CB Jr, Schifrin BS: Prenatal monitoring. In Aladjem S, Brown AK (eds): Perinatal Intensive Care. St Louis, CV Mosby Co, 1977, p 155.

Mendenhall HW, O'Leary JA, Phillips KO: The nonstress test: the value of a single acceleration in evaluating the fetus at risk. Am J Obstet Gynecol 136:87, 1980.

Miller FC, Skiba H, Klapholz H: The effect of maternal blood sugar levels on fetal activity. Obstet Gynecol 52:662, 1978.

Modanlou HD, Freeman RK, Ortiz O, et al: Sinusoidal FHR pattern and severe anemia. Obstet Gynecol 49:537, 1977.

Murata Y, Martin CB Jr, Ikenoue T, et al: Fetal heart rate accelerations during the course of intrauterine death in chronically catheterized rhesus monkeys. Am J Obstet Gynecol 144:218, 1982.

Myers RE, Mueller-Heubach E, Adamsons K: Predictability of the state of fetal oxygenation from the quantitative analysis of the components of late deceleration. Am J Obstet Gynecol 115:1083, 1973.

Parer JT: Normal and impaired placental exchange. Contemp Ob/Gyn 7(2):117, 1976.

Platt LD, Eglinton GS, Sipos L, et al: Further experience with the fetal biophysical profile. Obstet Gynecol 61:480, 1983.

Pose SV, Castillo JB, Nora-Rojas EO, et al: Test of fetal tolerance to induced uterine contractions for the diagnosis of chronic distress. In Perinatal Factors Affecting Human Development. Washington, DC, Pan American Health Organization, 1969, p 96.

Poseiro JJ, Mendez-Bauer C, Pose SV, et al: Effect of uterine contractions on maternal blood flow through the placenta. In Perinatal Factors Affecting Human Development. Washington, DC, Pan American Health Organization, 1969, p 161.

Ray M, Freeman RK, Pine S, et al: Clinical experience with the oxytocin challenge test. Am J Obstet Gynecol 114:1, 1972.

Read JA, Miller FC: Fetal heart rate acceleration in response to acoustic stimulation as a measure of fetal well-being. Am J Obstet Gynecol 129:512, 1977.

Resnik R, Huddleston JF, Freeman RK, et al: NST or CST? What's best for spotting the high-risk fetus? Contemp Ob/Gyn 19(4):92, 1982.

Richards DS: Determinants of fetal heart rate response to vibroacoustic stimulation in labor. Obstet Gynecol 71(4):535, 1988.

Rochard F, Schifrin BS, Goupil F, et al: Nonstressed fetal heart rate monitoring in the antepartum period. Am J Obstet Gynecol 126:699, 1976.

Schifrin BS: Antepartum fetal heart rate monitoring. In Gluck L (ed): Intrauterine Asphyxia and the Developing Fetal Brain. Chicago, Yearbook, 1977, p 205.

Scott DB, Kerr MG: Inferior vena caval pressure in late pregnancy. J Obstet Gynaecol Br Commonw 70:1044, 1963.

Smith CV: Intrapartum assessment of fetal well-being:

a comparison of fetal acoustic stimulation with acid-base determinations. Am J Obstet Gynecol 155(4):726, 1986.

Smith CV, Phelan JP, Broussard P, Paul RH: Fetal acoustic stimulation testing. III. Predictive value of a reactive test. J Reprod Med 33(2):217, 1988.

Smith CV, Phelan JP, Platt LD, et al: Fetal acoustic stimulation testing. II. A randomized clinical comparison with the nonstress test. Am J Obstet Gynecol 155(1):131, 1986.

Spellacy WN: Human placental lactogen in high-risk pregnancy. Clin Obstet Gynecol 16:298, 1973.

Varner MW, Hauser KS: Human placental lactogen and other placental hormones as indicators of fetal well-being. Clin Obstet Gynecol 25:673, 1982.

Vintzileos AM, Campbell WA: Fetal biophysical profile scoring: Current status. Clin Perinatol 16:661, 1989.

Zlatnik FJ, Varner MW, Hauser KS: HPL: physiologic and pathophysiologic observations. Obstet Gynecol 54:314, 1979.

# CHAPTER 6

# Ultrasound In Pregnancy

Jean Claude Veille, Marty Deviney, and Regina Hanson

Ultrasound, first used as a sonar device during World War I to detect enemy submarines, is the preferred method in obstetrics for imaging the fetus. Ultrasound is composed of short bursts of high-frequency sound waves transmitted into the body. The transmitted waves are reflected by body tissues and processed electronically to form an image on a monitor. Ultrasound has become one of the most important technologies in modern obstetrics.

## Definition

Sounds that are audible to the human ears are in the frequency of 16 to 20,000 cycles per second or hertz ($H_z$). Ultrasound has a frequency of 1 to 20 million cycles per second (1 to 20 megahertz [MHz]). These sounds are undetectable by the human ear. The frequency of ultrasounds used for diagnostic purposes in obstetrics is between 1 and 5 MHz. These high-frequency ultrasounds are obtained by using an alternating current on a piezoelectric crystal. The net result is the production of high-frequency waves. This mechanical energy is then transmitted to a part of the human body as high-frequency sounds, which bounce off tissues and reflect back to the piezoelectric crystal. These signals are integrated and displayed on the oscilloscope (Kremkau, 1989). Finally, all of the points are translated into images (Safety standard for diagnostic ultrasound equipment, 1983). Factors that are implicated in ultrasound are frequency of sound, the wave length of sound, the propagation speed (i.e.,

speed with which a wave moves through a medium), and the amplitude and intensity of the wave (Kremkau, 1989).

## FACTORS INFLUENCING ULTRASOUND EXAMINATION

Impedance is the product of the density of the tissue studied and the velocity at which the sound travels in this tissue. The greater the density or the stiffness of the tissue, the greater its impedance. By the same token, the greater the propagation speed of the sound, the greater the impedance. Gas-containing bowel has a low propagation speed, whereas it is higher in lungs (made of solid and gas). Even though the density of the tissue is the major determinant of the acoustic impedance in the human body, sound velocity in the tissue studied also seems to influence the quality of the ultrasound. The elasticity of the tissue also influences the velocity of the sounds and thus the quality of the images (Smith, 1977).

## TYPES OF ULTRASOUND EQUIPMENT

There are two main types of ultrasound equipment: static and real time.

Static scanners (grey scale contact scanners) produce a series of static images as the ultrasounds make contact back and forth with the mother's abdomen.

Real-time scanners (sector or linear-array scanners), depending on the sweep of the ultrasounds that are emitted, are either sectorial (pie-shaped) or linear (rectangular in shape). Both of these transducers produce two-dimensional images of the examined area automatically and continually. The linear or curvilinear array is best for pregnancies in the second or third trimesters because of the size of the abdomen at this time. The sector transducer is small and thus can cover a smaller area of the abdomen. Its use is preferred to evaluate the lateral walls of the pelvis (to find follicles or small tumors) or for the uterus in early pregnancy.

## SAFETY OF ULTRASOUND

No clinically significant adverse side effects have been reported in humans. Ultrasounds have been considered safe when used at the intensities currently used for diagnosis. Biologic effects from ultrasounds have been experimentally observed. Theoretic risks include absorption heating, cavitation, and microstreaming.

**Heat.** The most straightforward and best understood mechanism of action of ultrasound on biological systems is temperature rise due to absorption of sound in the medium. The temperature rise depends on the heat generated (ultrasound intensity) (Gross et al, 1986). The diagnostic ultrasound instruments used at present in obstetrics do not produce a significant temperature rise in tissue. This led most authorities in the field to conclude that "in judicious clinical utilization of calibrated ultrasonic equipment of current designs there is no danger of hyperthermic teratogenicity in man" (Kremkau, 1989).

**Cavitation.** Acoustic cavitation is the oscillation of small gaseous or vaporous bubbles subjected to the pressure variations of an acoustic wave. This includes the growth and the eventual collapse of the bubble when it reaches a certain size. The terms stable cavitation and transient cavitation have been given respectively to such phenomena. The bubble collapse associated with transient cavitation results in high temperatures and pressure gradients. Though such phenomena have been observed in plants, the occurrence of cavitation in mammalian soft tissues is not well documented even with pulsed-echo diagnostic ultrasound.

**Microstreaming.** Microstreaming is a term used to describe the flow of a liquid in a well-defined pattern in the vicinity of a nonuniformly oscillating bubble. Because it occurs only very close to the bubble, it is called microstreaming. Such flow can, in turn, produce shear forces that cause stretching, twisting, and disruption of the cells (Kremkau, 1989).

In humans, a study by Stark and associates (1984) failed to demonstrate a significant difference in conductive and nerve measurements of hearing, visual acuity and color vision, cognitive function, and complete and detailed neurologic examination between 425 children exposed to diagnostic ultrasound and 381 matched control children. It is important to realize that overexposure to anything may be deleterious to an organism, and thus, a prudent approach to ultrasound is needed; ultrasound should be used when indicated, the output of the instrument should be minimized, and the exposure time should be kept to a minimum if possible.

There are no experimental data showing that heating, cavitation, or microstreaming occur in any significant way in the human tissue under diagnostic ultrasound during an obstetric ultrasound (Kremkau, 1989).

# Indications for Obstetric Ultrasound

Routine ultrasound for all pregnant women remains controversial. Some health care professionals see pregnancy as an indication for ultrasound. Others believe that a scan is indicated only for the reasons listed in Table 6–1. Routine scanning was not advocated by a task force on ultrasounds (Consensus Conference, 1984), nor by the Section of Obstetrical and Gynecological Ultrasound of the American Institute for Ultrasound in Medicine. Three recent studies have suggested otherwise and have found some benefits of routine ultrasound screening (Rosendahl and Kivinen, 1989; Warsof et al, 1983; Warsof et al, 1986). Guidelines have been developed for antepartum obstetric ultrasound examination, as put forward by the Joint Task Force Group on Training for Diagnosis in Obstetrical and Gynecological Ultrasound (Diagnostic ultrasound imaging in pregnancy, 1984).

1. To determine fetal viability when an abortion or intrauterine demise is suspected

**Table 6–1**
INDICATIONS FOR OBSTETRIC
ULTRASOUND EXAMINATIONS

Estimation of gestational age (by multiple
    parameters)
Evaluation of fetal growth (for growth retardation or
    macrosomia)
Placental localization when vaginal bleeding occurs
Determination of fetal lie
Fetal number confirmation
Adjunct to all amniocenteses
Uterus size/clinical dates discrepancy
Estimation of fetal size in breech presentation
Suspected congenital anomaly
Pelvic masses
Suspected hydatidiform mole
Adjunct to cervical cerclage
Suspected ectopic/abdominal pregnancy
Adjunct to special procedures, such as fetoscopy and
    intrauterine transfusion
Fetal demise
Uterine pathology (e.g., leiomyoma or bicornuate
    uterus)
Postpartum evaluation of uterus and adnexae
Intrauterine contraceptive device localization
Ovarian follicle development surveillance
Evaluation of postdate pregnancy
Fetal activity studies to assess fetal well-being
Monitoring intrapartum labor and delivery events
    (e.g., version/extraction of second twin)
Evaluation of amount of amniotic fluid (when
    oligohydramnios or polyhydramnios is suspected)

2. To determine gestational age when there is a consistent discrepancy between clinical findings and the patient's data (Fig. 6–1)

3. Elevated maternal serum alphafetoprotein value; a level II ultrasound should be an integral part of any maternal serum alpha-fetoprotein (MSAFP) program

4. To locate the placenta if there is vaginal bleeding or if the fetus is in an unstable lie

5. To evaluate gestation at any stage if there is a discrepancy between uterine size and dates

6. Prior to amniocentesis or percutaneous umbilical blood sampling (PUBS)

7. To monitor fetal growth when intrauterine growth retardation is suspected

8. When multiple gestation is suspected

9. To determine fetal size in breech presentation

10. To evaluate amniotic fluid quantity

11. To rule out fetal congenital anomalies

12. To evaluate post-term pregnancy

13. As an adjunct to special procedures, such as intrauterine transfusion, chorionic villi sampling, placental aspiration, percutaneous umbilical blood sampling

14. To evaluate possible molar pregnancy

15. To evaluate pelvic masses during pregnancy

A. Equipment

- Real-time or a combination of real-time and static scanners
- Never solely a static scanner
- Transducer should be appropriate frequency (i.e., 3–5 MHz)

B. Documentation

I. Guidelines for first trimester scans record:
   a. location of the gestational sac
   b. accurate gestational age (crown-rump length and/or parietal diameter)
   c. presence or absence of fetal life
   d. number of fetuses should be reported
   e. evaluation of the uterus (including the cervix) and adnexal structures

II. Guidelines for second and third trimester scans record:
   a. fetal life, number, and presentation
   b. estimation of the amount of amniotic fluid (stage of pregnancy must be taken into account)
   c. placental location and its relationship to the internal os
   d. assessment of gestational age and growth, which should be done by a combination of biparietal diameter (or head circumference), femur length, and abdominal circumference (Table 6–2) (see Fig. 6–1).

   Biparietal diameter should be done at the level of the cavum septum pellucidum, and the thalamus and/or cerebral peduncles.

   Abdominal circumference should be at the level of the junction of the umbilical vein and portal sinus.
   e. evaluation of the uterus and adnexal structures. Any ultrasound study should also include the following fetal anatomy:
      - cerebral ventricle
      - spine, four limbs
      - stomach
      - urinary bladder
      - umbilical cord insertion site
      - kidneys
      - four-chamber heart
      - bowel

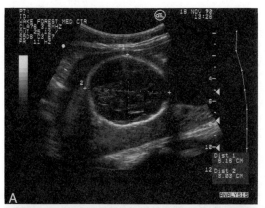

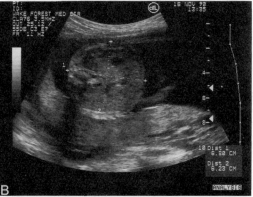

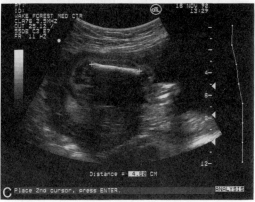

**Figure 6–1.** *A,* Typical measurements of the biparietal and occipitofrontal diameters. *B,* Biparietal diameter may be affected by fetal position and oligohydramnios. Head circumference is a better indicator of fetal head biometry than either one of the two measurements. *C,* Femur length determination. Linear scan should be used on the most proximal femur in order to avoid artifacts.

Table 6–3 lists some of the anomalies that can be detected by ultrasound.

The American Institute for Ultrasound in Medicine (Official guidelines and statements on obstetrical ultrasound, 1985) has devel-

**Table 6–2**
ROUTINE STAGE I ULTRASOUND: APPROPRIATE MEASUREMENTS AT VARIOUS GESTATIONAL AGES

| Age | Measurement |
| --- | --- |
| <12 weeks | Crown-rump length |
| | Gestational sac mean diameter |
| 12–24 weeks | Biparietal diameter |
| | Femur length |
| ≥24 weeks | Biparietal diameter |
| | Occipitofrontal diameter |
| | Anteroposterior abdominal diameter |
| | Transverse abdominal diameter |
| | Femur length |

oped Guidelines for Minimum Post Residency Training in Obstetrical and Gynecological Ultrasounds.

"It is recommended that a minimum of three months' experience in obstetrical and gynecological ultrasound or its equivalent be obtained." More specifically this should include:

1. one month of supervised and documented training in an established ultrasound facility. This should include basic physics, technique, performance, and interpretation

**Table 6–3**
COMMON REPRESENTATIVE ANOMALIES DETECTABLE WITH DIAGNOSTIC ULTRASOUND

| **CNS and Skull** | **Spine** |
| --- | --- |
| Hydrocephaly | Meningomyelocele |
| Anencephaly | Spina bifida |
| Holoprosencephaly | **Abdomen** |
| Microcephaly | Omphalocele |
| Encephalocele | Gastroschisis |
| Arachnoid cysts | Atresias of bowel |
| Vein of Galen aneurysm | Renal agenesis |
| Cystic hygroma | (unilateral or |
| Craniosynostosis | bilateral) |
| Agenesis of corpus | Ascites |
| collosum | Bladder outlet |
| **Thorax** | obstruction |
| Diaphragmatic hernia | Ovarian cysts |
| Pleural effusions | Hydronephrosis |
| Pericardial effusions | Hydroureter |
| Hypoplastic heart | Persistent cloaca |
| Arrhythmias | **Limbs** |
| Teratomas | Short-limbed dwarfism |
| Esophageal atresia | Osteogenesis imperfecta |
| Ventricular septal defects | (I–IV) |
| Valvular atresias | Phocomelia |
| Congenital cystic | Thanatophoric dysplasia |
| adenomatoid | Achondroplasia |
| malformation | |
| Lung sequestration | |
| Bronchogenic cysts | |

2. at least 2 months of practical experience or its equivalent ($\geq$ 200 examinations) prior to the offering of services as a physician with competence in the use of diagnostic ultrasound

The NAACOG (1991a) recommends that before assuming expanded responsibilities in the performance of ultrasound examinations, nurses should "evaluate the scope of practice as defined by their state or area and the regulations of the licensing and accrediting bodies for the agency or institution in which they practice. Relevant issues that should be considered include the types of ultrasound examinations to be performed; educational preparation and clinical practicum under appropriate supervision needed to establish competency; and risk management, liability, and other legal issues." Competency should be validated before the nurse assumes responsibility for ultrasound examinations. "In addition, policies, procedures, and protocols must be developed that direct and guide nurses in the performance of ultrasound examinations" (NAACOG, 1991a, 1991b).

# Vaginal Ultrasound

Transvaginal ultrasound (TVS) has been a new, exciting, and progressive development in imaging. The close proximity of the probe to the pelvic structures has resulted in the ability to evaluate the pelvic anatomy in greater detail and to diagnose intrauterine pregnancy at an earlier gestational age. The frequency of the vaginal probe is in the order of 5 to 10 MHz, which accounts for the increase in the resolution (Official guidelines and statements on obstetrical ultrasound, 1985; Timor-Tritsch et al, 1988; Cullen et al, 1989).

TVS is well tolerated by most patients, because it alleviates the need for the previously required full bladder. Furthermore, it circumvents the great difficulty often encountered in obese patients because of the increased depth the ultrasounds have to travel. Depending on the indication, vaginal ultrasound can be used alone or, if an intraabdominal process is suspected, in conjunction with the transabdominal scan. In the case of suspected ectopic pregnancy, transabdominal scanning should be performed. The idea of the transvaginal probe entering the vagina may be of concern to some patients. Allowing the patient to introduce the probe may decrease her anxiety and allow a more comfortable insertion of the probe.

## INDICATIONS FOR TRANSVAGINAL ULTRASOUND

A partial list of clinical indications is tabulated below. This list will probably become obsolete as probes improve and as the image of the anatomy becomes even clearer in future years. For now, transvaginal scanning is best used for

1. Establishing early pregnancy, because fetal heart rate motion can be seen by this technique as early as the 5th to 6th week of gestation (Fig. 6–2).
2. Determining ectopic pregnancy and free fluid in the cul-de-sac and correlating that with $\beta$-hCG levels.

Nyberg correlated the levels of $\beta$-hCG and early pregnancy findings using vaginal ultrasound (Nyberg et al, 1985). A $\beta$-hCG level of greater than 1000 mIU/ml (IRP) should have a gestational sac. With a level of 7200 mIU/ml (IRP), a yolk sac should be seen. Finally, a gestational sac, an embryo, and heart activity should be imaged at a level of at least 10,800 mIU/ml. Using TVS, absence of a gestational sac with $\beta$-hCG at or greater than 1000 mIU/ml or absence of a yolk sac with a level at or greater than 7200 mIU/ml, strongly suggests the diagnosis of ectopic pregnancy (Table 6–4).

There are two methods for reporting the level of $\beta$-hCG. The first, International Reference Preparation kit measures the pure form of the hormone. The Second International Standard is not as pure a method. It is important to know which method is the standard method of reporting in one's own laboratory before comparing ultrasound findings and $\beta$-hCG levels. As a rule, the Second International Standard levels are roughly half the International Reference Preparation levels.

3. Monitoring follicular growth (size) during ovulation induction and ova retrieval (Hull et al, 1986).
4. Evaluating the abnormal pregnancy (i.e., blighted ovum, missed or incomplete abortion, pseudosac of gestation, molar pregnancy) (Nyberg et al, 1983).

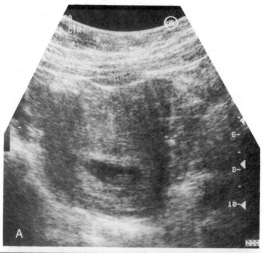

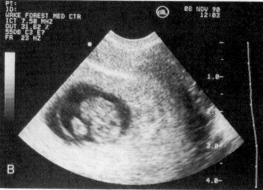

**Figure 6–2.** *A,* Abdominal ultrasound of an early pregnancy. *B,* Same patient using vaginal ultrasound. Early intrauterine pregnancy. At this stage, variability in dating pregnancy is minimal (± 2–4 days).

5. Evaluating adnexal pathology, such as tubo-ovarian abscess or hydrosalpinx (Herrmann et al, 1987).

6. Diagnosing uterine abnormalities, like fibroids, uterine malformation, or even bladder abnormalities.

7. Visualizing retained products of conception.

8. Diagnosing fetal abnormalities, placental location, or even vasa previa. TVS has been used to diagnose anencephaly at 10 weeks, hydranencephaly, omphalocele and gastroschisis as early as the 14th week of gestation (Brown et al, 1989; Bulie et al, 1987). As TVS evaluation improves, ultrasound embryography may allow for earlier detection of normal and abnormal fetal development.

9. Evaluating certain second or third trimester pregnancies as a supplement to the abdominal scan.

In certain patients, the lower uterine segment is very difficult to see, and thus, the fetal structures in this part of the uterus may be difficult to observe. Depending on the fetal presentation, TVS is very helpful in imaging the head anatomy, the lower fetal spine, and the sacrum, especially for small meningoceles and meningomyeloceles (Ayers et al, 1988; Farine et al, 1988; Benacerraf and Estroff, 1989; Hilpert and Kurtz, 1990).

The cervix can be seen with the use of the TVS when transabdominal scanning fails to give an adequate imaging of this structure.

Placental location can be difficult to ascertain using transabdominal scans; in such cases, TVS is very helpful. In order to better visualize the lower uterine segment and the cervix using TVS, the transducer should be introduced farther than the middle of the vagina.

Even in vaginal bleeding, TVS can be used carefully. As noted earlier, the vaginal probe should be inserted carefully to the middle of the vagina. Using the TVS scanning approach, the diagnosis of placenta previa or low-lying placenta can be made reliably.

**Table 6–4**

CORRELATION BETWEEN BETA hCG AND TRANSVAGINAL ULTRASOUND FINDINGS

| Beta hCG = *IRP (mIU/ml)<br>( ) = 2nd IRS | †GS | ††YS | **Embryo/Heart Beat** |
|---|---|---|---|
| <1000 (<500) | +/− | 0 | 0 |
| 1000–7200 (500–3600) | + | +/− | +/− |
| 7200–10,800 (3600–5400) | + | + | +/− |
| > 10,800 (> 5400) | + | + | + |

Adapted from Bree RL, Edward M, Bohm-Velez M, et al: Transvaginal sonography in the evaluation of normal early pregnancy: Correlation with HCG level. AJR, 153:75–79, 1989.
* International Reference Standards
† Gestational sac
†† Yolk sac

## TECHNIQUE AND ORIENTATION

The examination can be performed either with the patient in a lithotomy position, to get a free angulation of the probe, or with the patient's pelvis elevated by towels, cushions, or a folded pillow. This pelvic tilt is optimal to image the pelvic structures. An examination table with stirrups is ideal in our own setting.

Methods of probe insertion vary from one institution to the next. In a radiology department, the probe is most often inserted by the patient. If the sonographer is male, a female assistant should be present during the scan.

Water-soluble gel should be placed on the tip of the transducer to allow better sound wave transmission. A protective sheath should be placed over the transducer. A condom, a sterile glove, or any other cover should be used. The tip of the transducer should be lubricated, and then gently introduced into the vagina. Gentleness should be used during the scanning to avoid pain and trauma to the vaginal fornices. Slow withdrawal of the probe often brings the area of interest into focus.

The probe initially should be inserted with the reference point of the transducer pointing toward the symphysis pubis. This technique gives a view of the pelvic structures in the sagittal plane. Even though the patient has emptied her bladder, residual urine is almost always present. This can be used as a landmark for anatomic orientation. The long axis of the uterus should be seen. Depending on the type of probe used, manipulation of the transducer will vary. In the end-firing transducers, rotation from one plane to the next can easily be accomplished. With the off-axis or tilted transducers, rotation of the transducer has to be associated with an actual repositioning of the transducer, in order to properly see the area of interest.

The pelvic structures are observed by rotating the probe 90 degrees to one side and to the next. The adnexae can be seen by pointing the transducer to the right and to the left in either the sagittal or the coronal plane and sweeping the area to localize the ovaries. The bowel may often be mistaken for the ovaries; however, peristalsis easily differentiates the two structures.

The future of the vaginal ultrasound is an exciting one. With the use of color Doppler flow, funic (cord) presentation or vasa praevia, can now be documented. The vaginal probe can also be used in the second and third trimester to document low-lying placenta. As instrumentation becomes more refined and endovaginal scanning more cost effective, vaginal scanning will become a routine technique both in the private office and in the hospital setting.

# Ultrasound and Congenital Abnormalities

High-resolution ultrasound allows better delineation of the fetal anatomy and, as such, offers in utero diagnosis of the major congenital anomalies. Most series report an incidence of sonographically detected major abnormalities of approximately 1 percent. About one third of these anomalies are detected before the 21st week of gestation. The most frequent congenital anomalies are those of the central nervous system (CNS), the genitourinary system, the gastrointestinal tract, abdominal wall defect, diaphragmatic hernia, and musculoskeletal. Other miscellaneous abnormalities can also be observed.

**CNS.** Ventriculomegaly is the most frequently detected CNS malformation, followed by anencephaly, encephalocele, meningocele, posterior fossa abnormalities, and holoprosencephaly and hydranencephaly.

With the efficacy of maternal screening for neural tube defect with alpha-fetoprotein determination, approximately 3 percent of all screened pregnancies require further ultrasound evaluation. Spina bifida can be difficult to diagnose with ultrasound. The appearance of the cranium in the second trimester is often a clue to an open neural defect. The parietal bones of the skull are often pulled inward, giving it a lemon-like shape (Vergani et al, 1987; Nyberg et al, 1988; Filly, 1988; Gabbe et al, 1988; Nicolaides et al, 1986) (Fig. 6–3). As a rule, there is dilatation of the lateral ventricles with a downward drop of the choroid plexus as the ventriculomegaly increases. The posterior fossa is often shallower and even obliterated, resulting in the "banana" sign (see Fig. 6–3) (Benacerraf, 1985). This sign describes the appearance of the elongated cerebellum in the presence of an open tubal neural defect.

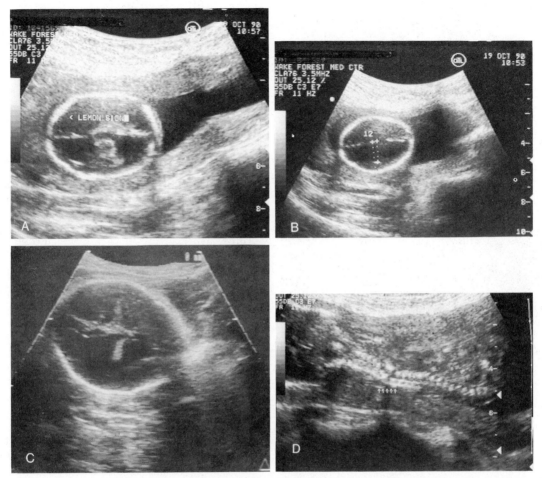

**Figure 6–3.** *A,* Scalloping of the frontal bones, associated with open tubal neural defect. "Lemon" appearance. *B,* Ventriculomegaly—increased in ventricular-hemispheric ratio (V/H). *C,* Downward displacement of the choroid plexus. The choroid angle normally should be at or less than 22 degrees with midline. *D,* Major open tubal neural defect at the level of the thoracic spine. Note the abnormal curvature of the spine due to the abnormal development of the vertebral bodies.

A careful ultrasound examination needs to be performed at all times; however, in the face of a significant elevated MSAFP, a more extensive and detailed CNS and spinal examination by experienced personnel is necessary. If the ultrasound is normal but the MSAFP is elevated, we recommend an amniocentesis, because a small sacral defect can be missed even in the most experienced hands.

**Soft Tissue Abnormalities.** Nuchal edema has been reported to be associated with chromosome abnormality, especially trisomies 21 and 13. The edema takes on the appearance of a posterior cystic mass, often divided by a septum in the detection of open tubal neural defects (Chervenack et al, 1983).

Cystic hygroma on the other hand, are multiloculated posterior cervical cystic masses. The multiple cystic masses are often associated with Turner's syndrome (45 XO), and with hydrops fetalis (Seeds et al, 1982).

Teratomas are common germ cell tumors originating most often from the presacral area (Hobbins et al, 1982). The sacrococcygeal teratoma is the most frequent region affected by such abnormalities, but occasionally, teratomas have been described in the neck, the mouth, or the rest of the spine (Fig. 6–4).

**Skeletal Abnormalities.** Disorders of the limbs are usually associated with congenital or acquired disorders. When looking for skeletal abnormalities in the fetus, one needs to document not only the size of the bone, but

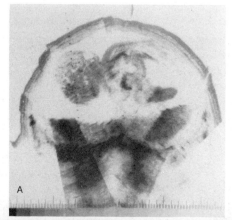

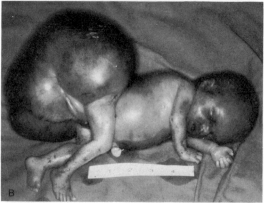

**Figure 6–4.** *A,* Sacrococcygeal teratoma. *B,* Gross findings at delivery of patient with sacrococcygeal teratoma.

also its brightness and whether or not there is a deformity or fracture of the bone. The femur is the bone that is used to estimate gestational age during the second and third trimesters. As such, it is the first indication of any skeletal abnormality. If the femur length falls below 2SD of the gestational age in a patient that is sure of her last menstrual period, the possibility of skeletal dysplasia should be entertained. A family history is often important in the prenatal detection of such anomalies, because the majority of these disorders are inherited through either an autosomal recessive (25 percent probability) or a dominant mode (50 percent probability). Once the femur is suspected to be short, the ratio of the biparietal diameter to the femur length should be evaluated. If this is found to be abnormal, the other bones should be measured. Frequently, skeletal abnormalities are associated with deformities of the skull and thorax as well as with polyhydramnios. Some skeletal dysplasias like achondroplasia may not become apparent until the 21st week of gestation and may be missed if the patient is evaluated during the early part of the pregnancy. Serial studies may be necessary in such a case.

## LETHAL SHORT-LIMBED CHONDRODYSPLASIA

The detection in utero of lethal skeletal dysplasia is often helpful in obstetric management. Conditions associated with lethal skeletal dysplasia are achondrogenesis, homozygous achondroplasia, thanatophoric syndrome, asphyxiating thoracic dystrophy, chondroectodermal dysplasia, chondrodysplasia punctata camptomelic syndrome, and short rib polydactyly syndrome (Hobbins et al, 1982).

1. *Thanatophoric* (Greek word meaning "death bringing") *dysplasia* is associated with short, bowed limbs and macrocephaly. The coronal views of the skull show a "cloverleaf" skull with a prominent forehead. The chest is usually short, and there is severe growth retardation often associated with polyhydramnios (Fig. 6–5). There is a lack of the usual caudal widening of the spinal canal. Most infants suffering from the condition die soon after birth (Mahony et al, 1985).

2. *Achondrogenesis* is a very short limb syndrome that is always lethal. In the homozygous form of achondroplasia, the chest is also small and polyhydramnios is present; however, the long bones do not have such striking shortening. Most infants are stillborn or die shortly after birth (Golbus et al, 1977).

3. *Achondroplasia* is associated with small limbs, small vertebral bodies with short pedicles, and macrocephaly.

4. *Osteogenesis imperfecta* is an autosomal dominant disorder that is associated with osteoporosis, which results in bowing or fracture of the long bones. This condition has been reported in utero before the 20th week of gestation. The ribs may occasionally show multiple fractures (Hobbins et al, 1982).

**Genitourinary.** Renal agenesis is often difficult to detect because of the marked oligohydramnios. Hydronephrosis is the most frequent renal abnormality (Hadlock et al, 1981). Fetal kidneys are easily seen on a transverse scan on either side of the spine (Fig. 6–6). As a rule, the size of the kidneys'

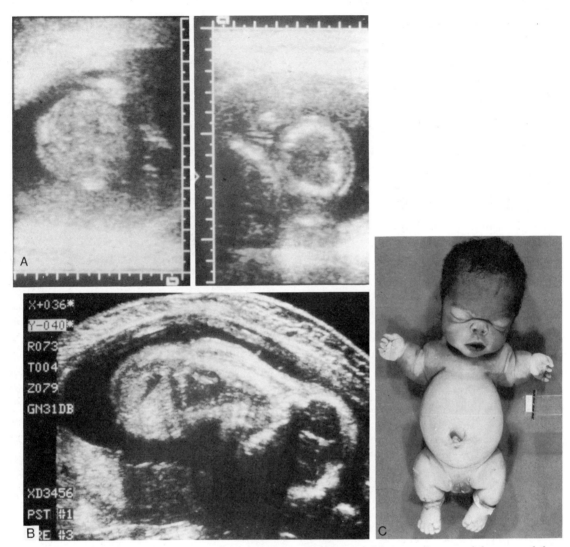

**Figure 6–5.** *A*, ABD (*left*) Thanatophoric dysplasia is demonstrated by protuberant abdomen; polyhydramnios is a frequent association. Chest (*right*). Thanatophoric dysplasia is demonstrated by narrow thorax with short ribs. *B*, Small chest compared with the abdomen. This chest/abdomen discrepancy is usually associated with lethal skeletal dysplasias. *C*, Thanatophoric dysplasia (most common form of neonatal dwarfism): proximal limb shortening, narrow thorax, prominent abdomen, thickened skin, macrocephaly. Death usually occurs in utero or during the first few hours of life.

circumference is about 30 percent of the size of the abdominal circumference. The fetal bladder is usually seen after the 18th to 20th week. Failure to find the bladder after 1 hour of scanning suggests abnormal renal function. By the same token, observation of the bladder after the 16th week almost always rules out renal agenesis or nonfunctioning polycystic kidneys. Enlarged fetal adrenals often have been mistaken for fetal kidneys and need to be included in the differential diagnosis of renal agenesis. When the fetus is in a breech position, transvaginal ultrasound may be very helpful in assessing the fetal bladder and even the fetal kidneys.

Oligohydramnios and enlarged solid kidneys suggest infantile polycystic kidneys (Potter type 1). This is an autosomal recessive disorder that carries a 25 percent recurrence risk for siblings. There is varying ability to observe the fetal bladder.

In multicystic dysplastic kidneys (Potter type 2), this abnormality of the renal architecture is replaced by multiple cysts varying in size from less than one to several centimeters. There is usually oligohydramnios,

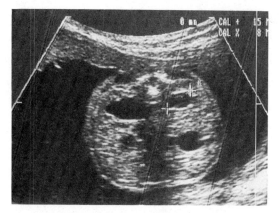

**Figure 6–6.** Bilateral mild hydronephrosis. Usually normal and found in male fetus. Amniocentesis might occasionally be considered to rule out chromosome anomalies.

and there is failure to observe the bladder if the problem is bilateral (Fig. 6–7).

Obstructive uropathy may result in varying ultrasound findings depending on the level of obstruction. For example, posterior urethral valve obstruction results in overdistended fetal bladder with or without a thickened bladder wall and a bilateral hydronephrosis (Fig. 6–8). Urethral atresia results in oligohydramnios, but a variable amount of amniotic fluid is seen in the posterior urethral valves (Copel et al, 1987). Ureteropelvic junction obstruction is usually unilateral; it is associated with hydronephrosis and dilated renal calices. Malformations of the kidneys, the gastrointestinal (GI) tract, and the cardiovascular system are often associated with ureteropelvic junction (Fig. 6–9).

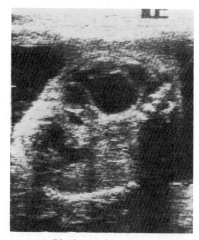

**Figure 6–7.** Unilateral multicystic kidney.

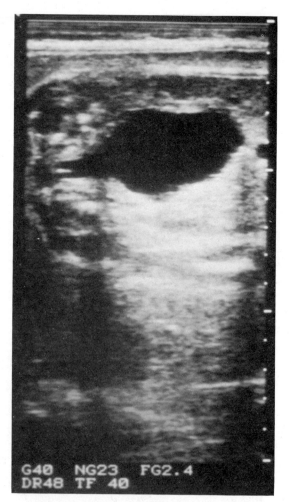

**Figure 6–8.** Posterior urethral obstruction.

## ABDOMINAL WALL DEFECT

*Congenital diaphragmatic hernia* is a rare finding. Classically, the abdominal contents protrude into the chest cavity. On initial scanning, the heart may be displaced anteriorly and the stomach cavity goes above the diaphragm. Most of the defects are posterior (foramen of Bochdalek) or anterior (foramen of Morgagni). Defects of the central portion of the diaphragm are usually associated with major protrusion of the abdominal contents into the thorax, including the liver and the spleen. These infants often succumb because of severe pulmonary hypoplasia. Extracorporeal membrane oxygenation has shown some improvement in the outcome of these infants.

*Omphalocele* occurs more frequently than diaphragmatic hernias and is usually due to

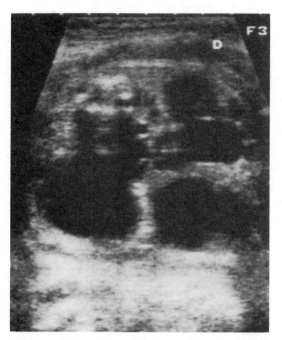

**Figure 6–9.** Unilateral ureteropelvic junction (UPJ) obstruction resulting in an important hydroureter and dilated renal calices.

a failure of the internalization of the abdominal contents. This is often associated with chromosome anomalies (trisomies 13, 18, and 21), and these infants often have cardiac anomalies (atrioventricular septal defects or ventricular septal defects). Large defects are usually repaired in multiple stages using a silo made of synthetic materials such as Teflon.

*Gastroschisis* is an abdominal defect usually located to the right of the umbilical cord.

The cord insertion is usually normal and should be seen in order to be sure of the diagnosis. There are usually no covering membranes around the herniated bowels. It is not unusual to find that there is some form of bowel atresia or malrotation. In the majority of cases, there is no association with fetal chromosome anomalies (Fig. 6–10).

## Imaging the Fetal Heart

Echocardiography has become a useful tool for imaging the fetal heart in utero, enabling the operator to diagnose cardiac anomalies and cardiac arrhythmias. The heart is located on the left side of the thorax. No standard views to observe the fetal heart have been published to date. Standardized views of the heart are needed in order to ensure accurate information and to avoid the risk of misdiagnosis. The apical four- or five-chamber view needs to be documented (Fig. 6–11) (Copel et al, 1988). In most patients, this is obtained at the 18th week of gestation and later. Using the four-chamber view of the right and left ventricles, the atrioventricular valves and both atria should be seen easily. The right ventricle is slightly larger than the left due to the fetal cardiovascular hemodynamics (Veille et al, 1990). The moderator band can be identified in the right ventricle. The tricuspid valve insertion points are seen closer to the apex of the heart than is the mitral valve. The eustachian valve can be seen within the right atrium.

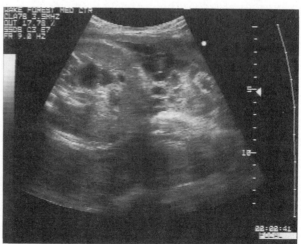

**Figure 6–10.** Gastroschisis. Free bowel loops are seen outside of the abdominal wall.

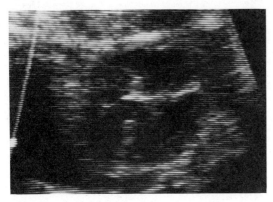

**Figure 6–11.** Four chambers of the fetal heart. Interventricular septum is seen; the atrioventricular values are shown.

The interatrial septum can be seen flapping into the left atrium during the cardiac cycle. The inferior vena cava is located on the right side of the vertebral spine. The aorta is on the left and is easily identified by its pulsation. The inferior vena cava can be traced into the anatomic right atrium. The right atrium is recognized by its connection to the superior vena cava and inferior vena cava. The eustachian valve at the inferior vena cava insertion site further supports its identification. The right ventricle has a moderator band connecting the right ventricle anterior wall to the septum. The right ventricle also has a coarser trabecular pattern. The short-axis view usually identifies the right outflow tract (pulmonary artery), which wraps around the aorta. The pulmonary veins often are difficult to see. The ballooning of the left atrium helps to visualize the pulmonary vein. The presence of the infundibulum in the outflow tract almost always indicates that the ventricle is the morphologic right ventricle, regardless of its anatomic site. The tricuspid valve goes with the morphologic right ventricle, and the mitral valve goes with the morphologic left ventricle.

**Cardiac Defects.** The apical four-chamber view of the heart often detects major anomalies of the fetal heart. In complex cardiac anomalies, a knowledge of anatomic locations of the different chambers of the heart may not be adequate for the diagnosis of congenital heart disease in utero. This is why a clear understanding of anatomic landmarks is essential to the proper recognition of different morphologic chambers. With the detection of a major congenital heart defect, a

karyotype should be performed to rule out major chromosomal anomalies (Lewis et al, 1983).

Most major cardiac anomalies have been diagnosed, or at least suspected, in utero.

*Large atrial septal defects* (ASD) either of the secundum or the primum type can be diagnosed using the apical or subxiphoid view. Most of these defects have an excellent prognosis and do not cause cyanosis in the newborn period. When a single or common atrium is found, it becomes important to identify the pulmonary venous drainage, because it might be abnormal. This is often difficult to assess in utero as the cardiac output to the fetal lung is markedly decreased.

*Ventricular septal defects* (VSD) may be difficult to see unless they are large. Depending on the location of the ventricular septal defect, four types can be identified: membranous, muscular, inlet, and outlet. The prognosis varies with the severity of the defect, but in general, small ventricular septal defects are acyanotic and well tolerated. The membranous ventricular septal defects are difficult to see in utero unless they are large. The muscular ventricular septal defects result in an echo drop out in the muscular part of the intraventricular septum and carry an excellent prognosis (Lewis et al, 1983). The inlet ventricular septal defects are usually associated with anomalies of the atrioventricular canal and have been associated with Down's syndrome. The best view to diagnose this defect is the four-chamber view. The outlet or infundibular ventricular septal defects are usually associated with other major cardiac defects such as a tetralogy of Fallot, a truncus arteriosus, or a double-outlet right ventricle. These are usually cyanotic defects, and the prognosis varies with the associated lesion.

**Anomalies of the Ventricles.** Poor development of the ventricles results in cyanotic lesions that carry a guarded prognosis.

1. *Hypoplastic left ventricles* have a poor prognosis even after surgery. Treatment options represent ethical dilemmas (Veille et al, 1989). The ventricle, the ascending aorta, the mitral, and the aortic valves are usually small and difficult to observe. Coarctation of the aorta can occasionally be associated with hypoplastic left ventricle (Fig. 6–12A).

2. *Hypoplastic right ventricle* carries a better prognosis than that of the left side. Usually, there is a small ventricle, small tricus-

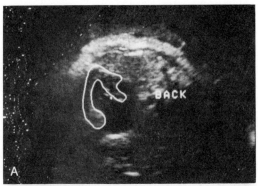

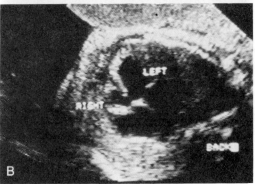

**Figure 6–12.** *A,* Hypoplastic left ventricle (HLV). The ventricular cavity closest to the back, in most instances, is the left ventricle. Hypoplastic left heart syndrome includes not only the HLV but also aortic atresia and hypoplasia of the ascending aorta. *B,* Hypoplastic right ventricle. Usually better tolerated than HLV. Associated with hypoplastic tricuspid valve and ventricular septal defect.

pid valve, and a small pulmonary valve. Newborns are cyanotic, and a real emergency can occur when the ductus arteriosus closes. Pulmonary blood flow stops or is markedly impaired. Most patients survive the initial palliative surgery and have a long-term survival (Fig. 6–12B) (Allan et al, 1985).

3. Atrialization of the right ventricle is the downward displacement of the septal and posterior leaflets of the tricuspid valve (Ebstein's anomaly) (Hirschklau et al, 1977). In some cases, there is a positive maternal history of lithium ingestion during the first trimester of the pregnancy. The prognosis for these infants depends on the degree of the downward displacement of the tricuspid valve.

4. *Truncus arteriosus* or a single outlet of the ventricle is a condition in which only one vessel arises from both ventricles. A large ventricular septal defect is usually associ-

ated with this condition. Heart failure develops early in the neonatal life, and the long term prognosis is often guarded.

5. *Double outlet right ventricle* is a condition in which both of the great vessels came out of the right ventricle. This cardiac anomaly is frequently associated with other fetal anomalies and chromosome abnormalities, especially trisomy 13.

## Doppler Ultrasound in Obstetrics

Doppler application has become another useful modality in assessing fetal well-being. Doppler study has been an accepted technology in confirming fetal heart rate. Recently it has been used to assess the umbilical artery and uteroplacental circulation. When an ultrasound wave of a known frequency strikes a moving target, such as moving red blood cells within a vessel, the reflected signal retrieved by the transducer has a different frequency. The difference in frequency is termed the Doppler shift. Doppler instrumentation is capable of intercepting the reflected ultrasound and computing the Doppler frequency shift signal. The frequency shift signal reflects the velocity with which the red blood cells are moving. Blood flow moving toward the transducer is displayed above the zero line. Blood flow moving away from the transducer is displayed below the zero line. When obtaining such Doppler signals from the mother's abdominal wall, results can be significantly different if there are significant maternal or fetal breathing movements.

Doppler study has been used to qualitatively and quantitatively evaluate blood flow through structures. Using a continuous wave, all blood motion along the Doppler beam is analyzed. Thus, a spectrum of different velocities is received and displayed. Pulsed-wave Doppler is best to study blood velocity in a small area or range. Such instrumentation makes pulsed-wave Doppler suitable for the study of blood flow across the different cardiac chambers and valve areas, as these have different velocities (Veille et al, 1991).

**Doppler Ultrasound of the Umbilical Artery.** To obtain a pulsed Doppler wave, the umbilical cord is visualized using two-dimensional scanning and the Doppler sample is placed over the umbilical artery. Pulsed-wave Doppler or continuous Doppler ultrasound may be used to obtain such signals. The continuous Doppler ultrasound lacks the precision of the pulsed-wave Doppler. Its cost, however, is much less than the continuous pulsed-wave Doppler. Both types of equipment have been shown to give similar values for the umbilical artery waveforms. The Doppler sample has been shown to vary depending on which part of the umbilical cord is interrogated. The free-floating part of the umbilical cord is an acceptable sampling site. Different values of the umbilical artery waveforms have been reported if obtained at the fetal, midportion, or the placental end of the umbilical cord (Trudinger and Giles, 1989). We have found that an acceptable landmark for obtaining a Doppler signal from the umbilical artery is its placental site insertion. Using this landmark, we have found that the signals are easily reproducible and easily identified (Veille et al, 1991). The normal flow pattern is a rapid upstroke during systole with a gradual decline during diastole. Under normal conditions, flow still occurs during diastole. Absent diastolic, or even reversed diastolic flow, is considered abnormal and has been associated with poor fetal outcome (Fig. 6–13) (Rochelson, 1989).

**Doppler Ultrasound of the Ductus Arteriosus.** Indomethacin has been the subject of a renewed interest as an alternate treatment to premature labor. The risks of primary pulmonary hypertension, premature closure of the ductus arteriosus in utero, and neonatal congestive heart failure in these infants rarely have been reported after the ingestion of indomethacin in the third trimester. Doppler can monitor the peak flow velocity of red blood cells passing through the ductus. As the ductus decreases its lumen, peak flow increases. If the peak flow through the ductus is at or greater than 140 cm/sec, this suggests partial vasoconstriction, and the medication should be discontinued (Moise et al, 1987). As a general rule, peak flow velocity through the ductus should be monitored frequently after the institution of such medication. In our laboratory, the flow is monitored every 2 to 3 days. The assessment of the amniotic fluid is also closely monitored, as indomethacin has been

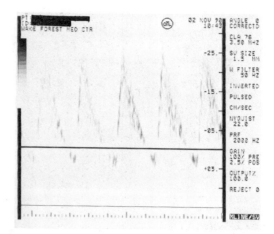

**Figure 6–13.** Umbilical artery Doppler study. This illustrates a reverse flow pattern during diastole, which has been associated with significant perinatal morbidity and mortality.

reported to cause oligohydramnios after prolonged use.

**Doppler Ultrasound of the Uterine Artery.** The Doppler waveform displays high diastolic velocities with highly disturbed systolic turbulent velocities. The degree of diastolic flow increases during normal pregnancies, and failure of this pattern to appear (i.e., absence of a diastolic notch in the waveform at the end of systole) has been reported with fetal growth retardation. As a result of these findings, it has been suggested that uterine artery Doppler tracings may be helpful in the screening of pregnancies at risk for fetal growth retardation, uteroplacental insufficiency, and pregnancy-induced hypertension (Campbell et al, 1986).

**Doppler Ultrasound and Fetal Arrhythmias.** Doppler study can be used to evaluate fetal irregular rhythms. The pulsed-wave Doppler sample volume can be easily placed at the tips of the atrioventricular valves. The signals that result identify the atrial contraction (i.e., inflow) and the ventricular contraction (i.e., outflow), making the analysis of the abnormal rhythm much easier to determine (Reed et al, 1987). Management of these fetal arrhythmias differ depending on the type of premature contractions one is dealing with. Most of the premature atrial contractions are well tolerated in utero, and further Doppler evaluation during the course of the pregnancy is not essential as long as the cardiac anatomy is normal; however, frequent fetal ultrasounds are necessary to rule out the presence of ascites, pleural, or pericardial effusion. Premature ventricular contractions are, however, more ominous because they can easily result in significant tachyarrhythmias that may result in cardiac failure. As such, premature ventricular contractions (PVCs) are monitored by Doppler ultrasound at least every 1 to 2 weeks. As a general rule, most of the fetal arrhythmias are well tolerated in utero and have a tendency to improve in the neonatal life. Tachyarrhythmias should be treated in utero with either digitalis and/or a β-blocker. Such treatment needs to be monitored closely by frequent Doppler and M-Mode ultrasound. Maternal pulse also must be monitored.

Bradyarrhythmias (i.e., fetal heart rate between 60 to 80 beats per minute) are usually well tolerated in utero. Doppler and/or M-Mode are essential for the correct diagnosis and to avoid doing an emergency delivery of an often premature infant. Collagen vascular disease in the mother, with circulating antibodies that cross the placenta, often do cause such blocks (Veille et al, 1985). It is essential here to rule out major congenital heart defects, especially those involved with a disruption of the conducting system. It may be difficult to get a readable tracing with electronic fetal monitoring, however, biochemical assessment of the acid-base status can be made by repeatedly finding scalp pH during the active phase of labor once the cervix has gone beyond 2 to 3 cm. It is not unusual for these infants to receive the placement of a permanent pacemaker because the heart block is often permanent.

## Use of Ultrasound in the Labor and Delivery Suite

Many labor and delivery suites are now equipped with an ultrasound machine. Most of these machines have a linear and a vaginal sector transducer. Some of the indications for scanning in the labor and delivery area are listed below.

1. Document fetal position in the premature pregnancy, in which the patient's habitus make clinical evaluation difficult.
2. Document the size, the position, and the number of fetuses in a patient who has an enlarged uterus.

3. Document placental location in cases of sudden vaginal bleeding. A careful ultrasound examination documents placenta previa and avoids the need for a "double-set up" which is an examination performed in the operating room with all the essential equipment necessary for urgent cesarean section, if the placenta is clearly away from the cervical os. The diagnosis of abruptio placenta may also be made with ultrasonic examination. Ultrasound may also be useful in the case of postpartum hemorrhage to determine the presence of retained placental tissue. At times, the authors have found ultrasound to be helpful to see the curette or the suction cannula during a postpartum hemorrhage, especially if the uterus is very flaccid or infected.

4. Estimate fetal weight and head to body ratio in cases of very premature fetuses, breech fetuses, or macrosomic infants. Some authors have advocated the vaginal delivery of frank or complete breech if the estimated fetal weight is between 2000 and 3000 g. Ultrasound may be useful during external cephalic version of either a singleton or a second twin, in case of either a transverse lie or a breech presentation.

5. Besides monitoring both fetal hearts during the delivery of twins, ultrasound enhances manipulation of internal podalic version in guiding the operator's hand through the intact membranes.

6. Determine fetal age prior to the use of tocolytics. In general, if a biparietal diameter of at least 9.2 cm, a femur length of at least 7.4 cm, and a grade-3 placenta are documented on ultrasound, the chance of the infant's developing hyaline membrane disease is small. If the gestational age is at or greater than 35 weeks of gestation, most institutions would not use intravenous tocolytic agents.

7. Diagnosis of intrauterine demise by real-time ultrasound is the method of choice.

8. Amniocentesis can be performed safely through ultrasound guidance. This especially becomes important when there has been premature rupture of the membranes and the amniotic fluid is decreased. Ultrasound can precisely guide the operator successfully to a small pocket of amniotic fluid. PUBS and intrauterine transfusion are ren-

**Table 6–5**
BIOPHYSICAL PROFILE

| Biophysical Variable | Normal (score = 2) | Abnormal (score = 0) |
| --- | --- | --- |
| Fetal breathing movements | One or more episodes of ≥ 30 sec in 30 min | Absent or no episode of ≥30 sec in 30 min |
| Gross body movements | Three or more discrete body/limb movements in 30 min (episodes of active continuous movements considered as single movement) | Two or less episodes of body/limb movements in 30 min |
| Fetal tone | One or more episodes of active extension with return to flexion of fetal limb(s) or trunk; opening and closing of hand considered normal tone | Either slow extension with return to partial flexion or movement of limb in full extension or absent fetal movement |
| Reactive fetal heart rate | Two or more episodes of acceleration of ≥15 bpm and of ≥15 sec associated with fetal movement in 20 min | Less than 2 episodes of acceleration of fetal heart rate or acceleration of <15 bpm in 40 min |
| Qualitative amniotic fluid | One or more pockets of fluid measuring ≥1 cm in two perpendicular planes | Either no pockets or a pocket <1 cm in two perpendicular planes |

From Manning FA, Morrison I, Lange IR, Harman CR, Chamberlain PFC: Fetal biophysical scoring: selective use of the nonstress test. Am J Obstet Gynecol 156:709, 1987.

dered significantly easier when assisted by continuous ultrasound guidance.

9. Demonstration of fetal anomalies in patients that have little or no prenatal care. It is important to document such anomalies that are incompatible with life, such as anencephaly.

10. Amniotic fluid volume determination can be assessed by real-time ultrasound in the labor and delivery area. If oligohydramnios is documented, especially in a postdate pregnancy (greater than 42 weeks), the pregnancy is at risk for intrapartum complications. A biophysical profile can easily be assessed in the labor and delivery area if there is any doubt about fetal well-being (Table 6–5). The combination of fetal breathing movements, gross body movements, muscle tone, amniotic fluid volume, and fetal heart rate tracing, constitutes a biophysical profile. A score of 8 on a 10 point scale is reassuring of fetal well-being, as long as the amniotic fluid remains normal (Manning et al, 1987).

11. We have found ultrasound in the labor and delivery area to be useful prior to a cesarean section when the placenta is known to be anterior and previa. As such, ultrasound may help the surgeon make an uterine incision avoiding the placenta.

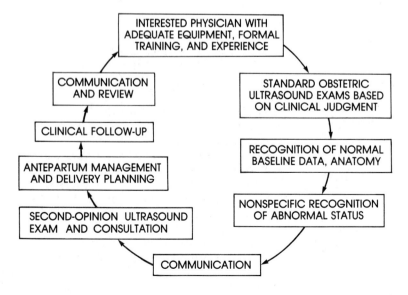

**Figure 6–14.** Diagram showing the ideal functioning of regionalized ultrasound consultation.

12. Finally, in the postpartum period curettage, the use of continuous ultrasound helps localize not only the tip of the currette, so as to avoid uterine perforation, but also helps in securing an empty uterine cavity.

A real-time ultrasound unit on or in close proximity to the delivery floor is an integral part of the antenatal tests offered during normal and abnormal pregnancies. As such, it is essential to properly teach and educate all health personnel that may have to use ultrasound in obstetrics and gynecology and to establish standards to assure the proper usage of such technology. As ultrasound expands into most practitioners offices, the schematic representation (Fig. 6–14) drawn by the late Charles W. Kohler, M.D. in the last edition of this book seems ever so true and "bears witness to" the great judgment and foresight of our late colleague.

### Acknowledgment

Special thanks are extended to Dr. L. Nelson for his expert comments in reviewing this manuscript and Marie King, RDMS, for providing some of the illustrative cases.

## References

Allan LD, Crawford DC, Anderson RH, Tynan M: Spectrum of congenital heart disease detected echocardiographically in prenatal life. Br Heart J 54:523, 1985.

Ayers JWT, DeGrood RM, Compton AA, et al: Sonographic evaluation of cervical length in pregnancy: diagnosis and management of preterm cervical effacement in patients at risk for premature delivery. Obstet Gynecol 71:939, 1988.

Benacerraf BR, Estroff JA: Transvaginal sonographic imaging of the low fetal head in the second trimester. J Ultrasound Med 8:325, 1989.

Benacerraf BR, Barss VA, Laboda LA: A sonographic sign for the detection in the second trimester of the fetus with Down's Syndrome. Am J Obstet Gynecol 151:1078, 1985.

Bree RL, Edwards M, Bohm-Velez M, et al: Transvaginal sonography in the evaluation of normal early pregnancy: correlation with HCG level. AJR 153:75, 1989.

Brown DL, Emerson DS, Shulman LP, et al: Sonographic diagnosis of omphalocele during 10th week of gestation. AJR 153:825, 1989.

Bulie M, Podobnik M, Korenic B, et al: First trimester diagnosis of low obstructive uropathy: an indicator of initial renal function in the fetus. J Ultrasound Med 10:537, 1987.

Campbell S, Pearce JMF, Hackett G, et al: Qualitative assessment of uteroplacental blood flow: an early screening test for high risk pregnancies. Obstet Gynecol 68:649, 1986.

Chervenack FA, Isaacson G, Blackemore KJ, et al: Fetal cystic hygroma. Cause and natural history. N Engl J Med 309:822, 1983.

Consensus Conference: The use of diagnostic ultrasound imaging during pregnancy. JAMA 252(5):669, 1984.

Copel JA, Pilu G, Green J, Hobbins, Kleinman CS: Fetal echocardiographic screening for congenital heart disease: the importance of the four-chamber view. Am J Obstet Gynecol 157:648, 1987.

Copel JA, Cullen M, Green JJ, Mahoney MJ, Hobbins JC, Kleinman CS: The frequency of aneuploidy in prenatally diagnosed congenital heart disease: an indication for fetal karyotyping. Am J Obstet Gynecol 158:409, 1988.

Cullen MT, Green JJ, Reece A, Hobbins JC: A comparison of transvaginal and abdominal ultrasound in visualizing the first trimester conceptus. J Ultra Med 8:565–69, 1989.

Diagnostic ultrasound imaging in pregnancy. National Institutes of Health Consensus Development Conference Consensus Statement 5:1, 1984.

Farine D, Fox HE, Jakobson S, et al: Vaginal ultrasound for diagnosis of placenta previa. Am J Obstet Gynecol 159:566, 1988.

Filly R: The "lemon" sign: a clinical perspective. Radiology 167:573, 1988.

Gabbe S, Mintz MC, Menutti MT, McDonnell AE: Detection of open spina bifida by the lemon sign: pathologic correlation. J Clin Ultrasound 16:399, 1988.

Golbus MS, Hall BD, Filly RA, et al: Prenatal diagnosis of achondrogenesis. J Pediatrics 91:464, 1977.

Gross DR, Williams AR, Wagner-Mann C, McCord F, Miller DL: Thermal and heart rate response to ultrasonic exposure in the second and third trimester dog fetus. J Ultra Med 5:507, 1986.

Hadlock FP, Deter RL, Carpenter R, et al: Review. Sonography of fetal urinary tract anomalies. AJR 137:261, 1981.

Herrmann UJ Jr, Locher GW, Goldhirsch A: Sonographic patterns of ovarian tumors: prediction of malignancy. Obstet Gynecol 69:777, 1987.

Hilpert PL, Kurtz AB: The role of transvaginal ultrasound in the second and third trimesters. Semin Ultrasound CT MR 11(1):59, 1990.

Hirschklau MJ, Sahn DJ, Hagan AD, et al: Cross-sectional echocardiographic features of Ebstein's anomaly of the tricuspid valve. Am J Cardiol 40:400, 1977.

Hobbins JC, Bracken MB, Mahoney MJ: Diagnosis of fetal skeletal dysplasia with ultrasound. Am J Obstet Gynecol 142:306, 1982.

Hull ME, Moghissi KS, Maygar DM, et al: Correlation of serum estradiol levels and ultrasound monitoring to assess follicular maturation. Fertil Steril 46:42, 1986.

Kremkau FW. Doppler Ultrasound: Principles and Instruments, Philadelphia, WB Saunders Co, 1990.

Kremkau FW: Diagnostic Ultrasound: Principles, Instruments, and Exercises, 3rd ed. Philadelphia, WB Saunders Co, 1989.

Lewis AB, Wells W, Lindesmith GG: Evaluation and surgical treatment of pulmonary atresia and intact ventricular septum in septum in infancy. Circulation 67:1318, 1983.

Mahony BS, Filly RA, Callen PW, et al: Thanatophoric dwarfism with cloverleaf skull: a specific antenatal sonographic diagnosis. J Ultrasound Med 4:151, 1985.

Manning FA, Morrison I, Lange IR, Harman CR, Chamberlain PFC. Fetal biophysical profile scoring: selective use of the nonstress test. Am J Obstet Gynecol 156:709, 1987.

Moise KJ, Huhta JC, Sharif DS, et al: Detection and quantitation of constriction of the fetal ductus arteriosus by Doppler echocardiography. Circulation 75:406, 1987.

NAACOG: Committee on Practice: The Nurse's Role in Ultrasound. Committee Opinion. Washington, DC, September, 1991a.

NAACOG: Standards for Nursing Care of Women and Newborns (4th ed). Washington, DC, 1991b.

Nicolaides KH, Campbell S, Gabbe SG, et al: Ultrasound screening for spina bifida: cranial and cerebellar signs. Lancet 2:72, 1986.

Nyberg DA, Filly RA, Mahony BS, et al: Early gestation: correlation of hCG levels and sonographic identification. AJR 144:954, 1985.

Nyberg DA, Laing FC, Filly RA, et al: Ultrasonographic differentiation of the gestational sac of early intrauterine pregnancy from the pseudogestational sac of ectopic pregnancy. Radiology 146:755, 1983.

Nyberg DA, Mack LA, Hirsh J, Mahony BS. Abnormalities of fetal cranial contour in sonographic detection of spina bifida: evaluation of the "lemon sign." Radiology 167:387, 1988.

Official guidelines and statements on obstetrical ultrasound. American Institute for Ultrasound in Medicine 1985, 1–10.

Reed KL, Sahn DJ, Marx GR, et al: Cardiac Doppler flows during fetal arrhythmias: physiologic consequences. Obstet Gynecol 70:1, 1987.

Rochelson B: The clinical significance of absent enddiastolic velocity in the umbilical artery waveforms. Clin Obstet Gynecol 32:692, 1989.

Rosendahl H, Kivinen S: Antenatal detection of congenital malformations by routine ultrasonography. Obstet Gynecol 73(6):947, 1989.

Safety standard for diagnostic ultrasound equipment. Suppl J Ultra Med 2(4):S1–S50, 1983.

Seeds JW, Mittelstaedt A, Cefalo RC, et al: Prenatal diagnosis of sacrococcygeal teratoma: an anechoic caudal mass. J Clin Ultrasound 10:193, 1982.

Smith RP: Basic physics of ultrasound. Clin Obstet Gynecol 20(2):231, 1977.

Stark CR, Orleans M, Haverkamp AD, Murphy J: Short- and long-term risks after exposure to diagnostic ultrasound in utero. Obstet Gynecol 63(2):194, 1984.

Timor-Tritsch IE, Farine D, Rosen MG: A close look at early embryonic development with the high-frequency transvaginal transducer. Am J Obstet Gynecol 159(3):676, 1988.

Trudinger BJ, Giles WB: Clinical and pathologic correlations of umbilical and uterine artery waveforms. Clin Obstet Gynecol 32:669, 1989.

Veille JC, Ben Ami M, Sivakoff M: Ranged gated pulsed Doppler of the umbilical artery in human fetuses during normal pregnancies. Am J Perinatol 8:269, 1991.

Veille, JC, Sivakoff M, Mahowald MB: Ethical dilemmas in fetal echocardiography. Obstet Gynecol 73:710, 1989.

Veille JC, Sivakoff M, Nemeth M: Evaluation of the human fetal cardiac size and function. Am J Perinatol 7:54, 1990.

Veille JC, Sunderland C, Bennett RM: Complete heart block in a fetus associated with maternal Sjogren's syndrome. Am J Obstet Gynecol 151:691, 1985.

Vergani P, Ghidini A, Sirtori M, et al: Antenatal diagnosis of fetal acrania. J Ultrasound Med 6:715, 1987.

Warsof SL, Pearce JM, Campbell S: The present place of routine ultrasound screening. Clin Obstet Gynecol 10(3):445, 1983.

Warsof SL, Cooper DJ, Little D, Campbell S: Routine ultrasound screening for antenatal detection of intrauterine growth retardation. Obstet Gynecol 67(1):33, 1986.

. . . . . . . . . . . . . . . . . . . . . . . . . . . . . . . . . . . . .

# CHAPTER 7

# Perinatal Infections

Sebastian Faro and Joseph G. Pastorek II

Infection continues to be a major problem for the high-risk team, even though a plethora of antimicrobial agents are available. The practitioner must be familiar with those potential pathogenic microorganisms that exist in the environment, as well as with the patient's endogenous microflora. There must also be a basic understanding of both the mechanisms of action and the strengths and weaknesses of individual classes of antibiotics. All antibiotics, especially the newer broad-spectrum antibiotics, can exert selective pressure on microorganisms, thereby selecting out resistant strains. The obstetrician is further challenged because it is often difficult to make a diagnosis of an acute infection, because some infections may be chronic or asymptomatic. The pregnant female poses a special problem in that the presence of the fetus often prohibits the use of many antimicrobial agents.

## Viral Infections

### AIDS (HIV INFECTION)

#### Epidemiology

In 1981, the first cases of a mysterious disease began to be reported in homosexual men. These patients were suffering from a multitude of unusual infections and rare malignancies that commonly affected only immunocompromised individuals. After the medical technocracy was brought to bear on this strange disease, initially termed the acquired immunodeficiency syndrome (AIDS), it was discovered that the culprit was a human retrovirus.

The epidemic of AIDS has progressed exponentially since 1981. The first patients with the disease included homosexual men, hemophiliacs, and, inexplicably, Haitian immigrants. It became apparent that viral transmission was by sexual contact in the homosexuals, via contaminated blood in the hemophiliacs, and perhaps by sexual contact in the Haitian population. At any rate, as the decade wore on, the disease became more widespread and transmission characteristics changed.

As of 1990, over 100,000 deaths attributable to AIDS had been reported in the United States. Over 40,000 new cases are diagnosed yearly. However, the populations affected and the modes of transmission are now changing. It is predicted that in the 1990s, AIDS will be one of the five leading causes of death in young women. Currently, 14 percent of individuals who die from AIDS are women. Clearly, homosexual men, though still a majority, are not the predominant target of the virus that they once were.

In the 1990s, the AIDS virus is being transmitted predominantly through heterosexual activity, parenteral drug abuse, and perinatal transmission. Recent increases in cases of pediatric AIDS, not including children with hemophilia, underscore the third factor. As any disease spreads through the female population, it invariably appears in the fetus and the newborn.

## Microbiology

The clinical syndrome of AIDS is caused by a small, human retrovirus called human immunodeficiency virus, type I (HIV-I or simply HIV). A similar virus, HIV-II, has been identified in Africa as a cause of clinical AIDS, but it has yet to be reported in the United States in any significant numbers. Previous nomenclature for HIV included HTLV-III (human T-lymphotrophic virus, type III) in the United States and LAV (lymphadenopathy-associated virus) in Europe. Each of these labels was descriptive of the virus' favorite target (the T-lymphocyte) and clinical disease (originally the mysterious lymphadenopathy in homosexual men), but each has been superceded by the modern term HIV.

Retroviruses are small RNA viruses that are associated with the enzyme reverse transcriptase. This enzyme allows the virus to do something unique in the molecular biologic world—namely, form DNA from RNA, reversing the natural order of information flow. After the retrovirus attaches to the target cell, it enters the host and the reverse transcriptase catalyzes the transcription of viral-specific DNA from the original viral RNA. Thus, viral DNA effectively becomes the dominant genetic apparatus of the infected cell.

Retroviral diseases are commonly encountered in animals; feline leukemia is a well-known example. In humans, hairy cell leukemia is one recognized retroviral illness. Similar infections are described in other animal species.

## Infection

AIDS is a syndrome, not one specific disease. The underlying pathophysiology consists of the depletion of T-cells by HIV infection. The resultant immunodeficiency is the culprit in the host of different opportunistic infections that come into play in the clinically ill patient. The initial infection, interestingly, is merely a short-lived febrile illness with no unique characteristics.

A rough classification of HIV infection consists of four groups of patients listed later; a given patient travels from group I to group IV (and eventually dies) over a period of 5 to 10 years.

Group I     acute infection
Group II    asymptomatic
Group III   generalized lymphadenopathy
Group IV   other illnesses
          a. constitutional
          b. neurologic
          c. infectious
          d. malignant
          e. miscellaneous

The most well-publicized aspect of AIDS is the myriad of opportunistic infectious agents that strike the immunocompromised host. Some of the more common infectious agents include *Pneumocystis carinii*, atypical mycobacteria, cytomegalovirus and herpes simplex, *Cryptosporidium,* fungal infection (e.g., histoplasmosis), and extragenital candidiasis. The unusual neoplasms common in the AIDS patient include Kaposi's sarcoma, non-Hodgkin's lymphoma, and primary lymphoma of the brain.

The most common presentation of the HIV-infected obstetric patient is asymptomatic disease. The practitioner rarely, if ever, finds a pregnant patient suffering acute infection. More commonly, a gravida will present with pneumocystis pneumonia. Still, the vast majority of patients in this setting are asymptomatic.

Infection during pregnancy with HIV alone, in the absence of complicating infection or malignancy, does not seem to affect pregnancy outcome. However, approximately 30 percent of neonates will be infected before birth or in the peripartal period. Most of these will then go on to develop clinical AIDS before their second birthday. Uninfected neonates are at risk of contracting the disease from the mother through body fluid contact, including breast milk.

## Diagnosis

Because the majority of HIV-positive gravidas are asymptomatic, diagnosis is generally accomplished by detecting HIV-specific antibody in the patient's blood. The usual screening test performed by most clinical laboratories is an enzyme linked immunosorbent assay (ELISA) test with over 90 percent sensitivity and specificity. However, positive ELISA tests are verified with the Western blot assay.

Although occasional false-positive tests do occur, they are becoming a rarity with the refinement of the techniques. False-negative tests, on the other hand, can occur in patients shortly after their acute infection, before they develop significant antibodies; in cases in which this is suspected, sophisticated antigen tests are available to detect actual viral antigens in the patient's serum.

Neonatal diagnosis is complicated by the fact that maternal antibody, passively acquired transplacentally, will be present in the baby's blood for up to a year after birth. If it is desired, HIV-specific IgM may be sought, indicating fetal and neonatal infection; maternally derived antibody would be of the IgG class.

## Treatment

A cure for HIV does not exist. The asymptomatic patient, of course, does not necessarily need therapy, although treatment with antiretroviral drugs such as zidovudine (AZT) may be beneficial to patients with very low lymphocyte counts. Patients with adenopathy or full-blown AIDS need to be treated for their specific infection or malignancy, of course, as well as with AZT, for their HIV infection. Pregnant women should be treated in the usual fashion, with attention to the effects of any medication on the fetus.

There are studies underway investigating the use of AZT prophylactically during pregnancy, in an attempt to prevent the spread of HIV from the infected mother to her fetus. So far, there does not appear to be any major adverse effect of the drug on pregnancy.

The bleak picture of inadequate therapy highlights the advisability of prevention. It is important for all health care workers to stress to their patients the sexual transmissibility of HIV, as well as the possibility of transmission through blood (e.g., sharing needles for intravenous drug use). Also, screening of pregnant women for HIV allows preventive measures (e.g., avoidance of breastfeeding) to be taken with those 70 percent of uninfected infants born to HIV-positive women (see also Chapter 8).

## HERPES

### Epidemiology

Genital herpes has become one of the most common sexually transmitted diseases,

ranking in prevalence with gonorrhea and syphilis. The Centers for Disease Control estimate that there are approximately 300,000 new cases of genital herpes per year, occurring more frequently in the 15- to 24-year-old age group. Data collected from venereal disease clinics show that the ratio of gonorrhea to herpes is 10:1. However, data obtained from the UCLA Student Health Clinic indicated that genital herpes is more prevalent than gonorrhea, with a ratio of 1:10 (gonorrhea/herpes). These two sources of information imply that herpes may be more common among the middle and upper socioeconomic classes.

### Microbiology

Genital herpes is caused by either herpesvirus serotype I or serotype II (HSV-I or HSV-II). HSV-I and HSV-II both contain a central core of DNA that is surrounded by an icosahedral protein capsid. The protein capsid is enveloped by an impermeable membrane made up of lipids, polyamines, and glycoproteins. The two serotypes can be distinguished by serologic, biologic, and biochemical analysis.

These viruses are unique in that they have evolved to develop a complex relationship with their adult hosts. Humans are the only known natural host, and the virus can cause an active infection, a latent infection, or cell transformation.

### Infection

Genital herpes occurs either as a primary infection or as recurrent disease. Primary genital infection may be asymptomatic, mild, or severe. Inoculation of the host by the virus occurs by contact with infectious material, usually via sexual intercourse or orogenital sex. Vesicles appear at the site of inoculation (e.g., the vulva, vagina, or cervix) 2 to 10 days after inoculation. An individual with a primary infection may experience a prodrome of general malaise that precedes the development of genital lesions. Before the formation of vesicles, the area may become edematous, erythematous, and painful. Bilateral inguinal lymphadenopathy is common in those individuals who develop numerous lesions. The vesicles may be grouped close together and may coalesce to form large bullous lesions. The vesicles contain clear serum and tend to disrupt spontaneously, forming shallow ulcers with clean margins and red bases. If the vulva is not kept clean, the lesions easily become secondarily infected. The lesions persist for 7 to 21 days and resolve spontaneously. Viral shedding continues until the lesions become re-epithelialized. The patient with herpetic cervicitis and no other lesions does not experience pain; she may be totally asymptomatic or have a watery discharge.

During the symptomatic phase, the virus invades the epithelial cells, replicates, and ultimately destroys the host cell. On entering the host cell, viral DNA is exposed and host DNA-dependent RNA polymerase transcribes viral DNA, thereby coding for viral proteins and viral DNA, resulting in the synthesis of new herpesviruses. It is estimated that well over 100,000 copies of viral DNA are made per host cell, with approximately 20,000 being encapsulated, resulting in intact virus.

Resolution of the lesion is associated with the latent stage of the virus. Latency is thought to be accomplished by viral migration along sensory nerves, with ultimate residence in the sensory ganglion.

## Diagnosis

Approximately half the infants exposed to herpes during vaginal delivery will become infected. Approximately half of these infected infants will die, and half of the survivors will have severe sequelae.

Primary infection occurs in those individuals who have not been exposed to HSV-I or HSV-II. An individual can be primarily infected with HSV-I and HSV-II simultaneously. Clinical symptoms and signs of infection usually appear within 3 to 7 days after exposure; however, the incubation period may be 20 days. Lesions are usually multiple and are generally preceded by a prodromal phase characterized by headache, generalized aching, malaise, low-grade fever, paresthesia, and burning in the area where the vesicles are destined to appear. The patient may develop inguinal and pelvic lymphadenopathy, giving rise to pelvic and inguinal pain. Micturition may be accompanied by severe pain, resulting in urinary retention. Lesions may develop on the labia majora and minora, the perianal region, and the vaginal and ectocervical epithelium. The lesions appear as small vesicles, often in clusters, on an erythematous base. In moist areas such as the labial folds and introitus, the vesicles become unroofed within 48 hours and easily become secondarily infected (Fig. 7–1). Lesions on the drier areas of the vulva tend to remain vesicular for longer periods. The entire vulva may become edematous and erythematous.

If the cervix is involved, there may be a profuse watery discharge. The lesions may be few in number, usually appearing as small, erythematous, shallow ulcers. Occasionally, the cervix may be covered by a large, fungating, necrotic mass that may be mistaken for a malignancy. The lesions may last from 2 to 6 weeks. When healing has occurred, there is usually no residual scarring.

Recurrent episodes of genital herpes occur in approximately 66 percent of the patients during the first 12 months following the primary episode. Recurrent lesions are usually fewer in number, less severe, and restricted to small areas, and usually develop near the site of the primary lesions. Patients experiencing recurrent herpes may note a prodromal period beginning 24 hours before the appearance of lesions. The prodromal symptoms may consist of localized itching, burning, or hypersensitivity of the skin, as well as neuralgia and severe pruritus. Recurrent lesions may be minute and inconspicuous and, therefore, difficult to identify. The vesicles may become pustular and develop a crust. Reepithelization occurs in a few days to 3 weeks. Recurrences are less likely with HSV-I than with HSV-II. The frequency of recurrence tends to decrease with the passage of time.

The presumptive diagnosis of herpes can be established by Papanicolaou (Pap) smear, serology, or direct fluorescent antibody staining technique. A definitive diagnosis can be established only by isolation of the virus from a lesion. Fluid can be aspirated from a vesicle, or the base of an unroofed vesicle can be touched with a sterile swab and the specimen placed in transport medium. The specimen should be taken to the laboratory immediately or temporarily kept at 4° C. If it is to be stored for a prolonged period, it should be kept at −70° C. Rabbit kidney cells or similar tissue can be inoculated to determine if herpesvirus is present.

If the capability to culture HSV-I or HSV-II does not exist, then the Pap smear, fluorescent antibody studies, or antibody titer

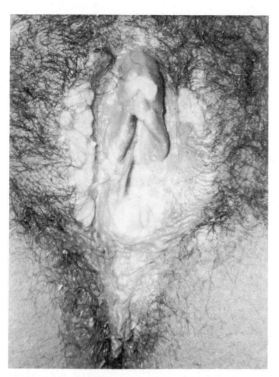

**Figure 7–1.** Herpes simplex type II. Large ulcerated lesions that have a thick purulent exudate. Lesions have become secondarily infected. Note white discharge exiting from introitus (patient also had *T. vaginalis* vaginitis).

determination can be done. The Pap smear or Giemsa stain can be used to detect the presence of multinucleated giant cells or intranuclear inclusions in host cells. These tests detect from 60 to 80 percent of genital infections. Serum antibody tests can be performed to determine if an acute infection has occurred; however, there is cross-reactivity between HSV-I and HSV-II. Antibody to HSV-I is usually acquired in childhood, and approximately 60 percent of pregnant women will have antibody to HSV-II; therefore, it is often difficult to establish the existence of an acute infection. Acute and convalescent sera should be obtained for determination of the presence of herpes antibody using paired sera. Herpes-specific IgM will remain elevated for several months.

The presence of type-specific antibody does not offer the patient protection against recurrent infection. Serum antibody determinations are of no value in the face of recurrent infection, because there is no elevation during the convalescent period.

## Treatment

The patient must be reassured that even though she has contracted a herpetic infection, she is not a social outcast; she can have a normal sex life and bear children, barring any infertility problem. The disease is manageable, and new agents are available that are promising.

The patient and her sex partner must be educated about herpes. They should be taught to recognize prodromal symptoms and signs of recurrent lesions. The male partner must also be made aware of how to examine himself. Patients should not engage in sexual activity if genital or oral lesions (Fig. 7–2) are present. Intercourse should be avoided for 10 to 14 days after the lesions subside.

When lesions are present, it is important that the vulva be kept clean and dry. If a vaginal discharge is present, this should be examined microscopically. Endocervical and urethral specimens should be obtained for the possible isolation of *Neisseria gonorrhoeae,* since sexually transmitted diseases tend to occur in conjunction. A serum venereal disease research laboratory (VDRL) test should also be obtained. If the lesion is solitary, or if there are only two to three lesions and they are not really painful, then a dark-field microscopic examination and Gram stain should be performed.

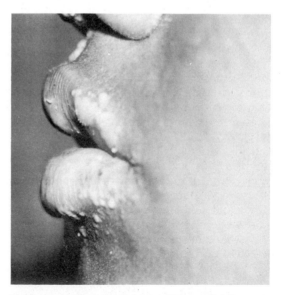

**Figure 7–2.** Herpes simplex. Note multiple vesicles on the lips; lesions are individual, and on upper lip have coalesced.

If the patient is having difficulty voiding, she should be advised to take sitz baths and void in the water. This will dramatically reduce the discomfort. If there is severe edema and urinary retention, a Foley catheter should be inserted. The vulva can be washed with povidone-iodine solution, which may also be used to douche, provided the patient is not pregnant. Such treatment will not facilitate resolution of the viral infection, but it will help reduce the possibility of secondary infection.

A number of treatment modalities have been tried, such as iodine, idoxuridine, neutral red dye and light, lysine, zinc, and 2-doxy-D-glucose; however, all have been shown to be worthless. Acycloguanosine (acyclovir [Zovirax]) and vidarabine are two newer agents that appear to be very promising. Acyclovir inhibits virus-specific thymidine kinase, blocking DNA synthesis. The drug has been shown to reduce the durations of lesions and viral shedding during acute primary infection. Acyclovir does not eliminate latent infection, but it can reduce the intensity of recurrent attacks.

Pregnant women with a history of herpes antedating the pregnancy, or who have their initial infection during the pregnancy, should be examined for the presence of lesions every week during the last month. (Routine culturing for herpes virus is of no value; to be beneficial, culturing would have to be done on a daily basis.) If there is clinical evidence of herpes when labor begins, the infant should be delivered by cesarean section. If the patient's amniotic membranes have been ruptured for up to 12 hours, cesarean section should still be considered. If the membranes have been ruptured for more than 12 hours, however, the patient should be allowed to deliver vaginally, if possible. The infant may then be treated with acyclovir.

If the patient has lesions on the abdomen, thigh, or buttock at the time she goes into labor, cervical and vulval specimens can be obtained for fluorescent antibody test. If the cervix and vulva are found to be free of virus, vaginal delivery should be attempted.

Postpartum management should be directed at preventing infection of the infant as well as all individuals coming in contact with the mother. Universal precautions should be maintained while caring for the mother and her infant. Premature and newborn infants are at risk for developing serious infection. If a patient understands the risks and wishes to handle her infant, she should cover all lesions, wash her hands, and put on a surgical gown and gloves. The infant should then remain with the mother and not be taken back to the nursery. All personnel should practice good aseptic technique while tending to patients with active herpes lesions. All bandages, dressings, perineal pads, and such materials, should be double-bagged and disposed of properly.

## RUBELLA

### Epidemiology

Rubella virus has no known animal vector. Transmission is from human to human, usually via the respiratory route. However, rubella is not as highly contagious as varicella or the rhinoviruses; therefore, a sizable population of susceptible individuals exists among unvaccinated women of childbearing age. This is perhaps the major reason for the high incidence of congenital rubella infection in an unvaccinated population.

### Microbiology

Rubella is a member of the family Togaviridae. It is an RNA virus with a characteristic protein capsid and lipoprotein envelope. Immunologically, rubella possesses a complement-fixing antigen and two precipitins. Of paramount medical importance is the hemagglutinating antigen on the viral envelope, which is the basis for laboratory antibody testing.

### Infection

Postnatal rubella infection is usually a benign disease. The hallmark of acute infection is the characteristic nonconfluent maculopapular rash that starts on the face and migrates caudally, lasting roughly 3 to 5 days. Desquamation may occur. In 30 percent of infections, however, the rash may be absent or clinically inapparent.

Concomitant findings include fever, malaise, posterior auricular and occipital adenopathy, and anorexia; arthritis and arthralgia also may develop, especially in adults. Viral shedding may occur up to 10 days before onset of the rash and for up to 15 days after its onset. The fact that the rash does not correspond with the peak viremia indicates that a possible immunologic mechanism is involved.

Maternal rubella infection in the absence of maternal immunity may be transmitted transplacentally with devastating results to the fetus, depending upon gestational age at the time of infection.

It is estimated that 50 to 90 percent of fetuses are affected by rubella if exposure occurs during the first trimester. Approximately one third of these cases result in spontaneous abortions, whereas the surviving affected fetuses may be severely compromised. Abnormalities such as deafness, psychomotor retardation, and microcephaly have been reported in offspring of mothers infected up to 21 weeks' gestation. A fetus exposed to rubella in the second or third trimester appears relatively safe. However, those exposed in the second or third trimester may develop subtle abnormalities that may be manifested later in life in a child who seemed normal at birth, such as childhood diabetes, thyroid disorders, precocious puberty, progressive panencephalitis, and "soft" neurologic defects.

## Diagnosis

Postnatal rubella infection is such a mild disease that clinical diagnosis is difficult. Many other viruses may cause similar signs and symptoms. The virus may be isolated from respiratory secretions or from the pharynx. Seroconversion, however, is the chief diagnostic modality. Hemagglutination inhibition is an easy-to-perform and sensitive method, commonly used in most laboratories. Hemagglutination inhibition antibody is long lasting and is therefore a useful indication of previous infection and immunity. It is first necessary to document acute infection conversion from negative to positive hemagglutination inhibition serology. If the initial (acute) sample is drawn too late, i.e., after hemagglutination inhibition antibodies have had time to develop, rubella-specific IgM may be measured, or complement-fixation antibodies may be used, because they arise later in the infection (4 to 8 weeks) than do hemagglutination inhibition antibodies.

The clinical manifestations of congenital (intrauterine) rubella infection (Table 7–1) are not unique to this virus. Therefore, docu-

**Table 7–1**

CLINICAL MANIFESTATIONS OF CONGENITAL RUBELLA INFECTION

| | |
|---|---|
| Intrauterine growth retardation | Seizures |
| Failure to thrive | Radiolucent long bone lesions |
| Cataracts | Bulging fontanelles |
| Glaucoma | CSF pleocytosis |
| Patent ductus | Deafness |
| Valvular lesions | Vestibular dysfunction |
| Septal defects | Mental retardation |
| Thrombocytopenic purpura | Micro-ophthalmia |
| Hepatosplenomegaly | Chorioretinitis |
| Hepatitis | Iridocyclitis |
| Motor delay | Chronic meningitis |

mentation of intrauterine fetal infection is derived from detection of rubella-specific IgM or viral isolation from the infant.

## Treatment

Prenatal rubella is treated symptomatically. Immune serum globulin may attenuate maternal symptoms but has not been proved to alter fetal infection. Immune serum globulin may be administered as a desperation measure (in the hope that it might alter fetal infection) should a woman decide against abortion after documented rubella infection early in gestation.

Immunization is the cornerstone of therapy. Vaccination is recommended at age 15 months for all children. Any nonimmune woman of childbearing age should be immunized if not pregnant, or vaccinated after delivery if susceptibility is discovered during pregnancy. It is recommended that a woman not become pregnant for 3 months following vaccination, because there is a theoretical risk to the fetus from the live-virus vaccine. In practice, however, no congenital rubella abnormalities have been documented in children exposed to vaccine *in utero,* although vaccine virus has been recovered from the conceptus in cases in which the mother opted for abortion.

Vaccination has reduced the incidence of congenital rubella syndrome in the United States. In the last several years, however, there has been a minor upswing in the annual prevalence of the disease due to deficient vaccination practices of modern American families. The Centers for Disease Control have recommended vaccination in preconceptual examination.

# CYTOMEGALOVIRUS

## Epidemiology

Cytomegalovirus (CMV) can be isolated from many body fluids, including blood, saliva, semen, breast milk, endocervical mucus, urine, and feces. In the United States, 0.5 to 2.5 percent of newborns may be infected at birth. In the neonatal period, 2 to 5 percent of infants are colonized with CMV by handling, breastfeeding, and other means of contact. By age 10 years, 10 to 30 percent of children show evidence of exposure to CMV. This figure rises to 20 to 50 percent for women during the childbearing years and 60 to 90 percent for individuals over 60 years of age.

## Microbiology

CMV is a member of the herpesvirus group, which includes herpes simplex virus types I and II, Epstein-Barr virus, and varicella-zoster virus, as well as numerous animal herpesviruses. CMV is a DNA virus that may invade the host's cells and insert its DNA into the host's nucleus, remaining latent only to be reactivated under the influence of, as yet, poorly understood stimuli.

Human CMV exists as many different serotypes, some quite antigenically diverse. Antigenic cross-reactivity usually exists between strains. Occasionally, a strain is rare enough to confound routine serologic tests. Additionally, a person may be primarily infected with one strain of CMV only to contract a separate strain of virus against which he or she has little or no protective antibody from the first infection. It is important to note that a woman may have more than one affected infant owing to infection by antigenetically different strains during different pregnancies.

## Infection

Primary CMV infection in adults is usually asymptomatic and clinically inapparent. Symptomatic primary infection in adults may take the form of a heterophil-negative mononucleosis syndrome, resembling Epstein-Barr virus infectious mononucleosis. There is usually less adenopathy and pharyngitis with CMV disease than with the latter infection; however, the epidemiology of the two syndromes is similar, with each being spread as a "kissing disease" among a fairly young population.

CMV infection may occur after blood transfusion. Seven percent of CMV seronegative individuals become seropositive following transfusion, resulting in a syndrome of fever, splenomegaly, and atypical lymphocytosis. Immunocompromised individuals, including transplant recipients, are at risk for a fulminating systemic form of the disease that may include chorioretinitis, encephalitis, and pneumonitis. A fatality rate of 80 percent or more is not uncommon. The source of the virus may be latent disease in the patient, transmission in the transplanted organ (especially with kidney transplants), or infection via blood transfusion.

Congenital CMV infection is a significant problem in newborn infants. Ninety-five percent of infants infected *in utero* are asymptomatic at birth. However, 5 to 10 percent of these infants go on to develop significant neurologic difficulties, such as hearing deficit, lower IQs, and chronic CMV shedding (usually up to 2 years, although cases of shedding for as long as 8 years have been reported).

In the minority of infants symptomatic from CMV infection at birth, the outlook is grave. There may be intrauterine growth retardation, jaundice, hepatosplenomegaly, microcephaly with severe mental retardation, chorioretinitis, and optic atrophy, intracranial calcification, seizures, and numerous other disorders. If the infant acquires CMV after birth, however, there is little ill effect other than occasional mild liver dysfunction, pneumonitis, and/or skin lesions.

## Diagnosis

Viral culture is the best method of viral isolation and identification. Nearly any body fluid may be cultured, and specimens may successfully be stored and transferred at 4° C (refrigerator temperature) for a week. Results must be interpreted cautiously, however. The virus isolated may be merely an agent of colonization, and not the organism responsible for the particular illness. Viral isolation from the amniotic fluid, however, is probably always significant, because the source is probably the fetal kidneys.

Serology for CMV is difficult to interpret. Although seroconversion in the face of characteristic clinical illness may make a good case for primary infection, there may be a significant number of false-positive and false-negative results, especially when different techniques are used. Other herpesviruses may cross-react with CMV. Also, if the infecting strain is antigenically distinct from the testing strains, there may appear to be no seropositivity. Additionally, viral shedding may wax and wane (as in pregnancy) with no change in antibody titer. In fact, the prevalence of CMV shedding in pregnant women increases with advancing gestational age.

## Treatment

Treatment for CMV is still essentially in the research stage. Chemotherapy with nucleic acid analogs has been shown to decrease viral shedding but not the clinical course in infected infants. Interferon has been shown to have little clinical benefit.

Active immunization with live attenuated strains (AD-169, Towne strain) has been shown to induce both humoral and cell-mediated immunity in volunteers. The risks of such vaccination (and colonization with live vaccine DNA virus) are as yet unknown. The subjects did not excrete virus, however. Passive immunization with large doses of human immune globulin has been anecdotally reported to help immunosuppressed patients with severe systemic disease. No extensive studies have conclusively documented consistent efficacy.

The mainstay of therapy is thus avoidance. Isolation of pregnant women from known CMV excretors seems to be indicated. However, the effect on the whole picture is probably minimal, because the virus seems to be a remarkably successful parasite living in a large reservoir of usually asymptomatic hosts, with no known animal vector to be controlled and no way to break the chain of transmission.

## VARICELLA-ZOSTER

### Epidemiology

Varicella (chickenpox) is a highly contagious disease, frequently occurring in children. Humans are the only natural host, and transmission is via droplets or direct contact. Zoster infections (shingles) may occur at any age but are more frequent in the older population. On reactivation of the varicella-zoster virus, migration occurs along a nerve, vesicles are produced along a well-demarcated dermatome, and the virus does not cross the midline.

Pregnant women who contract varicella infection during the first trimester have a 2 percent risk of having a child with congenital defects. However, data collected by the Collaborative Perinatal Research Study revealed a prevalence rate of only 1 in 7500 pregnancies. A total of 8 cases were found in 60,000 pregnancies, and none of these infants had evidence of congenital disease.

Sequelae from congenital infection include scarring from skin lesions, hypotrophy of limbs, atrophy of digits, psychomotor and growth retardation, and cortical atrophy. Maternal infection appearing in the last 4 days of gestation, including 48 hours postpartum, can result in severe, often fatal infection of the newborn.

### Microbiology

Chickenpox and herpes zoster are caused by the varicella-zoster virus, which is a member of the herpesvirus group. The varicella-zoster has a central core of DNA surrounded by a protein capsid that, in turn, is covered by a lipid-protein envelope. Unlike herpes simplex, there is only one serotype of the varicella-zoster virus.

### Infection

The incubation period following exposure to the varicella virus is from 12 to 18 days. A prodrome occurs in which the patient develops fever (from 38.3° to 39.4° C), myalgia, and malaise. Following the prodromal phase, a rash develops on the skin and mucous membranes that becomes vesicular. These vesicles appear in clusters and are pruritic. The exanthem is asynchronous in that all stages can be found—unlike variola, in which the lesions are synchronous.

The lesions seen in varicella and herpes zoster are indistinguishable; morphologically they are identical to the lesions seen in herpes simplex infection. The vesicles of varicella and herpes zoster are surrounded by an intense erythema of inflammation (Fig. 7–3) and contain straw-colored fluid. The vesicles of varicella appear in successive crops, first

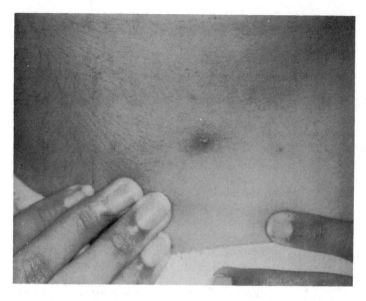

**Figure 7–3.** Varicella lesion. Note erythematous margin surrounding a pustule.

on the trunk, followed by the neck, face, and finally the extremities (Fig. 7–4). Vesicles appearing on the skin are usually painless, whereas those occurring on the tympanum, cornea, or mucous membranes are often painful. The rash may be mild or severe, as determined by the number of lesions.

The illness may be limited to several vesicles appearing in a simple crop, or the individual may experience recurring crops of lesions. Serious systemic disease may occur in the form of pneumonia, encephalitis, Reye's syndrome, glomerulonephritis, myocarditis, or thrombocytopenia.

Varicella pneumonia is an uncommon occurrence in children but occurs in up to 35 percent of adults who are infected with the varicella virus. Pulmonary symptoms begin with the onset of the exanthem. These may consist of nothing more than a mild, nonproductive cough that resolves spontaneously; in more severe cases, a high fever, chills, chest pain, nonproductive cough, hemoptysis, dyspnea, and cyanosis may develop. Approximately 10 percent of the patients who develop varicella pneumonia will have pleural effusions. Severely ill patients may also develop pulmonary edema, subcutaneous emphysema, secondary bacterial infection, and abscesses. Varicella pneumonia may result in pulmonary fibrosis and diffusion defects. The patient may develop calcific nodules that resemble healed tuberculosis lesions.

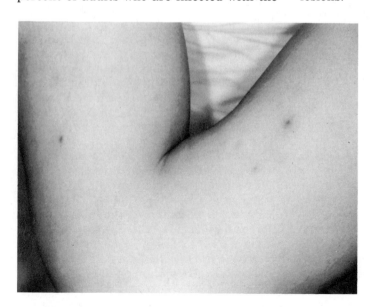

**Figure 7–4.** Varicella lesions that have formed a scab. Note also older healed lesions.

Varicella may involve the central nervous system, producing encephalitis, transverse myelitis, neuritis, and aseptic meningitis. Encephalitis is the most common neurologic complication, occurring more frequently in males than in females. Reye's syndrome (acute encephalopathy and visceral fatty degeneration) primarily occurs in children. The syndrome develops following many viral infections and may occur in up to 10 percent of the cases of varicella.

Congenital varicella is rare, and antepartum maternal infection has not been associated with an increase in fetal mortality or prematurity. Neonatal varicella occurring within the first 28 days of life is seen in 25 percent of neonates whose mothers acquire varicella 1 to 16 days before delivery. Approximately 20 percent of neonates who develop a rash 5 to 10 days after birth will die; however, no deaths have been reported among those infants who develop a rash within the first 4 days of life.

### Diagnosis

The diagnosis is usually made by the clinical presentation, especially if there has been exposure within the previous 3 weeks. Giemsa- or Wright-stained preparations from the base of a fresh vesicle will often reveal the presence of multinucleated giant cells characteristic of herpes and varicella-zoster infection. Direct fluorescent antibody staining of cellular material from a new vesicle is useful. Measurement of serum antibody, demonstrating a fourfold increase in varicella-zoster antibody titer, is useful, especially in mild or atypical cases. Complement-fixation antibodies appear within 4 days after the onset of the exanthem, and it is within this time period that acute-phase serum should be obtained; convalescent serum should be obtained 2 to 6 weeks later.

### Treatment

There is no specific therapy for varicella, and treatment is directed to alleviating the symptoms. Measures should be taken to prevent bacterial infection of the skin lesions; this can be achieved by having the patient bathe daily in warm water with an antibacterial detergent. Mild sedation and relief from pruritus can be accomplished by administering histamines.

In pregnant women with active varicella infection, signs and symptoms may be more severe than usual. In particular, varicella pneumonia may be quite deadly during pregnancy. Women with such an infection must be carefully watched, and if pulmonary decompensation is suspected, intensive care and intravenous acyclovir are indicated.

Varicella-zoster immune globulin administered within 3 days of exposure prevents varicella in normal children and attenuates the disease in compromised individuals. Disease may also be modified in exposed adults. Varicella-zoster immune globulin has not been shown to be of value in the treatment of pregnant women with varicella-zoster infection to prevent fetal infection, congenital defects, or abortion. However, many individuals recommend varicella-zoster immune globulin therapy for exposed pregnant women because it may attenuate any resultant maternal disease and because of its remote theoretic effect on fetal infection.

## HEPATITIS

There are three distinct viruses responsible for acute viral hepatitis: hepatitis A, also known as infectious hepatitis; hepatitis B, which is referred to as serum hepatitis; and non-A, non-B hepatitis, which was commonly referred to as post-transfusion hepatitis and is now known as hepatitis C. Hepatitis B is of major concern in pregnancy because of the possibility of genital infection and the risk of maternal chronic hepatitis.

### Epidemiology

It is estimated that the hepatitis A virus has an attack rate of approximately 80 cases per 100,000 population, with the highest frequency seen in individuals less than 20 years old. The hepatitis A antibody is present in approximately 24 to 64 percent of the adult population. The virus is transmitted by serum and feces, with the fecal-oral route being the most common.

Hepatitis B has been estimated to affect more than 300,000 individuals annually. The peak incidence occurs in the 15- to 24-year age group. The hepatitis B virus is prevalent among percutaneous drug users, individuals receiving blood transfusion, those requiring hemodialysis, and individuals who handle human blood, serum, and blood products. The virus can gain entrance to the body through any open skin or mucous membrane, or it may be transmitted via oral ingestion of infected material. The virus is hardy and may be transmitted on toothbrushes, baby bottles, toys, razors, eating utensils, or respirators and other equipment.

Hepatitis C has been observed more frequently over the last 10 years. The incidence is higher when blood is obtained from paid donors, though effective testing is now available to screen banked blood. However, it has been found that not all cases of hepatitis C are related to blood transfusions, but a route of transmission remains unknown.

## Microbiology

The hepatitis A virus is an RNA virus measuring 28 nm in diameter and is similar to the picornaviruses; the genome is a single strand of RNA enveloped by three polypeptides.

The hepatitis B virus is different from the hepatitis A virus. It is a DNA virus that measures 42 nm in diameter. The hepatitis B virus is antigenically complex. There are three main antigens, the surface antigen, $HB_sAg$; the core antigen, $HB_cAg$; and the "e" antigen, $HB_eAg$. The surface antigen ($HB_sAg$) is complex and consists of eight subtypes that are clinically important. The core antigen ($HB_cAg$) is associated with the Dane particle, which consists of the surface antigen, a lipid-containing outer envelope, and an internal nucleocapsid. The $HB_eAg$ is distinct from $HB_sAg$ and $HB_cAg$, and is present only in $HB_sAg$-positive sera.

## Infection

The incubation period for hepatitis A virus (HAV) is between 14 and 49 days, with a mean of 28 days. Infection with HAV results in lasting immunity against reinfection with HAV but offers no protection against hepatitis B or hepatitis C infection. The likelihood of percutaneous transmission of HAV occurring is low and is due to the relatively short incubation period and short duration of viremia. Approximately 2 to 3 weeks after infection, hepatitis A antigen ($HAA_g$) particles can be detected in feces. The titer of $HAA_g$ particles peaks coincidently with the elevation of serum glutamic-oxaloacetic transaminase (SGOT), and $HAA_g$ excretion becomes negative at about the time SGOT concentration peaks. Antibody to $HAA_g$ (anti-$HAA_g$) begins at approximately 5 weeks following infection and peaks at 8 weeks after infection. Anti-HA can be detected in the serum for many years following infection.

Hepatitis B infection may follow one of three courses: self-limited infection with transient serum surface antigenemia; self-limited infection without surface antigenemia; and persistent infection with chronic $HB_sAg$ carriage. Hepatitis B has an incubation period of 28 to 196 days. Individuals who develop a self-limited $HB_sAg$-positive infection usually have antigen detectable 42 to 84 days after infection. The $HB_sAg$ titer peaks at about 56 days after infection and begins to decline with the onset of clinical symptoms. Core antibody (anti-$HB_c$) becomes detectable with onset of clinical illness, and as the anti-$HB_c$ titer rises, the $HB_sAg$ titer falls. Serum antibody (anti-$HB_s$) becomes detectable approximately 2 to 3 weeks after $HB_sAg$ disappears. However, the anti-$HB_c$ rises and reaches its peak at this time and remains elevated for many years. Approximately 11 weeks following infection, $HB_eAg$ appears and the serum remains positive until the clinical illness resolves. Anti-$HB_e$ appears shortly after anti-$HB_s$ appears. Individuals with self-limited disease without surface antigenemia can manifest anti-$HB_s$ 24 to 84 days after exposure to HBV. The anti-$HB_s$ titer rises rapidly and may be detected for several years. Coincident with the rise in anti-$HB_s$, the serum becomes positive for anti-$HB_c$. Individuals who remain $HB_sAg$-positive for 20 weeks or longer are likely to develop persistent hepatitis and remain $HG_sAg$-positive indefinitely. Anti-$HB_c$ is present in all patients with persistent infection, and $HB_eAg$ is present in up to 50 percent of these individuals.

In hepatitis C, the time between transfusion and abnormal liver function is about 8 weeks. The infection results in manifestation of detectable antibodies, which are the target of much active research in the hope that hepatitis C will be as well understood as hepatitis B.

## Diagnosis

Clinically, it is not possible to distinguish between the various causes of viral hepatitis, although there may be subtle differences.

Initially the patient experiences fever, malaise, headache, anorexia, nausea, and vomiting. Patients who smoke usually develop an aversion to tobacco. The patient may develop hepatosplenomegaly, which is followed by scleral icterus, generalized jaundice, and pruritus, as well as cervical lymphadenopathy.

Prior to the onset of symptoms, the serum glutamic-pyruvic and serum glutamic-oxaloacetic transaminases (SGOT) become elevated, with the serum glutamic-pyruvic transaminase (SGPT) reaching greater than 1000 units/ml. The SGOT usually rises first and precedes the onset of jaundice by approximately 5 days, peaking prior to the onset of jaundice. The total serum bilirubin rarely exceeds 10 mg/100 ml and gradually falls over a 2- to 4-week period. The hematocrit and hemoglobin are usually not significantly affected. There may be a mild lymphocytosis. Urobilinogen and bilirubin are found in the urine.

The diagnosis of the specific viral hepatitis is established by the presence or absence of specific antigens or antibodies, or both, in conjunction with the clinical and laboratory findings. The diagnosis of HAV may be established on finding $HAA_g$ in the stool. However, a more common method is to demonstrate in serum the presence of acute antibody to hepatitis A antigen (anti-HA IgM) during the acute phase of the disease. The presence of anti-HA IgG in the absence of jaundice excludes HAV as the cause of illness. Serum should be obtained also during the convalescent phase and titers determined in conjunction with the initial specimen. A fourfold or greater rise in titer is indicative of active disease.

The diagnosis of hepatitis B can be established by serologic determination of $HB_sAg$, anti-$HB_s$, and anti-$HB_c$. Serum that is positive for $HB_sAg$ is indicative of active infection except in cases of conversion following blood transfusion. Serum that is positive for $HB_sAg$ and negative for anti-$HB_c$ in conjunction with the absence of $HB_sAg$ indicates past infection and immunity to HBV. Individuals who are seropositive for $HB_eAg$ are considered to be more likely to transmit infection.

Individuals who have $HB_sAg$-positive sera for greater than 20 weeks are at risk to develop persistent hepatitis. Chronic persistent hepatitis is usually asymptomatic. The SGOT and SGPT may be either persistently or intermittently elevated, and usually there is no jaundice. These patients have persistent mild hepatosplenomegaly and usually show no progression of their disease. However, patients with persistent hepatitis associated with chronic or episodic jaundice have chronic active hepatitis. These individuals have a guarded prognosis in that they may develop cirrhosis with hepatic failure and succumb to the disease.

Hepatitis C does not produce a detectable antigen or antibody in the patient's serum. The diagnosis is usually based on clinical findings, as well as the elevation of SGOT and SGPT and the absence of antibodies or antigens to HAV or HBV.

## Treatment

There is no specific therapy for acute viral hepatitis in either the nonpregnant or the pregnant patient. However, the liver of a pregnant patient in her second or third trimester is thought to be more susceptible to noxious liver stimuli. Therefore, if a pregnant patient is found to have a rising SGOT and SGPT, it is recommended that she be hospitalized with restricted activity until her liver functions begin to return to normal. Universal precautions should be followed to prevent transmission of the virus.

Immune globulin, immune serum globulin for hepatitis A exposure, and hepatitis B immune serum globulin (HBIG) should be administered shortly after exposure. Early administration of immune serum globulin or HBIG is capable of modifying or preventing the infection. HBIG should be given when direct exposure to HBV occurs via a needle stick or broken skin contact with blood, following sexual intercourse, or by exchange of saliva through kissing. The dosage of immune serum globulin is 0.02 ml/kg of body weight, with a repeat dose in 28 days. Prior to administering HBIG, blood studies should be obtained for measurement of SGOT and SGPT and presence of $HB_sAg$ and anti-$HB_s$. If the individual is negative for $HB_sAg$ and anti-$HB_s$, then HBIG should be administered. Sera should be obtained at 2 and 6 months after exposure for testing of SGOT, SGPT, $HB_sAg$, and anti-$HB_s$. Individuals who were initially positive for $HB_sAg$ and anti-$HB_s$ do not need HBIG.

Pregnant patients with antigenemia, i.e., those who are positive for $HB_sAg$ and $HB_eAg$, have a 90 percent chance of infecting their offspring. Infants born to these women should receive HBIG and be vaccinated. Mothers positive for $HB_sAg$ and anti-$HB_e$ have a 10 to 15 percent chance of infecting their infants; however, their infants should also receive vaccine and HBIG. $HB_sAg$-positive mothers should be advised not to breastfeed their infants. These women should be instructed in handwashing and other precautionary techniques to be used when coming in contact with their infants. There is no need to separate the infant and the mother; however, the infant should not be placed in the nursery with the other infants.

It is currently recommended that all pregnant women be routinely screened for $HB_sAg$ to identify those infants who need vaccinations at birth. Such a global screening and vaccination program should ideally prevent 90 percent or more cases of neonatal hepatitis B due to vertical transmission.

## MUMPS (PAROTITIS)

### Epidemiology

Humans are the only known natural host of mumps virus. The virus is spread via respiratory droplets, direct contact, or fomites. The peak contagious period is just prior to or during the initial attack of parotitis.

Ninety percent of mumps cases occur in individuals less than 14 years of age, although infants younger than 12 months old are usually protected by transplacentally acquired immunity. Women of childbearing age are unlikely to be susceptible, and the problem of prenatal exposure to mumps virus is not very common.

### Microbiology

Mumps is caused by a member of the paramyxovirus family, which includes the paramyxoviruses (mumps, parainfluenza, and Newcastle disease virus), the morbilliviruses (measles), and the pneumoviruses (respiratory syncytial virus). The virus consists of a nucleocapsid made up of a single strand of RNA surrounded by protein units that have RNA-polymerase activity. The nucleocapsid is surrounded by a complex envelope of glycoprotein, lipid, and nonglycosylated protein structures exhibiting various characteristic viral antigens.

### Infection

A nonspecific prodrome of fever, headache, malaise, and anorexia heralds the onset of clinical mumps after an incubation period of 2 to 4 weeks (usually 16 to 18 days). Parotid tenderness follows within a day or two. Over the next 2 or 3 days, the parotid glands enlarge rapidly, causing severe pain, with an accompanying fever as high as 40° C. Thereafter, signs and symptoms rapidly resolve over the next week or so.

Parotitis occurs in 60 to 70 percent of persons with mumps. Other salivary glands are affected perhaps 10 percent of the time. In addition, epididymo-orchitis may occur in up to 25 percent of postpubertal males and oophoritis in 5 percent of postpubertal females. The next most common manifestation of mumps is central nervous system infection. Approximately half of patients exhibit central spinal fluid (CSF) pleocytosis, whereas up to 10 percent have actual aseptic meningitis. Rarely encephalitis occurs.

Mumps infection during pregnancy has been a mildly controversial topic. Most reports of congenital malformations are anecdotal and not supported by findings of large cohort studies, which demonstrate a slight increase in fetal deaths associated with first-trimester maternal infection. Fetuses infected in the first trimester who do not abort are usually of low birth weight.

There is a suggestion that intrauterine mumps infection may be associated with endocardial fibroelastosis in the neonate. A high incidence of positive mumps skin test has been demonstrated in children with endocardial fibroelastosis. This is supported to some extent by chick embryo studies. However, because endocardial fibroelastosis and intrauterine mumps infection are both uncommon entities, the association is still very tenuous.

### Diagnosis

Mumps is commonly diagnosed by clinical examination. This is especially easy in cases of appropriate prodrome followed by obvious parotitis in a person with a history of exposure. If a case is atypical, or if extraparotid infection occurs that may be due to other viruses, virus may be isolated from saliva, urine, or CSF (if indicated) during the period from several days before until 4 to 5 days after the onset of clinical illness.

Serologic mumps testing demonstrates a fourfold rise in antibody titer, measured by hemagglutination inhibition, complement fixation, or neutralization tests. The hemagglutination inhibition test has a high rate of cross-reactivity with parainfluenza viral infections, and hence, must be used cautiously.

## Treatment

Therapy of mumps infection is purely supportive. There have been reports that injection of mumps immunoglobulin may reduce the incidence of orchitis in men. The patient should, of course, be isolated from susceptible individuals to prevent spread of the disease.

The cornerstone of mumps therapy is active immunization with live attenuated mumps virus vaccine. This is usually given to infants at age 15 months, in combination with measles and rubella vaccine. A single inoculation produces an antibody response in 95 percent of subjects. The vaccine should not be administered to pregnant patients, because it is a live virus.

## PARVOVIRUS B19 (FIFTH DISEASE)

### Epidemiology

The recently described parvovirus B19 is responsible for a ubiquitous and heretofore confusing exanthematous disease primarily infecting school-aged children. Classically, small epidemics occur, leading to an outbreak of absenteeism in local schools during winter and spring.

The virus is usually spread by droplet transmission, with an incubation period of approximately a week before viremia, which is followed by the characteristic rash. Among susceptible individuals, the transmission rate is roughly 30 to 50 percent, depending on the closeness of contact.

### Microbiology

Human parvovirus B19 is a small, single-stranded DNA virus of the family Parvoviridae. The virus was accidentally discovered in 1975, during laboratory studies of hepatitis B. (The nomenclature B19 is attributed to the virus' discovery as a contaminant in well #19 of the particular experimental run. The reader is therefore reassured that there are not parvoviruses B18, B20, and so on to worry about.) Genetic material is contained within an icosahedral protein coat. Some parvoviruses require coinfection with so-called helper viruses for replication. However, B19 does not have, as yet, a detectable helper virus.

### Infection

The usual syndrome of parvovirus B19, especially as it occurs in children, is the classic "fifth disease" or erythema infectiosum. A low-grade prodromal fever occurs about a week after exposure. Thereafter, the characteristic "slapped face" rash appears, giving way after several days to a more morbilliform or reticulate generalized rash. Subsequently, the rash may recur during periods of stress or exercise, lasting for a couple of weeks.

Adults with parvovirus infection tend to have a less extensive rash, exhibiting, rather, adenopathy and arthritis and arthralgia. Also, adults may experience several weeks of fatigue and depression after an acute infection.

Parvovirus B19 seems to have a particular predilection for erythroid cell lines, especially rapidly dividing cells. Apparently, this explains a particular manifestation of the disease in patients with a variety of hemolytic syndromes. If infected by B19, patients with sickle cell disease, hereditary spherocytosis, and other chronic hemolytic states often suffer acute aplastic crisis. Hematopoiesis is interrupted by the cytotoxic viral effect on rapidly proliferating erythroid precursors attempting to keep up with the patients' pathologically increased demand for red blood cell turnover.

Transplacental spread of parvovirus B19 is known to occur in roughly 33 percent of infected gravidas. Although the majority of infected fetuses are subsequently delivered without incident, fetal morbidity and mortality rates of 5 to 10 percent have been reported. In particular, a syndrome of nonimmune hydrops is present in many such cases, presumably owing to fetal aplastic crisis incited by the virus. The virus has been implicated as a cause of fetal myocardiopathy as well. Aside from fetal concerns, maternal illness is not appreciably different from B19 infection in the nonpregnant adult.

## Diagnosis

Parvovirus B19 may be isolated in laboratory culture or visualized by electron microscopy. Also, B19 DNA may be identified by DNA hybridization techniques. However, the most common and clinically relevant methods of diagnosis are clinical examination and serology.

Typical cases of fifth disease occurring in the course of a local epidemic usually present no diagnostic dilemma. However, for diagnostic accuracy or for academic purposes, or in the face of unconvincing clinical findings, B19-specific IgM antibodies may be measured. Although such antibody assays have been primarily available from the Centers for Disease Control, commercial laboratories are making such testing available in some areas.

Evidence of previous infection, and therefore immunity, may be documented by the measurement of B19-specific IgG antibodies. In most adult populations, 50 to 60 percent of individuals exhibit such immunity if tested. This is occasionally clinically relevant, especially if the patient is a pregnant woman who has been exposed to the virus.

## Treatment

The therapy of an otherwise uncomplicated case of fifth disease is supportive. No specific antiviral drugs exist as yet. Indeed, there is not even a B19 vaccine available. However, for patients suffering aplastic crisis due to parvovirus infection, blood product replacement is necessary.

The pregnant woman exposed to or contracting B19 infection poses little threat to herself; however, the fetus may be affected. Therefore, if available, the immune status of the mother is helpful in deciding whether or not she need worry about her exposure. On the other hand, mothers with clinical infection must be observed for evidence of fetal compromise.

A general protocol for longitudinally evaluating the fetus of an infected mother consists of serial ultrasonography beginning 2 to 3 weeks after maternal infection. If evidence of fetal hydrops is noticed (e.g., ascites, pericardial effusion), the infant is presumed to be severely anemic. If the fetus' gestational age is 34 weeks or older, delivery and postnatal transfusion are the usual course. However, in the fetus who is less than 34 weeks' gestation, intrauterine transfusion via funipuncture or paracentesis usually reverses the anemia and hydrops, allowing prolongation of the pregnancy and normal outcome.

As with any incurable viral disease, prevention of B19 infection is often the best form of therapy. It is difficult, however, to keep a patient away from suspect children for the duration of her pregnancy. This is certainly true if she has other children herself. School teachers in particular are often faced with the dilemma of a B19 outbreak among their pupils. Patients should be reassured that over half of them are already immune, and that the attack rate among susceptible individuals is about 33 percent. Therefore, the intrauterine transmission rate of roughly 33 percent places the statistical chance of fetal infection at less than 5 percent or so. And these infected babies are usually detectable by ultrasound and are amenable to therapy.

## CONDYLOMA ACUMINATUM

### Epidemiology

Warts in humans present either as condyloma acuminatum, verruca vulgaris, verruca plana, or verruca plantaris. The verruca varieties usually occur on the skin, whereas the condylomas tend to occur on mucous membranes. Although these lesions are seen worldwide and know no age, sex, or racial barriers, the obstetrician-gynecologist is the physician who usually treats patients with condyloma acuminatum. The specific concerns are the presence, number, and distribution of genital lesions, infection of the newborn, treatment of the pregnant patient, and possible long-term maternal sequelae.

### Microorganism

The human papillomavirus (HPV) belongs to the group papovaviridae, which causes condyloma acuminatum. The HPV is a small icosahedral DNA virus. The virus gains entrance to the host cell and enters the nucleus, gaining control of nucleic acid and protein synthesis. HPV can produce latent, chronic, and proliferative infection.

### Infection

Condyloma acuminatum is transmitted via direct contact, but fomites can also serve as a source of infection. However, the most common route of transmission is sexual intercourse. The incubation period is thought to be from 2 to 6 months.

The lesions begin as small verrucous or pyriform growths on the labia, fourchette, urethral meatus, vagina, cervix, perineum, or anus. The lesions may appear as flat or endophytic growths, with the verrucous form being the most easily recognized. Spread of the disease is accomplished by the formation of small seedling-like growths adjacent to the initial lesions. These verrucous-like growths enlarge, proliferate, and may coalesce to form large lesions that may replace the labia (Fig. 7–5). Proliferation is often associated with concomitant vaginitis, poor personal hygiene, use of oral contraceptives, pregnancy, and altered cell-mediated immunity. Condylomatous lesions occur more frequently in moist areas and thus have a predilection for mucosa or mucosa-like surfaces; they are rarely seen on the normally drier dermal areas.

Two problems have been raised in conjunction with condyloma acuminatum: the development of malignant change and the formation of laryngeal papillomatosis. Once the virus infects the cell, the host cell undergoes marked alterations, including alterations of the nucleus. An association has been made between the occurrence of cervical, vaginal, and vulvar carcinoma and condyloma acuminatum. Individual HPV types have been associated with dysplasia of these epithelial surfaces and frank squamous cell carcinoma. It is currently believed by many authorities that the vast majority of squamous cell cancers of the cervix arise due to HPV infection. The second problem that has surfaced is the development of laryngeal papillomatosis in offspring born to mothers with genital condyloma acuminatum at the time of delivery.

## Diagnosis

The greatest difficulty in making a diagnosis of condyloma acuminatum is realizing that not all lesions are exophytic, pyriform, or soft. The lesion may be flat or endophytic, and, therefore, may go unrecognized by the naked eye. The exophytic lesions are usually white, whereas the flat and endophytic lesions may not appear different from the surrounding tissue on gross examination.

The presence of condyloma acuminatum in the female should alert the physician to have her male partner examined. However, if the male patient is sent to a urologist who has no

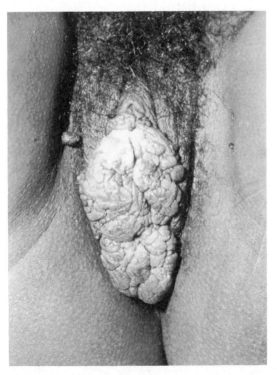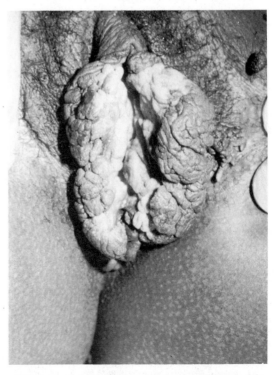

**Figure 7–5.** Condyloma acuminatum lesions have replaced the labia. This patient was delivered by cesarean delivery.

real interest in sexually transmitted diseases, he will conduct a gross examination that will more than likely be unrewarding. The male penis must be examined colposcopically, because the lesions are usually minute and are on the penile shaft. It should be remembered that if the female develops condyloma acuminatum, the virus must have been transmitted to her, and the most likely route is via sexual intercourse.

If the lesion becomes indurated or ulcerated or does not respond to treatment, a biopsy is warranted. If the lesions are flat, sessile, red or white, and generally do not resemble condylomata acuminata, a biopsy is indicated. It is important that the abnormal-appearing areas be biopsied before any treatment is begun, because agents such as podophyllin will cause atypical changes.

Often the only manifestation of genital HPV infection in women is the atypical or dysplastic Pap smear. Commonly, only routine colposcopy and biopsy alert the health care professional to the presence of HPV.

### Treatment

The pregnant patient with condyloma acuminatum poses several interesting challenges for the obstetrician. What modality should be used for treatment? Should the patient with genital condyloma acuminatum in labor be delivered by cesarean delivery?

The initial procedure in the treatment of the patient with condyloma acuminatum is the taking of a detailed sexual history. It is important to determine whether the patient practices oral-genital sex or anal intercourse, because the virus attacks any mucosal epithelium. If extragenital sites are involved but remain undetected, they will serve as foci for viral shedding.

If the pregnant patient has lesions on the cervix or vagina, they should *not* be treated with podophyllin. It should first be determined whether or not the lesions are secondarily infected. If they are, antibiotics should be employed. A culture should be obtained and Gram stained; commonly S. *aureus, S. epidermidis,* or perhaps a gram-negative bacterium is involved. An initial choice would be a first-generation cephalosporin. If there are a few small isolated lesions on the vulva, then podophyllin can be used. It should be noted that the chemical composition of podophyllin preparations varies from one batch to another. The half-life of podophyllin is from 1 to 4.5 hours. The toxic effects range from local irritation to acute systemic toxicity. The patient may experience dizziness, general weakness, emesis, diarrhea, hypotension, bradycardia, stupor, depressed respirations, progressive peripheral neuropathy, and depression of the bone marrow. Small lesions on the vulva, vagina, and cervix may be treated with either bichloracetic or trichloroacetic acid. The lesions in the pregnant patient are more vascular than in the nonpregnant patient, so if topical therapy is used, bleeding may occur. Small lesions on the vulva may be treated with electrocoagulation.

Patients who are pregnant tend to develop large cauliflower-like lesions that sometimes fill the vagina or replace the labia. In such cases, it is best to allow the patient to reach term and deliver by cesarean delivery. Following the pregnancy, the lesions will become reduced in size over a short period of time and can be managed more easily. Otherwise, cesarean delivery is reserved for the usual obstetric indications and *not* for prevention of fetal infection.

---

# Bacterial Infections

## SYPHILIS

### Epidemiology

Syphilis, caused by *Treponema pallidum,* continues to be a major sexually transmitted disease. The infection is transmitted by direct contact with an infected lesion, by accidental inoculation, or by blood transfusion from a syphilitic donor. Congenital syphilis occurs when there is maternal bacteremia, and *T. pallidum* crosses the placenta and infects the fetus.

Syphilis is most prevalent among those in the reproductive age group. The Centers for Disease Control estimate that there are probably more than 400,000 cases of untreated syphilis and only about 80,000 reported cases yearly.

### Microbiology

*T. pallidum* is a spiral bacterium that is 0.25 $\mu$m in diameter and up to 15 $\mu$m long.

The bacterium moves by an undulating motion as well as by a corkscrew-like rotation about its long axis. Identification of the bacterium is accomplished by dark-field microscopy of a serum sample obtained from a chancre, which enables the examiner to note the organism's morphology as well as its characteristic motion.

*T. pallidum* was once considered an anaerobic bacterium but is now known to use oxygen for growth and reproduction. The spirochetes require moisture and tissue for survival. The treponemes are destroyed by drying, water, heat, and disinfectants.

### Infection

*T. pallidum* gains entrance to the body through minute abrasions or by penetration of intact mucous membranes. Once the treponemes have entered the body, they enter the lymphatic and vascular systems. The incubation period from infection to development of the chancre is approximately 10 to 90 days and is dependent on the number of organisms present. An ulcerative lesion forms at the point of contact—usually the genital organs—but it may occur at other sites, such as the lips, oral mucosa, fingers, or anus.

### Diagnosis

The diagnosis of syphilis can be difficult at times. Syphilis has been referred to as the great mimic. There are three stages of syphilis—primary, secondary, and tertiary—which are related to the time of onset of the infection.

Primary syphilis is characterized by the appearance of a nontender, indurated, clean ulcer known as a chancre (Fig. 7–6). The ulcer contains numerous spirochetes and, therefore, is highly infectious. Primary syphilis is best diagnosed by the identification of spirochetes in serum obtained by scraping the surface of an ulcer, which is examined by dark-field microscopy. In the female patient, the primary chancre may go unnoticed because it is painless and may form between labial folds or on the cervix. Therefore a careful examination of the vulva, vagina, and cervix must be performed on all patients.

Secondary syphilis occurs after the spirochetes invade the tissues of the host—usually 8 to 10 weeks after the appearance of

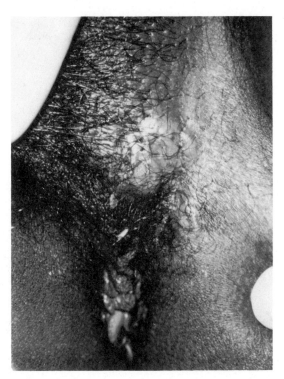

**Figure 7–6.** Primary chancre of syphilis. Note that ulcers appear clean with erythematous base.

the primary chancre, which generally disappears before the onset of secondary syphilis. The disease may affect every organ of the body, but the diagnosis is usually made on the basis of skin lesions. The cutaneous lesions may be varied, manifesting as macular, papular, papulosquamous, pustular, follicular, or nodular lesions (Fig. 7–7). It is because of this great variety of presentations that syphilis is referred to as the great mimic. The lesions often appear on the trunk and extremities as well as on the palms and soles (Fig. 7–8).

The patient may develop alopecia, which occurs in a random fashion, leaving patches of hair. The alopecia is temporary and resolves whether treatment is begun or not. In addition, the patient may develop symptoms of systemic illness. She may present with malaise, anorexia, headache, sore throat, arthralgia, and low-grade fever. She may also develop lymphodenopathy with large nontender, discrete lymph nodes.

Latent syphilis is categorized as either *early* latent syphilis, referring to disease of less than 4 years, or *late* latent syphilis, denoting disease of more than 4 years. Early latent syphilis is associated with relapses of

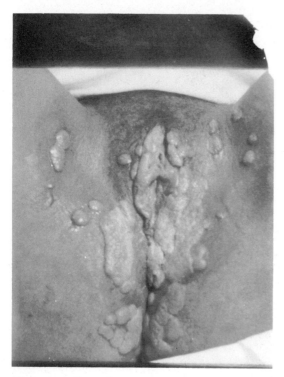

**Figure 7-7.** Secondary syphilis: anogenital condylomata lata.

mucocutaneous lesions if the patient is not treated and is infectious. Latent syphilis is present when the patient has serologic evidence of disease but has no clinical signs or symptoms of syphilis. She may or may not have a history of primary or secondary syphilis, and the cerebrospinal fluid may be normal. The diagnosis is established by obtaining positive results with the reagin serum test when repeated several times, together with a positive fluorescent treponemal antibody-absorption test. Diseases known to produce false-positive reagin tests, such as infectious mononucleosis, hepatitis, leprosy, systemic lupus erythematosus, rheumatoid arthritis, and sarcoidosis, should be ruled out. Late latent syphilis may be transmitted to a fetus *in utero* or to transfusion recipients.

Tertiary syphilis is a noninfectious destructive stage of the disease, manifested by gummatous (late benign) syphilis, cardiovascular syphilis, and neurosyphilis. The difficulty with this stage of the disease is that it can be present even though the serologic tests for syphilis are nonreactive. Gummatous syphilis is characterized by lesions that appear mainly on the skin but that may also develop in bone, liver, and the cardiovascular and central nervous systems. The cutaneous gummas appear as superficial nodules or punched-out ulcers. This stage of the disease appears in untreated individuals from 1 to 10 years after the initial lesions.

Cardiovascular syphilis occurs 10 or more years after the initial infection. The primary lesion is aortitis. The elastic tissue of the aorta is destroyed and replaced by fibrous tissue. The ascending and transverse segments of the aorta are primarily affected.

Neurosyphilis occurs within 5 to 35 years after the initial infection in untreated individuals. Early central nervous system involvement is usually asymptomatic. Because nontreponemal tests are nonreactive in one third of patients with neurosyphilis, a specific treponemal test should be done in patients suspected of having neurosyphilis. In asymptomatic neurosyphilis the cerebrospinal fluid is abnormal (i.e., >5 mononuclear cells/mm$^3$), total protein is >40 mg/100 ml, and there is a reactive (positive) Venereal Disease Research Laboratory (VDRL) test.

Neurosyphilis may present as a meningovascular and parenchymatous syphilis. Meningovascular syphilis includes meningitis

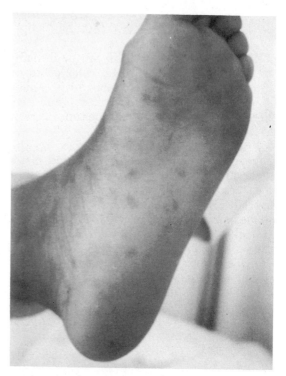

**Figure 7-8.** Rash of secondary syphilis: papular rash on sole of foot.

and central nervous system involvement resulting from cerebrovascular occlusion, infarction, and encephalomalacia. Parenchymatous syphilis includes syphilitic pareses and tabes dorsalis.

Pregnant women who contract syphilis may transmit the disease to their fetus at any time during the pregnancy. If the pregnant patient is untreated, approximately 25 percent of the fetuses will die *in utero,* 30 percent will die shortly after birth, and 40 percent of the survivors will develop late syphilis. The clinical manifestations of congenital syphilis can be divided into early disease (occurring before age 2) and late congenital syphilis (occurring after age 2). The earlier the onset of signs and symptoms, the poorer the prognosis. Active disease at birth is associated with a higher neonatal death rate.

Serologic diagnosis of syphilis can be established by reactive reagin or treponemal tests. The reagin tests are nontreponemal and are based on a modification of the Wasserman cardiolipin test; they include the following: VDRL test, rapid plasma reagin, automated reagin, and unheated serum reagin. The VDRL test and the rapid plasma reagin are the two most widely diagnostic nontreponemal tests employed in the United States. The treponemal tests use *T. pallidum* as the antigen and detect specific antitreponemal antibodies; these tests are performed for verification procedures. The standard test used today is the fluorescent treponemal antibody-absorption (FTA-ABS) test.

The nontreponemal reagin tests are the most commonly used diagnostic tests. The VDRL test becomes positive 1 to 3 weeks after the appearance of the primary chancre. The titer rises rapidly and reaches a peak dilution of 1 : 256. The titer then falls as the patient enters the latent stage of syphilis. After 10 to 20 years, the VDRL test begins to plateau and may remain at a dilution of 1 : 4 to 1 : 8. However, some individuals may develop nonreactive sera even in the absence of treatment. The FTA-ABS test becomes especially important in those individuals who are suspected of having syphilis but in whom the VDRL test is nonreactive. On the other hand, a positive VDRL test and a negative FTA-ABS test (i.e., a false-positive VDRL test) are often not indicative of any infection but of the presence of antiphospholipid antibodies such as lupus anticoagulant, which may cause adverse pregnancy outcome.

Therefore, false-positive VDRL tests indicate laboratory investigation in that direction, including a search for systemic lupus erythematosus and other collagen-vascular diseases.

## Treatment

Penicillin remains the treatment of choice for syphilis. Primary, secondary, and early latent syphilis can be treated with benzathine penicillin G, 2.4 million units given intramuscularly, or with aqueous procaine penicillin G, 4.8 million units, given as 600,000 units by intramuscular injection daily for 8 days. Patients who are allergic to penicillin can be treated with erythromycin, 500 mg orally 4 times daily for 15 days.

Late syphilis is best treated with benzathine penicillin G, 7.2 million units given in doses of 2.4 million units intramuscularly weekly for 3 weeks, or aqueous procaine penicillin G, 600,000 units intramuscularly daily for 15 days. Pregnant patients who are allergic to penicillin may be treated with erythromycin, 500 mg orally 4 times a day for 30 days. However, it is probably more effective to formally desensitize the mother with graduated oral doses of penicillin and then proceed with the usual benzathine penicillin therapy. The desensitization routine is generally done in the hospital (e.g., in labor and delivery as an outpatient) and takes roughly 4 hours. Of course, the patient is monitored for signs of anaphylactic reaction during this period.

Penicillin is highly effective in the treatment of syphilis; however, treatment failures do occur, and post-treatment follow-up is extremely important. Post-treatment follow-up is more important when an antibiotic other than penicillin is used. Individuals treated for primary and secondary syphilis should be monitored with quantitative VDRL measurements at 1, 3, 6, 9, and 12 months. Those patients with latent and late syphilis should be followed at 1, 3, 6, 9, 12, 18, and 24 months. Patients with primary syphilis who were adequately treated will have a negative titer within 2 years. Of those individuals with secondary syphilis, 25 percent will remain VDRL positive 2 years after treatment. In syphilis of less than 2 years' duration, the VDRL titer will decrease or stabilize at a low titer. Individuals with syphilis of more than 2 years' duration who are successfully treated will be seropositive and have a reactive VDRL test.

# TUBERCULOSIS

## Epidemiology

Tuberculosis results from infection by *Mycobacterium tuberculosis*. Transmission is by aerosolized droplets of liquid containing the bacteria, which are inhaled by a noninfected individual and taken into the lung. The bacteria become lodged in the alveoli, where they implant and cause infection.

Most individuals who contract tuberculosis are asymptomatic. Infected individuals are frequently detected by exhibiting a hypersensitivity reaction when subjected to intradermal injection of mycobacterial protein. In adults, the disease usually remains asymptomatic after the initial infection, and it is only years later that clinical signs and symptoms of infection occur. In recent years, with the increasing prevalence of AIDS cases, tuberculosis has been more common, especially in the inner cities where higher percentages of HIV-positive patients are found.

## Microbiology

*Mycobacterium tuberculosis* is an obligate aerobic, nonmotile, nonencapsulated, acid-fast bacillus. The bacteria do not readily take up stains and require heat to take up basic fuchsin dye. Once the bacteria are stained, they resist decolorization by alcoholic solution of mineral acids. The bacteria are slow-growing, requiring up to 24 hours to replicate. They are also resistant to desiccation and produce no endotoxin.

## Infection

Tuberculosis is primarily an infection of the pulmonary system. Infection of the female genital tract usually results from hematogenous dissemination from the pulmonary tract. However, if the gastrointestinal tract is the portal of entry, dissemination follows involvement of the lymphatics in the area of the cecum and terminal ileum. The fallopian tubes are the primary site of infection, which usually results in sterility. Approximately 2 to 5 percent of all cases of infertility are due to genital tuberculosis.

The pregnant patient with tuberculosis will most likely be asymptomatic. A noninfected pregnant or nonpregnant patient, who subsequently becomes infected, inhales droplets containing *M. tuberculosis*, which then become lodged on the surface of alveoli and are phagocytized by macrophages. It is within the macrophages that the bacteria multiply. Once the inflammatory response has begun, bacteria outside the macrophages also begin to reproduce and migrate into the pulmonary bloodstream, through which they are disseminated and may lodge anywhere in the body. Progression of the disease is noted by the development of tubercles and caseation necrosis.

Symptomatic patients may present with malaise, fatigue, loss of appetite, weight loss, and temperatures of 103° to 104° F (39.4° to 40° C). An increase in body temperature occurs in late afternoon and evening and is accompanied by night sweats. Patients in the initial stages of disease usually have no cough and produce little sputum. When the disease has progressed to the cavitary stage, the patient has a chronic cough and produces a mucopurulent sputum containing streaks of blood.

Congenital infection is rare but may occur following maternal bacillemia. Fetal infection follows thrombin formation in the intervillous spaces, which stimulates an inflammatory response in the adjacent placental tissue. Infection of placental tissue leads to fetal infection. The primary focus of infection in the congenitally infected fetus is the liver or regional lymph nodes.

## Diagnosis

The diagnosis of *M. tuberculosis* infection is established by isolating and identifying the bacteria. A tentative diagnosis can be established if typical acid-fast bacilli are found in smears of sputum. Infection may go unnoticed, because the primary infection is normally asymptomatic. The tuberculin skin test can be used as a screening procedure. A positive skin test indicates a history of tuberculosis and not necessarily active disease. The purified protein derivative skin test (PPD intradermal skin test, also known as the Mantoux test) is administered by injecting 0.1 ml in the dermis of a patient. A positive tuberculin reaction is characterized by an area of erythema and induration more than 10 mm in diameter forming within 48 hours. Patients with a positive PPD should have a chest roentgenogram if they are known converters or if the time of conversion is unknown and if the history or physical examination suggests disease.

## Treatment

Treatment of tuberculosis is based on the administration of one or more antibicrobial agents to prevent the growth of resistant organisms, and the therapy must be continued for a prolonged period of time. Chemotherapy for established or suspected active tuberculosis in the pregnant woman is similar to that in the nonpregnant woman. Prophylactic chemotherapy should be withheld during pregnancy and administered following delivery.

The recommended therapy regimen is isoniazid, 300 mg/day, plus ethambutol, 15 mg/kg/day. Isoniazid has been shown to be associated with a twofold increase in fetal malformations when administered to those with active disease. Pyridoxine should be administered concomitantly with isoniazid to prevent fetal neurotoxicity. Ethambutol is not contraindicated during pregnancy.

## LISTERIOSIS

### Epidemiology

Listeriosis is caused by *Listeria monocytogenes,* which is found in soil, water, sewage, and both domestic and wild animals, including birds, flies, ticks, and crustaceans. It is also transmitted via consumption of unpasteurized milk or contaminated meat. Approximately one third of the cases occur during pregnancy, and the disease can be transmitted transplacentally to the fetus. Infection in adults occurs most frequently in those over 40 years of age, and is associated with a mortality approaching 50 percent.

### Microbiology

*L. monocytogenes* is a gram-positive non–spore-forming bacillus. The organism is microaerophilic and motile, and causes hemolysis when grown on blood agar. When gram-stained in clinical specimens, the organisms may appear coccoid and are easily mistaken for gram-positive cocci. Listeria may be mis-

taken for *Corynebacterium, Erysipelothrix,* beta-hemolytic streptococci, or enterococci.

## Infection

Listeriosis is not manifested by any unique characteristics. The patient may be asymptomatic, have only genital colonization, or present with a flu-like or mononucleosis-like syndrome. Some patients present with high-spiking temperatures accompanied by back and flank pain. Others initially present with diarrhea and subsequently develop bacteremia. A patient may be totally asymptomatic but present with intrauterine fetal demise. If maternal infection is treated early, fetal infection may be averted.

Rupture of the amniotic membranes allows for ascending infection. Maternal fever is usually coincident with the onset of labor and the development of chorioamnionitis. In most instances, when the fetus is delivered and the uterus evacuated, the mother's clinical illness resolves. However, in some instances maternal infection may progress to meningitis. A careful history usually reveals that the meningitis was preceded by gastrointestinal disturbance or mild respiratory infection. Following the initial symptoms, the patient develops headache, myalgia, fever, chills, nausea, vomiting, and a stiff neck.

Fetal infection usually results in intrauterine death. Liveborn infants who were infected *in utero* frequently die within a week or two of birth. They develop cardiovascular collapse and respiratory as well as CNS complications.

## Diagnosis

Listeriosis is often not detected because of the lack of symptoms. Because *L. monocytogenes* is morphologically similar to *Corynebacterium,* cultures of the organism are frequently discarded under the assumption that they are diphtheroid contaminants. It would be beneficial to request that bacteriology laboratory personnel screen for listeria whenever culture arouses suspicion.

Gram-stained preparations that reveal small, short, gram-positive rods with rounded ends should arouse suspicion for listeria. The organism can be differentiated from other diphtheroids by its motility at 20° to 30° C. *L. monocytogenes* can be easily cultured from spinal fluid, blood, and urine.

## Treatment

*L. monocytogenes* is sensitive to penicillin, ampicillin, cephalothin, erythromycin, chloramphenicol, and tetracycline. Therapy should be continued for 2 weeks. The drug of choice is ampicillin, 40 to 60 mg/kg/day intravenously every 6 hours; or penicillin 300,000 units/kg/day, intravenously every 6 hours. Erythromycin, 60 mg/kg/day intravenously every 6 hours, may be used in patients who are allergic to penicillin. Asymptomatic colonization may be treated with ampicillin, 40 to 60 mg/kg/day orally every 6 hours. The isolates should be tested for antibiotic sensitivities, and patients should be recultured after therapy is complete.

## CHORIOAMNIONITIS

### Epidemiology

Chorioamnionitis is an infection of the chorion, amnion, and amniotic fluid. Approximately 1 percent of all pregnant women are at risk of developing chorioamnionitis, which is a major cause of perinatal as well as maternal morbidity and mortality. The histologic evidence of chorioamnionitis far exceeds the incidence of clinically manifested chorioamnionitis. In most fatal cases of fetal intrauterine bacterial infection, histologic chorioamnionitis can be demonstrated. Although chorioamnionitis is usually associated with premature rupture of the amniotic membranes, infection of the amniotic membranes and amniotic fluid has been demonstrated in patients with intact membranes.

Chorioamnionitis occurs most frequently in patients who are in labor and whose membranes have ruptured. Intrauterine infection may occur following amniocentesis or intrauterine transfusion; however, infection is most commonly due to the invasion of the uterine contents by members of the endogenous microflora of the lower genital tract. Organisms introduced from the external environment, such as *N. gonorrhoeae*, have also been implicated in chorioamnionitis.

### Microbiology

Infection is frequently caused by the bacteria that inhabit the genital tract; however, organisms such as *N. gonorrhoeae, L. mono-* *cytogenes,* herpes simplex virus, and cytomegalovirus have also been implicated in chorioamnionitis. Among the endogenous bacteria, *E. coli,* group B beta-hemolytic streptococci, anaerobic streptococci, and *Bacteroides* are frequently involved in chorioamnionitis. The isolation of *N. gonorrhoeae, L. monocytogenes,* group A or B beta-hemolytic streptococci, or *Staphylococcus aureus* should be considered evidence of pathogenesis.

### Infection

There are numerous gram-negative as well as gram-positive aerobic and anaerobic bacteria present in the lower genital tract. Many of these bacteria have the potential to be pathogenic. During pregnancy, the physiologic environment of the lower genital tract is altered, owing to the hormonal changes that affect the pH, glycogen level, and other local environmental parameters, and these changes, in turn, affect the normal bacterial flora with regard to growth and the ratio of one genus to another.

There are basically two barriers protecting the fetus against infection. The cervical mucus is a formidable barrier preventing the bacteria from advancing up the endocervical canal and thereby colonizing the amniotic membranes. The fetus and amniotic fluid are encased and protected by the amniotic membranes. Once the more pathogenic bacteria, such as *E. coli* or group B beta-hemolytic streptococci, advance up the endocervical canal, they may colonize the amniotic membranes and weaken them by enzymatic activity, thereby facilitating rupture or bacterial crossing of the membranes. Although the amniotic fluid contains bacterial inhibitors, the concentrations of these inhibitors in the second and early third trimesters are low, and, therefore, they may not effectively protect against the bacteria. In addition, the amniotic fluid contains glucose and amino acids, making it a good medium for the growth of bacteria.

Chorioamnionitis can lead to maternal or fetal infection. The fetus may become infected either by swallowing infected amniotic fluid, by inhaling the fluid, or by hematogenous spread from the placenta. If these organisms gain entrance to the lungs, the bacteria multiply in the intra-alveolar spaces, and the fetus develops an intra-alveolar pneumonia. If fetal infection begins with bacterial colonization of the fetal side of the placental circulation, venous vasculitis ensues and fetal septicemia may occur.

The development of chorioamnionitis with intact membranes has been reported with *L. monocytogenes,* group B beta-hemolytic streptococci, *E. coli,* and *Streptobacillus moniliformis.* In some instances, a hematogenous route is suspected, because the mother presents with a mild illness. However, in some instances the mother may be completely asymptomatic except for being in premature labor, and the site of origin of the bacteria is unknown.

Chorioamnionitis exposes both the mother and the fetus to serious infection. The fetus may develop pneumonia, sepsis, or meningitis. Women with chorioamnionitis who deliver vaginally are at relatively low risk of developing a postpartum infection, whereas those who deliver by cesarean delivery have a much greater risk of developing postpartum endometritis, peritonitis, septic pelvic vein thrombosis, sepsis, and dying.

## Diagnosis

The diagnosis of chorioamnionitis may be difficult to establish, especially during the initial stages, because the clinical diagnostic criteria are vague. The risk of maternal infection increases with the amount of time that has passed since the membranes have ruptured.

Initially, the patient may present in premature labor with intact membranes and no other findings. Often, these individuals are at less than 34 weeks' gestation, and tocolytic agents as well as corticosteroids are administered. It would be prudent to determine whether infection is present before embarking on such a course. Amniocentesis may be attempted in order to have the amniotic fluid Gram stained and cultured for aerobic and anaerobic bacteria. If bacteria are seen in the Gram-stained preparation, a tentative diagnosis of chorioamnionitis can be established. Bacterial growth is accompanied by the release of pyrogens and endotoxins that will cause maternal fever and tachycardia. This is also reflected in a rise in the fetal heart rate. Progression of the infection will be manifested by the development of uterine tenderness and a discharge that may be purulent or malodorous. The presence of a foul odor is characteristic of an anaerobic infection.

## Treatment

If amniotic fluid can be obtained via amniocentesis or by intrauterine aspiration, it should be cultured for aerobic and anaerobic bacteria. If fluid cannot be obtained, which is frequently the case when the membranes have ruptured, an endocervical specimen should be obtained for the culture and identification of *N. gonorrhoeae,* group B beta-hemolytic streptococci, *L. monocytogenes, H. influenzae,* and *Chlamydia trachomatis.*

Once the diagnosis is established, antibiotic therapy should be instituted. Many patients who deliver vaginally with mild chorioamnionitis have spontaneous resolution of their infection following delivery. However, whether the mother's infection is mild or severe, it is clear from recent studies that neonates fare better in the nursery if the mother is treated before delivery (Gibbs and Duff, 1991).

The newer broad-spectrum antibiotics, such as mezlocillin, piperacillin, ticarcillin, timentin (ticarcillin plus clavulanic acid), unasym (ampicillin plus sulbactum), and cefoxitin, are effective against gram-positive and gram-negative aerobic and anaerobic bacteria. Clavulanic acid and sulbactum are β-lactomase inhibitors, thereby increasing the spectrum of activity of ticarcillin and ampicillin. The addition of these β-lactamase inhibitors makes the parent antibiotic more effective against gram-negative facultative and obligate anabolic bacteria. These antibiotics have an advantage in that they may be used as single agents that have less serious toxicity than do combinations of antibiotics that include the aminoglycosides. Antibiotics cross the placenta and achieve peak levels in the fetal circulation within an hour after parenteral administration to the mother. Antibiotics also enter the amniotic fluid but at a slower rate. The concentration is often below therapeutic levels.

One very critical aspect in the management of chorioamnionitis is delivery of the fetus, because this drains the uterus of infected material and allows for treatment of the fetus. The tendency is to want to deliver the fetus immediately; however, this often means a cesarean delivery, which places the mother at a risk for serious postpartum infection. If the patient's labor is effective and she is making progress, and there is no evidence of fetal distress, then she should be allowed to deliver via the vaginal route, while being closely observed for the progression of infection during labor.

If the patient is not in active labor, or if she has a dysfunctional labor pattern or fails to make adequate progress, an attempt should be made to establish a good labor pattern. If this fails, or if there are additional obstetric indications, cesarean delivery should be performed. It should be pointed out that, as the infection progresses and the myometrium is invaded, the muscle loses its capacity to contract effectively and a dysfunctional labor ensues. These patients are also at risk for severe postpartum uterine atony. In the postpartum period, the patient may develop a serious endomyoparametritis, bacteremia, and sepsis. The patient who develops extensive infection, myometritis, and necrosis may require a cesarean hysterectomy.

## GENITAL MYCOPLASMAS

### Epidemiology

The actual epidemiology of the mycoplasmas is extremely difficult to delineate. It is known that these organisms inhabit the vagina and urethra and are sexually transmissible. However, carriage rates in asymptomatic women may be as high as 60 percent for *Mycoplasma hominis* and 80 percent for *Ureaplasma urealyticum*. Therefore, the exact relationship of carriage to disease, and the usual methods of spread, are nebulous.

### Microbiology

The mycoplasmas and *U. urealyticum* are bacteria that lack cell walls. They divide by binary fission and constitute one of the smallest groups of cellular microorganisms; highly pleomorphic, they can pass through filters that retain bacteria and are considered to be gram negative.

### Infection

Genital mycoplasma infection during pregnancy is thought to take the form of chorioamnionitis, postabortal fever, and postpartal fever. In some studies, however, women who were thought to have mycoplasma infections recovered even without antibiotics. Mycoplasmas have also been iso-

lated from the blood of pregnant women who were completely afebrile.

### Diagnosis

Both *U. urealyticum* and *M. hominis* may be grown on appropriate artificial media. A patient presenting with dysuria and pyuria, but with negative routine bacterial cultures, is a prime suspect for *Mycoplasma, Ureaplasma,* or *Chlamydia* urethritis. In the absence of the capability to culture for these organisms, treatment may be initiated empirically.

### Treatment

The mycoplasmas do not respond to the β-lactam antibiotics, since they have no cell walls. Tetracycline and related drugs are usually effective against most clinically important species. Erythromycin is effective against *U. urealyticum*, whereas lincomycin is effective against *M. hominis*. Erythromycin is the antibiotic of choice for the pregnant patient.

## CHLAMYDIA

### Epidemiology

A variety of diseases have been associated with *C. trachomatis*. Besides trachoma and neonatal conjunctivitis, lymphogranuloma venereum has long been known to be caused by certain serotypes of *C. trachomatis*. Recently, a syndrome of infant pneumonitis and several forms of urogenital infection have been described.

The common thread in many forms of *C. trachomatis* infection is genital carriage and sexual transmission. Asymptomatic male and female carriers probably serve as a reservoir and pass the organism by sexual contact. Further, genital carriage by the pregnant woman at parturition serves to colonize the infant, leading to conjunctivitis. If the infant's tracheal tree is similarly colonized, pneumonitis may result.

### Microorganism

*C. trachomatis* is a bacterium. It contains both DNA and RNA, divides by binary fission, stains gram negative, and is susceptible to antibiotics. It is an obligate intracellular parasite that depends on the host cell for a supply of ATP. *C. trachomatis* exists as multiple serotypes. Endemic trachoma is caused by types A, B, Ba, and C. Serotypes De, E, F, G, H, I, J, and K produce infant disease and the urogenital syndromes. Lymphogranuloma venereum is produced by the somewhat different, more invasive serotypes $L_1$, $L_2$, and $L_3$.

## Infection

Chlamydia preferentially infects columnar epithelial cells in the human, primarily because these cells have specific receptors that cause the chlamydial organism to bind to them. The human disease syndromes are, therefore, diseases of columnar epithelium.

Neonatal conjunctivitis has been associated with chlamydia, as well as with gonorrhea. The conjunctivitis usually begins within days of birth and is relatively self-limiting, unlike the progressive lesions of endemic trachoma. Colonization of the nasopharynx at birth may lead to the development of a characteristic diffuse pneumonitis in the infant that usually manifests by 4 to 6 weeks of age. In most cases, the mother harbors the organism in the endocervix.

The urogenital syndromes associated with *C. trachomatis* include cervicitis, epididymitis, and urethritis. Many cases of the acute urethral syndrome in women, as well as nongonococcal urethritis, are apparently caused by chlamydia. Another important site of chlamydial disease is the columnar epithelium of the fallopian tubes. Acute salpingitis is said to be a major complication of chlamydial colonization in some parts of the world.

The pregnant uterus is at risk for chlamydial infection. Chlamydial colonization increases the risk of pelvic infection after elective abortion. Severe puerperal infection associated with *C. trachomatis* has been reported after cesarean delivery, and a syndrome of late (up to 6 weeks) postpartum endometritis after vaginal delivery has been attributed to the organism.

Maternal cervical carriage of *C. trachomatis* has been reported to be as high as 23 percent in some groups of patients. Preliminary data suggest that pregnancies complicated by chlamydial infection may have a poor outcome (i.e., stillbirth, premature delivery, abortion) in up to 10 times the usual rate of cases.

## Diagnosis

Because chlamydia are intracellular parasites, they can be propagated only in cell culture. After suitable growth and processing, the cells are stained with iodine, enhancing the visibility of the intracellular inclusion bodies, which are then easily seen under the light microscope.

Chlamydial infection may occasionally be documented by a Giemsa or Wright stain of clinical materials. Also a Pap smear may reveal characteristic inclusions in exfoliated cells. Both of these methods are fraught with error and are not standard diagnostic techniques. Infection may be assumed to have occurred if acute and convalescent paired sera show a fourfold rise in titer.

Several rapid tests are available that enable the physician to make a diagnosis prior to the patient leaving the clinic. Abbott Laboratories has two tests, the Chlamydia Test Pack and Chlamydiazyme. There are also other rapid tests such as the Syva Monofluronescent Antibody test in addition to other tests. The Abbott rapid Chlamydia Test Pack can be performed in an office setting with the results obtained within 30 minutes. This type of test allows the physician to treat the patient during the initial visit, therefore making it unnecessary for the patient to return for treatment.

## Treatment

*In vitro* and *in vivo* studies have shown that *C. trachomatis* is sensitive to tetracyclines, erythromycin, sulfonamides, and rifampin. The Centers for Disease Control recommend therapy with tetracycline, 500 mg orally 4 times per day for 7 days in cases of urogenital disease. Doxycycline is administered as follows: 100 mg orally, twice daily for 7 days. Ofloxacin, is given in a dosage of 400 mg orally, twice daily for 7 days. Both doxycycline and ofloxacin, as well as other quinolines and tetracyclines, are contraindicated during pregnancy and for breast-feeding mothers. Erythromycin may be substituted for tetracycline and ofloxacin, 500 mg orally 4 times per day. Pregnant patients who cannot tolerate erythromycin can be treated with ampicillin, 500 mg orally four times per day for 7 days or amixicillin, 500 mg orally three times per day for 7 days. Individuals allergic to penicillin and who have gastric disturbance with erythromycin can be treated with clindamycin, 300 mg orally, three times per day for 7 days.

## GONORRHEA

### Epidemiology

Nearly 3 million cases of gonorrhea occur in the United States annually, an estimate based on the more than 1 million cases actually reported. The majority of cases of gonorrhea are contracted by sexual contact, including oral, genital, and rectal contact. Vertical transmission from mother to infant also may occur. The incidence of *N. gonorrhoeae* isolation during pregnancy varies from population to population and may range from less than 5 percent to over 15 to 20 percent.

### Microbiology

*N. gonorrhoeae* is a gram-negative coccus that classically occurs within leukocytes and in pairs in clinical specimens. The organism is grown on Thayer-Martin medium, with chocolate agar combined with various antibiotics added to inhibit overgrowth by other, less fastidious organisms. The gonococcus may be differentiated from the other *Neisseria* species, such as *N. meningitidis,* by carbohydrate fermentation tests.

There may be some relation between auxotype, antibiotic sensitivity, and clinical virulence among gonococci. Evidence indicates that the strains that are most likely to be invasive are also more likely to show antibiotic resistance and have fewer requirements for the various amino acids in auxotyping.

### Infection

*N. gonorrhoeae* infection during pregnancy usually consists of subclinical cervical colonization, because of blockage by the pregnancy of the usual route of access by the organism to the fallopian tubes. The gonococcus possesses surface receptors that allow it to attach to the surfaces of the columnar epithelium of the endocervix. The major areas of primary colonization of the body are the cervix, urethra, pharynx, rectum, and conjunctiva.

The pregnant woman with gonococcal cervical colonization is at risk for several different syndromes. Cervical inflammation and weakening of the neighboring fetal membranes may cause premature rupture of membranes and place the fetus at risk for premature delivery, or infection if delivery is delayed. During labor and delivery, chorioamnionitis and subsequent postpartum endomyoparametritis may develop, occasionally accompanied by bacteremia. In the era before antibiotics, deaths due to gonococcal sepsis, and such entities as gonococcal endocarditis, were common.

If the patient is colonized with *N. gonorrhoeae,* which remains relatively asymptomatic for a long period of time, she seems to be at risk for developing the syndrome known as disseminated gonococcal infection. Pregnant women seem to be especially at risk for disseminated gonococcal infection, possibly because they remain asymptomatically colonized; i.e., they are not likely to develop salpingitis. The main clinical presentation during pregnancy is infectional arthritis or tenosynovitis, accompanied by fever, malaise, and often a fine papular, erythematous rash, especially on the extremities. These women may be colonized by the organism on the cervix, urethra, rectum, or pharynx, or combinations thereof. However, it is difficult to isolate the gonococcus from the joint fluid or skin.

### Diagnosis

Clinical materials suspected of harboring *N. gonorrhoeae* should be immediately plated on Thayer-Martin medium and placed in an environment enriched with carbon dioxide, e.g., a candle jar, as soon as possible. Prolonged exposure to air or cold temperatures causes a decrease in yield. All clinical specimens should be Gram stained in an attempt to demonstrate the gram-negative diplococci that characteristically occur within polymorphonuclear leukocytes. This not only gives immediate information on which to initiate patient therapy but also serves to augment the results of formal cultures, should they fail to grow for the reasons mentioned above.

## Treatment

*N. gonorrhoeae* that does not produce penicillinase is still very sensitive to penicillin. The recommended therapy for uncomplicated urethritis or cervicitis is aqueous procaine penicillin, 4.8 million units intramuscularly in two divided doses, accompanied by probenecid, 1.0 g orally. Alternative therapy is ampicillin, 3.5 g orally at one sitting, or amoxicillin, 3.0 g orally; both of these agents are given with probenecid. The patient who is allergic to penicillin is usually treated with tetracycline or doxycycline; however, both of these are contraindicated during pregnancy. The penicillin-allergic pregnant woman with uncomplicated colonization should receive spectinomycin, 2.0 g intramuscularly.

Penicillinase-producing gonococci may be treated with ceftriaxone, 250 mg intramuscularly, given once. Alternative choices are spectinomycin, 2.0 g intramuscularly and either cefoxitin, 2.0 g intramuscularly, or cefotaxime, 1.0 g intramuscularly, each in combination with 1.0 g of oral probenecid. These regimens are often ineffective against pharyngeal colonization, however, Pharyngeal infection with penicillinase-producing strains may be treated with 9 tablets of trimethoprim-sulfamethoxazole (80 mg/400 mg), although it should be noted that trimethoprim has not been approved for use in pregnancy.

Pregnant patients with disseminated gonococcal infection must be hospitalized for initial therapy. Several treatment regimens may be used; aqueous crystalline penicillin, 10 million units intravenously per day until improvement, followed by amoxicillin or ampicillin, 500 mg orally four times a day for at least a week of total antibiotic therapy; or erythromycin, 500 mg orally four time daily for 7 days (for penicillin-allergic patients).

Neonatal ophthalmic prophylaxis may be accomplished with ocular deposition of 1 percent silver nitrate drops, tetracycline ointment, or erythromycin ointment. Systemic infection or actual conjunctivitis, however, should be treated with aqueous crystalline penicillin in appropriate newborn dosages or cefotaxime if the organism is known or thought to be penicillinase producing.

## POSTPARTUM ENDOMETRITIS

### Epidemiology

The vast majority of cases of postpartum endometritis occur following operative delivery, usually cesarean delivery. Although in most populations the endometritis rate following vaginal delivery is less than 5 percent, postcesarean endometritis rates may be as high as 60 to 80 percent in selected populations of patients.

Risk factors for postpartum endometritis include both endogenous factors, such as low socioeconomic status, anemia, and undernutrition (the "poor protoplasm" factors), and exogenous factors (usually associated with cesarean delivery), such as the use of general anesthesia and indwelling catheters. The risk factors for endometritis are listed in Table 7–2.

### Microbiology

Multiple bacteria are usually isolated from the uterine cavity of women with postpartum endometritis. Even when care is taken to prevent cervical and vaginal contamination, specimens usually contain three or more types of general bacteria. Both aerobes and anaerobes are isolated. Thirty percent of cases have only aerobic and 30 percent only anaerobic species isolated. The remaining patients have a mixed aerobic/anaerobic flora. The most frequently isolated bacteria are listed in Table 7–3.

**Table 7–2**
ENDOMETRITIS RISK FACTORS

Operative delivery
General anesthesia
Rupture of membranes (≥6 hours pre-op)
Multiple cervical exams
Prolonged labor
Indwelling catheter
Low socioeconomic status
Anemia
Poor nutrition
Cervicitis
Urinary tract infection
Amnionitis
Colonization (e.g., group B β-hemolytic streptococcus)

**Table 7–3**
BACTERIOLOGY OF ENDOMETRITIS

| Aerobes | Anaerobes |
| --- | --- |
| *Escherichia coli* | *Peptostreptococcus* spp. |
| *Proteus mirabilis* | *Peptococcus* spp. |
| *Streptococcus agalaciae* | *Bacteroides bivius* |
| *Streptococcus faecalis* | *Bacteroides desiens* |
| *Neisseria gonorrhoeae* | *Bacteroides* |
| *Klebsiella* spp. | *melaninogenicus* |
| *Citrobacter* spp. | *Bacteroides fragilis* group |
| | *Fusobacterium* |

## Infection

Bacterial colonization of the endometrial cavity following delivery is unavoidable. However, the magnitude of colonization—i.e., the numbers of organisms present—is related to the length of labor and the amount of time elapsed between rupture of the membranes and the time of delivery; another factor is the degree of manipulation involved in delivery (e.g., use of forceps, manual removal of placenta). In addition, impairment or destruction of natural defenses, such as by immunocompromise due to poor nutrition or by breech of tissue barriers due to cesarean delivery, aids in the establishment of infection rather than mere surface colonization.

Bacteria are likely to colonize and infect areas of the uterus that have been denuded or damaged, notably the placental attachment site and any cervical or lower segment lacerations and abrasions. Cesarean delivery introduces additional variables: the uterine incision, a foreign body (i.e., the suture material), tissue strangulation, and relative hypoxia.

If the development of endometritis is followed by extension of infection into myometrial tissues through lymphatics and large venous channels, endomyometritis is produced. Bacteria can further disseminate, via the same pathways, into the broad ligaments, paracervical tissues, and adnexae, resulting in endomyoparametritis. At any point in this progression, but depending in large part on host factors and the virulence of the bacteria, microorganisms may gain entry into the bloodstream (bacteremia).

If untreated or improperly treated, postpartum infection, especially endomyoparametritis, may progress to diffuse pelvic cellulitis, pelvic peritonitis, pelvic abscess, and on to disseminated intra-abdominal infection. In any stage of the disease after cesarean delivery, wound infection is not uncommon, in part, because many of the risks and predisposing factors are the same for the two entities.

## Diagnosis

Postpartum endometritis is not difficult to diagnose. Common initial findings include elevated temperature, mild to moderate tachycardia, and uterine tenderness. If pelvic peritonitis is present, lower abdominal rebound tenderness will be evident.

The initial examination is extremely important in the evaluation of a patient with fever during the puerperium. A general physical examination should be performed, with emphasis on the lungs (to rule out pneumonia, especially after general anesthesia) and the cardiovascular system (tachycardia, bounding pulse, weak pulse, elevated or decreased blood pressure). The general abdominal examination should be directed at the presence of rebound and direct tenderness, the size and firmness of the uterine fundus, and the status of the abdominal incision, if present. Specific attention should be directed to any incision that is overtly bloody or leaking any fluid (serum, pus), indurated, erythematous, or unusually tender. Needle aspiration of the wound may be attempted in an effort to locate a seroma, hematoma, or abscess in a suspicious wound.

Cultures should be obtained from the endometrium (with as little cervicovaginal contamination as possible), venous blood, catheterized urine specimen, wound exudate or discharge, if present, and sputum, if indicated. All specimens should be processed aerobically and anaerobically. It is important to remember that *N. gonorrhoeae* is a common puerperal pathogen in certain patient populations. In such persons, it is a good idea to plate all genital specimens on Thayer-Martin medium as well as on the routine media.

## Treatment

Postpartal endometritis is usually due to infection by the aerobic and anaerobic flora of the lower genital tract; therefore, antibiotic therapy should be directed against these bacteria. In the patient with moderate to severe infection, initial therapy with a broad-spectrum agent that has a reasonable anaerobic spectrum and also activity against the Enterobacteriaceae is recommended. Suitable antimicrobial agents are the second-generation cephalosporins, such as cefoxitin; third-generation cephalosporins, such as moxalactam, cefotaxime, and cefoperazone; and the expanded-spectrum penicillins, such as ticarcillin, mezlocillin, piperacillin, ticarcillin and clavulanic acid (timentin), and ampicillin and sulbactam (unasyn). In the case of a patient who is seriously allergic to penicillin, a combination regimen employing either clindamycin or metronidazole plus an aminoglycoside may be substituted. These combinations tend to be more difficult to use, because serum levels of aminoglycosides should be monitored to avoid toxicity.

Initial therapy with single antibiotic agents or the combinations listed above cures approximately 90 percent of patients with moderate to severe infection. Failures after treatment with the cephalosporin drugs or the combinations are often due to resistant strains of enterococci, requiring the addition of penicillin or ampicillin to effect cure. Failures with the expanded-spectrum penicillins are most often due to resistant gram-negative facultative organisms and respond to the addition of an aminoglycoside. Before adding any other antibiotics, however, the physician should thoroughly reexamine the patient to rule out abscess formation and document that persistent fever and other signs are truly due to continuing endometritis rather than to such entities as drug fever or septic pelvic vein thrombophlebitis.

## PNEUMONIA

### Epidemiology

Pneumonia may be caused by a number of infectious organisms, including viruses and bacteria. Most of these agents produce pneumonia in a sporadic manner, and as such, there are no true epidemiologic factors to discuss with respect to the organisms themselves. However, host condition is an important predisposition to the development of pneumonia.

Whether pregnant or not, certain groups of women of childbearing age are prone to develop pneumonia. Patients who are asplenic either iatrogenically or through autosplenectomy, as with sickle cell hemoglobinopathy, have a higher incidence of pneumonia due to encapsulated bacteria, notably *Streptococcus pneumoniae*. Patients from endemic areas have a higher risk developing active *Mycobacterium tuberculosis* pulmonary infection than have members of the usual population, as evidenced by the high incidence of this disease among Southeast Asian immigrants in this country in recent years. Finally, some studies, though not all, implicate pregnancy itself as the factor increasing the rate of pneumonia, especially some of the viral pneumonias such as varicella (chickenpox) pneumonia.

### Microorganism

The most common isolate in most studies is *S. pneumoniae*. Culture-negative pneumonia, i.e., presumed viral pneumonia, and pneumonia due to *Mycoplasma pneumoniae* are the other major categories. Other bacteria isolated less frequently include *Haemophilus influenzae*, *Staphylococcus aureus*, *M. tuberculosis*, and *E. coli*.

### Infection

Pneumonia, whatever the cause, is a clinical syndrome commonly defined by cough, sputum production, fever, and demonstration of either lobar consolidation or patchy infiltration of the lungs on the chest roentgenogram. Bacterial and viral pneumonias are generally classified by organism.

Pneumonia during pregnancy used to be associated with maternal mortality rates as high as 20 or 30 percent. Advances in antibiotics and medical support technology have decreased this rate to nearly zero in recent surveys. A concomitant rise in the level of neonatal intensive care has dropped the perinatal mortality rate from over 50 percent to less than 10 percent in infants delivered during the acute phase of the disease.

### Diagnosis

The woman who presents with fever, productive cough, and possibly dyspnea should be thoroughly examined. The chest should be auscultated and percussed in order to locate any areas of decreased breath sounds, rales or rhonchi, E to A changes, or percussive dullness. Pleural rubs also should be sought.

The heart should be auscultated carefully for rubs, gallops, or murmurs. Bacterial endocarditis is not so rare in pregnancy that it should not be suspected, nor should congestive heart failure be overlooked. Care must be taken not to confuse the rotation of the heart and physiologic murmur due to pregnancy with pathologic changes.

The abdomen and gravid uterus should be examined in the usual manner. The physician should be alert for any signs of premature labor. Fetal tachycardia may be the result of maternal fever. However, fetal tachycardia that is inconsistent with the mother's condition may signal chorioamnionitis, either secondary to maternal bacteremia or as a primary infection. The flanks should be examined for renal tenderness, because renal colic due to calculus or infection may mimic lower lobe pneumonia.

Laboratory examination should include a complete blood count with white cell differential, urinalysis to exclude pyelonephritis or calculus, and a chemistry panel to explore the liver transaminases and rule out acute hepatitis. Serum electrolytes should be measured, because fever, coughing, and the anorexia and nausea accompanying severe infection may cause dehydration and electrolyte disturbances.

If pneumonia is suspected, the physician should not hesitate to obtain posteroanterior and lateral chest roentgenograms, with the abdomen suitably shielded. The risk of radiation to the fetus is far outweighed by the risk of complications if a case of pneumonia is overlooked during pregnancy. If the chest x-ray study supports the diagnosis, efforts should be made to isolate the microorganism responsible.

A good tracheal sputum specimen should be obtained for Gram stain and culture and sensitivity testing. If the patient fails to raise sputum, or cannot give a sputum specimen correctly without too much oral contamination, a transtracheal specimen may be aspirated. In the healthy young woman, the trachea should normally be free of leukocytes and bacteria. Sputum or nasopharyngeal specimens may be cultured for viruses if viral infection is suspected and facilities are available.

Finally, blood for acute viral serology may be collected, as well as cold agglutinin titers if *M. pneumoniae* is considered.

## Treatment

Therapy for pneumonia during pregnancy is based on the organism suspected. The most common pathogen, *S. pneumoniae*, is still sensitive to penicillin in this country, although penicillin-tolerant strains are being reported around the world. Penicillin-allergic patients may be treated with erythromycin. If an individual is particularly susceptible to pneumococcal pneumonia because of splenectomy or some immune defect, trivalent pneumococcal vaccine may be administered for future protection. The vaccine is made from polysaccharide bacterial capsule and is not dangerous to the fetus, because there is no live virus. *M. pneumoniae* is best treated with erythromycin, whereas viral pneumonias are treated with supportive care and vigilance against bacterial superinfection.

## URINARY TRACT INFECTION

### Epidemiology

Asymptomatic bacteriuria during pregnancy occurs in up to 10 percent of gravidas, depending on the population examined. One of the more serious possible sequelae to asymptomatic bacteriuria is pyelonephritis, which develops in perhaps 40 percent of patients who have asymptomatic bacteriuria. Intermediate in degree of seriousness of urinary infection is cystitis, which is bacterial infection of the bladder wall with resultant inflammation.

Factors that predispose certain individuals to develop urinary tract infections during pregnancy are at least partially understood and include the following: a progesterone-induced decrease in ureteral motility, leading to relative ureteral distention; partial obstruction of the ureters by the enlarging uterus and the engorged pelvic vasculature; and somewhat decreased perineal hygiene. These all aid, to some extent, in the pathophysiologic course that may lead to infection.

### Microorganism

The bacterial species most frequently involved in urinary tract infection are members of the family Enterobacteriaceae. Most initial and uncomplicated urinary infections are due to *E. coli, Proteus mirabilis, Klebsiella pneumoniae,* and various species of *Citrobacter* and *Enterobacter.* Group B beta-hemolytic streptococci may also cause bacteriuria and infection in a small percentage of pregnant patients.

Patients who have been hospitalized, catheterized, or previously treated with antibiotics have a different bacterial flora. Hospital flora tend to consist of resistant gram-negative facultative organisms, including *Enterobacter* species, the pseudomonads (especially *Pseudomonas aeruginosa*), and *Serratia* species. The enterococci, which are notoriously resistant to cephalosporin antibiotics, are more commonly seen in patients following instrumentation of the urinary tract. It is important, therefore, for the patient's previous history to be considered as a factor in the discussion of the possible offending organisms in urinary infections.

## Infection

Asymptomatic bacteriuria is, by definition, a noninfection. The patient has no signs or symptoms of infection, other than a positive urine culture. Cystitis, on the other hand, may be an extremely symptomatic infection. Inflammation of the bladder wall and urethra causes the subjective symptoms of dysuria (pain when the bladder is full) and urinary incontinence resulting from irritability of the detrusor muscle. Occasionally, there may be flank discomfort, resembling that seen with pyelonephritis. Physical examination may reveal suprapubic tenderness, especially with the bladder full. If there is significant urethral involvement, the urethral meatus may be erythematous and swollen. The urinary sediment contains numerous polymorphonuclear leukocytes and bacteria, and occasionally blood.

The patient with pyelonephritis presents with high fever, occasionally to 104° F (40° C), tachycardia, and hypotension if significant bacteremia or bacterial toxemia has occurred. The flank on the side of the infected kidney is extremely tender to percussion. There may be associated nausea or vomiting.

Pyelonephritis may progress rapidly to gram-negative septic shock, leading ultimately to death. The kidney may develop microabscesses that eventually coalesce, resulting in nephric and perinephric abscess. Areas in the body seeded during the bacteremia may also develop infection and abscess.

One particular syndrome accompanying pyelonephritis in the pregnant woman is acute respiratory insufficiency. Apparently, bacterial substances or immunologic mediators cause "leaky capillaries" in the lungs, leading to a condition similar to adult respiratory distress syndrome, often aggravated by large volumes of intravenous fluids.

In the pregnant patient, untreated pyelonephritis often incites premature labor, as does any severe febrile illness during pregnancy. Hypotension decreases uteroplacental perfusion, leading to fetal compromise and myometrial irritability. However, even in women without overt pyelonephritis, i.e., those with asymptomatic bacteriuria or cystitis, there may be a higher rate of premature delivery and lower-birth-weight babies, although this is still a matter of some debate. Maternal anemia and decrease in renal function may occur with urinary infection during pregnancy, especially after pyelonephritis.

## Diagnosis

The cornerstone of diagnosis of urinary tract infection is the demonstration of bacteria in the urine. A clean-catch midstream urine specimen is considered colonized if more than 100,000 colonies of bacteria are recovered per milliliter of urine. Catheterized specimens, or specimens obtained by suprapubic bladder aspiration, are considered significantly colonized if any pathogenic bacteria are grown from the specimen.

The clinical diagnosis of either asymptomatic bacteriuria, cystitis, or pyelonephritis is made on the basis of the physical findings combined with the results of urinalysis. For instance, a patient who has many white blood cells and bacteria in a catheterized urine specimen and is spiking a temperature of 103° F (39.5° C) with severe right-sided pain is diagnosed as having acute pyelonephritis. A similar urinalysis in a patient with no fever or other symptoms, except dysuria and frequency, indicates cystitis. The diagnosis of asymptomatic bacteriuria is made when the patient has no signs or symptoms but urine culture reveals the presence of significant colonies of bacteria.

Occasionally, a patient with the signs and symptoms of acute pyelonephritis is found to have no pyuria on initial urinalysis. This is not uncommon in the patient who has partial obstruction of the ureter as a result of calculus or compression by the gravid uterus. In these cases, it is helpful to position the patient with her affected side up, e.g., on her left side if she has right flank pain, and collect another urine specimen for examination after the affected ureter has been allowed free drainage for 20 to 30 minutes. This maneuver often allows drainage of infected urine into the bladder and thus reveals the diagnosis.

### Treatment

Patients with asymptomatic bacteriuria should be started on a course of at least 7 to 10 days of oral antibiotic therapy to eradicate the organism colonizing the bladder and thus prevent possible future development of cystitis and acute pyelonephritis. The choice of antibiotic may be made based on culture results, because these are usually available at the time the diagnosis is made. Antibiotics that produce high urinary levels but that have little systemic effect, e.g., nitrofurantoin, are of use in these patients. It may be wise to save antibiotics that have greater systemic action for use in patients with pyelonephritis. After completion of the course of therapy, the urine should be recultured to document clearing of the bacteriuria.

Patients with cystitis during pregnancy should be treated with oral antibiotics for 10 to 14 days, again, to eradicate the bacteria and prevent future infection. If symptoms are severe, a bladder anesthetic, e.g., pyrimethamine, may be included for the first few days for symptomatic relief. The patient should be encouraged to increase oral fluid intake. The physician should review the results of the culture and sensitivity tests after 48 to 72 hours, in case the organism is resistant to the initial antibiotic prescribed. Antibiotics that give high urinary levels are also useful in treating cystitis during pregnancy. Reculture of the urine after the administration of therapy is mandatory.

Acute pyelonephritis in pregnancy is a serious disease, and patients with this entity should be hospitalized. Intravenous fluids should be given to prevent dehydration and to ensure good urine output. The mother's hemodynamic and respiratory status should be closely monitored for signs of deterioration. A large-bore intravenous line guarantees quick access in case the patient becomes shocky and unstable. Blood should be obtained initially for a complete blood count

and white cell differential, serum electrolyte studies, a chemistry profile, and for the isolation of bacteria. A catheterized urine specimen should be sent for urinalysis, culture, and sensitivity testing. The fetus should be monitored and any signs of premature labor noted, because chorioamnionitis often mimics pyelonephritis and vice versa. Sustained high maternal body temperature may have a deleterious effect on the fetus; therefore, acetaminophen should be given when the maternal temperature is greater than 102.2° F (39° C).

Initial antibiotic therapy should be based on the patient's clinical condition and the physician's experience with the antibiotic sensitivities of those organisms most often causing pyelonephritis at the particular institution. If the patient is in septic shock, antibiotics that provide coverage against urinary pathogens should be chosen. Combinations of a semisynthetic penicillin and an aminoglycoside, for example, would provide coverage against the pseudomonads, the coliforms, and the enterococci. In fact, synergy between these combinations of drugs has been documented for many of these pathogens.

If the patient is not in clinical shock, a single agent that is known to be active against most isolates clinically encountered in the particular institution is generally adequate. The physician must be aware of the sensitivity patterns of *E. coli, P. mirabilis,* the *Klebsiella* species, and the occasional streptococci encountered. In some institutions, drugs such as ampicillin may be adequate. In most institutions, antibiotic pressures have caused many of the *E. coli* and other organisms to become resistant to ampicillin as well as to ticarcillin and carbenicillin. *Klebsiella pneumoniae* is almost universally resistant to these drugs as well. In such cases, the first-generation cephalosporins, such as cephalothin, cefazolin, and cephapirin, may be successfully used to treat these infections.

After the patient has been on therapy for 48 to 72 hours, she should show signs of response, such as defervescence and decreasing pain. At this time, the urine should be sterile. Failure to respond to antibiotics may indicate a resistant organism or some urinary tract abnormality, such as total or partial obstruction of a ureter. Such patients need a more in-depth workup, which may include renal ultrasonography or one-shot intravenous pyelography. It is advisable to evaluate creatinine clearance in these patients to determine if any profound decrease in renal function has occurred.

If a patient is treated with and responds appropriately to antibiotics given for acute pyelonephritis, she may be switched to oral medication after being afebrile for approximately 48 hours. Ideally, the oral medication should be of the same type as the parenteral drug. The patient should complete a 14-day course of medication, and the urine should be recultured at the conclusion of the treatment course. Any patients with persistent bacteriuria, and patients who have had several different episodes of urinary tract infection during the pregnancy, should probably be put on suppressive therapy for the duration of the pregnancy and monitored closely.

# Parasitic Diseases

## TRICHOMONIASIS

### Epidemiology

The incidence of infection with *Trichomonas vaginalis* in women in the United States is estimated to be 3 million per year. The disease is more common in individuals with multiple sexual partners, and the incidence in female prostitutes is over 70 percent. Therefore, the argument for sexual transmission is very strong.

Trichomoniasis may also be acquired by nonvenereal means, since the organism may live for varying amounts of time in fresh water, semen, and urine, and even on toilet tissue, toilet seats, and damp wash cloths. The rate of infection, therefore, is expectedly high in institutionalized individuals, even when there is no sexual activity.

The newborn infant may acquire trichomoniasis by birth through an infected cervix and vagina. The infection in the neonate is short lived, however, because the organism cannot survive in the infantile, nonestrogenized vagina.

### Microbiology

*T. vaginalis* is a motile protozoan organism that is recognized in wet preparation by its characteristic twitching, caused by the five flagella that are distributed on the surface of the organism. The animal is anaerobic and ingests bacteria and erythrocytes by phagocytosis.

### Infection

Approximately 75 percent of women with *T. vaginalis* infection are symptomatic. The usual infection consists of a vaginitis/cervicitis, accompanied by a frothy, greenish discharge that may occasionally have a disagreeable odor. There may be an associated vulvitis. Dysuria and urinary frequency are not uncommon, and trichomonads may be seen in the bladder urine. Unusual features in the infection are inguinal adenopathy and lower abdominal pain resembling pelvic inflammatory disease. None of these factors is specific for trichomoniasis.

In recent reports, trichomoniasis during pregnancy has been implicated in premature labor and premature rupture of the membranes. Although the exact associations are still under academic scrutiny, it is clear that the organism is a significant gestational pathogen.

### Diagnosis

Demonstration of the organism from genital secretions is the method for diagnosis of trichomoniasis. Up to 60 to 70 percent of infections may be documented by microscopic examination of vaginal secretions. There are also many white cells and erythrocytes, depending on the amount of inflammation present. It is important that vaginal pool fluid be used, not endocervical mucus.

### Treatment

In the nonpregnant patient, metronidazole (Flagyl) is the drug of choice for trichomoniasis. Metronidazole given in a dose of 250 mg orally 3 times daily for 7 days cures roughly 95 percent of women. Those who fail therapy should be retreated, along with their sexual partner. A regimen of 2.0 g orally at one sitting gives reasonably comparable rates of cure. A single dose regimen is effective when the sexual partner is treated simultaneously. All patients treated for a sexually transmitted disease should be counseled as to prevention and should encourage their partner(s) to be treated. Metronidazole tolerance and resistance occasionally have been reported, however.

Metronidazole has been shown to be tumorigenic in laboratory animals given large doses for long periods of time. However, no adverse reports have been described in humans, other than mild nausea, bitter taste, and an Antabuse-like reaction if taken with alcohol. Still, use in pregnancy during the first trimester is probably contraindicated. During the last two trimesters, the use of metronidazole must be weighed against the risk from severe cervicitis, vaginitis, and prematurity complications. In lieu of metronidazole therapy, nonspecific local care, such as douches or suppositories, may be helpful, especially with some of the imidazole creams that have antitrichomonal activity.

## TOXOPLASMOSIS

### Epidemiology

Toxoplasmosis results from infection by the parasite *Toxoplasma gondii,* which is found in herbivorous, omnivorous, and carnivorous animals. The domestic cat is the only known animal known to shed oocysts. Therefore, cats serve as vectors of transmission to other animals and humans. Invertebrates that feed on feces can transport oocysts and thus serve as intermediate hosts. The disease can also be contracted by the ingestion of raw meat or by transplacental infection.

Toxoplasmosis occurs more frequently in tropical areas. In addition to geographical location being a factor, there is also an increased incidence of seropositivity with increasing age. Approximately 20 to 25 percent of women in the reproductive age group in the United States are seropositive for *T. gondii.* The incidence of primary infection in pregnancy is estimated to range between 0.5 and 1.5 percent, with a third of these women giving birth to infected neonates.

There is an inverse relationship between the time of infection in pregnancy and the incidence of fetal infection. Pregnant women who contract *T. gondii* in the first trimester transmit the disease to their fetuses in 15 percent of cases. If the disease is contracted in the second trimester, the incidence of fetal infection increases to 25 percent, and 60 percent of fetuses contract the disease if the

mother acquires it during the third trimester. However, the manifestations of congenital toxoplasmosis are more severe with earlier infection. Infection that occurs early in the first trimester may result in abortion, whereas infection acquired in the third trimester may be asymptomatic.

### Microorganism

*T. gondii* exists in three forms during its life cycle: trophozoites, tissue cysts, and oocysts. The trophozoite is the proliferative form, which invades the mammalian cells. Once within the host cells, the trophozoites multiply until the cells are disrupted, thereby liberating more trophozoites or tissue cysts.

Tissue cysts have an outer wall that protects against the host defense mechanisms. This form of the disease is the latent stage and may also serve to transmit the disease. Disruption of the cell wall results in the liberation of viable parasites that are capable of invading host epithelial cells.

Oocysts have been found only in members of the cat family. The cat ingests tissue cysts or oocysts, which enter the cat's gut; here, dissolution of the cyst wall occurs, releasing viable *T. gondii.* The parasite then invades the epithelial cells lining the intestine and begins the asexual phase of its life cycle. This is shortly followed by a sexual phase, which results in the formation of noninfectious unsporulated oocysts. These oocysts are shed in the cat's feces. Once outside the body, each oocyst undergoes sporogeny, forming two sporocysts. Each sporocyst matures, forming four sporozoites. Ingestion of the oocysts containing the sporozoites results in liberation of trophozoites, thereby completing the life cycle.

### Infection

Toxoplasmosis is a unique disease in that infection by *T. gondii* is often asymptomatic but may be fulminant. Infection acquired by the mother during pregnancy is often asymptomatic, but congenital infection can result in serious sequelae. The disease is seen in the following four forms: congenital, acquired, ocular, and in the immunocompromised patient. Infection in the adult is frequently asymptomatic, although the patient may present with lymphadenopathy, chorioretinitis, myocarditis, meningoencephalitis and a rash resembling the exanthem seen in typhus.

Toxoplasmosis acquired during pregnancy may range from asymptomatic to fatal acute fulminant disease. The most common manifestation during pregnancy is cervical lymphadenopathy, which may be associated with supraclavicular and inguinal lymphadenopathy. The patient may also have fever, myalgias, pharyngitis, and headache. The presentation mimics that seen in mononucleosis or cytomegalovirus infection. In addition, some individuals may have a rash similar to the exanthem seen in typhus; hepatosplenomegaly and an atypical lymphocytosis may also develop.

Congenital infection in the United States occurs in 1 in 500 to 1 in 3000 deliveries, depending on the geographic region. It should be emphasized that in certain areas of the country, there has been an influx of immigrants from tropical areas where the disease is more prevalent; therefore, special attention should be given to ensure that these patients are properly evaluated. The incidence of congenital infection varies, depending on the trimester during which the infection is acquired. Maternal infection acquired during the first trimester is associated with the lowest incidence of fetal infection but is likely to result in spontaneous abortion if the fetus contracts the illness. The highest risk of congenital infection occurs with maternal infection in the third trimester; as noted earlier, however, most newborns infected in the third trimester are asymptomatic and may suffer no sequelae. Others may develop retinochoroiditis, strabismus, blindness, epilepsy, and/or psychomotor or mental retardation months or years later. Infants born with clinical infection may present with retinochoroiditis, hydrocephaly or microcephaly, cerebral calcifications, convulsions, psychomotor retardation, fever, hepatosplenomegaly, jaundice, lymphadenopathy, and rash.

## Diagnosis

The diagnosis of toxoplasmosis may be established by isolation of *T. gondii* from body fluids and tissue specimens. This is not a practical method, however, because most institutions do not have the facilities for inoculating mice or tissue cultures. A second method is based on demonstration of trophozoites in tissue sections or smears. This is a difficult procedure in that trophozoites are not easily recognized. Fluorescent antibody techniques have been developed that facilitate the diagnosis and are easier to perform.

Serologic methods often have been used to establish the diagnosis of toxoplasmosis. The Sabin-Feldman dye test, the indirect fluorescent antibody (IFAT) test, and the indirect hemagglutination test (IHAT) are frequently used serologic tests. The IFAT and IHAT detect IgG antibodies. The Sabin-Feldman dye test serves as the standard to which all other tests are compared. The IFAT is the most widely used serologic test, and the IFAT and Sabin-Feldman dye test become positive 1 to 2 weeks after acute infection. In 6 to 8 weeks, titers of 1 : 1000 are reached that will decline in several months to titers of 1 : 4 to 1 : 64—with these low titers persisting for life.

Another useful serologic test is the IgM-fluorescent antibody test, which becomes detectable within 5 days after infection and disappears 3 to 4 months after infection. The presence in the fetus of IgM antibodies specifically directed against *T. gondii* indicates intrauterine infection, because IgM does not cross the placenta. In a patient suspected of acute toxoplasmosis, serum should be obtained for IgM-IFAT and IgG-IFAT antibodies. If the IgM-IFAT is 1 : 80 or if there is a serial two-tube rise in titer in specimens run in parallel, then the diagnosis of acute toxoplasmosis is established even in the absence of symptoms. The presence of a positive IgM-IFAT and a rising IgG-IFAT also establishes the diagnosis. A negative IgM-IFAT and a fixed IgG-IFAT titer do not indicate acute infection. However, a negative IgM-IFAT in the presence of a rising IgG-IFAT titer does indicate active disease. The IgG-IFAT titer may become fixed at 1 : 2400 for years.

Fetal infection, or lack thereof, has been demonstrated in recent years by sampling fetal blood by funipuncture. Large series of cases from France, where toxoplasmosis is quite common, have verified the utility of this method of diagnosis (Daffos et al, 1985). Recently, Knuppel (1992) has reported a case of maternal toxoplasmosis at 2 weeks of gestational age. The chorionic villus tissue obtained at 10 weeks' gestation demonstrated an early method to obtain fetal tissue for signs of fetal infection.

## Treatment

Whether or not to treat a pregnant woman with asymptomatic toxoplasmosis is a question that is confronted by many obstetricians. Originally it was thought that since the prognosis in untreated asymptomatic toxoplasmosis was good and that disease contracted during one pregnancy would confer immunity during subsequent pregnancies, treatment was not necessary. However, congenital toxoplasmosis may be asymptomatic at first, only to produce serious sequelae many years later. In addition, organisms have been isolated from abortuses, stillborns, and neonates who expired following delivery from women with chronic disease. *Toxoplasma* organisms have, on several occasions, also been recovered from the maternal blood in asymptomatic patients. Therefore, although rare, subsequent congenital infection may occur. It is probably best to have these patients practice some form of contraception for a year's duration or, if the patient is already pregnant, to discuss the risks of treatment and treat for fetal indications.

Individuals who contract the disease during the first trimester risk having a severely affected child if the pregnancy goes to term. If these individuals do not elect abortion, treatment of acute maternal toxoplasmosis appears to decrease the incidence of congenital toxoplasmosis. Treatment should be started with sulfadiazine, 1 g given orally 4 times a day for 28 days. Pyrimethamine (Daraprim), a folic acid antagonist, is contraindicated during the first trimester because it is teratogenic. Sulfadiazine should be discontinued at term, in order to prevent neonatal hyperbilirubinemia. In the second and third trimesters sulfadiazine should be administered in conjunction with pyrimethamine, administered orally in a dose of 25 mg daily for 28 days. Because pyrimethamine is a folic acid antagonist, folinic acid should be given concurrently in dosages of 2 to 10 mg per day, to prevent bone marrow suppression in the second and third trimesters.

Spiramycin, a macrolide antibiotic with reasonable activity against the parasite, is available from the Centers for Disease Control and is relatively harmless in pregnancy. Fetal cure is not guaranteed with any drug, however, and retreatment postnatally is often warranted.

In an attempt to prevent acquired and congenital toxoplasmosis, patients should be advised to eat meat that has been thoroughly cooked. Uncooked meat should be kept frozen at 20° C for 24 hours to kill cysts. Fruits and vegetables should be thoroughly washed. Pregnant women should avoid contact with cats and should not change the cat litter. This is especially true for cats that go outdoors and occasionally kill and eat wild animals.

# Nursing Considerations in Perinatal Infections

Women who have perinatal infections need emotional as well as physical support. Emotional support involves helping the mother and her family to understand her disease and its ramifications, which in some cases may include the need to isolate the mother from her baby. Good education should be part of this support, especially if the mother has been newly diagnosed with herpes. She will need to understand the importance of cesarean section and what herpes means to her and her sexual partner. The mother may also need supportive care for her physical symptoms, because she may not feel well during her labor and delivery.

Generally speaking, when a woman with a perinatal infection is discharged from a room, it should have a thorough terminal cleaning. This includes not only antepartum, postpartum, and labor rooms but also delivery and recovery rooms. If possible, these mothers should be allowed to labor and deliver, and perhaps recover, in the same room.

Universal precautions should be in effect in every hospital to protect employees and patients from infections. Universal precautions do not take the place of good handwashing, which is necessary to prevent other infectious diseases. The Occupational Safety and Health Association (Federal Register, 1991) has developed guidelines to decrease employee exposure to blood and body fluids. These include intravenous systems that do not require needles, protective re-capping devices, suction machines, and protective eyewear with side shields.

Universal precautions now in effect in hospitals protect the caregiver from potential contamination. However, specific isolation, such as enteric precautions or respiratory precautions for women with chickenpox,

**Table 7—4**
MANAGEMENT OF PERINATAL INFECTIONS

| Infection | Antepartum and Intrapartum Recommendations | Postpartum Recommendations | Breastfeeding* |
|---|---|---|---|
| Herpes—oral and vaginal | (1) Good handwashing<br>(2) Rooms should be cleaned in accordance with universal precautions | (1) Rooming-in OR<br>(2) Separate mother and baby so baby does not take infection back to nursery from mother<br>(3) Good staff handwashing<br>(4) Good maternal handwashing when handling baby<br>(5) Terminal cleaning of recovery room and postpartum room | Yes, with good maternal handwashing |
| Rubella | (1) Strict isolation during disease<br>(2) Terminal cleaning of antepartum, labor, and delivery rooms | (1) Isolate baby from mother<br>(2) Strict isolation<br>(3) No pregnant women to attend patient | May breastfeed after infectious period<br>Pump breast and discard milk to preserve lactation until that time |
| Cytomegalovirus (CMV) (if diagnosed as active) | (1) Strict isolation during disease<br>(2) Terminal cleaning of antepartum, labor, and delivery rooms | (1) Isolate baby from mother<br>(2) Strict isolation<br>(3) No pregnant women to attend patient | May breastfeed after infectious period<br>Pump breast and discard milk to preserve lactation until that time |
| Varicella-zoster | (1) Strict isolation during disease<br>(2) Terminal cleaning of antepartum, labor, and delivery rooms | (1) Isolate baby from mother<br>(2) Strict isolation<br>(3) No pregnant women to attend patient | May breastfeed after infectious period<br>Pump breast and discard milk to preserve lactation until that time |
| Hepatitis | (1) Enteric precautions<br>(2) Terminal cleaning of antepartum, labor, and delivery rooms | (1) Isolate baby from mother<br>(2) Enteric precautions<br>(3) Terminal cleaning of recovery room and postpartum room | May breastfeed after infectious period<br>Pump breast and discard milk to preserve lactation until that time |
| Mumps | (1) Strict isolation during disease<br>(2) Terminal cleaning of antepartum, labor, and delivery rooms | (1) Isolate baby from mother<br>(2) Strict isolation<br>(3) No pregnant women to attend patient | May breastfeed after infectious period<br>Pump breast and discard milk to preserve lactation until that time |
| Condyloma acuminatum | No restrictions | No restrictions | No restrictions |
| AIDS-HIV | (1) Universal blood and body fluid precautions<br>(2) Terminal cleaning of antepartum, labor, and delivery rooms | (1) Blood and body fluid precautions<br>(2) Other precautions depending on mother's accompanying infections | Discourage breastfeeding |
| Genital mycoplasmas | Unknown | Once treatment started, baby can be with mother | May breastfeed; however, this is dependent on antibiotic treatment<br>May breastfeed after antibiotic therapy is completed; pump breast and discard milk to preserve lactation until that time |

*Table continued on following page*

**Table 7–4**
MANAGEMENT OF PERINATAL INFECTIONS *Continued*

| Infection | Antepartum and Intrapartum Recommendations | Postpartum Recommendations | Breastfeeding* |
|---|---|---|---|
| *Chlamydia* spp. | Terminal cleaning of antepartum, labor, and delivery rooms | Once treatment started, baby can be with mother | May breastfeed; however, this is dependent on antibiotic treatment<br>May breastfeed after antibiotic therapy is completed; pump breast and discard milk to preserve lactation until that time |
| Gonorrhea | (1) Good handwashing<br>(2) Terminal cleaning of antepartum, labor, and delivery rooms | Once treatment started, baby can be with mother | May breastfeed; however, this is dependent on antibiotic treatment<br>May breastfeed after antibiotic therapy is completed; pump breast and discard milk to preserve lactation until that time |
| Postpartum endometritis | No restrictions | Isolate baby from mother until afebrile | May breastfeed; however, this is dependent on antibiotic treatment<br>May breastfeed after antibiotic therapy is completed; pump breast and discard milk to preserve lactation until that time |
| Pneumonia | (1) Good handwashing<br>(2) Terminal cleaning of antepartum, labor, and delivery rooms | Isolate baby from mother until afebrile | May breastfeed; however, this is dependent on antibiotic treatment<br>May breastfeed after antibiotic therapy is completed; pump breast and discard milk to preserve lactation until that time |
| Urinary tract infection (UTI) | No restrictions | No restrictions | May breastfeed; however, this is dependent on antibiotic treatment<br>May breastfeed after antibiotic therapy is completed; pump breast and discard milk to preserve lactation until that time |
| Trichomoniasis | No restrictions | No restrictions | May breastfeed; however, this is dependent on antibiotic treatment<br>May breastfeed after antibiotic therapy is completed; pump breast and discard milk to preserve lactation until that time |

**Table 7–4**
MANAGEMENT OF PERINATAL INFECTIONS *Continued*

| Infection | Antepartum and Intrapartum Recommendations | Postpartum Recommendations | Breastfeeding* |
|---|---|---|---|
| Toxoplasmosis | No restrictions | No restrictions | May breastfeed; however, this is dependent on antibiotic treatment<br>May breastfeed after antibiotic therapy is completed; pump breast and discard milk to preserve lactation until that time |

* **Note:** For mothers on antibiotic therapy, breastfeeding depends on the type of antibiotic used, because some are permissible and others are contraindicated during breastfeeding.

may be necessary. Emotional support for the isolated patient is a well-known need, because such patients start to feel separated from their families and even the staff. Furthermore, as noted, it is sometimes necessary to separate mothers from their babies, thus increasing the mother's frustration. In some instances, the babies can be isolated with the mothers in a rooming in setup. If the mother must be isolated from her baby, she should be encouraged to view her baby and to have pictures to promote bonding. Other family members should be enouraged to visit and handle the newborn frequently.

When the mother has a perinatal infection, the baby can usually be breastfed, provided that treatment has been started and the mother is afebrile. Advisability of breastfeeding also depends on the medication administered for treatment of the mother's infection (see Chapter 6). If breastfeeding is desired by the mother but con-

traindicated by her treatment, she can pump her breasts and discard the milk while she is receiving treatment. Once the medication is completed the mother can start to breastfeed her infant. Because HIV virus can be transmitted through breast milk, breastfeeding should be discouraged in mothers infected with HIV.

Table 7–4 gives more specific management for mothers with perinatal infections.

The Department of Labor and the Department of Health and Human Services have published recommendations for employer responsibilities to protect workers. These include:

1. Classification of work activity.
2. Development of operating procedures.
3. Provision of training and education.
4. Development of procedures to ensure and monitor compliance.
5. Redesign of the workplace.

**Table 7–5**
SUMMARY OF TASK CATEGORIZATION AND IMPLICATIONS FOR PERSONAL PROTECTIVE EQUIPMENT

| Joint Advisory Notice Category* | Nature of Task/Activity | Personal protective equipment should be: Available? | Worn? |
|---|---|---|---|
| I | Direct contact with blood or other body fluids to which universal precautions apply | Yes | Yes |
| II | Activity performed without blood exposure but exposure may occur in emergency | Yes | No |
| III | Task/activity does not entail predictable or unpredictable exposure to blood | No | No |

* US Department of labor, US Department of Health and Human Services. Joint advisory notice: protection against occupational exposure to hepatitis B virus (HBV) and human immunodeficiency virus (HIV). Washington, DC: US Department of Labor, US Department of Health and Human Services, 1987.

Once the employee has been classified as to his or her level of exposure, protective equipment should be available to the employer and to all category II and III employees (Table 7–5). Use of this equipment should be mandatory when category I activities are performed. Standard operating procedures should be developed for all activities that have a potential for exposure. Employees should not be expected to perform these activities until they have been educated about these policies. Dates of educational sessions should be maintained. The employees should monitor the availability of supplies and the level of compliance with universal precautions through the hospital's quality improvement program. This should include periodic reassessment of the program. Whenever possible, the hospital should indentify devices and other approaches that modify the work environment and reduce high-risk exposure (MMWR, 1989).

**Acknowledgment**

We would like to acknowledge Sandra Jackson, MT (ASCP) C.I.C. Infection Control Manager, Magee-Womens Hospital for her contributions.

# References

American College of Obstetricians and Gynecologists: Human immune deficiency virus infection. ACOG Technical Bulletin #123, Dec 1988.

American College of Obstetricians and Gynecologists. Perinatal herpes simplex virus infection. ACOG Technical Bulletin #122, Nov 1988.

Amstey MS: Current concepts of herpesvirus in women. Am J Obstet Gynecol 177:717, 1975.

Beasley RP, Hwang LY, Lin CC, et al: Hepatitis B immune globulin (HBIG) efficacy in the interruption of perinatal transmission of hepatitis B carrier. Lancet 2:388, 1981.

Benedetti TJ, Valle R, Ledger WJ: Antepartum pneumonia in pregnancy. Am J Obstet Gynecol 144:413, 1982.

Cassell GH, Cole BC: Mycoplasmas as agents of human disease. N Engl J Med 304:308, 1981.

Centers for Disease Control: 1989 Sexually Transmitted Diseases Treatment Guidelines. MMWR 38(5–8):1–40, 1989.

Chang TW: Rubella reinfection and intrauterine involvement. J Pediatrics 84:617, 1974.

Daffos F, Capella-Pavlovsky M, Forestier F: Fetal blood sampling in the umbilical cord using a needle guided by ultrasound: A study of 606 consecutive cases. Am J Obstet Gynecol 153:655, 1985.

Desmonts G, Couvreur J: Congenital toxoplasmosis: a prospective study of 378 pregnancies. N Engl J Med 290:1110, 1974.

Faro S: Hepatitis A, B and non-A, non-B in pregnancy. In Amstey MS (ed): Viral Infections in Pregnancy. New York, Grune & Stratton, 1984, pp 19–33.

Faro S: Sexually transmitted diseases. In Hale RN, Knueger JA (eds): Gynecology. New Hyde Park, New York, Medical Examination Publishing Co, 1983.

Faro S, Pastorek J, Aldridge K: Short course parenteral antibiotic therapy for pyelonephritis in pregnancy. South Med J 77:455, 1984.

Faro S, Sanders CV, Aldridge K: Use of single-agent antimicrobial therapy in the treatment of polymicrobial female pelvic infections. Obstet Gynecol 60:232, 1982.

Federal Register: Department of Labor. Occupational Safety and Health Administration (OSHA), 29 CFR Part 1910.1030 Occupational Exposure to Bloodborne Pathogens; Final Rule, December 6, 1991.

Gibbs RS, Duff P: Progress in pathogenesis and management of clinical intraamniotic infection. Am J Obstet Gynecol 164:1317, 1991.

Gibbs RS, Castillo MS, Rodgers PJ: Management of acute chorioamnionitis. Am J Obstet Gynecol 136:709, 1980.

Giles C, Brown JA: Urinary infection and anemia in pregnancy. Br Med J 2:10, 1962.

Gilstrap LC, Cunningham FG: The bacterial pathogenesis of infection following cesarean section. Obstet Gynecol 53:545, 1979.

Harris RE, Gilstrap LC: Prevention of recurrent pyelonephritis during pregnancy. Obstet Gynecol 44:637, 1974.

Heggie AD, Lumica G, Stuart LA, et al: Chlamydia trachomatis infection in mothers and infants. Am J Dis Child 135:507, 1981.

Knuppel RA: Personal communication, January, 1992.

Martin DH, Koutsky L, Eschenbach DA, et al: Prematurity and perinatal mortality in pregnancies complicated by maternal chlamydia trachomatis infections. JAMA 247:1585, 1982.

Miehinen M, Saxen L, Saxen E: Lymph node toxoplasmosis. Acta Med Scand 208:431, 1980.

Nahmias AJ, Josey WE, Naib ZM, et al: Perinatal risk associated with maternal genital herpes simplex virus infection. Am J Obstet Gynecol 110:825, 1971.

Pastorek JG: Hepatitis B. Obstet Gynecol Clin North Am 16(3):645, 1989.

Remington JS: Toxoplasmosis in the adult. Bull NY Acad Med 50:211, 1974.

Rodis JF, Hovick TJ, Quinn DL, et al: Human parvovirus infection in pregnancy. Obstet Gynecol 72:733, 1988.

Sargal S, Lunyk O, Larkee RPB, et al: The outcome in children with congenital cytomegalovirus infection. Am J Dis Child 136:896, 1982.

Sever JL: Infections in pregnancy; highlights from the collaborative perinatal project. Teratology 25:227, 1982.

Thurn J: Human parvovirus B19: historical and clinical review. Rev Infect Dis 10(5):1005, 1988.

# CHAPTER 8

# AIDS in Pregnancy

Hunter A. Hammill and Cathy Murtagh

The human immunodeficiency virus (HIV) presents a particular dilemma to the health care provider caring for an HIV-positive pregnant woman. The health care provider must be wary of many of the signs and symptoms associated with a normal pregnancy, yet frequently, these signs and symptoms are the early warning signals of progression of HIV disease. Perinatal transmission has been well documented at rates of 30 to 50 percent (Fallon et al, 1989; Hammill, 1989). How and when this occurs has yet to be clearly delineated owing to the lack of a definitive *in utero* test to evaluate HIV infection in the fetus. Other issues, such as the effect of pregnancy on the progression of HIV infection and the treatment of opportunistic infections and a dysfunctional immune system in pregnancy, are not clearly defined. The use of zidovudine (AZT, Retrovir) in pregnancy is controversial and recent clinical trials are ongoing.

This chapter explores the epidemiologic, social, and psychologic aspects as well as the immunologic recognition and recommended treatment of diseases associated with HIV infection during pregnancy.

## Epidemiology

**Statistics.** Since the discovery of HIV in March 1984, the morbidity and mortality of this virus in women and their children have taken a tremendous toll. The death rate for women quadrupled between 1985 and 1988 owing to HIV and acquired immunodeficiency syndrome (AIDS) (0.6 per 100,000 to 2.5 per 100,000). The death rate for black women was nine times greater than that for white women (10.3 per 100,000 to 1.2 per 100,000). Women of reproductive age (25 to 34 years of age) accounted for 14 percent of all HIV- and AIDS-related deaths (Chu et al, 1990). Between August, 1988 and July, 1990; the Centers for Disease Control reported 558 new AIDS cases in adolescents aged 13 to 19 years old. Twenty-three percent of these cases are in females (HIV/AIDS Surveillance, 1990). This frightening figure does not include the number of teenagers who are HIV positive. It is not surprising then that by 1991, HIV and AIDS have become two of the leading causes of death in women of reproductive age (Chu et al, 1990).

These projected trends in HIV and AIDS mortality do not fare well for the infants of these women. A recent study of 172 children diagnosed with perinatal HIV infection revealed that these children have a median survival rate of approximately 38 months once the child becomes symptomatic. Most of these children were symptomatic by a median age of 8 months (Scott et al, 1989).

The leading cause of death in both women and children who are HIV positive is the acquisition of an opportunistic infection secondary to a compromised immune system. Much of what is known about this process has been extrapolated from studies performed on other immunocompromised patients such as leukemics, organ transplant patients, and cancer patients. The primary opportunistic killer in HIV-positive women and children is *Pneumocystis carinii* pneumonia (Chu et al, 1990). Other frequently noted pathogenic agents responsible for death in women are cryptococcus and atypical mycobacterial infections (Chu et al, 1990). In children, candida esophagitis, recurrent bacterial infection, and encephalopathy are noted to be responsible for deaths related to HIV infection (Scott et al, 1989).

## Etiology and Pathogenesis

HIV is an RNA virus known as a retrovirus. A retrovirus implies that during the cycle of replication of the virus, the genetic information flows from RNA to DNA, reversing the classic direction of information flow (Kornfeld, 1989). HIV has, in general, three major structural components: RNA, a core, and an envelope. HIV is a virus enclosed by an envelope containing core proteins, genomic RNA, and the reverse transcriptase enzyme unique to retroviruses that allows the assemblage of DNA from the RNA template. The genome of HIV codes for the core proteins (gag), reverse transcriptase (pol), and the envelope glycoproteins (env) (Fallon et al, 1989; Kornfeld, 1989).

HIV has a selective tropism for the CD4 receptor site on lymphocytes. After attaching to the cell's CD4 receptor site, the virus fuses with the cell's membrane, enters the cell, and uncoats within the cytoplasm. After transcription of viral RNA to DNA, the DNA is incorporated into the host cell's DNA in a latent proviral form. From here, on activation of the host cell, the proviral DNA follows the usual sequence of genetic information flow and new HIV virions are released by budding through the plasma membrane (Fallon et al, 1989).

Abnormalities in the immune system are the result of the infection in the helper T lymphocytes; this produces profound defects in cellular immunity. Deficiencies in T cell numbers, as a result of cellular destruction and also qualitative defects in T-cell function, produce these defects. Lymphopenia is common in adults with AIDS, as is decreased ratio of help-inducer to suppressor-cytotoxic T lymphocytes (T4/T8 ratio) secondary to a reduction in T4 lymphocytes. The decrease in T-cell function increases the risk of susceptibility to neoplasms and opportunistic infections. Also, there is a depressed or absent skin sensi-

**Table 8–1**
IMMUNOLOGIC ABNORMALITIES ASSOCIATED WITH HIV INFECTION OF T4 CELL

**B Cells**
Spontaneous production of immunoglobulins (hypergammaglobulinemia)
Decreased response to specific antigens

**T Helper/Inducer Cells (CD4)**
Decreased in absolute number
Decreased response to antigen
Decreased "helper" activity for B cell immunoglobulin production
Decreased lymphokine production

**T Suppressor/Cytotoxic Cells (CD8)**
Normal to increased number of cells

**Monocytes/Macrophages**
Decreased chemotaxis
Decreased clearance of Ig-coated red blood cells and platelets
Defective antigen presentation
Increased production of Interleukin-1 and prostaglandin E2

From Harawi S: Epidemiology in pathology and pathophysiology of AIDS. *In* Harawi S, O'Hara C (eds): Pathophysiology of AIDS. St Louis, CV Mosby, 1989, p 5.

tivity reaction to mitogenic stimulation (anergy). Because T4 cells play a large role in B-cell activation, defects in humoral immunity occur, such as impaired antibody production, which increases the patient's susceptibility to bacterial infections (Table 8–1) (Fallon et al, 1989; O'Hara, 1989).

## Transmission

The transmission of HIV infection is limited, in general, to three modes: sexual contact, infected blood components and clotting factor concentrates, and through birth. The HIV virus is an RNA virus that grows in lymphocytes and monocyte/macrophages. It has an affinity for the CD4 receptor site, and it is conceivable that the virus could be recovered from any area where these cells are found. HIV has been isolated in a number of body fluids, such as sweat, urine, cerebrospinal fluid, saliva, tears, and semen. These findings are not necessarily significant, though, in that contact with saliva or tears has not been shown to result in infection (Harawi, 1989).

Certain behaviors and actions are considered high risk and are associated with HIV infection. Vaginal and anal intercourse and other sexual activities that disrupt mucous membranes, such as fellatio, cunnilingus, and anilingus with an HIV-infected individual, are associated with HIV transmission. Needle-sharing among intravenous drug abusers is a particularly high-risk behavior. Behavior not associated with transmission includes casual contact such as hugging or kissing. Also, HIV has not been shown to be transmitted by mosquitos, fomites, food, air, or water (Harawi, 1989).

## TRANSMISSION GROUPS

The current distribution of AIDS cases reflects the mode of transmission 5 to 10 years ago; that is, homosexual activity. Statistics, however, point to an ever-increasing role of heterosexual activity and intravenous drug abuse in the spread of HIV infection to women (Feinkind and Minkoff, 1988).

Substance-abusing women are particularly susceptible to HIV infection due to their at-risk behaviors. Needle-sharing and "survival sex" (trading sex for drugs) are life-threatening behaviors. Addicted women do not have the power to control the sexual expectations and preferences of their partners when they use their bodies to procure drugs (Karan, 1989). The lack of inhibition associated with alcohol and drug use contributes to the lack of self-control these women exhibit. Frequently, intravenous drug–abusing women are also in a poor state of physical health because of malnutrition, poverty, lack of health care, and the effects of drug and alcohol abuse. Many women have a poor health status in combination with practicing high-risk sexual behavior plus needle-sharing. This explains the Centers for Disease Control's reported 51 percent female AIDS cases between September, 1988 through September 1990 associated with intravenous drug abuse (HIV/AIDS Surveillance, 1990). The National Institute on Drug Abuse estimates that 8 million (15 percent) of the 56 million American women of reproductive age are substance abusers (Karan, 1989).

Heterosexual contact with males infected with HIV is the other predominant mode of transmission. The Centers for Disease Control report that of the 13,807 female cases of AIDS reported from September, 1988 through August, 1990, 4425 (32 percent) of these women had heterosexual contact with a male exhibiting high-risk behavior. Sixty-three percent had contact with a male intravenous drug abuser. Other contacts included sex with a bisexual male, sex with a person with hemophilia, sex with a person born in a pattern-II country, and sex with a transfusion recipient (HIV/AIDS Surveillance).

It is a reflection of the times that with increased sexual freedom, women have had the responsibility for safe sex transferred to them. Unfortunately, many young women fear rejection by their partners and, in their desire for intimacy, find it difficult to negotiate sexual practices (Karan, 1989). Also, with the advent of the birth control pill, there has been a notable shift away from the use of condoms. Contributing to the lack of use of condoms is the frequent complaint by the male partner of decreased sensuality. Along with the continuing increase in the rate of heterosexual spread of HIV infection, the authors believe the concurrent rise in other sexually transmitted diseases such as gonorrhea, herpes, chancroid, and syphilis, reflects the decrease in condom use.

Adolescent females make up another subset of HIV-positive women. The Centers for Disease Control report that 21 percent of known AIDS cases were in the 21- to 29-year-old age group. Because the average latency period between HIV-seropositivity and a diagnosis of AIDS is approximately 1 to 5 years, many of these particular women became HIV-positive as teenagers (Lawrence et al, 1990). Most of these adolescents contracted HIV infection either through sexual activity or intravenous drug use. Adolescents, with their perception of invincibility and their misconceptions and misinformation about high-risk behavior, are a particularly vulnerable group. Lawrence, Levy, and Rubinson evaluated 58 pregnant adolescents' perceptions of their ability to perform AIDS prevention behaviors. These adolescents had the most difficulty asking their sex partners about previous sexual experiences and about obtaining and using condoms (Lawrence et al, 1990).

Additionally, HIV may be transmitted to very young girls through the sexual abuse of children. The authors had the unfortunate task of delivering a 15-year-old, HIV-positive female recently. She had a history of having been prostituted for drugs by her mother since the age of 12. She subsequently became pregnant, at age 14, and she was found to be HIV positive.

## Identification

Although there is some controversy regarding history as the sole means of identifying patients for HIV infection, the authors do not advocate universal testing of all pregnant females. A thorough sexual history, including the number of partners in a lifetime, exposure to intravenous drug–abusing males, prostitution, sexually transmitted diseases, drug abuse, sexual abuse, and blood transfusions before 1985 warrants a discussion of possible HIV infection with the patient and an HIV screening test (Table 8–2). Currently, the enzyme-linked immunosorbent assay (ELISA) antibody and the Western Blot confirmation tests are used to diagnose infection.

## Testing

One of the concerns about testing is the controversy of screening select populations versus screening the entire population. With the application of universal precautions, there should be no difference in management of patients, whether or not they are identified as seropositive. However, misconceptions have arisen with the predictive value of a negative test in a high-risk population. For groups at high risk for AIDS, such as hemophiliacs, intravenous drug abusers, and partners of intravenous drug abusers, the prevalence of HIV-antibody testing positive is high. The predictive value of a negative test may be as low as 77 percent. Conversely, in a low-risk population, the predictive value of a positive test is less than 3 percent, so that at least 97 percent of the positive tests in the general population, when tested by a screening ELISA procedure, will be false-positives and not indicative of AIDS exposure to HIV (Sivak and Wormser, 1986). Additional concern has arisen about indeterminate Western Blot tests in the low-risk population. Currently, it is recommended that these tests be repeated in 6 months. It is estimated that with repeat testing, the rate of a false-positive Western Blot test would be 0.001 percent. New tests such as $p^{24}$ antigen may help clarify the Western Blot and the ELISA tests in the future. Current recommendations would suggest that all patients with a high-risk history be offered the possibility of testing. It has been suggested that premarital screening should be a means of preventing perinatal transmission; however, it is estimated that this would probably result in 350 false-positive tests and 100 false-negative tests and detect only 1/10 of 1 percent of individuals affected with HIV in the United States (Shapiro et al, 1989).

When the mother is identified as the index case, it has been suggested that all children born to this mother also should be tested. It has been the authors' experience that children up to 5 years of age may be tested and found to be seropositive. It has also been observed that the disease may skip a generation in large families and it may not affect every child.

### Table 8–2
#### INDICATIONS FOR HIV SCREENING IN OBSTETRIC PATIENTS

Intravenous drug user
Heterosexual partner drug user
History of prior cocaine use
Partner with history of sexually transmitted diseases and/or multiple partners
History of prostitution
History of no prior prenatal care, presenting late in pregnancy
History of probation, parole, or jail sentence
History of >5 sexual partners
History of bisexual partner
Received blood or blood products prior to 1985
Patient request

## Intervention

Intervention in this spiraling process must take the form of innovative outreach and education on the part of the health care provider. The health care provider must be well versed and comfortable in discussing sexual matters with his or her patients and must be willing to intervene on the behalf of the pregnant HIV-positive patient in a complex web of social, medical, ethical, and legal aspects. Women of reproductive age frequently turn to their obstetric or gynecologic health care provider for information. In fact, the OB/GYN health care provider may be the only health care provider in regular contact with women at risk. Frank discussions of sexual practices and birth control are necessary with the nonpregnant high-risk female. Women should be counseled early in pregnancy as to the probability of having an infected child and the availability of pregnancy termination. Many women, with the discovery of the positive serostatus in early pregnancy, do not elect to terminate the pregnancy, and many women may delay seeking prenatal care to a point in gestation in which termination is not possible (Fekety, 1989).

Unfortunately, women with the highest potential risk for HIV infection are often found in areas isolated by illiteracy, poverty, language barriers, and inaccessibility to health care (Taylor, 1989). It is this particular group of women who have incomplete or inaccurate and sometimes nonexistent knowledge regarding HIV infection and AIDS (Christiamo and Susser, 1989). The authors have found that these women benefit the most from innovative outreach. Frequently, the identifying index event is labor and delivery. By providing obstetric and gynecologic care in alternative settings (e.g., prison, drug rehabilitation centers, homes for unwed adolescent mothers, charity hospitals), we can identify an increasing number of HIV-positive pregnant women before delivery and initiate prenatal care. By using all available social service and medical resources, it is possible to track and audit these women and to provide them with standard prenatal care. The networking of the different available agencies is an art form in its orchestration, but one can coordinate services to the benefit of the patient. If the patient views the health care team as an advocate and resource tool, compliance with prenatal care is enhanced.

## Social and Psychologic Aspects: Special Obstetric Concerns

When a pregnant woman is identified as HIV positive, sensitivity should be given to the confidentiality of the patient's condition and, in particular, to the fact that social problems may develop when positive test results are known. The social stigma attached to a positive test result may result in a litany of social dilemmas that the health care provider is not prepared to deal with. As noted earlier, additional children within the woman's family may be seropositive. Unfortunately, not all school systems or communities are able to understand the true nature of transmission, and appropriate social services and health officials should be used to ensure confidentiality and support for the mother and her children.

Most of these women come from an environment of poverty, surrounded by drug abuse, illiteracy, and hardship. Even when these women first discover they are pregnant, they do not seek prenatal care as early as they should. The authors' experience has been that this population seeks out medical care at approximately 22 to 26 weeks' gestation. The woman begins to feel the baby move, and the uterus is enlarged enough so that she begins to show her pregnancy. Once she arrives seeking care, it is necessary to help her overcome the barriers she perceives to accessing health care for her to maintain compliance in her prenatal visits.

**Transportation.** Frequently, these women do not have any means of transportation for their visits. It has been the authors' experience that some patients do not know how they will get to the hospital when they go into labor; cab fare is too expensive and buses are not easily accessed, run too infrequently, or are too crowded for a pregnant woman with other children in tow. Although the Department of Human Services, welfare, and services such as the Red Cross offer some transportation assistance, their geographical areas are limited, the number of seats that one patient may occupy is limited, and their time limitations are very restrictive. Churches in the community have begun to network their volunteer organizations in an effort to help patients with HIV and AIDS. They may help by assisting one patient and ensuring that she gets her prenatal care and a ride to the hospital when labor begins. The health care provider should speak to the various church groups and let them know his or her needs in order to successfully develop a network of support for his or her patients.

**Living Environment.** Many pregnant HIV-positive women do not have stable living arrangements. Many women feel tremendous guilt and shame about the infection they have acquired. Some choose not to tell anyone of their seropositivity; others tell their family members, and frequently, the familial support is withdrawn, and these women are asked to leave the household. The dilemma the health care provider faces is the lack of facilities for pregnant women and their children. The best the health care provider has to offer is to assess each case individually and work closely with the social service agencies in locating housing for these patients.

**Nutrition.** Many communities have "stone-soup kitchens" available to patients with a diagnosis of AIDS, however, these services may not be available to women who are HIV positive. Many AIDS patients have problems with wasting and malabsorption, or they may be undernourished secondarily to their pregnancy and drug abuse. They may also feed their children before they feed themselves. These facilities provide food on a daily or weekly basis to eligible patients. The authors have found that many patients need supplemental feeding such as liquid supplement prescribed two to three times daily. The health care provider may also network with the social agencies and churches to try to arrange for more food in the house.

The multiple social and medical dilemmas of pregnant HIV-positive patients can be overcome with creative outreach and thorough networking with the available social agencies.

# Management of the HIV-Positive Pregnant Patient

Management should be undertaken with several goals in mind:

1. To be wary of nonspecific symptoms commonly attributed to normal pregnancy, which may be the harbingers of progression of HIV infection.

2. To attempt to decrease the risk of morbidity and mortality to the woman and her fetus of HIV-associated diseases and their treatments.

3. To attempt continued surveillance of the patient's social environment, being wary that a disruptive living environment can lead to antigenic stimulation due to malnutrition, infection, and depression.

# ANTEPARTUM MANAGEMENT

The initial assessment of the HIV-positive pregnant woman should include an evaluation of her medical and social needs. The immediate needs of a woman who has been informed she is HIV-positive are "support and counseling" (Minkoff, 1987). Issues of concern to her are those of death and transmission of the virus to her infant. Psychologic support in the form of counseling and education should be ongoing. Other issues that may arise after the initial visit are transmission of the virus to sexual partners, safe sex, testing of sex partners, and health concerns. The initial medical evaluation should include a surveillance of the maternal immune system as well as laboratory tests to detect other immunologic problems indirectly evidenced. Because HIV infection is a sexually transmitted disease, screening cultures for other sexually transmitted diseases should be done. These include reactive plasma reagin (RPR) for syphilis evaluation, hepatitis B surface antigen, chlamydia and gonorrhea cultures, skin testing for anergy with purified protein derivative (PPD), and candida control. Specific serologies for cytomegalovirus and Epstein-Barr virus should be performed. It may be helpful to culture for cytomegalovirus, since in the carrier state of the mother, this may be an early marker for infants that are more predisposed to cytomegalovirus infections. In addition to these tests, a complete blood count (CBC) with differential and an absolute T-cell count should be performed and repeated every trimester. (Table 8–3)

It should be stressed that past fears about the transmission of HIV through the administration of the RhoGAM preparation have been alleviated in recent studies (Physicians Desk Reference, 1991). Owing to the way the immunoglobulin is prepared, transmission of HIV through this route cannot be accomplished. RhoGAM is safe; it does not transmit HIV infection, and under no circumstances should it be withheld (Wofsy, 1988).

Initial ultrasound evaluation should also be performed and repeated every trimester for intrauterine growth retardation, congenital abnormalities, and placental problems. This population of mothers is at risk for complications, including prematurity, low birth weight, and fetal distress, that are frequently seen in drug-abusing mothers and mothers of low income. Prospective studies

## Table 8–3
### PRENATAL LABS AND CULTURES

**Prior to Delivery/One Time**
HIV antibody—p$^{24}$ antigen
RPR*
PAP†
Hepatitis B surface antigen
Chlamydia culture, gonorrhea culture
HSV‡ titer, Rubella titer
Toxoplasmosis serology
Skin tests—PPD§, *Candida*
CMV‖ culture (cervix and womb)

**Every Trimester**
CBC¶, diff, platelet, and T helper/
suppressor
Immunoglobulin
Ultrasound of fetus

---

\* RPR = reactive plasma reagin
† PAP = Papanicolaou's smear
‡ HSV = herpes simplex virus
§ PPD = purified protein derivative
‖ CMV = cytomegalovirus
¶ CBC = complete blood count

suggest that HIV-positive infants and their noninfected counterparts have no significant difference in the rate of these complications. An ultrasound study should include assessment of the biparietal diameter, head circumference, the abdominal circumference, femur length, and amniotic fluid volume estimates.

## INTRAPARTUM MANAGEMENT

A concern of health care providers is that during labor, owing to contamination, they may be exposed to an increased risk of contracting HIV. The Centers for Disease Control have published guidelines for prevention of HIV infection in the health care setting that include the basic universal precautions concept (Centers for Disease Control, 1987). New Occupational Safety and Health Association (OSHA, 1991) guidelines have mandated new controls to decrease health care workers' exposure to blood and body fluids. The Centers for Disease Control recommend that blood and body fluid precautions be consistently used for *all* patients, regardless of their bloodborne infection status. They recommend that protective barriers be used when handling any blood or body fluids; this includes the use of gowns, gloves, masks, and protective eyewear, as the setting indicates (MMWR, 1987). In addition, it should be stressed that the use of gloves, protective

eyewear, and repellent gowns has been recommended for vaginal and cesarean deliveries (Minkoff, 1987). Gloves should also be worn when handling the infant. It has been the authors' personal experience that even with a vaginal delivery, all participants should wear masks. Though there have been no cases of AIDS transmission to the health care provider by the splashed amniotic fluid, wearing a mask is still recommended. Furthermore, it should be stated that all practitioners who have the privilege of assisting women at the time of delivery encourage their patients by shouting at them to push. Because most health care providers cannot restrain themselves from such encouragement, masks should be worn. There are no data to suggest that a cesarean section would prevent transmission of the virus, and it should be carried out for obstetric or medical indications only. Again, universal precautions should be adhered to and certain practices such as pointing with one's finger in the incision when one's assistant has a sharp instrument should be discouraged to prevent accidents. It has also been the authors' practice to cut the needle off before tying knots, to further prevent accidental needle sticks. It is also important that the pediatrician be notified of the mother's infection prior to the delivery so he or she can also adhere to universal precautions. Currently, for HIV-positive women in the United States, breastfeeding is not recommended. It has been reported that breast milk has the virus present, and it is recommended that, even with the initial colostrum, breastfeeding not be performed by the mother (Wofsy, 1988).

## POSTPARTUM CONSIDERATIONS

Before the delivery of the child, the health care provider arranges for the pediatric follow-up. The pediatric group is notified, and the patient meets with the team before her delivery. This ensures close pediatric supervision after delivery. The health care provider also counsels the parents before delivery regarding the serostatus of their infant. It is necessary to inform them that 100 percent of the babies born to HIV-positive women have positive results when a blood test is performed at birth; this is secondary to the passage of maternal antibodies to the infant. Also, only 30 percent of infants born to HIV-positive women are truly HIV positive; and the infants' serostatus cannot be determined until 3 to 6 months after birth. Of those infants who are HIV-positive, 90 percent die by the age of 4, without therapy. Thus, the emphasis is on close pediatric follow-up and the importance of arranging pediatric care before the delivery.

## SPECIAL THERAPEUTIC CONSIDERATIONS IN HIV-POSITIVE PATIENTS

There are several controversies surrounding HIV-positive patients as to when therapy should be initiated, especially in the asymptomatic patient. The rationale for the use of zidovudine (Retrovir or AZT) is based on clinical trials, and the recommendations of the FDA advisory committee on new drug applications are for all adult, HIV-positive patients without symptoms and with CD4 cell counts of 500 or less to receive treatment with zidovudine. Earlier, management included treatment for patients with CD4 counts less than 200. The current recommendations state that Retrovir be started in dosages of 500 mg/day in asymptomatic patients. Prior recommendations had prescribed dosages of 200 mg q 4 hr. The monitoring of patients on Retrovir in the nonpregnant state is summarized:

1. Monitor CBC and clinical status q 2 weeks for 4 to 8 weeks until the patient is stabilized on Retrovir
2. Monitor CBC q 1 month
3. Monitor CD4 periodically, and when CD4 level approaches 200, consider PCP prophylaxis
4. Watch for pneumocystis pneumonia (PCP) and other complications of immune CD4 dysfunction
5. Start counseling concerning opportunistic infections and other complications of HIV disease as CD4 level approaches 200

In the summer of 1989, Burroughs Wellcome Company reviewed the results of standard lifetime carcinogenicity bioassays of AZT in animals. Oral AZT was administered on a daily basis at three different dosages to mice and rats and to 60 males and 60 females of each species for periods of 18 and 20

months. Histologic examination revealed vaginal carcinoma in five female mice in the highest dose group. Two other mice in this group and one in the middle dose group had a benign vaginal tumor. There were also 2 of the 60 female rats in the highest dose group that had vaginal carcinomas. It is believed, currently, that the predictive value for humans of these animal models is limited and that these drugs should still be prescribed for humans owing to the fact that the potential effectiveness outweighs the risks. Further murine studies are planned, particularly to study transplacental carcinogenicity (Schuman et al, 1990). A phase I pharmacokinetic study of AZT use during pregnancy reports plasma levels similar to those of nonpregnant patients. The AZT levels (90 minutes after the dosage) were 0.43 mmol in maternal plasma and 0.48 mmol in infant plasma. This suggests that AZT freely crosses the placenta (Schuman et al, 1990).

Prophylaxis studies have indicated that trimethoprim-sulfamethoxazole (Kaplan et al, 1986), pyrimethamine and sulfidoxime (Fischl et al, 1988), and pentamidine may decrease the incidence of PCP (Madoff et al, 1986; Karaffa et al, 1986). Trimethoprim-sulfamethoxazole is a category C drug. Cleft palates have been reported in rodents; however, in a study of 186 human pregnancies, there was no significant increase in congenital abnormalities.

Aerosolized pentamidine isethionate (Nebu-Pent) has reduced PCP by 50 to 70 percent at a dosage of 300 mg q 4 weeks (Leoung et al, 1990). The aerosol form may be better tolerated with less toxicity of hypoglycemia, renal, and other metabolic side effects. The use of PCP agents in pregnancy produces some concerns. There should be some awareness that Bactrim may interfere with folic acid metabolism. The controversy of this report is that, at present, the uninfected versus the infected fetus cannot be distinguished, and two thirds of the babies treated may be HIV negative. The dilemma of the mother's need for therapy when her T cells are low versus the production of unwanted side effects on the fetus is still unresolved (Table 8–4).

The demographics of HIV infection are rapidly changing. Heterosexual contact and intravenous drug use are the predominant modes of transmission in women. Women most susceptible to HIV infection are those who are of reproductive age. This fact repre-

**Table 8–4**
DRUGS THAT MAY BE NECESSARY FOR TREATMENT OF HIV-INFECTED
PREGNANT WOMEN

| Problem | Drug/Dose | FDA Category | Side Effects |
|---|---|---|---|
| **CD4 count <200** | Zidovudine 100 mgPO q 4 h (Retrovir/AZT) (Note: patient taking AZT should not take acetaminophen or probenecid—can elevate blood levels of AZT by interfering with excretion) | C | Anemia, GI upset, nausea, vomiting, headache, fatigue, pruritus |
| ***Pneumocystis carinii*** Acute | Trimethoprim-sulfamethoxazole 15–20 mg/kg, 75–100 mg/kg PO, or IV × 14–21 days in 3–4 daily doses or | C | Drug fever, nausea, rash, bone marrow suppression |
| | Pentamidine 3–4 mg/kg/day IV | C | Nephrotoxicity, nausea, hypotension, hypoglycemia, marrow suppression |
| Prophylaxis | Aerosolized pentamidine 300 mg q monthly | C | May have less toxicity since not absorbed systemically |
| | Trimethoprim (5 mg/kg), sulfamethoxazole 20 mg/kg, PO (1DS) q 3 × wkly | C | Interferes with folic acid metabolism |
| ***Toxoplasma encephalitis*** | Pyrimethamine 25 mg + Folic acid 15 mg + | C | Thrombocytopenia, neutropenia |
| | Sulfadiazine 4–6 g/day, PO q d, or 3–5 × wkly | C | Acute renal failure, thrombocytopenia |

(Patients who respond to primary therapy with the above-mentioned drugs should be given lifelong suppressive therapy. Also, for patients allergic to sulfonamides, Clindamycin, 900 mg TID, can be used)

| Problem | Drug/Dose | FDA Category | Side Effects |
|---|---|---|---|
| ***Candida*** | Clotrimazole troche 30–50 mg | B | Mild transaminase elevation, dental caries secondary to dextrose component |
| | or Nystatin suspension 3 MU | B | Diarrhea, nausea, vomiting |
| | or Ketaconazole 200–400 mg PO BID | C | Nausea, hepatotoxicity, rash, adrenal suppression |
| **Herpes** Cutaneous | Acyclovir 200 mg PO q 4 h for 10–14 days | C | Rash, nausea, diarrhea, vertigo |
| Disseminated | Acyclovir 15 mg/kg/day IV × 7 days | C | Nephrotoxicity, headache, marrow suppression, encephalopathy |

sents a poor forecast for the infants born to these women. Opportunistic infections remain the principal cause of death in HIV-infected women and children.

Transmission is secondary to certain behaviors and actions. Continued education by health care providers can help intervene in the spread of HIV. Health care providers must be able to comfortably examine and discuss sexual issues with the female patient in order to disseminate information.

The pregnant HIV-positive woman presents a particular challenge to the health care provider in terms of medical, social, and ethical issues. The health care provider must be alert to signs and symptoms of HIV progression, which can be masked by the pregnancy. Most importantly, the HIV-infected obstetric patient needs to be identified early in pregnancy. Continued outreach and programs that can break through the barriers of illiteracy, poverty, and language differences are needed to allow women access to care. Alternative care sites are ideal for identifying at-risk populations.

The management of an HIV-positive obstetric patient brings many issues of controversy to the health care provider. Abortions, alternative sexual lifestyles, drug use in pregnancy, testing issues, and protection of health care providers are only a few of the problems associated with an HIV-positive woman. Health care providers must understand the fundamental nature of the disease, recognize areas of intervention, and be committed to providing care to a most difficult population.

## References

AIDS Research Exchange, National Institute of Allergy and Infectious Disease. Washington, DC, US Department of Health and Human Services, Summer, 1990.

Centers for Disease Control: Recommendations for prevention of HIV transmission in health care settings. MMWR 36(25), 1987.

Christiamo A, Susser I: Knowledge and perceptions of HIV infection among pregnant women. J Nurse Midwifery 34(6):318, 1989.

Chu SY, Buehler JW, Berkelman RL: Impact of human immunodeficiency virus epidemic on mortality in women of reproductive age in the United States. JAMA 204(2):225, 1990.

Fallon J, Eddy J, Wiesner L, Pizzo P: Human immunodeficiency virus infection in children. J Pediatr 114:1‑27, 1989.

Feinkind L, Minkoff HL: HIV in pregnancy. Clin Perinatol Jun; 15(2):189, 1988.

Fekety S: Managing the HIV-positive patient and her newborn in a CNM service. J Nurse Midwifery 34(5), 1989.

Fischl MA, Dickinson GM, LaVoie L: Safety and efficacy of sulfamethoxazole and trimethoprim chemoprophylaxis for Pneumocystis carinii pneumonia in AIDS. JAMA 259:1185, 1988.

Hammill HA: AIDS during pregnancy. In Faro S, Gilstrap L (eds): Infections and Pregnancy. New York, Alan R Liss, 1989.

Harawi S: Epidemiology in pathology and pathphysiology of AIDS. In Harawi S, O'Hara C (eds): Pathophysiology of AIDS. St Louis, CV Mosby, 1989, p 5.

HIV/AIDS Surveillance. Washington, DC, US Department of Health and Human Services, July 1990.

Kaplan LD, Wong R, Wofsy C, et al: Trimethoprim-sulfamethoxazole prophylaxis of Pneumocystis carinii pneumonia in AIDS. Paris, Second International Conference on AIDS, 1986, no 53. Abstract.

Karaffa C, Rehm S, Calabrese L: Efficacy of monthly pentamidine infusions in preventing recurrent Pneumocystis carinii pneumonia (PCP) in AIDS patients. Washington, DC, 26th Interscience Conference on Antimicrobial Agents and Chemotherapy, 1986, no 224. Abstract.

Karan L: AIDS prevention and chemical dependence. Treatment needs of women and their children. J Psychoactive Drugs 21(4):395, 1989.

Kornfeld H: HIV and T-lymphotropic virus In Harawi S, O'Hara C (eds): Pathophysiology of AIDS. St Louis, CV Mosby, 1989, p 37

Lawrence L, Levy S, Robinson L: Self-efficacy and AIDS prevention for pregnant teenagers. J Sch Health, 60(1):19, 1990.

Leoung G, Montgomery AB, Feigal DW, et al: Aerosolized pentamidine prophylaxis therapy for Pneumocystis carinii pneumonia (PCP) in AIDS patients. Data on file, Lyphomed, Inc. 1990.

Madoff LC, Scavuzzo D, Roberts RB: Fansidar secondary prophylaxis of Pneumocystis carinii pneumonia in AIDS patients. Clin Res 34:524A, 1986.

Minkoff HL: Care of pregnant women infected with human immunodeficiency virus. JAMA 258:2714–2717, 1987.

MMWR (Morbidity and Mortality Weekly Report) Update: Universal Precautions for Prevention of Transmission of Human Immunodeficiency Virus, Hepatitis B Virus, and Other Bloodborne Pathogens in Health Care Settings. 37(24):377–382, 1988.

MMWR (Morbidity and Mortality Weekly Report) Increase in Primary and Secondary Syphilis—United States. 36(25), 1987.

Occupational Safety and Health Administration (OSHA): Occupational Exposure to Blood Borne Pathogens. Federal Regulation 29 CFR, PART 1910.1030, December, 1991.

O'Hara C: The lymphoid and hematopoietic systems. In Harawi S, O'Hara (eds): Pathophysiology of AIDS St. Louis, CV Mosby, 1989, p 135.

Schuman P, Jaufman R, Crane L, Philpot D: Pharmacokinetics of zidovudine during pregnancy. San Francisco, Sixth International Conference on AIDS, June 23, 1990, p 94. Abstract.

Scott GB, Hutto C, Makuch RW, et al: Survival in children with perinatally acquired human immunodeficiency virus type I infection. N Engl J Med 321 (26):1791, 1989.

Shapiro CN, Shulz SL, Lee NC, Dondero TJ et al: Review of human immunodeficiency virus infection in women in the United States. Obstet Gynecol 74(5):801, 1989.

Sivak SL, Wormser GP: Predictive value of a screening test for antibodies to HTLV-III. Am J Clin Pathol 85:700–703, 1986.

Taylor P: Impact of AIDS on women's lives and implementation for nurse-midwifery practice. J Nurse Midwifery 34(5):273, 1989.

Wofsy C: Prevention of HIV transmission. In Sande M (ed): The Medical Management of AIDS. Philadelphia, WB Saunders Co, 1988, p. 35.

1991 PDR, publisher Edward Barhart, Medical Economics, Data p. 1131.

· · · · · · · · · · · · · · · · · · · · · · · · · · · · · · · · · ·

# CHAPTER 9

# Medications in Pregnancy

William Rayburn and Donald Marsden

Among the most deeply rooted fears of the pregnant woman is the concern that her baby may be malformed. One of the first questions she asks after the birth is usually "Is the baby normal?", and at the earliest opportunity she will generally examine the baby herself for reassurance. But for at least 3 percent of mothers, such fears are realized by the delivery of a child with a major congenital abnormality. When such an event occurs it is natural for the mother, her family, and her attendants to seek a cause or explanation. For untold centuries, the only explanations were divine retribution for actual or imagined sins, witchcraft, or the imprint on the fetus of traumatic events affecting the mother during gestation.

The recognition that drugs, radiation and other environmental agents are potentially teratogenic is relatively recent, yet it has captured the imagination of the public at large and the medical and legal professions in particular. Increased awareness of the risks of drug use in pregnancy raises the prospect of more sensible and controlled patterns of demand and use. On the other hand, it has spawned a flood of chiefly anecdotal reports in the medical and lay press, incriminating, on often dubious grounds, a wide range of drugs in the production of an equally wide range of abnormalities.

Some authors advocate therapeutic nihilism, an attitude that is encouraged by the package inserts in a large proportion of currently available medications carrying such disclaimers as "the safety of this drug for use in pregnancy has not been established." These statements greatly increase the medicolegal hazards of prescribing medications without clarifying the medical risks. The end result could easily be a situation in which even potentially lifesaving drugs are withheld for fear of teratogenesis, and the pregnant woman and her child become deprived of therapy (Shirkey, 1968). Attention has also been drawn to a tragic postscript that may follow the birth of a malformed baby, in which distortion or misinterpretation of available information regarding teratogens can lead to litigation-produced pain, disease, and suffering affecting the whole family, medical attendants, and attorneys.

Although teratogenic effects are the most publicized concern related to prescribed drug use in pregnancy, there are a number of other important considerations. The physical and physiologic changes of pregnancy affect the absorption, distribution, metabolism, and excretion of medications. For example, plasma levels of ampicillin achieved after a given oral or intravenous dose of ampicillin in pregnancy are significantly lower than those in the same women in the nonpregnant state, even when corrected for weight changes (Philipson, 1977). The potential therapeutic connotations of such changes are readily apparent. Medications used during pregnancy and labor may affect parameters used to assess fetal well-being, without necessarily compromising the fetus. For example, narcotics given to a woman during labor can temporarily reduce the fetal heart rate beat-to-beat variability. The potential for neonatal depression from opiates and tranquilizers used in labor is well known. Although this list of factors that have a bearing on drug use in pregnancy is far from complete, it highlights the importance of considerations other than teratogenicity in decision-making.

It is the aim of this chapter to present the problems in perspective, to summarize the current state of knowledge relating to various commonly used medications, and to help the reader develop a rational approach to prescribed drug use in pregnancy.

Establishing the appropriate plan of medication management for the pregnant woman requires collaboration among all members of the perinatal team, as well as the cooperation of family members. This collaborative effort involves education and counseling, perhaps including genetic counseling, for those patients taking medications for preexisting medical diseases. Education is also necessary for patients who will be taking medications they have never taken before, including explanations of how to administer the medication, the necessity for taking it, and any adverse effects that may be anticipated. This education should include the entire family, because the medication regime, its use, including disposal of syringes when used, and side effects may influence the family's lifestyle.

## Medications as Teratogens

(Table 9–1)

### HISTORICAL ASPECTS

The ancient belief that a pregnant woman's experiences impressed themselves on the fetus, producing congenital abnormalities, is accepted in varying degrees by segments of contemporary society. As recently as the 18th century, malformed infants (and often their mothers) were burned as "products of witchcraft or bestiary" (Tuchmann-Duplessis, 1975). (The role of drugs in teratogenesis was suggested in the early 18th and 19th centuries by committees of the Royal College of Physicians and British Parliament, which reported that infants of alcoholic women had a "starved, shriveled, and imperfect look" [Woollam, 1980].)

For the first half of this century, congenital defects in humans were believed to be genetic in origin. Environmental teratogens were thought to be excluded by a "placen-

**Table 9–1**
THE TERATOGENIC STATUS OF
VARIOUS MEDICATIONS

**Proven Teratogens**
  Alcohol (as in alcohol abuse)
  Androgenic hormones
  Cytotoxic agents
    *High risk:* Folate antagonists, e.g., methotrexate;
              Alkylating agents, e.g., busulfan
              cyclophosphamide
    *Lesser risk:* All others
  Diethylstilbestrol
  Radioiodine
  Thalidomide
  Therapeutic radiation
  Warfarin
  *Cis* retinoic acid
**Probable Teratogens**
  Lithium
  Phenytoin
  Quinine
  Trimethadione
  Valproic acid
**Possible Teratogens**
  Barbiturates
  Chloroquine
  Estrogens
  Primidone
  Progestagens

tal barrier." In 1935, it was shown that anophthalmia in pigs was not inherited but was due to deficiency of vitamin A (Hale, 1935). Transplacental viral teratogenesis was recognized in 1941 with the description of part of the now classic congenital rubella syndrome (Gregg, 1941). Simultaneous reports from Australia (McBride, 1962) and Germany (Lenz, 1961) of thalidomide-induced abnormalities, most notably phocomelia, demonstrated the fallibility of the "placental barrier." That a supposedly harmless sedative left 5000 grossly deformed infants in Germany alone, and thousands more worldwide, led to intense research into teratogenesis, undermined faith in the medical profession and drug industry, and changed our attitudes regarding prescribing medicine in pregnancy. In 1971, transplacental carcinogenesis was described when diethylstilbestrol (DES) was found to be responsible for an "epidemic" of vaginal adenocarcinoma (Herbst et al, 1971), which was subsequently recognized to be only a relatively uncommon part of a syndrome of genital tract abnormalities in both sexes (Herbst, 1981). The effects of DES are not usually recognized before puberty, a reminder that teratogenicity may not become apparent for many years.

Important though animal and laboratory studies are, "reliable predictability of human teratogenic potential . . . is not possible other than by long term assessment . . . in humans" (Stern, 1981). Such studies are difficult to initiate and execute, yet they are crucial.

## INCIDENCE AND CAUSES OF CONGENITAL ANOMALIES

It is generally accepted that at least 3 percent of newborns have birth defects requiring therapy, one third of them life-threatening. With long-term follow-up the overall rate reaches 7 to 10 percent (Shepard and Fantel, 1981), varying according to standards of observation, definitions of "defect," and racial factors.

Wilson (1973) believed 25 percent of birth defects to be due to genetic or chromosomal factors, 10 percent to environmental factors, and 65 percent to unknown factors. More recently, multifactorial inheritance has been blamed for 30 percent of congenital defects, mendelian inheritance or chromosomal disorders for 20 percent, and drugs and environmental agents for 8 percent, with 42 percent being of unknown etiology (Holmes, 1980). It is important to recognize that the proportion of congenital abnormalities resulting from genetic or chromosomal factors is much greater than that arising from medications. Nevertheless, medications may play some role in the sizable category of defects of unknown origin. Thalidomide and DES are unusual teratogens, producing, in a high proportion of exposed fetuses, easily recognized abnormalities that rarely occur spontaneously. More subtle agents may produce abnormalities in a small proportion of cases or increase the incidence of relatively common anomalies.

Teratogenic effects can be species-specific: rats, mice, and rabbits are immune to thalidomide, whereas primates and humans are sensitive. Within a species, genetic factors affect susceptibility to various teratogens. Differing genetic strains of mice vary greatly in the incidence of both spontaneous and cortisone-induced cleft palates (Fraser and Fainstat, 1951). Many genetically controlled factors, such as palatal closure rate, predispose or protect different strains of mice from medication-induced cleft palate (Fraser, 1980). Susceptibility to medication-induced neural tube defects is genetically controlled in mice (Cole and Trasler, 1980). Further-more, fetal mice within the same uterus have different sensitivities to maternally administered teratogens, related to enzyme production controlled by a single gene (Nebert and Shum, 1980).

## DETERMINING THE TERATOGENIC POTENTIAL OF MEDICATIONS

Animal tests are the first wall of defense against teratogenesis. One limitation is variations in sensitivity from one species to another. Dosage is an important consideration: The mother must survive, and there may be only a narrow dose range between the safe dosage and fetotoxic dosages that result in teratogenesis. Massive doses of saline or sucrose are teratogenic in animals (Shepard, 1973). The production of congenital malformations in experimental animals still is an art, and the application of the results to humans is complex. As Blake (1982) has stated, "There are so many examples of inconsistency between results of animal teratogenic studies and the human experience that a credibility gap has developed." The future may lie in testing medications in cell, organ, or even embryo cultures.

Information regarding teratogenicity in humans may be derived from case reports, controlled or uncontrolled retrospective studies, or prospective studies. All are important, but the most valuable are prospective studies of large populations, which monitor drug exposure and include careful follow-up of the infants.

Retrospective studies usually involve taking a group of women delivering infants with congenital abnormalities, matching them with a control group delivering normal infants, and comparing drug use. This method allows study of small numbers of patients, whereas a prospective study may involve, for example, following as many as 10,000 pregnancies in order to gain data on 50 neural tube defects. The problem with retrospective studies is memory bias, with "the control mother forgetting and the mother of the malformed child embroidering events that the latter may blame for her misfortune" (Leck, 1978). This problem can seriously bias the results of retrospective studies and produce spurious associations between birth defects and pregnancy events. An example of recall bias is a Finnish study of congenital central nervous system abnormalities. In this study, several drugs apparently related to the defects when one control group was used were found to bear no significant relationship to the defects when another control group was used (Granroth, 1978). All who have seen the often desperate attempts of parents of children with congenital abnormalities to find a cause for the abnormalities understand how easily false assumptions can be made. Most frequently, such false assumptions are made linking the use of commonly used drugs with uncommon anomalies.

It is suggested that a national register of birth defects should be established, which would indicate changing incidence rates and allow prospective studies of etiologic factors. Difficult though such a project would be to initiate and maintain, it holds the greatest hope for satisfactory monitoring of teratogens.

## RELATIVE AND ABSOLUTE RISKS

Virtually all congenital abnormalities associated with intrauterine medication exposure also occur spontaneously in the general population. Thalidomide and diethylstilbestrol are unusual in that they affect a very high proportion of exposed fetuses and produce distinctive abnormalities that occur at a very low frequency in the unexposed population. Most suspected teratogens appear to produce small increases in incidence of more common abnormalities; hence the concept of relative risk.

Heinonen and coworkers define the relative risk of a medication producing an abnormality as "the ratio of the rate of a defect in exposed children to the rate in non-exposed children" (Heinonen et al, 1977). This approach offers information on the magnitude of the association and allows one to estimate the reduction in risk if a drug is not used. It is important to keep in mind a number of factors when considering teratogenic risks. First, it is easier to recognize the teratogenic effect of a commonly used drug producing a rare anomaly than the effect of a rarely used drug producing a commonly seen abnormality. Second, the impact of a teratogen depends on *absolute* risk as well as *relative* risk. For example, a drug with a relative risk of 3 produces a threefold increase in abnormalities in infants of users compared with those of nonusers. But if the incidence of the abnormality in the unexposed population is 1 in

1000, the incidence in the exposed population is still predicted to be only 3 in 1000. Even when *relative* risks are high, *absolute* risks may be low. Few medications had relative risks higher than 2 in the study of Heinonen and colleagues (1977). This is not to diminish the significance of the damage done to affected children but rather to emphasize the importance of considering risk-to-benefit ratios when prescribing medications in pregnancy.

## EXTENT OF MEDICATION USE IN PREGNANCY

Pregnant women consume a large variety of medications. The Collaborative Perinatal Project considered medications taken from the time of conception to 48 hours before labor and excluded vitamins, iron, antacids, and intravenous fluids. The mean number of medications used was 3.8, with less than 6 percent of all the women studied taking no medications at all. Furthermore, the study extended from 1958 to 1965, a period that included the thalidomide "epidemic"; yet, throughout the time of the study, drug use by pregnant women increased, making it clear that "publicity directed to avoiding unnecessary use of drugs during pregnancy was a failure" (Heinonen et al, 1977).

The most commonly used medications are antipyretic analgesics, antimicrobials, antinauseants, and antihistamines. A pregnant woman and the high-risk team must weigh the potential benefits of any medication against possible risks. Our present knowledge makes the risks of most agents difficult to predict; thus, all that can be hoped for is the avoidance of thoughtless or frivolous prescribing of medications in pregnancy.

# Problems in Prescribing Medications in Pregnancy

It is beyond the scope of this chapter to discuss all of the situations involving the prescription of medications that can arise in pregnancy. Rather, the aim of this section is to discuss principles and offer guidelines for prescribing medications for chronic medical disorders during pregnancy.

Ideally, each person should be counseled before conception about the risks and benefits of the underlying medical condition and accompanying medications therapy. Medications prescribed for chronic medical disorders during pregnancy may not necessarily be the ideal choice for the nonpregnant patient, but they should be the ones used most often and thought to be the least harmful during intrauterine exposure. Unless the medication or metabolite is of large spatial configuration or molecular weight, umbilical cord serum concentrations become nearly comparable to those of the mother as exposure to the medication is continued during pregnancy. Information is limited about comparative trials of medications used to treat medical disorders during pregnancy because of insufficient patient numbers and ethical dilemmas in undertaking randomized or double-blind investigations during pregnancy.

General principles of therapy in pregnancy are the same as in the nonpregnant state. A healthy mother is more likely to deliver a healthy infant. To maintain therapeutic concentrations in the expanded intravascular volume during pregnancy, the medication may need to be given in a higher dose or with greater frequency. Symptoms of pregnancy may mimic side effects or toxic reactions of medications. Prenatal vitamins containing iron and folic acid should be prescribed to women with chronic medical disorders during pregnancy. Antibiotics, the most commonly prescribed medications during pregnancy, may affect the metabolism of other medications through the normal bacterial flora. Antacids and kaolin-pectin may impair absorption of oral medications.

## CHRONIC HYPERTENSION

A challenge to the obstetrician is to choose the medication that offers the maximum safety for the fetus and therapeutic response for the mother. Many medications have been used, but few randomized clinical trials have been undertaken (Lubbe, 1990). Home blood pressure monitoring has been especially useful in our practice, because so many women whose blood pressures are elevated in the clinic are within a more acceptable range at home.

The most commonly used antihypertensive medication during pregnancy is methyldopa (Aldomet), a false neurotransmitter. Maternal sedation, a rare hemolytic anemia, and a positive Coombs' test are the only significant maternal adverse effects. Fetal effects are thought to be negligible. The second antihypertensive of choice during pregnancy is usually hydralazine (Apresoline). This peripheral vasodilator may cause maternal tachycardia, palpitations, a lupus-like syndrome, and headaches, but no adverse effects on the fetus have been associated with long-term use.

Beta-adrenergic blocking agents, most notably propranolol (Inderal), may also serve as second-line medications for treating chronic hypertension. Initial reports of an increased incidence of fetal growth retardation, bradycardia, hypoglycemia, and neonatal respiratory distress are likely exaggerated (Lindheimer and Katz, 1985). Less information is available about the newer and more selective beta-blocking medications. These more selective beta-adrenergic blocking agents (atenolol, metoprolol [Lopressor], labetalol [Normodyne, Trandate]) are as effective as propranolol but pose the risk of acute hypotension if started initially during pregnancy.

Thiazide diuretic therapy should not be used during pregnancy in order to avoid metabolic disturbances and thrombocytopenia in the mother and fetus. A decreased maternal intravascular volume has been associated with diuretic therapy, and short-term therapy using large doses may diminish uteroplacental perfusion and lead to a greater incidence of fetal demise.

Angiotensin-converting enzyme (ACE) inhibitors such as captopril (Capoten, Capozide) and enalapril (Vasotec) are becoming commonly used in reproductive-aged women. Hypotensive effects are concerns presented with the use of these agents, as with the calcium channel blockers (nicardipine [Cardene], verapamil [Calan, Isoptin, Verapamil]), which may also lead to heart failure and atrioventricular block (Hanssens, 1991). Drugs with central sympatholytic action, such as clonidine (Catapres), are often very helpful as first-line oral antihypertensive medications during the immediate postpartum period. Insomnia and rebound hypertension after discontinuation are potential problems (Dunagen and Redner, 1989).

The same antihypertensives used before pregnancy should be resumed after delivery.

Breastfeeding should not be discouraged. Allowing the patient to monitor her own blood pressure continues to be useful under these circumstances.

## ANTICONVULSANT THERAPY

Epileptic women should be discouraged from becoming pregnant when seizures are difficult to control. If the mother has idiopathic grand mal seizures, she should be advised that the risk of her child developing epilepsy is approximately 2 to 5 percent (Dalessio, 1985).

An attempt should be made to withdraw anticonvulsants from the patient over several months before pregnancy if she has been seizure-free for several years and has a normal electroencephalogram. If the woman is not pregnant and is taking a combination of anticonvulsants, an attempt should be made to observe whether or not the seizures can be controlled with only one agent, preferably phenobarbital. However, the patient should be maintained on as many medications as are necessary to control her seizures, because a seizure with hypoxia is of greater concern than is teratogenicity (Meadow, 1991). Trimethadione (Tridione) and valproic acid (Depakene) should be avoided in women during the reproductive-age years because of definite teratogenic concerns. Carbamazepine (Tegretol) is commonly used in reproductive-aged women with grand mal seizures. Despite reports of safety, it may present an increased risk of minor craniofacial abnormalities, digital hypoplasia, and developmental delays.

If the patient is first seen during pregnancy and is well controlled on her current regimen, anticonvulsant agents should not be withdrawn, because this may result in the patient developing status epilepticus. The mother should be advised that the risk of fetal anomalies is increased two- to threefold (8 percent overall) when taking anticonvulsants, and that certain agents present increased risk of mental retardation. Excessive weight gain and sudden fluid retention may increase the risk of seizures.

Patients should be advised that there is a 50 percent risk that a grand mal seizure disorder will worsen during pregnancy, and that this risk is even higher if the woman recently has had frequent seizures (Dalessio,

1985). Serum levels of anticonvulsants should be measured monthly during pregnancy, with adjustments in dosage to keep serum levels in a low-to-normal therapeutic range. Pregnant epileptics receiving phenytoin (Dilantin) or phenobarbital should be given prophylactic oral folic acid (1 mg daily) throughout gestation. This dose is found in standard prenatal vitamins. Vitamin K (5 to 10 mg daily) may be helpful during the last 2 months of pregnancy to prevent a neonatal coagulopathy.

Anticonvulsants should be administered parenterally during labor to prevent intrapartum or postpartum seizures. Infants of mothers receiving phenobarbital should be observed carefully for generalized depression or withdrawal symptoms. There is no contraindication to breastfeeding for mothers taking anticonvulsants as long as the infant shows no signs of generalized depression.

## ASTHMA

Asthma is one of the most common medical disorders in pregnancy, with a reported prevalence of 1 percent. Many medications are available for the control of asthma, and therapy in pregnancy differs little from that in the nonpregnant state. Many patients can be treated solely with intermittent inhalation administration of the $\beta$-2 adrenergic agonists (metaproterenol, terbutaline, or albuterol) through metered-dose inhalers. During short periods of wheezing, two deep inhalations every 4 to 6 hours should be employed.

If intermittent inhalation therapy does not suffice, oral methylxanthine therapy should be initiated. The most common of these phosphodiesterase inhibitors is theophylline; 200 to 400 mg bid of a long-acting preparation is a standard daily maintenance dose. Theophylline (Primatene, Slo-Phyllin, Theo-Dur) clearance is often reduced during late pregnancy (Carter et al, 1986). For optimal effects, the dosage should be adjusted to maintain therapeutic serum levels between 10 and 20 mg/ml. Methylxanthines inhibit the force but not the frequency of uterine contractions, and their use is associated with a theorized risk of prolonged gestation or abnormally long labor (Greenberger and Patterson, 1985). They also accelerate the development of fetal pulmonary maturity because of the phosphodiesterase inhibiting property.

If these women still experience respiratory symptoms, oral beta-adrenergic agents should be used. Several preparations are available, but oral terbutaline, at a dose of 2.5 to 5.0 mg 2 to 3 times daily, is standard. These agents exert their bronchodilating effect by stimulating the $\beta$-2 receptors in bronchial smooth muscle, leading to an increased production of cyclic AMP. Because these medications may also inhibit premature labor, there is a theorized risk of prolonged gestation and desultory labor.

Corticosteroids may be started if the patient remains refractory to the above-mentioned therapeutic regimens. Varying doses from 60 to 100 mg of prednisone as a single daily dose are recommended, with clinical improvement usually seen within 6 hours of therapy. The dosage usually is tapered over 5 days to 2 weeks. Women receiving oral corticosteroid therapy for more than a few days should receive intravenous hydrocortisone (100 mg every 6 hours) during labor and delivery and immediately postpartum (Greenberger and Patterson, 1985).

Breastfeeding should be encouraged, because newborn infants inherit a tendency toward asthma and allergies. The exclusive use of breastfeeding for at least six months may delay the onset of these allergic problems in the child. Less than 4 percent of ingested theophylline appears in breast milk. Inhaled bronchodilators have minimal systemic absorption and, therefore, are probably not secreted in breast milk (Carter et al, 1986).

## INFLAMMATORY BOWEL DISEASE

Inflammatory bowel disease usually begins in adolescence or early adulthood. Neither ulcerative colitis nor Crohn's disease is associated with decreased fertility nor is the problem exacerbated during pregnancy. Therapy begins with modification of diet to avoid lactulose and some fruits and vegetables. Because of an increased requirement during pregnancy, calcium intake may need to be supplemented with Os-Cal, one or two tablets three times daily. Codeine and Imodium are not likely to be associated with any increased fetal risk and may be used judi-ciously for persistent diarrhea. Corticosteroids are usually employed for patients who fail to respond to the above-mentioned measures. They exert their beneficial effect by accumulating in the inflamed bowel tissue and producing a dose-related inhibition of the inflammatory response. However, research into the efficacy of corticosteroids for preventing recurrences in quiescent ulcerative colitis has yielded conflicting results (Willoughby, 1980). Exposure to any of these medications during breastfeeding should not pose a threat to the infant.

Corticosteroids may be administered either orally or as retention enemas in cases of distal colitis. Prednisone in a daily dose of 40 mg is used initially. A single daily dose is preferable to multiple-dose therapy, and most patients experience therapeutic response in 1 to 2 weeks. The dosage is then generally reduced to allow for 4 to 8 weeks of total therapy.

Sulfasalazine (Azulfidine) is also frequently used alone or in combination with corticosteroids for the treatment of inflammatory bowel disease. This medication is split by the bacteria to form 5-aminosalicylate and sulfapyridine. Sulfasalazine has been proved to be effective for treatment of both acute ulcerative colitis and acute Crohn's disease. The body of evidence suggests that prolonged therapy to prevent recurrences is of little benefit (Nielsen et al, 1984). Potential maternal side effects include nausea, anorexia, vomiting, diarrhea, and dizziness. Because sulfasalazine inhibits absorption of folate in the small bowel, folate supplementation is required during pregnancy. This medication crosses the placenta, and cord blood concentrations have been reported to be approximately half those of simultaneously obtained maternal plasma concentrations (Mogadam et al, 1981). No teratogenic effect or jaundice has been attributed to the use of this medication, however. Sulfasalazine is also secreted in breast milk, with concentrations approaching 30 percent of the simultaneous maternal serum concentrations (Mogadam et al, 1981). No adverse neonatal effects have been reported with its use.

Azathioprine (Imuran) is an immune antagonist that is sometimes used in these patients. Most studies have not demonstrated a significant beneficial effect for this anti-inflammatory agent during acute inflammation. It may be beneficial for the prevention of recurrences, but there is considerable controversy regarding this issue. Furthermore, little information has been published about azathioprine and the treatment of inflammatory bowel disease during pregnancy and breastfeeding.

## MIGRAINE HEADACHES

Migraine headaches are very common among women of childbearing age, and relationships to menstruation and oral contraceptive use have been described. Most authors have noted a decrease in the frequency of migraine attacks during pregnancy, especially after the first trimester (Somerville, 1977). The administration of ergot alkaloids for their vasoconstricting properties at the earliest indication of an attack forms the cornerstone of drug therapy in nonpregnant individuals. Most authors recommend that these agents be avoided during pregnancy because of their oxytocic effect. This recommendation may be more emotional than scientific, because several preparations are available that contain ergotominetartrate, which is devoid of oxytocic effects. Ergot alkaloids are also relatively contraindicated in the breastfeeding mother, because of associated neonatal vomiting, diarrhea, and blood pressure disturbances.

Simple analgesics such as acetaminophen (Tylenol) and codeine are generally used for primary therapy during pregnancy. Propranolol (Inderal), 20 mg bid, may be used if analgesics are unsuccessful. In addition to propranolol therapy, chlorpromazine (Thorazine) may be useful for acute attacks in a dose of 25 to 50 mg every 6 to 8 hours; for chronic migraines, a dose of 25 mg three times daily is suggested. Amitriptyline (Elavil, Triavil) also may be useful before sleep in patients with coexisting depression. No reports are available about the use of combinations of analgesics, sedatives, and caffeine or sympathomimetic amines (such as Midrin or Fiorinal) during pregnancy. Little is known about the safety of monoamine oxidase (MAO) inhibitors, calcium channel blockers, and low-dose ergot preparations for prophylaxis for recurrent headaches (Tengborn et al, 1989). Intermittent continuation of these drugs during breastfeeding is likely to be safe.

## THROMBOEMBOLIC DISEASES

Thromboembolic disorders have long concerned obstetricians because of the risk of maternal death due to pulmonary embolism. The frequency of thrombophlebitis during labor, delivery, and the puerperium has been reported to be four to six times that in the nonpregnant state (Le Clerc and Hirsh, 1988). Impedance plethysmography is more reliable than Doppler ultrasonography, and venography should generally be used to confirm the diagnosis.

Because of the potential teratogenic effect and late fetal complications associated with warfarin (Coumadin) therapy, most authors recommend heparin for anticoagulation during the antepartum period. An initial bolus of 70 U/kg followed by an infusion of 1000 to 2000 U/h is recommended. Intravenous therapy should be continued for 7 to 10 days.

Following initial therapy, a moderate dose of approximately 10,000 units of subcutaneous heparin every 12 hours is necessary, with adjustments to maintain a midinterval aPTT 1.5 to 2 times the control value. The provision of a 5-ml bottle of concentrated heparin (40,000 U/ml) allows for easier self-administration. Intravenous heparin followed by oral warfarin for 3 months is recommended for women who develop thrombotic phenomena during labor or the puerperium. During labor, the commonly used therapy is continuing minidose heparin (8000 U twice daily) with the omission of a single dose when delivery is imminent. Breastfeeding is safe, although ecchymosis or a hematoma may develop around the nipple.

Persons who have experienced a prior thromboembolic episode have a 5 to 12 percent risk of recurrence during a subsequent pregnancy (Badracca and Vessey, 1974). Minidose prophylactic heparin (8000 U twice daily) is often recommended, especially from the 34th gestational week until the patient is fully ambulatory postpartum (Howell, 1983; Dahlman et al, 1989). Bone demineralization is a possibility with prophylactic minidose heparin during pregnancy for some unknown reason, especially when the medication is used for more than 20 weeks (de Swiet, 1983). Thrombocytopenia occurs in approximately 20 percent of cases, is usually mild, and is dose- and duration-dependent.

Streptokinase and urokinase have been used to lyse clots in patients with thromboembolic disease. Because of the significant risk of hemorrhage, these medications are contraindicated during the antepartum and postpartum periods, with the rare exception of a person at risk for death from pulmonary embolism who did not respond to heparin therapy.

## COLLAGEN VASCULAR DISORDERS

Rheumatoid arthritis and systemic lupus erythematosus are the most common collagen vascular disorders and, perhaps, the most amenable to therapy. Although many women experience exacerbations in the postpartum period, few cases actually develop *de novo* during pregnancy. Exacerbation of lupus nephritis is a particularly dangerous complication, however, and may be difficult to differentiate from preeclampsia.

Salicylates form the first line of drug therapy for rheumatoid arthritis and may be helpful for the control of minor symptoms in patients with systemic lupus erythematosus (Lavin, 1991). These agents exert their therapeutic benefit by blocking prostaglandin synthetase through the inhibition of cyclooxygenase. Enteric-coated acetylsalicylate (aspirin) is the preferred preparation in daily doses of 650 to 1300 mg every 4 to 6 hours. Salicylates cross the human placenta. Although a few reports have suggested an increased risk of fetal malformations, the overwhelming body of evidence has demonstrated no teratogenic effect. Because of the inhibiting properties of prostaglandin, the length of gestation has been reported to be longer, the incidence of postdatism higher, and the duration of labor more prolonged for mothers who have been treated with salicylates. Possible but unlikely effects of salicylate use are premature closure of the ductus arteriosus and pulmonary hypertension in the newborn, resulting from prostaglandin inhibition observed with other prostaglandin agents. Maternal salicylate ingestion has been associated with neonatal platelet dysfunction, and an increased frequency of intracranial hemorrhage compared with untreated controls has been reported among neonates of mothers who had ingested the medication.

Other nonsteroidal anti-inflammatory agents are frequently used in the treatment of rheumatoid arthritis. Some authors have reported the occurrence of fetal pulmonary hypertension, presumably from the antiprostaglandin effects of these agents on the ductus arteriosus. Although other investigators have not observed this problem, most authorities suggest that these agents are contraindicated during pregnancy.

Systemic corticosteroids are seldom indicated for the treatment of rheumatoid arthritis, but they form the mainstay of drug therapy for systemic lupus erythematosus. These medicines are prescribed in the lowest doses to minimize symptoms and prevent recurrence. A daily dose of 20 to 40 mg of prednisone may be used for flare-ups with no major organ involvement. If major organs are involved (nephritis, cerebritis, vasculitis), the daily dose should be increased to 40 to 80 mg. The only known controlled study of the use of corticosteroids in pregnant patients with lupus erythematosus revealed that those who received medication had fewer exacerbations and a lower incidence of perinatal mortality than those who did not receive the drug therapy (Kitzmiller, 1978).

A number of other agents, including gold, immunosuppressive medications, and penicillamine, have been used to treat selected patients with collagen vascular disorders (Lavin, 1991). Because of a lack of knowledge regarding potential fetal effects or the substantial suggestion of fetal risk, most authorities recommend that these agents be avoided during pregnancy except in life-threatening situations or when more traditional agents have failed.

## CARDIAC DISEASE

Heart disease has been found in 1 to 4 percent of pregnancies and remains the fourth leading cause of maternal death in the United States (Lavin, 1992). As a result of pregnancy-induced physiologic changes, demands on the functional capacity of the heart increase markedly. Labor and delivery are particularly worrisome periods, because these patients have difficulty maintaining adequate cardiac output in light of acute increases in afterload and acute decreases in preload. Hypertension, fluid overload, and hypotension secondary to blood loss or regional anesthesia should be avoided.

Cardiac glycosides are steroid or steroid-glycoside structures commonly used for their positive inotropic and antiarrhythmic properties. Digoxin is the most commonly used. Unless a loading dose is employed, several days of oral therapy are required to reach a steady blood state. The usual digitalizing dose is 0.25 to 0.5 mg orally or intravenously in 0.25 mg increments at 4- to 6-hour intervals, or 1.0 to 1.5 mg orally in divided doses. The maintenance dose is 0.125 to 0.375 mg daily. Monthly tests of digoxin (Lanoxin) levels are recommended, because toxicity occurs frequently with any of these preparations. Maternal manifestations include rhythm disturbances, nausea, vomiting, headache, and neurologic imbalances. The primary use of cardiac glycosides during pregnancy is for treatment of pulmonary congestion unresponsive to rest and diuretic therapy. The agents may also be used for treatment of maternal supraventricular tachycardia, atrial fibrillation, and atrial flutter; occasional reports of successful fetal therapy for tachycardia have been limited by maternal toxicity. No adverse fetal effects have been reported, and the concentration in breast milk is low, with clinical effects on the infant probably minimal.

Arrhythmias may occur during pregnancy in women with pre-existing congenital myocarditis or ischemic cardiac disorders. The cardiac glycosides and $\beta$-adrenergic blockers (primarily propranolol) are the agents most widely used (Rotemensch et al, 1989). Major indications for propranolol are any evidence of coexisting hypertension, premature atrial and ventricular beats, supraventricular and ventricular tachycardias, and reduction in ventricular response to atrial fibrillation or flutter. Propranolol is also useful for the reduction of cardiac output and pulse pressure when aortic dissection is a concern for women with coarctation of the aorta and Marfan's syndrome. Verapamil, a calcium channel blocker originally developed to treat angina, may also be useful for supraventricular tachycardia. Cardiovascular side effects in the mother are a concern, and little information is available about the use of verapamil for treating cardiac disease in pregnancy and during breastfeeding.

Pregnant women who have undergone mechanical prosthetic valve placement are at an increased risk for thromboembolic phenomena and require chronic anticoagulation. Heparin therapy is the preferred form of anticoagulation, with a subcutaneous dose of 150 to 250 U/kg given every 12 hours to achieve an anticoagulation level of 1.5 to 2 times control values (aPTT 60 to 90 sec). One or two doses may be given before delivery using a minidose (5000 U every 12 hours). Heparin therapy may be reinstituted 6 hours following delivery and continued for 48 to 72 hours.

Women with valvular or several forms of congenital heart disease are at increased risk to develop bacterial endocarditis if they experience bacteremia. The incidence of bacteremia following parturition has been reported as 0 to 5 percent (Lavin, 1991). Because the effect of developing bacterial endocarditis may be devastating, investigators suggest antibiotic prophylaxis at the time of labor and delivery. In cases of penicillin allergy, vancomycin (1.0 g intravenously over 1 h) with gentamicin is a worthwhile choice for prophylaxis; in non-allergic patients ampicillin (2.0 g intramuscularly or intravenously) and gentamicin (1.5 mg/kg intramuscularly or intravenously) are usually prescribed before and 6 hours after the procedure. Routine prophylaxis for an uncomplicated vaginal delivery remains controversial and may lead to unwarranted fetal drug exposure and predisposition to bacterial endocarditis from resistant organisms. Most authorities recommend antibiotic prophylaxis if special risks such as chorioamnionitis or cesarean section are present. Once a woman begins breastfeeding, she should have minimal exposure to antibiotics.

## DIABETES

Care for the diabetic pregnant woman requires a proper understanding of anticipated insulin therapy changes. Attempts to maintain strict glucose control should begin before conception. Oral hypoglycemic agents have no role during pregnancy. Most persons are already accustomed to using the standard rapid-acting (regular; 4 to 12 h duration) and intermediate-acting (NPH, Lente;

14 to 28 h duration) insulin preparations. Regardless of metabolic control and duration of diabetes, average daily insulin requirements are expected to increase approximately twofold (Rayburn and Zuspan, 1985). The only times in which insulin doses may decrease would be during early gestation, because of inadequate caloric intake from nausea, and during the third trimester, when placental insufficiency is most likely.

Daily self-monitoring of fasting and postprandial glucose values should be performed using reflectance glucometers. In late gestation, insulin is usually administered two or three times each day, with a mixture of regular and intermediate acting (preferably NPH) U-100 insulins. Experience with insulin infusion therapy during pregnancy has been limited to those with brittle diabetes requiring more than three daily doses of insulin.

Most diabetic women require an average of 1 unit of continuous intravenous regular insulin (range 0 to 2 U) per hour during induction of labor. Insulin adheres to containers and to plastic infuser lines; therefore, insulin-containing fluid from the intravenous unit should be run through the tubing and discarded before the infusion starts to the patient. A low dose of intermittent regular insulin may be given instead when a cesarean section is anticipated. Insulin demand is expected to drop precipitously after delivery. The total insulin requirement has been found to be two thirds of the prepregnancy dose at the third postpartum day and approximately the same as that before pregnancy by the end of the first postpartum week.

Biosynthetic recombinant DNA human insulin is not immunogenic and, thus, should be prescribed to women who acquire glucose intolerance for the first time during pregnancy. Gestational-onset diabetic women are eligible for insulin therapy if diet therapy is inadequate. The usual initial daily dose of 0.5 to 0.7 U/day of insulin in divided morning and evening doses of NPH and regular insulin should be started as early in gestation as possible to minimize the risk of the fetus becoming large for gestational age (Gabbe, 1992). Once insulin is begun, principles for managing the diabetic pregnancy are the same as those for already insulin-dependent women. Insulin doses should be

unaffected by breastfeeding, and no insulin crosses into the breast milk and is absorbed in the infant's gut.

## THYROID DISEASE

Medical therapy of hyperthyroidism is the primary form of treatment during pregnancy. A subtotal thyroidectomy is best reserved for patients who fail on medical management because of poor compliance, severe disease, or the need for excessive antithyroid medication. Prescribed medications are intended to decrease the amount of circulating thyroid hormones (antithyroid medications) and to relieve severely bothersome maternal symptoms such as ($\beta$-adrenergic blocking medications). The two principal antithyroid preparations, propylthiouracil and methimazole (Tapazole), are thiourea derivatives that prevent the iodination of tyrosine by inhibiting the oxidation of iodide to iodine. The placenta is permeable to each drug, but propylthiouracil is preferable to methimazole, because transfer of the latter is less rapid (Hollingsworth, 1989). The response of hyperthyroidism to therapy is governed by the long time needed to deplete thyroid stores that may persist until 3 to 6 weeks after beginning therapy. Adjustment of daily doses should be based on relief of symptoms and circulatory levels of free $T_4$, which should be maintained within an upper-normal or slightly elevated range. Daily doses exceeding 300 mg should be avoided because of potential fetal thyroid effects. Agranulocytosis has been reported in 1 in 500 cases. Fetal goiter formation has been reported in up to 10 percent of all infants of treated mothers and is dependent on the dose and duration of *in utero* exposure (Hollingsworth, 1989). Neonatal hypothyroidism is short lived, lasting only a few days. Long-term intellectual development in exposed infants has not been compared with that of their siblings. Presumably, insignificant amounts of propylthiouracil reach the suckling infants, and no changes in their serum $T_4$, $T_3$, TSH or resin $T_3$ uptake levels is to be anticipated.

Patient complaints during pregnancy may overlap with symptoms of hypothyroidism. Low free $T_4$ levels and elevated TSH levels have been reported to be associated with an increased risk of infertility and unfavorable perinatal outcomes. It is recommended that thyroid supplementation should be continued during pregnancy if laboratory evidence exists, and the patient continues to exhibit symptoms. Levothyroxine (Synthroid) is the preferred drug, because it is the most physiologic replacement, being $T_4$ alone rather than a combination of $T_3 : T_4$. Thyroid supplements do not pass through the placental barrier in appreciable amounts and should have no effect on the autonomous fetal thyroid-pituitary function (Mestman, 1980). The usual nonpregnant daily dose is 0.1 to 0.2 mg, which may need to be increased slightly during pregnancy (Mandel, 1990). The only major complication is overdosage, and the dose of levothyroxine would be such that the TSH level is less than 10 mU/ml. Measurement of serum thyroxine levels may produce falsely higher results during maintenance thyroxine therapy.

## ANTIBIOTICS

Antibiotics are the most commonly prescribed medications during pregnancy. No increased risk of malformations, specifically or overall, has been reported with first trimester exposure, nor is a short-term course of antibiotics thought to adversely affect the fetus during the second and third trimesters. Ampicillin remains the most commonly prescribed antibiotic. Cephalosporins are also thought to be safe. Less is known about synthetic penicillins and third-generation cephalosporin. Erythromycin crosses the placenta negligibly and, therefore, would not be effective in treating the fetus. Metronidazole (Flagyl) has not been reported to be associated with any increased risk of malformations. Its use during pregnancy should be limited to cases of severe infection during the second and third trimesters. No adequate or well-controlled studies in pregnant women have been undertaken using the broad-spectrum bactericidal quinolones.

Although rare, hemolysis is associated with nitrofurantoin (Macrodantin), but hyperbilirubinemia is not thought to be a concern with the use of this medication. Sulfonamides are thought to be associated with a greater risk of hemolytic anemia, thrombocytopenia, and hyperbilirubinemia. Their use during pregnancy should be avoided.

Staining of deciduous teeth (enamel hypoplasia) associated with tetracyclines is not reported to result from first trimester exposure; instead, this finding is associated with the development of adult teeth, which does not begin until the second half of pregnancy.

## Summary

This chapter is comprehensive but not complete. The aim is to emphasize principles of medication administration in pregnancy, using specific medications or diseases as examples of the problems involved. Several texts are more useful for information regarding specific drugs (Berkowitz et al, 1986; Briggs et al, 1990; Rayburn et al, 1992).

It must be recognized that there can be no final word on the safety of the vast majority of medications in pregnancy. As already mentioned, the chance of most congenital abnormalities being drug induced is far less than the chance of a genetic causation. Furthermore, few known teratogens affect more than a small proportion of exposed fetuses. Before ascribing teratogenic potential to a medication already used by a pregnant woman, or a congenital abnormality to a medication she used, physicians and other health personnel should consider the uncertain state of our knowledge and the load of anxiety and guilt that the mother must carry if she believes her actions have adversely affected her baby. In particular, we must not hide the state of our ignorance behind a false cloak of certainty.

Medications should never be used without good reason, and this is especially true in pregnancy, when the health of both a mother and a fetus are involved. But the health and safety of the mother and her baby are interrelated, and pregnant women must not be denied necessary medications simply because of their pregnancy.

"Ultimately, to deal effectively with the problem of drug effects in pregnancy, [we] must continue to become better informed and alert to the potential dangers of all agents . . . to supply the appropriate medication when needed, and to withhold it when not needed. . . . Only in this way can the risk of fetal drug toxicity be minimized and the optimal health of both mother and fetus ensured" (Barber, 1981).

# References

Anderson VE: Genetic Counseling for Epilepsy. *In* Commission for the Control of Epilepsy and its Consequences: Plan for Nationwide Action on Epilepsy, Vol 2. Washington, DC, US Dept Health, Education and Welfare, 1978, p 141.

Badracca M, Vessey M: Recurrence of venous thromboembolic disease and the use of oral contraceptives. Br Med J 1:215, 1974.

Barber HRK: Symposium on drugs in pregnancy: introduction. Obstet Gynecol 58:15, 1981.

Berkowitz RL, Coustan DR, Mochizuki TK: Handbook for Prescribing Medications During Pregnancy, 2nd ed. Boston, Little, Brown & Co, 1986.

Blake DA: Requirements and limitations in reproductive and teratogenic risk assessment. *In* Niebyl JR: Drug Use in Pregnancy. Philadelphia, Lea & Febiger, 1982.

Briggs G, Bodendorfer T, Freeman R, et al: Drugs in Pregnancy and Lactation. Baltimore, Williams and Wilkins, 3rd ed, 1990.

Carter BL, Driscoll CE, Smith GD: Theophylline clearance during pregnancy. Obstet Gynecol 68:555, 1986.

Cole WA, Trasler DG: Gene-teratogen interaction in insulin-induced mouse exencephaly. Teratology 22:125, 1980.

Dahlman TC, Hellgren MS, Blomback M: Thrombosis prophylaxis in pregnancy with use of subcutaneous heparin adjusted by monitoring heparin concentration in plasma. Am J Obstet Gynecol 161:420, 1989.

Dalessio DV: Seizure disorders during pregnancy. N Engl J Med 312:559, 1985.

de Swiet M: Prolonged heparin therapy in pregnancy causes bone demineralization. Brit J Obstet Gynaecol 90:1129, 1983.

Dunagen W, Redner W (eds): Manual of Medical Therapeutics, 26th ed. Boston, Little, Brown & Co, 1989.

Fraser FC: Animal models for craniofacial disorders. Prog Clin Biol Res 46:1, 1980.

Fraser FC, Fainstat TD: Production of congenital abnormalities in the offspring of pregnant mice treated with cortisone. Progress report. Pediatrics 8:527, 1951.

Gabbe SG: Definition, detection, and management of gestational diabetes. Obstet Gynecol 67:121, 1992.

Golbus MS: Teratology for the obstetrician: current status. Obstet Gynecol 55:269, 1982.

Granroth G: Defects of the central nervous system in Finland. III. Diseases and drugs in pregnancy. Early Hum Dev 2:147, 1978.

Greenberger P, Patterson R: Management of asthma during pregnancy. N Engl J Med 312:897, 1985.

Gregg NM: Congenital cataract following German measles in the mother. Trans Ophthalmol Soc Aust 3:35, 1941.

Hale F: The relation of vitamin A to anophthalmos in pigs. Am J Ophthalmol 18:1087, 1935.

Hanssens M, Keirse M, Vankelecom F, van Assche F: Fetal and neonatal effects of treatment with angiotensin-converting enzyme inhibitors. Obstet Gynecol 78:128, 1991.

Hartz SC, Heinonen OF, Shapiro S, et al: Antenatal exposure to meprobamate and chlordiazepoxide in relation to malformations, mental development, and childhood mortality. N Engl J Med 292:726, 1975.

Hawe P, Francis HH: Pregnancy and thyrotoxicosis. Br Med J 2:817, 1962.

Heinonen OP, Slone D, Shapiro S: Birth Defects and Drugs in Pregnancy. Littleton, MA, Publishing Sciences Group, 1977.

Herbst AL: Diethylstilbestrol and other sex hormones during pregnancy. Obstet Gynecol 58:35S, 1981.

Herbst AL, Ulfelder H, Poskanzer DC: Adenocarcinoma of the vagina. Association of maternal stilbestrol therapy with tumor appearance in young women. N Engl J Med 284:878, 1971.

Hollingsworth D: Endocrine disorders of pregnancy. *In* Creasy, R and, Resnik (ed): Maternal-Fetal Medicine: Principles and Practice, 2nd ed. Philadelphia, WB Saunders Co, 1989.

Holmes LB, quoted by Knuppel RA: Recognizing teratogenic effects of drugs and radiation. Contemp Obstet Gynecol 15:171, 1980.

Howell R: The risks of antenatal subcutaneous heparin prophylaxis: a controlled trial. Brit J Obstet Gynaecol 90:1124, 1983.

Kitzmiller J: Antoimmune disorders: maternal, fetal, and neonatal risks. Clin Obstet Gynecol 21:385, 1978.

Lavin J: Pharmacologic therapy for chronic medical disorders during pregnancy. *In* Rayburn W, Zuspan F (eds): Drug Therapy in Obstetrics and Gynecology, 3rd ed. St Louis, CV Mosby, 1992.

Le Clerc J, Hirsh J: Venous thromboembolic disorders. *In* Burrow GN, Ferris TF (eds): Medical Complications during Pregnancy. 3rd ed. Philadelphia, WB Saunders, 1988, pp 204–223.

Leck I: Backwards and forwards in search of teratogens. Early Hum Dev 2:203, 1978.

Lenz W: Thalidomide and congenital abnormalities. Lancet 2:1358, 1961.

Lindheimer MD, Katz AI: Hypertension in pregnancy. N Engl J Med 313:675, 1985.

Lubbe WF: Treatment of hypertension in pregnancy. J Cardiovasc Pharmacol 16 (Suppl 7): S110, 1990.

Mandel SJ, Larsen P, Seely E, Brent C: Increased need for thyroxine during pregnancy in women with primary hypothyroidism. N Engl J Med 323: 91, 1990.

Meadow R: Anticonvulsants in pregnancy. Arch Dis Child 66:62, 1991.

McBride WA: Thalidomide and congenital abnormalities. Lancet 1:45, 1962.

Mogadam M, Dobbins W, Konelitz B, et al: Pregnancy and inflammatory bowel disease: effect of sulfasalazine and corticosteroids on fetal outcome. Gastroenterology 80:72, 1981.

Nebert DW, Shum S: The murine *Ah* locus: genetic differences in birth defects among individuals in the same uterus. Prog Clin Biol Res 46:173, 1980.

Niebyl JR, Blake DA, Freeman JM, et al: Carbamazepine levels in pregnancy and lactation. Obstet Gynecol 53:139, 1979.

Nielsen OH, Adreasson B, Bondesen S, et al: Pregnancy in Crohn's disease. Scand J Gastroenterol 19:724, 1984.

Philipson A: Pharmacokinetics of ampicillin during pregnancy. J Infect Dis 136:370, 1977.

Rayburn W, Zuspan F (eds): Drug Therapy in Obstetrics and Gynecology, 3rd ed. St Louis, CV Mosby Co, 1992.

Rayburn WF, Lewis R, Piehl E: Changes in insulin requirements during pregnancy. Am J Perinatol 2:271, 1985.

Robertson RT, Allen ML, Bokelman DL: Aspirin: teratogenic evaluation in the dog. Teratology 20:313, 1979.

Ross S, Burke RG, Sites J, et al: Placental transmission of chloramphenicol (chloromycetin). JAMA 142:1361, 1950.

Rotemensch H, Lessing J, Donchin Y: Clinical pharmacology of antiarrhythmic drugs in the pregnant patient. *In* Elkayam U, Gleicher N (eds): Cardiac Problems in Pregnancy: Diagnosis and Management of Maternal and Fetal Disease, 2nd ed. New York, Alan R Liss, 1989, pp 227–244.

Saxen I: Associations between oral clefts and drugs taken during pregnancy. Int J Epidemiol 4:37, 1975.

Shepard TH: A Catalog of Teratogenic Agents. Baltimore, The Johns Hopkins Press, 1973.

Shepard TH: Teratogenicity from drugs—an increasing problem. *In* Disease-A-Month, June 1974, Chicago, Year Book Medical, 1974.

Shepard TH, Fantel AG: Teratology of therapeutic agents. *In* Iffy L, Kaminetzky HA (eds): Principles and Practice of Obstetrics and Perinatology. New York, John Wiley & Sons, 1981, p 461.

Shirkey HC: Editorial comment: therapeutic orphans. J Pediatr 72:119, 1968.

Somerville B: A study of migraine in pregnancy. Neurology 22:224, 1977.

Stern L: In vivo assessment of the teratogenic potential of drugs in humans. Obstet Gynecol 58:3S, 1981.

Tengborn L, Bergqvist D, Matzsch T, et al: Recurrent thromboembolism in pregnancy and puerperium. Is there a need for thromboprophylaxis? Am J Obstet Gynecol 160:90, 1989.

Tuchmann-Duplessis H: Drug effects on the fetus. Sydney, Adis Press, 1975, p 6.

Urowitz M, Gladman D: Rheumatic disease. *In* Burrow GN, Ferris TF (eds): Medical Complications during Pregnancy, 3rd Ed. Philadelphia, WB Saunders, 1988, 499–525.

Willoughby C, Truelove S: Ulcerative colitis and pregnancy. Gut 21:469, 1980.

Wilson JG: Environment and Birth Defects. New York, Academic Press, 1973.

Woollam DHM: Teratogens in everyday life. The Milroy Lecture, 1980. J Roy Coll Phys London 14:213, 1980.

. . . . . . . . . . . . . . . . . . . . . . . . . . . . . . . . . . .

# CHAPTER 10

# Substance Abuse in Pregnancy

Marsha E. Kaye and Ira J. Chasnoff

## Prevalence

The problems of substance abuse during pregnancy have been noted for thousands of years. Soranus of Ephesus (first or second century AD) cautioned against drinking alcohol during pregnancy.

*The seed when attached must be nourished, and takes food from the substance containing blood and pneuma which is brought to it. But in drunkenness and indigestion all vapor is spoilt and the pneuma too is rendered turbid. Therefore, danger arises, lest by reason of the bad material contributed, the seed too changes for the worse. Furthermore, the satiety due to heavy drinking hinders attachment to the uterus.*

Between the 1800s and 1960s the medical literature only alluded to adverse effects of alcohol on pregnancy (Keith et al, 1988). No specific outcomes were identified until Lemoine (1968) and Jones and colleagues (1973) described fetal alcohol syndrome. This brought public attention to the possible teratogenic effects of recreational drugs used during pregnancy. Around the same time, neonates suffering from withdrawal who had been exposed to narcotics (heroin and methadone) were described (Finnegan et al, 1975).

The use and abuse of drugs during pregnancy occur more frequently than is generally realized (Schnoll, 1986). It has been reported that as many as 60 percent of pregnant women use some medication (Schnoll, 1986). The drugs used are primarily over-the-counter analgesics, antinauseants, tranquilizers, and sedatives. These drugs are often used before a woman knows she is pregnant.

Moreover, during the past decade, the use of illicit drugs during pregnancy has increased at alarming rates, with cocaine and marijuana often being the drugs of choice. This reflects the pattern of abuse among the general population, with an estimated 30 million Americans having tried cocaine and 5 million using it on a regular basis (Abelson and Miller, 1985).

Prior to the widespread use of cocaine in the United States, a survey of women enrolled in a Chicago hospital obstetric clinic showed only a 3 percent incidence of sedative-hypnotics in the mothers' urine (Chasnoff et al, 1984). But in 1988, Frank and associates (1988) reported a 28 percent use of marijuana and a 17 percent use of cocaine in pregnant women at Boston City Hospital. The Illinois Department of Children and Family Services reported a 78.8 percent increase in cocaine-exposed babies being born over the same period a year before (Silverman, 1989).

A nationwide survey of 36 hospitals by Chasnoff (1989) reported an overall incidence of illicit substance use among pregnant women of 11 percent, with a range of 0.4 to 27 percent. Illicit substances included in this survey were cocaine, heroin, methadone, amphetamines, phencyclidine (PCP), and marijuana (Chasnoff, 1989). However, marijuana and cocaine use were documented more frequently than other illicit substances.

Most of these studies include data collected from hospital-based populations serving urban populations composed of women of lower socioeconomic status. However, substance use during pregnancy is not limited to this socioeconomic level. A study by Chasnoff and colleagues (1990) found in Pinellas County, Florida, an overall rate of 13.35 percent of pregnant women using illicit substances, with no significant difference between women of different socioeconomic backgrounds.

The pregnant substance abuser is easily overlooked; she volunteers little information, and often there is denial and fear of a social stigma. In addition, many health care professionals still lack knowledge of perinatal addiction, and those providing care to the middle and upper classes of society refrain from obtaining a substance abuse history, thereby protecting their patients. Subsequently, drug abuse in pregnancy is one of the most frequently missed diagnoses (Chisum, 1986) in maternal and child health.

Health care workers are faced with increasing numbers of mothers and infants affected by illicit substances. There is an increased incidence of spontaneous abortion, labor and delivery complications, and behavioral and neurologic effects that impair the development of infants and children. We must accept the challenge of recognizing substance abuse in pregnant women in all socioeconomic, ethnic, and racial groups. We must provide appropriate medical, obstetric, nursing, and chemical dependence services. The infants born to these mothers also require long-term assessment, evaluation, and appropriate intervention as specific needs are identified.

## Prenatal History

To help identify a pregnant substance abuser and prevent the untoward effects on the mother and fetus, a thorough history and assessment of the physical appearance and behaviors of a pregnant woman should be performed at the initial interview. The history must include medical, obstetric, social, and substance abuse information. Adequate time should be allotted for this crucial initial contact. It is important to establish a trusting relationship in order to ascertain a detailed history, so that appropriate treatment, referral, and education can be provided.

## PHYSICAL APPEARANCE AND BEHAVIORS

The pregnant substance abuser often appears untidy, physically exhausted, and disoriented. She may display defensive, avoidance or hostile behavior during the interview (Chisum, 1990). Her pupils may be extremely dilated or constricted. Needle marks, abscesses, edema of the extremities, and inflamed or indurated nasal mucosa may be present (Chasnoff, 1987). She may emit an odor consistent with recent alcohol intake.

Often, the pregnant woman has poor weight gain and her uterine size does not correlate with her stated gestational age. Noting the physical appearance of a pregnant woman is particularly useful in identifying an intravenous substance abuser because the physical signs of chemical dependence are visible. Typically, the heroin abuser presents to a health care provider either intoxicated or exhibiting signs of withdrawal. Although there are intermittent periods of alertness, the heroin abuser is either "up" (elated) or "down" (depressed). She may be drowsy or lethargic with pinpoint pupils, or she may be anxious, tearing, perspiring, and complaining of nausea. In more severe cases, agitation, vomiting, diarrhea, and complaints of cramping may be present.

The first prenatal visit may be late in the pregnancy. Many substance-abusing women have irregular menstrual cycles. Amenorrhea occurs most frequently with heroin addiction but has been reported with methadone and cocaine use. Pregnant substance abusers have decreased awareness of bodily changes, and missed menses may be interpreted as the result of drug use (Daghestani, 1988). Thus, they are often unaware of their pregnancy status until many weeks into the pregnancy. Reasons for eventually seeking health care include anxiety about delivery and fear of complications of drug use. Even after seeking health care, poor compliance is a recurring problem.

## MEDICAL HISTORY

The purpose of the medical history is to help identify effects of the substance abuse. A history with the following problems may be a clue that a woman is a substance abuser: bacteremia, hepatitis, pancreatitis, pneumonia, cellulitis, cirrhosis, sexually transmitted diseases, recurrent urinary tract infections, and acquired immunodeficiency syndrome (AIDS); heart palpitations; acute hypertension; seizures; sleep disturbances; extreme exhaustion; depression; and suicide attempts (Chisum, 1990).

## SOCIAL HISTORY

Substance-abusing women often come from families with alcoholism or medical problems related to drug abuse (Chisum, 1990). Family violence, incarceration, or removal of other children from the home is often found. Homelessness is a recurring problem. These women have chaotic lifestyles and lack social and family support. Prostitution is a common means that drug-abusing women use to support their drug habit. Feelings of isolation, powerlessness, shame, and guilt prevail (Chisum, 1990). Typically, the pregnant substance abuser has low self-esteem and a poor self-image. She may express ambivalence, anger, or apathy toward her pregnancy.

## OBSTETRIC HISTORY

The obstetric history should include past and current pregnancy information. The past obstetric history may provide useful information, because many women have been substance abusers for several years prior to the current pregnancy.

Past obstetric complications, such as spontaneous abortion, premature labor, abruptio placentae, meconium-stained amniotic fluid, fetal death, birth of a low-birth-weight infant, sexually transmitted diseases, spotting or vaginal bleeding, cramping, and an inactive or hyperactive fetus, are often noted in the history (Chisum, 1990).

With the current pregnancy, early contractions, poor weight gain, poor nutritional status, sexually transmitted diseases, spotting or vaginal bleeding, and an inactive or hyperactive fetus continue to be noted.

## SUBSTANCE ABUSE HISTORY

A substance abuse history should be a routine part of the prenatal history. The approach of the health care professional toward the patient has a great impact on what information the patient is willing to disclose. It is important to maintain a sincere, empathetic, non-judgmental, matter-of-fact approach that promotes an open dialogue. Asking open-ended questions elicits more detailed information. The reason for obtaining such a history should be clearly stated. Health care professionals are concerned about the health and well-being of the mother and newborn. Decreasing medical and obstetric complications for the mother and reducing infant morbidity and mortality are primary goals. The substance abuse information is important in order to provide the best possible care for mother and infant.

A thorough substance abuse history includes all forms of drug use and abuse and the amount, duration, frequency, route of administration (oral, smoking, intravenous use), and setting of abuse, such as crack houses or shooting galleries. Patterns of illicit drug abuse can vary and may include occasional, weekend use only, monthly binges, and daily dependence. These patterns may change as the pregnancy progresses, especially at times of greater stress. Street availability may also affect the frequency and type of drug used. As a result, a woman may use more than one drug at different times or in combination during the pregnancy. In addition, many illicit substances have variable concentrations of the actual drug, and agents such as sugar, quinine, amphetamines, procaine, strychnine, and boric acid may be added.

The substance abuse history (Table 10–1) is most effective when the interview begins with cigarettes, and proceeds to questions concerning over-the-counter medication, prescribed medication, alcohol (beer, wine, wine coolers, mixed drinks, hard liquor), marijuana, and other illicit drugs. Information about the partner's abuse of drugs should be included. This information may help the health care professional understand more completely the patient's lifestyle. A systematic approach, such as the one described, is often less threatening to the patient.

When obtaining the initial history, each month of gestation should be explored, beginning with the month before the last menstrual period and also noting the earliest exposure (Chisum, 1990). Periods of abstinence and admission to drug treatment programs should be noted. With each prenatal visit an

**Table 10–1**
DRUG ABUSE HISTORY SEQUENCE

Cigarettes
Over-the-counter medication
  Cough or cold medication
  Diet pills
  Sleeping aids
Prescribed medication
Alcohol
  Beer
  Wine
  Wine coolers
  Mixed drinks
  Hard liquor
Illicit drugs
  Marijuana (pot, grass, reefer, weed, THC, or hash)
  Cocaine (crack, freebase, coke, snow)
  Narcotics (heroin, methadone, Demerol)
  Stimulants (speed, amphetamines)
  Depressants (barbiturates such as Nembutal or
    Seconal; sedatives such as Valium, Librium,
    Quaalude)
  Hallucinogens (PCP, LSD, peyote, Ecstasy)

THC = Delta 9-tetrahydrocannabinol
PCP = Phencyclidine
LSD = Lysergic acid diethylamide

updated substance abuse history should be reviewed.

Most substance abusers use more than one drug. Common combinations include any of the following: cocaine, alcohol, marijuana, and cigarettes. Each drug should be individually reviewed, including all forms of alcohol. Illicit drugs have many names and are more prevalent in different areas in the United States. Health care professionals should be aware of the drugs in their area and their street names and obtain a complete substance abuse history for each substance. The following are examples of questions in various categories that may be used when eliciting a substance abuse history.

● **Cigarette Use**
  ○ How many cigarettes do you smoke daily?
  ○ How often did you smoke cigarettes last month?
  ○ Have you ever smoked more?

● **Over-the-Counter Medication**
  ○ How often have you taken over-the-counter medications since you have known you were pregnant?
  ○ What drugs did you take?
  ○ Were the drugs prescribed for you?

● **Prescribed Medication**
  ○ How often have you taken prescribed medication since you've known you were pregnant?
  ○ What drugs did you take?
  ○ Were the drugs prescribed for you?
  ○ How many did you take?

● **Alcohol**
  ○ Beer: How many times a week do you drink beer?
    How many cans each time?
    Do you ever drink more?
  ○ Wine: How many times a week do you drink wine?
    How many glasses each time?
    Do you ever drink more?
  ○ Liquor: How many times a week do you drink liquor?
    How many drinks each time?
    Do you ever drink more?
  ○ Has your drinking changed during the past year?

● **Illicit Drug Use (such as cocaine)**
  ○ How often did you use cocaine before you knew you were pregnant?
  ○ How often did you use cocaine since you've known you were pregnant?
  ○ How do you use it?
  ○ How much cocaine do you use?
  ○ Do you ever use more?
  ○ Where are you when using cocaine?

## PERINATAL PHARMACOLOGY

The placenta was once commonly believed to act as a protective barrier against drugs and other substances for the fetus. However, all drugs used during pregnancy cross the placenta to some extent. The effect of the drug depends on several factors such as route of administration, molecular weight, and lipid solubility.

Drugs that affect the central nervous system and cross the blood-brain barrier (such as alcohol, opiates, cocaine, sedatives, and hypnotics) are lipophilic and have a low molecular weight, which allows the drugs to pass through the placenta. Intravenous and intranasal routes of administration bypass maternal liver metabolism and allow drugs to enter the fetal circulation directly.

Some drugs may accumulate in the fetus because the fetal liver is not fully developed and cannot metabolize the substance adequately. Also, excretion by the kidney may be delayed because of the immature renal function. The fetus is most susceptible to the potential teratogenic effects of drugs during the first 8 weeks of gestation (Abrams, 1982). Drugs that may cause damage to the fetus should be avoided, especially at this critical time. However, the substance abuser is often unaware of her pregnant state.

## Maternal Complications

### MEDICAL COMPLICATIONS

Lifestyle, nutritional status, patterns of prenatal care, and patterns of drug abuse are factors that influence pregnancy outcomes. Inadequate or poor prenatal care, especially with the opiate- or cocaine-addicted pregnant woman, is common. Anemia is frequently noted, and nutritional status is frequently poor, depending on the length of addiction. One study found that the prepregnancy weight was significantly lower in substance abusers than in nonusers, reflecting the inadequacy of the diet (Frank et al, 1988). Infections such as hepatitis, urinary tract infections, and sexually transmitted diseases are common findings (Chasnoff et al, 1987;

Connaughton et al, 1977; Frank et al, 1988; Pelosi et al, 1975). If a woman is an intravenous drug user, subacute bacterial endocarditis, cellulitis, bacteremia, and phlebitis may occur during her pregnancy, or she may have a past history of these illnesses. AIDS is becoming more frequent among this group of women. Table 10–2 lists the medical complications that are found among pregnant substance abusers.

If a health care provider obtains a positive history of medical complications that may be associated with substance abuse, it is imperative that other obstetric risk factors associated with substance abuse and use of illicit substances be explored.

### OBSTETRIC COMPLICATIONS

Obstetric complications are frequent, especially in women who do not seek adequate prenatal care. Table 10–3 lists obstetric complications observed in chemically dependent women.

Cocaine may cause damaging effects to the mother and fetus throughout the pregnancy. Cocaine acts as a stimulant on the peripheral nervous system and inhibits the reuptake of dopamine and norepinephrine at nerve terminals, thereby increasing circulating levels of these catecholamines. As a result, hypertension; tachycardia; vasoconstriction, including placental vasoconstriction; and uterine contractions occur. These pharmacologic actions of cocaine may be linked to the occurrence of spontaneous abortion among pregnant cocaine users.

A study by Chasnoff and associates (1985) compared the incidence of spontaneous abortion among four groups of women: cocaine users only, cocaine and opiate users, opiate users only, and nonusers. These patients all admitted to having been substance abusers

**Table 10–2**
MEDICAL COMPLICATIONS

Anemia
Poor dental hygiene
Cardiac disease
    Subacute bacterial endocarditis
    Myocardial infarctions and ischemia
    Arrhythmias
Cerebrovascular accidents
Hypertension
Infections
    Bacteremia
    Cellulitis
    Hepatitis—chronic and acute
    Phlebitis
    Pneumonia
    Septicemia
    Sexually transmitted diseases
        Congenital warts
        Chlamydia
        Herpes
        Syphilis
        Acquired immunodeficiency syndrome
    Urinary tract infections

**Table 10–3**
OBSTETRIC COMPLICATIONS

Abortion
Abruptio placentae
Breech presentation
Eclampsia
Intrauterine death
Intrauterine growth retardation
Meconium-stained amniotic fluid
Postpartum hemorrhage
Preterm labor and delivery
Premature rupture of membranes

during their pregnancies (except for the non-users). Thirty-eight percent of women who were using only cocaine had a history of spontaneous abortion; 46 percent of women who were using cocaine and opiates had such a past history, but only 16 percent of women who were using opiates alone had a past history of spontaneous abortion. The group of nonusers had a significantly lower previous history of spontaneous abortion.

Frank and associates (1988) reported that cocaine users were significantly more likely than nonusers to have had a previous spontaneous abortion. In this study, 30 percent of pregnant cocaine users had a past history of a spontaneous abortion. Hadeed and Siegel (1989) found a 25 percent incidence of spontaneous abortion among cocaine users.

In the third trimester, abruptio placentae is more likely to occur among pregnant cocaine users than among nonusers. One study by Chasnoff and associates found a 17.3 percent incidence among cocaine users compared with a 1.3 percent incidence in a group of pregnant women taking methadone. Bingol and colleagues (1987) found an 8 percent incidence of abruptio placentae, all resulting in stillbirth, and Hadeed and Siegel (1989) found a 10.7 percent incidence compared with a 1.7 percent incidence among nonusers. A more recent study by Chasnoff and associates (1989) compared the incidence of abruptio placentae in women who used cocaine throughout the pregnancy with women who abstained after the first trimester. A 15 percent incidence of abruptio placentae occurred in the group of women who used cocaine throughout the pregnancy, and a 9 percent incidence occurred in the group of women who stopped using cocaine. This difference did not reach statistical significance. The authors postulated that there is damage done to the placenta and uterine vessels early in pregnancy that increases that risk of this obstetric complication (Chasnoff et al, 1989).

Preterm labor and delivery are other obstetric complications of cocaine use (Chasnoff et al, 1987; MacGregor et al, 1987). Meconium-stained amniotic fluid and intrauterine growth retardation occur more frequently among infants exposed to cocaine than infants not exposed to drugs (Bingol et al, 1987; Chasnoff et al, 1989; Chasnoff et al, 1987; Hadeed and Siegel, 1989). However, if a cocaine user seeks early prenatal care and continues to receive adequate obstetric care, some obstetric complications are less frequent. Chasnoff and associates (1989) found a decrease in preterm delivery as well as improved intrauterine growth and birth weight among women who abstained from cocaine use in the second and third trimesters.

Obstetric complications from heroin, as with cocaine, occur with great frequency. Preterm delivery has been reported to be as high as 30 to 56 percent (Perlmutter, 1967; Stone et al, 1971), spontaneous abortion 14 percent (Pelosi et al, 1975), and stillbirth 5.1 percent (Pelosi et al, 1975). Abruptio placentae has a wide range of occurrence (between 3.2 percent and 16 percent) (Chasnoff et al, 1985; Connaughton et al, 1977; Pelosi et al, 1975). These percentages are lower than those in women who abuse cocaine during pregnancy. Premature rupture of membranes has been reported to occur in 11 to 21 percent of women who use heroin during their pregnancy (Connaughton et al, 1977; Pelosi et al, 1975); preeclampsia occurs in 10 to 15 percent meconium-stained amniotic fluid in 33 percent, and intrauterine growth retardation in as high as 50 percent (Finnegan, 1975). However, the earlier studies did not distinguish between preterm infants with low birth weights and small-for-gestational-age infants. Other obstetric complications include an increased incidence of breech presentations, thrombophlebitis, and postpartum hemorrhage.

However, if a woman is placed on methadone treatment, obstetric and neonatal complications are substantially decreased, especially when a woman is on a low dose. Several studies (Blinick et al, 1976; Stimmel and Adamsons, 1976; Strauss et al, 1974) compared women enrolled in a methadone maintenance program with a group of nonusers and found no difference in obstetric complications.

The effect of marijuana use on pregnancy has been difficult to demonstrate, because a large number of marijuana users also use other illicit substances. However, a study by Greenland and colleagues (1982) found that marijuana users were more likely to have a precipitous labor and meconium-stained amniotic fluid. Although not statistically significant, marijuana users exhibited poor weight gain, suspected intrauterine growth retardation, and prolonged or arrested labor.

# Management of the Chemically Dependent Pregnant Woman

## MULTIDISCIPLINARY APPROACH

The pregnant substance abuser has a multitude of health care issues that need to be evaluated. Health care interventions should begin as soon as possible during pregnancy and continue beyond the birth of the infant. The multidisciplinary treatment team should include an obstetrician and/or nurse mid-wife, obstetric and pediatric staff nurses, a therapist (clinical psychologist, social worker, or psychiatric nurse specialist), a pediatrician and/or nurse practitioner, and a developmental psychologist. In addition, referrals should be established whenever necessary with a psychiatrist, an infectious disease physician for HIV-positive women and infants, a nutritionist, a physical therapist for the infant, and home health nursing services.

Services may be provided in an inpatient or outpatient treatment setting. Routine and high-risk obstetric care, psychiatric treatment for dual diagnoses, addiction counseling, social service referral, and health education in all aspects of addiction and pregnancy should be included. The care of the pregnant substance abuser must focus on her special needs. Prenatal education, Lamaze instruction, nutrition, and routine baby care also must be included.

The infant should receive routine health care, anticipatory guidance, and immunizations, as outlined by the American Academy of Pediatrics. In addition, evaluation by a developmental psychologist should be integrated into a routine schedule, especially for infants with a history of alcohol and cocaine exposure, to help identify early developmental delays.

This comprehensive health care approach requires integration of all services, and a case manager is often required. The goals are to lessen the effects of substance abuse on pregnancy and the newborn, promote ad-diction recovery, and improve the mother-infant relationship.

## PRENATAL LABORATORY EVALUATION

In addition to the routine obstetric assessment and evaluation, special considerations must be taken into account when providing health care to pregnant substance abusers (Table 10–4). A urine sample for a toxicology screen should be administered at each prenatal visit. As many as 60 percent of pregnant substance abusers continue to use illicit substances during their pregnancy, even when enrolled in a chemical dependence program (Chasnoff, 1988a). A positive result helps identify a fetus at risk, and the information may be used to encourage additional involvement with psychosocial services.

Sexually transmitted diseases such as gonorrhea, syphilis, and chlamydia infection are common and must be screened for and treated appropriately. AIDS testing with the enzyme-linked immunosorbent assay (ELISA) confirmed by Western Blot should be offered to all drug-using women. However, women with a history of the following high-risk factors should be counseled and strongly encouraged to have HIV testing performed:

1. A history of intravenous drug use;
2. A sexual partner (past or present) with a history of intravenous drug use;
3. Sexual contact (past or present) with bisexual males;
4. A history of prostitution; and
5. Having received a blood transfusion prior to 1985.

If the initial testing is negative but the woman has answered affirmatively to any of the above-mentioned high-risk factors, HIV testing should be repeated at routine intervals during the pregnancy (such as every 3 months). Hepatitis B is a common infection found among substance abusers. If a pregnant woman has acute or chronic viral hepatitis during pregnancy, she can transmit the infection to her infant. Therefore, hepatitis B screening should be performed on all substance-abusing women.

Ultrasound examinations help establish fetal growth patterns and are useful in evaluating fetal status. Ultrasounds are often

Table 10–4
PRENATAL LABORATORY TESTS

| Type of Test | Initial Visit | 15–19 Weeks | 26–28 Weeks | 30–34 Weeks | 36 Weeks |
|---|---|---|---|---|---|
| Blood | | | | | |
| Alpha fetoprotein | | * | | | |
| Antibody screen | * | | | | |
| Blood type | * | | | | |
| CBC | * | | | | |
| Coombs' test | * | | | | |
| ELISA (HIV Screen) | * | | | | |
| Hepatitis B profile | * | | | | |
| Rh determination | * | | | | |
| Rubella titer | * | | | | |
| Serology | * | | | | |
| Sickle cell prep (if indicated) | * | | | | |
| 1 hour postprandial blood glucose | | | * | | |
| RPR | * | | | | |
| Urine | | | | | |
| Urine toxicology | * | * | * | * | * |
| Urinalysis | * | | | | |
| Urine culture | * | | | | |
| Vaginal smears | | | | | |
| Pap | * | | | | |
| Chlamydia culture | * | | | | |
| Gonorrhea | * | | | | |
| Ultrasound | | | | | |
| Dating | * | | | | |
| Level II | | *(20 wk) | | | |
| Growth | | | | | * |

recommended initially to help determine dates, at 20 weeks' gestation to assess the presence of congenital anomalies, and at 36 weeks' gestation if intrauterine growth retardation is suspected.

## USE OF METHADONE

If a pregnant woman is an opiate user, methadone should be prescribed to replace the illicit substance. Methadone reduces the use of street opiates by blocking withdrawal and craving. The use of methadone has several advantages. It is a long-acting drug (lasting approximately 24 hours) and maintains a steady blood level. It does not cause euphoria, and the highs and lows of the heroin cycle are not present. It may be given orally, is obtained legally, and is inexpensive. Methadone has a lower risk of teratogenic effects than street opiates, often contaminated with other substances. Methadone use may also lessen the risk of AIDS if the pregnant woman is an intravenous drug user.

When they were first put into use, metha-

done treatment programs placed women on high doses of methadone (80 to 120 mg/day). The rationale for this therapy was to create a tolerance to prevent the addict from getting her usual "high" if heroin was also used (Keith et al, 1986). However, the higher dose of methadone produced a more severe and prolonged period of abstinence for the newborn, compared with withdrawal symptoms from infants exposed to heroin. Women are now placed on low doses of methadone (5 to 40 mg/day); the lowest possible dose without inducing craving or withdrawal is optimal. If the maintenance dose is too low, the woman will obtain other illicit substances to alleviate the withdrawal symptoms.

When a pregnant opiate user enters a methadone program, a detailed history of the amount of the opiate used in the past 24 hours is the most accurate way to determine the average amount used. It is also important to be aware of the current amount of street heroin in each bag. When this information is known, the initial methadone dose should be approximated. Methadone is given once a day by mouth. However, if oral administration is not possible, intramuscular injection may be used every 8 to 12 hours. The patient needs to be assessed daily at the onset of treatment. Signs of withdrawal or intoxication should be noted and dose adjustments made. Progressive signs of intoxication are miosis, drowsiness, decreased rate and depth of respirations, bradycardia, hypotension, hypothermia, and coma (Fultz and Seney, 1975).

There is some controversy as to the safety of detoxification during pregnancy. Detoxification is defined as medically supervised withdrawal with methadone from a state of physical dependence on opiate drugs (Fultz and Seney, 1975). The concern of the detoxification process during pregnancy is the possibility of spontaneous abortion, preterm labor, or fetal withdrawal. One study by Zuspan and associates (1975) measured epinephrine and norepinephrine in amniotic fluid as a means of measuring fetal homeostasis in a pregnant woman who was being detoxified from methadone in the third trimester. These catecholamines were 8 to 10 times higher than normal during attempted detoxification. The patient's dose was then increased, and the epinephrine and norepinephrine levels returned to normal. However, experience with one program during a 3-year period demonstrated that methadone doses may be lowered during pregnancy without harm to the fetus or mother (Schnoll, 1986). The detoxification was begun in the second trimester, once the mother was stabilized and continued through the third trimester. The advantage of this type of treatment is that it decreases the withdrawal symptoms of the newborn after birth. When the dose of methadone is reduced, a gradual reduction is recommended. The pregnant woman should be informed that the dose will be changed, but the amount or rate of reduction should not be disclosed (Schnoll, 1986). Any signs of withdrawal or evidence of fetal distress indicate an alteration in the rate of withdrawal (Schnoll, 1986).

No other maintenance drugs have been used in pregnant women who abuse other substances, such as alcohol, stimulants, or sedatives. Women must be encouraged to remain abstinent and receive addiction counseling.

All substance-abusing women should receive education on the effects of drug abuse on the mother and fetus and the general risk factors of substance abuse. Each drug she is abusing must be reviewed in detail. A combi-nation of oral and written information such as pamphlets and diagrams is helpful; films and demonstrations add to the quality of education. During the education sessions, women often begin to express their feelings of guilt. Emotional support by the health care staff is imperative. The woman must be encouraged to express her feelings and fears, an important step toward recovery.

## LABOR AND DELIVERY

The management of a pregnant substance abuser during labor and delivery may be complicated. If a woman is using drugs such as marijuana or cocaine, identification may be difficult because no physical evidence may be present. Often, the drug history is unknown. However, if a woman presents in labor with no prenatal care, and needle marks or other physical characteristics of substance abuse, the patient should be questioned as to her involvement with illicit drugs during her pregnancy. Urine should be obtained for a toxicology screen. The urine screen should also be obtained in each woman with a known history of drug use during pregnancy to help establish her chemical dependence status and provide appropriate intervention. Typically, the pregnant woman addicted to heroin comes to the labor and delivery area intoxicated from a recent drug administration and well into her labor and requests discharge shortly after delivery, in order to avoid withdrawal or craving. Frequently, she leaves the hospital against medical advice. However, withdrawal symptoms may be observed while the pregnant heroin user is in labor, delivery, or postpartum. Early withdrawal symptoms may include restlessness, lacrimation, diaphoresis, rhinorrhea, and yawning. Symptoms of more severe withdrawal include increased respiration, heart rate, and blood pressure; vomiting; diarrhea; and abdominal pain.

To prevent or stabilize heroin withdrawal during labor, methadone should be administered intramuscularly. Methadone also should be given to the woman who is receiving methadone as chemical dependence treatment if she has not received her daily dose that day. Oral administration may be used if the woman is not vomiting or having other symptoms that would contraindicate an oral dose.

Once the patient is stabilized on methadone, routine methods of anesthesia or analgesia may be used for pain reduction during labor and delivery. Real pain is experienced in pregnant substance abusers as with nonusers. However, if signs of withdrawal or intoxication are present, the following medications should be used with caution: morphine, meperidine, and hydromorphone (Keith et al, 1988). Pentazocaine must be avoided because it acts as a narcotic antagonist and may cause acute withdrawal in an individual (Fultz and Senay, 1975). Table 10–5 lists the signs and symptoms of opiate withdrawal. Continuous electronic fetal heart monitoring should be considered during labor because of the frequency of meconium passage and heart rate abnormalities.

## POSTPARTUM CARE

Routine postpartum care should be provided for the mother as well as continuation of methadone if she is an opiate user. Continuation with chemical dependence treatment should be strongly encouraged. Even those women who have stopped using illicit substances during their pregnancy have a high rate of relapse. One chemical dependence program found 56 percent of women had relapsed in the first month postpartum and 69 percent by the second month (Chandler). If the mother was initially identified as chemically dependent during her labor and delivery, psychosocial services and chemical dependence counseling should be provided and appropriate referrals made.

### Table 10–5
#### SIGNS AND SYMPTOMS OF MATERNAL OPIATE WITHDRAWAL

| Early | Late |
|-------|------|
| Craving for drugs | Aching in bones and muscles |
| Thirst | Regurgitation |
| Anxiety | Diarrhea |
| Restlessness | Elevated blood pressure |
| Lacrimation | Hyperpyrexia |
| Tremors | Hyperventilation |
| Hot or cold flashes | Tachycardia |
| Diaphoresis | Abdominal girth |
| Nausea | Cramps |
| Yawning | Seizures |
| Miosis | |

From Keith L, Donald W, Rosner M, et al: Obstetric aspects of perinatal addiction. *In* Chasnoff IJ (ed): Drug Use in Pregnancy: Mother and Child. Lancaster, PA, MTP Press, 1986, p 35.

Close observation of the infant for effects of drug exposure is necessary. A urine sample for toxicology should be obtained on the infant as soon after delivery as possible.

The mother should be encouraged to "room in" with her infant. The mother needs to understand the effects of drug exposure and the special needs of her newborn. Drug-exposed infants may be difficult to handle. They are often irritable, difficult to feed, and cry when stimulated. They may have difficulty with eye-to-eye contact that impairs the attachment process. The mother and infant need much time together while supportive services are made available. Many drug-exposed infants are discharged with their mother within 48 hours and may not have adequate support systems at home. Delays in hospital discharge should be limited to those infants who fail to gain weight, feed poorly, have seizure activity that requires stabilization, or whose home environment and the mother's ability to care for her infant are assessed as unsuitable for acceptable growth and development.

## NEONATAL EFFECTS

Infants exposed prenatally to illicit substances such as cocaine, opiates, marijuana, and alcohol are at risk for a variety of physical and developmental abnormalities, including prenatal and postnatal growth retardation, congenital anomalies, and neurobehavioral problems. Some of these abnormalities appear at birth, whereas others may not appear until months or even years later.

### Cocaine

Cocaine-exposed infants tend to be shorter, have lower birth weights, and smaller head circumferences compared with infants born to nonusers (Bingol et al, 1987; Chasnoff et al, 1987; Hadeed and Siegel, 1989; Zuckerman et al, 1989). In addition, these infants have a slightly lower gestational age. One study (Chasnoff et al, 1989) found that the mean gestational age in cocaine-exposed infants was $38.0 \pm 0.7$ weeks as opposed to 40 weeks in a drug-free group. This particular group of cocaine-exposed infants was exposed throughout the pregnancy. In comparison, infants who were born to women who abstained from cocaine after the first trimester did not differ from drug-free control group members in their mean gestational age (Chasnoff et al, 1989).

Congenital anomalies, especially of the genitourinary tract, have been reported. However, as yet, no specific pattern of malformation has been found to be associated with cocaine exposure during pregnancy (Dixon et al, 1990). The most commonly reported anomalies are hydronephrosis, cryptorchidism, and hypospadias (Chasnoff et al, 1988). Other anomalies include ambiguous genitalia, atresia, and renal and ureteral agenesis (Chasnoff et al, 1988; Chavez et al, 1989). Cerebral infarction has been reported in two infants whose mothers used large amounts of cocaine in the 48 to 72 hours prior to delivery (Chasnoff, 1988a; Chasnoff et al, 1986). Limb reduction defects, cardiac anomalies (atrial and ventricular septal defects), gastrointestinal defects (ileal atresia, prune belly syndrome, gastroschisis), and cranial defects (encephalocele, exencephaly, partial bone defects) have also been reported in cocaine-exposed infants (Chasnoff et al, 1989; Chasnoff et al, 1988; Chavez et al, 1989; Hoyme et al, 1990). It has been suggested that these anomalies occur as a result of fetal vascular disruption (Hoyme et al, 1990). Cocaine acts as a stimulant on the central nervous system, which causes generalized vasoconstriction, hypertension, and tachycardia leading to hemorrhage and infarction.

Muscle tone abnormalities are characteristic of cocaine-exposed infants. At birth, these infants are frequently in overly extended postures and demonstrate poor quality of movement, such as tremulousness (Schneider and Chasnoff, 1987). When holding an infant upright to assess weightbearing, the legs are often held stiffly and arching in extension may be observed. There is very little head lag, which normally would be present in drug-free infants.

By the time cocaine-exposed infants reach four months of age, they tend to lie excessively in extended positions when supine, have stiff and jerky movements of their extremities, and are less able to round their buttocks and kick reciprocally (Schneider at al, 1989). When held in an upright position, these infants have stiff extension of hips, knees, and ankles. Normal 4-month-old infants have very active lower extremities, often flexing their legs in order to play with their knees

and feet. With weightbearing, they hold a relaxed position and use both flexor and extensor muscles. As the cocaine-exposed infant gets older, delays in sitting have been observed. These delays may be due to the overuse of extensor muscles and decreased use and strength in the flexor and abdominal muscles.

Cocaine-exposed neonates exhibit a high degree of irritability and tremulousness and are difficult to console. Griffith describes cocaine-exposed infants as fragile because they have very low thresholds for over-stimulation, often maintain a hyperexcitable state, and require much assistance to calm down (Griffith, 1988). The Brazelton Neonatal Behavioral Assessment Scale (NBAS) (Brazelton, 1984) has been used to assess the neurobehavioral effects of drugs on newborns. This tool is usually administered between the third and 30th day of life with repeated assessments during this period of time. Orientation and state control are the primary dimensions affected.

Orientation is defined as the ability to interact actively with the environment by attending to and responding to visual and auditory stimuli presented either alone or simultaneously (Griffith, 1988). A newborn not exposed to drugs typically follows stimuli visually and becomes alert to sounds and tries to locate those sounds. By 1 month of age, normal infants continue to respond to visual and auditory stimuli and may do so for long periods of time (Griffith, 1988). However, a cocaine-exposed infant is different. Many of these infants have difficulty tracking stimuli and often actively look away from the stimulus (gaze aversion). Those infants who begin to respond appropriately cannot maintain the interaction. Signs of distress are observed, which may include crying, yawning, sneezing, color changes, increased respirations, disorganized motor activity, and frantic gaze aversion.

State control is defined as the ability to move through the different states of arousal (sleep state, drowsy state, alert and responsive state, agitate state, and crying state) in a smooth, consecutive manner, beginning with the sleep state, during a NBAS examination (Griffith, 1988). The cocaine-exposed infant tends to move from one state to the other abruptly and responds inappropriately to the amount of stimulation offered (Griffith, 1988). Griffith has observed four different patterns of state control. The first pattern is the infant who pulls down into a sleep state in response to the first stimulation and remains asleep; the second is the infant who cannot be awakened at all, although he may whimper, change colors, and thrash about; the third is the infant who moves abruptly from a sleep state to crying; and the fourth is the infant who uses both sleeping and crying to shut himself or herself off from the stimuli (Griffith, 1988).

At 1 month of age, state control has improved in cocaine-exposed infants, but is still significantly below that of drug-free newborns (Griffith, 1988). The first-mentioned infants can maintain an alert, responsive state but only for short periods of time.

The NBAS examination demonstrates that these infants require close observation and assessment by health care professionals, parents, and other caretakers as to the types of everyday activity and stimulation that cause the infants to be overloaded and exhibit distress signals. Sucking and feeding difficulties that have been observed may be a result of overstimulation.

The mother-infant attachment process may be affected by excessive crying, irritability, and inability to maintain eye-to-eye contact. The mother often feels exhausted, inadequate, rejected, and sometimes even hostile toward her infant. The feelings may escalate the already present feelings of guilt, worthlessness, and depression. This situation may predispose the mother to neglect or physically abuse her child, who is so difficult to handle.

It is important to educate parents and other caretakers on the special needs and behaviors of these infants. The types of stimulation that overload the infants, distress signs, and comforting measures should be routinely discussed. Swaddling, using a pacifier, and vertical rocking are methods used with much success to calm infants (Table 10–6). The first measures should be swaddling with a blanket and using a pacifier; in addition, slow, smooth vertical rocking–keeping the infant facing away, supporting the head, and flexing the knees–will aid in calming the infant. Removing accessory noise and light from the environment may be necessary. Once the infant is calm, the parent or caretaker may begin to offer either visual or auditory stimuli but not both.

The goal is to learn how to stimulate and interact with the infant without over-

**Table 10–6**
STEP BY STEP APPROACH TO COMFORT INFANT

1. Avoid a frantic cry state—stop interaction and allow recovery if early distress signs (yawning, hiccoughs, sneezing, gaze aversion, color changes, frowns) occur.
2. If infant is unable to gain control, swaddle and offer pacifier.
3. If irritability continues, hold infant close and rock vertically.
4. Once infant is calm interact with infant by offering one stimulus at a time—initially, voice or face.
   a. infant may require swaddling or a pacifier to maintain alert, responsive state;
   b. observe for distress signs.
5. Gradually increase the amount of play.
6. When infant maintains a calm state, unwrap and allow to move around.

From Griffith DR: The effects of perinatal cocaine exposure on infant neurobehavior and early maternal-infant interactions. *In* Chasnoff IS (ed): Drugs, Alcohol, Pregnancy and Parenting. Boston, Kluwer Academic Publishers, 1988, pp 105–113.

stimulating him or her. Keeping an infant as calm as possible and as often as possible allows the infant to respond more appropriately to his or her environment. One concern of many parents and caretakers is that they will spoil their children by holding the infant and responding to every cry. It must be emphasized that the earlier the infant is comforted, the more quickly the infant will calm down. These infants have special needs that require special types of handling.

Speech and learning delays are suspect in cocaine-exposed infants. Many children reaching school age who are found to have learning disabilities have a positive history of cocaine exposure by retrospective clinical review. Many studies on perinatal cocaine use are recent, with no long-term follow-up results. It is important for researchers of early cocaine effects to determine the significance of these findings for school-aged children through prospective studies on the long-term effects of cocaine. Specific assessments may be needed to provide earlier interventions so that learning problems may be lessened or avoided.

## Opiates

Prenatal exposure to narcotics such as heroin and methadone can result in low birthweight, small head circumference, and short stature in the infants (Blinick et al, 1976; Chasnoff et al, 1986; Fulroth et al, 1989;

Lifschitz et al, 1985; Pelosi et al, 1975). Follow-up studies through the preschool years have found that these children catch up in weight and length; however, head circumference measurements remain smaller than in drug-free infants (Lifschitz et al, 1985; Chasnoff et al, 1986).

At birth, neonatal withdrawal is the most characteristic finding of the narcotic-exposed infant (Table 10–7). The acute signs of withdrawal present within 3 to 4 days of birth and persist for 2 to 3 weeks after delivery. Chasnoff (1988b) reports a subacute form of withdrawal that lasts from 4 to 6 months, with a peak at approximately six weeks of age. The onset and severity of withdrawal depend on the type of drug used, the amount and frequency of use, and when it was used by the mother prior to delivery. Neonatal withdrawal symptoms have been reported to occur in 21 to 85 percent of infants born to mothers using narcotics. However, infants whose mothers receive 20 mg or less of methadone usually have very mild symptoms. The most common signs of neonatal withdrawal are high-pitched cry, tremulousness, sweating, frantic sucking, abrasions on the elbows and knees, vomiting, and diarrhea. The tremors are flailing as opposed to fine tremors exhibited by the cocaine-exposed infants. Seizures have been noted but are rare.

Other signs of withdrawal include low-grade fever, hypertonicity, restlessness, yawning, sneezing, rhinorrhea, tachypnea, and mottling of skin. The subacute signs and symptoms of withdrawal that have been reported include hypertonia, hyperflexia, and feeding and sleep problems. When assessing for neonatal withdrawal symptoms, other problems such as hypoglycemia, hypocalcemia, hyperthyroidism, CNS hemorrhage, birth anoxia, and sepsis may appear and should be considered.

Treatment of narcotic withdrawal for most newborns should be supportive. As previously mentioned, comforting techniques to calm the irritable cocaine-exposed infant work extremely well. However, if the newborn has feeding difficulties, cannot gain weight, or has excessive vomiting, diarrhea, or seizures, pharmacologic treatment is indicated.

The three drugs most commonly used include paregoric, diazepam, and phenobarbital. Paregoric (anhydrous morphine) is given in amounts sufficient to control symptoms and then gradually withdrawn (Sweet, 1982). The advantage of using this drug is that these infants exhibit better feeding behaviors and weight gain than infants treated with diazepam or phenobarbital. However, it may take a day or two to reach its effective blood level, and it is gradually withdrawn over a long period of time. Because it is only given orally, paregoric cannot be used if the newborn is vomiting.

Diazepam acts promptly in neonatal withdrawal, but it may be associated with depressed sucking, bradycardia, and respiratory depression; late-onset seizures have occurred after cessation of treatment (Chasnoff, 1986b). Phenobarbital may be given orally or intramuscularly and is effective in controlling seizures. Phenobarbital sedates the newborn and quiets him or her; however, it too, may cause sucking impairment and does little to control vomiting and diarrhea. Blood levels should be followed closely, and slow tapering of the dose should begin once the infant is stabilized for a few days.

## Alcohol

Infants exposed to alcohol during pregnancy may or may not be easy to detect. At birth, some newborns may display withdrawal symptoms, such as restlessness, irritability, tremulousness, hypotonicity, and hyperactivity. Only a small percentage have the stigmata of fetal alcohol syndrome, which include three specific parameters: (1) prenatal and postnatal growth retardation; (2) central nervous system effects, most commonly mental retardation; and (3) facial anomalies.

The face of an infant with fetal alcohol syndrome displays a thin upper lip, long flattened philtrum, flattening of the maxillary area, micro-ophthalmia and/or short

**Table 10–7**
SIGNS OF NEONATAL WITHDRAWAL

| More Common | Less Common |
|---|---|
| Abrasions of elbows and knees | Hypertonicity |
| Diarrhea | Low-grade fever |
| Frantic sucking | Mottling of skin |
| High-pitched cry | Restlessness |
| Sweating | Rhinorrhea |
| Tremulousness | Seizures |
| Vomiting | Sneezing |
| | Tachypnea |
| | Yawning |

palpebral fissures, flattened nasal bridge, and a short nose. Infants with only one or two of these characteristics are considered to have fetal alcohol effects. Without the recognizable facial features, some infants with fetal alcohol effects may go undetected for months until abnormal growth and delayed developmental patterns become apparent. Even with early recognition of these delays, the fetal alcohol syndrome infants do not catch up as they mature; these children remain below the average height and weight and with small head circumferences.

Children exposed to alcohol *in utero* may exhibit mild to moderate delays in social and fine and gross motor development. Some children are severely delayed in intellectual development; however, the average IQ is 65 (Clarren and Smith, 1978; Jones et al, 1973; Lemoine et al, 1968; Streissguth et al, 1978). One study (Streissguth et al, 1978) found that the more severe the physical characteristics, the more intellectually impaired the children were. As these children got older, some of the facial features became less apparent, although intellectual growth continued to be affected. In addition, behavioral problems such as hyperactivity, distractibility, and short attention spans were frequent findings (Streissguth, 1979).

Other physical findings associated with perinatal exposure to alcohol include cardiac (atrial and ventricular septal defects) and ocular defects (estropia, blepharophimosis, myopia, strabismus); ear malformations, such as incomplete development of the superior helix; nail hypoplasia; hirsutism; diastasis recti; labial hypoplasia; hemangiomas; aberrant palmar creases; pectus excavatum; and limited joint movements (Ernhart et al, 1987; Golden et al, 1982; Hanson et al, 1976; Jones et al, 1973).

Fetal alcohol syndrome is usually seen in children born to alcoholics who drank heavily for years prior to becoming pregnant and during their pregnancies. Heavy drinking is defined as 45 alcoholic drinks or more per month or one ounce of absolute alcohol per day. Studies have found that increasing alcohol consumption is related to an increase in facial anomalies (Ernhart et al, 1987) and other associated congenital anomalies of fetal alcohol exposure (Ouellette et al, 1977). Studies on moderate drinking also have shown some teratogenic effects (Davis et al, 1982; Hanson et al, 1978; Ouellette et al, 1977). The question that arises is, How little alcohol consumption can cause damage to the fetus? As yet, no safe level of alcohol has been determined; therefore, it is recommended that women abstain from all alcoholic products for the duration of their pregnancy.

## Marijuana

Effects of marijuana on the fetus have been difficult to ascertain. Most women who smoke marijuana during pregnancy use other illicit substances as well. Therefore, it is difficult to isolate one factor causing specific abnormalities. In addition, studies on fetal effects of marijuana have been largely inconsistent. Some studies have found lower birth weights and decreased length associated with marijuana use (Hingson et al, 1982; Zuckerman et al, 1989). Other studies were unable to demonstrate these findings (Fried et al, 1984; Linn et al, 1983). Congenital anomalies were reported in one study but did not reach statistical significance (Linn et al, 1983). Yet another study found that women who smoked marijuana during pregnancy were five times more likely than nonusers to deliver an infant with features compatible with fetal alcohol syndrome (Hingson et al, 1982).

One study found that length of gestation was shorter in substance abusers than in nonusers, especially among heavy marijuana users. The gestational age was reduced by 0.8 week in women who smoked six or more marijuana cigarettes per week, even when other factors such as cigarette smoking and alcohol use were controlled analytically (Fried et al, 1984). However, the study with the largest number of women enrolled (12,825) found no association between shortened gestational age and marijuana use (Linn et al, 1983). It is evident that more research must be conducted to understand perinatal effects of marijuana. At the present time, no firm conclusion can be made.

## NEONATAL MANAGEMENT

Any newborn whose mother has a known or suspected history of substance abuse during her pregnancy must have a urine sample collected for toxicology as soon as possible after delivery. A positive urine screen will confirm drug exposure in the 2 to 3 days prior to delivery. A thorough review of the mother's medical, obstetric, and social histories should be obtained to help understand the potential risks and to develop strategies to provide appropriate health care.

The mother should be informed of the urine toxicology screen, its importance in evaluating the status of her infant, and its implications for the child's health. Some states require reporting for child abuse if an infant has a positive urine toxicology result or any physical signs of drug withdrawal. Because of the overwhelming number of drug-exposed infant cases being reported, investigations often begin after the mother (and infant) are discharged from the hospital. It is the practice of some hospitals to keep the infant in the hospital for several weeks, until the investigation and recommendations are complete.

This practice may cause more difficulties because of maternal-infant separation. The mother may not have the opportunity to learn about her infant's needs and how to care for him or her. The attachment process is hindered, which later may lead to abuse and neglect. Thus, whenever possible, the mother and infant are discharged together, especially if adequate support systems are available. In either situation, the multidisciplinary team of physicians, nurses, and therapists must continue to evaluate and provide appropriate services and referrals to the mother and the newborn.

Education is paramount in helping mothers and other caretakers of drug-exposed infants. Discussion of the neonatal effects of substance abuse and treatment recommendations such as special comforting measures, length of hospitalization, and medication must be accomplished prior to hospital discharge. Assessment of the mother-infant interaction and discussion of the mother's feelings toward her newborn should be a routine part of postpartum care.

Home health nursing services are used to eliminate the gap between hospital discharge and the first pediatric visit. Nursing services include assessment of neonatal withdrawal symptoms and other effects of drug exposure, feeding patterns, and the maternal-infant interaction. Observing the feeding process may provide much of this information. The infant's weight is obtained to monitor growth, and the nurse reinforces comforting measures, reviews routine infant care, and provides support and encouragement to the mother.

Drug-exposed infants often have been observed to have feeding patterns different from those of nonexposed infants. Drug-exposed infants feed more frequently and take smaller amounts at each feeding for several weeks. Therefore, demand feeding is the only feeding schedule that should be given for these infants. However, if the infant is preterm and unable to suck or gain weight, nasogastric feedings at frequent intervals may be necessary.

Another nutritional concern is hypoglycemia due to the high rate of preterm delivery, small for gestational age births, and feeding difficulties in drug-exposed infants. Screening for hypoglycemia should be a routine consideration in the first 24 to 48 hours after delivery.

Feeding choices are not always optional for the chemically dependent woman. The promotion of breastfeeding for these women must be done with caution owing to the high rate of relapse in the early postpartum months. Virtually all drugs present in the maternal circulation are transferred to breast milk, and adverse effects on the newborn may result. Cocaine intoxication was reported in a 2-week-old infant who presented to a pediatric emergency room with extreme irritability (Chasnoff et al, 1987). Other physical findings include hypertension, tachycardia, vomiting, diarrhea, tremulousness, high-pitched cry, dilated pupils with a poor response to light, increased sucking reflex, increased deep tendon reflexes, and marked lability in mood. Milk samples were found to be negative for cocaine use and its metabolites 36 h after the mother's last cocaine use, and the infant's urine sample was negative by 60 hours after the last breastfeeding (Chasnoff et al, 1987).

A woman who is drug free for at least 3 months prior to her delivery (confirmed by urine toxicology screening tests) and who demonstrates motivation to remain drug free should be encouraged to breastfeed, if she desires. A mother on methadone maintenance therapy also may be encouraged to breastfeed without much restriction, especially if she is given a low dose (< 40 mg/day). Methadone is considered compatible with breastfeeding by the American Academy of Pediatrics (Committee on Drugs, 1989). The presence of methadone in breast milk may even reduce the infant's withdrawal symptoms from the drug. Every mother must be made aware of the dangers of illicit drug ingestion through breast milk and given specific instructions on feeding alternatives if she relapses.

The first pediatric health care visit ideally should be within 1 to 2 weeks after hospital discharge to assess drug effects, feeding difficulties, weight gain, and mother-infant interaction, and to continue to provide education and support to the mother to maintain the health and well-being of her infant. Referrals for periodic developmental assessment should be considered, especially with alcohol- and cocaine-exposed infants, because of the developmental delays often observed. The routine well-child schedule, including immunizations, is the same as with non–drug-exposed infants.

Substance abuse during pregnancy is widespread in this country, involving women of all socioeconomic, racial, and ethnic groups. The drugs of choice are cocaine and marijuana, and most abusers use several drugs.

Substance abuse during pregnancy may have severe consequences for the mother and the infant, which may be reduced or possibly prevented with early prenatal intervention involving several health care disciplines. It is important for health care providers to recognize the problem; incorporate a complete history as part of routine obstetric care; and provide education, treatment, and referral services for all women.

Health care of the pregnant substance abuser should not end with the birth of her infant, because most women continue to use illicit substances, which will ultimately affect the health and overall quality of life for herself and her infant. Drug-exposed infants deserve long-term evaluation. Our understanding of the effects of drug exposure is limited to the newborn period through the preschool years. More research must be conducted, especially in the area of growth and development in school-aged children.

# References

Abelson HI, Miller JD: A decade of trends in cocaine use in the household population. National Institute of Drug Abuse Research Monograph Series, 61:35, 1985.

Abrams CA: Cytogenetic risks to the offspring of pregnant addicts. Addict Disease 2, 63–77, 1982.

Bingol N, Fuchs M, Diaz V, Stone RK, Gromisch DS: Teratogenicity of cocaine in humans. Pediatr 110(1):93–96, 1987.

Blinick G, Wallach R, Jerez E, Ackerman BD: Drug addiction in pregnancy and the neonate. Obstet Gynecol 125(2):135–142, 1976.

Brazelton TB: Neonatal Behavioral Assessment Scale. Philadelphia, JB Lippincott Co, 1984.

Chandler J: National Association of Perinatal Addiction Research and Education, Chicago, IL (unpublished data).

Chasnoff IJ: Drug use and women: establishing a standard of care. Ann Acad Sci 562:208–210, 1989.

Chasnoff IJ: Cocaine: effects on pregnancy and the neonate. In Chasnoff IJ (ed): Drugs, Alcohol, Pregnancy and Parenting, Boston, Kluwer Academic Publishers, 1988a, pp 97–113.

Chasnoff IJ: Newborn infants with drug withdrawal symptoms. Pediatr Rev 9(9):273–277, 1988.

Chasnoff IJ: Perinatal effects of cocaine. Contemporary Obstetrics and Gynecology, May 1987, pp 163–179.

Chasnoff IJ, Burns KA, Burns WJ: Cocaine use in pregnancy: perinatal morbidity and mortality. Neurotoxicol Teratol 9:291–293, 1987.

Chasnoff IJ, Chisum GM, Kaplan WE: Maternal cocaine use and genitourinary tract malformations. Teratology 37:201–204, 1988.

Chasnoff IJ, Landress HJ, Barrett ME: The prevalence of illicit drug or alcohol use during pregnancy and discrepancies in mandatory reporting in Pinellas County, Florida. N Engl J Med 322(17):1202–1206, 1990.

Chasnoff IJ, Lewis DE, Squires L: Cocaine intoxication in a breast-fed infant. Pediatrics 80(6):836–838, 1987.

Chasnoff IJ, Burns KA, Burns WJ, Schnoll SH: Prenatal drug exposure: effects on neonatal and infant growth and development. Neurobehav Toxicol Teratol 8(4):357–263, 1986.

Chasnoff IJ, Burns WJ, Schnoll SH, Burns KA: Cocaine use in pregnancy. N Engl J Med 313:666–69, 1985.

Chasnoff IJ, Bussey ME, Savich R, Stack CM: Perinatal cerebral infarction and maternal cocaine use. J Pediatr 108(3):456–459, 1986.

Chasnoff IJ, Griffith DR, MacGregor SN, et al: Temporal patterns of cocaine use in pregnancy. JAMA 261(12):1741–1744, 1989.

Chasnoff IJ, Schnoll SH, Burns WJ, et al: Maternal nonnarcotic substance abuse during pregnancy: effects on infant development. Neurobehav Toxicol Teratol 6(4):277–280, 1984.

Chavez GR, Mulinare J, Cordero JF: Maternal cocaine use during early pregnancy as a risk factor for congenital urogenital anomalies. JAMA 262(6):795–798, 1989.

Chisum GM: Nursing interventions with the antepartum substance abuser. J Perinat Neonat Nurs 3(4):22–33, 1990.

Chisum GM: Recognition and initial management of the pregnant substance abusing woman. In Chasnoff IJ (ed): Drug Use in Pregnancy: Mother and Child. Lancaster, PA, MTP Press, 1986, pp 17–22.

Clarren SK, Smith DW: The fetal alcohol syndrome. N Engl J Med 298(19):1063–1067, 1978.

Committee on Drugs, American Academy of Pediatrics: Transfer of drugs and other chemicals into human breast milk. Pediatrics 84(5):924–936, 1989.

Connaughton JF, Reeser D, Schut J, Finnegan LP: Perinatal addiction: outcome and management. Am J Obstet Gynecol 129:679–686, 1977.

Daghestani AN: Psychosocial characteristics of pregnant women addicts in treatment. In Chasnoff IJ (ed): Drugs, Alcohol, Pregnancy and Parenting. Boston, Kluwer Academic Publishers, 1988, pp 7–16.

Davis PJ, Partridge JW, Storrs CN: Alcohol consumption in pregnancy: how much is safe? Arch Dis Child 57(12):940–943, 1982.

Dixon S, Bresnahan K, Zuckerman B: Cocaine babies:

meeting the challenge of management. Contemporary Pediatrics, June 1990, pp 70–92.

Ernhart CB, Sokol RJ, Martier S, et al: Alcohol teratogenicity in the human. A detailed assessment of specificity, critical period and threshold. Am J Obstet Gynecol 156(1):33–39, 1987.

Finnegan LP: Narcotics dependence in pregnancy. Psychedelic Drugs 7(3):299–311, 1975.

Finnegan LP, Connaughton JF, Kron RE, Emich JP: Neonatal abstinence syndrome: assessment and management. *In* Harbison RD (ed): Perinatal Addiction. New York, Spectrum Publications, 1875, pp 141–158.

Frank DA, Zuckerman BS, Amaro H, et al: Cocaine use during pregnancy: prevalence and correlates. Pediatrics 82(6):888–95, 1988.

Fried PA, Watkinson B, Willan A: Marijuana use during pregnancy and decreased length of gestation. Am J Obstet Gynecol 150(1):23–27, 1984.

Fulroth R, Phillips B, Durand D: Perinatal outcome of infants exposed to cocaine and/or heroin in utero. Am J Dis Child 143:905–910, 1989.

Fultz JM, Senay EC: Guidelines for the management of hospitalized narcotic addicts. Ann Intern Med 82: 815–818, 1975.

Golden NL, Sokol RJ, Kuhnert BR, Bottoms S: Maternal alcohol use and infant development. Pediatrics 70(6):931–934, 1982.

Greenland S, Staisch KJ, Brown N, Gross SJ: The effects of marijuana use during pregnancy. Am J Obstet Gynecol 143(4):408–413, 1982.

Griffith DR: The effects of perinatal cocaine exposure on infant neurobehavior and early maternal-infant interactions. *In* Chasnoff IJ (ed): Drugs, Alcohol, Pregnancy and Parenting. Boston, Kluwer Academic Publishers, 1988, pp 105–113.

Hadeed AJ, Siegel SR: Maternal cocaine use during pregnancy: effect on the newborn infant. Pediatrics, 82(2):205–210, 1989.

Hanson JW, Jones KL, Smith DW: Fetal alcohol syndrome, experience with 41 patients. JAMA 235(14): 1458–1460, 1976.

Hanson JW, Streissguth AP, Smith DW: The effects of moderate alcohol consumption during pregnancy on fetal growth and morphogenesis. J Pediatr 92(3):457–460, 1978.

Hingson R, Alpert J, Day N, et al: Effects of maternal drinking and marijuana use on fetal growth and development. Pediatrics 70(4):539–546, 1982.

Hoyme, HE, Jones KL, Dixon DS, et al: Prenatal cocaine exposure and fetal vascular disruption. Pediatrics 85(5):743–747, 1990.

Jones KL, Smith DW, Ulleland CN, Streissguth AP: Malformation in offspring of chronic alcoholic mothers. Lancet 1:1267–1271, 1973.

Keith L, Donald W, Rosner M, Mitchell M, Bianchi J: Obstetric aspects of perinatal addiction. *In* Chasnoff IJ (ed): Drug Use in Pregnancy: Mother and Child. Lancaster, PA, MTP Press, 1986, pp 23–41.

Keith LG, MacGregor SN, Sciarra JJ: Drug abuse in pregnancy. *In* Chasnoff IJ (ed): Drugs, Alcohol, Pregnancy and Parenting. Boston, Kluwer Academic Publishers, 1988, pp 17–46.

Lemoine P, Harousseau H, Borteyru JP: Les enfants de parents alcooliques: anomalies observies. Quest Med, vol 25, 1968, pp 476–482.

Lifschitz MH, Wilson GS, Smith EO, Desmond MM: Factors affecting head growth and intellectual function in children of drug addicts. Pediatrics 72(2):269–274, 1985.

Linn S, Schienbaum SC, Monson RR, et al: The association of marijuana use with outcome of pregnancy. Am J Public Health 73(10):1161–1164, 1983.

MacGregor SN, Keith LG, Chasnoff IJ, et al: Cocaine use during pregnancy: adverse perinatal outcome. Am J Obstet Gynecol 157(3):686–690, 1987.

Mills JL, Graubard BI: Is moderate drinking during pregnancy associated with an increased risk for malformations? Pediatrics 80(3):309–314, 1987.

Newman RG, Bashkow S, Calko JD: Results of 313 consecutive live births of infants delivered to patients in New York City Methadone Maintenance Treatment Program. Am J Obstet Gynecol 121(2):233–237, 1974.

Ouellette EM, Rosett HL, Roseman NP, et al: Adverse effects on offspring of maternal alcohol abuse during pregnancy. N Engl J Med 297(10):528–530, 1977.

Pelosi MA, Frattarola M, Apuzzio J, et al: Pregnancy complicated by heroin addiction. Gynecol Obstet 45(5):512–515, 1975.

Perlmutter JF: Drug addiction in pregnant women. Am J Obstet Gynecol 99:569–572, 1967.

Schneider JW, Chasnoff IJ: Cocaine abuse during pregnancy: its effects on infant motor development–a clinical perspective. Topics in Acute Care and Trauma Rehabilitation, July 1987, pp 59–69.

Schneider JW, Griffith DR, Chasnoff IJ: Infants exposed to cocaine in utero: implications for developmental assessment and intervention. Infants and Young Children 2(1):25–36, 1989.

Schnoll SH: Pharmacologic basis of perinatal addiction. *In* Chasnoff IJ (ed): Drug Use in Pregnancy: Mother and Child. Lancaster, PA, MTP Press, 1986, pp 7–16.

Silverman S: Scope, specifics of maternal drug use, effects on fetus are beginning to emerge from studies. JAMA 261(12):1688–1689, 1989.

Stimmel B, Adamsons K: Narcotic dependency in pregnancy: methadone maintenance compared to use of street drugs. JAMA 235(11):1121–1124, 1976.

Stone ML, Salerno IJ, Green M, Zelson C: Narcotic addiction in pregnancy. Am J Obstet Gynecol 109:716–723, 1971.

Strauss ME, Andresko M, Styker JC, Wardell JN, Dunkel LD: Methadone maintenance during pregnancy: pregnancy, birth, and neonatal characteristics. Am J Obstet Gynecol 120(7):895–900, 1974.

Streissguth AP: Fetal alcohol syndrome: where are we in 1978? Women Health, 4(3):223–237, 1979.

Streissguth AP, Herman CS, Smith DW: Intelligence, behavior and dysmorphogenesis in the fetal alcohol syndrome. A report on 20 patients. J Pediatr 92(3):363–367, 1978.

Sweet A: Narcotic withdrawal syndrome in the newborn. Pediatr Rev 3(9):285–291, 1982.

Weiner L, Gunilla L: Clinical prevention of fetal alcohol effects–a reality. Alcohol Health and Research World, 1987, pp 60–63, 92–93.

Zuckerman B, Frank DA, Hingson R, et al: Effects of maternal marijuana and cocaine use on fetal growth. N Engl J Med 320(12) 762–768, 1989.

Zuspan FP, Gumpel JA, Mejia-Zelaya A, et al: Fetal stress from methadone withdrawal. Am J Obstet Gynecol 122(1):43–46, 1975.

# CHAPTER 11

· · · · · · · · · · · · · · · · · · · · · · · · · · · · · · · · · · ·

# Nutrition in Pregnancy

William N. P. Herbert, Janice M. Dodds, and Robert C. Cefalo

The importance of proper nutrition during pregnancy is receiving increased attention as perinatal care shifts from crisis to preventive care. All members of the health care team require current scientific information to adequately assess the patient's nutritional status and to encourage her to eat a nutritionally adequate diet. Many patients are unaware of the importance of good food selection practices during pregnancy and often follow fad weight control schemes or substitute multivitamin and mineral supplements for a nutritionally adequate diet. They also may not be aware of the increased tendency for ketosis with overnight or daytime fasting during pregnancy. Preferably, education on nutrition should begin prior to pregnancy, because a woman with good nutritional habits and normal body weight prior to conception has distinct advantages during the course of pregnancy.

This chapter discusses nutritional considerations relating to obstetric care. It provides (1) a review of nutritional requirements during pregnancy; (2) a discussion of obstetric complications that have important nutritional interrelationships; (3) a section on special situations, e.g., multiple gestation, that require nutritional adjustments; (4) techniques for the assessment of nu-

tritional status; and (5) methods for intervention when nutritional guidance is required.

## Nutritional Requirements During Pregnancy

### MATERNAL GROWTH AND ENERGY NEEDS

The total energy requirement of pregnancy is estimated to be 55,000 kcal (Committee on Nutritional Status During Pregnancy and Lactation, 1990). These calories must be added to the number of calories needed to fulfill the nutritional requirements of the woman that are unrelated to her pregnancy, which vary with her age and physical activity. Table 11–1 contains the recommended dietary allowances (RDA) for calories, protein, vitamins, and minerals during gestation, as proposed by the Food and Nutrition Board (National Academy of Sciences, 1989).

The actual increase in energy needs varies through the course of pregnancy, with a greater demand in the second and third trimesters than in the first. The Food and Agriculture Organization, a division of the World Health Organization, recommends that the caloric intake be increased by 150 kcal/day during the first trimester and 350 kcal/day thereafter. These are general recommendations and do not reflect individual variation with physical activity.

Much of the material in this chapter has been developed for presentation at the Intensive Course in Maternal Nutrition supported by the March of Dimes Birth Defects Foundation, White Plains, New York. Drs. Herbert and Cefalo have served as directors of this course.

# FETAL GROWTH AND ENERGY NEEDS

Glucose has traditionally been considered the sole energy source for the fetus, but, as noted in the review by Moghissi (1978), amino acids may be important for fetal aerobic metabolism. In general, amino acid concentrations are higher in fetal plasma than in maternal plasma (Ghadimi and Pecora, 1964). The capacity of the placenta to transfer both glucose and amino acids increases throughout pregnancy.

The maternal contribution of protein to the fetus is not limited to placental transfer. Passage of proteins from the mother into the amniotic fluid enables the fetus to swallow, hydrolyze, absorb, and use certain amino acids (Gitlin, 1974).

## MATERNAL WEIGHT GAIN

### Prepregnancy Weight

Next to gestational age, a woman's weight prior to pregnancy and the amount of weight gained through pregnancy are the two strongest determinants of the infant's birth weight. A comprehensive review of weight relationships in pregnancy showed that less than 5 percent of women whose prepregnant weight was 64 kg (140 lb) or greater delivered an infant at term weighing less than 2500 g, regardless of the amount of weight gained during pregnancy (Eastman and Jackson, 1968). Moreover, less than 2 percent of women whose weight gain during pregnancy exceeded 14 kg (30 lb) delivered term infants weighing less than 2500 g, regardless of prepregnant weight. Maternal height does not appear to be a significant factor in regard to birth weight.

### Amount of Weight Gain During Pregnancy

Although the optimal amount of weight gain during pregnancy is not known, the amount of weight added through pregnancy has been studied repeatedly. An accurate weight measurement of pregnant women at each visit is critical in order to give pertinent

**Table 11–1**
RECOMMENDED DIETARY ALLOWANCES

| Females | | Nonpregnant | | | | Pregnant |
|---|---|---|---|---|---|---|
| | | **11–14 Years** | **15–18 Years** | **19–24 Years** | **25–50 Years** | |
| WEIGHT | Pounds | 101 | 120 | 128 | 138 | |
| HEIGHT | Inches | 62 | 64 | 65 | 64 | |
| ENERGY | Calories | 2200 | 2200 | 2200 | 2200 | 2500 |
| PROTEIN | (g) | 46 | 44 | 46 | 50 | 60 |
| *Fat-Soluble Vitamins* | | | | | | |
| Vitamin A | ($\mu$g RE) | 800 | 800 | 800 | 800 | 800 |
| Vitamin D | ($\mu$g)[b] | 10 | 10 | 10 | 5 | 10 |
| Vitamin E | (mg $\alpha$-TE) | 8 | 8 | 8 | 8 | 10 |
| *Water-Soluble Vitamins* | | | | | | |
| Vitamin C | (mg) | 50 | 60 | 60 | 60 | 70 |
| Folacin | ($\mu$g) | 150 | 180 | 180 | 180 | 400 |
| Niacin | (mg NE) | 15 | 15 | 15 | 15 | 17 |
| Riboflavin | (mg) | 1.3 | 1.3 | 1.3 | 1.3 | 1.6 |
| Thiamin | (mg) | 1.1 | 1.1 | 1.1 | 1.1 | 1.5 |
| Vitamin $B_6$ | (mg) | 1.4 | 1.5 | 1.6 | 1.6 | 2.2 |
| Vitamin $B_{12}$ | ($\mu$g) | 2.0 | 2.0 | 2.0 | 2.0 | 2.2 |
| *Minerals* | | | | | | |
| Calcium | (mg) | 1200 | 1200 | 1200 | 800 | 1200 |
| Phosphorus | (mg) | 1200 | 1200 | 1200 | 800 | 1200 |
| Iodine | ($\mu$g) | 150 | 150 | 150 | 150 | 175 |
| Iron | (mg) | 15 | 15 | 15 | 15 | 30[c] |
| Magnesium | (mg) | 280 | 300 | 280 | 280 | 300 |
| Zinc | (mg) | 12 | 12 | 12 | 12 | 15 |

[a] Retinol Equivalent (RE) = 5 International Units (IU).
[b] $\mu$g = 40 IU.
[c] The use of an oral iron supplement is recommended.
Data from Recommended Dietary Allowances, 1989. Food and Nutrition Board, National Academy of Sciences, National Research Council, Washington, DC.

guidance during prenatal care. The body mass index provides a more accurate picture of weight status by relating the woman's weight to her height. The index is defined as weight/height$^2$. This can be computed in metric units (kilograms and meters) or in pounds and inches. Because none of the weight-for-height classification schemes has been validated against pregnancy outcome, any cutoff points are arbitrary for women of reproductive age. The cutoff points in Table 11–2 generally correspond to 90, 120, and 135 percent of the 1959 Metropolitan Life Insurance Company's weight-for-height standards—the standards that have been in most common use in the United States.

Previous recommendations of weight gain between 10 to 12 kg (22 to 26 lb) recently have been revised. The Committee on Nutritional Status during Pregnancy and Lactation recommends that different amounts of weight be added during pregnancy depending on the patient's prepregnancy weight status. Using the body mass index, it is suggested that women of normal prepregnant weight gain 11.5 to 16 kg (25 to 35 lb); underweight women should gain more, 12.5 to 18 kg (28 to 40 lb); and overweight women less, 7 to 11.5 kg (15 to 25 lb), as shown in Table 11–2.

It has taken many years for practitioners to abandon the unfounded notion that limiting weight gain prevents toxemia of pregnancy. Also, many weight-conscious women fear obesity following pregnancy. It is important that health care providers help women, who are often highly motivated to keep in good health during pregnancy, to understand the importance of adequate weight gain.

## Pattern of Weight Gain

Possibly more important than the actual amount of weight added during pregnancy is the rate at which the additional increase in weight occurs. During the first trimester, a total gain of 1.4 kg (3 lb) is recommended. Thereafter, a steady gain of about 1 lb/week is suggested.

Although weight gain beyond the first trimester is essentially linear, the use of the additional weight changes as pregnancy advances. During the second trimester, the majority of additional weight is used in expansion of the maternal components (uterus, breasts, blood volume, fat deposition). In the

**Table 11–2**

RECOMMENDED TOTAL WEIGHT GAIN RANGES FOR PREGNANT WOMEN*, BY PREPREGNANCY BODY MASS INDEX (BMI)†

| Weight-for-Height Category | Recommended Total Gain | |
|---|---|---|
| | kg | lb |
| Low (BMI < 19.8) | 12.5–18 | 28–40 |
| Normal (BMI of 19.8 to 26.0) | 11.5–16 | 25–35 |
| High‡ (BMI > 26.0 to 29.0) | 7–11.5 | 15–25 |

\* Young adolescents and black women should strive for gains at the upper end of the recommended range. Short women (<157 cm, or 62 in) should strive for gains at the lower end of the range.

† BMI (body mass index) is calculated using metric units.

‡ The recommended target weight gain for obese women (BMI > 29.0) is at least 6.0 kg (15 lb).

Reprinted with permission from: Nutrition During Pregnancy, © 1990, National Academy Press, Washington, DC.

third trimester, the products of conception (fetus, placenta, and amniotic fluid volume) predominantly account for the increase in weight (Hytten and Leitch, 1971).

Use of a weight gain grid (Fig. 11–1) as a part of the prenatal health care record emphasizes the recommended pattern of weight gain to the patient and helps health care providers monitor her continuing weight gain status as pregnancy advances. Such weight gain grids are available for under-, normal, and overweight women as well as for adolescents.

## Components of Weight Gain

The products of conception and the maternal response to gestation share equally in the distribution of total weight gain. At term, products of conception account for approximately 5 kg (11 lb), and the maternal compensatory changes represent approximately 4 kg (9 lb) (Table 11–3). Therefore, on the average, only weight gain in excess of 9 kg (20 lb) is considered additional weight gain, a portion of which represents fat deposition in preparation for lactation.

## Postpartum Weight Change

During the first week following delivery, the average overall decrease in weight is approximately 9 kg (20 lbs), reflecting the weight gain just outlined. During the second to the twelfth postpartum weeks, an additional 3 to 4 kg (6 to 8 lb) is generally lost. The majority of women lose virtually all of the weight gained during pregnancy, especially if they breastfeed. An average residual weight gain of about 2 lb occurs after each pregnancy, but some patients retain considerably more (Greene et al, 1988).

## SPECIFIC NUTRIENTS

### Protein, Carbohydrates, and Fats

The pregnant woman must increase her dietary intake of *protein* to provide for enlargement of her blood volume, uterus, breasts, and placenta. Fetal protein synthesis requires adequate placental transfer of amino acids. Based on protein accumulation, as estimated from the nitrogen content of the fetal and maternal compartments, approximately 1 kg of protein is needed through the course of pregnancy. To provide this amount, approximately 10 g of additional protein must be consumed daily. Based on nitrogen balance studies, however, the estimated additional need in pregnancy may be greater. As shown in Table 11–1, it is recommended that pregnant women consume 60 g of protein daily, compared with 44 to 50 g when they are not pregnant.

Although it has been stated that a large nitrogen storage, in excess of the requirements of the fetal and maternal compartments, occurs during pregnancy, evidence indicates that the degree of nitrogen storage meets but does not exceed metabolic demands (Johnstone et al, 1981).

Regardless of the amount of maternal protein intake, total serum protein levels decline during pregnancy. After a steady decrease during the first two trimesters, the concentrations approach the nonpregnant levels as late pregnancy is reached. This decline in serum proteins is selective— alpha globulins and beta globulins increase, whereas gamma globulins and albumin decrease.

*Carbohydrates* are also a primary energy source, both for the mother and for the fetus. As long as total caloric needs are met, pregnancy does not impose any specific requirements for additional carbohydrates. Adequate energy intake from a combination of carbohydrate and fat food sources is necessary for protein use and to spare use of protein as an energy source.

For both mother and fetus, glucose and fatty acids provide the main sources of energy, with additional supply from deaminated amino acids. Glucose is the prime fuel on which the fetus heavily depends in order to achieve adequate tissue protein synthesis and conversion of fat to glycogen. Near term, the fetal glucose use rate is estimated to be 7 mg/kg/min (30 g of glucose a day), as compared with the adult consumption of 2 to 3 mg/kg/min.

*Fat* storage accounts for one half of the total energy costs of pregnancy and occurs primarily between the 20th and 30th weeks of gestation (Hytten and Leitch, 1971). Fat in the diet is a concentrated source of needed calories. Fat also is a carrier of the essential fat-soluble vitamins A, D, and E, all of which have an increased requirement during pregnancy.

### Vitamins

A nutritionally adequate diet meets essentially all of the recommended daily allowances for vitamins listed in Table 11–1. Unfortunately, dietary sources of nutrients are often not adequately stressed and are replaced with the widespread prescription of multivitamin supplementation during gestation. It is important that pregnant women be made aware that multivitamin supplementation cannot substitute for a nutritionally adequate daily diet offering the array of nutrients that interact with the essential macronutrients and micronutrients.

### Water-Soluble Vitamins

*Folate* is important for the growth of maternal, fetal, and placental tissues because of its role in DNA synthesis. Fetal demands, impaired maternal absorption, and defective use are related to the increased folate requirements during pregnancy (Kitay, 1969).

Frank megaloblastic anemia is uncommon, despite the fact that one fourth of gravidas are deficient by nonpregnant standards. Folate deficiency has been thought to be associated with a number of abnormalities of pregnancy, including abruptio placentae, congenital malformations, abortion, and pregnancy-induced hypertension. A number of investigators have refuted these claims, however, and at the present time, folate deficiency seems associated only with megalo-

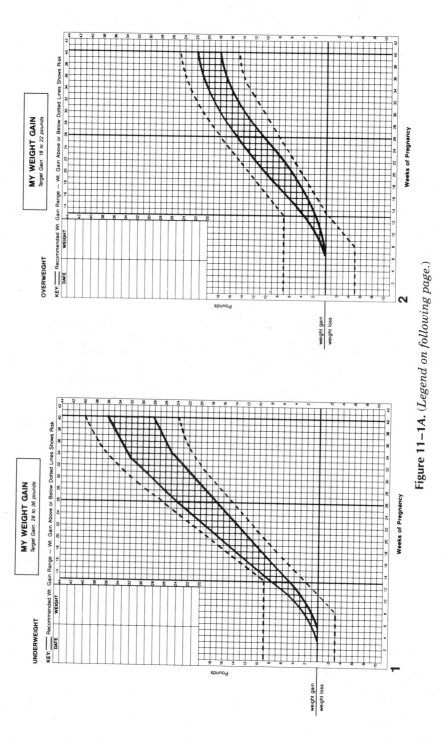

**Figure 11–1A.** (*Legend on following page.*)

184

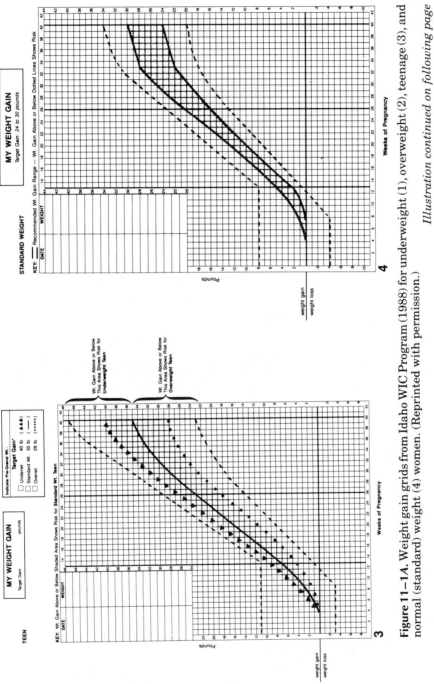

*Illustration continued on following page*

**Figure 11–1A.** Weight gain grids from Idaho WIC Program (1988) for underweight (1), overweight (2), teenage (3), and normal (standard) weight (4) women. (Reprinted with permission.)

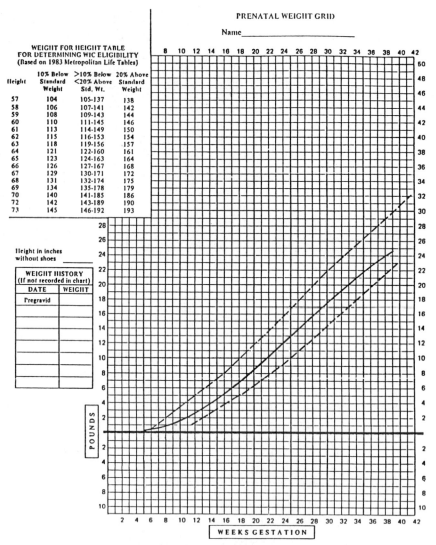

**WEIGHT FOR HEIGHT TABLE FOR DETERMINING WIC ELIGIBILITY**
(Based on 1983 Metropolitan Life Tables)

| Height | 10% Below Standard Weight | >10% Below <20% Above Std. Wt. | 20% Above Standard Weight |
|---|---|---|---|
| 57 | 104 | 105-137 | 138 |
| 58 | 106 | 107-141 | 142 |
| 59 | 108 | 109-143 | 144 |
| 60 | 110 | 111-145 | 146 |
| 61 | 113 | 114-149 | 150 |
| 62 | 115 | 116-153 | 154 |
| 63 | 118 | 119-156 | 157 |
| 64 | 121 | 122-160 | 161 |
| 65 | 123 | 124-163 | 164 |
| 66 | 126 | 127-167 | 168 |
| 67 | 129 | 130-171 | 172 |
| 68 | 131 | 132-174 | 175 |
| 69 | 134 | 135-178 | 179 |
| 70 | 140 | 141-185 | 186 |
| 72 | 142 | 143-189 | 190 |
| 73 | 145 | 146-192 | 193 |

Height in inches without shoes

**WEIGHT HISTORY**
(If not recorded in chart)

| DATE | WEIGHT |
|---|---|
| Pregravid | |

**Figure 11–1** *Continued B.* Weight gain grid from Georgia WIC (Georgia Dietetic Association, 1987). Lower dashed line is recommended gain for overweight women; upper dashed line is recommended gain for underweight women. (Reprinted with permission. From Nutrition During Pregnancy, © 1990, National Academy Press.)

blastic anemia (Pritchard and MacDonald, 1980). The offspring of mothers with megaloblastic anemia have normal hemoglobin levels (Pitkin, 1976).

The recommended daily increase of folate is 400 $\mu$g. Green leafy vegetables, liver, kidney, other meats, eggs (not raw), and nuts are good dietary sources.

The value of routine supplementation of folate is unclear, but the administration of folic acid is necessary for certain patients who are at special risk of developing folate deficiency. Patients with multiple fetuses, hemoglobinopathies and other chronic he-

molytic anemias, and those taking diphenylhydantoin (Dilantin) should be supplemented with 1 mg of folate daily throughout pregnancy.

*Vitamin $B_{12}$* deficiency during pregnancy is rare, because fetal needs total 50 $\mu$g, a small fraction of the maternal store of 3000 $\mu$g. However, patients who are vegans, eating no animal protein foods, do require supplementation during gestation (Leader et al, 1981).

*Vitamin $B_6$* (pyridoxine) concentrations decrease in both plasma and cellular elements of the blood during pregnancy. However, ad-

Table 11–3
COMPONENTS OF WEIGHT GAIN DURING PREGNANCY

| Products of Conception | | Maternal Response to Gestation | |
|---|---|---|---|
| Fetus | 7.5 lb | Enlarged uterus | 2.5 lb |
| Placenta and membranes | 1.5 lb | Increased blood volume | 3.5 lb |
| Amniotic fluid | 2.0 lb | Increased breast size | 1.0 lb |
| Subtotal | 11.0 lb | Increased extracellular fluid | 2.0 lb |
| | | Subtotal | 9.0 lb |
| | *Total:* 20 lb | | |

Data from Pritchard JA, MacDonald PC (eds): Williams Obstetrics, 16th ed. New York, Appleton-Century Crofts, 1980.

verse effects are difficult to demonstrate clinically (Pitkin, 1976). Because of its important role in the metabolism of proteins, the need for vitamin $B_6$ increases during pregnancy to accommodate the greater protein intake. A daily intake of 2.2 mg, which is 0.6 mg above the nonpregnant intake, is suggested to meet this increased demand. Liver, meats, fish, eggs (not raw), cabbage, bananas, corn, whole wheat, and rolled oats are good dietary sources.

*Vitamin C* (ascorbic acid) is essential for normal cell integrity and growth. The RDA for vitamin C during pregnancy is 70 mg, which represents an increase of 10 mg over the nonpregnant recommendation. Citrus fruits, strawberries, cantaloupe, dark green leafy vegetables, raw cabbage, and green peppers are among the best dietary sources. Paradoxically, intake exceeding 1 g daily has been reported to lead to neonatal scurvy, apparently as a result of conditioning the fetus to an elevated level of vitamin C (Cochrane, 1965).

## Fat-Soluble Vitamins

*Vitamin A* is necessary for normal cellular growth, especially for epithelial cells. To provide adequate Vitamin A for fetal storage, the recommended daily requirement during pregnancy is 800 μg retinol equivalents (RE), unchanged from the nonpregnancy recommendation. Well-nourished adults maintain hepatic stores of vitamin A sufficient to meet requirements for several months. Dietary sources of vitamin A are liver, milk (whole or fortified low-fat or nonfat), dark green leafy and deep yellow vegetables, and yellow fruits. Excessive intake of vitamin A in megavitamin supplements has been associated with increased intracranial pressure and congenital malformations in offspring (Rosso, 1980).

*Vitamin D* is important in regulating the metabolism of calcium and phosphorus. As the need for these minerals increases throughout pregnancy, vitamin D requirements also rise. The recommended daily allowance during pregnancy is 10 μg daily, compared with 5 to 10 μg daily in the nonpregnant state. Exposure to sunshine can provide adequate vitamin D; milk fortified with vitamin D is a good food source. Excessive intake through high-potency supplements has been associated with adverse fetal effects, including aortic stenosis, hyperparathyroidism, and other congenital anomalies (Leader et al, 1981).

*Vitamin E* is evidently found in sufficient quantities in most diets, because deficiency in humans is rare. Specific functions for vitamin E are unclear, but it is believed to have a significant role in fatty acid metabolism. Neonatal hemoglobinopathies have been reported with vitamin E deficiency in the newborn. The RDA for vitamin E during pregnancy is 10 mg tocopherol equivalents, an increase of 2 mg over the nonpregnant daily recommendation.

## Minerals

Pregnancy increases the demand for most minerals, but the need for routine supplementation of multiple minerals, widely practiced by the public and many health care providers, lacks substantiation. With the exception of iron, a nutritionally adequate diet should amply supply the needs of pregnancy for most women.

## Iron

Although the primary function of iron is in hemoglobin synthesis and function, iron is involved in many enzyme systems relating to a variety of metabolic processes.

The total iron need during pregnancy has been determined to be between 800 and 1000 g, depending on whether or not maternal excretion, which through pregnancy totals about 200 mg, is calculated in the amount. Approximately 500 mg of this total iron requirement is necessary to accommodate the expanded maternal blood volume, which occurs in varying degrees in all pregnant women. Another 300 mg is necessary to supply fetal needs.

The blood volume increases by about 50 percent in pregnancy, with the increase being disproportionate between red cells and plasma. About three fourths of the 1500- to 2000-ml increase in blood volume is due to an elevation in plasma volume, whereas the red cell mass increases by about one third. The hematocrit, which represents the proportion of the total blood composed of cells, decreases as a reflection of these changes.

Whether or not a woman receives iron supplementation, the hematocrit declines slightly through pregnancy, reaching a nadir at about 32 weeks. Thereafter, it increases to approach the prepregnant level. This fact has clinical value—for normal patients whose initial hematologic evaluation does not suggest iron deficiency, the most appropriate time to reassess the iron status is at about 32 weeks, when the hematocrit is expected to be at its lowest point. Largely because of blood loss with menses, the average iron store in young adult women has been estimated to be 270 mg. It is of interest to note that, in a group of apparently healthy young adult nursing students, about one fourth were found to have *no* stainable iron in their bone marrow (Pritchard and Scott, 1970).

Besides stored iron, the other source of iron is through the diet. The average daily adult diet contains 10 to 12 mg of iron, considerably less than the 15 mg recommended for women of childbearing age. In pregnancy, 30 mg daily is recommended. The best dietary sources of iron are liver, red meats, seafood, nuts, legumes, green leafy vegetables, and whole grain and iron-fortified cereals. Iron in the heme form, as in animal foods, and adequate vitamin C (ascorbic acid) in the diet facilitate iron absorption.

Because of the difficulty in obtaining sufficient iron from the diet, iron is the one nutrient supplement usually prescribed for women during pregnancy. It is important to understand that it is the amount of *elemental iron,* not the *iron salt,* that is important. Various salt forms yield different amounts of elemental iron—a 300-mg tablet of ferrous sulfate and a 300-mg tablet of ferrous fumarate each provides approximately 65 mg of elemental iron; the same dosage of ferrous gluconate provides approximately half this amount.

Side effects of iron supplements are common and troublesome. Nausea and epigastric pain (indigestion) occur in up to 20 percent of patients, constipation in 10 percent, and diarrhea in 5 percent. These effects are primarily the result of iron absorption rather than the type of preparation. Therefore, total lack of side effects may indicate insufficient absorption. Although absorption is maximal when an iron supplement is taken on an empty stomach, ingestion of the iron supplements with meals tends to decrease the side effects described.

Iron toxicity in adults is rare, but infants and young children are particularly prone to its toxic effects, and ingestion of as few as 3 to 5 iron tablets can have catastrophic results. It may be difficult for the mother to have iron tablets readily available for her use, yet away from small children. Childproof safety caps are strongly recommended.

Oral iron supplements make the stool dark green or almost black in color. Determining a patient's recent compliance concerning intake of the iron supplement includes inquiring as to stool color and performing a rectal examination.

Although the fetus has long been thought to be an effective parasite in terms of meeting its iron needs, more recent evidence suggests that iron stores of offspring of iron-deficient mothers are lower than those of offspring whose mothers had adequate iron intake throughout gestation (Fenton et al, 1977). Neonatal serum iron levels are not decreased with maternal iron deficiency.

The majority of iron transferred to the fetus occurs in the last trimester, and it is during this time that fetal iron stores are developed. For this reason, premature infants have diminished stores of iron. Two thirds of the iron transported to the fetus is incorporated into hemoglobin, and the remainder is stored as ferritin in the fetal liver for use in the first year of life (McFee, 1979).

## Calcium

Calcium is necessary for the development of bones and teeth and is also important in maintenance of cell membrane permeability, the coagulation process, and neuromuscular excitability. During pregnancy, the maternal serum concentration of calcium decreases slightly because of a decline in albumin concentration, to which about half of the blood calcium is bound. Calcium absorption is actually increased and excretion decreased during gestation (Villar and Belizán, 1986).

The total fetal demand for calcium is estimated to be 30 g, mostly required in the later stages of pregnancy (Hytten and Leitch, 1971). Because the total calcium content of an adult is estimated to be 1100 to 1200 g, the fetal need represents a small fraction of that available, and deficiency is extremely rare in developed countries.

Because of the increased calcium need during pregnancy, it is recommended that the daily calcium intake be changed for some women from 800 to 1200 mg in the nonpregnant state to 1200 mg daily during pregnancy. One quart of milk contains this amount of calcium, along with 400 units of vitamin D. Cheese, other dairy products, and calcium supplements are other sources.

## Other Minerals

*Phosphorus* is primarily combined with calcium in bone formation. The total fetal need of approximately 20 g represents about 3 percent of the total maternal content of phosphorus (Hytten and Leitch, 1971). The RDA for phosphorus is 1200 mg daily during pregnancy. Its widespread availability makes deficiency unlikely.

*Sodium* metabolism is strongly influenced by pregnancy, as a result of significantly increased glomerular filtration and increased renal tubular reabsorption. To provide the estimated 750 mEq of sodium to compensate for pregnancy, a daily increase of 3 mEq is recommended. Because the average adult diet contains 100 to 300 mEq, this additional sodium need presents no difficulty. The previous practice of restricting sodium during pregnancy is now discouraged.

*Zinc* is essential for growth of all tissues, because it is involved in many major metabolic pathways. Congenital malformations, particularly of the central nervous system, and iron deficiency anemia have been reported with zinc deficiency (Moghissi, 1978). An increase in zinc intake from 12 mg/day when the woman is not pregnant to 15 mg/day during pregnancy is suggested.

*Iodine* requirements are increased during pregnancy to provide sufficient iodine to the fetus and to compensate for the increased renal loss that occurs during pregnancy. A balanced diet plus use of iodized salt is recommended to avoid neonatal cretinism. Conversely, excessive iodine intake may suppress fetal thyroid function.

*Potassium* concentration does not change substantially during pregnancy, and no disorders peculiar to pregnancy are related to its metabolism.

---

# Obstetric Complications with Nutritional Interrelationships

## CONDITIONS COMMON IN PREGNANCY

### Anemia

**Iron Deficiency Anemia.** As noted in the discussion of iron use during pregnancy, the plasma volume increases to a greater extent than does the red blood cell mass, resulting in a decline in the hematocrit. This dilutional effect, most marked in the early third trimester, may be compounded by the nutritional deficiencies of iron and folic acid. Anemia is defined as a hematocrit of less than 30 percent or a hemoglobin concentration of less than 10 g/dl at any time during pregnancy (Pritchard and MacDonald, 1980). The majority of cases of anemia in pregnancy are due to iron deficiency, but folate deficiency is also seen. Infection (most commonly pyelonephritis), acute blood loss, hemoglobinopathies and other hereditary hemolytic anemias, thalassemia, and hypoplastic anemia are other causes.

With iron deficiency, a stained smear of the peripheral blood may show the characteristic microcytic and hypochromic appearance of the red blood cells, but these findings are often absent. Likewise, the mean cell volume, typically decreased with iron deficiency, may be within the normal range. Determination of serum iron and total iron-binding capacity, with a ratio of less than 15 percent being indicative of iron deficiency, has been used to assess iron status. However, very recent iron intake will elevate the serum iron and lead to erroneous conclusions. More recently, serum ferritin has been used to measure iron status. Small amounts of this storage form of iron in serum reflect total iron stores. A level of less than 12 ng/ml suggests deficiency.

The objectives of treatment of anemia are to correct the anemia and to replenish stores. Treatment of iron deficiency anemia consists of prescribing a diet high in food sources of iron, protein, and vitamin C, along with approximately 180 mg of elemental iron taken orally daily. This is provided by three tablets of ferrous sulfate or ferrous fumarate, because each tablet of these iron salts contains approximately 60 mg of elemental iron. Ferrous gluconate may be used, but the number of tablets may need to be increased to provide the necessary iron. Doses in excess of 180 to 200 mg daily do not result in more rapid blood cell production and may cause significant side effects. Correction of anemia does not occur faster with parenteral than with oral iron.

Response to treatment is rapid, but is less than the response seen in the nonpregnant state. Larger basophilic, polychromatophilic red blood cells can be seen in a stained smear of peripheral blood 10 to 14 days after initiation of treatment. The hematocrit rises slowly thereafter at a rate of 1 to 2 percentage points per week. Once the anemia is corrected, continued supplemental iron—e.g., 120 mg daily—is recommended throughout the remainder of pregnancy and for 4 to 6 weeks thereafter.

When there is an apparent lack of response to prescribed iron, patient compliance should be thoroughly determined. As noted earlier, iron ingestion should cause the stool to become dark green or almost black, and therefore stool color is helpful information in determining the patient's iron intake.

**Megaloblastic Anemia.** Folic acid deficiency is almost always responsible for megaloblastic anemia during pregnancy, because the increasing demand for this vitamin may exceed dietary intake and stores are consumed. The sequence of events following folate deficiency has been evaluated (Table 11–4) (Herbert, 1962). Characteristic megaloblastic changes in bone marrow occur relatively late in the process. An erythrocyte folate level of less than 150 ng/ml indicates deficiency of this vitamin. A serum folate value of less than 4 ng/ml also suggests folate deficiency, but the increasing plasma volume with pregnancy may make this test less diagnostic during this time (Kitay, 1980).

**Table 11–4**
SEQUENCE OF ALTERATIONS FOLLOWING EXPERIMENTAL FOLATE DEPRIVATION

| Event | Weeks After Onset Of Folate Deprivation |
|---|---|
| Low concentration of serum folate | 3 |
| Hypersegmentation of neutrophil nuclei in peripheral blood | 7 |
| Elevated urinary FIGLU* excretion | 14 |
| Low folate in erythrocytes | 16 |
| Macro-ovalocytosis | 18 |
| Megaloblastic marrow (florid) | 19 |
| Anemia | 19 |

Data from Herbert V: Experimental nutritional folate deficiency in man. Trans Assoc Am Phys 75:307, 1962.
* formiminoglutamic acid.

Treatment of folate deficiency is with oral folate at a dose of 1 mg daily. Response is rapid and first noted as an increase in the reticulocyte count several-fold over the reticulocyte level of 1.5 to 2.5 percent seen in normal pregnancy. In the absence of other factors, the rise in hematocrit is approximately 1 percentage point per day after 1 week.

It is important to remember that folate and iron deficiencies may frequently coexist in pregnancy. Therefore, characteristic hematologic indices may be lacking. For example, the macrocytic changes of folate deficiency may be offset by the microcytic cells indicative of iron deficiency. Other indices may also be misleading—serum iron may be elevated in patients who are both iron and folate deficient because of inefficient erythropoiesis. With folate therapy, however, the serum iron may decrease dramatically as proper iron use occurs.

Most cases of anemia during pregnancy can be prevented by stressing good nutrition. Supplementation with iron and possibly folate will ensure adequate intake of these substances. If anemia is identified, attention to diet and simple iron and folate treatment should precede extensive hematologic evaluation, because the vast majority of cases of anemia are due to inadequate intake of these two important nutrients.

## Hyperemesis Gravidarum

Nausea and occasional vomiting during the first trimester usually do not interfere with nutrition. Simple treatment includes the taking of small, frequent meals, emphasizing easily tolerated carbohydrates (crackers, baked potato) and taking liquids between meals rather than with food. However, persistent hyperemesis can result in a severe physiologic disturbance, leading to dehydration, electrolyte imbalance, ketoacidosis, nutritional depletion, and hypovitaminosis. These complications may require hospitalization for sedation, antiemetics, and replacement of fluids, electrolytes, and vitamins. In severe cases, total parenteral nutrition may be necessary.

## Underweight and Poor Weight Gain

Women who enter pregnancy at a weight below the standard for height or women who experience poor weight gain risk increased rates of prematurity, low-birth-weight infants, and infants with low Apgar scores. The presence of anemia, a history of maternal smoking, and/or poor weight gain in the low-prepregnancy-weight patient markedly increases the incidence of low-birth-weight infants.

The objective of a nutrition and weight gain program in pregnancy is to help ensure the most favorable outcome for both the mother and her infant. The patient should be guided toward a planned goal, beginning with an estimate of her desirable weight, an assessment of her nutritional status, and an estimate of what would constitute an adequate weight gain for her.

Optimal fetal growth is dependent on the nutritional status of the mother not only during pregnancy but for many years prior to conception. Ideally, underweight women should attain their appropriate weight prior to pregnancy.

## Pica

As early as the sixth century AD there were accounts of peculiar food and nonfood cravings, or pica. The variety of nonfood substances consumed includes laundry starch, clay, ashes, and ice. The propensity of pregnant women for this condition has been singled out as particularly strong, yet research has failed to reveal the underlying etiology (Luke, 1979). A strong and persistent link between this nutritional problem and iron deficiency has been demonstrated, but the exact relation between the two conditions remains unclear. Some suggest that the anemia is a result of the pica; others suggest that it is the cause.

One way in which pica is thought to cause iron deficiency anemia is through the binding of dietary iron, rendering it unusable for the body. In particular, clay with high cation exchange capacity is found to be effective in blocking iron absorption. Magnesium oxide also has been found to be extremely effective in preventing iron absorption in this way. Because cravings have been reported for antacids, some of which contain magnesium, the cation exchange capacities may have some clinical significance in relation to iron absorption.

Unusual cravings in some women have been eliminated by the treatment of iron deficiency anemia. With serum iron values above 70 $\mu$g/dl, the unusual cravings may disappear.

Culture and tradition seem to play a significant role in the condition of pica. Women take clay and other substances such as corn starch, flour, and baking soda in order to relieve nausea, prevent vomiting, relieve dizziness, cure swollen legs, and relieve headaches. In some cultures, it is even believed that ingestion of these substances will result in a beautiful child, whereas failure to have the cravings satisfied is popularly thought by some to cause birthmarks. Others have hypothesized that pica represents an unconscious endeavor to compensate for certain nutritional deficiencies.

Diet counseling should include an open discussion about pica and food cravings. Discussion of a nutritionally adequate diet can include suggestions for foods to substitute for nonfoods. Nonfat dry milk powder has been found to be an acceptable alternative to laundry starch for some women.

## ASSOCIATED MEDICAL DISORDERS

### Diabetes

**Diabetes Mellitus.** Changes in maternal glucose level and other metabolites are due not only to use by the fetus but also to the action of placental hormones on carbohydrate metabolism. Estrogen, progesterone, and lactogen antagonize the effects of insulin at the cell wall. In addition, placental lactogen is lipolytic, which increases the circulating levels of fatty acids.

As pregnancy progresses, despite the anti-insulin hormonal setting, carbohydrate homeostasis and normal glucose tolerance are maintained in most patients. This is accomplished by an increased maternal secretion of insulin. Hyperinsulinemia has been observed in response to an intake of both glucose and certain amino acids. Although there is an increase in immediate postprandial insulin levels, the fasting level of insulin is reduced because of the fasting hypoglycemic tendency that persists throughout pregnancy.

Caring for a woman with diabetes during pregnancy represents a great challenge. Close teamwork among several health care providers is necessary for the greatest likelihood of a successful outcome. It is clear that perinatal outcome is greatly improved when optimal care is given.

Diabetes and pregnancy may interact in two ways. Evidence of glucose intolerance may appear in a pregnant woman not previously known to be diabetic, or a known diabetic may become pregnant. The patient diagnosed as having diabetes during pregnancy must be counseled carefully and promptly about the management of this disorder and its impact on pregnancy. The previously diagnosed diabetic who becomes pregnant must adjust to the metabolic changes of pregnancy described earlier. The importance of preconceptional counseling and optimal control of the diabetes cannot be overemphasized, because evidence suggests that the incidence of congenital anomalies in the offspring of diabetics may be increased in women whose diabetes is poorly controlled near the time of conception (Kitzmiller et al, 1991).

**Gestational Diabetes.** Gestational diabetes is defined as carbohydrate intolerance that is diagnosed at any time during pregnancy and disappears by the sixth week postpartum. It occurs in approximately 2 to 3 percent of pregnancies. Perinatal mortality rates are approximately doubled in pregnancies complicated by *undiagnosed* gestational diabetes; these rates may be significantly reduced by identification and close monitoring of such pregnancies. Usually, the diagnosis of gestational diabetes is made by a screening test. All pregnant women should be screened. Screening is generally carried out at 26 to 28 weeks' gestation. However, a screening test should be performed at the first prenatal visit if there are any risk factors, such as maternal age of 25 or older, a family history of diabetes mellitus, or a history of a large baby (greater than 4 kg [9 lb]), stillborn, or neonatal death. An O'Sullivan screening test using a 50-mg oral glucose load (Glucola) should normally yield a plasma glucose level 1 hour later of less than 140 mg/dl (O'Sullivan et al, 1973). The patient need not be fasting. If the screening result is greater than or equal to 140 mg/dl, a 3-hour oral glucose tolerance test (OGTT) is recommended. A nonfasting plasma glucose over 200 mg/dl on screening or a fasting greater than 105 mg/dl is indicative of diabetes mellitus.

The diagnosis of gestational diabetes requires that two or more of these tests have abnormal values (fasting level greater than 105 mg/dl; at 1 hour, greater than 190 mg/dl; at 2 hours, greater than 165 mg/dl; at 3 hours, greater than 145 mg/dl). If only one value is abnormal, repeat testing at about 32 weeks' gestation may be indicated. Table 11–5 outlines the accepted plasma glucose levels during pregnancy. Approximately 15 to 20 percent of gestational diabetics will develop overt diabetes mellitus with abnormal fasting and postprandial glucose values.

**Dietary Management of Diabetes.** The cornerstone of the management of all types of diabetes mellitus is a meal plan providing consistent dietary intake to control blood glucose. The principles of diet management are based on three general concepts of balance:

1. *Energy Balance*—consistent intake of calories providing the energy needed to

**Table 11–5**
STANDARDS FOR ORAL GLUCOSE TOLERANCE TEST IN PREGNANCY

|  | Plasma mg/dl | Whole Blood mg/dl |
|---|---|---|
| Fasting | 105 | 90 |
| 1 hr* | 190 | 165 |
| 2 hr* | 165 | 145 |
| 3 hr* | 145 | 125 |

* Post glucose ingestion.
Plasma values are approximately 14 percent higher than corresponding whole blood values.
Glucose load is 100 g.
For proper interpretation, carbohydrate intake for each of the 3 days preceding the test should exceed 300 g. One candy bar each day helps to ensure that this requirement is met.
Data from O'Sullivan JB, Mahan CM: Criteria for the oral glucose tolerance test in pregnancy. Diabetes 13:278, 1964.

maintain ideal maternal and fetal weight gain.

2. *Nutrient Balance*—the proper ratio of macronutrients (carbohydrate, protein, fat) to meet energy needs and micronutrients (vitamins and minerals) to meet nutritional needs.

3. *Distribution Balance*—consistent distribution of the macronutrients throughout the day, to balance with activity levels, and insulin when prescribed, in order to avoid hypoglycemia and yet provide a sustained availability of glucose.

**Energy Balance.** During pregnancy, the total daily energy requirement is governed by the maternal and fetal metabolic needs, which on the average will require 2000 to 2400 kcal or approximately 30 to 35 kcal/kg of ideal body weight.

### Nutrient Balance

*Carbohydrate.* Contrary to what was formerly believed, carbohydrates should not be disproportionately reduced in a diet prescribed for managing diabetes. Approximately 50 percent of the total number of calories, with a minimum intake of 250 g daily, should be provided by carbohydrates. The greater proportion of the carbohydrate calories should be obtained from complex carbohydrate foods, such as starchy vegetables and cereals, which are digested and absorbed slowly, with the lesser amounts coming from the simple sugars, as in fruits. Large intakes of concentrated sweets that are quickly digested and absorbed result in greater fluctuation of blood glucose.

*Protein.* Proteins are important in controlling diabetes. The diet of a pregnant woman with diabetes should contain approximately 1.5 to 2.0 g of protein per kilogram of body weight per day, or approximately 100 to 125 g/day. Approximately 25 percent of the total calories should be derived from protein foods.

*Fat.* Fat needs of the diabetic woman during pregnancy are not primary, so the amount of fat should be kept at moderate levels. Thus, 60 to 80 g of fat, or approximately 30 percent of the total calories consumed, may come from fat. An effort should be made to keep a 1:1 ratio between saturated and polyunsaturated fats.

*Fiber.* A diet high in soluble fibers may be useful in the management of diabetes mellitus. Dietary fiber has been defined as the portion of plant material taken in the diet that is resistant to digestion by the secretions of the gastrointestinal tract. As such, fiber remains in the stomach and the small bowel for longer periods of time than does the digestable fraction of food. Fiber increases the volume of bowel contents and might also simultaneously influence general metabolism by altering the rate of absorption from the stomach; this may decrease glucose levels, reduce postprandial hypoglycemia, and diminish insulin requirements (Anderson, 1981).

Fibers may be water soluble or water insoluble. The substances that are generally thought of as being fibrous are most often high in cellulose content and predominantly insoluble. The soluble fibers are generally categorized biologically as gums, mucilages, and storage polysaccharides. Soluble fibers are the substances with the greatest likelihood of altering the absorption nutrients. The fiber content of the diet can be increased by using greater quantities of whole grain breads and cereals, raw fruits, vegetables, and legumes (Anderson and Ward, 1975).

**Distribution Balance.** The most important aspect of diet for a pregnant diabetic is consistency of mealtimes and time between meals, as well as caloric content of the diet. It is usually desirable to find the patient's preferred eating and exercising patterns and try to adjust insulin to them. To tailor an appropriate insulin schedule, meals should be eaten at the same time each day and be consistent in calories, protein, and carbohydrates. The caloric intake may be divided into three meals and one bedtime snack, using approximately 2/7 of the total calories for each meal and 1/7 for the snack. Some diabetics, especially those who are overweight, may require one to two additional snacks in order to maintain euglycemia. The carbohydrate calories (50 percent of the total calories) are divided about equally for each meal, with an allowance of about 10 percent for snacks. If urinary acetone spillage occurs, then 100 calories in the form of carbohydrate are added to the next meal or snack. If morning fasting acetonuria persists despite increasing the evening snack by 100 calories, then a snack, such as 8 ounces of skim milk, is added at about 3:00 AM. Alternative snacks containing a combination of protein and complex carbohydrate are also appropriate (Couston et al, 1980; Gabbe, 1981; Williams, 1989). If the patient's insulin is adjusted in the hospital, allowances should be made concerning her exercise when she returns to her usual schedule at home.

The patient should be seen approximately every 1 to 2 weeks during her prenatal course. At each visit a fasting and a 2-hour postprandial plasma glucose is obtained, and appropriate adjustments are made.

**Weight Gain.** The weight gain goals depend on the woman's body mass index. An obese woman should gain no more than 7 to 11.5 kg (15 to 25 lbs); patients of average weight may gain 11.5 to 16 kg (25 to 35 lbs); and a lean patient may gain 12.5 to 18 kg (28 to 40 lbs).

**Insulin Therapy in Diabetes.** Women with gestational diabetes should check their blood glucose several times a day to ensure that their diet is adequate to maintain a fasting and preprandial blood glucose level of 90 to 100 mg/dl and a 2-hour postprandial blood glucose of less than 120 mg/dl. If these goals are not attained, the patient should be given insulin. Patients requiring insulin prior to pregnancy often need frequent adjustment throughout gestation. In the pregnant insulin-dependent diabetic, the goal of therapy is to maintain a fasting plasma glucose level of 80 to 100 mg/dl and a 2-hour postprandial level of 120 to 140 mg/dl, which are levels associated with the least perinatal mortality and morbidity. In practical terms, insulin dosage is readjusted if the fasting plasma glucose is more than 100 mg/dl or if any 2-hour postprandial value is more than 140 mg/dl. Efforts are made to avoid large fluctuations of plasma glucose during the day (Jovanovic and Peterson, 1980).

After 20 weeks' gestation, most pregnant diabetics are treated with combinations of intermediate- and short-acting insulins, with dosages split between morning and evening. Patients take insulin prior to breakfast and dinner each day, using a mixture of intermediate-acting (NPH or Lente) and short-acting (regular) insulin. The fasting plasma glucose reflects the intermediate-acting insulin given at dinnertime on the preceding day, the 2-hour postprandial morning plasma glucose reflects the regular insulin given that morning, and the late afternoon plasma glucose value reflects the morning intermediate-acting insulin dose. If an evening glucose can be obtained, it reflects the pre-dinnertime, short-acting insulin. In this manner the various components of the day's

insulin doses can be adjusted to maintain optimal goals of glucose control.

The detailed management of the pregnant diabetic patient is covered in Chapter 26.

### Essential Hypertension and Chronic Renal Disease

In about 30 percent of patients with hypertension during pregnancy, elevated blood pressure will persist after pregnancy and is characterized as hypertension of unknown etiology. When chronic renal disease and hypertension coexist, urinary protein loss may be as high as 5 g/day. If the losses become massive, serum proteins could fall to levels at which their reduced osmotic pressure will allow water to move into extravascular spaces and cause generalized edema. Usually, dietary protein supplements are not necessary, because the urinary losses constitute only 5 to 7 percent of the total protein intake.

The general dietary recommendations for essential hypertension with chronic renal disease include a well-balanced diet containing a mixture of essential nutrients (Luke, 1979). Sodium restriction to about 5 g/day may be indicated in patients with essential hypertension. If diuretics are used, it should be acknowledged that potassium as well as sodium may be lost, and the patient should be counseled as to good dietary sources of potassium. These include bananas, orange or grapefruit juice, prunes, potatoes, raisins, and peanuts. It should be remembered that excessive protein intake by patients with impaired glomerular filtration may be hazardous, in that the blood urea level may become elevated.

### Cardiac Disease

The two important factors in the nutritional support of pregnancy complicated by heart disease are (1) energy balance in relation to weight control and (2) careful control of sodium intake. The usual pattern of weight gain should be encouraged. Although sodium is a necessary mineral for the health of the pregnant woman, a woman with heart disease is vulnerable to cardiac failure and should restrict her sodium intake to 5 g/day. A diet providing much less than this amount is unpalatable and is associated with a very low rate of patient compliance. This general level of sodium intake can be achieved by (1) omitting salty foods such as salt-cured meats or fish, salted snacks and crackers, pickles, relishes, and condiments, and (2) light use of salt in cooking and none added to food at the table. The nutritionist can assist the patient in planning meals, selecting suitable food, reading food package labels for sodium content, and seasoning food with lemon juice, herbs, and spices rather than with salt.

## Maternal Phenylketonuria

Because of the success of past treatment of this disorder, many women with phenylketonuria (PKU) are intellectually normal and are entering into the reproductive age. Since 1957, concern has increased over children born to women with PKU (Dent, 1957). A maternal phenylalanine level above 20 mg/dl is toxic to the developing fetus. The maternal PKU syndrome consists of offspring without evidence of PKU having microcephaly, severe mental retardation, congenital heart disease, and intrauterine growth retardation. It is important that guidelines be established for counseling these young women about diet during their reproductive life. However, uncertainty still exists about the relationship among maternal PKU, diet adequacy, hyperphenylalaninemia, and developmental problems in the fetus. Some believe that the low phenylalanine diet must begin prior to the onset of pregnancy.

The outcome of 34 pregnancies in which dietary therapy was aimed at lowering maternal phenylalanine concentration in an attempt to avoid fetal damage was reported (Lenke and Levy, 1982). The data indicated that most women with PKU have pretreatment phenylalanine blood levels of 20 mg/dl or greater. During dietary treatment in pregnancy, the levels of phenylalanine were generally maintained between 4 and 12 mg/dl. There was some relation between protection of the fetus and how early in pregnancy treatment was begun, as well as how effectively the blood level of phenylalanine was controlled. When good dietary control was achieved before conception, 2 of 2 offspring had normal test results for intelligence and no congenital defects were noted. When the diet was started in the first trimester, only 36 percent (4 of 11) of the infants appeared to be

normal. The percentage of normal infants when treatment was begun in the second or third trimester was 13 percent (2 of 16) and 50 percent (2 of 4), respectively. The available data tend to support initiation of dietary therapy *prior to conception* for best results.

The low-phenylalanine diet prescribed for maternal PKU is similar to that administered to children who are treated for this disorder. It consists of a specifically designed dietary supplement containing protein free of the amino acid, phenylalanine, plus vegetables, fruits, and some specially prepared bread or dessert products. Routine recommendation of prenatal vitamins *should be avoided,* because vitamins are supplied in the dietary preparations. As noted earlier, an excess of vitamins could be harmful to the fetus.

Specifically, the dietary management of maternal PKU should (1) provide sufficient, but not excessive, phenylalanine (250 to 500 mg/day) (the specific prescription of patients' individual tolerances is estimated through monitoring of serum phenylalanine levels); (2) provide 50 g/day of protein during the first half of pregnancy and 100 g/day during the second half; (3) meet the appropriate caloric needs of both mother and fetus, with needs for the former determined by age, prepregnancy weight, and physical activity.

## Inflammatory Bowel Disease

*Regional enteritis* is associated with infertility in one third of patients. However, it may have no significant adverse effects on pregnancy once achieved. In one study, only about 10 percent of the patients with inflammatory bowel disease had an exacerbation during pregnancy (those patients with colonic involvement may be more prone to flare-ups in pregnancy). On the other hand, 24 percent of pregnancies were associated with relapses postpartum, which were attributed to the sudden decrease in hormone concentration (Wong et al, 1981).

Also, *ulcerative colitis* is associated with infertility in 10 percent of patients. The majority of pregnancies in women with ulcerative colitis result in live births; however, 20 percent of these patients show an exacerbation of the disease during pregnancy. As in patients with regional enteritis, there is a significant risk of exacerbation postpartum.

In pregnant women, the management of

inflammatory bowel disease is essentially the same as it is in nonpregnant women. The aims are to maintain good nutrition and to correct anemia or electrolyte imbalances. The diet of pregnant women with inflammatory bowel disease should be supplemented by oral administration of iron, folic acid, other vitamins, and by intramuscular administration of vitamin $B_{12}$. Nutritional support may involve total parenteral nutrition (TPN) in severe episodes; successful perinatal outcome has been reported (Herbert et al, 1986; Martin et al, 1985).

## Special Situations

### MULTIPLE PREGNANCY

Theoretically, the nutritional needs of the woman with more than one fetus should increase because she has both a larger volume and a greater fetoplacental mass. Studies to date indicate that weight gain during a twin pregnancy is higher than the weight accounted for by the additional mass of the second conceptus. However, it is not possible to draw conclusions about the components of the additional weight gain. A total weight gain of 16 to 20.5 kg (35 to 45 lbs) is recommended (Committee on Nutritional Status During Pregnancy and Lactation, 1990).

As mentioned previously, patients with multiple gestations should be supplemented with 1 mg of folate daily throughout pregnancy to prevent folate deficiency.

### ADOLESCENT PREGNANCY

Nutritional studies of pregnant adolescents indicate that the nutritional needs of those who conceive before their longitudinal growth is completed are greater than for girls who are 4 or more years postmenarchal. For pregnant adolescents between the ages of 15 and 18, the recommended allowance is 1.5 mg protein/kg/day; for younger girls, 1.7 mg/kg/day is suggested. The adolescent's needs for some vitamins and minerals are also increased. There are no differences in the recommended intake for adults and adolescents of vitamins A, E, $B_{12}$, and folic acid, and of the minerals magnesium, iron, iodine, and zinc (see Table 11–1).

## Assessment of Nutritional Status

Ideally, a nutritional assessment prior to conception should be performed. This approach allows the identification of any weight problems, other nutritional inadequacies, or metabolic alterations that require treatment or correction. In addition, the importance of adequate food intake and weight gain to a successful pregnancy outcome is stressed.

During pregnancy, the additional and changing nutritive demands require that nutritional assessment be an integral part of all prenatal care. Each prenatal patient should have an assessment at her first prenatal visit, with periodic reviews thereafter.

A more meticulous assessment should be made for those women who, because of age, health condition, education, or socioeconomic status, are at greater risk of nutritional deficiency. These include:

- Adolescents who are less than 4 years postmenarchal, who are still undergoing their own linear growth, and who, therefore, are superimposing these nutrient requirements on the nutrient demands of pregnancy.
- Women who are underweight at the onset of pregnancy, with underweight being defined as below 90 percent of the standard weight for height.
- Women with a history of frequent conceptions—i.e., more than two conceptions within the past 2 years.
- Women with a history of low-birthweight infants (weighing under 2500 g).
- Women with a history of anemia.
- Women with a poor reproductive history, e.g., those who have experienced spontaneous abortions or perinatal loss.
- Women with chronic or infectious diseases that can negatively influence their nutritional status, such as diabetes, hypertension, gastrointestinal disorders (nausea, vomiting, diarrhea, intestinal bypass), allergies, cardiovascular disease, kidney disease, liver disease, and tuberculosis.
- Women with a history of substance abuse, such as habitual smoking, excessive alcohol intake, or other drug abuse.

- Women with a history of unusual dietary practices, including pica, macrobiotic diet, strict vegetarianism (vegans), anorexia nervosa, and bulimia.
- Women in families with insufficient income to purchase a nutritionally adequate diet and/or those who are living in housing without adequate facilities to store and prepare a varied diet.

## HISTORY

Much of the data needed for nutritional assessment are found in the patient's medical, family, and social history, which should be included in the prenatal health care record. Pertinent information includes:

- Present age
- Age at menarche
- Previous obstetric history
  —Parity and outcome
  —Weight gain in previous pregnancies
  —Length of interconceptional period
- Weight history
- Diagnosed illnesses, including chronic diseases and infections (including parasitic infections)

## DIETARY EVALUATION

Dietary information must be collected in order to assess nutrient intake. This includes data on the variety of environmental, psychosocial, and economic factors that influence food choices, as well as a pattern of usual or current food choices. One should also note the kinds and amounts of foods consumed, how these foods are prepared, and the timing of meals and snacks. Some of the influencing factors that must be investigated are as follows:

- Usual appetite, as well as any problems with nausea and vomiting during pregnancy.
- Regular or irregular eating habits and patterns of meals and snacks.
- Which family member is responsible for planning meals and buying and preparing food, including this person's knowledge of nutrition and attitude regarding meeting individualized nutritional needs.
- Usual food budget and expenditures for food and how many people are fed. Other sources of food, such as available food from a garden, meals provided at employment site, food gifts, or meals provided by parents and others, should also be taken into account.
- Whether housing and available equipment are in working order to store, refrigerate, and prepare a variety of foods.
- Use of vitamin or mineral supplements, weight-control medications, diuretics, laxatives, antacids, and so on.
- Food dislikes, intolerances, or allergies.
- Food or nonfood cravings (pica) during pregnancy.
- Cultural, ethnic, or religious practices that influence food choices.

Current food intake information must be obtained both in order to evaluate the nutritional adequacy of the patient's diet and for use as a starting point in counseling the patient on proper nutrition and diet. The simplest method for obtaining this information is a 24-hour recall, in which the patient is asked to list all the foods she has eaten during the last 24 hours. Questions should be open-ended. Probing questions are used to determine methods of food preparation, amounts of food, and whether added food items, such as salad dressings, spreads on breads, toppings, sauces, gravies, and sweeteners, were used. Questions also need to be asked to be sure all beverages taken with and between meals are listed.

The patient's eating pattern may vary on weekends or holidays or at different times of the month depending on social activities, changes in schedule, availability of paycheck, welfare allowance, or food stamps. It is advisable to ask the patient to provide a usual eating pattern if it is believed the intake during the preceding 24 hours is not typical. A sample form for eliciting, summarizing, and evaluating a day's dietary intake is shown in Figure 11–2.

There are limitations to the validity of dietary intake information, owing to time constraints, variations in the skills of interviewers, variations in the memory and motivation of patients, and difficulty in accu-

24-HOUR TYPICAL FOOD INTAKE                    SUMMARY

Name:_____ Interviewer:_____

Date:_____

| | | | | | Protein-Rich Foods | Milk and Milk Products | Cereal Products | Vitamin C–Rich Foods | Leafy Green and Yellow Vegetables | Other Fruits & Vegetables |
|---|---|---|---|---|---|---|---|---|---|---|
| TIME | PLACE | FOOD EATEN | PREPARATION | AMOUNT | | | | | | |
| | | | | | | | | | | |

RECOMMENDATIONS AND FOLLOW-UP:

| ASSESSMENT: | | | | | | |
|---|---|---|---|---|---|---|
| Servings eaten | | | | | | |
| Servings needed | 4 | 4 | 3 | 1 | 2 | 1 |
| Addition suggested | | | | | | |

**Figure 11–2.** Typical food intake (per 24-hour period). (Adapted from Nutrition During Pregnancy and Lactation, California Department of Health, 1975.)

rately interpreting information concerning the variety of food eaten by any individual. The greatest value of dietary assessment is to identify gross inadequacies in major food sources of nutrients and to use the patient's own dietary pattern as the basis for remedial diet counseling.

Another commonly employed dietary assessment tool, used to supplement the 24-hour or usual dietary intake listing, is a Food Frequency checklist (Fig. 11–3), which provides insight into the range of foods the patient eats and gives some indication of how often a particular food is consumed. Similar foods are usually grouped together according to the commonly used Daily Food Guide or Four Food Groups. The Food Frequency checklist generally differentiates foods that are habitual in the patient's diet from those rarely or never eaten. For example, if the patient rarely or never consumes milk or milk products, a suboptimal intake of calcium, riboflavin, and vitamin D might be assumed. The Food Frequency checklist does not provide information on amounts or time of eating. Although it is a rather subjective assessment, it is useful as a basis for nutrition education.

FOOD FREQUENCY CHECKLIST

Name: _____    Date: _____

For each food checked EATEN, write the appropriate number of times eaten in a week (e.g., if eaten daily, number would be 7 – if a food is eaten once a month, put 1/4). A space is provided at the end to add other foods eaten regularly. Any food not eaten regularly should be checked in the DO NOT EAT column.

| FOOD | TIMES EATEN PER WEEK | DO NOT EAT |
|---|---|---|
| PROTEIN RICH FOODS | | |
| Eggs | | |
| Chicken, Turkey | | |
| Beef, Veal, Lamb | | |
| Pork, Ham | | |
| Liver | | |
| Fish, Shellfish | | |
| Luncheon Meat | | |
| Hot Dogs, Sausage | | |
| Dried Beans, Peas | | |
| Soybeans, Tofu | | |
| Peanut Butter, Nuts | | |
| MILK & MILK PRODUCTS | | |
| Milk (fluid, dried, canned) | | |
| Yogurt | | |
| Cheese (cottage, etc.) | | |
| Ice Cream, Pudding, Custard | | |
| CEREAL PRODUCTS | | |
| Wholegrain Bread | | |
| Enriched White Bread | | |
| Rolls, Biscuits, Muffins, Bagels | | |
| Crackers, Pretzels | | |
| Pancakes, Waffles | | |
| Pasta, Spaghetti, Noodles | | |
| Rice, Grits | | |
| Cereal, cooked | | |
| Cereal, ready-to-eat | | |
| Tortillas | | |

| FOOD | TIMES EATEN PER WEEK | DO NOT EAT |
|---|---|---|
| VITAMIN C RICH FOODS | | |
| Orange, Grapefruit, Tangerine or Juice | | |
| Tomato (sauce or juice) | | |
| Cantaloupe | | |
| Strawberries | | |
| DARK GREEN OR YELLOW FRUITS & VEGETABLES | | |
| Greens (beet, collard, kale, turnip, mustard) | | |
| Broccoli | | |
| Peppers (green or red) | | |
| Spinach | | |
| Salad Greens (dark green) | | |
| Carrots | | |
| Sweet Potato | | |
| Winter Squash | | |
| Apricots | | |
| Other Fruits & Vegetables | | |
| Potatoes | | |
| Green/Wax Beans | | |
| Corn | | |
| Peas | | |
| Apples | | |
| Bananas | | |
| Pears | | |
| FATS | | |
| Bacon, Salt Pork | | |
| Butter, Margarine | | |
| Cooking Fat, Oil | | |
| Salad Dressing | | |

| FOOD | TIMES EATEN PER WEEK | DO NOT EAT |
|---|---|---|
| MISCELLANEOUS | | |
| Cakes, Cookies, Pies | | |
| Sweet Rolls, Doughnuts | | |
| Candy | | |
| Soft Drinks, Koolade | | |
| Coffee, Tea, Cocoa | | |
| Wine, Beer, Cocktails | | |
| Sugar, Honey, Syrup | | |
| Jam, Jelly | | |
| Chips (potato or corn) | | |
| ANY OTHER FOODS EATEN REGULARLY | | |

**Figure 11–3.** Food frequency checklist.

199

## PHYSICAL EXAMINATION

Indicators of nutritional deficiencies may be observed in the hair, face and neck, eyes, lips, gums, teeth, arms, hands, and lower extremities. Some examples of physical signs of nutrient deficiencies that might be observed in a malnourished, pregnant, or lactating woman are listed in Table 11–6.

It should be recognized that clear-cut physical signs of malnutrition are not frequently observed in the United States; therefore, subclinical signs may be easily confused with conditions unrelated to nutrition. Any signs that might be clues to malnutrition should be incorporated into the routine physical examination and analyzed by the health professionals involved in the patient's nutritional assessment.

## LABORATORY TESTS

Biochemical tests are useful in assessing nutritional status in that they provide objective and precise measurements of nutrient concentrations in tissues, blood, or urine. Some problems in interpretation occur in pregnancy because of the alterations in physiology and the lack of established norms for specific time periods throughout pregnancy. However, the laboratory tests provide baseline data for monitoring nutritional status.

It is generally recommended that hematocrit or hemoglobin and possibly serum folic acid be monitored for all pregnant women initially and in each trimester. Monitoring of serum vitamin $B_{12}$ is desirable for women who are total vegans and who do not eat any animal protein foods. Serum albumin and total serum protein are suggested when a patient's diet appears to be consistently low in protein, calories, or both. According to in-dividual needs, tests of other vitamin levels may also be performed.

Routine testing for blood glucose and urine glucose and ketones is recommended for women with either preexisting or gestational diabetes. Guidelines for criteria for laboratory evaluation of nutritional status are shown in Table 11–7.

## ANTHROPOMETRIC ASSESSMENT

The simplest and most common measure of growth during pregnancy is weight gain. The accuracy of height and weight measures are increasing in importance because data on outcomes in pregnancy are more strongly associated to the weight gain a woman achieves during pregnancy. These measures are the least invasive, so they are regularly collected during the pregnancy. Weight should be measured consistently with light street clothing, shoes off, and heavy coats and outer wraps off. Height should be measured with a measuring board or the measuring surface with feet slightly apart. Shoulders, buttocks, and heels should touch the measuring surface. With the person looking straight ahead, slide the headboard firmly down to the head, with the eyes level with the indicator, read the height. The height will not change during pregnancy except with adolescent girls, whose height should be measured on each visit.

The rate of weight gain should be monitored as carefully as the total weight gain. The Prenatal Weight Gain Grid, shown in Figure 11–1, provides a visual reference for the health care professionals to compare each patient's weight gain with the currently recommended pattern. An excessive or sudden weight gain that greatly exceeds this rate is usually caused by fluid retention. Sudden or continuous weight loss should

### Table 11–6
#### PHYSICAL SIGNS OF NUTRITIONAL DEFICIENCIES

| Site | Finding | Deficiency |
|------|---------|------------|
| Generalized | Significant nondependent edema | Protein |
| Tongue | Filiform papillary atrophy | Iron/folate |
| Thyroid gland | Diffusely enlarged and visible | Iodine |
| Skin (upper arms) | Follicular hyperkeratosis | Vitamin A |
| Gums | Diffusely swollen, red, interdental papillae in a clean mouth | Vitamin C |
| Lips | Angular fissures and cheilosis | Riboflavin |

Data from ACOG: Assessment of Maternal Nutrition. Chicago, The American College of Obstetricians and Gynecologists, 1978.

Table 11–7

GUIDELINES FOR CRITERIA FOR LABORATORY EVALUATION OF NUTRITIONAL STATUS
IN PREGNANCY

| Test | Acceptable For Pregnancy | Deficient For Pregnancy |
|---|---|---|
| Hemoglobin | 11.0 + g/100 ml after 6 months | <9.5 g/100 ml |
| Hematocrit (packed cell volume) | 33 percent | <30 percent |
| Serum folic acid | 6 ng/ml | <3 ng/ml |
| Serum albumin | 3.5 g/100 ml | <3 g/100 ml |
| Total serum protein | 6.5 g/100 ml | <2.5 g/ml |
| Serum vitamin $B_{12}$ | 200 pg/ml | <80 pg/ml |
| Thiamine in urine | 50 $\mu$g/g creatinine | <21 mg/g creatinine |
| Riboflavin in urine | 90 $\mu$g/g creatinine | <30 $\mu$g/g creatinine |

Adapted from Christakis G (ed): Nutritional Assessment in Health Programs. Washington, DC, American Public Health Association, 1973.

trigger concern about severe nutritional or other health problems and should prompt an assessment for intrauterine growth retardation. The grid is also useful for patient education, to point out any weight loss or inappropriate weight gain.

For the woman who is underweight at conception, with underweight defined as less than 90 percent of standard weight for height, the initial weight is plotted to indicate the deficit, and a greater weight gain is recommended 12.5 to 18 kg (28 to 40 lbs). For women who are grossly obese at the onset of pregnancy, a weight gain of about 7 to 11.5 kg (15 to 25 lb) is recommended (Committee on Nutritional Status During Pregnancy and Lactation, 1990).

## Nutritional Intervention

Nutritional assessment identifies and specifies each woman's need for nutrition education and diet counseling. The Recommended Dietary Allowances of the Food and Nutrition Board of the National Research Council, National Academy of Sciences, provides the frame of reference (see Table 11–1). For pregnant women with adequate income and low-risk pregnancies, nutrition education should focus on providing most of the recommended nutrients through food. Because it is difficult for most American women to consume sufficient iron and folic acid in food, the use of daily supplements of iron (60 to 120 mg) and folic acid (400 to 800 $\mu$g) may be recommended. Women who are allergic to milk or who cannot tolerate milk or milk products may also require a calcium

supplement, and diet counseling for these women should ensure that adequate calories, protein, and riboflavin are obtained from sources other than dairy products. The focus of individual and group nutrition education is on the basic diet for normal pregnancy and recommendations for desirable weight gain. Pregnant women should be advised regarding their nutritional needs for breastfeeding (Table 11–8). They should also be given information to make an informed choice regarding methods of infant feeding.

A vegetarian diet can provide the nutrients necessary in pregnancy if it is correctly balanced. If dairy products are included in the diet, it is relatively easy to meet pregnancy needs; however, if all animal products are excluded from a woman's diet, referral to a nutritional professional for regular nutrition assessment and monitoring is needed. The protein may be poor if vegetable sources are not balanced and calories may be low because of a lower fat intake and increased high-bulk foodstuffs. These dietary practices can lead to a vitamin $B_{12}$, calcium, riboflavin, and vitamin D deficiency; iron and zinc may also be low. Vitamin $B_{12}$ may be supplemented to 2 $\mu$g/d and vitamin D to 10 $\mu$g if deficient in the diet.

Federal, state, and local officials, as well as nongovernmental health agencies, have developed food guides to interpret recommended dietary allowances into practical food groups. The Dietary Guidelines authorized by the Departments of Agriculture and Health and Human Services are appropriate for pregnancy. They recommend a variety of foods, moderation in fat and sodium, emphasis on complex carbohydrates and fruits and vegetables, and maintaining ideal body weight. In pregnancy, the lean meat for iron

## Table 11-8
### RECOMMENDED DIETARY ALLOWANCES FOR LACTATION

| Age | Body weight (kg) | Energy* (kcal) | Energy* (mega j) | Protein*† (g) | Vitamin A‡§ (μg) | Vitamin D¶ (μg) | Thiamin‡ (mg) | Ribo flavin‡ (mg) | Niacin‡ (mg) | Folic acid‖ (μg) | Vitamin B12‖ (μg) | Ascorbic acid‖ (mg) | Calcium** (g) | Iron‖†† (mg) |
|---|---|---|---|---|---|---|---|---|---|---|---|---|---|---|
| Adult woman (moderately active) | 55.0 | 2200 | 9.2 | 29 | 750 | 2.5 | 0.9 | 1.3 | 14.5 | 200 | 2.0 | 30 | 0.4-0.5 | 14-28 |
| Pregnancy (later half) | | +350 | +1.5 | 38 | 750 | 10.0 | +0.1 | +0.2 | +2.3 | 400 | 3.0 | 50 | 1.0-1.2 | ‡‡ |
| Lactation (first 6 months) | | +550 | +2.3 | 46 | 1200 | 10.0 | +0.2 | +0.4 | +3.7 | 300 | 2.5 | 50 | 1.0-1.2 | ‡‡ |

*Energy and Protein Requirements. Report of a Joint FAO-WHO Expert Group, FAO, Rome, 1972.

†As egg or milk protein.

‡Requirements of vitamin A, thiamin, riboflavin, and niacin. Report of a Joint FAO-WHO Expert Group, FAO, Rome, 1965.

§As retinol.

‖Requirements of ascorbic acid, vitamin D, vitamin B12, folate and iron. Report of a Joint FAO-WHO Expert Group, FAO, Rome. 1970.

¶As cholecalciferol.

**Calcium requirements. Report of a Joint FAO/WHO Expert Group, FAO, Rome, 1961.

††On each line the lower value applies when over 25 percent of calories in the diet come from animal foods, and the higher value when animal foods represent less than10 percent of calories.

‡‡For women whose iron intake throughout life has been at the level recommended in this table, the daily intake of iron during pregnancy and lactation should be the same as that recommended for nonpregnant, nonlactating women of childbearing age. For women whose iron status is not satisfactory at the beginning of pregnancy, the requirement is increased, and in the extreme situation of women with no iron stores, the requirement can probably not be met without supplementation.

and protein and green vegetables for folic acid need to be eaten regularly. Selecting recommended amounts of standard servings from a given food group is easier and more realistic for most women than calculating amounts of nutrients in foods.

A daily food guide suggested for the pregnant woman is shown in Table 11-9. This is the basic food guide suggested to evaluate the nutritional adequacy of the pregnant woman's diet and to help her develop a meal plan that will meet her nutritional needs for pregnancy.

Although the Daily Food Guide, adapted for pregnancy, provides a useful teaching tool, dietary counseling should also involve an exchange between the health professional and the patient, so that the patient can achieve the recommended diet within the constraints of her own individual lifestyle, food preferences, meal patterns, and socioeconomic situation.

Health professionals who conduct nutrition assessment should identify patients with more complex nutritional problems who require more individualized, in-depth counseling, follow-up, and referral. Women with severe nutritional deficiencies or weight problems, with concomitant medical conditions requiring dietary modifications, with unusual eating patterns, or with emotional problems that affect their eating behavior should be referred to a registered dietitian. The dietitian can provide detailed diet counseling and follow-up with continued monitoring of the woman's nutritional status at each prenatal visit. Registered dietitians are generally available in Level III perinatal centers, major medical centers, community hospitals, local or state public health departments, and private practice.

For women who are unable to afford the recommended diet, all nutrition counseling must include assistance with obtaining adequate food. Most health agencies now participate in the Special Supplemental Food Program for Women, Infants and Children (WIC). Pregnant and lactating women, certified by health professionals as meeting nutritional risk and low-income criteria, receive supplemental foods to ensure availability of a quart of milk, an egg, a serving of iron-fortified cereal, and a serving of vitamin C–rich fruit juice each day. These

## Table 11-9
### DAILY FOOD GUIDE*

| Food Group | Minimum Number of Servings Recommended During Pregnancy |
|---|---|
| Milk and milk products | 4 |
| Meat, fish, poultry, eggs, dried beans, peas and lentils | 4 |
| Leafy green vegetables | 1-2 |
| Vitamin C source | 1 |
| Other fruits and/or vegetables | 1-2 |
| Whole grain or enriched breads and cereals | 3 |

* The Recommended Dietary Allowance (RDA) for calories is not meant to be achieved by this food guide.

foods provide useful nutrient-dense foods supplemental to a basic nutritious diet, but assume the woman has access to the other components of a nutritionally adequate diet, including needed sources of calories and protein. Women in need of basic food and financial assistance must be referred to the official social services or human service agency administering public assistance (e.g., Aid to Families with Dependent Children) and advised on how to apply for food stamps. For emergency food, many communities now have food banks. Private agencies, such as the Salvation Army and many churches and missions, also provide emergency food or meals.

Another useful community resource is the Expanded Food and Nutrition Education Program of the Cooperative Extension Service. Trained program aides, supervised by a professional home economist, assist young mothers in their homes in learning more about meal planning, food purchasing and preparation, and management of their food budget and food stamps.

The nutritional assessment identifies malnutrition and nutritional risk factors and provides the data for ongoing nutritional care and monitoring during pregnancy and lactation. Nutritional intervention should be provided as indicated. Follow-up, support, and evaluation of the outcome of nutritional care must be provided by the physician and nurse and should include referral to the registered dietitian or public health nutritionist and appropriate community resources. To be effective, nutrition services must accommodate the patient's financial and general living situation, as well as be accessible and individualized. For middle- and upper-income women, the emphasis is on nutritional assessment and nutrition education, with in-depth diet counseling for those identified as at high nutritional risk because of complicating medical or emotional problems or lack of knowledge. For low-income women, an added risk is inability to purchase recommended foods. For these women, assistance in obtaining nutritious food and providing money for food is an urgent component of nutritional intervention.

### Acknowledgment

Acknowledgment is given to Mildred Kaufman, RD, MS, for her contribution to the first edition.

## References and Recommended Reading

Abrams BF, Laros RK: Prepregnancy weight, weight gain, and birth weight. Am J Obstet Gynecol 154:503, 1986.

ACOG (American College of Obstetricians and Gynecologists): Nutrition in Maternal Health Care. Chicago, 1974.

ACOG (American College of Obstetricians and Gynecologists) and The American Dietetic Association: Assessment of Maternal Nutrition. Chicago, The American College of Obstetricians and Gynecologists.

Anderson JW: Fiber, carbohydrates, and diabetes. Nutrition and the MD 7:1, 1981.

Anderson JW, Ward K: High carbohydrate, high fiber diets for insulin-treated men with diabetes mellitus. Am J Clin Nutr 32:2312, 1975

Barnes FEF (ed): Ambulatory Maternal Health Care and Family Planning Services, Policies, Principles, Practices. Washington, DC, American Public Health Association, 1978.

Burrow GN, Ferris TF: Medical Complications During Pregnancy, 2nd ed. Philadelphia, WB Saunders Co. 1982.

California Department of Health: Nutrition During Pregnancy and Lactation. Sacramento, CA, California State Department of Public Health, 1975.

Christakis, G. (ed): Nutritional Assessment in Health Programs. Washington, DC. American Public Health Association, 1973.

Cochrane WA: Symposium on nutrition: overnutrition in prenatal and neonatal life: a problem? Can Med Assoc J 93:893, 1965.

Committee on Nutritional Status During Pregnancy and Lactation. Washington, DC, Food and Nutrition Board, Institute of Medicine, National Academy Press, 1990.

Couston DR, Berkowitz RL, Hobbins JL: Higher metabolic control of overt diabetes mellitus in pregnancy. Am J Med 68:895, 1980.

Davies NT, Williams RB: Zinc balance during pregnancy and lactation. Am J Clin Nutr 30:300, 1977.

Dent CE: Relationship of biochemical abnormality to development of mental defect in PKU. Report of 23rd Ross Conference, Columbus, OH, 1957.

Dietary Guidelines for Americans. Home and Garden Bulletin No 232, US Department of Agriculture, US Department of Health and Human Services. Washington, DC: Government Printing Office, 1990.

Eastman NJ, Jackson E: Weight relationships in pregnancy. Obstet Gynecol Surv 23:1003, 1968.

Fenton V, Cavill I, Fisher J: Iron stores in pregnancy. Br J Haematol 37:145, 1977.

Fuhrmann K, Reiber H, Semmler K, et al: Prevention of congenital malformation in infants of insulin-dependent diabetic mothers. Diabetes Care 6:219–223, 1983.

Gabbe SG: Optional diabetes control. Contemp Obstet Gynecol 18:105, 1981.

Garden AN: Nutritional Management of High Risk Pregnancy. Reference Manual, Berkeley, CA, Society for Nutrition Education, 1981.

Ghadimi H, Pecora P: Free amino acids of cord plasma as compared with maternal plasma during pregnancy. Pediatrics 33:500, 1964.

Gitlin D: Protein transport across the placenta and protein turnover between amniotic fluid and maternal and fetal circulations. *In* Moghissi KS, Hafez

ESE (eds): The Placenta: Biological and Clinical Aspects. Springfield, IL, Charles C Thomas, 1974, pp 151–191.

Greene GW, Smiciklas-Wright H, Scholl TO, Karp RJ: Postpartum weight change: how much of the weight gained in pregnancy will be lost after delivery? Obstet Gynecol 71:701–707, 1988.

Herbert V: Experimental nutritional folate deficiency in man. Trans Assoc Am Phys 75:307, 1962.

Herbert WNP, Seeds JW, Bowes WA, Sweeney CA: Fetal growth response to total parenteral nutrition in pregnancy. J Reprod Med 31:263–266, 1986.

Hytten RE, Leitch I: The Physiology of Human Pregnancy, 2nd ed. Oxford, Blackwell Scientific, 1971.

Ingardia RJ, Fischer JR: Pregnancy after jejunoileal bypass and the SGA infant. Obstet Gynecol 52:215, 1978.

Johnstone FD, Campbell DM, MacGillivray I: Nitrogen balance studies in human pregnancy. J Nutr III:1884, 1981.

Joint FAO/WHO Ad Hoc Expert Committee: Energy and Protein Requirements. Geneva, WHO, 1973.

Jovanovic L, Peterson CM: Management of pregnancy, insulin-dependent diabetic woman. Diabetes Care 3.63, 1980.

Kelly AM, MacDonald DJ, McDougall AN: Observations on maternal and fetal ferritin concentrations at term. Br J Obstet Gynaecol 85:338, 1978.

Kitay DZ: Folic acid deficiency in pregnancy. Am J Obstet Gynecol 104:1067, 1969.

Kitay DZ: Anemia. In Queenan JT (ed): Management of High Risk Pregnancy. Oradell, NJ, Medical Economics Co, 1980, Chapter 28.

Kitzmiller JL, Gavin LA, Gin GD, et al: Preconception care of diabetes: glycemic control prevents congenital anomalies. JAMA 265(6): 731–736, 1991.

Lawrence RA: Breastfeeding: A Guide to the Medical Professional. St. Louis, CV Mosby, 1989.

Leader A, Wong KH, Deitel M: Maternal nutrition in pregnancy. Part I: A review. CMA Journal 125:545, 1981.

Lenke RR, Levy HL: Maternal phenylketonuria—result of dietary therapy. Am J Obstet Gynecol 142:548, 1982.

Mandel HG: Fat-soluble vitamins. In Goodman LS, Gilman A (eds): The Pharmacological Basis of Therapeutics, 5th ed. New York, Macmillan, 1975, p 1574.

Martin R, Trubow M, Bistrian BR, et al: Hyperalimentation during pregnancy: a case report. JPEN 9:212, 1985.

McFee JG: Iron metabolism and iron deficiency during pregnancy. Clin Obstet Gynecol 22:800, 1979.

Moghissi KS: Maternal nutrition in pregnancy. Clin Obstet Gynecol 21:297, 1978.

Naeye RL: Weight gain and the outcome of pregnancy. Am J Obstet Gynecol 121:724, 1978.

National Academy of Sciences: Recommended Dietary Allowances. Washington, DC, 1989.

O'Sullivan JB, Mahan CM: Criteria for the oral glucose tolerance test in pregnancy. Diabetes 13:278, 1964.

O'Sullivan JB, Mahan CM, Charles D, et al: Screening criteria for high-risk gestational diabetic patients. Am J Obstet Gynecol 116:895, 1973.

Pitkin RM: Nutritional support in obstetrics and gynecology. Clin Obstet Gynecol 19:489, 1976.

Pritchard JA, MacDonald PC (eds): Williams Obstetrics, 16th ed. New York, Appleton-Century-Crofts, 1980.

Pritchard JA, Scott DE: Iron demands during pregnancy. Iron deficiency–pathogenesis–clinical aspects–therapy. New York, Academic Press, 1970, p 173.

Rosso P: Nutritional factors affecting intrauterine growth and development. In American Society for Parenteral and Enteral Nutrition: Syllabus: Nutrition for Growth and Development. Chicago, 1980, pp 61–66.

Steel JM, Johnstone FD, Smith AF: Five years experience of a "pre-pregnancy" clinic for insulin-dependent diabetics. Br Med J 285:353–358, 1982.

Villar J, Belizán JM: Calcium during pregnancy. Clin Nutr 5(2):55–62, 1986.

Vong KH, Leader A, Dutel M: Maternal nutrition in pregnancy. Part II: Previous gastrointestinal operation and bowel disorder. CMA Journal 125:550, 1981.

Williams SR: Nutritional therapy in special conditions of pregnancy. In Worthington-Roberts B, Williams SR (eds): Nutrition in Pregnancy and Lactation. St. Louis, CV Mosby Co, 1989.

Worthington-Roberts BS, Williams SR (ed): Nutrition in Pregnancy and Lactation. St. Louis, CV Mosby Co, 1989.

# CHAPTER 12

# Placental Pathology

Trevor Macpherson

The placenta is functionally a maternal-placental-fetal unit dependent on the integrity of separate but interactive components. The maternal component results in the efficient delivery of blood to and from the intervillous space via uteroplacental vessels that undergo physiologic changes unique to pregnancy. The placenta contributes to the development, maturation, and function of the chorionic villous tree to permit optimal exchange between the intervillous space and the fetal circulation across the terminal villi. The fetus contributes to the delivery of fetal blood to and from the villous tree via the large chorionic plate vessels and the umbilical cord.

This section presents indications for placental examination and placental disorders that are important to look for when perinatal outcome is poor. Discussion of the placental pathology considers disorders of placentation, maternal blood supply, the villous tree, fetal placental blood flow, umbilical cord and membranes, and multiple pregnancy. The focus is on the macroscopic appearance of abnormalities, maternal associations, and perinatal outcome.

## Placental Examination

It is not necessary nor is it practical for every placenta to be examined for pathology, but in the circumstances listed in Table 12–1, it is essential to the full evaluation of these maternal or fetal events. The decision to submit the placenta for examination is based on the clinical indications listed in Ta-

ble 12–1 and careful gross examination of the placenta in the delivery room to identify those abnormalities readily identified in this manner. Along with observation, it is important to palpate the placenta for firm nodules that require section and further evaluation.

## GROSS EXAMINATION

### Fetal Membranes

The examination of the placenta begins by restoring the membranes to their intrauterine relationships and identifying the maternal and fetal surfaces. The umbilical cord insertion and the fetal membranes identify the fetal surface, and the site of rupture of the membranes usually locates the portion of membranes overlying the cervical os in a vaginal delivery. The membranes not covering the placental disc are examined for opacity, discoloration, incompleteness, attachment at the placental margin for placenta extrachorialis (placental disc extending beyond the rim of membrane attachment), exposed fetal vessels in the membranes that might result in vasa praevia, and wartlike nodules of amnion nodosum.

### Umbilical Cord

The cord length and diameter are measured; the number of vessels is determined; and the cord is examined for constriction, knot, hematoma, edema, torsion, velamentous insertion, and discoloration. When determining the number of vessels, the cord must be examined at least 5 cm from its in-

**Table 12–1**

INDICATIONS FOR PLACENTAL EXAMINATION
BY PATHOLOGY

Perinatal death
Preterm delivery (less than 37 weeks' gestation)
Fetal growth deviation
  Intrauterine growth retardation
  Macrosomia
Perinatal asphyxia
Maternal hemorrhage
  Placenta previa
  Abruption
Hydrops fetalis
Post-term pregnancy
Infection
Multiple pregnancy for
  Vascular anastomoses for transfusion syndrome
  Placental growth discordance
  Chorionicity
Amniotic fluid deviations
  Polyhydramnios
  Oligohydramnios
Congenital anomalies of fetus
Maternal disease
  Pregnancy induced hypertension
  Essential hypertension
  Diabetes mellitus
  Collagen disease
Placental weight deviation

the placenta to detect firm areas not seen by observation of the maternal surface alone.

## Indications for Placental Examination

Table 12–1 lists the indications for placental examination by pathology that apply at Magee-Womens Hospital. Table 12–2 summarizes the important placental and cord lesions that may contribute to perinatal morbidity and mortality. Several comprehensive texts and chapters are available by various authors (Beaconsfield and Birowood, 1982; Benirschke and Kaufmann, 1990a; Chard, 1986; Fox, 1978; Fox, 1987; Gersell et al, 1987; Kohler, 1987; Macpherson and Szulman, 1990; Naeye and Tafari, 1983; Perrin, 1984; Pratola and Wilkin, 1985; Ramsey, 1987; Rushton,

sertion into the placenta, because umbilical arteries may branch close to the placenta. Cord length charts by gestational age have been published (Naeye, 1985a).

## Placental Disc

**Fetal Surface.** The placenta is best weighed with cord and membranes trimmed around the disc. The fetal surface is normally of steel-blue shiny appearance and is examined for meconium staining, opacity, and yellow discoloration of chorioamnionitis; warty nodules of amnion nodosum associated with oligohydramnios; thrombosis of fetal vessels; amniotic bands or missing amnion; subamniotic hemorrhage; and subchorionic hematoma. The yolk sac remnant is noted as a small yellow-white oval nodule about 0.3 cm at its widest point. Firm, yellow plaques of subchorionic fibrin may be seen.

**Maternal Surface.** This surface is normally tan, without any obvious lesions. It is abnormal when it is pale, has adherent blood clot, or has depressed areas caused by a removed blood clot. Calcification is often present as white flecks. Infarcts are recognized as firm red (recent) or yellow (old) lesions, the extent of which must be determined by section of the placenta. It is essential to palpate

**Table 12–2**

PLACENTAL AND CORD LESIONS THAT MAY
CONTRIBUTE TO PERINATAL MORBIDITY
AND MORTALITY

| **Placenta** |
| --- |
| ***Disorders of Maternal Vasculature*** |
| Infarction |
| Retroplacental hematoma |
| Maternal floor infarction |
| ***Inflammatory Lesions*** |
| Infection (chorioamnionitis/villitis) |
| ***Disorders of Placentation*** |
| Placenta accreta |
| Placenta membranacea |
| Circumvallate placenta |
| Placenta previa |
| Vasa praevia |
| ***Villous Abnormalities*** |
| Delayed villous maturity |
| Chronic villitis of unknown etiology |
| Villous edema |
| ***Fetoplacental Vessels*** |
| Fetal artery thrombosis (severe) |
| Intervillous thrombus |
| ***Miscellaneous*** |
| Twin-to-twin transfusion syndrome |
| Amnion nodosum |
| Early amnion rupture |
| **Cord** |
| Knot |
| Torsion |
| Constriction |
| Hematoma |
| Velamentous insertion |
| Funisitis |
| Short cord |
| Long cord |
| Single umbilical artery |
| Cord rupture |
| Cord entanglement |

1991; Russell, 1987). The pathologist plays a key role in recognizing these lesions, including the time during pregnancy that they exert their influence (Macpherson, 1985; Macpherson et al, 1986; Naeye, 1977a, Naeye, 1986; Naeye, 1987b; Naeye and Peters, 1987; Niswander et al, 1984).

# General and Developmental Features

## ABNORMAL PLACENTATION

Several abnormalities of placentation have maternal and fetal consequences, including antepartum and postpartum hemorrhage, preterm delivery, fetal hemorrhage, and compression of exposed fetal vessels. (Fox, 1978; Fox, 1987). The extent of maternal antepartum bleeding determines the fetal risk, although low birth weight is related to the still poorly understood effects of certain placentation disorders on fetal growth. With *placenta membranacea* (Fig. 12–1), the entire fetal membranes are covered with villous tissue to form a very thin (0.5 cm) placenta. Complications include placenta previa, which is inevitable because the placenta covers all of the membrane, antepartum hemorrhage, postpartum hemorrhage, preterm delivery,

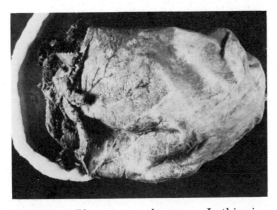

**Figure 12–1.** Placenta membranacea. In this view of the placenta from the fetal surface note that villi cover the entire gestational sac. The delivery of the infant occurred through villous tissue. (Used with permission from Macpherson TA, Szulman AE: The placenta and products of conception. *In* Silverberg SB (ed): Principles and Practice of Surgical Pathology, 2nd ed. New York, Churchill Livingstone, 1990.)

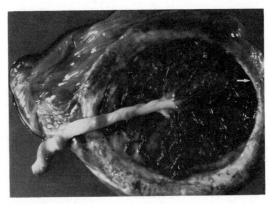

**Figure 12–2.** Circumvallate placenta. In this view of the placenta from the fetal surface, the ridge of membranes formed at the point of attachment to the chorionic plate is seen (*arrow*). The fetal membranes are attached around the placental disc inside rather than at the edge of the chorionic plate of the placental disc.

low birth weight, and increased perinatal mortality (Janovski and Granowitz, 1961; Pryse-Davies et al, 1973).

In *placenta extrachorialis,* the chorionic plate is smaller than the basal plate, which results in an exposed ridge of villous tissue around the edge of the placenta. The two variants of placenta extrachorialis are placenta circummarginata, with a flat rim of membrane attachment, and placenta circumvallata (Fig. 12–2), with a folded back ridge of membranes. These entities occur in partial and complete forms, with the complete circumvallate variant being complicated by antepartum hemorrhage, preterm delivery, and low birth weight. The extent of these complications determines the influence on perinatal outcome (Benson and Fujikura, 1969; Fox and Sen, 1972; Scott, 1960; Torpin, 1966). In *accessory* and *multilobed placentation,* fetal risk is from fetal hemorrhage caused by vasa praevia or fetal vessel compression caused by fetal parts; in these conditions, evidence of fetal hemorrhage should be sought (Fujikura et al, 1970; Torpin and Hart, 1941). The *ring-shaped* placenta has a central absence of villous tissue that may be interpreted as a missing portion. *Placenta previa* is a clinical condition without distinct morphologic features after delivery. In some instances, associated retroplacental hematoma occurs. *Placenta accreta* is important because it may cause retained placenta, uterine inversion, or postpartum bleeding, and it may require a hysterectomy. It is a difficult diagnosis to make with certainty in the absence of a hysterectomy. The clinical features of placenta accreta have been well described by Fox's review of 622 cases (Fox, 1972; Fox, 1978). Patients with a previous cesarean section are at risk for this condition. Placenta extrachorialis is the only abnormality that occurs with any degree of frequency, but all are readily recognized at delivery on gross examination of the placenta.

## PLACENTAL WEIGHT

Placental weight percentile graphs have been developed according to race and gestational age (Naeye, 1987a). Measurement of accurate weight is only possible after removal of the umbilical cord, membranes, and adherent blood clot. Retained fetal blood volume ranges from 25 to 270 g, even with maximal cord drainage (Garrow and Howes, 1971), whereas weight loss of the stored fresh placenta after delivery is from 4 percent in 12 hours to 10 percent after 48 hours (Lemtis and Hadrich, 1974), and these features are considered by some to render placental weight values invalid (Fox, 1978). However, despite these variables, placental weight does have certain clinical and morphologic associations. Low placental weight may occur with pregnancy-induced hypertension, essential hypertension, and congenital anomalies, whereas heavy placentas are more common with extensive villous edema, diabetes mellitus, hydrops fetalis, severe maternal anemia, fetal anemia, and blood clot caused by intervillous thrombus or subchorionic bleeding. Extremes of abnormal placental weights serve, therefore, to alert the pathologist to seek an explanation from several maternal or morphologic associations. The fetoplacental ratio may provide additional information in evaluating placental weight (Molteni et al, 1978).

---

# Lesions Involving Maternal Uteroplacental Vasculature

Adequate maternal blood flow into the intervillous space is essential for normal placental function and fetal well-being. The establishment and maintenance of this flow is dependent on the establishment of dilated funnel-shaped intradecidual and intramyometrial segments of the maternal spiral arteries. This physiologic change is induced by intravascular cytotrophoblast invasion of the intradecidual (early first wave) and then intramyometrial (second wave at 14th to 20th week) portions of the maternal spiral arteries (Brosens et al, 1967; Sheppard and Bonnar, 1974, Sheppard and Bonnar, 1976). It is now well established that the second wave of intravascular cytotrophoblast invasion does not occur in patients who will develop preeclampsia (Brosens and Renaer, 1972; DeWolf et al, 1980; Robertson et al, 1975; Sheppard and Bonnar, 1976). When this physiologic change is incomplete, the absence of the funnel-shaped, dilated spiral arteries results in what can now be termed maternal uteroplacental vascular insufficiency—that is, reduced perfusion of the intervillous space by maternal blood. This change is not an all-or-nothing phenomenon but occurs to varying degrees in these vessels. This term should replace the term placental insufficiency because, in many instances, the placenta responds to reduced intervillous flow by increasing its efficiency via accelerated villous maturation. It is important to appreciate that the pathology of the maternal vessels cannot be accurately evaluated in vessels of the decidua vera, that portion normally available for examination in the separated placenta. Placental site biopsy tissue is required to accurately study the physiology and pathology of these important maternal vessels. This procedure is generally not performed except, for example, at cesarean section when intrauterine growth retardation is present.

Disorders recognized on the maternal side of the placenta include infarction, retroplacental hematoma, marginal hematoma, and maternal floor infarction.

## INFARCTION

Infarction (Fig. 12–3) is the most easily recognized lesion that results from maternal uteroplacental vascular insufficiency with narrowing and occlusion of maternal vessels. Infarctions are seen grossly on the maternal and cut surface as clearly defined firm nodules, being dark red when recent and brown-yellow through white when old. The nature

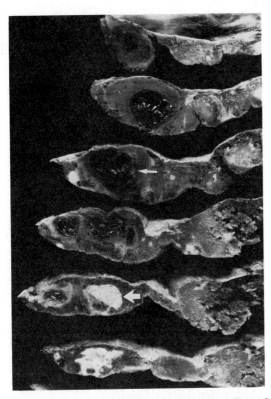

**Figure 12–3.** Infarction. This cross-section view of the placenta with the fetal surface along the top shows multiple infarcts of both recent (*small arrow*) and old (*large arrow*) origin. These lesions are present not only at the placental margin but also more centrally as indicated on the right of this section.

and extent of infarction is only determined by cross section of the entire placenta. The extent of infarction should be expressed as a percentage of the placental volume. Infarcts occur in about 25 percent of uncomplicated pregnancies but are most common in pregnancy-induced hypertension (34 to 60 percent), essential hypertension (27 to 70 percent), and systemic lupus erythematosus (Baramowsky et al, 1980; Fox, 1967a; Fox, 1978; Fox, 1987; Naeye and Tafarin, 1983; Wentworth, 1967). The extent of infarction often correlates with the severity of the maternal disorder for preeclampsia and essential hypertension, but severe placental can occur when lupus erythematosus is not severe in the mother. In fact, extensive infarction in the absence of hypertension should alert the clinician to the possibility of lupus erythematosus in the mother. Infarcts represent the most severely compromised regions of a placenta that has an overall reduction of in-

tervillous blood supply. Therefore, as little as 5 to 10 percent of centrally located placenta infarction is associated with an increase in perinatal mortality and morbidity, including intrauterine growth retardation, fetal hypoxia, intrauterine fetal death, and neonatal mortality and morbidity (Naeye, 1977b; Wigglesworth, 1964). In the Collaborative Perinatal Study (CPS) of the National Institute of Neurological and Communicative Disorders and Stroke, true infarction was responsible for 2.4 stillbirths/1000 births (Naeye, 1977b).

## RETROPLACENTAL HEMATOMA

Retroplacental hematoma (Fig. 12–4), clinically often presenting as abruptio placentae (Gruenwald et al, 1968), is easily recognized on the maternal surface as an adherent blood clot causing compression of adjacent villi, sometimes with resultant infarction. Early lesions cause decidual necrosis, giving the decidua a red color. Cross section shows significant compression of villi, indicating that the extent of placental compromise is greater than the surface percentage alone. Like infarction, retroplacental hematoma should be expressed as a percentage of placental volume. Retroplacental hematoma occurs in about 4.4 percent of pregnancies but is increased threefold in patients with preeclampsia (Fox, 1978), whereas those with Hemorrhage, Elevated Liver enzymes and Low Platelets (HELLP) syndrome have an incidence as high as 20 percent (Sibai et al, 1986). In one third of the cases, a retroplacental hematoma occurs in the absence of the clinical signs and symptoms of

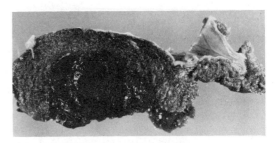

**Figure 12–4.** Retroplacental hematoma. This cross section of the placenta with the fetal surface along the top shows a large retroplacental hematoma, which compresses the adjacent rim of placenta tissue.

abruption; the reverse is also true (Fox, 1978). Maternal smoking, advanced maternal age, acute chorioamnionitis, and cocaine abuse are associated with retroplacental hematoma (Acker et al, 1983; Chasnoff et al, 1985; Paterson, 1979). Other recognized but rare causes include trauma, amniocentesis, hydramnios, systemic lupus erythematosus, and sudden decompression of the uterus (Naeye, 1987b, Naeye et al, 1979). In a large study from Sweden involving 894,619 births over 9 years, multiple pregnancy, male infants, maternal age less than 20 years, and three or more pregnancies were associated with an increased incidence (Karegard and Gennser, 1986).

Adverse perinatal outcome with retroplacental hematoma correlates with the size of the lesion and the severity of accompanying disorders such as preeclampsia, systemic lupus erythematosus, and infarction. Perinatal mortality is increased by retroplacental hematoma, with a perinatal mortality rate of 3.9/1000 births in the CPS (Karegard and Gennser, 1986; Naeye et al, 1979, Naeye et al, 1977). At Magee-Womens Hospital, it is the third most common cause of perinatal mortality, accounting for 8 percent of perinatal deaths, a percentage similar to the study from Sweden (8.6 percent) (Karegard and Gennser, 1986). In this latter study, the perinatal mortality rate from retroplacental hematoma was 20.2 percent. Along with fetal hypoxia caused by placental separation, the association of preterm delivery with retroplacental hematoma also contributes to poor perinatal outcome. In addition, maternal risk is higher from an increased cesarean section rate (74.6 percent in the Swedish study) and disseminated intravascular coagulation in severe cases (Karegard and Gennser, 1986).

## MARGINAL HEMATOMA

Apart from causing antepartum hemorrhage, this lesion is of little clinical significance because it does not cause compression or a significant loss of functioning placental tissue. It occurs most frequently in low-lying placentas, when the placental disc margin is less than 10 cm from the internal cervical os (Fox, 1978; Pratola and Wilkin, 1985).

## MATERNAL FLOOR INFARCTION

This lesion was recognized in 1970 (Benirschke, 1990b) and occurred in 0.5 percent of placentas in the CPS with 17 percent of the fetuses being stillborn for a perinatal mortality rate of 0.8 stillbirths/1000 births (Naeye 1985b, Naeye, 1987b). The term infarct, here, is misleading because maternal floor infarction is not a true infarct but a heavy deposition of fibrin along the decidual plate with associated atrophy of the entrapped villi. Maternal floor infarction can recur in subsequent pregnancies. It is a cause of recurrent early and late pregnancy loss and intrauterine growth retardation, and may be associated with an elevated maternal serum alphafeto protein level (Clewell and Manchester, 1983; Katz et al, 1987; Nickel, 1988); its etiology is uncertain.

# Miscellaneous Lesions of Maternal Origin

## PERIVILLOUS FIBRIN DEPOSITION

Perivillous fibrin deposition (Fig. 12–5) in the intervillous space is present in up to 22 percent of term placentas and is reduced in preterm deliveries, preeclampsia, essential hypertension (12 percent), and diabetes mellitus (6 percent) (Fox, 1967b; Fox, 1978; 1987; Moe, 1969). There is no pregnancy factor associated with an increased incidence of this lesion. Recognized as a plaquelike, usually peripheral, often hard, characteristically mottled lesion with a brown-yellow color, it has an ill-defined border that distinguishes it from an infarct. Associated fibrin and normal villous tissue account for the mottled appearance and indistinct border. The reduced incidence of perivillous fibrin deposition in hypertension indicates that it is not due to reduced maternal blood flow into the intervillous space but rather increased flow with resultant turbulence, eddies, stasis, and thrombosis. Perivillous fibrin deposition usually does not contribute to poor perinatal outcome unless it renders more than 40 percent of the placenta nonfunctional.

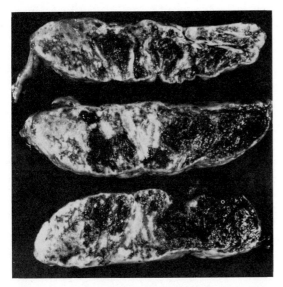

**Figure 12–5.** Perivillous fibrin deposition. This cross section of the placenta with the fetal surface along the top of the upper two and bottom of the lower section shows the placental parenchyma with the mottled irregular diffuse distribution of perivillous fibrin deposition (white areas) most prominent at the placental edge.

## SUBCHORIONIC FIBRIN DEPOSITION (PLAQUES)

These triangular plaques are noted on the fetal surface as firm nodules and are sometimes associated with progressive fresh thrombus. Subchorionic fibrin deposition is considered to have the same cause as perivillous fibrin deposition but in a different location, without entrapment of significant proportions of chorionic villi. It is of no known clinical significance (Fox, 1978; Fox, 1987).

## MASSIVE SUBCHORIONIC THROMBUS (BREUS' MOLE)

This laminated thrombus beneath the chorionic plate does not contain villi and is believed to consist of maternal blood. It is sometimes extensive and may form a transplacental thrombus (sometimes known as Breus' mole) (Fig. 12–6). It is now considered a possible cause rather than result of fetal death and abortion, as demonstrated by its occurrence in liveborn infants (Shanklin and Scott, 1975). The cause of the maternal bleeding is not known, although maternal venous obstruction from the intervillous space has been suggested. The mechanism of perinatal loss is unknown (Hart, 1902). Preterm delivery is a common association, but no definite conclusion is possible on the contribution of this lesion to perinatal mortality (Fox, 1978).

## SEPTAL CYSTS AND CALCIFICATION

Septal cysts are commonly associated with diabetes mellitus and rhesus disease and are often striking when the placenta is cross sectioned. These septal cysts are not associated with poor perinatal outcome. Calcification is rarely seen prior to 32 weeks' gestation and does not contribute to poor perinatal outcome.

---

# Disorders of Fetoplacental Circulation

## INTERVILLOUS THROMBUS

Defined as a villous-free nodular focus of coagulated blood in the intervillous space, these multiple, usually small, laminated lesions are a mixture of fetal and maternal blood (Devi et al, 1968; Kaplan et al, 1982) and are notable for their association with

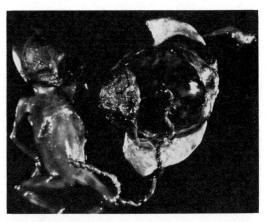

**Figure 12–6.** Breus' mole. This macerated congested fetus is attached to a placenta with a large subchorionic hematoma (Breus' mole) occupying a large portion of the placenta.

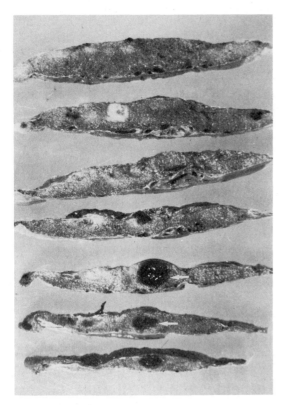

**Figure 12–7.** Intervillous thrombus. This cross section of the placenta with the fetal surface along the top shows several distinct circumscribed recent intervillous thrombi (*arrows*). A few old infarcts are also noted (white areas).

rhesus disease and possible increased incidence in preeclampsia and ABO incompatibility (Batcup et al, 1983). Sometimes detected as a soft nodule on palpation, intervillous thrombi are seen on a section of the placenta as either small mulberry-like lesions, when fresh (Fig. 12–7), or as organized laminated thrombi, when older. They indicate fetomaternal hemorrhage, which occurs in small amounts in 15 to 30 percent of women during pregnancy (Fox, 1978; Wentworth, 1964). Because most of these lesions are small, their clinical significance is not clear and they are not known to be associated with any adverse perinatal outcome.

## SUBAMNIOTIC HEMATOMA

Subamniotic hematoma is usually a fresh lesion seen on the fetal surface and is caused by bleeding from cord traction (Fox, 1978). Organized lesions have been described in association with low birth weight but these

findings are not widely accepted and, thus, this lesion is not a factor in perinatal outcome (DeSa, 1971).

## FETAL ARTERY THROMBOSIS

Thrombosed chorionic plate vessels (Fig. 12–8) are recognized on the fetal surface as firm, distended arteries that are superficial to the veins. Thrombus is easily seen on section of the vessel and occurs in about 4.5 to 10 percent of term placentas, with an increased incidence in diabetes mellitus (Driscoll, 1965; Fox, 1966). Thrombus results in a distinct, well-demarcated triangular pale zone of placental parenchyma of normal spongy appear-

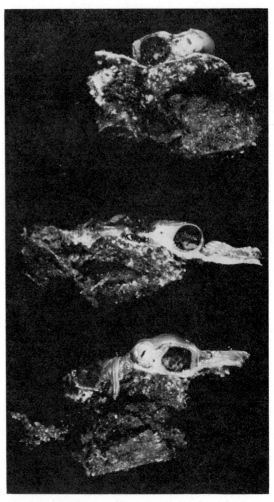

**Figure 12–8.** Fetal artery thrombus. This cross section of the placenta with the fetal surface along the top shows an organized fetal vessel thrombus distending a chorionic plate vessel.

ance and consistency, recognized only on section of the placenta. The pale appearance is a result of absence of fetal blood in villi with villous stromal fibrosis and increase in syncytial knots recognized microscopically in older lesions. In the absence of other pathology, 50 percent or more of the villi must be involved to be clinically significant. This extent of involvement can occur but is very rare (Fox, 1986). The cause of this lesion is not established.

# Histological Abnormalities of Chorionic Villi

Fox (1987) has developed an approach to villous changes described as abnormalities of villous maturation and differentiation, changes secondary to reduced maternal uteroplacental blood flow, changes secondary to reduced fetal villous blood flow, and abnormalities of uncertain pathogenesis. The examination of most of these conditions is more appropriate to a pathology text, and only villous maturation, villitis, villous edema, and hemorrhagic endovasculitis are discussed in this chapter.

## VILLOUS MATURATION AND DIFFERENTIATION

Normal villous maturation proceeds from stem villi (first trimester) to intermediate villi (second trimester) through terminal villi (30 weeks' gestation to term) (Kaufmann et al, 1979). This maturation results in an increased villous surface area—up to sixfold, between 20 and 40 weeks (Aherne, 1975)—by a reduction in villous size, a decrease in villous stromal density, and an approximation of fetal vessels to the intervillous space. This approximation of fetal and maternal compartments is essential for exchange of nutrients between mother and fetus. Accelerated maturation is associated with pregnancy-induced hypertension and essential hypertension, and placental weight is often low in these cases. Maternal smoking has been associated with accelerated maturation by ultrasound criteria (Pinette et al, 1989).

## DELAYED VILLOUS MATURATION

Delayed villous maturation, referred to as villous immaturity or dysmaturity, results in chorionic villi that are large for gestational age, with increased stromal density and paucity of fetal vessels close to the intervillous space at the periphery of the villi. It is associated with diabetes mellitus, rhesus disease, maternal severe anemia, congenital syphilis, and congenital anomalies of the fetus (Fox, 1978) and occurs in the absence of any maternal disorder. It has a decreased incidence in preeclampsia and essential hypertension. When the delayed maturation involves almost all villi, it is associated with a high incidence of fetal hypoxia and growth retardation (Becker, 1975). These adverse effects on the fetus are not seen in all instances, which makes interpretation difficult in individual cases. The etiology of delayed villous maturity is not known. At Magee-Womens Hospital, delayed villous maturity is the only abnormal feature noted in some fresh stillbirths at or near term and must be considered an important factor in perinatal morbidity and mortality; in particular, this condition should be sought in the placenta from late unexpected fresh stillbirths.

## CHRONIC VILLITIS

Chronic villitis is associated with hematogenous infections predominantly of viral etiology, with fetal outcome dependent on the extent of villous damage and fetal infection (Altschuler and Russell, 1975; Fox, 1981; Russell, 1987; Russell, 1979; Russell and Altschuler, 1974; Russell et al, 1980). Most cases of chronic villitis, however, are not due to infection but to "villitis of unknown etiology" (Knox and Fox, 1984; Russell et al, 1980). This lesion has been classified into various histologic types, and fetal outcome is dependent on the extent of villous damage, with more than 30 percent of villi being destroyed before the perinatal mortality rate is increased (Russell, 1980). The prevalence of this villitis varies from 8 to 14 percent and is associated with an increased stillbirth rate and intrauterine growth retardation (Altschuler and Russell, 1975; Knox and Fox, 1984). In the CPS, stillbirth was three times more common when villitis was present and 63 percent more frequent than expected in neonates with body weights in or below the 10th percentile (Naeye and Tafari, 1983). Others have confirmed this increased rate of perinatal mortality (Althabe and Labarrere, 1985; Redline and Abramowsky, 1985; Russell, 1980).

Chronic villitis of unknown etiology occurs in association with preeclampsia and chronic hypertension, leading to speculation that immunologic mechanisms of the semiallograft of pregnancy may be etiologic factors (Labarrere and Althabe, 1986; Labarrere and Althabe, 1987). It also means that some cases that are called villitis may be ischemic lesions caused by reduced intervillous blood flow. This is further supported by seeing infarction and villitis in the same placenta. When intrauterine growth retardation is present, it may therefore be caused by this reduced uteroplacental blood flow rather than or in addition to the chronic villitis. Chronic villitis of unknown etiology is an important contributor to adverse perinatal outcome that can recur in a subsequent pregnancy (Labarrere and Althabe, 1987; Russell et al, 1980).

## ACUTE VILLITIS

Acute villitis is sometimes seen as part of acute infection and is caused by bacterial organisms (Russell, 1987). Apart from severe infections, it is rare to find this condition with chorioamnionitis. When acute villitis and intervillitis are seen, characteristically with microabscesses, *Listeria monocytogenes* infection should be suspected. The consequences of acute villitis are related to the degree of fetal infection rather than the acute villitis itself.

## VILLOUS EDEMA

Villous edema is associated with diabetes mellitus, rhesus incompatibility, preeclampsia, placental infections such as syphilis, toxoplasmosis, and cytomegalovirus, as well as with chorioangioma (Fox, 1978). There have been three studies of villous edema in the absence of the above-mentioned associations. Alvarez and colleagues (1972) performed a morphometric study on term placentas and showed reduction of the intervillous space. They concluded that higher

perinatal mortality might be caused by reduced maternal intervillous blood flow and compromised fetal oxygen supply. Naeye and associates (1983) examined placenta selected for pregnancy complications and found that edema was rare before 22 weeks' gestation and most frequent between 22 and 32 weeks' gestation; this condition decreased progressively thereafter. A strong correlation with chorioamnionitis and antenatal hypoxia in preterm infants and a high predictive value for neonatal deaths was found. Compression of villous capillaries by edema was postulated as causing fetal hypoxia by reducing fetoplacental blood flow. Shen-Schwarz and associates (1989) examined 1925 consecutive unselected singleton placentas and found an overall incidence of villous edema in 13 percent—an incidence of 25 percent in preterm placentas and 11 percent at term. Villous edema was generally more severe in preterm placentas. Villous edema was significant in term infants with increased fetal and neonatal death, but there was no association with chorioamnionitis. These authors concluded that it was difficult to distinguish the immature villi from villous edema, which might explain their different conclusions about preterm infants.

## HEMORRHAGIC ENDOVASCULITIS

Hemorrhagic endovasculitis was originally described by Sander (1980), who found an incidence of this lesion in 19 percent of selected placentas referred to the Michigan Placental Registry and who associated it with intrauterine fetal death (Sander et al, 1985). This compares with data from an unselected group of placentas, in which the condition was found in 13 of 1925 cases (0.6 percent) with minimal immediate clinical importance (Shen-Schwarz et al, 1988). Other reports have found this lesion increased in placentas from intrauterine fetal deaths (Rayburn et al, 1985; Rayburn et al, 1989). The demonstration that similar changes occur in placental tissue culture under hypoxic conditions raises the possibility that this lesion occurs after fetal death or as part of agonal events preceding fetal death (Silver et al, 1988). This feature is particularly relevant in interpreting reports of hemorrhagic endovasculitis, being the only placental abnormality found in the placenta of some stillbirths (Jaffe et al, 1985). It has been suggested that this lesion is caused by obstruction or cessation of fetal blood flow, with the wide spectrum of histologic changes dependent on whether the obstruction is primarily of arterial or venous origin. It is still not clear what causes hemorrhagic endovasculitis or what its role is in producing adverse perinatal outcome. Histologically, the lesion shows varying degrees of fetal vessel occlusion, with thrombi, fetal red cells throughout the vessel wall and in the villous stroma, and vascular endothelial proliferation. Surrounding villi usually show increased stromal density.

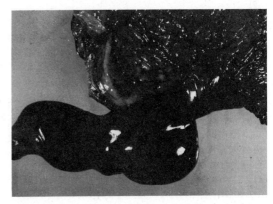

**Figure 12–9.** Umbilical cord hematoma. The fusiform umbilical cord hematoma is seen near the placental attachment.

## Umbilical Cord Abnormalities

The umbilical cord is the life line of the fetus, and several abnormalities and complications contribute to poor perinatal outcome. These include short cord, long cord, cord hematoma, cord knots, torsion, stricture, thrombus, insertion into the membranes, and single umbilical artery.

A *short cord* (≤ 32 cm) (Gardiner, 1922) can cause cord rupture or delay in delivery in the second stage of labor (Rayburn et al, 1981). In animal studies, reduced fetal movements result in a short cord (Moessinger et al, 1982) and the CPS showed that short cord doubled and even tripled the predictive value of low Apgar scores, several neonatal neurologic abnormalities, low IQ, and neurologic abnormalities in older children (Naeye, 1985a). Other rarer causes occur with abdominal wall defects (Grange et al, 1987).

A *long cord* (≥ 100 cm) is associated with true knots, cord compression from fetal entanglement, and cord prolapse (Rayburn et al, 1981). Knots and prolapse are particularly increased in monoamniotic monochorionic twins and with polyhydramnios (Naeye, 1987b).

*Cord hematoma* (Fig. 12–9) is a rare event that is claimed to cause fetal death either from blood loss or compression of cord vessels by confined hematoma (DeSa, 1984). This lesion is more common in late pregnancy. The origin of bleeding is usually venous, but arterial rupture does occur. Injection studies assist in determining the origin of bleeding (Macpherson, 1982). The etiology of this lesion and its exact mechanism of causing fetal death is uncertain.

*True cord knots* occur in less than 1 percent of placentas and may account for 8 to 11 percent of cases of perinatal mortality (Fox, 1978; Naeye, 1987b). Cord edema, thrombosis, grooving, and narrowing are morphologic changes that indicate the presence of knot tightness sufficient to cause obstruction to blood flow. Without these factors, the knot is incidental.

Cord *stricture* and *torsion* are rare but can cause fetal death and are generally seen within the first 3 cm of the fetal end of the cord (Ghosh et al, 1984; Gilbert and Zugibe, 1974). Amniotic bands are important to exclude.

*Thrombosis* of the cord is usually seen in association with other cord complications of cord knot, hematoma, torsion, stricture, or prolapse but can occur as an isolated event. There have been reports of cases that did not result in fetal death (Eggens and Bruinse, 1984; Hoag, 1986; Wolfman, 1983).

*Cord edema,* seen in diabetes mellitus, preterm delivery, and rhesus incompatibility, is of uncertain importance (Fox, 1978).

*Cord cysts* and *tumors* need to be large enough to compromise cord blood flow to be of significance, and such events are very rare (DeSa, 1984).

*Velamentous insertion* and *insertio funiculi furcate* cord insertion are the only two conditions with perinatal consequences. With velementous insertion, the fetal vessels are exposed in the membranes not attached to the placental disc; whereas in insertio funiculi furcate, the fetal vessels are exposed in membranes over the placental disc area between the end of the umbilical cord and the placental disc. In these instances, the cord is at risk for fetal hemorrhage or compression due to unprotected fetal vessels in the membranes.

*Single umbilical artery* is important because of its association with congenital anomalies in 50 percent of cases, although only half of these have major functional or cosmetic effects (Benirschke and Brown, 1955; Froehlich and Fijikwa, 1973; Froehlich and Fujikura, 1966; Soma, 1979). Anomalies are often multiple; and genitourinary, cardiovascular, musculoskeletal, central nervous system, and gastrointestinal anomalies are most frequent. A persistent vitelline artery, rather than an umbilical artery, is seen in cases of sirenomelia (Talamo et al, 1982). An association with caucasians, diabetes mellitus, maternal hypertension, and smoking has been reported (Froehlich and Fujikura, 1966). A single umbilical artery is, in and of itself, not a cause of fetal hypoxia.

# Placental Membranes

## CHORIOAMNIONITIS

Chorioamnionitis is the morphologic evidence that bacteria have gained access to the amniotic fluid; this is recognized grossly in advanced cases as opaque, dull yellow, sometimes malodorous membranes. In the early stages, the membranes may appear normal. Histologically, it is recognized by the presence of neutrophils infiltrating to varying degrees through the chorionic plate into the membranes. In the most advanced degree, the membranes are densely infiltrated throughout their full thickness by inflammatory cells. The most reliable site for diagnosis is the chorionic plate section of the placenta, which is taken where this plate is very thin and free of subchorial fibrin or blood clot. Inflammation may also be less accurately detected when squamous metaplasia is present. Acute chorioamnionitis is present in at least 20 percent of placentas and is associated with preterm labor, fetal and neonatal infection, and intrauterine hypoxia (Naeye and Peters, 1978a; Naeye and Ross, 1982; Naeye and Tafari, 1983).

Intrauterine (fetal and placental) infection occurs, in order of frequency, via ascending (transcervical), hematogenous (transplacental), external (transabdominal), or internal (transfallopian) routes (Blanc, 1981). Chorioamnionitis has received much attention in the literature and is not comprehensively reviewed here (Bejar et al, 1981; Blanc, 1981; Lauweryns et al, 1973; Miller et al, 1980; Naeye and Peters, 1978; Naeye and Ross, 1982; Pankuch et al, 1989; Russell, 1979) (see Chapters 7 and 21). Although fetal and neonatal infections such as pneumonia occur, the major contributors to perinatal morbidity and mortality are prematurity and antepartum hypoxia that leads to respiratory distress. An association of chorioamnionitis and abnormal fetal heart tracing has been reported. Fetal compromise was considered to be due to either the increased metabolic demands made on the fetus or from vasoconstriction of umbilical cord vessels from the accumulation of thromboxanes and prostaglandins in amniotic fluid (Salafia et al, 1989). This study, however, did not confirm fetal hypoxia with umbilical cord gas data.

Most cases of chorioamnionitis are caused by ascending bacterial infections that reach the amniotic fluid through the membranes adjacent to the cervical os (Blanc, 1981). In most cases, membranes are intact, and membrane rupture can no longer be considered to be a prerequisite for ascending infection, although the incidence of chorioamnionitis increases after 6 hours of membrane rupture. The bacteria isolated are generally normal inhabitants of the birth canal and elicit an inflammatory response seen in the membrane roll, chorionic plate, and umbilical cord (Blanc, 1981). There is some relationship between the duration of infection and the extent of neutrophil migration through the chorionic plate. In the first 24 to 48 hours, neutrophils marginate and adhere to the underside of the chorionic plate (stage 1), penetrate the plate in the next several days (stage 2), and eventually reach the amnion (stage 3) (Naeye, 1987b). The correlation with positive placental cultures and chorioamnionitis is high—70 percent—when sampling is adequate to accurately identify fastidious anaerobes (Naeye, 1987b).

The clinical significance of chorioamnionitis is not only the risk of fetal infection but, more importantly, associated prematurity and its consequences. The numerous organisms associated with chorioamnionitis result in prostaglandin production via the release of phospholipase A2 (Mitchell, 1986). Human fetal membranes and uterine decidua contain large amounts of esterified arachidonic acid, which represent about 20 percent of fatty acids in fetal membranes. Phospholipase A2 cleaves arachidonic acid from the structural lipids present in fetal membranes and decidua and initiates the prostaglandin cascade. This cascade is now considered to be one of the mechanisms initiating preterm labor.

Factors predisposing a woman to chorioamnionitis with intact membranes include reduced antimicrobial activity of amniotic fluid, which is markedly reduced in patients of low socioeconomic status (Pankuch et al, 1984). Premature rupture of membranes exposes the amniotic cavity to ascending infection, but the rupture itself might be initiated by chorioamnionitis due to weakening of membrane structure following membrane damage by inflammation (Naeye and Ross, 1982b, Naeye, 1987b).

A major hindrance in understanding and managing chorioamnionitis has been the lack of accurate detection prior to delivery. At Magee-Womens Hospital, only 25 percent of patients with chorioamnionitis are symptomatic; the other 75 percent are diagnosed after delivery on examination of the placenta. The recent report on the 87 percent predictive value of a positive leukotactic response for histologic chorioamnionitis, as compared with predictive values of 33 percent (Gram's stain), 53 percent (amniotic fluid culture), 40 percent (gas liquid chromatography), and 60 percent for all three, holds promise for detection of chorioamnionitis prior to delivery (Pankuch et al, 1989). Chorioamnionitis is an important factor in causing preterm birth, fetal hypoxia, low Apgar score, respiratory distress, and neonatal infection including pneumonia, otitis media, and meningitis. Placental examination is a useful means of establishing the diagnosis of chorioamnionitis with certainty.

*Umbilical cord inflammation* occurs in association with chorioamnionitis as angiitis in 6.6 percent of cases and funisitis in 3.7 percent of cases, and on occasion, from changes due to cord prolapse (Fox, 1978). The cord surface may be opaque and yellow. Angiitis refers to inflammation in the wall of any blood vessel, whereas funisitis indicates extension of inflammation into the surrounding Wharton's jelly. Cord inflammation indicates prolonged and often severe infection

and that the fetus was alive at the time of intrauterine infection because an inflammatory response of the cord is only possible from a live fetus.

## AMNION NODOSUM

Recognized as small wartlike papillary surface nodules on the fetal membranes (Fig. 12–10), this lesion is caused by attachment of fetal squames and skin debris to the membranes from prolonged contact between fetal skin and the membranes due to oligohydramnios. Reduced amniotic fluid can result from oliguria due to congenital urinary tract anomalies or from amniotic fluid loss following prolonged rupture of membranes or intrauterine fetal death. At least 3 weeks or more of oligohydramnios is required for this lesion to occur. It is clinically significant when it is associated with severe pulmonary hypoplasia that causes respiratory distress, particularly when not due to prematurity.

## EARLY AMNION RUPTURE

Early amnion rupture initiates a sequence (Jones, 1988) of fetal anomalies that result from the mechanical effects of fetal containment (Miller et al, 1981), constriction by amniotic bands (Torpin, 1965), or aberrant amniotic bands and sheets that disrupt normal morphogenesis, particularly of the craniofacial and abdominal wall regions (Jones, 1988). It is important to recognize this lesion as a sequence and not focus on any one of several major defects that occur, particularly

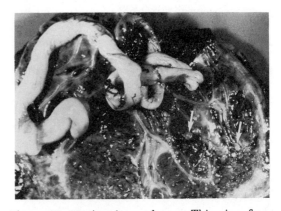

**Figure 12–10.** Amnion nodosum. This view from the fetal surface shows multiple small wartlike lesions of amnion nodosum (*arrows*).

central nervous system anomalies that might be misdiagnosed as anencephaly (Jones, 1988). Umbilical cord stricture may also result from these bands, as may a short umbilical cord, when associated with an abdominal wall defect. The placenta shows a spectrum of changes from simple amniotic bands to large amnion defects of the surface. An association with amniocentesis has been made in animals (Moessinger et al, 1981).

### Meconium Staining

Meconium staining is present in up to 20 percent of deliveries (Naeye and Tafari, 1983) and is noted in association with acute chorioamnionitis, premature rupture of membranes, abruptio placentae (Naeye, 1987b), and more recently, with cocaine use (Mastrogiannis et al, 1990). Cocaine has also been associated with low birth weight, growth retardation, premature rupture of membranes, and abruptio placentae (Mastrogiannis et al, 1990). Meconium alone is not an indicator of fetal hypoxia, which would need additional confirmation by other monitors of fetal condition. Its value in placental examination is that the morphologic changes and location of pigment correlate with the duration of meconium exposure (Miller, 1985). Meconium staining can occur within 1 hour of exposure and is in the chorionic plate within 3 hours. The earliest change of the amnion (pseudostratification) is followed by epithelial disorganization and cell degeneration in 12 hours and even complete necrosis (Miller, 1985). The evaluation of the length of time meconium has been present cannot be performed with absolute certainty in vivo. In vitro studies have established that amnion changes occur within 1 hour, and that within 12 hours, meconium pigment is present deep in the membrane layer within macrophages (Miller, 1985). However, the biologic variability of maternal response and the different concentrations of meconium limit making a direct correlation between in vitro and in vivo circumstances.

# Nontrophoblastic Placental Tumors

Nontrophoblastic tumors can be classified as primary or secondary, with secondary tumors of either fetal or maternal origin.

Hemangioma and teratoma are the two primary tumors.

*Chorioangioma* occurs as a well-circumscribed firm tumor located near the chorionic plate and varies in color, depending on the amount of contained blood. Chorioangioma has an incidence of about 1 percent (Wallenburg, 1971). Large chorioangiomas are clinically associated with fetal anomalies (hemangiomas), polyhydramnios, fetal hydrops, cardiomegaly, congestive heart failure, newborn anemia, and newborn thrombocytopenia (Battaglia and Woolevor, 1968; Wallenburg, 1971).

*Teratomas* are rare and may represent an abnormal twin. Secondary tumors usually present as tumor masses in the intervillous space and have been recently summarized in tabular form (Macpherson and Szulman, 1990).

## TWIN PLACENTATION

The twin placenta is subject to all the entities that involve the singleton placenta, and all such lesions should be documented. In addition, examination of the twin placenta can clarify or confirm several clinical concerns such as the number and size of gestational sacs, dichorionic versus monochorionic placentation, vascular anastomoses in twin-to-twin transfusion syndrome, and fetus papyraceous or fetus compressus. Twins are classified as monozygous or dizygous, with monozygous twins originating from division of a fertilized single ovum and dizygous twins originating from fertilization of two separate ova by two separate sperms.

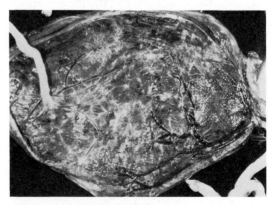

**Figure 12–11.** Monochorionic monoamniotic twin placenta. The fetal surface view of this twin placenta shows a single amniotic sac. There is no dividing membrane.

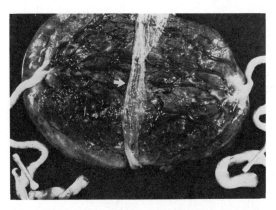

**Figure 12–12.** Monochorionic diamniotic twin placenta. The fetal surface of this twin placenta shows two amniotic sacs. A thin translucent dividing membrane is present (*arrow*) that contains two layers of amnion. There is no chorion present in the dividing membrane.

Placentation, on the other hand, is classified according to the number of gestational sacs and the structure of the dividing membrane when more than one sac is present. A single sac without a dividing membrane is a *monochorionic monoamnionic placenta* (Fig. 12–11), and the twins are monozygous. When two sacs are present, the twins are definitely diamniotic, and the only challenge is to distinguish between monochorionic diamnionic and dichorionic diamnionic placentation. If chorion is absent from the dividing membrane by histology, then the twins are *monochorionic diamnionic* (Fig. 12–12). If chorion is present in the dividing membrane, then the twins are *dichorionic diamnionic* (Fig. 12–13). Monochorionic twins are monozygous, whereas dichorionic twins can be either monozygous or dizygous, the distinction between the two is not possible on placental evaluation. Thus, twin zygosity can only be determined from the monochorionic placenta, unless of course, the twins are of opposite sex.

From the clinical perspective, it is the monochorionic twin rather than the monozygous one that is important. This group has a higher perinatal morbidity and mortality rate than singletons and dichorionic twins, mainly owing to prematurity, cord complications, and twin-to-twin transfusion syndrome. When the placenta is monochorionic, vascular anastomoses are generally present, but these are extremely rare when the placenta is dichorionic. Injection study is conveniently performed using a Micropaque gelatin mixture (Macpherson, 1982). Vascular

anastomoses can have several consequences including twin-to-twin transfusion syndrome; the acardiac variant, twin reversal arterial perfusion syndrome (TRAP) (Van Allen et al, 1983); fetus papyraceous; and fetus compressus. Vascular anastomoses may occur artery to artery, vein to vein, or vein to artery, with the artery to artery type being the most common but with few consequences. Important anastomoses are those that occur via a cotyledon supplied by the arterial tree from one twin and that drain unidirectionally to the venous tree of the other, thereby forming the so-called third circulation. The twin transfusion syndrome is seen in 15 to 30 percent of monochorionic twins and is probably due to the extent that this third circulation is present (Rausen et al, 1965; Strong and Corney, 1967). With chronic twin-to-twin transfusion syndrome, the donor twin is generally pale, has a lower body weight and organ size (especially the heart), and is anemic, whereas the recipient is plethoric, heavier, has a larger heart, and is polycythemic. These parameters are sometimes reversed because of a change in the direction of blood flow in late pregnancy, an entity accurately termed "acute twin-to-twin in utero transfusion" (Bendon et al, 1989). Interestingly, the twin-to-twin transfusion syndrome is rare in monoamnionic twins, and it has been suggested that the degree of vascular communication might be so extensive as to constitute a single circulation (Benirschke and Kaufmann, 1990a). There have been reports of vascular anastomoses in

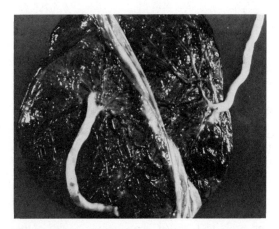

**Figure 12–13.** Dichorionic diamniotic twin placenta. The fetal surface view of this twin placenta shows two amniotic sacs. In comparison with Figure 12–12, however, the dividing membrane is thick and opaque, since it contains two layers of chorion as well as two layers of amnion.

dizygous twins. Fetus papyraceous is identified as a flattened, mummified, and paper-like fetus that might be seen as fetus compressus, a nodule in the placental membranes (Fig. 12–14) that may show a fetal skeleton by radiology or histology. When a twin "disappears" very early in pregnancy, a nodule of perivillous fibrin may be all that remains. (Bardawil et al, 1988; Jauniaux et al, 1988).

As mentioned previously, perinatal mortality and morbidity is more frequent in multiple gestation when compared with singletons, particularly in monochorionic twins. In the CPS study, the mortality rate was 191/1000 for monozygous twins compared with 75/1000 for dizygous twins (Naeye et al, 1978b). Monochorionic twins are a major contributor to perinatal morbidity and mortality, accounting for a greater proportion as certain causes of death in singletons are being reduced. When twin-to-twin transfusion is present, fetal mortality can be as high as 70 percent and can account for 34 percent of monochorionic twin deaths (Timmons and de Alvarez, 1963). The overall mortality rate for twins is as high as 14 percent (8.9 percent for dichorionic twins, 25.9 percent for monochorionic twins, and 50 percent for monoamniotic twins) (Benirschke and Kaufmann, 1990a). Cord complications contribute significantly to the high mortality rate in monoamniotic twins (Timmons and de Alvarez, 1963). The increased rates of morbidity and mortality in twins in general is due to prematurity, chorioamnionitis, cord complications of knotting, entanglement and prolapse, abruptio placentae, and the twin-to-twin transfusion syndrome (Naeye, 1987b; Naeye et al, 1978; Perrin, 1984). Evaluation of the twin placenta contributes to the determination of zygosity, the identification of vascular anastomoses, the recognition of an absorbed twin, and the diagnosis of any of the other placental findings seen with singletons.

Placental examination is an important part of the evaluation of an adverse perinatal outcome. There are several abnormalities that have functional consequences that contribute to or explain perinatal events; these abnormalities need to be distinguished from those that are incidental. Those lesions that compromise maternal blood flow into the intervillous space are among the most important causes of perinatal morbidity and mortality and intrauterine growth retardation. Some lesions are unique to the twin placenta.

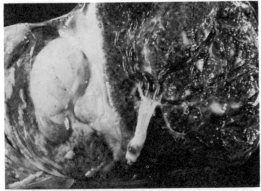

**Figure 12–14.** Compressed twin in placental membranes. The left edge of the picture shows a distinct oval nodule overlying thin atrophic placental tissue. A radiograph and tissue section revealed the autolysed tissue and skeleton of a fetus (twin). Alongside is the attached placenta and umbilical cord of the surviving twin. (Used with permission from Macpherson TA, Szulman AE: The placenta and products of conception, In Silverberg SB (ed): Principles and Practice of Surgical Pathology, 2nd ed. New York, Churchill Livingstone, 1990.)

## References

Acker D, Sachs BP, Tracey KJ, Wise WE: Abruptio placentae associated with cocaine use. Am J Obstet Gynecol 146:220–221, 1983.

Aherne A: Morphometry. *In* Gruenwald P (ed): The Placenta and its Maternal Supply Line. Lancaster, MTP Press, 1975, pp 80–97.

Althabe O, Labarrere C: Chronic villitis of unkown etiology and intrauterine growth retarded infants of normal and low ponderal index. Placenta 6:369–373, 1985.

Altschuler G, Russell P: The human placental villitides: a review of chronic intrauterine infection. Cur Top Pathol 60:64–112, 1975.

Alvarez H, Sala MA, Benedetti WL: Intervillous space reduction in the edematous placenta. Am J Obstet Gynecol 112:819–820, 1972.

Baramowsky CR, Vegas ME, Swinehart G, Gyves MT: Decidual vasculopathy of the placenta in lupus erythematosus. N Engl J Med 303:668–672, 1980.

Bardawil WA, Reddy RL, Bardawil LW: Placental consideration in multiple pregnancy. Clin Perinatol 15:13–40, 1988.

Batcup G, Tovey LA, Longster G: Fetomaternal blood group incompatibility studies in placental intervillous thrombosis. Placenta 7:449–553, 1983.

Battaglia FC, Woolevor CA: Fetal and neonatal complications associated with recurrent chorangiomas. Pediatrics 41:62–66, 1968.

Beaconsfield R, Birowood G: Placenta—The Largest Human Biopsy. Oxford, Pergamon, 1982.

Becker V: Abnormal maturation of villi. *In* Gruenwald P (ed): The Placenta and its Maternal Supply Line. Lancaster, MTP, 1975, pp 232–243.

Bejar R, Curbelo V, Davis C, Gluck L: Premature labor: II bacterial sources of phospholipase. Obstet Gynecol 57:479–482, 1981.

Bendon RW, Siddiqi T: Acute twin-twin in utero transfusion. Pediatr Pathol 9:591–598, 1989.

Benirschke K, Brown WH: A vascular anomaly of the umbilical cord: the absence of one umbilical artery in the umbilical cords of normal and abnormal fetuses. Obstet Gynecol 6:399–404, 1955.

Benirschke K, Kaufmann P: Pathology of the Human Placenta. New York, Springer-Verlag, 1990a.

Benirschke K, Kaufmann P: Pathology of Maternal floor infarction. *In* Pathology of the Human Placenta, 2nd ed. New York, Springer Verlag, 1990b, pp 406–411.

Benson RC, Fujikura T: Circumvallate and circummarginate placenta: unimportant clinical entities. Obstet Gynecol 34:799–804, 1969.

Blanc WA: Pathology of the placenta, membranes and umbilical cord in bacterial, fungal and viral infections in man. *In* Naeye RL, Kissane JM, Kaufmann N (eds): Perinatal Disease. Baltimore, Williams & Wilkins, 1981, pp 67–132.

Brosens I, Renaer M: On the pathogenesis of placental infarcts in pre-eclampsia. Br J Obstet Gynaecol 79:794–799, 1972.

Brosens I, Dixon HG, Robertson WB: Fetal growth retardation and the arteries of the placental bed. Br J Obstet Gynaecol 84:656–663, 1977.

Brosens I, Robertson WB, Dixon HG: The physiologic response of the vessels of the placental bed to normal pregnancy. J Pathol Bacteriol 93:569–579, 1967.

Chard T: The Human Placenta. Clin Obstet Gynecol 13:421–663, 1986.

Chasnoff IJ, Burns WJ, Schnoll SH, Burns KA: Cocaine use in pregnancy. N Engl J Med 313:666–669, 1985.

Clewell WH, Manchester DK: Recurrent maternal floor infarction: a preventable cause of fetal death. Am J Obstet Gynecol 147:346–347, 1983.

DeSa DJ: Diseases of the umbilical cord. *In* Perrin EVDK (ed): Pathology of the Placenta. New York, Churchill Livingstone, 1984, pp 121–139.

DeSa DJ: Rupture of foetal vessels on placental surface. Arch Dis Child 46:495–501, 1971.

Devi B, Jennison RF, Langley FA: Significance of placental pathology in transplacental hemorrhage. J Clin Pathol 21:322–331, 1968.

DeWolf, F, Brosens I, Renaer M: Fetal growth retardation and the maternal arterial supply of the human placenta in the absence of sustained hypertension. Br J Obstet Gynecol 87:678–685, 1980.

Driscoll SG: The pathology of pregnancy complicated by diabetes mellitus. Med Clin North Am 49:1053–1067, 1965.

Eggens JH, Bruinse HW: An unusual case of fetal distress. Am J Obstet Gynecol 148:219–220, 1984.

Fox H: General pathology of the placenta. *In* Fox H (ed): Obstetrical and Gynecological Pathology, Vol 2. New York, Churchill Livingstone, 1987, pp 972–1000.

Fox H: Pathology of the placenta. Clin Obstet Gynecol 13:501–519, 1986.

Fox H: Placental involvement in maternal systemic infection. Perspect Pediatr Pathol 6:63–81, 1981.

Fox H: Pathology of the Placenta. Philadelphia, WB Saunders, 1978.

Fox, H: Placenta accreta, 1945–1969. Obstet Gynecol Surv 27:475–490, 1972.

Fox H, Sen DK: Placenta extrachorialis: a clinicopathological study. J Obstet Gynaecol Br Commonw 79:32–35, 1972.

Fox H: The significance of placental infarction in peri- natal morbidity and mortality. Biol Neonatorum 11:87–105, 1967a.

Fox H: Perivillous fibrin deposition in the human placenta. Am J Obstet Gynecol 98:245–251, 1967b.

Fox H: Thrombosis of fetal arteries in the human placenta. J Obstet Gynaecol Br Commonw 73:961–965, 1966.

Froehlich LA, Fijikwa T: Follow-up of infants with single umbilical artery. Pediatrics 52:22–29, 1973.

Froehlich LA, Fujikura J: Significance of a single umbilical artery. Report from the collaborative study of cerebral palsy. Am J Obstet Gynecol 94:274–279, 1966.

Fujikura T, Benson RC, Driscoll SG: The bipartite placenta and its clinical features. Am J Obstet Gynecol 107:1013–1017, 1970.

Gardiner JP: The umbilical cord: normal length: length in cord complications: etiology and frequency of coiling. Surg Gynecol Obstet 34:252–256, 1922.

Garrow JS, Howes SF: The relationship of the size and composition of the human placenta to its functional capacity. J Obstet Gynaecol Br Commonw 78:22–28, 1971.

Gersell DJ, Kraus FT, Riffle MB: Diseases of the placenta. *In* Kurman RJ (ed): Blaustein's Pathology of the Female Genital Tract, 3rd ed. New York, Springer-Verlag, 1987, pp 769–834.

Ghosh A, Woo JS, MacHenry C, et al: Fetal loss from umbilical cord abnormalities—a difficult case for prevention. Europ J Obstet Gynecol Reprod Biol 18:183–198, 1984.

Gilbert EF, Zugibe FT: Torsion and constriction of the umbilical cord: a cause of fetal death. Arch Pathol 97:58–59, 1974.

Grange DK, Arya S, Opitz JM, et al: The short umbilical cord. *In* Gilbert EF, Opitz JM (eds): The Genetic Aspects of Developmental Pathology. New York, Alan R Liss, Inc, 1987, pp 191–214.

Gruenwald P, Levin H, Yousem H: Abruption and premature separation of the placenta. The clinical and the pathologic entity. Am J Obstet Gynecol 102:604–610, 1968.

Hart DB: The nature of the tuberase fleshy mole. J Obstet Gynaecol Brit Emp 1:479–487, 1902.

Hoag RW: Fetomaternal hemorrhagé associated with umbilical vein thrombosis. Case report. Am J Obstet Gynecol 154(6):1271–1274, 1986.

Jaffe R, Siegal A, Rat L, et al: Placental chorioangiomatosis—a high risk pregnancy. Postgrad Med J 61:453–454, 1985.

Janovski NA, Granowitz ET: Placenta membranacea: report of a case. Obstet Gynecol 18:206–212, 1961.

Jauniaux E, Elkazen N, Leroy F, et al: Clinical and morphological aspects of the vanishing twin phenomenon. Obstet Gynecol 72:577–581, 1988.

Jones KL: Miscellaneous sequences: early amnion rupture sequence. *In* Jones KL (ed): Smith's Recognizable Patterns of Human Malformation. Philadelphia, WB Saunders, 1988, pp 576–583.

Kaplan C, Blanc WA, Celias J: Identification of erythrocytes in intervillous thrombi. A study using immunoperoxidase identification of hemoglobins. Hum Pathol 13:554–557, 1982.

Karegard M, Gennser G: Incidence and recurrence rate of abruptio placentae in Sweden. Obstet Gynecol 67:523–528, 1986.

Katz VL, Bowes WA, Sierkh AE: Maternal floor infarction of the placenta associated with elevated second trimester serum alpha-fetoprotein. Am J Perinatol 4:225–228, 1987.

Kaufmann P, Sen DK, Schweikhart G: Classification of human placental villi. J Cell Tissue Res 200:409–423, 1979.

Knox WF, Fox H: Villitis of unknown etiology: its incidence and significance in placentae from a British population. Placenta 5:395–402, 1984.

Kohler HG: Pathology of the umbilical cord and fetal membranes. In Fox H (ed): Obstetrical and Gynecological Pathology, Vol 2. New York, Churchill Livingstone, 1987, pp 1079–1116.

Labarrere C, Althabe O: Chronic villitis of unknown aetiology in recurrent intrauterine fetal growth retardation. Placenta 8:167–173, 1987.

Labarrere C, Althabe O: Chronic villitis of unknown aetiology and decidual maternal vasculopathies in sustained chronic hypertension. Eur J Obstet Gynecol Reprod Biol 21:27–32, 1986.

Lauweryns J, Bernat R, Lerut A, Detournay G: Intrauterine pneumonia, an experimental study. Biol Neonate 22:301–318, 1973.

Lemtis H, Hadrich G: Uber die Gewichtsabnahne des Mutterkuchens nach de Geburt und die Bedeutung fur den Quoteinten aus Plazenta-und Kindsgewicht. Geburtshilfe und Frauenheilkunde 34:618–622, 1974.

Macpherson TA: The role of the anatomical pathologist in perinatology. Semin Perinatol 9:257–262, 1985.

Macpherson TA: Angiographic evaluation of fetal vascular anomalies at autopsy in the fetus and neonate. Lab Invest 46:10, 1982.

Macpherson TA, Szulman AE: The placenta and products of conception. In Silverberg SB (ed): Principles and Practice of Surgical Pathology, 2nd ed. New York, Churchill Livingstone, 1990, pp 1825–1856.

Macpherson TA, Valdes-Dapena M, Kanbour A: Complications of perinatal care—the role of the perinatal pathologist. Semin Perinatol 10:179–186, 1986.

Mastrogiannis DS, Decavalas GO, Verma U, Tejani N: Perinatal outcome after recent cocaine usage. Obstet Gynecol 76:8–11, 1990.

Miller JM Pupkin MJ, Hill GB: Bacterial colonization of preterm labor. Am J Obstet Gynecol 136:796–804, 1980.

Miller ME, Graham JM Jr, Higginbottom MC, et al: Compression related defects from early amnion rupture: evidence for mechanical teratogenesis. J Pediatr 98:292–297, 1981.

Miller PW, Coen RW, Benirschke K: Dating the time interval from meconium passage to birth. Obstet Gynecol 66:459–462, 1985.

Mitchell MD: Pathways of arachidonic acid metabolism with specific application to the fetus and mother. Semin Perinatol 10:242–254, 1986.

Moe N: Depositions of fibrin and plasma proteins in the normal human placenta: an immunofluorescence study. Acta Pathol Microbiol Scand 76:74–88, 1969.

Moessinger AC, Blanc WA, Byrne J, et al: Amniotic band syndrome associated with amniocentesis. Am J Obstet Gynecol 141:588–591, 1981.

Moessinger AC, Blanc WA, Merone PA, et al: Umbilical cord length as an index of fetal activity: experimental study and clinical implications. Pediatr Res 16:109–112, 1982.

Molteni RA, Stanley JS, Battaglia FC: Relationship of fetal and placental weight in human beings: fetal/placental weight ratios at various gestational ages and birth weight distributions. J Reprod Med 21:327–334, 1978.

Naeye RL: How important is perinatal hypoxia as a cause of brain damage. JAMA. In press.

Naeye RL: Do placental weights have clinical significance? Hum Pathol 18:387–391, 1987a.

Naeye RL: Functionally important disorders of the placenta, umbilical cord, and fetal membranes. Hum Pathol 18:680–691, 1987b.

Naeye RL: When and how does antenatal brain damage occur? In Iffy L (ed): Second Perinatal Practice and Malpractice Symposium. New York, Healthmark Communications, 1986, pp 125–132.

Naeye RL: Umbilical cord length: clinical significance. J Pediatr 107:278–281, 1985a.

Naeye RL: Maternal floor infarction. Hum Pathol 16:823–828, 1985b.

Naeye RL: Causes of perinatal mortality in the US Collaborative Perinatal Project. JAMA 238:228–229, 1977a.

Naeye RL: Placental infarction leading to fetal or neonatal death: a prospective study. Obstet Gynecol 50:583–588, 1977b.

Naeye RL, Peters EC: Antenatal hypoxia and low IQ values. Am J Dis Child 141:50–54, 1987.

Naeye RL, Peters EC: Amniotic fluid infection with intact membranes leading to perinatal death: a prospective study. Pediatrics 61:171–177, 1978.

Naeye RL, Ross SM: Amniotic fluid infection syndrome. Clin Obstet Gynecol 9:593–607, 1982a.

Naeye RL, Ross SM: Coitus and Chorioamnionitis, a prospective study. Early Hum Dev 6:91–97, 1982b.

Naeye RL, Tafari N: Risk Factors in Pregnancy and Diseases of the Fetus and Newborn. Baltimore, Williams & Wilkins, 1983.

Naeye RL, Harkness WL, Utts J: Abruptio placentae and perinatal death: a prospective study. Am J Obstet Gynecol 128:740–746, 1977.

Naeye RL, Tafari N, Marboe CC: Perinatal death due to abruptio placentae in an African city. Acta Obstet Gynecol 58:37–40, 1979.

Naeye RL, Maisels J, Lorenz RP, Botti JJ: The clinical significance of placental villous edema. Pediatrics 71:588–594, 1983.

Naeye RL, Tafari N, Judge D, Marboe CC: Twins: causes of perinatal death in 12 United States cities and one African city. Am J Obstet Gynecol 131:267–272, 1978.

Nickel RE: Maternal floor infarction: an unusual cause of intrauterine growth retardation. Am J Dis Child 142:1270–1271, 1988.

Niswander KR, Henson G, Elbourne D, et al: Adverse outcome of pregnancy and the quality of obstetric care. Lancet 2:827–831, 1984.

Pankuch GA, Cherouny PH, Botti JJ, Appelbaum PC: Amniotic fluid leukotaxis assay as an early indicator of chorioamnionitis. Am J Obstet Gynecol 161:802–807, 1989.

Pankuch GA, Applebaum PG, Lorenz RP, et al: Placental microbiology and histology and the pathogenesis of chorioamnionitis. Obstet Gynecol 64:802–806, 1984.

Paterson MEL: The etiology and outcome of abruptio placentae. Acta Obstet Gynecol Scand 58:31–35, 1979.

Perrin EVDK: Pathology of the Placenta. New York, Churchill Livingstone, 1984.

Pinette MG, Loftus-Brault K, Nardi DA, Rodis JF: Maternal smoking and accelerated placental maturation. Obstet Gynecol 73:379–382, 1989.

Pratola D, Wilkin P: The placenta, umbilical cord, and amniotic sac. In Gompel C, Silverberg SG (eds): Pathology in Gynecology and Obstetrics, 2nd ed. Philadelphia, JB Lippincott, 1985, pp 435–452.

Pryse-Davies J, Dewhurst CJ, Campbell S: Placenta membranacea. J Obstet Gynaecol Br Commonw 80:1106–1110, 1973.

Ramsey EM: Development and anatomy of the placenta. *In* Fox H, (ed): Obstetrical and Gynecological Pathology, Vol 2. New York, Churchill Livingstone, 1987, pp 959–971.

Rausen AR, Seki M, Strauss L: Twin transfusion syndrome: a review of 19 case studies at one institution. J Pediatr 66:613–628, 1965.

Rayburn WF, Beynen A, Brinkman DL: Umbilical cord length and intrapartum complications. Obstet Gynecol 57:450–452, 1981.

Rayburn W, Sander C, Compton A: Histologic examination of the placenta in the growth-retarded fetus. Am J Perinatol 6:58–61, 1989.

Rayburn W, Sander C, Barr M Jr, Rygiel R: The stillborn fetus: placental histologic examination in determining a cause. Obstet Gynecol 65:637–641, 1985.

Redline RW, Abramowsky CR: Clinical and pathologic aspects of recurrent placental villitis. Hum Pathol 16:727–731, 1985.

Robertson WB, Brosens I, Dixon G: Uteroplacental vascular pathology. Eur J Obstet Gynaecol Reprod Biol 5:47–65, 1975.

Rushton DI: Pathology of the Placenta. *In* Wigglesworth JS, Singer DB (eds): Textbook of Fetal and Perinatal Pathology. Boston, Blackwell Scientific Publications, 1991, pp 161–219.

Russell P: Infections of the placental villi (villitis). *In* Fox H (ed): Obstetrical and Gynecological Pathology, Vol 2. New York, Churchill Livingstone, 1987, pp 1014–1029.

Russell P: Inflammatory lesions of the human placenta. III. The histopathology of villitis of unknown etiology. Placenta 1:227–244, 1980.

Russell P: Inflammatory lesions of the human placenta. I. Am J Diagn Gynecol Obstet 1:127–137, 1979.

Russell P, Altschuler G: The placental abnormalities of congenital syphilis. Am J Dis Child 128:160–163, 1974.

Russell P, Atkinson K, Krishnan L: Recurrent reproductive failure due to severe placental villitis of unknown etiology. J Reprod Med 24:93–98, 1980.

Salafia CM, Mangam HE, Weigl CA, et al: Abnormal fetal heart rate patterns and placental inflammation. Am J Obstet Gynecol 160:140–147, 1989.

Sander CH: Hemorrhagic endovasculitis and hemorrhage villitis of the placenta. Arch Pathol Lab Med 104:371–373, 1980.

Sander CH, Kinnane L, Stevens NG: Hemorrhagic endovasculitis of the placenta: a clinicopathologic entity associated with adverse pregnancy outcome. Comprehensive Therapy 11:66–74, 1985.

Scott JS: Placenta extrachorialis (placenta marginata and placenta circumvallata): a factor in antepartum hemorrhage. J Obstet Gynecol Brit Emp 67:904–918, 1960.

Shanklin DR, Scott JS: Massive subchorial thrombohematoma (Breus' mole). Br J Obstet Gynaecol 82:476–487, 1975.

Shen-Schwarz S, Macpherson TA, Mueller-Heubach E: The clinical significance of hemorrhagic endovasculitis of the placenta. Am J Obstet Gynecol 159:48–51, 1988.

Shen-Schwarz S, Ruchelli E, Brown D: Villous oedema of the placenta: a clinicopathological study. Placenta 10:297–307, 1989.

Sheppard BL, Bonnar J: The ultrastructure of the arterial supply of the human placenta in pregnancy complicated by fetal growth retardation. Br J Obstet Gynaecol 83:948–959, 1976.

Sheppard BL, Bonnar J: Scanning electron microscopy of the human placenta and decidual spiral arteries in normal pregnancy. J Obstet Gynaecol Br Commonw 81:497–511, 1974.

Sibai BM, Taslimi MM, el-Nazer A, et al: Maternal-perinatal outcome associated with the syndrome of hemolysis, elevated liver enzymes, and low platelets in severe preeclampsia-eclampsia. Am J Obstet Gynecol 155:501–509, 1986.

Silver MM, Yeger H, Lines LD: Hemorrhagic endovasculitis-like lesion induced in placental organ culture. Hum Pathol 19:251–256, 1988.

Soma H: Single umbilical artery with congenital malformations. Curr Topics Pathol 66:159–173, 1979.

Strong SJ, Corney G: The placenta in twin pregnancy. Oxford Pergamon Press, 1967.

Talamo TS, Macpherson TA, Dominguez R: Angiographic demonstration of vascular anomalies in sirenomelia—a case report. Arch Path Lab Med 106:347–348, 1982.

Timmons JD, de Alvarez RR: Monoamniotic twin pregnancy. Am J Obstet Gynecol 86:875–881, 1963.

Torpin R: Evolution of a placenta circumvallata. Obstet Gynecol 27:98–101, 1966.

Torpin R: Amniochorionic mesoblastic fibrous strings and amnionic bands: associated constricting fetal malformations or fetal death. Am J Obstet Gynecol 91:65–75, 1965.

Torpin R, Hart BF: Placenta bilobata. Am J Obstet Gynecol 42:38–49, 1941.

Van Allen MI, Smith DW, Shepard T: Twin reversed arterial perfusion (TRAP) sequence: a study of 14 twin pregnancies with acardius. Semin Perinatol 7:285–293, 1983.

Wallenburg HCS: Chorangioma of the placenta: thirteen new cases and a review of the literature from 1939 to 1970 with special reference to clinical complications. Obstet Gynecol Surv 26:411–425, 1971.

Wentworth P: Placental infarction and toxemia of pregnancy. Am J Obstet Gynecol 99:318–326, 1967.

Wentworth P: A placental lesion to account for foetal hoemorrhage into the maternal circulation. J Obstet Gynaecol Br Commonw 71:379–387, 1964.

Wigglesworth JS: Morphological variations of the insufficient placenta. J Obstet Gynaecol Br Commonw 71:871–884, 1964.

Wolfman WL, Purohit DM, Sally ES: Umbilical vein thrombosis at 32 weeks' gestation with delivery of a living infant. Am J Obstet Gynecol 146:468–470, 1983.

# CHAPTER 13

. . . . . . . . . . . . . . . . . . . . . . . . . . . . . .

# Maternal Adaptations to Pregnancy

Mildred G. Harvey and Michael L. Moretti

A multitude of maternal physiologic changes begin in the first week of gestation and continue to unfold throughout pregnancy, labor, delivery, and puerperium. These maternal adaptations influence the function of practically every organ system in the maternal body as adjustments are made for the growing uteroplacental-fetal unit. Hormones, both ovarian and placental, govern the majority of these adaptations, either directly or through secondary effects. A few of the alterations are caused by the presence and mechanical effects of the enlarging uterus and growing fetus.

An understanding and an appreciation of the normal adaptations to pregnancy facilitate management but are essential for the management of the high-risk and complicated pregnancy. This chapter focuses on those physiologic changes that have an impact on the major organ systems in a way that creates a high-risk status when the pregnant woman is unable to make the necessary adaptations or may contribute to her high-risk condition.

---

## Cardiovascular System

The maternal cardiovascular system makes profound adjustments to meet changing maternal needs as well as to promote the growth and development of the utero-placental-fetal unit. A thorough understanding of this system during gestation is of extreme importance (Table 13–1).

## HEART

As the uterus enlarges progressively, the diaphragm is elevated, displacing the heart to the left and upward. This process results in a slight anterior rotation so that the apex beat is more often heard in the fourth intercostal space rather than the fifth intercostal space and is heard lateral rather than medial to the midclavical line (Walters and Lim, 1975).

### Heart Rate

Heart rate increases during pregnancy, with the major increase occurring in the last trimester. Clark and associates (1989) report a 17 percent increase in heart rate over nonpregnant levels. The increase usually begins at about 8 weeks' gestation (Capeless and Clapp, 1989). Heart rate returns to prepregnant levels by 6 weeks' postpartum (Walters and Lim, 1975).

### Heart Sounds

Cutforth and MacDonald (1966) reported the results of serial phonocardiograms as follows:

1. An increased loudness is present in both components of the first heart sound beginning from 12 to 14 weeks' gestation and lasting until 2 to 4 weeks' postpartum.

2. An exaggerated splitting of the first heart sound between the closure of the mitral and tricuspid valves is usually heard.

**Table 13–1**
CARDIOVASCULAR CHANGES DURING PREGNANCY

| Parameter | Change | Magnitude of Change |
|---|---|---|
| Cardiac output | increase | 40 to 50 percent |
| | | ↑ 22 percent by 22 weeks |
| | | ↑ 43 percent by 36 to 38 weeks |
| | | ↑ additional 22 percent in labor |
| Blood volume | increase | 45 percent (1500 ml) |
| Plasma volume | increase | 45 to 50 percent (1200 to 1300 ml) |
| RBC mass | increase | 20 to 30 percent (250 to 450 ml) |
| Albumin concentration | decrease | 10 g/liter |
| Colloid osmotic pressure (COP) | decrease | |
| Arterial blood pressure | decrease | greatest in second trimester, |
| | | return to pregnant level by term |
| Venous pressure | unchanged | in upper extremities |
| | increase | in lower extremities |
| SVR | decrease | 21 percent |
| PVR | decrease | 34 percent |
| Heart | | displaced to left and upward, |
| PMI | | located fourth ICS and lateral |
| Rate | increase | 10 to 15 BPM (17 percent) |
| Sounds | | exaggerated splitting first sound |
| | | third sound present |
| | | systolic murmur present |
| ECG | | flattening of T wave |

3. Approximately 90 percent of pregnant women have longer intervals between the first (mitral) and second (tricuspid) components of the first heart sound.

4. No changes are noted in the second heart sound until after 30 weeks' gestation. As the uterus enlarges and there is reduced diaphragmatic movement with respirations, the interval between the aortic and pulmonic valve closures is more constant with respirations.

5. Eighty to 90 percent of pregnant women exhibit a third heart sound by the 20th week of gestation. This sound usually disappears by the eighth postpartum day.

6. A fourth heart sound may be heard by auscultation in less than 5 percent of pregnant women.

7. More than 95 percent of pregnant women develop a systolic murmur at about 22 weeks' gestation. This murmur is heard best along the left sternal border.

Two types of functional murmurs may be heard during pregnancy: a pulmonary systolic murmur, heard loudest at the right intercostal space, and a supraclavicular systolic murmur that is produced by blood flow in the brachiocephalic trunks. The hyperdynamic state predisposes the pregnant woman to these functional murmurs.

## Electrocardiogram

The size of the heart may increase because of both hypertrophy and dilatation. In addition, there is a leftward deviation of the heart secondary to the upward lift of the diaphragm by the enlarging uterus. Thus, electrocardiogram findings later in pregnancy include a left axis deviation with nonspecific ST-T wave changes. The most constant change in the electrocardiogram during pregnancy is flattening of the T wave (Walters and Lim, 1975). Occasionally, benign atrial and ventricular premature beats occur.

## CARDIAC OUTPUT

Cardiac output (defined as the volume of blood expelled by the left ventricle in a unit of time) reflects the magnitude of the demands on the cardiovascular system and is the most important factor to be considered in assessment of this system. Four factors govern cardiac output: preload, afterload, contractility, and heart rate (Yeomans and Hankins, 1989). Preload is the volume of blood in the ventricle at the end of diastole or end diastolic volume. Afterload is defined as ventricular wall tension during ejection and is dependent mainly on vascular resistance: systemic vascular resistance for the left ventricle and pulmonary vascular resistance for the right ventricle.

Contractility is synonymous with the inotropic state of the heart and is governed by the Frank-Starling Law of the heart. This law states that the greater the length of the muscle before contraction, the greater the tension is developed, resulting in increased contractility up to the point of failure (Yeomans and Hankins, 1989).

Heart rate also affects cardiac output, as evidenced by the mathematical equation:

$$CO = HR \times SV$$

Stroke volume (SV) is composed of preload, afterload, and contractility. Increasing the heart rate increases cardiac output up to a point, but an increase beyond a critical level results in the reduced time for adequate diastolic filling. The result is decreased diastolic filling with reduced stroke volume and reduced cardiac output.

## Changes in Pregnancy

Cardiac output has been reported to increase 40 to 50 percent at rest during gestation. Clark and associates (1989) used pulmonary artery catheterization (Swan-Ganz catheter) to assess cardiac output in the left lateral recumbent position. Using the thermodilution technique, 10 healthy primipara patients were studied between 36 to 38 weeks' gestation. This study found cardiac output to increase 43 percent during pregnancy.

The first study of cardiac output changes during pregnancy was done by Lindhard in 1915 (Ueland and Ueland, 1986), using a nitrous oxide technique with a reported 50 percent increase in cardiac output. Since that time, numerous investigators have researched this variable, using more refined and sophisticated technology as it has become available. All reported that cardiac output increased during pregnancy but differed as to the extent and pattern of this increase. Ueland and associates (1969) used the dye dilution technique in 11 normal women in three different stages of pregnancy: late second trimester, early third trimester, and at term. They reported a 40 percent increase in cardiac output. The increase begins very early in pregnancy with a 22 percent increment by 8 weeks'

gestation (Capeless and Clapp, 1989). Nearly all of the increase is achieved by the end of the second trimester of pregnancy. This level is maintained until term if measured in the left lateral recumbent position.

The increase in cardiac output in early pregnancy is attributed mainly to an augmented stroke volume secondary to an expanded blood volume with a concomitant increase in end diastolic volume (Capeless and Clapp, 1989). Late pregnancy shows an additional increase in the cardiac output as the increased heart rate exerts an effect (Katz et al, 1978).

It is important to note that any measure of cardiac output during pregnancy is particularly sensitive to positional changes because of the effects of the gravid uterus on aortal caval flow. When the cardiac output is measured in supine recumbency, there is a significant fall in the cardiac output. This is especially evident in the late third trimester. When measured in the supine position, cardiac output may reach nonpregnant values (Ueland et al, 1969). This decline in cardiac output in the supine recumbency position late in pregnancy is due to occlusion of the inferior vena cava by the gravid uterus that results in a decreased venous return to the heart (Kerr, 1965). This occlusion of the vena cava can result in maternal hypotension and bradycardia, and it is recognized as the supine hypotensive syndrome.

## Changes During Labor

Much of our knowledge about hemodynamics during labor is derived from the research of Ueland and Hansen (1969a, 1969b); who studied cardiovascular changes in 23 laboring women in the supine position without sedation or regional anesthesia. Newer studies have corrected for the variables of maternal posture and the influence of pain. Lee and colleagues (1989) studied hemodynamics in laboring women in the left decubitus position with epidural anesthesia. M-mode and pulsed-Doppler echocardiography were used to noninvasively evaluate the consequences of uterine contractions on cardiac output. The researchers found an 11 percent increase in cardiac output with uterine contractions due to an increase in left ventricular stroke volume caused by the autotransfusion of uteroplacental blood with contractions. The intrauterine pressure increased with each contraction and eliminated the shunt of blood to the uteroplacental-fetal unit. Therefore, cardiac preload augmentation occurs with uterine contractions, and cardiac output is increased 11 percent. Robson and associates (1987) used Doppler and cross-sectional echocardiography to report similar increases. They reported a basal cardiac output increase of 12 percent toward the end of labor. The increased preload from the repetitive uterine contractions of labor, with resultant increase in cardiac output, increases the risks for women with borderline cardiac reserve or cardiac disease to develop congestive heart failure at this time.

Adequate pain relief during labor with conduction anesthesia can help to prevent significant changes in the maternal heart rate due to catecholamine release caused by pain. Lee and associates (1989) reported that when laboring patients receive epidural anesthesia, cardiac output increases only 11 percent over antepartum levels, whereas increases as high as 80 percent over antepartum values have been reported in patients receiving only local anesthesia for the labor and delivery process (Ueland and Hansen, 1969b). The lower cardiac output in those patients receiving epidural anesthesia has been attributed to diminished catecholamine release resulting from the relief of pain. In addition, the sympatholytic effect that causes peripheral vasodilatation reduces preload and thus cardiac output.

Elective cesarean delivery may eliminate the increase in cardiac output that accompanies uterine contractions and the bearing down efforts, but cannot prevent the significant increment that increases with delivery. Immediately after delivery of the fetus and placenta, the uterus contracts and shunts blood from the uterine vessels into the systemic circulation. Pressure of the heavy gravid uterus is now relieved, and the vena cava shunt is eliminated. This results in an increased venous return to the heart, thereby increasing the preload with approximately 1000 ml of blood. This creates an autotransfusion at the time of delivery (Lee et al, 1989). A decrease in heart rate often ensues because cardiac output can be maintained with a decreased rate. A bradycardia may last for a few days until diuresis eliminates the extra volume. Cardiac output returns to almost prepregnancy levels within a week after delivery (Monheit et al, 1980).

## CARDIAC WORKLOAD

Increased cardiac output during gestation results in an increased workload on the maternal heart. Cardiac workload is proportional to the cardiac output and mean arterial pressure. There is no significant change in mean arterial pressure during late pregnancy (Clark et al, 1989). Therefore, the basal cardiac workload will increase proportionally as the cardiac output increases. If the cardiac output increases 43 percent, the basal cardiac workload will increase 43 percent.

Exercise and physical activity cause an additional increase in heart rate and, therefore, add to the basal workload of the heart. Lotgering and colleagues (1984) found that, in early pregnancy, the energy cost of exercise for the pregnant woman is not greater than for the nonpregnant woman. However, they also found that, in late pregnancy, the energy cost of exercise increases owing to the pregnant woman's extra weight, greater cardiac demand, and greater ventilatory response to exercise. Artal and colleagues (1986) compared weight-bearing exercise (treadmill) and non–weight-bearing exercise (bicycle). They found non–weight-bearing exercise created less workload than weight-bearing exercise.

## BLOOD VOLUME

Maternal blood volume increases rapidly during normal pregnancy, with a 22 percent increase by 8 weeks' gestation (Capeless and Clapp, 1989). Expansion of total circulating blood volume continues to increase progressively to a maximum of 45 percent by 32 to 34 weeks' gestation and that level is maintained until delivery. Blood volume then begins to fall and returns to the prepregnant level within 2 to 3 weeks postpartum (Hytten and Leitch, 1971; Metcalfe et al, 1981). Venous dilatation, due to the action of progesterone on the smooth muscle in the wall of the vessels, accommodates the increased volume of blood, or blood volume expansion occurs to compensate for this increase in vascular capacity (Metcalfe et al, 1981).

Although the degree of hypervolemia that accompanies pregnancy varies from person to person, the above-mentioned pattern of change is consistent (Pritchard, 1965). When changes in total blood volume are plotted against gestational age, it is very similar to the curve demonstrating changes in cardiac output throughout pregnancy. The hypervolemia is produced to meet the metabolic demands of the uteroplacental-fetal unit to protect the mother and, therefore, the fetus against impaired venous return and decreased cardiac output as the mother continues her usual daily activities that involve numerous position changes. It also prepares the mother for the normal blood loss that accompanies delivery and early puerperium.

The average increase in total blood volume for a singleton pregnancy is 1500 ml; this represents a 48 percent increase in blood volume (Pritchard, 1965). Maternal hypervolemia for twin gestations is greater than for singleton pregnancies (Rovinsky and Jaffin, 1965), with a progressive rise that reaches a level of 28 percent above prepregnancy values at 21 to 24 weeks' gestation to a peak increase of 59 percent at 37 to 40 weeks' gestation. Triplet pregnancies show an even greater increase. The expansion in total blood volume results from an increase in both plasma volume and red blood cell mass.

## Plasma Volume

The increase in plasma volume begins at 6 to 8 weeks' gestation and reaches a plateau by approximately the 32nd week. The plasma volume level is maintained until delivery (Lund and Donovan, 1967; Metcalfe et al, 1981). This increase measures 1200 to 1300 ml greater than nonpregnant plasma volume (Hytten and Leitch, 1971).

Plasma volume regulation and transcapillary fluid balance are the result of many complex mechanisms. The increased levels of estrogens and progesterones during gestation increase plasma renin activity and aldosterone levels to promote sodium retention and an increase in total body water. Tubular sodium reabsorption rises with gestation, and 500 to 900 mEq of sodium are retained along with an increase of 6 to 8 liters of total body water, two thirds of which is extracellular (Lindheimer and Katz, 1975).

The extracellular fluid volume includes the plasma volume and the interstitial fluid volume. The fluid transport between the plasma and the interstitial compartment takes place at the capillary level across the semipermeable capillary membrane. Normally, there is a net capillary filtration pressure, and the filtration rate is balanced by an equal lymph flow. Any change in the hydrostatic pressures, the colloid osmotic pressure, or the lymph flow influences the transcapillary fluid transport and therefore both plasma volume and interstitial fluid volume.

During normal pregnancy, the plasma albumin concentration is reduced about 10 g/l below the prepregnant level (Fadnes and Oian, 1989), a result of a progressive decrease to the early third trimester and then a slower decrease until term. This produces a reduction in the colloid osmotic pressure. Colloid osmotic pressure describes the ability of the intravascular space to retain fluid owing to large molecules that set up an osmotic gradient. Albumin and globulin are the major components in the plasma that influence colloid osmotic pressure. Such a reduction in the colloid osmotic pressure should lead to a movement of fluid from the intravascular compartment to the interstitial compartment; yet, this does not occur. A steady state is maintained by the balance of the reduced peripheral resistance versus the increase in capillary pressure (Valenzuela, 1989). Mean colloid osmotic pressure values of 25.4 mm Hg have been reported for nonpregnant ambulatory adults. In pregnancy, there is a steady decline in the colloid osmotic pressure until approximately 36 weeks' gestation; mean values at term are reported to be 22.4 mm Hg. There is a further decline postpartum, with values as low as 15.4 mm Hg being reported. Under certain pathologic conditions, such as preeclampsia, the colloid osmotic pressure is further decreased (Cotton, 1984).

During normal pregnancy, pulmonary capillary wedge pressure does not increase significantly from the nonpregnant state (Clark et al, 1989), regardless of higher stroke volume. Ventricular dilatation occurs instead to accommodate the marked increased volume.

## Red Cell Volume

Red cell mass increases during pregnancy but at a disproportionate amount and rate to the increase in plasma volume. The increase in red cell mass begins later and continues longer than the increase in plasma volume, and the progressive increase is at a slower rate than plasma volume increase. The increase in red cell mass is 20 to 30 percent, with levels of 250 to 450 ml greater than the nonpregnant red cell mass. This expansion is due to an increase in red cell production, not by prolongation of red cell life (Pritchard, 1965). The plasma volume increase is 45 to 50 percent, whereas red cell volume increase is only 20 to 30 percent. This produces a hemodilution state with a decrease in hemoglobin and hematocrit values. A physiologic anemia occurs even in women with normal iron and folate stores (Hytten and Leitch, 1971). The anemia is most pronounced at the time when plasma volume reaches its plateau and is less pronounced as erythropoiesis continues without further expansion of plasma volume in the last weeks of pregnancy. The stimulus for increased erythropoiesis is probably a fall in tissue oxygen tension in the kidney (Metcalfe et al, 1981).

## ARTERIAL BLOOD PRESSURE

Arterial blood pressure measurement is a common cardiovascular study performed during pregnancy; therefore, the establishment of normal values is of great importance to detect pathologic states (Villar et al, 1989). Maternal position alters blood pressure readings. Blood pressure is highest when the pregnant woman is standing or seated, somewhat lower when she is supine, and lowest when she is in the lateral position. There is also a difference of 10 to 12 mm Hg in blood pressure between the superior and inferior arms in the lateral recumbent position. The superior arm has the lower reading, and the dependent arm has the higher reading, owing to hydrostatic principles. Consistency in blood pressure measurements is necessary to determine actual changes.

Because of the increased blood volume of pregnancy, the diastolic pressure may be difficult to determine because the Korotkoff's phase 5 (the point the sound disappears) may continue all the way down. When present, the Korotkoff's phase 4 (the point of muffling) needs to be included in the documentation of the blood pressure reading (e.g., 120/60/12) (Villar et al, 1989).

During pregnancy, blood pressure falls somewhat in the first trimester, reaches its lowest levels in the second trimester, and rises toward the prepregnancy level during the last four weeks of pregnancy. The systolic pressure decreases 5 to 10 mm Hg from the nonpregnant value, and the diastolic arterial pressure, as determined by Korotkoff's phase 4, decreases progressively to nearly 10 to 15 mm Hg by 28 to 32 weeks' gestation. Thus, there is an increase in pulse pressure (Wilson et al, 1980).

### Venous Pressure

Venous pressure in the upper extremities remains unchanged during pregnancy. However, there is a progressive increase in venous pressure in the lower extremities as pregnancy advances. This increase in lower extremity pressure is due to the hydrostatic forces involved when the pelvic veins and inferior vena cava are compressed by the enlarging uterus and the increased blood volume (Brinkman, 1989).

The venous bed becomes more prominent during pregnancy than in the nonpregnant state owing to the vasodilation. The enlarged superficial veins are readily seen over the pregnant woman's body. Venous compliance increases to accommodate the hemodynamic adaptations. This compliance peaks in the third trimester. The increased compliance produces a decrease in the velocity of venous blood flow that may lead to venous stasis (Brinkman, 1989). It is not possible to define the exact mechanism for the increase in venous capacitance during pregnancy. Progesterone has a relaxing effect on the smooth muscle of the venous system, and there are animal data to suggest that pregnancy may alter the elastic properties of the venous walls; therefore, it is likely that multiple mechanisms contribute to the changes in the venous capacitance during pregnancy.

Dependent edema commonly occurs during the last half of pregnancy as a result of two physiologic actions. One mechanism is the increased venous pressure in the lower extremities that results when the pregnant woman stands or sits upright, which increases the compression of the major vessels by the gravid uterus. The second mechanism is the decrease in colloid oncotic pressure that occurs during normal pregnancy. These two actions facilitate fluid shift from the capillaries to the extravascular space, resulting in dependent edema (Pritchard and MacDonald, 1980).

This pedal edema worsens during the day, when the gravida is busy with daily activities, and is greatly alleviated after a night's rest in the lateral position. This position eliminates the uterine compression of major veins, and the extravascular fluid is mobilized into the circulation.

## SYSTEMIC AND PULMONARY RESISTANCE

Systemic vascular resistance is decreased 21 percent and pulmonary resistance decreases 34 percent by 36 to 38 weeks' gestation (Clark et al, 1989). Two factors are responsible for the decline in systemic vascular resistance. One is the effect of progesterone on the vascular walls to dilate the peripheral blood vessels. The other factor is the uteroplacental circulation, with its low pressure network that uses a large portion of the maternal circulation (Hytten and Leitch, 1971).

The placental vascular bed is a low-resistant network that requires a large percentage of the maternal cardiac output. Early in the second trimester, trophoblastic invasion of the walls of the spiral arteries in the placental bed converts the uteroplacental circulation to a low-resistant network that uses a large percentage of the maternal cardiac output. In human pregnancy, uterine blood flow is estimated to be 700 ml.

The decrease in pulmonary vascular resistance is due to low-resistant vessels in the lung beds. The decrease is 34 percent, which is dramatic compared with the nonpregnant state (Clark et al, 1989). The decrease occurs as vascular tone of the vessels in the lungs decreases and the presence of high progesterone levels results in vasodilation.

---

# Respiratory System

Respiration involves two mechanisms: the first is the exchange of oxygen from inhaled air to the circulating blood in the pulmonary capillaries for carbon dioxide to be exhaled; the second mechanism includes oxygen use and carbon dioxide elimination on the cellular level.

Anatomic and physiologic adaptations are necessary during gestation so that a functional system exists to supply adequate oxygen and the elimination of carbon dioxide.

Oxygen consumption increases progressively because fetal oxygen needs multiply with growth, and maternal oxygen requirements surge in response to accelerated metabolism and growth in the maternal body.

## DEFINITIONS

The following lung volumes and lung capacities are commonly measured in respiratory physiology:

1. *Vital capacity*—the maximum volume of gas that can be expired after a maximum inspiration. Does not include the residual volume.
2. *Tidal volume*—the volume of gas that is exchanged with each breath.
3. *Minute ventilation*—the volume of gas expired per minute.
4. *Functional residual capacity*—the volume of gas that remains in the lungs at the end of a normal expiration (Expiratory reserve volume plus residual volume).
5. *Inspiratory capacity*—the maximum volume of air that can be inspired from the resting expiratory level.
6. *Residual volume*—the volume of gas remaining in the lungs at the end of maximal expiration. Does not include the anatomic dead space of the trachea and bronchial tree.
7. *Inspiratory reserve volume*—maximum amount of air that can be inspired, beyond the normal tidal inspiration.
8. *Expiratory reserve volume*—maximum amount of air that can be expired from the resting end-expiratory position.
9. *Resting end-expiratory position*—the position of the chest at the end of quiet expiration.

## ANATOMIC CHANGES

During normal pregnancy, capillary engorgement in the nose, nasopharynx, larynx, and tracheobronchial tree occurs as a result of the increased blood supply to peripheral tissues. Nasal congestion is common, nosebleed occurs easily, and edema of the larynx can produce voice changes (Bonica, 1967). Care must be exerted when manipulating the upper airway, because too forceful suctioning, forceful placement of airways, or careless laryngoscopy may result in bleeding and trauma (Gutsche, 1979). When endotracheal intubation is performed, a 6.5 to 7.0 cuffed endotracheal tube is used rather than the usual 8 mm cuffed endotracheal tube, because the area of the false cords is usually swollen (Gutsche, 1979).

The diaphragm rises about 4 cm above the nonpregnant level, causing a decrease in the length of the lungs (Cunningham, 1989). To compensate for this shortening of the lungs, the rib cage flares out progressively as pregnancy advances so that the transverse and anteroposterior diameters of the chest increase by 2 cm. The substernal angle widens 50 percent, from 70 degrees in the first trimester to 105 degrees at term (Bonica, 1967); the thoracic cage circumference increases 5 to 7 cm. These changes permit the maintenance of overall normal volume in the lungs during pregnancy. These alterations in chest configuration begin early in gestation, before mechanical upward pressure of the uterus is possible, suggesting that it is caused by hormonal mechanism. During gestation, breathing is more diaphragmatic than costal as compared with the nonpregnant state. The effect of the elevation of the diaphragm on the lungs is counterbalanced by four factors: (1) the compensatory broadening of the chest wall, (2) the change from abdominal to thoracic breathing, (3) the relaxation of smooth muscle in the tracheobronchial tree, and (4) the increase in minute ventilation. "Diaphragmatic excursion is not impeded by the enlarging uterus, but actually increases 1 to 2 cm." (Gabbe, 1986).

## VENTILATIONS

Tidal volume, respiratory rate, and minute volume all increase during early pregnancy. Dead space does not change. Residual volume, expiratory reserve volume, and functional residual capacity consistently decrease. Closing capacity and closing volume remain unaltered.

The progressive increase in minute ventilation begins in the first trimester of pregnancy and is about 50 percent above prepregnancy levels by the end of gestation. This increase is accomplished mainly by an increase in tidal volume, which increases from 450 to 600 ml/min over nonpregnant values. The rise in respiratory rate from 14 to 16 breaths/min also contributes to this effect (Bonica, 1967). This increase in respiratory rate is mediated by progesterone, which

stimulates the respiratory center. Increased ventilation is necessary to meet the demands for the increase in oxygen consumption and to increase the elimination of carbon dioxide.

The increase in alveolar ventilation causes the arterial carbon dioxide tension to fall to 32 mm Hg by the third month and remain unaltered through the duration of pregnancy. Maternal alkalosis is prevented by the compensatory decrease in serum bi-carbonate of about 4 mEq/l (from 26 to 22 mEq/l). Hyperventilation in labor, especially in the transition phase when pain becomes more severe, may result in maternal hypocapnia (Gutsche, 1979). Hyperventilation that lowers the maternal $Paco_2$ produces a concentration gradient across the placenta to facilitate the elimination of fetal carbon dioxide (Pritchard and MacDonald, 1980). Thus the transplacental oxygen transfer is regulated by a change in the oxygen affinity of the maternal and fetal hemoglobin (double Bohr effect). This maximizes oxygen exhange from the maternal and fetal circulation, and therefore, the amount of oxygen released to the fetal tissue at any given maternal $Pao_2$ is increased (Bauer et al, 1969).

During active labor, transition, and the pushing efforts in the second stage, ventilation may increase as much as 300 percent compared with the nonpregnant state (Gutsche, 1979). Hyperventilation during this part of labor is a response to pain. Pain relief, such as epidural anesthesia or appropriate breathing techniques taught in a prepared childbirth class, can help prevent maternal alkalosis during these stages of labor.

The rapid, deep breathing that accompanies gestation enhances gas anesthesia. This type of breathing facilitates a more rapid induction and recovery from inhalation anesthesia (Bonica, 1967).

## LUNG VOLUMES

A summary of lung volume changes is provided in Figure 13–1 (Bonica, 1967). Changes primarily involve functional residual capacity.

### Functional Residual Capacity

Functional residual capacity progressively decreases during gestation as the enlarging uterus elevates the diaphragm (Baldwin,

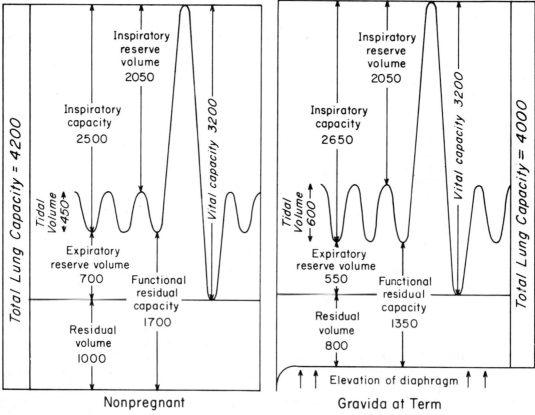

**Figure 13–1** Pulmonary volumes and capacities during pregnancy, labor, and postpartum period. (Reproduced with permission from Bonica, J. J.: Principles and Practice of Obstetric Analgesia and Anesthesia. Philadelphia, FA Davis, 1967, p 24.)

1977). The functional residual capacity is the volume of gas that mixes with the inhaled air with each breath. Tidal volume increases 40 percent during pregnancy, whereas functional residual capacity decreases 20 percent. Therefore, an increased volume of inhaled air is mixed with a smaller volume of residual air in the lungs. This accomplishes a more efficient mixing and exchange of the gases.

The decrease in functional residual capacity lowers oxygen reserve in the pregnant woman; hypoxia occurs rapidly, even with only a short period of apnea. The diminished functional residual capacity is of interest to the anesthesiologist attending the obstetric patient. Because of the diminished oxygen stores in the lungs and increased total body consumption, the rate and magnitude of the decreases in the $PaO_2$ in an apneic pregnant patient are greater than those in a nonpregnant patient.

## Airway Resistance

Increased airway resistance does not accompany this reduced functional residual capacity with less distended lungs. Usually, lungs that are less distended produce smaller airways with smaller lumina. However, the increased progesterone levels that occur with the gravid state relax the bronchial smooth muscle so that decreased airway resistance results (Bonica, 1967).

## Vital Capacity

Although functional residual capacity decreases during gestation, the inspiratory capacity increases so that vital capacity remains unchanged during pregnancy (Bonica, 1967). A decrease in vital capacity during pregnancy may indicate that a pulmonary or cardiovascular problem exists and that further study is indicated.

## OXYGEN CONSUMPTION

Oxygen consumption increases progressively as pregnancy advances, both at rest and during exercise. Numerous studies have found that oxygen consumption increases 20 percent during the last weeks of pregnancy when the gravida is at rest (Baldwin et al, 1977; Hytten and Leitch, 1971; Pernoll et al, 1975). The fetus and placenta use approximately half of this increase in oxygen consumption; the maternal body (including the uterus, breasts, cardiovascular system, respiratory system, and renal system) uses the other half. Oxygen consumption increases proportionally in multiple gestation (Hytten and Leitch, 1971). Additional oxygen is required during labor so that there is a 300 percent increase with each uterine contraction during the last part of the first stage of labor. Pushing efforts require an additional 200 percent increase in oxygen consumption (Gutsche, 1979).

### EXERCISE

The current interest in physical fitness has extended to the pregnant state. Numerous studies have explored the capacity for exercise during gestation. Artal and associates (1986) found that during treadmill testing in late pregnancy, pregnant women could not increase oxygen consumption as much as before their pregnancy. Clapp (1989) reported on treadmill testing before, during, and after pregnancy. Results were

1. The efficacy of low-to-moderate intensity treadmill exercise in physically active women is improved in early pregnancy.
2. The increased efficiency is masked in later pregnancy by the effects of weight gain.
3. The degree of efficiency is enhanced throughout pregnancy in women who continue a regular exercise program at or above a basic conditioning level.

Short-term exercise does not appear to cause adverse effects in the fetus. Changes in uterine blood flow caused by maternal exercise are compensated for by the increased oxygen extraction capacity of the placenta and fetus (Lotgering et al, 1984).

# Hematologic System

## PLASMA VOLUME AND RED BLOOD CELL MASS

During normal pregnancy, maternal plasma volume increase is detectable at 6 weeks' gestation (Lund and Donovan, 1967). After this time, levels rise rapidly and reach a peak at about 32 to 34 weeks' gestation. A plateau is then maintained until delivery (Lund and Donovan, 1967). The mean rise in plasma volume is 1200 ml (Hytten and Leitch, 1971) to 1500 ml (Lund and Donovan, 1967)— a 25 percent increase. In twin gestations, the increase is greater than in singleton pregnancies, from 1500 ml (Hytten and Leitch, 1971) to 2000 ml (Rovinsky and Jaffin, 1965).

The plasma volume increase of 40 percent and the red cell volume increase of only 20 percent is disproportionate and produces a decreased packed cell volume, or hematocrit, during pregnancy. A so-called physiologic anemia of pregnancy results. This physiologic anemia is greatest at 32 to 34 weeks' gestation, when plasma volume reaches its peak. The hematocrit may improve after this time as the plasma volume plateaus, and red cell volume is still increasing.

Red blood cell volume begins to increase at about 10 weeks' gestation, and increases steadily until term. The mean rise in red cell volume is approximately 400 ml, which is a 20 percent increase (Lund and Donovan, 1967). Iron supplementation during pregnancy makes a significant difference in red cell volume. Hytten and Leitch (1971) reported an increase in red cell volume of 250 ml when no iron supplementation was used, whereas the increase in red cell volume was 400 to 500 ml with iron supplementation. As with plasma volume, red cell volume increases more in multiple than in singleton pregnancies (Rovinsky and Jaffin, 1965).

Red cell counts decrease from nonpregnant values of $4.6 \times 10^6/mm^3$ to $3.88 \times 10^6/mm^3$ at 36 weeks' gestation (Meyer, 1983). The increase in red blood cell mass is a result of increased production of red blood cells and not prolongation of red cell life. The mean age of circulating maternal red blood cells is younger because the rate of red blood cell production exceeds that of destruction (Fleming, 1975). Red blood cells are largest when released from the bone marrow; therefore, an increased number of young red blood cells takes up more space or volume than old red blood cells and explains the increase in red blood cell volume in the presence of a decrease in the number of red blood cells.

This type of red blood cell also has an increased concentration of 2,3-diphosphoglycerate, which produces a decreased affinity for oxygen, facilitating the dissociation of oxygen from hemoglobin for placental transfer to fetal hemoglobin (Bauer et al, 1969). Hemoglobin and hematocrit decrease 15 percent with an overall hematocrit in the second trimester of 33.4 percent (range 31.9 to 36.5 percent) and 33.8 percent in the third trimester (range 31.9 to 36.5 percent) (Anderson, 1989). Although at higher altitudes such as Denver, Colorado, prepregnancy values as well as pregnancy values would be higher.

## WHITE BLOOD CELLS

The total white blood cell count increases considerably during gestation as a result of an increase in neutrophil polymorphonuclear leukocytes (Fleming, 1975). During the first trimester, the mean white blood cell count is 9500/mm³, with a normal range of 3000 to 15,000/mm³. During the second and third trimesters, the mean increases further to 10,500/mm³, with a range of 6000 to 16,000/mm³. During labor, the count may rise to 20,000 to 30,000/mm³ in the noninfected patient (Pitkin and Witte, 1979). The count returns to nonpregnant levels by the end of the first week postpartum.

## PLATELETS

In normal pregnancy, there is a significant fall in the platelet count after 31 weeks' gestation accompanied by a significant rise in mean platelet volume (Fay et al, 1983). Although there is a progressive decline in the platelet count throughout pregnancy and a rise in the platelet count in the early puerperium, the count remains within the normal range for the nonpregnant state of 150,000 to 400,000/mm³ (Pitkin and Witte, 1979). The mean platelet count in early pregnancy (< 20 weeks' gestation) is 257,000/mm³. In late pregnancy (> 35 weeks' gestation), the mean count is 260,000/mm³ (Gerbasi, 1990).

## BLOOD COAGULATION

Blood is hypercoagulable during pregnancy. The serum fibrinogen concentration increases from 300 mg/dl to 480 mg/dl. This change may be hormonally mediated by the estrogen stimulation of the liver to increase fibrinogen production. The concentration of Factor VII (proconvertin), Factor VIII (antihemophilic globulin), Factor IX (Christmas factor), and Factor X (Stuart-Prower factor) are increased. The levels of Factors XI and XIII decrease, however, probably because of consumption at the placental site. Prothrombin time, partial thromboplastin time, and bleeding time remain essentially within normal limits. In pregnancy, there is a progressive inhibition of fibrinolysis. Plasminogen levels remain the same, but the activity of plasminogen activator decreases. This leads to a delay in fibrinolysis. Fibrin split products increase only slightly during gestation, with no evidence of a generalized fibrinolysis (Meyer, 1983).

# Renal System

The renal system adapts to the demands of pregnancy by undergoing remarkable anatomic and physiologic changes that produce two potential problems: the increased risk of urinary tract infection and erroneous interpretation of diagnostic test results.

## ANATOMIC CHANGES

The kidneys enlarge during gestation as a result of the increase in renal blood flow and renal vascular volume. There is also some hypertrophy of the kidneys (Beydoun, 1985). The renal calyces, pelves, and ureters dilate to produce a physiologic hydroureter of pregnancy. This dilatation begins in the first trimester, as early as the 10th week of gestation, before the enlarging uterus has grown enough to produce mechanical compression. This suggests that a hormonal influence is involved in dilatation. Dilatation continues throughout pregnancy and into puerperium (Hytten and Leitch, 1971).

The mechanism or etiology of the pregnancy-associated hydronephrosis has been ascribed to multiple causes and includes the external compression exerted by the gravid uterus as well as hormonal influences on the renal collecting system. Microscopic changes that occur in the ureters during pregnancy include hyperplasia of the longitudinal smooth muscle and inflammatory edema (Lindheimer and Katz, 1975). Sala and Rubi (1967) studied ureteral contractility during gestation and found that in both pregnant and nonpregnant women, the ureters contract rhythmically with prolonged periods of relaxation. This contractility does not diminish during gestation. A decrease in the mean contractile pressure in the lower part of the ureter has been observed during pregnancy.

The dilation of the urinary collecting system in the second half of pregnancy increases the dead space or capacity of the ureters. The entire collecting system may have a volume of 200 ml in late pregnancy. This potential dead space can have a significant effect on evaluation of changes in renal function during pregnancy. In addition, increased volume contained in the dilated ureters and renal pelvis results in a slowing of the flow of urine. Stasis of urine occurs, predisposing the gravida to urinary tract infections (Hytten and Leitch, 1971). Postpartum resolution occurs rapidly, within weeks of delivery (Beydoun, 1985).

The sequence of the development of pyeloureteral dilatation is as follows;

1. Increased levels of sex hormones produce thickening of the lower part of the ureter and softening of the upper part.
2. Mild dilatation of the upper portion of the ureters occurs.
3. Pregnancy progresses; partial ureteral compression results.
4. Further dilatation develops.
5. Inflammatory edema ensues.

### Bladder

The tone of the bladder progressively decreases during gestation because of the effects of progesterone on smooth muscle. Capacity is doubled by term to more than a liter (Beydoun, 1985). Estrogen stimulation produces moderate hyperplasia and muscular hypertrophy in the trigone area. The bladder is displaced anteriorly and superiorly by the enlarging uterus and hyperemia of the organs in the pelvis.

Decreased bladder tone can result in incompetence of the vesicoureteral valve, which creates a reflux from bladder to ureters (Beydoun, 1985). The edema and hyperemia in the bladder, along with the decreased tone, predispose the pregnant woman to asymptomatic bacteriuria. The bacteriuria can ascend to the ureters via the vesicoureteral reflux.

Diagnostic procedures of the urinary bladder are more difficult during pregnancy because of the anterior and upward displacement of the bladder that changes the bladder surface from a normal convex into a concave one. There is a resultant lengthening of the urethra (Beydoun, 1985). Pressure from the uteroplacental-fetal unit on the bladder can interfere with the drainage of blood and lymph from the bladder base. This makes the bladder base edematous, easily traumatized, and susceptible to infection (Davidson, 1985).

## PHYSIOLOGIC CHANGES

Effective renal plasma flow is used as an index of renal blood flow. Effective renal plasma flow increases markedly and early during gestation, with mid-pregnancy increments reaching 60 to 80 percent, followed by a significant fall in the third trimester (Dunlop, 1981; Hytten and Leitch, 1971). Effective renal plasma flow increases to 75 percent over nonpregnant values to a mean value of 840 ml/min by 16 weeks' gestation, when a small decline in effective renal plasma flow occurs (Dunlop, 1981) that is not related to posture (Ezimokhai et al, 1981).

### GLOMERULAR FILTRATION RATE

The glomerular filtration rate (GFR) is most accurately determined by the evaluation of inulin clearance. Inulin is cleared only by the glomerulus, whereas creatinine is excreted by the tubules as well as the glomerulus. Therefore, endogenous creatinine clearance is usually higher than the actual GFR. Inulin clearance to determine the GFR is the preferred method of measurement for researchers, who must know exact amounts. However, the evaluation of endogenous creatinine clearance is an easier test to perform and is used clinically to determine the approximate GFR, unless a disease condition is present that will give grossly false results. In renal compromise states, creatinine clearance values may show false urine concentration when urine creatinine clearance is in fact low and serum creatinine is elevated. In normal physiologic states, creatinine clearance and inulin clearance show comparable ranges (Brinkman, 1989).

The GFR begins to increase early in the first trimester of pregnancy, reaching a peak of nearly 40 percent above nonpregnant levels by 20 weeks' gestation. Thereafter, the increase in GFR is slow for the remainder of pregnancy, with no more than an additional 10 percent increase, so that a total increase of 50 percent over nonpregnant levels occurs.

As a result of the increased GFR and renal plasma flow (RPF), the renal clearance of many substances is elevated during gestation, with a corresponding decrease in serum values. Endogenous creatinine clearance is greatly increased during pregnancy. Values of 150 to 200 ml/min are normal during gestation. Serum creatinine levels decrease from the nonpregnant level of 0.8 mg/dl to 0.7 mg/dl by the end of the first trimester and to 0.5 to 0.6 mg/dl in the latter weeks of pregnancy (Cruikshank and Hays, 1986). The blood urea nitrogen level decreases to values of 8 to 9 mg/dl during pregnancy because of the increased GFR (Cruikshank and Hays, 1986). Serum uric acid levels decrease in early pregnancy, reaching the lowest levels of 2.0 to 3.0 mg/dl by 24 weeks' gestation. After this time, uric acid levels begin to rise and reach nonpregnant levels by the end of gestation (Lind et al, 1984).

Immediately after delivery, 24-hour creatinine clearance increases profoundly to parallel the increased blood volume of autotransfusion that occurs in the fourth stage of labor. The marked diuresis that accompanies early puerperium eliminates the extra fluid, and creatinine clearance values return to nonpregnant levels by the sixth day postpartum (Davidson, 1985).

## RENAL TUBULAR FUNCTION

### Glucose

Glycosuria occurs frequently in normal pregnancy and may even occur with normal blood glucose levels. Glycosuria is thought to be a result of the greatly increased GFR in pregnancy combined with the inability of the renal tubules to increase reabsorption at the same rate of increase in GFR. The tubular maximum for glucose reabsorption does not change during pregnancy; thus, excess glucose is excreted in the urine (Davidson, 1985).

### Amino Acids

Aminoaciduria occurs frequently during gestation and may reach 2 g/day of amino acids in the urine. This is a result of the increased GFR combined with inability of the tubules to increase resorption. Three distinct patterns of amino acid excretion are present during pregnancy (Brinkman, 1989):

1. Excretion of glycine, histidine, threonine, serine, and alanine begins to increase in early pregnancy and doubles by 16 weeks' gestation. The excretion continues to increase until delivery.
2. Concentrations of lysine, cystine, taurine, tyrosine, and phenylalanine and excretion of leucine increase in the first half of pregnancy, then decrease in the last half.
3. Excretion of asparagine, glutamic acid, methionine, isoleucine, ornithine, and arginine is unchanged with pregnancy.

### Water Metabolism

During gestation, volume homeostasis must occur to meet the increased needs of the developing uteroplacental-fetal unit as well as the additional growth in the gravida body. To accomplish this, the retention of the following is necessary (Hytten and Leitch, 1971):

2 liters water
290 mEq sodium
155 mEq potassium
1.2 liters amniotic fluid
700 ml water in the uterus
300 ml water in the placenta
400 ml water in the breasts

increased electrolytes

1500 ml increased blood volume that contains:

    150 mEq sodium

    60 mEq potassium

extracellular fluid compartment expands 1.5 liters

The normal kidney has an almost unlimited ability to control water and electrolyte balance (Davidson, 1985). Early in pregnancy, the plasma osmolarity decreases 10 mOsm/kg $H_2O$ to 270 to 280 mOsm/kg $H_2O$. These values correspond to hyperhydration values in the nonpregnant woman.

## Sodium

The increase in glomerular filtration rate and renal plasma flow causes an increased natriuresis in pregnancy. Approximately 20,000 to 30,000 mmols of sodium may be filtered through the kidneys of a pregnant woman. If all of the filtered sodium is allowed to be excreted in the urine, the pregnant patient may rapidly develop circulatory collapse. Indeed, the pregnant woman gains 4 to 6 mmols of sodium/day to be stored in the fetal and maternal unit. Sodium metabolism in normal pregnancy is delicately balanced to facilitate a gradual accumulation of 900 to 1000 mEq of sodium, which is distributed to the fetus, placenta, and maternal vascular interstitial space (Lindheimer, 1980).

The changes in tubular resorption represent the largest renal adjustment that occurs during gestation (Davidson, 1985). Plasma sodium decreases slightly during gestation as a result of water retention in excess of solute (Brinkman, 1989).

Factors that promote sodium excretion during pregnancy are increased GFR, elevated progesterone levels, increased antidiuretic hormone, decreased plasma albumin, and decreased vascular resistance. Sodium resorption is promoted by increased concentrations of aldosterone, estrogens, cortisol, placental lactogen, and prolactin.

## POSTURE

The supine position decreases sodium excretion. The upright position causes extracellular shifts to the legs, producing a relative decrease in central blood volume. This results in the release of renin by the kidney to increase angiotensin production, which then stimulates aldosterone secretion. Aldosterone enhances renal tubular resorption of sodium to reduce urinary excretion of sodium and water. The supine position exaggerates this response (Pritchard and MacDonald, 1980).

Both supine and upright positions cause a reduction in renal blood flow and GFR and, thereby, a reduction in the excretion of water and sodium. The supine position can cause compression of the inferior vena cava and descending aorta by the gravid uterus. The upright position can cause compression of the common iliac veins by the uterus. Thus, venous return from the legs is reduced in both positions, producing decreased cardiac output and a drop in blood pressure. Compensatory renal vasoconstriction with decreased renal blood flow ensues. Glomerular filtration is reduced, and thus the excretion of water and electrolytes is reduced (Pritchard and MacDonald, 1980).

## RENIN-ANGIOTENSIN-ALDOSTERONE

All components of the renin-angiotensin-aldosterone system are elevated during gestation. Aldosterone concentrations increase early in pregnancy through the end of pregnancy. Increase in renin substrate shows a similar pattern. Increased amounts of renin substrate result in elevated levels of angiotensin I and II (Wilson et al, 1980). The normal pregnant woman has a markedly reduced sensitivity to the hypertensive effects of angiotensin. The main response during pregnancy to the elevated levels of angiotensin is to stimulate increased aldosterone production and thereby promote sodium resorption. The exact cause of the elevations in the components of this system is unclear. The increases may be a response to the volume expansion and elevated concentrations of progesterone and estrogen or perhaps primary pregnancy changes in themselves.

## Bicarbonate

Urinary excretion of bicarbonate increases during pregnancy as a result of the hyperventilation and hypocapnia that accompany the pulmonary adaptations of pregnancy.

This produces a slight increase in the urine pH (Ueland and Ueland, 1986).

## Protein

Protein excretion in the urine increases during gestation. Proteinuria is not considered significant until protein excretion exceeds 300 mg in 24 hours (Davidson, 1985).

## Vitamins

Excretion of several water-soluble vitamins increases with gestation. Urinary excretion of folate and vitamin $B_{12}$ is also increased in pregnancy.

## DIURNAL PATTERN

During the day, when the pregnant woman is upright and undertaking her usual daily activities, a large amount of fluid is retained as dependent edema develops. Urine concentration increases as the day progresses. At night, especially if resting in the lateral position, the fluid is mobilized into the systemic circulation and excreted. Nocturia occurs, and urine concentration decreases. During gestation, evening urine specimens are more accurate for urine concentration tests to determine tubular function (Ueland and Ueland, 1986).

# Gastrointestinal System

## APPETITE

The appetite increases to provide nutrients for mother and fetus. The increase begins early in the first trimester, in the absence of morning sickness or nausea, and persists throughout pregnancy. Pregnant women who eat according to appetite will increase their daily food intake. There are many myths associated with food cravings and aversions during pregnancy (Hollingsworth, 1985). (See also Chapter 11, Nutrition in Pregnancy.)

## METABOLIC CHANGES

Profound metabolic changes in the maternal body are necessary for growth and devel-opment of the fetus and to buffer it from internal and external environmental stresses. Higher levels of circulating insulin, relative fasting and nocturnal hypoglycemia occur in normal pregnancy (Hollingsworth, 1985). Maternal metabolic homeostasis continues in the presence of high serum levels of placental lactogen, estrogens, progesterone, adrenocorticotropic hormone, cortisol, and lipids.

## WEIGHT GAIN

Additional energy is needed during pregnancy to compensate for the increased maternal metabolism and for fetal growth and development. Weight gain represents energy intake to offset energy expenditure. The recommended weight gain of the normal gravida at term is between 25 and 35 pounds (Pitkin, 1976). However, the pattern of weight gain is more important than the total weight accumulated. Pitkin (1976) found that calorie expenditure is not evenly distributed during gestation, because it increases only slightly during the first nine weeks then increases fairly sharply and continues increasing constantly until term. This pattern results in a steady caloric expenditure during the last 30 weeks of gestation, so that the cumulative energy cost of pregnancy has been calculated as 75,000 kcal or 300 kcal/day (Pitkin, 1980). The usual pattern shows a gain of approximately 3 pounds for the first trimester, followed by a steady gain of 1.0 lb/week during the second and third trimesters. An adequate weight gain is most important. The underweight gravida is at high risk of having a low-birth-weight infant, as is the woman with inadequate weight gain during pregnancy (Pitkin, 1976). Abrams and Parker (1990) reported that a higher maternal weight gain than currently recommended is correlated with good outcomes.

## CARBOHYDRATE METABOLISM

The rise in serum levels of estrogen and progesterone stimulate increased glycogen storage. Increased insulin secretion then occurs with increased use of peripheral glucose, and the normal fasting blood glucose level decreases. Glucose and amino acids are continuously transferred from the maternal circulation to the fetus for growth and development. Plasma insulin levels fall throughout the day (Felig, 1977). Normal pregnant women maintain a very narrow euglycemic range, with a mean 24 h plasma glucose level of 84 ± 10 mg/dl, with marked hyperinsulinemia (Felig, 1977).

## PICA

Pica, the craving for nonnutritive foods, may occur during pregnancy. A careful history to identify pica is advised for pregnant women with a poor weight gain or refractory anemia (Cruikshank and Hays, 1986). The craving for non-nutritive foods seems to be the result of cultural influences rather than hunger. The practice is most common among the indigent population, especially in the Southern states in the United States. In this area, the ingestion of starch, either laundry or cornstarch (amylophagia), and clay (geophagia) are the most common forms of pica. In the United Kingdom, the most common form of pica is ingestion of coal. Soap, toothpaste, and ice pica have also been reported in numerous areas of the world (Cruikshank and Hays, 1986). Early studies suggested that pica may be triggered by iron deficiency anemia, because women with severe iron-deficiency anemia crave these nonfood substances. It is controversial whether or not iron deficiency in anemic pregnant women is the cause or effect of the anemia. Ingestion of some clay, especially Turkish clay and to a lesser extent clays from Mississippi and Georgia, impairs iron absorption, according to a study by Minnich and associates (1968). Talkington and associates (1970) found that Texas clays and Argo Gloss Starch did not significantly reduce iron absorption (Cunningham, 1989).

## TASTE AND SMELL

The pregnancy-induced hyperemia of the mucous membranes of the nasopharynx produces a more acute sense of taste and smell. Previously inoffensive odors are now offensive, especially those of fried foods, coffee, and perfumes. These offensive odors can precipitate nausea and vomiting in the early weeks of pregnancy. The acute sense of taste that develops during pregnancy can contribute to the nausea during the first trimester but then adds to the enjoyment of food after the nausea subsides.

## NAUSEA AND VOMITING OF PREGNANCY

Nausea, with or without vomiting, is common in early gestation; it has been reported in 70 percent of pregnancies (Cruikshank and Hays, 1986). Typically, onset is between 4 and 8 weeks' gestation, continuing to about 14 to 16 weeks' gestation. Symptoms vary from a slight nausea on awakening, in some women, to persistent and frequent vomiting throughout the day, in other women. Morning sickness may appear at any time of the day, but it is most common in the morning.

The cause of the nausea and vomiting of pregnancy is not fully understood. Relaxation of the smooth muscle of the stomach is a probable factor, as well as elevated levels of sex steroids and human chorionic gonadotropin. However, there does not seem to be as strong a correlation between maternal serum human chorionic gonadotropin levels and the degree of nausea and vomiting (Soules et al, 1980).

Relief measures include reassurance, psychologic support, avoidance of those foods that trigger nausea, and frequent small meals. Helpful suggestions are to eat a dry carbohydrate food, such as crackers, before arising in the morning or to consume something sweet (fruit or fruit juice) and to avoid spicy foods with strong odors. The gravida is encouraged to discover what works best for her so she can cope until the symptoms disappear after the first trimester.

Hyperemesis gravidarum is a pernicious form of nausea and vomiting of pregnancy and is associated with weight loss, ketonemia, electrolyte imbalance, dehydration, and possible hepatic or renal damage (Cruikshank and Hays, 1986). This condition can be life threatening for both the mother and fetus. Hospitalization with parenteral replacement of fluids, electrolytes, and calories may be necessary, as is the ruling out of underlying disease, such as pyelonephritis, pancreatitis, cholecystitis, or hepatitis.

## STOMACH

The enlarging uterus alters the position of the stomach thereby altering the angle of the gastroesophageal junction. The lower esophageal sphincter may then be displaced into the thorax, which causes incompetence of the gastroesophageal Pinchcock mechanism. Therefore, the pregnant woman is prone to passive regurgitation and aspiration during general anesthesia or unconsciousness from any cause (Gutsche, 1979). Tone and motility of the stomach are decreased because of the relaxing effects of progesterone on smooth muscle. Reduced emptying time of the stomach further increases the risk of pulmonary aspiration. Gastric acid secretion undergoes changes. The reduced incidence and improvement of peptic ulcer disease during pregnancy have been attributed to reduced acid secretion during pregnancy (Hytten and Leitch, 1971). Gastric acid secretion is probably reduced in the first and second trimesters, but in the third trimester, it is significantly increased over nonpregnant values (Murray et al, 1957). Hunt and Murray (1958) reported a significant increase in gastric acid secretion during lactation.

Studies show that parturients having an overnight fast still have greater than 25 ml of gastric fluids with a pH less than 2.5, and are at high risk for aspiration and the development of acid aspiration syndrome (Gutsche, 1979). Antacids may be prescribed during labor, or prior to delivery, especially if general anesthesia is administered for cesarean delivery, to decrease the risk for acid aspiration syndrome if aspiration of gastric content occurs.

### Heartburn

Heartburn is a painful, retrosternal burning sensation that is caused by regurgitation of acidic gastric contents into the esophagus. This regurgitation results from the upward displacement of the stomach by the enlarging uterus, relaxation of the lower esophageal sphincter by progesterone, and delayed gastric emptying time. Increased intra-abdominal pressure compounds the problem (Ueland and Ueland, 1986). Relief measures include smaller, more frequent meals, waiting at least 2 hours after eating before lying down, and bland (rather than spicy) foods. Antacid preparations may be prescribed.

### SMALL AND LARGE INTESTINES

The elevated progesterone levels during pregnancy produce decreased tone and motility of the entire gastrointestinal tract, including the small and large intestines. Constipation is a common problem because of the decreased motility of the colon, increased water absorption from the colon, and mechanical pressure from the gravid uterus (Cruikshank and Hays, 1986). Relief measures include a high fiber diet, adequate fluid intake, exercise, and good bowel habits. Flatulence can occur as a result of the decreased motility in the intestinal tract, along with the mechanical pressure of the enlarging uterus. Relief measures include the avoidance of gas-forming foods, increased activity, and regular bowel habits.

### Hemorrhoids

Hemorrhoids are a common problem in late pregnancy and early puerperium. Many factors contribute to the development of hemorrhoids. The general pelvic hyperemia that occurs during pregnancy, accompanied by mechanical obstruction of the venous return to the heart, produces venous engorgement and increased pressure on the hemorrhoidal vein. Constipation and straining because of hard stools, in the presence of venodilation, aggravate the situation. Hemorrhoids can be especially severe after a prolonged second stage of labor, when extended pushing efforts have been necessary (Ueland and Ueland, 1986). Preventing constipation does much to prevent hemorrhoids. Relief measures include hot sitz baths followed by application of a local anesthetic ointment, avoidance of standing still or sitting for long periods of time, and relieving pressure by propping the legs up several times during the day. The condition usually improves rapidly following delivery.

## Hepatic System

Liver size and morphology do not change during normal pregnancy. Blood flow to the liver does not change, nor are there specific histologic changes that characterize the liver during pregnancy. However, liver function is altered during gestation, as evidenced by alterations in values for liver function tests. In fact, many of the changes in serum values present during normal pregnancy would be suggestive of liver disease in the nonpregnant patient state (Bynum, 1977; Combes and Adams, 1972). Pregnant women frequently develop spider angiomata and palmar erythema owing to increased estrogen levels; these skin changes disappear after delivery.

Serum albumin and total protein levels decrease progressively during gestation. The albumin level of 4.3 g/dl in the nonpregnant state decreases to 3 g/dl during pregnancy. This decrease is due to the increase in plasma volume and hemodilution state of pregnancy. Total serum protein concentration falls during pregnancy but usually remains above 6 g/100ml. The decrease in total proteins is due to the decrease in albumin (Combes and Adams, 1972). Most of the globulins increase progressively throughout gestation. The decrease in serum albumin and increase in serum globulins cause a decrease in the albumin-to-globulin ratio (Combes and Adams, 1972).

Total serum alkaline phosphatase activity rises during pregnancy, so that by the end of pregnancy, values are 2 to 4 times greater than nonpregnant values. This increase is due to the heat-stable alkaline phosphatase isozymes from the placenta as well as maternal hepatic stores (Sadovsky and Zuckerman, 1965). This placenta enzyme appears during the first trimester and progressively increases until term. Levels are even higher with multiple gestation and preeclampsia (Tindall, 1975). Levels decrease gradually after delivery and reach prepregnancy values by 20 days postpartum (Sadovsky and Zuckerman, 1965).

Serum cholesterol levels are doubled by the end of pregnancy, along with the values of most other lipids (Tindall, 1975). The elevated estrogen levels of gestation stimulate an increase in the serum concentration of many proteins produced by the liver. Fibrinogen levels are increased 50 percent by the end of the second trimester. Ceruloplasmin concentrations increase in response to estrogen, as do the binding proteins for corticosteroids, sex steroids, thyroid hormone, and vitamin D (Cruikshank and Hays, 1986).

Values that are not altered during pregnancy are

1. Serum bilirubin does not exceed the upper limit of normal (0.1 mg/dl) values.
2. Serum transaminase values do not exceed normal nonpregnant values.
   a. Aspartate aminotransferase (AST, formerly SGOT)—pregnancy values are the same as nonpregnant.
   b. Alanine aminotransferase (ALT, formerly SGPT)—unchanged in normal pregnancy.
   c. 5-nucleotidase—unchanged.

3. Prothrombin time—unchanged.
   (Tindall, 1975)

Debate is still ongoing as to whether or not the serum y-glutamyltranspeptidase (GGT) is changed.

The dye Bromsulphalein (BSP) is used to study liver function because it is rapidly removed from the blood by the liver, conjugated with glutathione into the bile, and excreted. This ability of the liver to excrete BSP is decreased during gestation by 27 percent in the second half of pregnancy. The liver's capacity to store BSP increases during gestation by 122 percent; therefore, BSP retention can occur (Combes and Adams, 1972). Values for excretion and storage return to normal soon after delivery.

## CHOLESTASIS

Cholestasis is the retention and accumulation of bile in the liver because of excessive levels of sex hormones. Cholestasis can occur during pregnancy and is characterized by itching, jaundice, or both (Lunzer et al, 1986).

### Pruritus Gravidarum

Pruritus, secondary to cholestasis, can occur during pregnancy because of the high estrogen levels, producing a deposition of bile salts in the skin (Lunzer et al, 1986). Cutaneous itching results with varying levels of distress. Pruritus correlates with levels of bile salts in the serum (Bynum, 1977) and may precede jaundice by 2 to 3 weeks. Pruritus gravidarum usually occurs in the last trimester and disappears by 2 weeks postpartum. Relief measures include reassurance that the disorder will resolve itself after delivery. Frequent cornstarch baths, soothing ointments, and avoidance of perfumed soaps and toiletries are helpful. Oral administration of cholestyramine has been found helpful to reduce the discomfort (Lunzer et al, 1986).

## GALLBLADDER

There is a progressive increase in size of the gallbladder during pregnancy because the gallbladder moves into a horizontal position and is compressed by the enlarging uterus (Bartoli et al, 1984). Gallbladder function is altered during gestation because the gallbladder becomes hypotonic and distended. Fasting gallbladder volume in late pregnancy is increased 50 percent. Emptying is slowed and incomplete because the residual volume left in the gallbladder after a meal is larger during pregnancy than in the nonpregnant state (Radberry et al, 1989). Causative factors include the smooth muscle relaxation of progesterone and trophic factors that induce gallbladder hypertrophy (Radberry et al, 1989).

Cholesterol gallstone formation is more common in women than in men in all populations. The incidence increases even more for pregnant women and women taking steroid contraceptives. Although ovarian hormone increases the saturation of bile with cholesterol, abnormal gallbladder function during pregnancy further contributes to the formation of cholesterol gallstones (Bartoli et al, 1984). Pregnancy increases the risk of cholesterol-gallstone formation because the gallbladder is not completely emptied and is left with a large residual volume, which can lead to retention of cholesterol crystals (Braverman et al, 1980).

There are many physiologic adaptations to pregnancy, the majority of which occur early in gestation. A firm understanding of these changes is important to any member of the obstetric team who is caring for the pregnant patient.

## References

Abrams B, Parker JD: Maternal weight gain in women with good pregnancy outcome. Obstet Gynecol 76(1):1, 1990.

Anderson HM: Maternal hematologic disorders. In Creasy RK, Resnik R (eds): Maternal-Fetal Medicine: Principles and Practice, 2nd ed. Philadelphia, WB Saunders Co, 1989.

Artal R, Wiswell R, Romen Y, Dorey F: Pulmonary response to exercise in pregnancy. Am J Obstet Gynecol 154:378, 1986.

Baldwin GR, Moorthi DS, Whelton JA, MacDonnell KF: New lung functions and pregnancy. Am J Obstet Gynecol 127(3):235, 1977.

Bartoli E, Calonaci N, Nenci R: Ultrasonography of the gallbladder in pregnancy. Gastrointest Radiol 9:35, 1984.

Bauer C, Ludwig M, Ludwig I, Bartels H: Factors governing the oxygen affinity of human adult and foetal blood. Respir Physiol 7:271, 1969.

Beydoun SN: Morphologic changes in the renal tract in pregnancy. Clin Obstet Gynecol 28(2):245, 1985.

Bonica JJ: Principles and Practice of Obstetric Analge-sia and Anesthesia. Vol 1. Fundamental Considerations. Philadelphia, FA Davis Co, 1967.

Braverman DZ, Johnson ML, Kern JR F: Effects of pregnancy and contraceptive steroids on gallbladder function. N Engl J Med 302(7):362, 1980.

Brinkman CR III: Biologic adaptations to pregnancy. In Creasy RK, Resnik R (eds): Maternal-Fetal Medicine: Principles and Practice, 2nd ed. Philadelphia, WB Saunders Co, 1989.

Bynum TE: Hepatic and gastrointestinal disorders in pregnancy. Med Clin N Am 61(1):129, 1977.

Capeless EK, Clapp JF: Cardiovascular changes in early phase of pregnancy. Am J Obstet Gynecol 161(6):1449, 1989.

Clapp JR III: Oxygen consumption during treadmill exercise before, during, and after pregnancy. Am J Obstet Gynecol 161(6):1458, 1989.

Clark SL, Cotton DB, Lee W, et al: Central hemodynamic assessment of normal term pregnancy. Am J Obstet Gynecol 161(6):1439, 1989.

Cotton DB, Gonik B, Spillman T, et al: Intrapartum to postpartum changes in colloid osmotic pressure. Am J Obstet Gynecol 149(2):174, 1984.

Combes B, Adams RH: Disorders of the liver in pregnancy. In Assali NS, Brinkman CR III (eds): Pathophysiology of Gestation. Volume 1. Maternal Disorders. New York, Academic Press, 1972.

Cruikshank DP, Hays PM: Maternal physiology in pregnancy. In Gabbe SG, Niebyl JR, Simpson JL (eds): Obstetrics: Normal and Problem Pregnancies. New York, Churchill Livingstone, 1986.

Cunningham FG, MacDonald PC, Gant NF: Williams Obstetrics. Norwalk, Appleton & Lange, 1989.

Cutforth R, MacDonald CB: Heart sound and murmurs in pregnancy. Am Heart J 71(6):741, 1966.

Davidson JM: The physiology of the renal tract in pregnancy. Clin Obstet Gynecol 28(2):257, 1985.

Dunlop W: Serial changes in renal haemodynamics during normal human pregnancy. Br J Obstet Gynaecol 88:1, 1981.

Ezimokhai M, Davidson JM, Phillips PR, et al: Nonpostural serial changes in renal function during the third trimester. Br J Obstet Gynaecol 88:465, 1981.

Fadnes HO, Oian P: Transcapillary fluid balance and plasma volume regulation: a review. Obstet Gynecol Surv 44(1):769, 1989.

Fay RA, Hughes AO, Farron NT: Platelets in pregnancy: hyperdestruction in pregnancy. Obstet Gynecol 61(2):238, 1983.

Felig P: Body fuel metabolism and diabetes in pregnancy. Med Clin N Am 61(1)43, 1977.

Fleming AF: Haematological changes in pregnancy. Clin Obstet Gynaecol 2(2):269, 1975.

Gabbe SG, Niehyl JR, Simpson JL (eds): Obstetrics: Normal and Problem Pregnancies. New York, Churchill Livingstone, 1986.

Gerbasi FR, Bottoms S, Farag A, Mammen EF: Changes in hemostasis activity during delivery and the immediate postpartum period. Am J Obstet Gynecol 162(5):1158, 1990.

Gutsche BB: Maternal physiologic adaptations during pregnancy. In Schnider SM, Levinson G (eds): Anesthesia for Obstetrics. Baltimore, Williams & Wilkins, 1979.

Hollingsworth DR: Maternal metabolism in normal pregnancy and pregnancy complicated by diabetes mellitus. Clin Obstet Gynecol 28(3):457, 1985.

Hunt JN, Murray FA: Gastric function in pregnancy. J Obstet Gynecol Br Emp 65:78, 1958.

Hytten FE, Leitch I: The Physiology of Human Pregnancy, 2nd ed. Oxford, Blackwell Scientific Publications, 1971.

Katz R, Karliner JS, Resnik R: Effects of a natural volume overload state (pregnancy) on left ventricular performance in normal human subjects. Circulation 58:434, 1978.

Kerr MG: The mechanical effects of the gravid uterus in late pregnancy. J Obstet Gynaecol Br Commonw 72:513, 1965.

Lee W, Rokey R, Miller J, Cotton D: Maternal hemodynamic effects of uterine contractions by M-mode and pulsed-Doppler echocardiography. Am J Obstet Gynecol 161(4):974, 1989.

Lees MM, Taylor SH, Scott DB, et al: A study of cardiac output at risk throughout pregnancy. J Obstet Gynaecol Br Commonw 74:319, 1967.

Lind T, Godfrey KA, Otum H: Changes in serum uric acid concentrations during normal pregnancy. Br J Obstet Commonw 91:128, 1984.

Lindheimer MD: Current concepts of sodium metabolism and use of diuretics in pregnancy. Contemp OB/GYN 15:207, 1980.

Lindheimer MD, Katz Al: Renal changes during pregnancy: their relevance to volume homeostasis. Clin Obstet Gynaecol 2(2):345, 1975.

Lotgering FK, Gilbert RD, Lonzo L: The interactions of exercise and pregnancy: a review. Am J Obstet Gynecol 149:560, 1984.

Lund CJ, Donovan JC: Blood volume during pregnancy. Am J Obstet Gynecol 98(3):393, 1967.

Lunzer M, Barnes P, Byth K, O'Halloran M: Serum bile acid concentrations during pregnancy and their relationship to obstetric cholestasis. Gastroenterol 91:825, 1986.

Metcalfe J, McAnulty JH, Ueland K: Cardiovascular physiology. Clin Obstet Gynecol 24(3):693, 1981.

Meyer JE: Clinical chemistry. In Abrams RS, Wexler P (eds): Medical Care of the Pregnant Patient. Boston, Little, Brown, & Co, 1983.

Minnich V, Okcuoghi A, Tarcon V, et al: Pica in Turkey, II. Effect of clay upon iron absorption. Am J Clin Nutr 21:78, 1968.

Monheit AG, Cousins L, Resnik R: The puerperium: anatomic and physiologic adjustments. Clin Obstet Gynecol 23(4):973, 1980.

Murray FA, Eishine JP, Fielding J: Gastric secretion in pregnancy. J Obstet Gynecol Br Emp 64:373, 1957.

Pernoll ML, Metcalfe J, Schlenker TL, et al: Oxygen consumption at rest and during exercise in pregnancy. Respir Physiol 25:285, 1975.

Pitkin R: Nutritional support in obstetrics and gynecology. Clin Obstet Gynecol 19(3):489, 1976.

Pitkin R: Nutritional requirements in normal pregnancy. Diabetes Care 3(3):472, 1980.

Pitkin RM, Witte DL: Platelet and leukocyte count in pregnancy. JAMA 242(24):2696, 1979.

Pritchard JA: Changes in blood volume during pregnancy and delivery. Anesthesiol 26(4):393, 1965.

Radberry G, Asztely M, Cantor P, et al: Gastric and gallbladder emptying in relation to the secretion of cholecystokinin after a meal in late pregnancy. Digestion 42:174, 1989.

Robson SC, Dunlop W, Boys RJ, Hunter S: Cardiac output during labor. Br Med J 295:1169, 1987.

Rovinsky JR, Jaffin H: Cardiovascular hemodynamics in pregnancy: blood and plasma values in multiple pregnancy. Am J Obstet Gynecol 93(1):1, 1965.

Rubler S, Damani PM, Pinto ER: Cardiac size and performance during pregnancy estimated with echocardiography. Am J Cardiol 40:534, 1977.

Sadovsky E, Zuckerman H: An alkaline phosphatase specific to normal pregnancy. Obstet Gynecol 26(2):211, 1965.

Sala NL, Rubi RA: Ureteral function in pregnant women. II. Ureteral contractility during normal pregnancy. Am J Obstet Gynecol 99(2):228, 1967.

Soules MR, Hughes CL, Garcia JA, et al: Nausea and vomiting of pregnancy. Role of human chorionic gonadotropin and 17-hydroxyprogesterone. Obstet Gynecol 55:696, 1980.

Talkington KM, Gant NF, Scott DE, Pritchard JA: Effect of ingestion of starch and some clays on iron absorption. Am J Obstet Gynecol 108:262, 1970.

Tindall VR: The liver in pregnancy. Clin Obstet Gynaecol 2(2):441, 1975.

Ueland K, Hansen JM: Maternal cardiovascular dynamics. II. Posture and uterine contractions. Am J Obstet Gynecol 103(1):1, 1969a.

Ueland K, Hansen JM: Maternal cardiovascular dynamics. III. Labor and delivery under local and caudal analgesia. Am J Obstet Gynecol 103(1):8, 1969b.

Ueland K, Novy MJ, Peterson EN, Metcalfe J: Maternal cardiovascular dynamics. IV. The influence of gestational age on the maternal cardiovascular response to posture and exercise. Am J Obstet Gynecol 104(6):856, 1969.

Ueland K: Maternal cardiovascular dynamics. VII. Intrapartum blood volume changes. Am J Obstet Gynecol 126(6):671, 1976.

Ueland K, Ueland FR: Physiologic adaptations to pregnancy. In Knuppel RA, Drukker JE (eds): High-Risk Pregnancy: A Team Approach. Philadelphia: WB Saunders Co, 1986.

Valenzuela GJ: Is a decrease in plasma oncotic pressure enough to explain the edema of pregnancy? Am J Obstet Gynecol 161(6):1624, 1989.

Villar J, Pepke J, Markush L, et al: The measuring of blood pressure during pregnancy. Am J Obstet Gynecol 161(4):1019, 1989.

Walters WAW, Lim YL: Blood volume and haemodynamics in pregnancy. Clin Obstet Gynaecol 2(2):301, 1975.

Wilson M, Morganti AA, Zervoudakis J, et al: Blood pressure, the renin-aldosterone system and sex steroids throughout normal pregnancy. Am J Med 68:97, 1980.

Yeomans ER, Hankins GDV: Cardiovascular physiology and invasive cardiac monitoring. Clin Obstet Gynecol 32(1):2, 1989.

# CHAPTER 14

· · · · · · · · · · · · · · · · · · · · · · · · · · · · · · · ·

# Psychosocial Implications of High-Risk Pregnancy

Jane M. Murphy and Deborah Robbins

Pregnancy presents profound social and psychologic adaptive challenges to women and their families. Even an uncomplicated pregnancy has been described as a psychobiologic crisis in which the individual physiologic and psychologic equilibrium is disrupted, family and work roles are altered, and important interaction patterns between parents and baby are established. There is now considerable freedom of choice regarding pregnancy and the interpretation of the meaning of pregnancy in light of the currently changing roles of women in society. In the current climate, the social and psychologic implications of high-risk pregnancy take on even greater significance because pregnancy and parturition are increasingly viewed as requiring less medical intervention. Indeed, if pregnancy per se is an adaptive challenge, the high-risk pregnancy presents even greater social and psychologic problems for both patients and practitioners.

The woman who has been diagnosed to be at risk during pregnancy experiences a wide variety of emotions, and the normal emotional changes of pregnancy may be intensified. The patient must deal with realistic fears for her own safety as well as for the life of her unborn child. Because expectations for pregnancy may not have included complications, the patient may be confused about what is actually happening to her body, may fear having an abnormal child, and may feel a loss of control over the pregnancy because her choices regarding pregnancy and childbirth have been limited by her complications. Such psychologic features of high-risk patients may affect the level of satisfaction and positive involvement in medical care. It is also clear that negative attitudes toward pregnancy leading to increased anxiety contribute to problems with delivery and later problems with the maternal-infant relationship (McDonald, 1968).

Thus, although specialized, intensive perinatal care has been shown to result in improved fetal and neonatal outcomes (Merkatz et al, 1978), it is equally clear that there must be attention to the psychologic as well as physical aspects of care for mothers who are particularly at risk for poor pregnancy outcomes. The long-term hospitalization of pregnant women, or prolonged bed rest, may lead to successful parturition and postnatal course but also may prove to be a hardship for other children in the family, place stress on the marriage, and lead to depression for the patient (Smith, 1979).

In short, although maternal and fetal mortality rates have declined as a result of specialized high-risk obstetric care, it has been suggested that morbidity rates for psychologic and social factors that affect both mothers and children have increased for iatrogenic reasons and that high-risk obstetric care may be a double-edged sword in which procedures designed to protect mothers and infants from physical damage simultaneously may create profound psychosocial problems (Cohen, 1979).

Clearly, if practitioners responsible for the complex management of high-risk pregnancies do not actively consider the psychologic and social implications of intensive testing, lengthy hospitalization, prolonged bed rest at home, and illness or disability superimposed on pregnancy, the results may be antithetical to the goal of care, which is to guide mothers and children toward the highest level of physical and emotional care (Merkatz et al, 1978). This chapter is dedicated to a better understanding of the problems of psychosocial adaptation by high-risk patients.

## Adaptations in Pregnancy

Although pregnancy usually is regarded as a period of great joy and anticipation, it is actually a time of complex interrelated changes in physiologic equilibrium and interpersonal associations. Contrary to popular folklore, even when pregnancies are planned, only slightly over half of primigravidas experience positive emotions about being pregnant and taking on the role of motherhood; many are told primarily negative anecdotes about labor and delivery, over half report decreases in social contacts, and all report negative feelings about body image brought about by physical changes. Clearly, pregnancy is a time of marked emotional upheaval (Bibring, 1959; Caplan, 1960; Deutsch, 1945; Merkatz et al, 1978). Pregnancy demands that a woman redefine herself in terms of her social roles, that she accept the pregnancy and the psychologic stresses attendant to it, develop an attachment to the fetus, and adapt to a relationship with the neonate after parturition.

The decision to become pregnant or the actual fact of pregnancy marks the beginning of an elaborate transition. Adaptations to pregnancy extend far beyond the acceptance of altered energy levels, the tendency toward decrements in social interaction, and in many cases, the adjustment to the expectation of future financial difficulties. For the first time, in some cases, a pregnant person must define herself as a "woman" rather than as a "girl." Relationships with parents, spouse, and friends, which have evolved slowly over time and provide both social support and psychologic equilibrium, are suddenly altered. Changes in sexuality and sexual activity and increased introversion and passivity characteristically occur from the middle of the second trimester onward,

reaching a peak between the 30th and 35th weeks. These factors, coupled with physiologic and hormonal changes that may cause alterations in energy level and mood, may significantly disrupt the family unit and its traditional patterns of activity. Such disruptions cause anxiety, not only for the pregnant woman but also for those with whom she interacts.

Pregnancy has been termed a life crisis, which implies that the changes that occur pervade all facets of a woman's life, including the somatic, psychologic, and social. The importance of psychologic variables in life crises is that changes are of such magnitude that an individual's coping style or basic personality may no longer be adaptive. The multilevel disequilibrium of a first pregnancy is a stress for which most women have no personal precedent and that results in anxiety. Despite outward appearances of adaptation, anxiety occurs with all expectant mothers regardless of other aspects of physical or emotional health. Patients, particularly those pregnant for the first time, often present to the physician or nurse with symptoms of overt, repressed, or displaced emotional conflicts.

The pregnant woman with one or more children has reported greater stress intensity regarding physical symptoms during pregnancy (Sammons, 1990). The multipara may find increased fatigue and concerns of the first-born child's acceptance of a sibling that may influence her adaptation to this pregnancy.

Pregnant women experience a myriad of psychologic symptoms including introversion, passivity, mood swings, mixed feelings, restlessness, nervousness, irritability, preoccupations, and depression. These appear with such frequency and intensity that there is a statistically higher-than-normal incidence of psychiatric problems diagnosed in pregnant women (Bibring, 1959). Paradoxically, as the pregnant woman strives to develop a degree of comfort with the many changes in social context and psychologic equilibrium, there often occurs a surfacing of old conflicts that were never adequately resolved in earlier developmental periods. For example, pregnant patients may experience conflicts of autonomy with their mothers, renewed rivalry with siblings, or active uncertainty about sexuality and disturbing fantasies about past relationships, each of which had been adequately dealt with prior to pregnancy but that now result in troubling family interactions or marital discord. Furthermore, problems of adjustment prior to pregnancy, such as marital discord, economic difficulties, poor self-concept, and neuroticism may be exacerbated by pregnancy.

In short, even in the most well-adjusted patients, life-crisis disturbances can create the clinical impression of more severe decompensation. In general, such disturbances prove to be transient, situational conflicts rather than serious long-term psychiatric problems, but anxiety allowed to go unallayed may lead to maladaptive mother-child interaction, which is of increasing concern because of the deleterious effects maladaptations are purported to have on the child's emotional and cognitive development (Klaus and Kennell, 1976).

To summarize, the pregnant woman must adapt to

- Altered physiology with associated changes in energy level and mood
- Changes in somatic configuration and body image
- Changing expectations and interactions with parents, spouse, and other significant individuals
- Conflicting overt and covert messages about motherhood, the mechanics of labor and delivery, and parenthood
- Personal fear, uncertainties, ambivalent feelings, and preoccupations
- Feelings of vulnerability, loss of autonomy, lack of precedents, and dependency

## Maladaptations in Pregnancy

Although most psychosocial adpatations to pregnancy are characterized by some degree of stress, severe psychopathology seldom is seen. Although behaviors and thoughts of maladaptation may occur, they are usually transient in nature. Many women simply have difficulty achieving the developmental milestones of adaptation to pregnancy and the neonatal period. It is important, nonetheless, that health practitioners be able to distinguish between those psychosocial features of pregnancy that may be troublesome but occur with great frequency and those that are indicative of more severe pa-

thology. In one sense, pregnancy can be viewed as a testing ground for mental health. Because of the great reorientation demanded by pregnancy, women with pre-existing psychiatric problems may show evidence of acute decompensation for which psychiatric collaboration is essential.

There are many signs and symptoms of psychosocial maladaptation to pregnancy. Many women express early ambivalence about being pregnant, but in some cases, denial of pregnancy persists well into the second trimester. Such problems with acceptance of pregnancy may be exhibited by a denial of body changes or, conversely, over-reaction to such changes. Clinically, the woman who persists in wearing regular fashions that hide pregnancy changes or who wears maternity clothes prior to physical need may be having some difficulty accepting the fact of pregnancy. Other signs of early ambivalence about pregnancy are frequent complaints about or preoccupations with vague personal, physical, and emotional problems during prenatal visits and an increased number of visits or contact with the health care provider. The woman exhibits maladaptive behavior when there is exclusion of normal concerns about the developing fetus.

Failure to develop a meaningful emotional affiliation with the growing fetus is a psychosocial maladaptation that occasionally is observed in obstetric practice. In this situation, mothers present with either a subnormal or a supernormal response to the first fetal movements and may express no interest in fetal heart tones, position of the fetus *in utero,* and so forth. These women also may show symptoms of regressive behavior, such as being demanding, uncooperative, provocative, hostile, passive, controlling, or disinterested in care. The clinician may get the impression that the mother is in competition with the fetus for attention and that she has strong needs to be cared for or treated because of multiple problems unrelated to the baby. Paradoxically, women who are having difficulty accepting pregnancy and developing a relationship with the growing fetus may present with extreme anxiety about the condition of the baby and are vigilant in looking for signs that something is wrong with the pregnancy. Ambivalence about names for the baby or speculation or fantasies about the baby's physical characteristics, when persisting well into pregnancy, may be similarly indicative of problems in adaptation.

An additional psychosocial maladaptation of pregnancy is failure to make adequate, concerted plans for postnatal care of the baby. The absence of family members or friends to help care for the baby or, at the other extreme, passivity and overreliance on family members, are signs of difficulty in adapting to pregnancy, as is unrealistic planning or inadequate preparation for managing the baby at home.

To summarize, obstetric practitioners are cautioned to be alert to the following conditions in their patients and should screen for them during office visits (Cohen, 1979):

- Deficiency or lack of maternal figure in the patient's life
- Chronic conflict with mother or other female relatives
- Previous birth of a damaged child or the presence of another child with emotional disturbances or behavioral disorders
- Chronic marital discord or acute discord if the conflict is in the area of childbearing or childrearing
- Little or no preparation for sexual experience, childrearing, or childbearing
- Reports of experiences that are feared will damage the baby
- Third-trimester behavior indicative of overt or disguised rejection of the pregnant state
- Absence of plans for care of the baby after birth

# Psychosocial Problems in High-Risk Pregnancy

In general, there are two major types of high-risk patients: (1) those who have chronic conditions that predispose them to problems in pregnancy and (2) those who become pregnant and only subsequently develop conditions that demand special care, which may include hospitalization. In either case, however, consideration must be given to important psychologic factors that affect total obstetric care. In the former case, when the pregnant patient has a pre-existing condition such as diabetes or past obstetric complications, there will be a history of adaptation to chronic disease that is of utmost importance. In the latter case, in which a woman becomes pregnant and only later develops complications, the unexpected superimposition of problems on pregnancy can be especially stressful.

## HIGH-RISK PATIENTS WITH PRE-EXISTING MEDICAL AND PSYCHOSOCIAL CONDITIONS

Patients with longstanding medical complications that place them at risk during pregnancy (such as diabetes mellitus, cardiac disease, chronic hypertension, sickle cell disease, or systemic lupus erythematosus) deserve special attention from the psychosocial perspective. For women with pre-existing problems, the best predictor of adaptation to high-risk pregnancy is their adaptation to the previous health problems. In patients whose chronic conditions result in a persistent negative self-image, there can be an exaggeration of the expected body image disturbances or a persistence of negative fantasies and fears about the unborn baby.

Some women who have pre-existing conditions to which they have not adapted psychologically (e.g., an adolescent with juvenile-onset diabetes who denies or minimizes the significance of her illness) may view pregnancy and having a baby as evidence of their normalcy (Merkatz et al, 1978). High-risk obstetric care for such a patient reinforces feelings of abnormality, but now, for reasons of both their pre-existing chronic illness and pregnancy. In younger patients who are grappling with issues of self-image, the pregnancy that they thought would be liberating in terms of the ambiguity of adolescence becomes, instead, an albatross that perpetuates normal feelings of inadequacy and, typically, leads either to dangerous denial of medical problems or to a regression to even greater dependency.

Unfortunately, the pregnant woman is not immune to battering. For some women, battering increases during pregnancy, and for others, it is initiated during pregnancy. It does appear that men who batter during pregnancy are more violent in general, and that physical battering during pregnancy has a greater potential for severe injury. Battering may be one of the most common complications of pregnancy. The role of the health care provider is to identify that the problem exists. All patients should be asked if they are a victim of domestic violence. Examples of direct questions to ask are: "Are you in a relationship with a person who threatens or physically hurts you?" "Many patients tell me that they have been hurt by someone close to them; could this be happening to you?" and "Are you being beaten or threatened?" In asking the question, the health care provider starts the process of healing by encouraging the patient to talk (Chez, 1990). The social service department should have a list of shelters and other resources that address domestic violence. There is a national domestic violence hotline available 24 hours a day, seven days a week to assist clients. That number is 1-800-333-SAFE.

Substance abuse has risen among pregnant women in recent years (MacGregor, 1989). Patients should have a clinical assessment, including physical appearance, a medical and obstetric history, and a substance abuse interview (Chasnoff, 1987) to identify the patient using illicit drugs or alcohol. A multidisciplinary team is imperative when working with the substance abusing pregnant woman and her family.

Such patients deserve the opportunity for counseling, not only to help them deal with their high-risk pregnancy but also to enable them to come to terms with their pre-existing conditions. Practitioners must strive to help these patient overcome the denial of their problems so that they will be more likely to endorse measures necessary to ensure both their health and the health of the fetus. In doing so, however, the physician, nurse, or other health care provider must be careful not to impose an overprotectiveness that will result in total rejection of the perinatal team recommendations or, at the other extreme, in creating dependency difficulties during hospitalization. (Also, see Chapter 10.)

## PATIENTS WITH PREGNANCY-INDUCED COMPLICATIONS

Unlike women with prediagnosed conditions who tend to have psychologic adaptations to high-risk pregnancy that mirror their adaptations to their chronic conditions, women with high-risk conditions discovered as a result of pregnancy characteristically exhibit signs of a classic grief reaction (Lindemann, 1944). Women in this situation must adapt to two stresses, (1) the stress of the pregnancy and (2) the newly diagnosed complication. Women who are unexpectedly confronted with the possibility of hospitalization or bed rest at home for complications during a pregnancy that was previously normal may react with symptoms of anger, disbelief, anxiety, fear, and depression, all of which may be misinterpreted by health care professionals. A period of time in which the patient tries to come to terms with an additional health problem is essentially a time of grieving for the loss of a formerly healthy self and for hopes of a normal pregnancy. There may be anger, particularly if the physiologic changes of pregnancy precipitated the emergent problem, coupled with guilt for having feelings of regret about having become pregnant or for wishing that pregnancy had not occurred.

Many women whose pregnancies precipitate medical problems experience phases similar to the grieving process associated with the death of a child. Davidson (1979) describes four stages of grief: (1) shock and disbelief, (2) searching and yearning, (3) disorganization and despair, and (4) resolution and reorganization. In the case of the high-risk patient, the grief reaction results from the "death" of the idealized, trouble-free pregnancy that the patient had expected to have. Although classified into stages, the psychologic reactions of these patients are seldom so mechanistic: stages may be skipped entirely, superimposed on one another, or experienced with varying intensity.

When a woman finds that she is at risk, she may feel stunned. The high-risk patient actually may be unaware of or unable to remember what she is told during this phase. Often, the shock phase is the patient's way of protecting herself against the news she has heard. In providing patient education, practitioners should be alert to this problem and be prepared to give explanations more than once without becoming frustrated. Written patient material should be provided to reinforce information. Rather than providing unsolicited information, it is more appropriate for practitioners to answer the patient's questions, thereby proceeding at the patient's own pace.

Expectant parents often feel helpless and may not want to believe what they are told in regard to medical problems. Women have reported feeling nothing or being overwhelmed by a feeling of numbness. As a symptom of the need for denying the existence of complications, patients may fail to keep medical appointments, may leave the hospital against medical advice, or may avoid discussion of their medical complication.

The medical history of the pregnant woman, her spouse, and family members may influence the level of confidence in the medical health care system, which also may influence the patient's compliance with the treatment plan.

During the searching and yearning phase of the grief process, the patient may ask "Why me?" She may believe she has failed in her role as a mother because she has developed a complication. Many women feel guilty, believing that something they did early in pregnancy caused their problems; they search through their entire pregnancy and their past personal and family medical histories, trying to establish causal explanations. Usually, their complications are unrelated to the variables they feel are the cause. Women sometimes feel that they are being punished for some act they may have committed years ago, or they may blame their problems on dietary indiscretions, arguments with their spouse, and so forth. Patients need to find reasons and need something or someone to blame for their predicaments. Often, a patient blames herself, feeling guilty about normal ambivalent feelings she might have had early in pregnancy.

During the disorganization and despair stage, women are characteristically insecure about decisions that have to be made. Patients become confused and disorganized at a time when much medical information regarding treatment decisions must be comprehended. Patients often feel isolated from friends and family who do not understand what they are going through. Helplessness and isolation breed feelings of anger, which are often directed toward health care professionals. Ultimately, most patients achieve some level of resolution as they begin to come to terms with the problems and reorganize their plans for the pregnancy. The intense emotions experienced at first begin to lessen, and patients will be better able to make informed decisions, but only if practitioners are able to understand the dynamics of grief

reactions and can help the patient avoid maladaptive countertransference reactions. The insensitive clinician who reacts to the patient's emotionality as a personal affront rather than as a symptom of adaptation may permanently compromise the therapeutic relationship.

Finally, couples often deal with their feelings independent of one another, which can cause increased emotional stress. Families should be encouraged to communicate their feelings so that they better understand how all members feel and become involved in the plan of care for the patient as much as possible. Practitioners must recognize when parents react differently and fail to communicate and must learn to treat the couple as the patient.

# Medical Care for the High-Risk Pregnant Woman

The nature of the diagnosis and the stage of pregnancy in which it is made affects the mode of treatment in high-risk obstetrics. Depending on the diagnosis and the time it is made, one of the following may occur: (1) the patient may be referred early in pregnancy to a Regional Perinatal Intensive Care Center (RPICC) for outpatient care by perinatologists who specialize in high-risk obstetrics; (2) during labor, the patient may be determined to be at high risk in a hospital that has inadequate facilities to care for a critically ill mother or premature or sick infant and may be transported to an RPICC; or (3) the patient may unexpectedly deliver a sick or premature infant, with the baby then transported to a regional center. In any of these situations, the expectant parents face a time of emotional turmoil and confusion.

## PATIENT-PRACTITIONER RELATIONSHIPS

Because the patient-physician relationship is very special in obstetrics, it is common for a patient to have invested a great deal of time and emotion in choosing her personal obstetrician. When a pregnant woman has been referred to an RPICC with a set of unfamiliar specialized practitioners, a mutually satisfying relationship with her former physician may be perceived as being lost, and she may even feel abandoned by her original obstetrician (Souma, 1979). Practitioners specializing in high-risk pregnancies and the relative inflexibility of high-risk care often are compared unfavorably with nurses and physicians with whom patients were previously more familiar.

If referred to an RPICC, the patient likely is cared for by several physicians and other health care professionals working as a team (Freeman, 1982). Teams typically include several physicians, nurses, social workers, dietitians, and other health care professionals. Team members have specialized areas of expertise and responsibility relating to the patient, and although the team concept is crucial to high-risk care, it can confuse the patient. It is important that each team member be introduced to the patient and that different responsibilities are clarified so that the patient understands each team member's role. Once the patient feels comfortable with the team concept, she can use the diversity of its members to her best advantage. Often, patients develop a special relationship with one team member and may feel more comfortable dealing with this person on a one-to-one basis. The team member closest to the patient may be better able to communicate her needs by acting as her advocate or case manager in the team setting.

Many regional referral centers have set up maternal-fetal intensive care units within labor and delivery. Continuity of care is achieved as opposed to what may be fragmented care delivered between the medical intensive care unit and labor and delivery staff. An obstetric critical care team is an essential component for tertiary care centers.

## DIAGNOSTIC TESTS AND PROCEDURES

High-risk care usually involves many diagnostic procedures with which patients may have little familiarity. Tests such as amniocentesis, ultrasonography, the nonstress test, and the glucose tolerance test can confuse and frighten a patient who does not understand their purposes. It is essential that patients be made familiar with the pro-

cedures so that they feel more comfortable. A problem occurs when symptoms are ominous to the obstetrician and demand special testing (such as elevated blood sugar, elevated blood pressure, or intrauterine growth retardation) but are unrecognized or are not considered significant by the patient. In such cases, patients do not feel ill, and it is quite common for friends and family members to minimize signs such as edema or high blood pressure by telling patients "That's exactly what happened to me during my pregnancy, and everything was fine!" Such patients, particularly if confronted with the additional burden of young children at home or the need to continue to work to support the family, may skip appointments, may be reluctant to undergo diagnostic procedures or to enter the hospital for a long period of antenatal care, and may even be resistant to the prescription of a special diet, medications, or treatments.

High-risk obstetric care also runs counter to current cultural trends that increasingly promote pregnancy and childbirth as natural and condemn the use of technology in the birth process. For this reason, there is resistance to high-risk care on the part of some women, and care should be taken to negotiate mutual understandings and expectations between patient and practitioner (Johnson, 1981). This involves careful elicitation by the clinician of the patient's explanatory model of her special condition and of her pregnancy in general, including the possible cause of the problem, onset of symptoms, pathophysiology, likely course of illness (chronicity, severity, outcome), and treatment. The following are examples of questions designed to elicit patient explanatory models (Kleinman et al, 1978):

1. What do you think has caused your problem?
2. Why do you think it started when it did?
3. What do you think your sickness does to you and your baby?
4. How does it do that?
5. What kind of treatment do you think you should receive?
6. What are the most important results you have to receive from this treatment?
7. What problems have been (or will be) caused by your condition?
8. What do you fear most about your sickness?

Persistence and patience in such questioning, even in the face of patient hesitancy, provides bases for comparing the perinatal team and patient expectations, identifying discrepancies that may cause clinical management problems, and planning patient education activities. (The wording may be changed to meet patient needs.)

## ADAPTATIONS TO HOSPITALIZATION

Hospitalization, which may be a major feature of high-risk obstetric care, is inherently stressful and represents an adaptive challenge to both the pregnant woman and her family (Volicer, 1974; Williams, 1974; Wu, 1973). Women who are at special risk during pregnancy may be hospitalized for extended periods to allow close medical supervision. Such antepartum patients face the difficult situation of being placed in the hospital when they are actually feeling well. For example, a diabetic patient who is pregnant may have to be hospitalized for monitoring and control of blood sugar, even though she is feeling normal. Similarly, a woman who has been confined to bed owing to premature labor may not feel ill. Under such circumstances, both the patient and the medical and nursing staff face unusual circumstances in that the staff may not be accustomed to caring for someone who feels so well, and the patient may not understand why she must stay in the hospital. "Hospitals are for sick people, and I'm not sick," often is heard on the antepartum floor.

Patients who perceive themselves as being healthy usually have problems adapting to hospitalization (Rosen, 1975), particularly because of boredom, restlessness, and irritation caused by adherence to the rules and regulations of the hospital. Again, extensive negotiation and explanation are needed to educate the patient and her family so that they better understand the reasons for hospitalization and are able to make an informed and more willing decision. From their end, practitioners must make an effort to make the patient's hospital stay more bearable by modifying traditional hospital procedures— for example, by discontinuing the taking of vital signs in the middle of the night; relaxing strict visiting hours; allowing the significant other to spend the night; allowing for passes out of the hospital; and allowing patients to decorate their room with furnishings from home such as a quilt, a favorite painting or picture, and a lamp, to make the hospital room more homelike. Hospitalization results in a loss of autonomy and of decision-making responsibility in pregnant patients. Moreover, it has been demonstrated that hospitalization does not become easier with the passage of time but that patients who are hospitalized for periods of greater than 2 weeks show increased distress as the hospital stay becomes extended (Merkatz, 1976). Indeed, hospitalization may heighten a sense of dependency, and regressive adaptations in pregnancy may become even more profound as a result of prolonged periods in the hospital setting.

Hospitalization also involves a loss of familiar territory, personal identity, privacy, and control, which can result in patients responding with overassertiveness or anger displaced toward hospital personnel, hospital routine, family members, and others. At any time, physicians, nurses, medical technicians, social workers, dietitians, food service personnel, and housekeepers may pass through the patient's room without warning or explanation. When patients are in semiprivate rooms, twice the usual number of interruptions occur. These interruptions should be coordinated, if possible, to limit the intrusion to the patients.

Many patients may be afraid of being in a hospital. Even today, hospitals often are viewed as places to die. Such fears may be especially acute for the patient who is referred from another hospital or community. Tertiary centers frequently have reputations of being depersonalizing (Boehm et al, 1979), a factor that may increase the patient's anxiety and influence her relationship with the health care team. Community education and close coordination with the referral source may help to alleviate some of these fears (Boehm et al, 1979; Oh et al, 1977; Souma, 1979). Many patients feel reassured if RPICC staff maintain contact with their own physician during the course of their hospitalizations. Phone calls and visits from referring hospital personnel can be beneficial.

Perhaps because of lengthy hospitalization, with its inherent isolation from family and friends, but also as a result of proximity and shared perspectives, a powerful patient subculture exists in many high-risk units that influences patient adaptation to hospitalization. Patients commonly compare treatment recommendations, special orders, and other features of care so that exceptions to rules or general routine for one patient quickly leads to similar requests from others. Poor outcome of delivery or diagnostic tests for one patient also are known to all patients quickly, as are other administrative problems on the unit. Both may lower satisfaction with care or raise new fears about being pregnant. Some accounts of adverse effects of hospitalization or diagnostic tests on patients may reach mythic proportions and be passed along from patient to patient until long after the woman who originally encountered the difficulties has been discharged from the hospital. It is common for patients to threaten to leave the hospital against medical advice on the basis of unrealistic fears generated by other patients. On the other hand, patients often are tremendously insightful about the concerns of other patients and can be valuable therapeutic allies. Practitioners should listen to patients, not just for what they are saying about themselves but for what they reveal about the social milieu of the hospital unit. When a poor outcome occurs in the unit, the other patients need much support and reassurance that that patient is different and a bad outcome is unlikely for their condition. If the patient has a similar problem, more reassurance is necessary for her and her family to understand the difference of her condition. Support groups involving the patient and her health care team member can be helpful in reducing many anxieties that exist in a high-risk antenatal unit.

The responses of patients and family members to long-term hospitalization are highly variable. Many patients become active participants in their own care, becoming self-reliant in the hospital, whereas others become extremely dependent, rebellious, or both. Difficulties can arise between the patient and the father if the latter resents the coming baby, whether on a conscious or subconscious level. In such cases, the resentment may be made worse by the woman's hospitalization, because the father blames the pregnancy for causing their separation and increasing his responsibilities at home. In other instances, the father may not resent the situation at all, but the patient nevertheless fears that such resentment exists. It is common for patients to become acutely agitated, demanding to be discharged immediately, because of fears that their partners are becoming permanently alienated by their absence. In any case, wide fluctuations in affect can be expected to occur in patients during hospitalization, but the absence of liability of affect, including depression, may be more alarming than its presence.

High-risk patients have been shown to express characteristic areas of distress during antenatal hospitalizations (Merkatz et al, 1978). The most frequently mentioned concerns are about the baby, personal health, children at home, outcome of pregnancy for the baby, and concern about spouse or mate. Less frequently verbalized areas of distress include being bothered by hospital regulations or routine, depression, concern about receiving inadequate information about plans for care, loneliness, unhappiness with the performance of health personnel, and dissatisfaction with food. Events usually thought of by health professionals as stressful during hospitalization, such as sleeping in a strange bed, disruption of eating habits, wearing hospital gowns, having to stay in bed all day, or using bedpans actually are considered least stressful by patients. On the other hand, patients are most frequently and severely stressed by such unfortunately common problems in hospitals as not being told their diagnosis, not knowing what illness they have, not getting pain medications when needed, and not knowing the reasons for or the results of diagnostic procedures.

Patients frequently complain about those things that are not actually very stressful, such as quality of food or the hospital routine, when they are actually concerned about the more stressful aspects of high-risk care. The astute clinician is alert for these displaced expressions of anxiety, which are much more likely to be reflections of uncertainty about diagnosis, treatment, personal health, family functioning, and so on. On the other hand, it is common for patients to have so many personal problems that the hospital represents a refuge to which they cling. One should interpret a certain level of patient complaining as a healthy symptom of adaptation.

### Effects On Family Life

One of the most difficult aspects of hospitalization is the separation of the patient from her family. She may be forced to leave her partner and children and be unexpectedly admitted to the hospital for an indeterminate period of time. The patient who has children at home often feels guilty because she is no longer able to fulfill her maternal responsibilities. Also, she already is attached to her children at home and may have little bonding to her unborn fetus. The health of her fetus may not be as important as the well-being of her children at home. She may become angry at the fetus who prevents her from being with her family and may appear unconcerned for her fetus as her concerns increase regarding her established family. Finding alternative caretakers for children may be difficult, and other adult family members may be forced to alter their daily routines to stay home and take care of children. Hospitalization of young primigravidas who have been living at home with their parents also are a source of worry and disruption. Hospitalization may be inherently stressful for young patients because it is their first time away from home and family.

Family members often feel left out in the medical setting. Bedside rounds typically are made when relatives are not in the hospital, and physicians and nurses who have primary responsibility for patients may not be available during visiting hours. Thus, family members who are concerned about the decisions that are being made are not always given needed information or included in the decision-making process and may have difficulty relating to the health care team. Their sense of isolation often is expressed in terms of resentment of the medical system and hostility toward high-risk practitioners. It also is common in such situations for family members to exert emotional pressure on patients to resist treatment. Working at cross-purposes with family members is best avoided by keeping them apprised of the issues and of progress in treatment.

## HOME CARE

Maintaining bed rest at home in lieu of hospitalization may be the patient's preference or the medicaid or insurance provider's recommendation. Bed rest may be a less expensive, practical, safe alternative to a prolonged hospital stay. (Dahlberg, 1988). Many high-risk obstetric patients may have a combination of several hospitalizations with bed rest at home. Home fetal monitoring, blood glucose testing, intravenous therapy, and home uterine monitoring are available for home use. Careful discharge planning is essential to assist in a smooth transition from hospital to home. Insurance or medicaid benefits should be investigated for home health benefits for reimbursement of nursing care, nurse's aid, or homemaker services to assist the patient in maintaining bedrest at home.

Community resources may be available to assist the patient and her family with additional needs such as child care, services delivered to the home, housekeeping, and laundry service. Telephone support groups for women on bed rest are becoming available in some communities. For example, the Confinement Line (703-941-7183) in Springfield, Virginia, offers telephone support, education, and a newsletter to pregnant women confined to bed rest.

Although the pregnant woman may decrease her activities in the home, it is unlikely she will be able to escape these tasks completely (Monahan, 1991). The pregnant woman and her family need clear instruction of her limitations; a bed rest checklist (Fig. 14–1) may assist in giving specific guidelines for activity levels.

## FINANCIAL CONSIDERATIONS

Finances are a common but often overlooked concern for most high-risk patients and their families. Practitioners often are naive about the subtleties of health care financing and may not realize that increased visits to the physician, numerous diagnostic procedures, and potentially lengthy hospitalizations for mother and baby often force patients and family members to quit jobs to adhere to health care management; others may be forced to seek additional employment to pay the bills. Financial burden and economic uncertainty increase anxiety about pregnancy and high-risk care. Some regional perinatal centers have special funding that may assist the patient in paying her bills. In any case, the family should be advised to consult hospital social workers or financial counselors to ensure that every possibility for assistance is explored. All members of the health care team should be aware of what financial assistance is available so that the

**Figure 14–1**
EXAMPLE OF A BED REST CHECKLIST.

### What is Bed Rest?

The term bed rest is a familiar one to mothers experiencing high-risk pregnancies, but they are often confused about the exact parameters of their limitations. Variabilities depend on each mother, the extent of her complications and even on the physician himself. This chart has been developed in an attempt to help mothers and their OB/GYNs mutually define needs in specific situations. Since variables change during each individual pregnancy, you may wish to make several copies of this chart, to be completed at various stages of your pregnancy.

# What Can I Do Right Now?

**Date**

**1. Activity Level**

Maintain a normal activity level _____

Slightly decrease activity level _____

Greatly decrease activity level _____

**2. Working Outside the Home**

Maintain my full-time job _____

Work part-time (how many hours?) _____

Work in my home (how many hours?) _____

Stop work completely _____

Why: _____

**3. Working Inside the Home**

Continue doing all housework _____

Decrease housework including: _____

  Heavy lifting (laundry, moving furniture, etc.)

  Preparing meals (standing on feet for _____ a prolonged period of time)

Vigorous scrubbing _____

  Other: _____

  Why: _____

**4. Child Care**

Care for other children as usual _____

No lifting children _____

Have another caretaker watch an _____ active toddler

Have permanent caretaker for children _____

  Why: _____

**5. Mobility**

Continue normal mobility _____

Limit mobility (sit down frequently) _____

Lie down each day (how many hours?) _____

Recline all day (propped up) _____

Lie down flat all day (on side?) _____

May walk stairs (how many times a _____ day?)

Stairs forbidden _____

Take a shower/wash hair _____

Eat lying down? Sitting up? Sitting at _____ table?

  Why: _____

**Date**

**6. Driving**

May drive a car _____

May be a passenger in a car _____ (frequency?)

May not ride in a car, except to doctor _____

  Why: _____

**7. Bathroom Privileges**

May use bathroom normally _____

Should actively avoid constipation _____

May not use bathroom (use bedpan) _____

  Why: _____

**8. Sexual Relations**

May continue normal sexual relations _____

Should limit relations _____ (maximum times a month?)

Should avoid sexual intercourse _____

Should avoid all types of relations _____ which stimulate female orgasm

Should abstain from sexual relations _____

  Why: _____

(See also Chapter 15)

**9. Maintenance of Pregnancy**

Should monitor fetal activity __ hours each day by hand, counting movements _____

Should drink wine each day _____ (When? How much?)

Should stop smoking cigarettes _____

Should abstain from alcohol _____

Should limit cigarette smoking (no. per _____ day?)

Should monitor fetus by uterine home monitoring (Termguard)__

Should take (drug)_____

  __times daily, dosage:_____

  Reason:_____

Should take (drug)_____

  __times daily, dosage:_____

  Reason:_____

Should follow these dietary rules:

  Plenty of: Protein, vegetables, fruits, calcium, other:

  _____

Date

Avoid: Excess salt, excess fats, junk food, spicy foods, other:

_____

Approximate number of calories a day:_____

## What Might I Expect in the Future?

1. Decrease in Activity Level _____
2. Limitations of Work _____
   Stop working completely _____
3. Decrease Housework _____
4. Need for childcare helper _____
5. Need to recline in bed _____
   Need to stay in bed (total bedrest) _____
6. Limit driving _____
   Stop driving _____
7. Limit sexual relations _____
   Abstain from sexual relations _____
8. Need to self-monitor fetal activity _____
9. Need to use uterine home monitoring (Termguard) monitor _____
10. Need to take labor-inhibiting drugs _____
11. Need to have a cervical stitch put in _____
12. Need to stay in hospital for some period of time _____
13. Need to have amniocentesis _____
14. Need to have sonograms/ ultrasounds _____
15. Need to visit OB/GYN more frequently than normal _____
16. Need to visit a High-Risk specialist _____
17. Need to have alpha-fetal protein levels done _____
18. Need to have blood sugar screening _____
19. Need to have a nonstress test _____
20. Need to have a stress test _____

## If Problems Arise and I Go into Premature Labor. . .

1. When should I contact my OB/GYN?_____
2. Where will I be hospitalized?_____
3. Where might I be transferred?_____
4. Name of OB/GYN at other hospital?_____
5. Where would my baby be hospitalized?_____
6. Could my husband be present at delivery?_____
7. Is there a possibility of a cesarean?_____

## Hospital Bedrest

**1. What position do I have to be in?** _____
Trendelenberg (head lowered) _____
On side (left or right?) _____

Date

**2. Do I have to use a bedpan?** _____

**3. Can I reach for things, or should I use a reacher?** _____

**4. Personal hygiene**
Can I take a shower? _____
Can I take a bath? _____
Do I have to take a bed sponge bath? _____
Can I get out of bed to wash my hair? _____

**5. Mobility** _____
Can I walk the halls? _____
Can I walk in my room? _____
Can I sit in the chair in my room? _____
Can I take a wheelchair to the lobby? _____
Can I take a wheelchair to the nursery? _____
Can I take a wheelchair to hospital support group meetings? (If applicable)

**6. Visitors**
When can my husband visit?_____
(If you do not have a husband:) Can I _____
   have another friend or relative visit
   at the times husbands are normally
   permitted to visit?
Who can visit? When?_____
Can my children visit? When?_____
How many people can visit at a time? _____
If I am admitted to the labor room, who can visit?_____
Who can be present in the delivery room?_____

**7. Consults**
If appropriate, may I see: _____
   a physical therapist _____
   an occupational therapist _____
   a neonatologist (about fetal development and/or a typical premie) _____
   a social worker _____
   an ophthalmologist
   a dermatologist _____

**8. Other directions:** _____

This chart was developed by Intensive Caring Unlimited, a Philadelphia/Southern New Jersey parent support group. Copies may be made without permission. Please address questions and comments to: Lenette Moses, ICU, 910 Bent Lane, Philadelphia, PA 19118.

social worker, physician, and financial counselors are not giving the patient mixed messages about available assistance. Also, the patient can make more rational decisions about health care options based on financial considerations. Such consultation has the secondary function of helping family members feel useful and needed, which reduces their frustration with hospitalization.

## PATIENT EDUCATION

Childbirth education classes have become an accepted practice in modern obstetric care and have been demonstrated to reduce anxiety in patients (Browne and Dixon, 1978). Unfortunately, many high-risk women are hospitalized precisely at the time when they would ordinarily be starting such classes. These classes should be made available for individualized teaching if they cannot go to classes. Because of the association between high-risk hospitalization and an increased need for care of newborns in a specialized neonatal intensive care unit (NICU), either for prematurity or an increased incidence of neonatal abnormalities, these topics should be an integral part of comprehensive high-risk patient education.

Routine tours or at minimum bedside teaching about the NICU, during which parents can receive detailed explanations in response to questions they may have, as well as an opportunity to become familiar with the staff, are recommended (Chappell, 1988). Indeed, many parents have fears about giving birth to a deformed fetus and, although visiting the NICU can be a frightening experience, reality is seldom as frightening as a patient's fantasies. A formalized NICU visitation program helps to allay anxiety prior to the birth, makes postnatal visitation by parents less traumatic, and may improve the collaboration of patients and staff in the care of babies in the NICU.

High-risk patients are also at increased risk for cesarean delivery, and they and their partners deserve specialized counseling and patient education to prepare them for this possibility. Although this is not always possible (e.g., in cases of unforeseen emergency cesarean deliveries), it is known that patients who have received special counseling are better able to feel a part of the decision-making process. Many hospitals also allow

fathers who have undergone prenatal classes to be in the delivery room during cesarean deliveries, an arrangement that can be of benefit to both the patient and her partner.

## Maternal-Infant Interaction

High-risk mothers are at a greater risk of being separated from their newborn children. It is crucial that time for some interaction between mothers and their infants be available, given evidence that the amount of contact between mother and infant following birth and the first days of life influences her attachment to and relationship with her baby (Brown, 1979; Klaus and Kennell, 1970; Klaus and Kennell, 1976; Seashore et al, 1973). This interaction may include showing the newborn to the parents before admission to the NICU, a visit with the parents before transport to another hospital, and still photographs or videos of the baby, especially if transported to another hospital.

Lynch (1975) suggests that interference with maternal-infant attachment relates to the perinatal experience and early ill health of the infant, and identifies the following five factors that were over-represented in the history of abused children when compared with their nonabused siblings: (1) abnormal pregnancy, (2) abnormal labor or delivery, (3) other separations, (4) illness in the mother in the first year of life, and (5) illness in the first year of life in the infant. Lynch concludes that "episodes of ill-health in vulnerable families during pregnancy, delivery, and early childhood put the parent/child bond at risk."

Barnet and coworkers (1969) suggest that mothers who have a longer period of less infant interaction experience differences in commitment to their infants, have less self-confidence in their ability to mother appropriately, and behave differently toward their infants than do mothers who have not been separated from their babies. They question whether or not separation might also produce effects on the infant to the extent that stimulation of the infant at home may be affected by the prior separation experience in the hospital.

Stern (1973) suggests that in trying to understand how parents can develop negative feelings resulting in child abuse or neglect, one must include the possibility that anticipatory grief, guilt over a child's condition at birth, or prolonged separation for intensive medical care may prevent positive emotions from developing and growing. When mothers have to be hospitalized for long periods of time, the mothers and their families may have negative feelings toward the baby for prolonging her stay in the hospital. Sometimes, mothers say that it is more important to be at home with their children than to stay in the hospital for the child that is not yet born. These feelings certainly can interfere with bonding.

In short, the responsibility not only for the health of women but also for their families lies with the obstetric staff in collaboration with those in pediatrics to develop and change hospital policies regarding childbirth and early separation of mother and infant. Klaus and Kennell (1976) found that visitation in the nursery posed no increased medical hazard. Weekly bacteriologic infectious disease surveillance showed that when more lenient visitation was allowed, there was no increase in the occurrence of infection; in fact, the number of cultures with potentially pathogenic organisms declined, and yet, some institutions still limit visitation.

Mothers should be encouraged to see and touch their infants as much as possible after birth. It has been shown that mothers have difficulty forming an attachment when they have been separated from their babies during the first hours of delivery. Klaus and Kennell (1976) suggest that many factors influence the behavior of the mother. It is important that the influence of hospital practices and the behavior of the health care team be a positive one in terms of providing as much interaction as possible between mothers and other family members with their infants.

# Summary and Recommendations

From the preceding discussion of psychosocial adaptations in high-risk pregnancy, a series of recommendations can be derived. If these recommendations are used, care of high-risk pregnant women should be more effective and mutually satisfying.

1. Conduct early psychosocial screening for factors such as conflict with maternal figures, poor outcome in previous pregnancies, marital discord, little or no preparation, sexual experience, childrearing or childbearing, persistent ambivalence or fears about pregnancy, or absence of realistic plans for the baby.

2. Because patients at risk are stressed more by uncertainty than by almost any other factor, elicit patient perceptions of their problems and share the rationale for therapy, what can be expected regarding hospitalization, the nature and results of diagnostic procedures, and the probabilities for a successful outcome to the pregnancy.

3. Because pregnancy is something that happens to the family, not just to the patient, focus intervention strategies on all members of the family. Assess family functioning, and include family members in the decision-making process and in activities such as financial planning. Anticipate potential problems, and assist family members in dealing with patient frustration, depression, and displaced anger. Be alert to the problem of family members' exerting pressure on patients to resist treatment.

4. Recognize that pregnancy, in general, and high-risk pregnancy, in particular, may be associated with psychologic disequilibrium. Differentiate those psychologic problems that are situational reactions (such as a grief reaction) from those that are manifestations of a chronic personality style. Request early mental health consultation in either case.

5. Modify hospital routines that are designed for acutely ill patients to better suit women who are basically feeling well but must be hospitalized for problems related to their pregnancy. For example, patients may be more comfortable wearing their own clothes, visiting privileges can be modified, passes out of the hospital can be arranged, and so forth. It also is advisable to encourage patients with extended antepartum hospitalization to decorate their rooms with familiar personal items. Staff should regard these rooms as "belonging" to the patients and be respectful of this territory.

6. Arrange for early psychosocial assessment and have a member of the health care team visit regularly but for brief periods. Such a person (sometimes referred to as a "no needle" person in pediatric settings) should not be involved in direct patient care. It is easier for patients to express their full range of feelings about treatment to such a

## HOME BLOOD GLUCOSE MONITORING

**WHY:** You will learn how to check your blood glucose (sugar) at home in order to determine if it is high or low. The goal is better diabetic control during pregnancy.

**WHEN:**
1. Do a Chemstrip test when you feel well in order to periodically check glucose levels.
   A. Do this in the morning beore you eat breakfast and before you take your insulin.
   B. Do another test before you eat supper.
2. Do a test when you have symptoms of high or low blood sugar.
3. Do a test if you feel sick (cold, flu).

We want you to keep a record of your blood glucose levels at home during the weeks be-tween each clinic visit. Record them on this graph. BRING A GRAPH OF BLOOD GLUCOSE LEVELS WITH YOU TO EACH CLINIC VISIT. THAT GRAPH SHOULD HAVE THE BLOOD GLUCOSE LEVELS ON IT FROM THE PRECEDING WEEK.

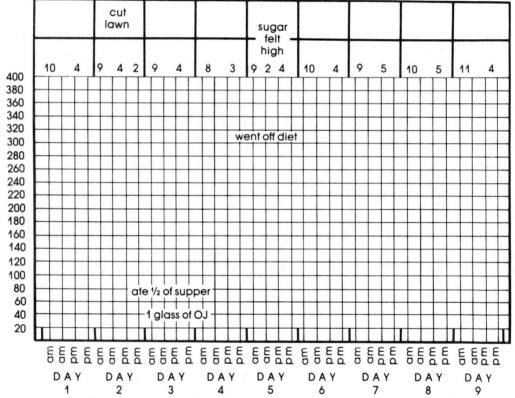

**Figure 14–2** Chart and instructions for self-monitoring of blood glucose levels. (Courtesy of Marian Lake and Tom Johnson, University of South Florida, Tampa, FL.)

person than to those who are figures of authority and on whom the patient feels dependent and vulnerable. It is also possible to use hospitalization as a catalyst for long-term psychotherapy, if indicated.

7. In a tertiary care center, recognize potential negative stereotypes patients have about such facilities and the possible prior emotional attachment to primary care obstetric practitioners. Consult regularly with referral sources and other providers of care to ensure continuity of nursing and medical care, both inpatient and outpatient, and regular high-risk care. Keep patients informed of this consultation and collaboration.

8. Provide childbirth education pro-

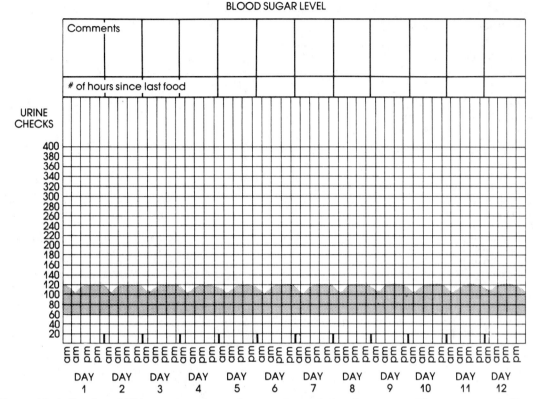

**Figure 14–2** *Continued* This portion shows the actual graph for the patient. The gray area indicates where the blood sugars should fall, making it easy for the patient to see if her blood sugars are in control.

grams for high-risk patients in the hospital, including tours of neonatal intensive care units and delivery rooms. Encourage participation of family members, and include educational preparation about both normal and cesarean deliveries. Also, educate patients about the team approach to high-risk care, and arrange for team members with special rapport to advocate for the patient in team meetings.

9. Because high-risk patients are in a compromised psychologic position in the hospital, in that their sense of control and expectations for pregnancy have been changed, afford patients as much control over care as possible. This can involve active decision-making, self-monitoring (such as blood glucose) (Fig. 14–2), and so forth.

10. In order to anticipate psychosocial reactions of high-risk patients, differentiate those who have a past history of a condition that places them at risk during pregnancy from those who after conception have developed complications demanding specialized high-risk care. In the former patients, the

best predictor of adaptation to high-risk care is their adaptation to prior conditions; in the latter patients, practitioners should expect the myriad of emotional responses that accompany any grief reaction. Some of these responses may be disconcerting, such as when denial or anger is directed personally toward a member of the hospital staff; however, these responses must be dealt with professionally.

11. The high-risk pregnant woman who is on bed rest at home needs assistance with referrals to community resources and, possibly, home health care. The patient and her family should be given clear discharge instructions for activity, sexual activity, child care, and employment.

12. Establish postnatal practices that maximize parent-infant interactions. Hospital routines and policies should allow the earliest possible interaction between parents and their infant. If interaction is not possible, still photographs and videos can be used to introduce and maintain the parent-child relationship.

# References and Recommended Reading

Adams C, Eyler FD, Behnke M: Nursing intervention with mothers who are substance abusers. Perinat Neonatal Nurs 3(4), 1990.

Arnold S, Brecht MC: Legislative issues affecting parenting: an overview of current policies. J Perinat Neonat Nurs 4(2):24–32, 1990.

Barclay RL, Barclay ML: Aspects of the normal psychology of pregnancy: the midtrimester. Am J Obstet Gynecol 125:207, 1976.

Barnet CR, Leiderman PH, Grobstein R, et al: Neonatal separation: the maternal side of interactions deprivation. Pediatrics 45:197, 1970.

Bechnard R: Organizational issues in the team delivery of comprehensive health care. Milbank Memorial Fund Quarterly 50:287, 1972.

Bibring G: Some considerations of the psychological processes in pregnancy. Psychoanal Study Child 14:113, 1959.

Blum L: Psychological Aspects of Pregnancy, Birthing and Bonding. New York, Human Services Press, 1980.

Boehm FH, Haire MF, Davidson K, et al: Maternal-fetal transport: inpatient and outpatient care. J Tenn Med Assoc November, pp 829–833, 1979.

Brazelton TB: The early mother-infant adjustment. Pediatrics 32:931, 1963.

Brown HA Jr: Improving Maternal Health from the Board Room. March of Dimes Foundation, White Plains, New York, 1990.

Brown MA: Social support during pregnancy: a unidimensional or multidimensional construct? Nurs Res 35(1):4–9, 1986.

Brown WA: Psychological Care During Pregnancy and the Postpartum Period. New York, Raven Press, 1979.

Browne JCM, Dixon G: Browne's Antenatal Care. London, Churchill Livingstone, 1978.

Bryce RL, Stanley FJ, Enkin MJ: The role of social support in the prevention of preterm birth. Birth 15:(1):19–24, 1988.

Cagan J, Meier P: A discharge planning tool for use with families of high risk infants. J Obstet Gynecol Neonatal Nurs 8:146, 1979.

Caplan G: Emotional implications of pregnancy and influences on family relationships. In Stuart H, Prugh D (eds): The Healthy Child. Cambridge, MA, Harvard University Press, 1960, pp 72–81.

Castille-Ahrens: The Rights of the Pregnant Employee. Small Business Reports. May, pp 64–67, 1990.

Chabon I: Awake and Aware: Participating in Childbirth Through Psychoprophylaxis. New York, Delacorte Press, 1966.

Chappell J: Thesis: University of Florida, Gainesville, FL, "Antepartum Orientation of High Risk Mothers to Neonatal Intensive Care Units: Effect on Maternal Anxiety Following Premature Birth," 1988.

Chasnoff I: Perinatal effects of cocaine. Contemporary OB/GYN 29:163–179, 1987.

Chez RA: NPA Bulletin, Battering in Pregnancy, 1990.

Cohen RL: Maladaptation to pregnancy. Semin Perinatol 3(1):15, 1979.

Connor GK, Denson V: Expectant fathers' response to pregnancy: review of literature and implications for research in high-risk pregnancy. J Perinat Neonat Nurs 4(2):33–42, 1990.

Dahlberg NL: A perinatal center based antepartum homecare program. J Obstet Gynecol Neonatal Nurs 17:1, 1988.

Davidson GW: Understanding Death of the Wished-For Child. Springfield, IL, OGR Service Corp, 1979.

Deutsch H: The Psychology of Women, Vol 2: Motherhood. New York, Grune & Stratton, 1945.

Flagler S, Nicoll L: A framework for the psychological aspects of pregnancy. NAACOG, Clinical Issues in Perinatal and Women's Health Nursing 1(3):267, 1990.

Freeman RK, Pescar SC: Safe Delivery: Protecting Your Baby During High Risk Pregnancy. New York, Facts on File, 1982.

Gabbe SG, Quilligan EJ: General obstetric management of the diabetic pregnancy. Clin Obstet Gynecol 24:91, 1981.

Glazer G: Anxiety and Concerns Among Pregnant Women. Res Nurs Health 3:107–113, 1980.

Gorsuch RL, Key MK: Abnormalities of pregnancy as a function of anxiety and life stress. Psychosom Med 36:352, 1974.

Grimm ER, Venet WR: The relationship of emotional adjustment and attitudes to the course and outcome of pregnancy. Psychosom Med 28:34, 1966.

Heaman M: Psychosocial Aspects of Antepartum Hospitalization. NAACOG's Clinical Issues in Perinatal & Women's Health Nursing 1(3):333–341, 1990.

Helfer RE, Kempe CH: Child Abuse and Neglect. Cambridge, MA, Ballinger, 1976.

Helton A: Battering During Pregnancy. Am J Nurs 86(8):910–913, 1986.

Hynan MT: The Pain of Premature Parents: A Psychological Guide for Coping. New York, University Press of America, 1987.

Johnson TM: Interpersonal skill in physical diagnosis. In Burnside J (ed): Physical Diagnosis: An Introduction to Clinical Medicine. Baltimore, Williams & Wilkins, 1981, pp 20–21.

Jones AC: Life change and psychological distress as predictors of pregnancy outcome. Psychosom Med 40:402, 1978.

Kane R: The interprofessional team as a small group. Soc Work Health Care 1:19, 1975.

Kemp VH: The psychological impact of a high-risk pregnancy on the family. J Obstet Neonat Nurs 15(3):232–236, 1986.

Kenner C: Caring for the NICU parent. J Perinat Neonat Nurs 4(3):78–87, 1990.

Kitzinger S: Sex before and after childbirth. Midwife and Health Visitor 8:315, 1972.

Klaus MH, Kennell JH: Mothers separated from their newborn infants. Pediatr Clin North Am 17:1015, 1970.

Klaus MH, Kennell JH: Parent-Infant Bonding. St Louis, CV Mosby Co, 1982.

Kleinman A, Eisenberg L, Good B: Culture, illness, and care: clinical lessons from anthropological and cross-cultural research. Ann Intern Med 88:251, 1978.

Lindemann E: Symptomatology and management of acute grief. Am J Psychiatry 101:141, 1944.

Lynch MA: Ill-health and child abuse. Lancet 2:317, 1975.

MacGregor SN, Keith LG: Substance abuse in pregnancy—A practical management plan. The Female Patient 14:61–67, 1989.

McCoy R, Kadowaki C, Wilks S, et al: Nursing management of breast feeding for preterm infants. J Perinat Neonat Nurs 1(1):42–55, 1988.

McDonald RL: The role of emotional factors in obstetric complications: a review. Psychosom Med 30:222, 1968.

McFarlane J: Battering during pregnancy: tip of the iceberg revealed. Women's Health 15(3):69–84, 1989.

McLendon MS: Home ambulatory uterine activity monitoring: a new tool in the management of women at risk for preterm birth. J Perinat Neonat Nurs 2(1):1–9, 1988.

Merkatz RB: Behavioral Responses of Hospitalized High Risk Maternity Patients. Unpublished thesis; Case Western Reserve University, Frances Payne Bolton School of Nursing, 1976.

Merkatz RB, Budd K, Merkatz IR: Psychologic and social implications of scientific care for pregnant diabetic women. Semin Perinatol 2:373, 1978.

Monahan PA, DeJoseph JF: The woman with preterm labor at home: a descriptive analysis. J Perinat Neonat Nurs 4:4, 1991.

Newberger E, et al: Pregnant Woman Abuse and Adverse Birth Outcome. Preterm Birth: Causes, Prevention, and Treatment, 2nd ed. Elmsford: Pergamon, 1990.

Novak JC: Facilitating nurturant fathering behavior in the NICU. J Perinat Neonat Nurs 4(2):68–77, 1990.

Oh W, Cowett RM, Clark S, et al: Role of an educational program in the regionalization of perinatal health care. Semin Perinatol 1:279, 1977.

Parad HJ: Crisis Intervention: Selected Readings. New York, Family Service Association of America, 1965.

Penticuff JH: Psychologic implications in high-risk pregnancy. Nurs Clin of North Am 17:69–78, 1982.

Plovnik M, Fry R, Tubin I: Managing Health Care Delivery: A Training Program for Primary Care Physicians. Cambridge, MA, Ballinger, 1978.

Rosen EL: Concerns of an obstetric patient experiencing long-term hospitalization. J Obstet Gynecol Neonatal 4:15, 1975.

Rubin I, Plovinick M, Fry R: Improving the Coordination of Care: A Program for Health Team Development. Cambridge, MA, Ballinger, 1975.

Sammons LN: Psychological aspects of second pregnancy. NAACOG, Clinical Issues in Perinatal and Women's Health Nursing 1(3):317–325, 1990.

Schwartz NL, Schwartz LH: Vulnerable Infants. New York, McGraw-Hill, 1977.

Seashore MJ, Leifer AD, Barnett CR, et al: The effects of denial of early mother-infant interaction on maternal self-confidence. J Pers Soc Psychol 26:367, 1973.

Smith DH: Psychologic aspects of gynecology and obstetrics. Obstet Gynecol Ann 8:457, 1979.

Souma ML: Maternal transport behind the drama. Am J Obstet Gynecol 134:1904, 1979.

Stern D: The effect of the infant on its care giver. *In* Lewis M, Rosenbloom LA: Origins of Behavior: The Effect of the Infant on Its Care Giver. New York, Wiley, 1974.

Taylor PM: Parent-Infant Relationships. New York, Grune & Stratton, 1980.

Tylden E: Psychological problems during pregnancy. Midwife and Health Visitor 8:311, 1972.

Volicer BJ: Patients' perception of stressful events associated with hospitalization. Nurs Res 23:235, 1974.

Waldron JA: Stress, adaptation and coping in a maternal-fetal intensive care unit. Soc Work Health Care 10(3):75–89, 1985.

Weinberg JS: Body image disturbance as a factor in the crisis situation of pregnancy. J Obstet Gynecol Neonatal Nurs 7:817, 1978.

Williams F: The crisis of hospitalization. Nurs Clin North Am 9:37, 1974.

Wolking S, Zajicek E: Pregnancy: A Psychological and Social Study. London, Academic Press, 1981.

Wu R: Behavior and Illness. Englewood Cliffs, NJ, Prentice-Hall, 1973.

# CHAPTER 15

. . . . . . . . . . . . . . . . . . . . . . . . . . . . . . . .

# Sexual Intimacy During Pregnancy

Barbara C. Rynerson and Deitra L. Lowdermilk

Sexuality is influenced by physiologic, psychologic, and sociocultural processes. An individual's sexuality includes sexual identity (internal feelings as well as overt sexual expression), gender roles, and sexual response. Sexual intimacy is a vital component of relationships—it is a medium for expressing love, fulfilling a basic human need, experiencing pleasure, and procreating.

Contraceptive technology currently offers couples choices about whether and when to conceive a child. Parenthood is a major developmental phase in which the couple experiences numerous adjustments. For most couples, it is an exciting and eagerly anticipated time, one that commonly results in significant adult growth. As with other important developmental periods in human life, however, parenthood also brings stresses and struggles with which the couple must cope. Adapting to parenthood is a complex task for each parent, both individually and as a couple, especially with a first pregnancy. Considering the stresses and adjustments that the couple must go through, it is not at all surprising that sexual intimacy during pregnancy can be a problem (Dameron, 1983; Osofsky, 1980; White and Reamy, 1982). Health care professionals, however, often have failed to include sexual intimacy as an important aspect of the life of the pregnant couple (Guana-Trujillo and Higgins, 1987), and objective information for counseling couples on issues of sexual intimacy during pregnancy is meager (Wilkerson and Bing, 1988). Factors that introduce risk to the pregnancy and the viability of the fetus produce additional concerns. Kemp and Page (1986) define high-risk pregnancy, in broad terms, as "any psychologic or physiologic condition having a potentially negative impact on the pregnancy." This chapter reviews some contemporary issues regarding sexual intimacy and pregnancy, including risk factors, and offers suggestions for assisting couples toward a positive and rewarding pregnancy experience.

## Intimacy and the Pregnant Couple

The numerous variables to be considered concerning both pregnancy and the expression of sexual intimacy provide a complex context in which to promote a couple's healthy adaptation. Current literature frequently refers to the pregnant couple, which shifts the focus in the childbearing process from the woman to the couple (or family). The concept of the pregnant couple implies active involvement of the father in all phases of pregnancy and childbirth. The practice of Lamaze and child delivery in birthing centers, in which fathers assist in the process of labor and delivery, illustrates this extensive involvement. However, in an exploratory study of 20 first-time expectant fathers, May (1980) found that the men exhibited one of three patterns of behavior: observer, in which the man has an emotional distance from the pregnancy; expressive, in which the man displays high emotional involvement and full participation; and instrumental, which emphasizes the man's task, manager, and caretaker functions in relation to the pregnancy and lies somewhere between detachment and full involvement. Health care professionals, however, frequently perceive fathers as androgynous and highly involved in the pregnancy experience (Sherwen, 1987). Thus, in order to counsel pregnant couples, health care professionals must overcome stereotyping and become attuned to the individual preferences of different couples. A complete understanding of sexual intimacy in the pregnant couple also must include such aspects of the relationship as the couple's gender role orientations, the degree of the father's involvement, and the couple's usual pattern of sexual expression.

Gender role behaviors may be masculine (instrumental, aggressive, independent); feminine (expressive, gentle, dependent); or androgynous (in which masculine and feminine characteristics exist in the same individual). Individuals with strict masculine or feminine role orientations display more inflexible, stereotypical, sex-typed behaviors. Sherwen (1987), summarizing the research on individuals of androgynous role orientation, notes that these individuals are more adaptable and enjoy increased satisfaction from sexual behaviors and relations. The ways in which role orientation may affect pregnancy and sexual expression are noted by Woods and Dery (1984), who point out that although sexual intercourse for many couples may be initiated by either partner, the pattern is altered during pregnancy. Physiologic and psychologic processes often lead to the woman's loss of sexual interest during the first trimester, and she may fall into a sex-role pattern of greater passivity or even reject the sexual advances of her mate. In response, the man may feel a need to adopt a more masculine role in initiating sexual activity, which may elicit guilt related to his feelings about the pregnancy in general. Feldman and Aschenbrenner (1983), in describing the qualities of androgynous couples during the course of pregnancy, indicate that both men and women increase in feminine role behavior and instrumental personality traits.

In addition to affecting gender role behavior, pregnancy has an impact on a couple's intimacy. The ways in which a couple expresses sexual intimacy are highly individual and are carried out in the context of cultural, societal, and religious beliefs and values. Although the act of intercourse is a form of communication, dialogue and nonverbal gestures are important in enhancing the meaning and pleasure of the experience for both partners. Verbal expression promotes understanding of the partner's needs and desires and serves to allay the fears and doubts that frequently pervade a sexual relationship. Both partners experience a number of feelings related to the act of intercourse, including feelings of harmony and unity with one another, caring and tenderness, and a sense of trust and belonging from which others are excluded. The expression of sexual intimacy, therefore, involves much more than intercourse. These important aspects of intimacy, as well as intercourse itself, are affected by the physiologic and emotional changes that the couple experience during pregnancy.

Ideally, the decision to become pregnant is made in the context of the couple's security and mutual readiness to assume responsibility for another person. As noted by Phillips and Anzalone (1982):

*The significance, the experience, and the joy of pregnancy as preparation for parenthood will all be enhanced if the expectant parents are in love and out of that love participate with each other in the growth process of their unborn child.*

## INTIMACY FOR THE PREGNANT WOMAN

Physiologic and emotional changes in the woman during each trimester of pregnancy influence her sexual response cycle, as well as the desirability and frequency of coital activity. Table 15–1 summarizes these changes.

During the first trimester, increased blood volume results in swollen tissues and, in particular, vasocongestion in the breasts and pelvic region. Breast tenderness, instead of being erotic, may result in discomfort if the breasts are stimulated during foreplay. Vaginal irritation and discomfort may be felt on penile penetration. Other symptoms experienced by the woman include gastric distress, nausea and vomiting, fatigue, urinary frequency, and constipation, all of which diminish sexual desire and responsiveness (Bennett, 1984; Wilkerson and Bing, 1988). For example, the tendency for the pregnant woman to have nausea and increased sensi-

Table 15–1.
EFFECTS OF PREGNANCY ON SEXUAL RESPONSE

| | First Trimester | Second Trimester | Third Trimester | Postpartum | Experience of Father |
|---|---|---|---|---|---|
| Physical Changes | Nausea, vomiting Heartburn, gastric distress Fatigue, sleepiness Pelvic vasocongestion Breast tenderness | General feeling of well-being Increased vascularity of breasts, labia, and vagina | Fatigue, insomnia Braxton Hicks contractions Increased physical discomfort Enlarged abdomen Leg cramps Leaking milk from the breasts Increased fetal size and weight | Fatigue and exhaustion caused by steroid starvation Thin vaginal mucosa and absent rugae Decreased vaginal lubrication Pain and swelling from tissue trauma Stretch marks Bulging abdomen Cracked nipples | May experience couvade syndrome Emotional upheavals may be manifested as physical complaints such as headache, backache |
| Emotional Adaptations | Ambivalent about pregnancy Labile emotions Alterations in body image Anxious and worried about parental responsibilities | May be introverted and passive Increased dependency needs Increased feelings of femininity May be conflict and guilt about pregnancy May be frequent emotional highs and lows | Feels less desirable because of body size or may feel more "womanly" Worry about premature labor May feel inhibited, vulnerable, and exposed Anxious about labor and delivery | Fear of pain during coitus Fear of damage to episiotomy and pelvic structures Negative body image Excitement or guilt over sexual stimulation of breast feeding | May reflect pregnant mate's mood swings Impregnation affirmation of masculinity Adjusting to becoming a father Conflicting role concept of partner and wife versus maternal role Feeling left out of mother-infant relationship— loneliness Jealousy |
| Sexual Response | Libido unchanged or decreased Vasocongestion causes a more pronounced orgasmic platform Glandular hyperplasia facilitates lubrication response | Libido unchanged or increased Increased interest in sex because of physical discomfort subsiding Relief from pressure to conceive; no longer fears getting pregnant | Decreased libido Dyspareunia and discomfort during coitus Positions for intercourse may need to be altered | Resume coitus four to six weeks or when comfortable Decreased libido related to fatigue and physical discomfort Delayed sexual response Dyspareunia Easily distracted during lovemaking by infant's needs | Anxiety about harming fetus Repelled or attracted by partner's appearance Feelings of virility maintain interest in active sexual practices Distraction of infant's needs may interfere with lovemaking |

Adapted from Mueller LS: Pregnancy and Sexuality. JOGN Nurs 14(4):289–294, 1985.

tivity to odors may result in decreased sexual interest or pleasure. Her partner's normal breath or body odors at the end of the day may repel the woman or even make her nauseated.

Labile emotional responses related to an increased need for rest and sleep, as well as to the ambivalence characteristic of pregnancy, may affect sexual intimacy in varying ways. Wilkerson and Bing (1988), among others, discuss the normalcy of anxiety or ambivalence related to concerns about planned or unplanned pregnancy, the timing of the pregnancy, impending parental responsibilities, family relationships, financial circumstances, and other social issues. Ambivalence toward sexual activity also may result from fear of harming the fetus or mother, causing premature labor, or inducing a miscarriage. A study by Savage and Reader (1984), however, like many other studies, found that intercourse (including orgasm) up to term did not negatively affect the outcome of pregnancy.

The second trimester of pregnancy is described as a more comfortable period than the first trimester. The increased vascularity and engorgement of the breasts, labia, and vagina lead to heightened sexual tension and more intense orgasms. As the fetus grows, the woman may feel a sense of well-being as her body becomes a source of happiness and pleasure for both partners. Many women become more aware of the uterus and its increasing size; they are distinctly aware of the presence of the baby in the uterus during intercourse. The uterus may contract during coitus, and tonic contractions may occur during orgasm, with a slowing of fetal activity and then a compensatory time of hyperactivity. Transient bradycardia in the fetus has been noted during these episodes with no apparent ill effects (Goodlin et al, 1972; Masters and Johnson, 1966). These changes in fetal activity, however, may make it difficult for the woman to feel sexually relaxed.

The interplay of physical discomfort and emotional factors may have a considerable impact on sexual intimacy during the third trimester. The discomfort produced by abdominal size, heartburn, leg cramps, Braxton Hicks contractions, weight, position of the fetus, milk leaking from the breasts, and the more intense uterine contractions with orgasm may diminish sexual interest and activity (Wilkerson and Bing, 1988). However, pelvic congestion and the intensity of Braxton Hicks contractions cause the sexual experience and orgasm to be heightened in some women, and some even find themselves orgasmic for the first time during pregnancy. Other women may find themselves distracted by the contractions and, thus, less able to enjoy intercourse. Especially during a first pregnancy, women may worry about whether intercourse and the accompanying contractions will cause them to go into labor prematurely. In subsequent pregnancies, some women become more comfortable about the normalcy of intercourse in pregnancy and report that the heightened contractions are pleasurable and an enjoyable part of the sexual experience.

During the later months of pregnancy, other issues may arise. For example, some women feel particularly embarrassed about their appearance. They may feel awkward, obese, bloated, and conscious of swelling around the vaginal area. It may be difficult for them to find a position in which intercourse is easy and comfortable. Women who previously felt at ease in their sexual experiences and in their nudity during intercourse may now feel more inhibited, vulnerable, and exposed.

The most significant impact on the desire phase of the sexual response cycle comes from the woman's feelings about body image. A positive image—feeling attractive and more womanly—may increase a woman's desire for intercourse and make her feel closer and more loving toward her mate. In the Hite (1987) report, one woman described her pregnancy as a profound and maturing experience, and she loved seeing her body get larger. Conversely, a negative image—feeling fat, unattractive, and unappealing—may elicit tenseness and decrease sexual interest (Mueller, 1985).

Generalized pelvic vasocongestion, copious vaginal lubrication, and the enlargement of the labia minora in pregnancy frequently contribute to a marked increase in sexual interest during the excitement phase. Increased vascularity may also shorten this phase for the pregnant woman (Engel, 1990; Mueller, 1985).

The marked, localized vaginal engorgement increases throughout the gravid state; during sexual stimulation, the rate of orgasmic platform development increases. Because of the vasocongestion and increased muscle tension, women report heightened arousal and responsiveness in the plateau phase. The sexual tension may increase the frequency and attainment of orgasm during the first and second trimesters. Uterine spasms lasting as long as a half hour, rather than orgasmic contractions, may occur during the third trimester; therefore, resolution is prolonged, because vasocongestion is not relieved completely by orgasm (Engel, 1990; Masters and Johnson, 1966; Mueller, 1985).

Although the reports concerning sexual intercourse during the first two trimesters of pregnancy vary considerably, a number of studies indicate that, in general, as pregnancy progresses, there is a gradual decrease in sexual interest, satisfaction with sexual activity, and frequency of coitus—with a more apparent decline in the third trimester (Engel, 1990; Holtzman, 1976; Lumley, 1978; Masters and Johnson, 1966; Solberg et al, 1973; Wilkerson and Bing, 1988). During the first trimester, the woman may not be aware of her pregnancy and, therefore, may experience no changes in sexual arousal or activity. Reports also indicate a general increase in sexual interest and activity in the second trimester (Masters and Johnson, 1966). It has been suggested that hormonal fluctuations may influence the changes in sexual desire and behavior reported during pregnancy. Ford and Beach (1951) found that hormonal influences increased eroticism in animals; in humans, however, the woman's generalized loss of libido increases consistently during the latter stages of pregnancy (Solberg et al, 1978).

In contrast to these general findings, many women report an increased desire for sex at various times during pregnancy. The desire may be related to relief from pressure to conceive, loss of fear of getting pregnant, elimination of the need to use contraception, increased awareness of the woman's body, pregnancy as proof of womanhood, celebration of the couple's accomplishment, or the physiologic alterations of pregnancy (Engel, 1990; Fogel and Rynerson, 1991). One woman reported being the happiest in her marriage during her first pregnancy and said that while on vacation together, during the seventh month, the couple made love more than they did on their honeymoon (Hite, 1987). Many women, whose physicians recommended coital abstinence beginning at times ranging from early pregnancy to 2 to 8 weeks before the estimated date of confinement, did not comply (Solberg et al, 1978; Guana-Trujillo and Higgins, 1987). This noncompliance may indicate continuing needs and desires for sexual intercourse.

As pregnancy progresses and the woman's uterus enlarges, some of the sexual techniques that the couple have used and enjoyed in the past may have to be modified to decrease awkwardness and facilitate deep penile penetration. For example, most couples usually find that intercourse in the so-called missionary position (i.e., with the man on top of the woman) is very uncomfortable. This problem, however, is not universal, and some couples report relatively little difficulty with this position even in late pregnancy. However, some couples may find alternative positions helpful (Fig. 15–1). If the couple can be flexible and patient with one another, they usually can find positions that do not seem awkward and are comfortable for both partners.

Within the general psychologic, social, and cultural context for alterations in patterns of sexual activity during pregnancy, there is a wide range of individual variability. As previously mentioned, the anxiety that couples experience emanates from a variety of sources. Conflict and guilt may play an important role if sexual activity is considered to be primarily for procreation (Colman and Colman, 1971).

Many women may decrease their sexual

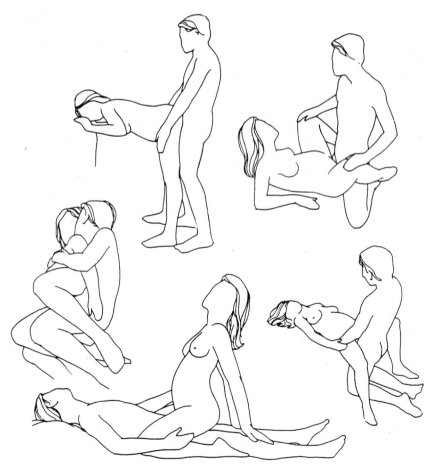

**Figure 15–1.** Alternate positions for intercourse during pregnancy. (From Wilkerson NN and Bing E. Sexuality. *In* Nichols FH and Humenick SS (eds): Childbirth Education: Practice, Research and Theory. Philadelphia, WB Saunders Co, 1988. p 384.)

activity during pregnancy because they see themselves as less attractive. The woman who attracted her partner as a young, slender, sexy lover is now uncertain about how he will react to her with the physical changes that occur during pregnancy. This perception may cause the woman to feel preoccupied, and her partner may feel isolated and lonely. Both may feel uncertain and insecure, with a pregnancy reawakening old doubts and introducing new pressures. Each partner may feel cut off from the other. The woman may even become annoyed with her partner if he seems more concerned about himself and his sexual desires and less concerned than she about the baby growing inside her. Because she recognizes that she is shifting into the new role of a mother as well as a wife, the pregnant woman with increased sexual desires may wonder if she is normal or worry about whether her partner will think she is abnormal. She sometimes believes that pregnant women are not supposed to enjoy sex, and that she should focus solely on impending motherhood. As pregnancy becomes a reality, it may awaken conflicts a woman has about dependency needs, reminding her of rivalries with her mother or siblings, which may influence her relationship with her husband. In addition, some women may feel that a pregnant woman should be a traditional Madonna-like figure for whom sex is dirty and inappropriate. During intercourse, some pregnant women imagine that they are impure and that both they and their partners are doing something wrong. Psychologically, pregnancy is influenced by how a woman perceives her pregnancy and its representative body changes, how she handles new stress, how she adjusts to changes in her relationship with her partner, and finally, her dependency needs.

The age of the woman may influence her feelings about pregnancy as well. Wilkerson and Bing (1988) report that as women delay childbearing to further develop their identities and careers, they may bring to the childbearing process a more stable relationship with the infant's father and a more mature sense of self. Other women may feel they are trapped by their pregnancy, which evokes negative feelings about society's expectations for the woman to produce a child or children. Thus, they may find pregnancy less enjoyable (Colman, 1983). When pregnancy occurs early in a marriage, before the couple has had time to experience the vari-

ances in normal sexual expression, it is difficult to put the sexual problems of pregnancy into perspective (Fader, 1989).

All cultures have a myriad of rituals and sanctions associated with both sexuality and pregnancy that may affect the way a woman responds sexually during pregnancy. Ford and Beach (1951) collected sexual data from 60 societies, all of which had an increase of taboos against sex in the last trimester of pregnancy. However, all but two of the societies that prohibited sex during all or most of pregnancy were polygamous, and therefore, other sexual outlets were available for the male partner. In contrast to these taboos against sex during pregnancy, in Liberian culture, it is believed that the woman will not have a healthy baby unless sexual activity is continued throughout pregnancy.

Perkins (1979) found that the rate of sexual activity declined at a lesser rate than would be expected by the decline of sexual interest on the woman's part, suggesting her willingness to participate for her partner's sake. Such willingness also may be influenced by rumors of men's infidelity during their partners' pregnancy.

For professionals, the task in counseling women about their sexuality and pregnancy is nearly overwhelming. The first priority is to *inquire* about any concerns the woman may be experiencing. Sexual intercourse in pregnancy is not a topic women usually bring up spontaneously. Dispelling myths and citing research about potential dangers, and especially lack of danger, is very important if the woman is to make informed choices. There is no conclusive evidence that intercourse throughout normal pregnancy and puerperium is harmful to either mother or fetus; in fact, women who exhibit a high interest in sexual activity prior to pregnancy are more likely to maintain higher levels of interest during pregnancy and postpartum periods (Guana-Trujillo and Higgins, 1987).

The physical and emotional upheavals of pregnancy make effective communication between the couple mandatory. The woman whose mate is particularly unexpressive may wish to include him in visits to the health professional for some objective information as well as to encourage him to be clearer about his desires and concerns.

The woman may feel pressured to continue sexual activity to meet her partner's needs. She may need support and encouragement as she helps him understand that, when intercourse is uncomfortable or prohibited, what she needs most is caring, gentleness, closeness, and reaffirmation of love through other means of expression than sexual intercourse. She may make every effort to meet his needs in a similar fashion, and he may be having difficulty with means of sexual expression other than intercourse. The woman also may need assistance in learning or feeling more comfortable with alternate modes of sexual expression such as massage, mutual masturbation, and oral sex (Engel, 1990).

## INTIMACY FOR THE FATHER-TO-BE

Research on intimate behaviors in men during pregnancy is scant, and in many reports, the sample populations were men who were experiencing difficulty; thus, the findings may have been negatively biased. Although there is much information about the physical and psychologic effects of pregnancy on men, the specific influences of pregnancy on sexual practices are elusive.

The numerous adjustments of the expectant father are related to both the reordering of his role and relationships in preparation for fatherhood and his responses to the physical and emotional changes of his mate's pregnant state. Several authors note that masculine attitudes toward intimacy and pregnancy may be a reflection of the woman's mood swings and the way she reacts to the physical changes of pregnancy (Fader, 1989; Wilkerson and Bing, 1988). Mueller (1985) suggests that a man has difficulty coping with his mate's labile emotions as well as her increased dependency on him. Because pregnancy is likely to increase the dependency needs of the expectant father as well, he may feel unable to respond to the demands placed on him by the woman.

Influences on the male partner's intimacy behaviors related to becoming a father include a myriad of emotions and perceptions. Although social and technologic changes in contemporary society have fostered greater integration of the father in the pregnancy and birth process, a defined role during pregnancy is still lacking for the father. Also, the man may feel abandoned because of the expectant mother's self-preoccupation and lack of involvement in his life (Fader, 1989).

Valuing the pregnancy as well as holding a sense of accomplishment that his sperm

has united with an egg are positive experiences for the man. Feelings of virility maintain his interest in active sexual practices throughout his mate's pregnancy. According to Hangsleben (1983) and Lemmer (1987), both acceptance of the pregnancy and a favorable adjustment to fatherhood are related to marital adjustment and are likely to sustain sexual relations. Some men report increased sexual desire during pregnancy related to feeling excited by their pregnant partners, experiencing emotional closeness, intimacy, and happiness (Reamy and White, 1985). In a review of nursing research on expectant fathers, Lemmer (1987) indicates that emotional involvement in the pregnancy correlates with readiness for fatherhood and notes that men tend to become more protective and nurturing of their mates during pregnancy. These caring behaviors tend to enhance intimacy in the relationship.

However, the wide range of feelings that men experience in relation to expectant fatherhood also may have a negative influence on their sexual responsiveness throughout the pregnancy. The feelings most commonly reported are ambivalence, especially in early pregnancy; loneliness; fear of intercourse; guilt, because their mate is seen in the mothering role rather than the wife role; worry; anxiety; and jealousy (Lemmer, 1987; Mueller, 1985; Wilkerson and Bing, 1988). In a review of sexuality and pregnancy, Reamy and White (1985) noted the following potential influences on the man's decreased sexual desire: fear of harming the pregnant woman or fetus; being repelled by the pregnant body; believing that sex with a pregnant woman is immoral; fearing that somehow the fetus would be an observer to sexual activity and could hurt the man's penis; and the need to withdraw from the wife while dealing with the stresses of pregnancy himself. As a means of seeking comfort and relief, men may engage in extramarital affairs. Often an affair during his partner's pregnancy is the man's first affair, and it usually terminates with delivery (Masters and Johnson, 1966; Osofsky and Osofsky, 1980).

Pregnancy may reawaken the man's emotions concerning his family of origin, resulting in some anxiety and ambivalence about fatherhood, which may affect his sexual responsiveness. The psychologic processes of fantasies and dreams help the man to resolve conflicts, re-establish kinships, and affirm his own paternal identity. Men who are aware of their emotions often are more empathic and invested in their wives (Sherwen, 1987). In addition to working through their emotions, both men's fantasies and affairs during pregnancy may, in part, be an attempt to protect their partners from confusing and hurtful emotions. If the man becomes involved in a relationship with another woman, he can avoid some of the feelings and inhibitions that arise from his repulsion of a pregnant body and sexual involvement with his "wife-mother."

As a result of the pressures and complex emotions that arise during pregnancy, some men may experience symptoms known as couvade. In some cultures, couvade refers to the rituals a man performs during his partner's pregnancy in order to protect the pregnant woman from evil spirits and pain. However, its current meaning in Western society, as defined by Shapiro and Nass (1986), is a psychogenic disorder in which the man experiences and expresses physical symptoms of pregnancy. These authors indicate that couvade has somatic and psychologic characteristics ranging from brief, minor symptoms to gross psychotic responses. The research reviews of Lemmer (1987) and a study of 81 expectant fathers by Clifton (1985) attest to the reality of couvade. The men in these studies complained of a wide variety of symptoms, including headache, irritability, nervousness, weight gain, gas pains, backaches, restlessness, colds, and depression. Significant factors influencing the man experiencing physical distress include being of an ethnic minority, having had children previously, having had health problems the year prior to pregnancy, low income, and greater emotional involvement in the pregnancy. Couvade experiences are discussed in the literature as both the man's identification with the pregnant woman and as a physical expression of anxiety (Bogren, 1983). There is no evidence of couvade affecting sexual intimacy, but it seems reasonable that for those men experiencing symptoms, there would be additional stress in the intimate relationship.

Assisting the "pregnant man" to cope with his many concerns may be difficult for two reasons: first, because there is no physiologic manifestation of pregnancy, there is less natural opportunity to interact with the man; second, traditional male role orientation as well as the man's perplexity over what he experiences considerably reduce his ability to communicate needs and concerns. Although there is lack of clarity and consistency about the many issues involved in male sexual intimacy during pregnancy, there are adequate data to support the premise that men's needs and desires for information are as great or greater than the pregnant woman's. Health care professionals must be creative in inviting men to share their concerns, and they must be sensitive to the discomfort and vulnerability the men may feel. For example, nurses and other health care providers may initiate and publicize open forums for expectant fathers in which experts address pertinent sexual issues, followed by a question-and-answer period. This type of intervention is a means of reaching the men by overtly acknowledging that their concerns are real. Other possible interventions would be expectant father support groups and provision of some evening hours in which men could make appointments for discussing individual dilemmas.

Accurate information about the woman's physiology of pregnancy and dispelling myths about sexual intimacy in both partners are priorities in talking with men. Men also need to understand that some of what they are experiencing is normal and universal, particularly the fears they have of harming the pregnant woman or the fetus. Encouragement and permission to share whatever is of concern to the men decreases their anxieties and allows them increased freedom of participation in the entire pregnancy and birth process while they maintain their sexual interactions. At the same time, health care professionals must recognize and accept some men's desires for less emotional involvement and assist these men in expressing intimacy and support toward their partners to the extent that they feel comfortable.

The course of pregnancy is a natural time for men to explore and affirm their own identity in becoming parents. For many men, talking openly with their partners, as well as with their fathers and male friends, enhances this process. However, when awareness of unresolved conflicts about a man's own family or about his partner's role as wife and mother results in dysfunctional anxiety, short-term psychologic assistance should be encouraged.

Although affairs during pregnancy occur, prolonged extramarital affairs signal real trouble in the relationship unrelated to the pregnant state. Men involved in prolonged extramarital affairs may be fleeing from the responsibility of family commitment and may not seek professional counseling. If they are ambivalent about whether or not they want to become a father and truly love their partners, they may be more amenable to seeking marital counseling. The health professional should assist the couple in engaging a sensitive and enlightened counselor.

As Bogren (1983) observed, 20 percent of the men in his study experienced couvade in spite of their information about and involvement in the pregnancy. Helping these men to better understand their own psychologic processes and physical manifestations in response to their partners' pregnancy at least could prevent the syndrome's interference in the intimate relationship.

Another important assessment to be made by health professionals is the man's potential for violent behavior toward the pregnant partner. Unrecognized rage and jealousy may be manifested in aggressive or emotionally abusive acts by the man during this time, even without any prior history of violent behavior. Protection of the pregnant woman and the fetus is a top priority, and health professionals are obligated to assist the woman in this endeavor by any means acceptable to her. Therefore, if the relationship is to continue peacefully, the man must be encouraged to be accountable for his own behavior and seek counseling.

# Complications

Some authors have speculated as to the safety of sexual practices during pregnancy. Some have suggested that the decreased interest in coitus during pregnancy is caused by a subconscious "holding back" of orgasm to prevent harm to the baby. Others have suggested that couples avoid intercourse because they fear causing miscarriage or congenital anomalies. Recent fears about AIDS and other sexually transmitted diseases and their potential risks to the mother and neonate are also reasons given by couples for avoiding sexual intercourse during pregnancy. However, most authors are of the opinion that coitus and orgasm are *not* harmful to the normal pregnant woman or her

fetus (Connell et al, 1981; Mills et al, 1981; Perkins, 1979; Reamy et al, 1982; Turnbull and Chamberlain, 1989). However, there are some concerns regarding coitus, orgasm, and breast stimulation in cases in which high-risk situations exist or are likely to develop, for example, bleeding; repeated fetal wastage; premature labor; incompetent cervix; premature rupture of the membranes; infection, including sexually transmitted diseases; and multiple gestation. In these situations, sexual activity may be limited. The rest of this section discusses sexual activity in relation to specific complications of pregnancy and long-term hospitalization of the high-risk pregnant patient.

## BLEEDING AND FETAL WASTAGE

In the first trimester, bleeding may occur as a prelude to spontaneous abortion. Couples should avoid intercourse if abdominal cramps or vaginal bleeding occur following coitus (Turnbull and Chamberlain, 1989). In cases of threatened abortion, abstinence of sexual activity is commonly advised, although it may have no effect on the outcome. However, intercourse could increase the chance of infection if the cervix is dilated (Woods and Esposito, 1987). Some couples who engage in sexual intercourse and experience spontaneous abortion may associate sexual activity with causing the abortion. Encouraging these couples to abstain from sexual activity until the bleeding resolves may help them avoid feelings of guilt.

If there have been repeated spontaneous abortions, it is imperative that the products of conception be studied for anomalies, genetic abnormalities, infection, or placental defects. If the miscarriages were the result of any of the above factors, further gynecologic assessment may be indicated. The conditions that produced the risk may be correctable or not likely to cause problems in the current pregnancy. Intercourse does not affect the outcome in most of these situations; the factors should be evaluated and discussed with the patient. A blighted ovum miscarriage is a statistical risk in any pregnancy, occurring in 1 out of every 10 pregnancies. Again, coitus and orgasm do not affect this outcome. If, however, factors such as congenital uterine anomalies or fibroid distortions rather than embryonic death are the cause of bleeding and first-trimester abortion, it is best to counsel against intercourse and orgasm (Grover, 1977). Resolution of these problems between pregnancies may be wise.

Often, a woman becomes pregnant soon after suffering the loss of a previous pregnancy. This pregnancy can cause stress on the marital relationship. The woman often is more concerned about the pregnancy than the relationship with her spouse. She may not want to engage in sexual activities, because she associates intercourse with the previous loss. The man may perceive that the woman is rejecting or punishing him. If these feelings are unresolved, a permanent change in the relationship could occur (Woods and Esposito, 1987). Health care professionals need to encourage the couple to share their concerns and feelings. If the couple decides not to engage in sexual activity after discussing their concerns, they should be supported in their decision. However, as the pregnancy progresses, milestones such as fetal heart tones and fetal movement may encourage the couple to accept the pregnancy and again enjoy sexual activities.

In the second and third trimesters, bleeding can be caused by uterine anomalies, placental abruption, or placenta praevia, or it may be of unknown origin. Naeye (1981a) studied the association between coitus and antepartum bleeding from placental abruption and antepartum bleeding of unknown origin. He found that there was an association between these two types of bleeding and coitus (orgasm not identified) that was independent of other factors, such as hypertension, smoking and placental infarcts that cause abruption, although he was unable to show a causal relationship between coitus and antepartum bleeding.

Placenta praevia is mentioned in the literature as a reason for avoiding intercourse during pregnancy. It is not clear whether this avoidance is advised only in cases in which there is active bleeding. However, because of the possibility that contact of the penis against the lower uterine segment may cause disruption of the placenta and bleeding, intercourse should probably be avoided by all patients with placenta praevia. Contractions during orgasm may also cause bleeding and should be avoided. If the placenta migrates away from the cervix, intercourse may be resumed; this is dependent on the location of the placenta and the physician's discretion.

## PREMATURE LABOR

It has been documented that, throughout pregnancy, uterine contractions occur with and without orgasm (Chayen et al, 1986; Fox et al, 1970; Goodlin et al, 1972; Goodlin et al, 1971; Perkins, 1979), especially in the last 2 months of pregnancy, when the uterus is more sensitive to stimuli of all types. Sexual intercourse has been identified as a positive risk factor for preterm labor for more than 25 years. In a study by Goodlin (1969), 55 percent of women who were orgasmic reported painful uterine contractions, pains of the back or pelvis, or pressure or round ligament type of pain after orgasm. Fox and coworkers (1970) measured uterine contractions during intercourse and orgasm. They found that regular uterine contractions occurred during coitus, irrespective of orgasm, which were interrupted by more irregular, sometimes tonic, contractions during orgasm. The regular contractions returned after orgasm. Perkins (1979) described varying percentages of women who had contractions during sexual activity. Oxytocin may play a part in initiating these contractions. Fox and coworkers (1970) found that there were small amounts of oxytocin in the peripheral bloodstream within 1 minute after orgasm. A pressure gradient exists between the vagina and uterus after female orgasm, which may also play a part in uterine irritability. Perkins (1979) also reported that multiparous patients perceived uterine irritability more readily than did nulliparous patients during coitus. However, most authors agree that these contractions during coitus and orgasm are not strong enough to initiate labor (Masters and Johnson, 1966; Pugh and Fernandez, 1953; Rayburn and Wilson, 1980; Wagner et al, 1976). Many of these authors recommend that unless intercourse is uncomfortable, it need not be discontinued in the normal pregnancy.

Several studies have been conducted to try to determine whether there is a relationship between coital or orgasmic contractions and premature labor. Goodlin (1969) found that there was an increased incidence of orgasm in those women delivering prematurely. However, this group also had a 3-times higher incidence of history of premature labor than did the control group delivering at term. In 1971, Goodlin again found a relationship between increased orgasm and premature delivery. In that study, Goodlin asked four women at term to try to initiate labor with orgasm, and three were successful in starting labor shortly after orgasm.

One of the problems with the comparison of frequency of coitus and orgasm in relationship to premature labor is that the frequency of sexual activity is higher in the second than in the third trimester. Thus, although many women have more sexual activity in the second trimester, few go into premature labor at that time. Goodlin (1971) found that many women who abstained from coitus, for fear that penetration would harm the baby, continued to achieve orgasm by other means. However, Wagner (1976), in a small matched study sample of a larger study group, noted that a higher frequency of mothers of premature infants had, in the first trimester, experienced one or more of the following: (1) a higher frequency of orgasmic coitus; (2) orgasm from noncoital stimulation; (3) multiple orgasms; and (4) a greater frequency of cramps and contractions following coitus than did mothers of nonpremature infants. Wagner questioned whether orgasm in early pregnancy could significantly affect the developing fetus so as to cause preterm birth. It should be noted that when this matched study group of mothers of premature infants was compared with the entire study, there was no statistically significant relationship between orgasm and prematurity.

Perkins (1979) found no adverse associations between orgasm and onset of labor. In fact, he found that orgasmic patients consistently had a lower percentage of early deliveries. Perkins also reported that the type of stimulation used to achieve orgasm was not important, except that masturbation was consistently associated with a lower risk of prematurity throughout pregnancy. Rayburn and Wilson (1980) found no relationship of coital activity with orgasm to the delivery of premature infants.

Brustman and colleagues (1989) reported a fivefold increase in uterine activity immediately following intercourse in a group of women previously treated for preterm labor in their current pregnancy. This increase did not occur in the control group of low-risk pregnant women. Both groups were monitored in the home with home uterine tocodynamometric systems. Despite these findings, the investigators did not offer recommendations to restrict sexual activity in pregnant women at risk for preterm labor.

Based on these studies, restriction of sexual activity for the woman at risk of preterm labor may be seen as a common but not universal recommendation. The focus of obstetric and public health practitioners and policy makers on prevention of preterm labor must include continued investigation into the advisability of unrestricted coitus during pregnancy. Until this issue is resolved, abstention from coitus and orgasm continues to be recommended for cases of

1. A poor reproductive history
2. Arrested premature labor in the present pregnancy, until the fetus reaches maturity
3. A prior *unexplained* premature delivery
4. Incompetent cervix or early ripening of the cervix on vaginal examination.

Two other factors—seminal fluid and breast stimulation—should be considered in relation to premature labor. Seminal fluid, rich in prostaglandins and enzymes, has been implicated as a possible initiator of labor. Lavery and Miller (1981) reported that the short-term exposure to the prostaglandins that occurs with ejaculation is not enough to cause premature labor. Anderson and Fuchs (1984) report a positive association of seminal prostaglandin and female orgasm with uterine contractile activity and suggest restriction of sexual activity for the woman with a high-risk pregnancy. Iams and associates (1988) also advise couples at risk to use condoms during coitus to decrease effects of prostaglandin on uterine contractility.

Breast stimulation has been used to initiate labor at term and is widely used in contraction stress testing. It has been known to cause uterine activity and even hyperstimulation (Chayen and Kim, 1988; Lipitz et al, 1987). Initiation of premature labor by breast stimulation has not been reported in the literature, but Iams and associates (1988) recommend that women at risk for preterm labor avoid breast stimulation if contractions are noted during this activity.

Stress has been identified as a factor in the initiation of preterm labor (Herron et al, 1982; Omer et al, 1986; Kemp and Hatmaker, 1989; Richardson, 1987). It would seem that sexual proscription would add to the life stress of pregnancy itself and might, therefore, actually increase the risk of premature labor. Also, many couples who are unable to abstain from their sexual activities acquire feelings of guilt from their lack of abstinence, especially if complications arise, and this creates further stress. Therefore, it would behoove practitioners to assess the situation carefully before proscribing sexual activities for the couple. Robertson and Berlin (1986) suggest some alternative means of sexual expression. Also, it should be remembered that sexual activities can be resumed when fetal maturity is achieved (as determined by lecithin-sphingomyelin (L/S) ratio).

As a final note regarding premature labor, it would be interesting to compare cervical changes in those women who have contractions during coitus, those who have contractions during coitus and orgasm, and those who do not have any contractions. This information might be helpful in making recommendations regarding sexual activities.

## RUPTURE OF THE MEMBRANES AND INFECTION

There have been several theories on the cause or causes of premature rupture of the membranes (PROM), including poor nutrition, cigarette smoking, coitus, parity, prior surgery to the cervix, and infection (Naeye, 1982). (See also Chapter 21.) In regard to coitus, it is believed that the contractions that occur during orgasm are not strong enough to cause PROM. In the laboratory, both normal and prematurely ruptured membranes usually resist pressures generated as high as those of labor (Al-Zais et al, 1980; Danforth and Hull, 1958; Embrey, 1954; Lavery and Miller, 1979). Most of the strength of the membranes is found in a zone of connective tissue beneath the amnion. It has been noted that the membranes may rupture along areas of membrane abnormalities, leaving the normal membrane areas intact. Artal and associates (1979) postulated that damage is caused by enzymatic depolymerization of the collagen fibers. Acute infection–releasing proteolytic enzymes or the collagenase-like enzymes in seminal fluid are possible mechanisms for this damage. However, Lavery and Miller (1981) found that seminal fluid acting alone does not appear to weaken the membranes. Naeye (1979) reported finding coitus combined with infection as a mechanism for PROM, although his methods have been criticized because of his definition of infection found in the placenta. Because intercourse is more frequent in the second trimester, this may skew the data toward an association between more frequent coitus and PROM (Herbst, 1979; Perkins, 1983).

Naeye's (1982) findings suggested that previous cervical damage may cause harboring of bacteria, which predisposes to PROM; his report included a recommendation for further studies in this area. Other sources suggest that coitus can increase risk by increasing the number of vaginal bacteria, but this theory has not been proved (Iams et al, 1988). Toth and associates (1988) suggest that infections that cause preterm labor may be attributed to a prepregnancy infection of the uterus (i.e., pelvic inflammatory disease) and that having more than one sex partner also increases the risk of PROM. The authors reported a study that correlated increased number of bacteria in the cervix with coitus. Development of amnionitis also has been associated with high titers of immunoglobin G (IgG) antisperm antibody, which is indicative of a bacterial infection in males (Toth et al, 1988). These findings suggest pregnant women who engage in sexual activity with more than one partner may be at higher risk of developing an infection that can invade the placental membranes, placenta, and amnionic fluid.

## SEXUALLY TRANSMITTED DISEASES

Sexually transmitted diseases in the prenatal period are now receiving more attention than ever. Failure to prevent and identify sexually transmitted diseases during pregnancy can lead to complications such as abortion, stillbirth, preterm labor, infertility, and maternal and neonatal infections (Wilson, 1988). More than 20 infectious diseases are noted to be sexually transmitted diseases, and pregnant women are not immune to any of them (Benoit, 1988). Couples need to be aware of risk factors associated with sexually transmitted diseases and safe sexual practices that may prevent transmission of infection. This information should be provided in early prenatal contacts.

Risk factors include a history of or current diagnosis of sexually transmitted diseases, drug use, sexual activity with multiple partners, or partners who are likely to have sex with multiple partners (Centers for Disease Control, 1989; McGregor et al, 1989). Unprotected sexual activity with infected partners can lead to sexually transmitted diseases, therefore, the pregnant woman should be counseled with her sexual partners about the risk of maternal and neonatal infections as well as prevention and treatment. Use of latex condoms provides considerable, but not complete, protection against human immunodeficiency virus (HIV) and other sexually transmitted diseases, such as gonorrhea, syphilis, genital herpes, chlamydia, and trichomonas (Centers for Disease Control, 1989; Cunningham et al, 1989; Mcheus, 1988). Condoms with spermicide (nonoxynol 9) may increase protection, and their risk of use in pregnancy has not been documented (Goldsmith, 1989; Smith et al, 1990). Some authors suggest the use of condoms for the entire 9 months of pregnancy as prophylaxis against sexually transmitted diseases; however, other sources advise the use of condoms or abstinence only when an infection is present and active or when lesions are present (e.g., in cases of herpes or condylomata) (Centers for Disease Control, 1989; MacGregor, 1989). Other means of sexual intimacy should be encouraged, especially near term (Dowen and Dillon, 1985).

## OTHER COMPLICATIONS

Some authors suggest abstinence from sexual activities when *uterine anomalies* (e.g., fibroids) are present that might cause uterine irritability or decrease uterine capacity (Grover, 1977). If there are recurrent problems, surgery between pregnancies may resolve the situation.

Because *multiple gestation* increases uterine size and may cause uterine irritability, some researchers recommend that coitus and orgasm be avoided (Connell et al, 1981; Rayburn and Wilson, 1980). Neilson and Mutambira (1989) studied the effects of coitus on precipitation of preterm labor in women pregnant with twins and found that there was no significant difference in reports of coital activity in those who delivered preterm and those who delivered at term. Based on these findings, the investigators do not discourage coital activity.

Another area of concern is whether there is *fetal distress* during orgasm. Goodlin and colleagues (1971) measured one patient for uterine pressure and fetal heart tones during female orgasm. They noted decelerations of the fetal heart rate and questioned whether fetal distress was present. (From the tracings in the article, the fetal decelerations appeared to be mild variables.) Grudzinskas (1979) reported that women who were sexually active during the last 4 weeks of pregnancy had an increase of meconium-stained fluid and their newborns had lower 1-minute Apgar scores. He questions whether there is a temporary compromise in fetal circulation associated with uterine contractions. Chayen and associates (1986) reported a study of fetal heart rate changes and uterine activity during intercourse in normal pregnant women whose pregnancies ranged from 28 to 40 weeks. A variety of fetal heart rate patterns, including ominous patterns, were seen on monitor tracings, and increased fetal activity was reported by the women. Fetal bradycardia with recovery was noted in some cases, suggesting transient hypoxia. Despite these findings, the investigators do not give specific advice about coitus during pregnancy but suggest that further study is needed.

There is one notoriously dangerous sexual activity during pregnancy, the practice of *insufflating air* into the vagina under pressure during cunnilingus. Sudden maternal deaths have been reported during this activity secondary to air embolism (Bernhardt et al, 1988).

## EFFECTS OF LONG-TERM HOSPITALIZATION

For many women who develop complications during pregnancy, hospitalization is used as a strategy to manage the high-risk pregnancy and to preserve maternal and fetal well-being. The psychosocial effects of hospitalization on the woman and her partner have been reported in the literature, but issues of sexuality have not been addressed specifically (Kemp and Page, 1986; Loos and Julius, 1989; White and Ritchie, 1984;

Williams, 1986). Kemp and Page (1986) reported that antepartum hospitalization caused increased stress in the woman because of separation from her home and family. The authors suggested measures such as flexible visiting hours and policies that would promote opportunities for family interaction. Loos and Julius (1989), in a study of hospitalized prenatal women, reported that loneliness was a consistent phenomenon experienced by the patients as a result of separation from significant others and a lack of intimate privacy. Women in the study reported missing their partners' touch and being alone with their partners. The emotions and concerns of the partner of the hospitalized woman have not been addressed in the literature. Studies to identify these concerns are needed. (See also Chapter 14.)

## Postpartum Sexual Activity

There is little scientific data that recommends when the couple should resume sexual intercourse after delivery. Studies have varied considerably, from reports that coitus was resumed as early as 2 weeks postpartum to as late as 3 months postpartum (Masters and Johnson, 1966; Robson and Kumar, 1981; Sapire, 1986; Turnbull and Chamberlain, 1989; Walbroehl, 1986). Women reported that resumption depended on the degree of discomfort, when the bleeding stopped, the presence of an episiotomy or lacerations, and whether the delivery was vaginal or cesarean. Multiparas reported resumption earlier than primiparas. Although earlier studies reported resumption of sexual activity to occur earlier in breastfeeding mothers (Falicov, 1973; Kenney, 1973; Masters and Johnson, 1966), results of a more recent study by Fischman and associates (1986) found no significant differences in postpartum sexual activity between breastfeeding and nonbreastfeeding women.

Little attention to sexual adjustment of new parents is reported in the literature, particularly for fathers. Studies have reported men's concerns related to the increased demands of work and home and feelings of exclusion from the mother-infant interactions, especially if the woman is breastfeeding (Fischman et al, 1986; Walbroehl, 1986). Walbroehl (1986) reported

that problems with sexuality for the male may develop as a result of the man's role during delivery; if he was not prepared for the blood and the woman's appearance during delivery, the sexual image of the woman could be affected.

Breastfeeding has been identified as another possible negative influence on sexuality for the male. Studies have reported that males have developed feelings of sexual inadequacy, latent homosexuality, incestuousness, and jealousy (Jordan, 1986; Liebenberg, 1969). The man may see the woman being sexually stimulated by breastfeeding and feel left out, jealous, or inadequate, especially if the woman does not want to engage in sexual activity. The male also may compare his wife to his mother and feel that this may be incest.

A decrease in sexual activity and enjoyment for up to 1 year has been reported in several studies of postpartum women. Women may experience sexual dysfunction as a result of exhaustion, sleepless nights, the perception that there is not enough time in the day to get everything done, the demands of the newborn, and dissatisfaction with body image (Fischman et al, 1986; Hampson, 1989; Walbroehl, 1986). Breastfeeding has been reported to cause sexual arousal for the woman. Studies describe sucking as sexually stimulating because the accompanying uterine contractions simulate an orgasmic feeling. However, decreased vaginal lubrication caused by decreased estrogen and elevated prolactin have been reported to cause dyspareunia, leading to decreased sexual activity (Fischman et al, 1986; Walbroehl, 1986). Dyspareunia from vaginal trauma including episiotomy has also been reported.

Couples who have experienced an unplanned cesarean delivery may express feelings of failure; these feelings can lead to stress in the sexual relationship (Walbroehl, 1986). Likewise, a couple who experiences a loss of an infant or who has an infant in the neonatal intensive care unit can also suffer stress in their sexual relationship. The woman may have decreased sexual desire if she feels like a failure for the loss or the preterm birth. Although engaging in sexual intercourse is a way couples can rebuild their intimate relationship after delivery, it also can be viewed as the cause of the loss or why the infant is ill (Woods and Esposito, 1987).

Counseling is important to guide couples through this stressful time and to help them to feel comfortable in resuming their sexual activities. Couples should be informed that use of water soluble lubricants or perineal massage may prevent or decrease dyspareunia. Couples who are breastfeeding need to expect milk leakage during sexual activity. Couples should plan time alone together on a regular basis to promote communication and intimacy. Teaching and counseling, prenatally and postnatally, can make the resumption of a sexual relationship easier.

## Recommendations

Research seems to indicate that sexual activity is normal and safe during pregnancy. However, in the presence of (1) bleeding in general, and specifically with placenta previa; (2) a poor reproductive history secondary to factors that could be influenced by coitus; or (3) cervical changes, abstinence from coitus, orgasm, and, perhaps, breast stimulation is recommended. Clinicians should be careful not to interfere with the couple's sexual activities or to give them information that would make them feel guilty or frustrated and angry when this is not needed. If there have been previous miscarriages or other problems, couples may decide temporarily to discontinue sexual activities. These patients should be supported in their decision. As the pregnancy progresses, they may be encouraged to resume intercourse.

Clinicians should counsel patients as to when they can resume intercourse, i.e., when bleeding has stopped or when the fetus reaches maturity (as determined by L/S ratio).

The couple should be counseled together, especially when abstinence is recommended, to avoid conflict and so that appropriate recommendations can be made. Tenderness and cuddling can be advised, and nongenital sexual play and gratification can be discussed. When recommendations are made, they should be very specific: Don't just say, "No sex." For example, if complications are related to penile penetration, other sexual activities discussed previously can be suggested. If the complication is related to uterine contractility, the use of condoms or abstinence from orgasm may be advised. If sexual activity for the woman is contraindicated, she may want to continue pleasing her partner through oral or manual stimulation (Cohn, 1982).

The couple should be encouraged to explore broader aspects of their physical and emotional relationship during abstinence. Often pamphlets such as "Some Things About Sex in Pregnancy," by Ann Hager can help in counseling the couple throughout pregnancy. Taking an initial sexual history can be helpful. This history can be updated as the pregnancy continues, with counseling to the couple on both physical and emotional needs. New parenting is an ideal time for the expression of love. The couple's sexual relationship can help them to maintain intimacy as a couple as the new baby, especially in the primipara, changes the family structure.

## References and Recommended Readings

Al-Zais NS, Bov-Resli MN, Goldpink G: Bursting pressure and collagen content of fetal membranes and their relation to premature rupture of the membranes. Br J Obstet Gynaecol 87:227, 1980.

Anderson LF, Fuchs F: Sexual activity and preterm birth. In Fuchs F, Stubblefield PG (eds): Preterm Birth, Causes, Prevention, and Management. New York, Macmillan & Co, 1984.

Artal R, Burgeson RE, Hobel CJ, et al: An in vitro model for the study of enzymatically mediated biomechanical changes in the chorioamniotic membranes. Am J Obstet Gynecol 133:656, 1979.

Bennett EC: The first trimester. JOGN Nurs 13(2Supp):93–96, 1984.

Benoit JA: Sexually transmitted diseases in pregnancy. Nursing clinics in North America. 23(4):937–945, 1988.

Bernhardt R, Goldmann RW, Thombs PA, Kindwall EP: Hyerbarci oxygen treatment of cerebral air embolism from orogenital sex during pregnancy. Crit Care Med 16:762, 1988.

Bogren LY: Couvade. Acta Psychiatr Scand 68:55–65, 1983.

Brustman LE, Raptoulis M, Langer O, et al, Changes in patterns of uterine contractility in relationship to coitus during pregnancy at low and high risk for preterm labor. Obstet Gynecol 73(2):166–168, 1989.

Centers for Disease Control: 1989 Sexually transmitted disease treatment guidelines. MMWR supplement 38(S-8), 1989.

Chayen B, Kim Y: Results of 317 contraction stress tests with controlled nipple stimulation using an electric breast pump. J Reprod Med 33(2):214–216, 1988.

Chayen B, Tejani H, Verma U, Gordon G: Fetal heart rate changes and uterine activity during coitus. Acta Obstet Gynecol Scand 65:853–855, 1986.

Clifton F: Expectant fathers at risk for couvade. Nur Res 35:290, 1985.

Cohn SD: Sexuality in pregnancy. Nurs Clin North Am 17(1):91–98, 1982.

Colman AD, Colman LL: Pregnancy: The Psychological Experience. New York, Herder & Herder, 1971.

Colman LL: Psychology of pregnancy. *In* Sonstegard L, Kowalski K, Jennings B (eds): Women's Health. Vol 2. New York, Grune & Stratton, 1983.

Connell EB, Butler J, Goodlin R: What do you advise patients concerning the safety of sexual relations during pregnancy? Med Aspects Human Sex 15:91, 1981.

Cunningham FG, MacDonald PC, Gant NF (eds): Williams Obstetrics. Norwalk, CT, Appleton & Lange, 1989.

Dameron G: Helping couples cope with sexual changes pregnancy brings. Contemp Obstet Gynecol 21:23, 1983.

Danforth DN, Hull RW: The microscopic anatomy of the fetal membrane with particular reference to the detailed structure of the amnion. Am J Obstet Gynecol 75:536, 1958.

Dowen RH, Dillon M: Herpes infection in pregnancy. NAACOG Update Series 3(4):1–7, 1985.

Embrey MP: On the strength of the foetal membranes. Br J Obstet Gynaecol 61:793, 1954.

Engel NS: The maternity cycle and sexuality. *In* Fogel CI, Lauver D (eds): Sexual Health Promotion. Philadelphia, WB Saunders, 1990.

Fader KB: Sex during pregnancy. Glamour 87(2):64–69, 1989.

Falicov CJ: Sexual adjustment during first pregnancy and postpartum. Am J Obstet Gynecol 117:991, 1973.

Feldman S, Aschenbrenner B: Impact of parenthood on various aspects of masculinity and femininity: a short term longitudinal study. Dev Psychol 19(2):1278–1289, 1983.

Fischman S, Rankin EA, Soeken KL, Lenz ER: Changes in sexual relationship in postpartum couples. JOGN Nurs 15(1):58–64, 1986.

Fogel CI, Rynerson BC: Sexuality Concerns. *In* Cohen S, Kenner C, and Hollingsworth A (eds): Maternal, Neonatal, and Women's Health Nursing. Springhouse, PA: Springhouse Corporation, 1991.

Ford C, Beach F: Patterns of Social Behavior. New York, Perennial (div of Harper & Row), 1951.

Fox CA, Wolff HS, Baker A: Measurement of intravaginal and intra-uterine pressures during human coitus by radiotelemetry. J Reprod Fertil 22:243, 1970.

Goldsmith MF: Pregnancy Dx? Rx may now include condoms. JAMA. 261(5):678–79, 1989.

Goodlin RC: Orgasm and premature labour. Lancet 2:646, 1969.

Goodlin RC, Keller D, Raffin M: Orgasm during late pregnancy; possible deleterious effects. Obstet Gynecol 38:916, 1971.

Goodlin RC, Schmidt W, Greevy DC: Uterine tension and fetal heart rate during maternal orgasm. Obstet Gynecol 39:125, 1972.

Grover JW: Coitus during pregnancy for women with a history of spontaneous abortion. Med Aspects Human Sex 5:113, 1977.

Grudzinskas JG: Does sexual intercourse cause fetal distress? Lancet 2:692, 1979.

Guana-Trujillo B, Higgins PG: Sexual intercourse and pregnancy. Health Care for Women International, 8:339–348, 1987.

Hager A: Some Things About Sex and Pregnancy. Publication available through Ann Hagar, 8240 Margaret Lane, Cincinnati, OH 45240, 1981.

Hampson SJ: Nursing intervention for the first three postpartum months. JOGN Nurs 18(2):116–122, 1989.

Hangsleben KL: Transition to fatherhood: an exploratory study. JOGN Nurs 12(4):265–270, 1983.

Herbst AL: Coitus and the fetus. N Engl J Med 301:1235, 1979.

Herron MA, Katz M, Creasy RK: Evaluation of a preterm birth prevention program: preliminary report. Obstet Gynecol 59:452, 1982.

Hite S: Women and Love. New York, Alfred A Knopf, 1987.

Holtzman L: Sexual practices during pregnancy. J Nurse Midwife 6:21, 1976.

Iams JD, Johnson FF, Creasy RK: Prevention of preterm birth. Clin Obstet Gynecol 31(3):357–359, 1988.

Jordan PL: Breastfeeding as a risk factor for fathers. JOGN Nurs 15(2):94–97, 1986.

Kappy A, Cetrulo CL, Knuppel RA, et al: Premature rupture of the membranes: a conservative approach. Am J Obstet Gynecol 134:655, 1979.

Kemp V, Hatmaker D: Stress and social support in high-risk pregnancy. Res Nurs Health 12(5):331–336, 1989.

Kemp V, Page CK: The psychosocial impact of a high-risk pregnancy on the family. JOGN Nurs 15(3):232–236, 1986.

Kenny JA: Sexuality of pregnant and breastfeeding women. Arch Sex Behav 2:215, 1973.

Lavery JP, Miller CE: Deformation and creep in the human chorioamniotic sac. Am J Obstet Gynecol 134:366, 1979.

Lavery JP, Miller CE: Effect of prostaglandin and seminal fluid on human chorioamniotic membranes. JAMA 245:2425, 1981.

Lemmer C: Becoming a father: a review of nursing research on expectant fatherhood. Matern Child Nurs J 16(3):261–75, 1987.

Liebenberg B: Expectant fathers. Child and Family 8:165–177, 1969.

Lipitz S, Barkai G, Rabinovinci J, Mashiach S: Breast stimulation test and oxytocin challenge test in fetal surveillance: a prospective randomized study. Am J Obstet Gynecol 151(5):1178–1181, 1987.

Loos C, Julius L: The client's views of hospitalization during pregnancy. JOGN Nurs 18(1):52–56, 1989.

Lumley J: Sexual feelings in pregnancy and after childbirth. Aust N Z J Obstet Gynecol 18:114, 1978.

Masters WH, Johnson VE: Human Sexual Response. Boston, Little, Brown & Co, 1966.

May KA: A typology of detachment/involvement styles adopted during pregnancy by first-time fathers. West J Nurs Res 2(2):445–453, 1980.

McGregor JA, French JI, Spencer NE: Prevention of STDs in women. Obstet Gynecol Clinics of North America 16(3):679–687, 1989.

Meheus A: Sexually transmitted pathogens in mother and newborn. Ann N Acad Sci 549:203–212, 1988.

Mills JL, Harlap S, Harley EE: Should coitus late in pregnancy be discouraged? Lancet 2:136, 1981.

Mundsley RF, Brix GA, Hinton NA, et al: Placental inflammation and infection a prospective bacteriologic and histologic study. Am J Obstet Gynecol 95:648, 1966.

Mueller LS: Pregnancy and sexuality. JOGN Nurs 14:289, 1985.

Naeye RL: Factors that predispose to premature rupture of the fetal membranes. Obstet Gynecol 60:93, 1982.

Naeye RL: Coitus and antepartum haemorrhage. Br J Obstet Gynaecol 88:765, 1981a.

Naeye RL: Safety of coitus in pregnancy. Lancet 2:686, 1981b.

Naeye RL: Coitus and associated amniotic fluid infection. N Engl J Med 301:1198, 1979.

Naeye RL, Peters EC: Causes and consequences of premature rupture of fetal membranes. Lancet 1:192, 1980.

Naeye RL, Ross S: Coitus and chorioamnionitis: a prospective study. Early Hum Dev 6:91, 1982.

Neilson JP, Mutambira M: Coitus, twin pregnancy, and preterm labor. Am J Obstet Gynecol 160(2):416–418, 1989.

Omer H Friedlander D, Palti Z, Shekel I: Life stresses and premature labor. Psychosom Med 48(5):362–369, 1986.

Osofsky HL, Osofsky JO: Answers for New Parents: Adjusting to Your New Role. New York, Walker Publishers, 1980.

Perkins RP: Adverse pregnancy outcome and coitus. Obstet Gynecol 26:399, 1983

Perkins RP: Sexual behavior and response in relation to complications of pregnancy. Am J Obstet Gynecol 134:498, 1979.

Phillips CR, Anzalone JT: Fathering: Participation In Labor and Birth. St Loius, CV Mosby Co, 1982.

Pugh WE, Fernandez FL: Coitus in late pregnancy. Obstet Gynecol 2:636, 1953.

Rayburn WF, Wilson EA: Coital activity and premature labor. Am J Obstet Gynecol 137:972, 1980.

Reamy K, White SE: Sexuality in pregnancy and the puerperium: a review. Obstet Gynecol 40(1):1–13, 1985.

Reamy K, White SE, Daniell WC, Levine ES: Sexuality and pregnancy: a prospective study. J Reprod Med 27:321–327, 1982.

Richardson P: Women's important relationships during pregnancy and the preterm labor event. West J Nurs Res 9(2):203–222, 1987.

Robertson PA, Berlin PH: The Premature Labor Handbook: Successfully Sustaining Your High Risk Pregnancy. Garden City, NY, Doubleday & Co, 1986.

Robson KM, Kumar R: Maternal sexuality during first pregnancy and after childbirth. Br J Obstet Gynecol 88:882, 1981.

Sapire KE: Conception and sexuality in health and disease. Isando, South Africa, McGraw-Hill, 1986.

Savage W, Reader F: Sexual activity in pregnancy. Midwife, Health Visitor and Community Nurse 20(11):398–402, 1984.

Shapiro S, Nass J: Postpartum psychosis in the male. Psychopathology 19(3):138–142, 1986.

Sherwen LN: Psychosocial Dimensions of the Pregnant Family. New York, Springer Publishing Co, 1987.

Smith LS, Lauver D, Gray PA Jr: Sexually transmitted disease. In Fogel CI, Lauver D (eds): Sexual Health Promotion. Philadelphia, WB Saunders Co, 1990.

Solberg DA, Butler J, Wagner NN: Sexual behavior in pregnancy. In Lopiccolo J, Lopiccolo L (eds): Handbook of Sex therapy. New York, Plenum, 1978.

Solberg D, Butler J, Wagner N: Sexual behavior in pregnancy. N Engl J Med 288:1098, 1973.

Toth M, Witkin S, Ledger W, Thaler H: Role of infection in the etiology of preterm birth. Obstet Gynecol 71(5):723–726, 1988.

Turnbull A, Chamberlain G (eds): Obstetrics. Edinburg, Churchill Livingstone, 1989.

Wagner N, Butler J, Sanders J: Prematurity and orgasmic coitus during pregnancy: data on a small sample. Fertil Steril 27:911, 1976.

Walbroehl GS: Sex and pregnancy current concepts. Compr Ther 12(11):3–5, 1986.

White S, Reamy K: Sexuality and pregnancy: a review. Arch Sex Behav 11:429, 1982.

White M, Ritchie CK: Psychological stressors in antepartum hospitalization: reports from pregnant women. Matern Child Nurs J 13(1):47–57, 1984.

Wilkerson NN, Bing E: Sexuality. In Nichols FH, Humenick SS (eds): Childbirth Education: Practice, Research and Theory. Philadelphia, WB Saunders Co, 1988.

Williams ML: Long-term hospitalization of women with high-risk pregnancies. JOGN Nurs 15(1):17–21, 1986.

Wilson D: An overview of sexually transmitted diseases in the perinatal period. J Nurse Midwifery 33(3):115–125, 1988.

Woods JR, Esposito JL (eds): Pregnancy loss: medical therapeutics and practical considerations. Baltimore, Williams & Wilkins, 1987.

Woods NF, Dery GK: Sexuality during pregnancy and lactation. In Woods NF (ed): Human Sexuality in Health and Illness. St Louis, CV Mosby Co, 1984.

**PART II**

Complications and
Delivery

# CHAPTER 16

# Labor

Roy H. Petrie and Athanasia M. Williams

Following fertilization, embryogenesis, organogenesis, and a period of growth and development, the fetus reaches a point at which a nonconfined and separate life is undertaken. Mammals deliver their offspring through a process of rhythmic contractions in the muscular portion of the reproductive tract known as labor. In humans, labor is generally described as that interval from the onset of regular rhythmic uterine contractions, initiating the movement of the fetus down the genital tract, through the time when the fetus is expelled from the mother and assumes its independent life as a neonate.

Reproduction is the ultimate of all biologic functions, and as such, it occupies a central drive and effort to maintain the population. The maintenance of the species by procreation generally requires multiple attempts at procreation by any one member of the species to replace that member. The reproductive process is a wasteful process in terms of the number of conceptions that take place compared with the number of offspring that reach maturity. This wastefulness is evident in the lower species, and on careful scrutiny, it is also true in humans. It has been estimated that as few as 50 percent of all human conceptions reach the age of 1 year. During labor, enormous maternal, fetal, and neonatal changes are experienced, and an evaluation and analysis of this process is necessary. After biologic and other considerations are analyzed, medical management processes are designed to correct steps that previously have yielded damage and loss. These prescribed medical processes result in improved outcome in human reproduction.

## Embryology

During the third week of fetal development, the intraembryonic mesoderm divides into three distinct parts: (1) the paraxial portion, which ultimately forms the somites; (2) the lateral plate, which forms the somatic and splanchnic mesoderm, or the layers lining the coelom; and (3) the intermediate megsoderm, which connects the paraxial portion and the lateral plate. The intermediate mesoderm at the cervical region loses contact with the somites and segmentally forms small cell clusters known as nephrotomes. The nephrotomes grow laterally and caudad, and develop a lumen. In the thoracic, lumbar, and sacral areas, the intermediate mesoderm loses contact with the coelomic cavity, segmentation disappears, and the nephrogenic cords form excretory tubules. This process represents the genesis of the three different and yet slightly overlapping renal systems embryologically noted in the human. The development of the urinary and genital systems is an interconnecting and intertwining saga that explains all of the basic anatomic relationships found in the adult.

The pronephros, which is located in the cervical region, is the first of the renal systems to develop. The pronephros is replaced by the mesonephros in the thoracic and lumbar regions, which in turn is replaced by the metanephros in the lower lumbar and sacral regions. During the fourth embryonic week, genital ridges are noted on each side of the midline of the intermediate mesodermal plate, between the mesonephros and the dorsal mesentery. By the sixth embryonic week, both male and female embryos have two pairs of genital ducts: the wolffian, or mesonephric, duct and the müllerian, or paramesonephric, duct (which runs parallel to the wolffian duct). In the female, the müllerian duct forms the primary skeleton of the internal female genital system; the upper part forms the fallopian tube, or oviduct, and the lower parts comes together, fuses, and forms the uterus and upper vagina. Although the wolffian duct becomes the primary genital duct in the male, it disappears for all practical purposes in the female (Arey, 1965).

## Anatomy

### THE UTERUS

The uterus is a slightly flattened, pear-shaped, muscular organ that lies between the vagina below and the fallopian tubes above. The opening to the uterus from the vagina is through the cervical os. The cervix is attached to the body, or corpus, of the uterus. The fallopian tubes enter the uterus laterally through the cornua; the area above the cornua is known as the fundus. The cervix is constructed of connective tissue that tapers into muscular tissue as the body of the uterus is approached. The connective tissue of the cervix includes elastin (Leppert et al, 1982), and it is that part of the uterus that dilates during labor to allow the fetus to move from the uterine cavity down the vagina to the outside. The uterine wall is composed of muscle tissue that runs in all directions, in order to control bleeding and exsanguination after delivery.

In the very young and very old woman, the uterus is small, perhaps no larger than an adult large thumb. During a woman's reproductive years, the body and fundus of the uterus enlarge to accommodate the implantation of the fertilized ovum (embryo); further enlargement takes place throughout the uterus, but particularly in the muscular portion, in order to allow for the growth of the fetus during the developmental process. Uterine size and growth are under the control of hormones. The uterus has a peritoneal covering for that portion found in the peritoneal cavity and is lined with endometrium.

The urinary bladder is anterior to the cervicovaginal junction, and the rectum of the bowel is posterior to the cervical ligaments. The utero-ovarian, or infundibulopelvic, ligament is attached to the uterus from the lateral side wall to the upper lateral one third of the uterus, and the cardinal ligaments connect the area just at the junction of the body and cervix to the side wall, thus forming the base of the broad ligament. Supporting each side of the uterus is the broad ligament, the superior boundary of which is the round ligament. The uterosacral ligament connects the posterolateral aspect of the cervicouterine junction with the sacral vertebrae (Fig. 16–1). Blood is supplied to the uterus primarily through the utero-ovarian artery, the uterine artery, and the superior or cervical branch of the vaginal artery (Fig. 16–2).

## Uterine Activity and the Onset of Labor

The etiology of the onset of labor is unknown, although a considerable amount of information regarding the onset of labor has been acquired in the past few years. There are a number of theories that deal with the onset of labor and the control of labor. For example, it is known that prior to the onset of labor, the maternal estrogen to progesterone ratio generally shifts in favor of estrogen. It is further known that the predominance of estrogen and the formation of the prostaglandins from arachidonic acid result in an inflammatory reaction similar to that which is seen with an infection (Mitchell, 1983). It is interesting to speculate that this inflammatory environment provides a biochemical-biophysical source of stimuli that provoke and alter action potentials that may be required to initiate individual muscle cells to contract.

It has been known for some time that the posterior pituitary octapeptide oxytocin causes the term or near-term uterus to respond with contractions, whereas the non-gravid uterus or the uterus early in gestation does not respond to oxytocin (Petrie, 1981). As the uterus grows near to term, and especially after the onset of uterine activity, the uterus may become sensitive to oxytocin. Oxytocin receptors in the myometrium

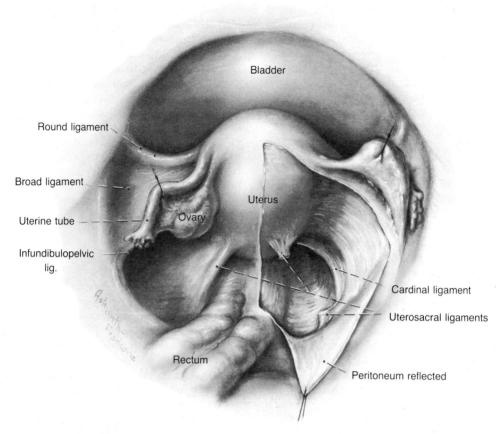

**Figure 16–1.** Ligaments of the female pelvis. (From Jacob SW, Francone C, Lossow WJ: Structure and Function in Man, 5th ed. Philadelphia, WB Saunders Co, 1982.)

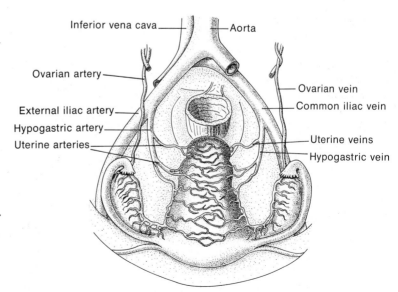

**Figure 16–2.** Blood supply of uterus and ovary. (From Moore ML: Realities in Childbearing, 2nd ed. Philadelphia, WB Saunders Co, 1983.)

have been identified (Soloff and Swartz, 1973; Soloff et al, 1977), and it has been demonstrated that more functional oxytocin receptors are available as pregnancy and labor progress (Fuchs et al, 1981). Concomitant with the rise in the number of oxytocin receptor sites that become available is the formation of apparent cellular communication routes or myometrial gap junctions. Garfield and Hayashi (1981) have demonstrated the specialized cell-to-cell contacts that are thought to lower impedence to current flow between cells. Gap junctions are present in increased number as parturition approaches and as labor ensues. The release of arachidonic acid from the fetal membranes and the formation of the prostaglandins, particularly $F_{2a}$ and the $E_2$ fraction, clearly establish that these compounds are intimately involved as uterine stimuli in the initiation of uterine activity and the continuation of labor.

Unfortunately, the relationship of the prostaglandins and oxytocin in the initiation, maintenance, and regulation of labor is as yet unclear. Myometrial prostaglandin $F_{2a}$ receptors have been identified, and their presence has been demonstrated in impending parturition and throughout labor (Hartelendy and Linter, 1982). Hall (1957) and Rusu and associates (1966) have demonstrated that, in pregnancy, the serum magnesium level falls. With the onset of either preterm or term labor, a further fall in serum magnesium level is identified. The myometrial contraction can be expressed by the following chemical equation:

$$\text{actin} + \text{myosin} + \text{ATP} + \text{calcium} \rightarrow$$
$$\text{a contraction response}$$

It is obvious that the control of calcium flow may enable the obstetrician to control labor. The $\beta_2$-sympathomimetic agents are thought to regulate calcium by altering cyclic AMP control, and magnesium probably displaces calcium.

It appears that, as the fetus reaches term, the uterus is being prepared biochemically and physiologically to perform its function: hormone levels shift; microscopic anatomic changes occur; hormones are formed; hormones are released; the myometrium is prepared initially to act independently at a cellular level; and as the process ensues, the majority of the myometrium acts in unison as a singular muscular effort. The exact etiology of the onset of spontaneous labor is as yet unknown; however, it is clear that there may be multiple physiologic, biochemical, and pharmacologic avenues by which labor may ensue, and correspondingly, there may be multiple avenues by which the onset of uterine activity leading to labor may be blocked.

It is interesting to construct an analogy between the onset of labor and the starting of an automobile engine. There are many ways in which an automobile may be started—by turning an ignition key, by pushing the automobile with another automobile, by "cross wiring" an ignition system, and so on. There are also several conditions that must be met to start an automobile, such as the proper fuel being available in the carburetor and sufficient amounts oxygen for the combustion of the fuel. By the same token, it is known that several conditions can cause labor. Labor is more likely to ensue as a result of overdistension of the uterus, as occurs with twin gestation; a Ferguson's reflex (a cervical reflex), which causes the generation of uterine activity; cervical dilatation; rupture of the membranes, if conditions in the myometrium are right, including the correct hormone relationship being present either from a maternal, fetal, or exogenous source; and infection or an electric stimulus, which may provoke sufficient uterine activity to initiate labor. Once sufficient uterine activity, from whatever source, has been generated to initiate labor, the process usually proceeds on its own, as the running of the automobile engine continues once it has been started.

# Normal Considerations of Labor

Normal considerations of labor should include the "Four Ps." Traditionally, there have been "Three Ps": Power, Passage, and Passenger. Recently, however, a fourth "P" has been added: Psyche (Moore, 1980).

## POWER (UTERINE ACTIVITY)

In the strict clinical sense, labor is defined as rhythmic uterine contractions that result in cervical effacement and dilatation with descent of the presenting fetal part.

In labor, repeated rhythmic uterine contractions provide a setting in which, during the course of each contraction, there is the possibility that the intramyometrial pressure may exceed the intravascular blood pressure; this would partially or completely interrupt blood flow to the placenta and the intervillous space, where maternal red cells unload oxygen and take on a new supply of carbon dioxide from the fetal red cells. Normally, the human fetus has sufficient reserve to tolerate this intermittent interruption in carbon dioxide-oxygen exchange. However, in instances of reduced placental surface, excess uterine activity, lowered maternal blood pressure, and increased fetal demands, the fetal tolerance may be exceeded and the Krebs' cycle can no longer supply all of the fetus' needs for energy in the form of adenosine triphosphatase (ATP), because of insufficient oxygen. At this point, the anaerobic glycolytic pathway is used for the production of ATP. As a result, lactic acid will be formed, which has the potential to cause nervous system damage and, in turn, may lead to fetal death. Thus, hypoxia, which causes acidosis and asphyxia, is a potential result of the labor process.

In order to reduce the potential for fetal and neonatal damage or death, it is necessary to monitor the labor process and its divisions. Thus, normal limitations and normal fetal tolerances can be established as guidelines for appropriate management. Although this concept appears simple, it was not until the last quarter to half century that any meaningful consideration of these aspects of labor was undertaken.

In the United States, until recently, once the myometrium had been surgically incised, as in a hysterotomy for the performance of a cesarean section or removal of uterine fibroids, it was considered dangerous to allow the patient to undergo term labor for fear of rupture of the uterus. It was known that, on occasion, the uterus did tolerate labor well and many women delivered vaginally when labor was unexpected and rapid. Moreover, in other parts of the world, it was common to allow labor when the surgical incision into the uterus was low at the junction of the fibrous or uterine segment with the muscular uterine fundus.

By the late 1970s through early 1980s, the cesarean section rate had risen 30 to 40 percent, in some instances, from the 2 to 3 percent rate of the 1950s. At the present time,

efforts are being made to reduce the cesarean section rate. One of the major areas chosen to attempt to reduce the cesarean section rate was the repeat cesarean section. A number of health care professionals in several cities proposed vaginal birth after cesarean section. In the late 1970s and early 1980s, a number of publications advocated a trial of labor in those patients with a prior low transverse cesarean section (Lavin et al, 1982; Murphy, 1976; Saldana et al, 1979). Initially, a trial of labor was used when there had been one prior low transverse cervical cesarean section. Papers were published reporting that a vaginal delivery could be achieved after two or more prior cesarean sections (Farmakides et al, 1987; Lawson et al, 1987).

When the type of cesarean section (low transverse versus vertical) is unknown, a vaginal delivery after cesarean section could be achieved safely (Beall et al, 1984). From a review of extensive literature on the subject, it appears that even in the presence of cephalopelvic disproportion at a prior cesarean section, between 60 and 80 percent of these gravidas can safely deliver vaginally after a prior cesarean section. Some investigators (Horenstein and Phelan, 1985) have advocated the judicious use of oxytocin when it is indicated for dysfunctional labor, and have demonstrated that the drug can be used safely. Recently, previous contraindications to vaginal birth after cesarean section have been studied; one of these includes appropriately selected labor with a large or macrosomic fetus that safely followed a prior cesarean section (Flamm and Goings, 1989).

Several years' experience supports the belief that vaginal delivery following a cesarean section is reasonably safe and often can be managed in a manner similar to that used in normal patients. Health care professionals treating patients in labor need to be aware of potential problems and be prepared to resort to immediate cesarean section for early uterine scar dehiscences. (Refer to Chapter 19 for more information on cesarean delivery.)

## EVALUATION AND QUANTITATION OF UTERINE ACTIVITY AND LABOR PROGRESS

The concept of force in relation to action is vital to the current study of labor. In labor, the force of the uterine contraction is measured and compared with the effects of that force on the cervix and fetus, as measured by cervical effacement and dilatation and descent of the presenting fetal part (labor).

The uterus differs in two parts during labor: the actively contracting upper segment becomes thicker as labor advances; the lower portion (lower uterine segment and cervix) is rather passive and develops into a much thinner walled muscular passage for the fetus. The upper passage contracts, retracts, and expels the fetus. In response to the force of contractions of the upper segment, the lower uterine segment and cervix dilate and thereby form a greatly expanded, thinned-out muscular and fibromuscular tube through which the fetus can pass.

With each contraction, the uterus changes shape. The ovoid uterus becomes elongated simultaneously with a decrease in the horizontal diameter. This produces a straightening of the fetal vertebral column, which presses the upper fetal pole firmly against the uterine fundus, whereas the lower fetal pole is driven downward into the pelvis. During this lengthening of the uterus, the longitudinal uterine fibers are drawn tight, pulling the lower segment and cervix upward over the lower fetal pole. This effect on the lower uterine segment and cervix is important to cervical dilatation and effacement. Although they are not essential for successful labor and delivery, the round ligaments can contract and pull the uterus forward.

It is essential to measure and compare uterine contractions (uterine activity) and the progress of labor in the form of temporal measurements of progress of labor as evidenced by cervical dilation and effacement with fetal descent. When uterine activity is compared with labor progress over an interval of time, normal ranges and expectations for each of these components and for the two integrated together can be established. This can be demonstrated in a labor curve.

## Methods of Uterine Activity Analysis

At the present time, there are three available methods of evaluating and quantitating uterine contractions: (1) timing and palpation, (2) external tocography, and (3) internal monitoring.

### Timing and Palpation

It is easy to time the frequency of contractions. This can be done by measuring from the onset of one contraction to the onset of subsequent contractions; likewise, it is relatively easy to make a crude measurement of a contraction's duration simply by timing the interval from the onset to the end of the contraction. Estimating the intensity of a uterine contraction is somewhat more difficult; however, by placing one's hand on the abdomen overlying the gravid uterus, one can palpate uterine contractions and estimate whether the contraction is mild, moderate, or strong. Once a uterine contraction reaches a point of being palpated and appreciated as being painful by the patient, the intensity of the contraction probably has reached approximately 40 mm Hg. For many clinical applications, particularly when attempting to establish whether true labor has begun, this form of analysis may be sufficient, despite the fact that it is rather subjective.

To palpate a contraction properly, it is necessary to leave one's hand on the fundus for a period of time, when the fundus is both in the relaxed and contracting states. Generally, one must palpate the uterus during a few contractions to properly evaluate uterine function. Because all uteri have some degree of tone throughout labor, a determination of the intensity of each contraction can be made only by comparing it with that patient's resting tone or with the tone between contractions.

### External Tocography

External tocography is a more accurate method of monitoring uterine activity, in which a tocodynamometer transducer (tocotransducer) is placed on the abdomen, overlying the gravid uterus in a position so that changes in the curvature of the abdomen that result from uterine contractions can be measured and recorded on a graph. Thus, the onset of a contraction can be measured more accurately, as can the duration of the contraction. However, the exact beginning and end of the contraction may be difficult to define, especially if the patient is moving around in the bed. (Defining the end of the contraction may be crucial to the recognition of deceleration patterns.) The evaluation of intensity of the uterine contraction is semiquantitative using this method of evaluation, owing to placement of the transducer and movements of the mother and fetus. Palpation should be used in conjunction with the tocotransducer to evaluate uterine intensity and resting tone. This form of analysis of uterine activity is currently used in labor until the fetal membranes are ruptured and the internal pressure of uterine activity analysis is initiated.

In the placement of the external transducer, it is important to remain with the patient during a few contractions to ensure that the tocotransducer is situated in the proper position. If the patient complains of pain or the health care professional is able to palpate increased tone in the uterus and it is not recording on the graph, the transducer must be moved to record contractions. External monitoring does not demonstrate the intensity of contractions. In an obese patient, a mild-appearing contraction can actually be a very strong one, whereas the reverse may be true in a thinner patient. Therefore, manual palpation of the contractions should be done in conjunction with use of a tocodynamometer. In this era of natural childbirth, the practitioner may encounter patients who do not want to be monitored during labor. It is important to discuss and explain the reasons for monitoring with all monitored patients, ideally during pregnancy rather than when the patient arrives in the delivery suite, so that the patient is well informed when the monitor is used.

### Internal Monitoring

The third form of uterine activity analysis is performed with the use of an intrauterine catheter inserted transcervically into the amniotic cavity to measure pressure. By this method, the frequency, duration, and intensity of the uterine contraction can be monitored. A number of methods of plotting uterine activity have been developed (Fig. 16–3) (Miller et al, 1976). Using the total area under the uterine pressure curve, Miller and associates (1976) and Huey and associates (1976) have demonstrated the normal amount of uterine activity required to achieve delivery in a large number of nulliparous and multiparous patients, as shown in Figures 16–4 and 16–5. By itself, the measurement of uterine contractions can indicate only whether a normal or an abnormal amount of uterine contractions is being generated by a given patient. This measurement contributes minimally to the overall clinical evaluation of labor. This form of uterine activity analysis is currently available on some fetal monitoring units. The measurement of uterine activity and the progress of labor is of considerable benefit in the evaluation and management of labor.

MONTEVIDEO UNITS

Average 1 x Frequency / 10 min

ALEXANDRIA UNITS

Average 1 x Frequency / 10 min
x Average duration (min)

ACTIVE PLANIMETER UNITS

Area under active pressure curve
x 10 min

TOTAL PLANIMETER UNITS

Area under entire curve
x 10 min

AVERAGE RATE OF RISE

Intensity / Tr

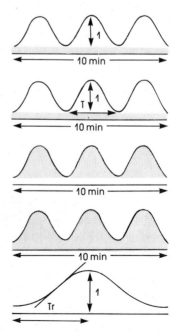

**Figure 16–3.** Alternative methods for the quantitation of frequency, duration, and intensity of the uterine contractions. (From Miller FC, Yeh S-Y, Schifrin BS, et al: Quantitation of uterine activity in 100 primiparous patients. Am J Obstet Gynecol 124:308, 1976.)

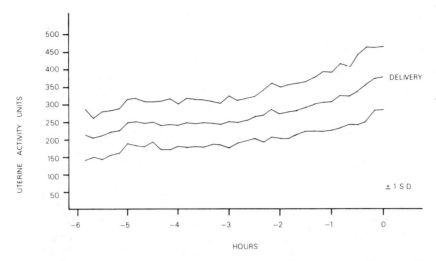

**Figure 16–4.** Mean uterine activity units for 100 patients (nulliparas) plotted every 10 minutes for 6 hours preceding delivery. (From Miller FC, Yeh S-Y, Schifrin BS, et al.: Quantitation of uterine activity in 100 primiparous patients. Am J Obstet Gynecol 124:308, 1976.)

If a satisfactory external recording of fetal heart rate and uterine activity has been achieved, internal monitoring may not be necessary. However, if only a poor tracing is recorded, or if a VBAC is being observed, or oxytocin is being administered, it is recommended to avail oneself of the additional information that internal monitoring can provide. Because kinking and clogging of a catheter can occur, periodic flushing with sterile water or saline should be performed when indicated to ensure the patency of the catheter and the accuracy of the information received. Closed and precalibrated intrauterine pressure catheters are commercially available. Recalibration problems and initial cost may prohibit their use on a large scale. On some of the closed catheters, ele-

vated resting tones have been noted. Hydrostatic pressure, from internal placement of the sensor, causes changes in pressure with position change. One company recommends obtaining a baseline reading in all positions and then comparing later pressures to the earlier baseline levels. Dual lumen catheters are now available to continue measuring intrauterine pressure while fluid is inserted for amnioinfusion.

## PLOTTING LABOR PROGRESS

Friedman's (1954) system of labor analysis, on which our current concepts of labor management and evaluation are based, in-

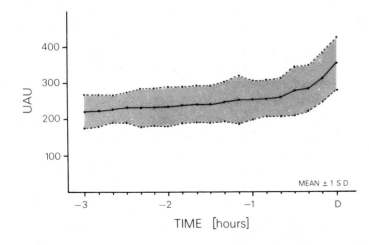

**Figure 16–5.** Mean uterine activity units for 149 patients (multiparas) plotted every 10 minutes for 3 hours preceding delivery. (From Huey JR, Al-Hadjiev A, Paul RH: Uterine activity in the multiparous patient. Am J Obstet Gynecol 126:682, 1976.)

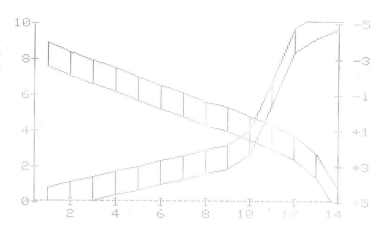

**Figure 16–6.** The S-shape projected nulliparous labor curve (one of 48 computer-generated labor curves available showing standard deviation) appropriately adjusted for parity, medication status, membrane status, and onset of labor for this nullipara. The curve from the upper left downward shows the station descent with standard deviation. (Courtesy of Henry R Rey and Dr Roy H Petrie, Columbia University, New York.)

troduced the practice of evaluating labor by plotting cervical dilatation and effacement with descent of the presenting fetal part against time. Clinically, the station of the presenting part (distance above or below the interischial spine plane) and the cervical dilatation are graphed on the vertical axis according to the elapsed time. Thus, a characteristic S-shaped curve will result for a normal labor. Normal S-shaped labor curves have been established for both the nullipara and multipara, as demonstrated in Figures 16–6 and 16–7. Figures 16–8 and 16–9 demonstrate normal patients meeting labor goals. During the past 20 or 30 years, the use of this graph to record labor progress has enabled the obstetrician to evaluate labor more logically than in the past. As a result,

subsequent comparisons between neonatal outcome and the progress of labor have enabled obstetricians to make advances in neonatal salvage and the quality of neonatal life based on this factor alone. When these evaluations are compared with uterine activity and the fetus' tolerance of labor from an analysis of fetal heart rate data, considerable improvement in fetal and neonatal salvage and quality of life is possible.

Characteristically, when labor is analyzed by the comparison of cervical dilatation and descent of the presenting part against elapsed time, three periods of labor are identified. The first period runs from the onset of contractions and minimal cervical dilatation until the point at which approximately 3 cm of cervical dilatation are achieved (latent

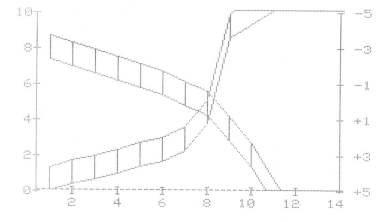

**Figure 16–7.** The S-shape projected multiparous labor curve appropriately adjusted for parity, medication status, membrane status, and onset of labor for this multipara. (The wide band indicates standard deviation.) The curve from the left corner downward indicates the station descent with standard deviation. (Courtesy of Henry R Rey and Dr Roy H Petrie, Columbia University, New York.)

STANDARD FRIEDMAN CURVES

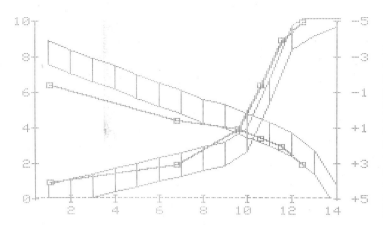

**Figure 16–8.** The actual labor data for a nullipara who met most of her projected labor guideline goals and experienced a normal nulliparous labor. The lines connecting the boxes represent the patient's actual dilatation and station changes. The wide bands indicate standard deviation for dilatation and station. (Courtesy of Henry R Rey and Dr Roy H Petrie, Columbia University, New York.)

phase) or until a point at which rapid changes should be expected in cervical dilatation, which generally occurs at about 3 to 4 cm of dilatation (active phase). The latent phase may take from a few to many hours. Most conservative obstetricians now consider that the latent phase of labor is prolonged after approximately 20 hours and then may be associated with an increased risk of fetal and neonatal damage and death. Once accelerated cervical dilatation begins, usually at about 3 to 4 cm, subsequent cervical dilatation with descent of the presenting part is rapid and usually falls within the 1 to 2 cm/h range. At approximately 8 cm, rapid cervical dilatation slows down, and the steepness of the cervical dilatation curve is diminished somewhat through delivery. Once complete cervical dilatation is accom-

plished, the interval to delivery may be short, as is usually seen in the multipara, or it can be longer—up to 1 or 2 hours normally in the nullipara. Many clinicians consider that as long as there is descent of the presenting part and the fetus demonstrates good health by appropriate fetal surveillance, the interval from complete cervical dilatation to delivery may actually reach two or more hours (Fig. 16–10) with no harm to the fetus (ACOG Technical Bulletin, 1991). A number of factors, including age, parity, position, duration of gestation, duration of labor, cervical maturity, medication, membrane status, and pelvic size, may affect the duration of the various stages of labor. From clinical analysis of the various stages of labor, it has been demonstrated that an advancement of cervical dilatation and effacement and de-

STANDARD FRIEDMAN CURVES

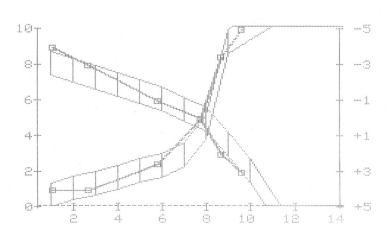

**Figure 16–9.** The actual labor data for a multipara who met most of her projected labor guideline goals and experienced a normal multiparous labor. The lines connecting the boxes represent the patient's actual dilatation and station changes. The wide bands indicate standard deviation for dilatation and station. (Courtesy of Henry R Rey and Dr Roy H Petrie, Columbia University, New York.)

**Figure 16–10.** A nullipara who reached complete full dilatation of the cervix at approximately 11 hours into the labor with prolonged or slow descent of the head. Note that the second stage of labor is over 3 hours; however, progress in descent is being made and the fetus is tolerating labor well as judged by fetal rate monitoring. A low or outlet forceps type of instrument-assisted delivery was subsequently accomplished. The lines connecting the boxes represent the patient's actual dilatation and station changes. The wide bands indicate standard deviation for dilatation and station. (Courtesy of Henry R Rey and Dr Roy H Petrie, Columbia University, New York.)

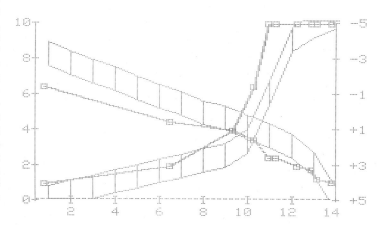

scent of the presenting part that is too rapid or too slow may have a deleterious effect on fetal and neonatal outcome.

As a patient is evaluated during labor, she should be informed as to how the labor is progressing and what this progress signifies. Not all patients are aware of what the physiologic changes are in labor, and this lack of knowledge can cause fear and anxiety that often are severe enough to obstruct the normal course of labor. An informed patient, on the other hand, can relax and, therefore, optimize the true potential of labor.

## Importance of an Integrated Evaluation

In the clinical evaluation and management of labor, it has been demonstrated by several investigators that age, parity, duration of pregnancy, cervical quality, position, and sedation and administration of other medications play an important role in the generation of uterine activity, and that the generation of uterine activity over time directly influences the "S-shape" labor curve that demonstrates the progress of

**Figure 16–11.** The average uterine activity units generated for each centimeter of cervical dilatation during the labors of 100 primiparas, demonstrating a progressive increase in the efficiency of uterine activity as labor advances. (From Miller FC, Yeh S-Y, Schifrin BS, et al: Quantitation of uterine activity in 100 primiparous patients. Am J Obstet Gynecol 124:308, 1976.)

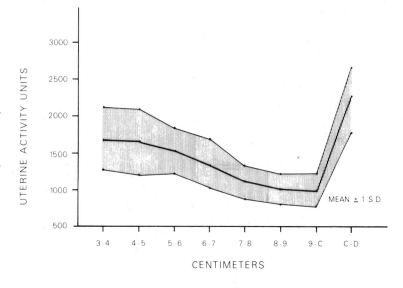

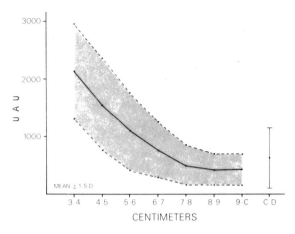

**Figure 16–12.** The average total uterine activity units generated for each centimeter of cervical dilatation during the labors of 149 multiparas, demonstrating a progressive increase in the efficiency of uterine activity as labor advances. (From Huey JR, Al-Hadjiev A, Paul RH: Uterine activity in the multiparous patient. Am J Obstet Gynecol 126:682, 1976.)

labor (Burnhill et al, 1962; Huey et al, 1976; Miller et al, 1976). Thus, it is important in managing labor to integrate both methods of monitoring labor: evaluation of uterine activity and the progress of labor over time. This allows evaluation of centimeters of progress and the amount of uterine activity required to achieve this progress, as depicted in Figures 16–11 and 16–12. Note that over time, decreased amounts of uterine activity are required to achieve cervical dilatation than were required earlier in the labor process. This is critical to the proper management of labor, especially when aggressive management may be needed. As long as the progress of labor is normal, less attention can be paid to the amount of uterine activity generated; however, if normal progress is not occurring, then the analysis of uterine activity may be important.

## DIFFERENTIATION BETWEEN TRUE AND FALSE LABOR

The consideration of definitions as well as that of the normal parameters of labor is essential to the proper analysis and management processes. For the purpose of this discussion, prodromal labor is defined as the erratic, nonregular to regular uterine contractions that are present prior to the establishment of the regular, rhythmic contraction pattern that is seen during the true labor process. False labor is the regular, rhythmic uterine contractions that simulate true labor but are not accompanied by either cervical dilatation and effacement or descent of the presenting part. In some cases, the

differentiation between true and false labor requires an interval of observation. During this observation period, after obtaining a brief monitoring strip to ensure the fetus' ability to tolerate the stress of the contractions, it is often helpful if a patient is encouraged to ambulate. Often, ambulation diminishes or totally eradicates false labor, whereas true labor increases in intensity. In true labor, ambulation can aid in the descent of the fetal presenting part, thereby making labor more effectual. The latent phase of labor is often confused with prodromal labor; however, the latent phase of labor is a slow, steady effacement and dilatation of the cervix that occurs from the time of the onset of contractions until the start of the active phase of labor. It is normal for labor in the primigravida to last between 8 and 12 hours from the onset of contractions through delivery. Various phases of labor are dependent on parity as well as age, duration of gestation, cervical ripeness, medications used, and so on.

## THE STAGES OF LABOR AND APPROPRIATE SUPPORT

For clinical consideration, labor is divided into three stages. The first stage of labor is the interval between the onset of contractions and the point at which full cervical dilatation is achieved. At this stage, a woman needs a great deal of support and encouragement from the intrapartum team as well as her coach. A patient needs to know where she is in the laboring process and how much more effort must be exerted until delivery.

With adequate knowledge and support, the patient can cope more effectively with the progressive intensity of her labor. An analgesic agent may be needed during this stage.

The second stage of labor lasts from the onset of full cervical dilatation through the delivery of the fetus. This stage can be the most difficult part of labor. In the second stage of labor, the main force that expels the fetus is intra-abdominal pressure created by contraction of the abdominal muscles simultaneous with forced respiratory efforts (i.e., pushing). Some clinicians are concerned by prolonged, repeated pushing efforts and encourage open glottal pushing to enhance the expulsion process. Minimal investigative efforts are available to evaluate this procedure. Chinese investigators are exploring the use of a insufflatable abdominal belt or corset to help shorten the second stage of labor (Gai and Zhao, 1992). After many hours of labor, it may be necessary for the exhausted patient to expend the most energy. She needs encouragement to summon all her strength to push as efficiently and forcefully as possible. Even the most prepared of patients can lose control at this time. It is necessary to encourage the patient to relax as much as possible and to reinforce use of the most effective positions and techniques for accomplishing her goal.

The third stage of labor is the interval from the delivery of the baby through the delivery of the placenta. At this point the fetus and mother are usually bonding. The patient still needs encouragement and help in handling her newborn infant. If the neonate cannot be with the mother, the mother and support person should be made aware of the infant's condition as soon as possible.

Some institutions classify a fourth stage of labor, defined as the first 1- to 2-hour interval following delivery of the placenta. It is during this interval that the recently delivered mother (parturient) is observed carefully for blood loss, proper uterine contaction, changes in blood pressure, and overall state of well-being. If the mother is in the recovery room with the newborn, this is an excellent opportunity to help the mother to examine her baby, to encourage continuation of bonding, to initiate breastfeeding and to allay any fears the mother may have for her baby's well-being.

## THE PASSAGE

The type of maternal pelvis may have an effect on labor. The gynecoid pelvis is considered the most satisfactory for normal labor; it allows effective uterine contractions and vaginal delivery. The wide pubic arch reduces perineal tears.

In women with an anthropoid pelvis, the fetal head is often in an occiput posterior position, and the woman may deliver with the fetus in that position. Usually, little difficulty is experienced with labor and delivery.

The android pelvis usually causes the fetal head to engage in a transverse or posterior position, and it may not rotate, which often results in the need to use forceps for rotation and delivery. Such a delivery may be difficult, causing stress to the fetus. Perineal tears are common because of the narrow pubic arch.

In a platypelloid pelvis, the fetus may never be able to enter the pelvis inlet because of the short anteroposterior, posterior sagittal, and anterior sagittal diameters. The outlook for the fetus is poor unless this pelvis shape is recognized and the fetus is delivered by cesarean section.

## THE PASSENGER

### Fetal Attitude

It is important to consider the anatomic relationship of the fetus to the mother. Fetal attitude is the relationship of the fetal limbs and head to its trunk and should be one of flexion. Threrefore, the fetus forms a compact, ovoid mass that accommodates itself well to the uterine cavity. To help determine this relationship, Leopold's maneuvers (examination of the fetus through the gravid uterus) (Fig. 16–13) can be helpful. However, in some instances, it is difficult to determine the relationship of the fetus to the mother, and the use of an additional evaluation technique, such as real-time ultrasound, can be immediately illuminating.

### Fetal Lie (see Fig. 16–13)

The fetus' vertebral column in relation to the maternal vetebral column is referred to as the lie. There is a longitudinal fetal lie

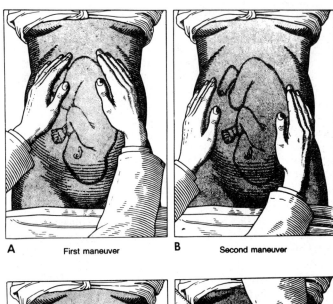

**A** First maneuver    **B** Second maneuver

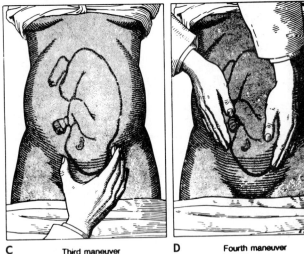

**C** Third maneuver    **D** Fourth maneuver

**Figure 16–13.** Leopold's maneuvers for determining (*A*) lie, attitude, and presentation of fetus; (*B*) position; (*C*) engagement; and (*D*) position and flexion. (From Pritchard JA, MacDonald PC: Williams Obstetrics, 16th ed. New York, Appleton-Century-Crofts, 1980.)

when the fetus' vertebral column is parallel to the maternal vertebral column. With a transverse lie, a fetus' vertebral column is at an approximately 90-degree angle to the maternal vertebral column. In cases of transverse lie, the extremities may be cephalad (extremities up) or caudad (extremities down). Some experienced obstetricians still deliver vaginally the appropriate fetus from a transverse lie when the extremities are down. With an oblique lie, the fetus' vertebral column is neither at right angles nor parallel to the maternal vertebral column but at some angle in between.

## Fetal Presentation (see Fig. 16–13)

It may be important to know and evaluate the type of fetal presentation (that part of the

fetus that is being applied to the cervix and will be delivered first). The most common type is the cephalic presentation. The cephalic presentation may be in varying degrees of flexion or extension. The most common cephalic presentation is the vertex, which presents the back of the head or the extreme form of flexion. The sinciput presentation is neither flexed nor extended. The brow presentation shows some degree of extension, and a face presentation is the extreme form of hyperextension.

The second most common presentation is the breech, of which there are three types: frank, in which the feet are extended fully toward the head; complete, in which the knees are bent; or footling, in which the feet present first. On occasion, there may be an acromial or shoulder presentation, and in

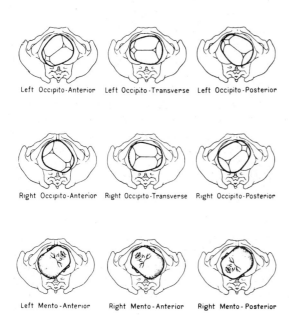

Left Occipito-Anterior    Left Occipito-Transverse    Left Occipito-Posterior

Right Occipito-Anterior    Right Occipito-Transverse    Right Occipito-Posterior

Left Mento-Anterior    Right Mento-Anterior    Right Mento-Posterior

Left Sacro-Anterior    Right Sacro-Anterior    Right Sacro-Posterior

**Figure 16–14.** Positions in relation to various presentations, with fetus viewed from below. (From Pritchard JA, MacDonald PC: Williams Obstetrics, 16th ed. New York, Appleton-Century-Crofts, 1980.)

rare instances, there may be a compound presentation such as an arm and leg, an arm and head, or some other combination of fetal parts.

### Fetal-Maternal Position (Fig. 16–14)

It is important to know the position of the presenting part in relationship to the maternal anatomy. Position is the relationship of the presenting part to one of the four quadrants of the maternal pelvis. The four quadrants are anterior, posterior, and lateral (right and left). In describing fetal position, the maternal symphysis is referred to as anterior and the sacrum as posterior, with the right maternal femur referred to as right and the left maternal femur, left. Therefore, in a vertex presentation, the occiput determines the fetal position to the mother. A left occiput anterior indicates that the occiput is to the

left of the maternal vertebral column and pointed toward the maternal symphysis. The same applies to breech presentations. A right sacrum posterior indicates that the fetal sacrum is directed to the right of the maternal vertebral column and pointed in the direction of the maternal sacrum.

With a face presentation, the position is determined by the fetal chin (mentum). A mentum posterior position indicates that the fetal mentum is directed toward the maternal sacrum. The persistent mentum posterior is one of the only positions that cannot be delivered safely at term vaginally; however, with proper progress in labor and rotation to a nonmentum posterior position, a safe vaginal delivery can be conducted. These relationships are important in determining whether or not labor will progress normally. When the fetus is askew, dysfunctional labor can ensue.

### THE PSYCHE

It has been suggested that there is more than a possibility of an interrelationship between difficulties during labor and delivery and sociocultural or psychologic factors. A relationship between anxiety and uterine dysfunction has been observed by obstetricians and nurses; women who reported more than average symptoms of muscle tension during pregnancy, and who demonstrated at the beginning of labor more than average physiologic and behavioral signs associated with anxiety, are more likely to develop physiologic disturbances related to uterine dysfunction.

Rosengren (1961) noted the relationship between a woman's tendency to take the sick role during pregnancy and the possibility of the same woman having difficulty during labor and delivery. His findings suggested that "the more a woman regarded herself as 'ill' during pregnancy, the greater was the likelihood of a longer period of active labor."

There is also a relationship between anxiety and pain. Several physiologic changes are initiated by anxiety. A major response to anxiety during labor is the production of epinephrine and norepinephrine: Epinephrine stimulates both $\alpha$ and $\beta$ receptors, whereas norepinephrine stimulates primarily alpha receptors. $\alpha$-Adrenergic receptor stimulation causes uterine vasoconstriction (as well as generalized vasoconstriction) and an increase in uterine muscle tone, leading to a decrease in uterine blood supply and an increase in both maternal blood supply and blood pressure. $\beta$-Adrenergic receptor stimulation causes vasodilatation and relaxation of uterine muscle. Because the uterine vessels are already fully dilated, the dilatation of other vessels reduces the flow of blood to the uterus. Decreased uterine blood flow may produce fetal bradycardia. Morishima and associates (1978) and Meyers and Meyers (1979), in animal studies, were able to produce fetal bradycardia by frightening monkey mothers.

Lederman and associates (1977) found that high epinephrine levels correlated with maternal anxiety and led to decreased uterine activity and longer labors. Newborn Apgar scores tend to be lower in those mothers demonstrating a high degree of anxiety. It would seem that anxiety may sometimes play a role in dysfunctional labor. It is very important, therefore, to assist mothers psychologically during their labor. This can be done by providing support, ensuring that her coach is present, encouraging the timid coach to participate more, and providing information to reduce anxiety.

# Exceptional Labor Circumstances

## DYSFUNCTIONAL LABOR

Labor does not always proceed as expected, nor does it fall within normal limits for all individuals in a given population. Many terms have been applied to this situation, such as failure to progress, clinical cephalopelvic disproportion, and various classifications of dystocia. It would be simpler, perhaps, and more appropriate to list all of these disorders of nonprogressive labor under the term dysfunctional labor, which could then be further defined as existing with excessive, normal, or subnormal amounts of uterine activity.

### Evaluation

Frequently, a review of the patient's history and/or a re-evaluation of the pelvis is needed in these cases, because the primary causes of a dysfunctional labor include in-adequate uterine activity, pharmacologic agents that reduce uterine activity, and even, perhaps, cephalopelvic disproportion. The effects of drugs on uterine activity are well known, and many of the sedative and narcotic drugs used during labor may reduce uterine activity to such a degree that inadequate progress of labor occurs. The use of oxytocin to augment labor by increasing uterine activity is discussed in Chapter 17. Potential bony disproportion between the fetus and the mother is always a consideration with dysfunctional labor, and it requires appropriate evaluation. A careful physical examination to evaluate and estimate fetal size in relation to pelvic size and space must be performed; clinical pelvimetry is considered the appropriate method of evaluation of potential cephalopelvic disproportion. (X-ray pelvimetry is still used at some centers but has fallen into disfavor in recent years, except in predelivery evaluation of the term breech presentation, in which it is still used.)

There is little reason to suspect that the generation of additional uterine activity will promote additional progress in labor in patients in whom the contraction pattern is essentially normal (contractions occurring every 2 to 3 minutes and lasting approximately 40 to 90 seconds, with an intensity of 40 to 90 mm Hg and a resting tone of 5 to 20 mm Hg) during the active phase of labor. If the fetus is tolerating the labor well, as evidenced by a normal fetal heart rate tracing, and uterine activity (i.e., contractions) has not reached this "normal" level, then an augmentation of the labor with oxytocin should be considered. In many cases of inadequate progress of labor, the condition may correct itself within 2 to 3 hours, and simply waiting and observing the patient for this period of time may be sufficient; however, many clinicians prefer a more aggressive form of labor management, with the use of oxytocin in the active phase. In some instances, such as when there is lack of progress of labor with otherwise normal appearing uterine contractions or when the patient is excessively tired, especially during the latent phase (very early first stage) of labor, the use of sedatives to rest the patient for a few hours is deemed appropriate.

### Delivery Considerations

Currently, many obstetricians clinically evaluate pelvic size by manual palpation.

The adequacy of the pelvis is also based on whether or not there is adequate uterine activity and normal progression of labor. Progress in labor is the final arbiter of pelvic adequacy. In the presence of an abnormal lie or presentation, such as a transverse lie or breech, the use of ultrasound scanning is considered the primary diagnostic tool, although x-ray pelvimetry is still considered an acceptable approach. Any abnormal presentation, whether a breech, transverse lie, oblique lie, or an aberrant form of the cephalic presentation, can be of major concern. At present, it has become almost axiomatic that all large fetuses that present in the breech position (> 3500 to 4000 g) should be delivered by cesarean delivery and in many institutions, all small fetuses presenting in the breech position (< 1750 g) are also delivered by cesarean delivery (Gimovsky and Petrie, 1982) in order to avoid the obvious problems of prolapsed cord and traumatic delivery. In some institutions, all fetuses in the breech position are delivered by cesarean delivery; however, other institutions maintain that it is unsafe to deliver term breech presentations of normal size (2 to 4 kg) from below (Gimovsky et al, 1981), especially with nulliparas with untested pelves. In cases of an oblique lie (with the fetal vertebral column crossing the maternal vertebral column at less than right angles), many institutions allow labor to continue with a cephalic presentation, with the expectation that the oblique lie will convert to a longitudinal lie. The oblique lie that may convert to a breech presentation is more likely to be considered an indication for cesarean delivery, especially by those institutions favoring this mode of delivery for breech presentation.

With the cephalic presentation, the head may be fully flexed, as with the vertex (occiput) presentation, or fully extended, with the face (mentum) presenting. Fetuses in all variants of cephalic presentation, with or without asynclitism (lateral deflexion of the head) to a more anteroposterior position in the pelvis, can be delivered vaginally from any position except for one: the mentum posterior. In the mentum posterior presentation, the fetal chin presents directly into the maternal sacral hollow with the fetal forehead coming under the symphysis pubis. Should the delivery occur from the mentum posterior position, insufficient room exists, and sufficient trauma will occur to a term-size fetus to bring about damage or death. To deliver the fetus with this type of presentation, rotation of the head must be achieved, either spontaneously, manually, or by forceps, so as not to deliver the baby in the direct mentum posterior position. In general, labor with presentations other than the vertex tends to proceed at a slightly slower rate, and descent is often retarded. The breech presentation constitutes only 2 to 4 percent of all term deliveries. With breech presentations, the largest part of the fetal body (the head) is delivered last, leaving an inadequate temporal opportunity for the fetal head to mold. Some investigators mandate that during the active phase of labor, to allow a breech to continue labor, the cervix must dilate at least 1 cm/h in the nullipara and 1 to 1 1/2 cm/h in the multipara (Gimovsky et al, 1981). The transverse lie, oblique lie, and the compound presentations are extremely uncommon, and there is a general trend toward delivery of all abnormal or uncommon presentations by cesarean delivery in order to avoid a prolonged labor and a traumatic delivery process.

## PREMATURITY AND POSTMATURITY

Prematurity represents the single largest cause of perinatal mortality and morbidity (Nochimson et al, 1980), and suspected prolonged gestation or postdatism is the single largest indication for antepartum fetal surveillance because of the inexactness of data regarding true gestational age (Yeh and Read, 1982). Both of these conditions require special management of labor, as do cases of intrauterine growth retardation (IUGR), diabetes, and preeclampsia.

Prematurity, prolonged gestation, IUGR, and a fetus of a severe preeclamptic or diabetic mother appear to be a divergent group to be given special consideration during labor and delivery. Nevertheless, the same physiologic considerations exist in each of these disorders to warrant special consideration during the evaluation of labor. The underlying principle is that each of these fetuses has the potential to be remarkably sensitive to hypoxia, stress, and trauma. The premature fetus has minimal reserves in the form of glycogen and body mass; the postdate fetus may be large and marginally oxygenated owing to a deteriorating biologic function of the placenta; the IUGR infant may be small, be poorly oxygenated, and have minimal amniotic fluid to cushion the stresses of labor. The diabetic infant, likewise, may be macrosomic or growth retarded, with marginal oxygenation and a high degree of sensitivity to the stresses of hypoxia and trauma. The fetus of a preeclamptic mother may have uteroplacental insufficiency as a result of the poor vascularization of the placental bed caused by the hypertension. This problem of poor vascularization may cause a decrease of oxygenation and consequent stress or distress to the fetus.

Because of the potential for respiratory distress syndrome, cord problems, and reduced biologic reserves, many centers tend to be very protective of these infants and observe fetal response to labor very carefully, with the aim of not allowing significant hypoxia or stress during labor. Generally speaking, a short, uncomplicated labor and delivery process is desired, and if this cannot be reasonably expected or achieved, an atraumatic cesarean delivery, in which hypoxia and asphyxia would be avoided, should be elected.

# The Delivery Process

Parturition, or delivery of the fetus, can occur from almost any maternal anatomic position. Depending on the culture and society, deliveries may take place from a squatting, sitting, reclining, or lounging position. In Western cultures and societies, two maternal delivery positions are most common: (1) the reclining position or its variant, the dorsolithotomy position, which allows greater anatomic access to the perineal area, and (2) the lateral Sims' position, in which the patient is lying on her side with her dependent leg slightly flexed and the superior leg elevated. The lateral Sims' position is frequently used when a spontaneous delivery is expected and additional perineal elasticity may be needed or, in the case of fetal distress, to position the mother off her back. This position can be easily accommodated in some birthing beds that provide support for the superior leg by reversing the normal position of the stirrup.

There are three delivery process techniques: (1) spontaneous vaginal delivery, (2) instrument-assisted vaginal delivery, and (3) cesarean section delivery. In spontaneous delivery, the presenting part is simply guided over the perineum with or without an episiotomy (incision into the perineum either obliquely or vertically) to allow additional delivery space. Instrument-assisted deliveries are of two types: (1) by the application of obstetric forceps around the face and head of the fetus, with downward traction to assist in the delivery process, and (2) by the application of a vacuum extractor device, in which negative pressure is applied on the fetal head with downward traction to assist in the delivery process. The decision as to which of these two types should be used is based on the relative position of the presenting part (usually the vertex) in the pelvic cavity, that is, the midcavity versus the outlet delivery. Engagement of the presenting part (vertex) occurs when the greatest diameter of the fetal vertex has successfully transversed the inlet of the pelvis; generally, this occurs when the leading part of the vertex has reached the level of the interischial spinal plane. This is called station zero. The point at which the fetal head is sufficiently low in the vagina to begin to distend the vulva in preparation for delivery, and the scalp is easily visible (as a 4- to 5-cm circle), is called crowning. Traditionally, when the fetal vertex is sufficiently low (usually 4 to 5 cm below the level of the ischial spine) to allow the easy application of forceps or a vacuum extractor, the procedure is called an outlet or low forceps delivery. The application of the vacuum extractor or the obstetric forceps at a level between station zero and station four (4 cm below the interischial spine plane) is known as a mid-cavity forceps or midforceps delivery. The American College of Obstetricians and Gynecologists (ACOG, 1989) has promoted a revised classification for the designation of this type of instrument-assisted delivery. This classification substitutes outlet forceps/vacuum for the traditional low forceps, as far as station is concerned, and defines low forceps/vacuum deliveries as those occurring greater than or equal to +2 station but not yet on the pelvic floor. The newer classification then defines a midforceps/vacuum application as occurring between 0 and +2 station. The differences appear to be subtle, and it is as yet unclear whether American obstetricians will adopt the opinions of the ACOG.

Deliveries that necessitate the application of an instrument at a level above station zero (floating) are not performed. In the past, such deliveries were performed and were termed high forceps. However, experience with instrument-assisted deliveries has demonstrated that the perinatal and maternal morbidity and mortality associated with high forceps deliveries is simply too great for them to be used, and a cesarean delivery should be performed instead. If an instrument-assisted delivery should be necessary, experience with instrument-assisted deliveries has demonstrated that there is no significant difference between the spontaneous vaginal delivery and the outlet type of instrument-assisted delivery. There may be an increase in perinatal morbidity and mortality and maternal morbidity with the use of traditional midforceps-assisted deliveries (Friedman, 1983). Many skilled obstetricians believe that the majority of cases of fetal morbidity and mortality associated with the midforceps delivery are noted in deliveries that require considerable manipulation and, in particular, rotation of the fetal vertex and delivery from some position other than one in which a direct application of the forceps to an occiput anterior or posterior is possible.

An instrument-assisted delivery of the outlet or low type may be elected in order to shorten the second stage of labor, or it may be indicated for one of several other reasons, including inability of the mother to adequately push the baby out, fetal distress, or excessive bleeding. The decision of whether to use forceps or the vacuum extraction method to assist delivery is often based on the obstetrician's background, training, and experience. The vacuum extractor functions by applying suction to the fetal scalp. The suction is formed under a latex or metal cup that is applied over the posterior fontanelle, with the sagittal suture pointing to the center of the cup. If the fetal occiput remains posterior or transverse, traction from the vacuum will usually allow the fetus to rotate on its own; the fetal head should not be rotated manually. In some cases in which there is minimal room for the application of forceps, a vacuum extractor device for delivery may be warranted. This method also decreases injury to the vagina, bladder, uterus, and bowel. Because the vacuum extraction does not press on the mother, it is less painful; however, inclusion of these tissues into the cup can cause maternal trauma. This should not happen with proper application of the device.

The major disadvantage of the vacuum extractor is the development of the chignon, an edematous, occasional ecchymotic area beneath the vacuum cup. In the majority of cases, this area regresses in 2 to 3 days. Small abrasions are sometimes seen around the rim of this area.

The use of the vacuum extractor has not been as popular in the United States as it has been in Europe. However, with the development of the latex cups, it has increased in popularity.

The therapeutic use of fundal pressure to assist in the expulsion of the fetal head at delivery is a source of considerable opinion among many obstetricians and nurses. There are few data bases in the literature to support the use or avoidance of therapeutic fundal pressure, although several widely read monographs and texts contain opinions regarding its use. When excessive force is not used and the pressure applied is therapeutic, most senior obstetricians find no contraindication to the use of fundal pressure and employ it in their practice when indicated; certainly, gentle fundal pressure is preferable to a traumatic forceps/vacuum instrument-assisted delivery. The crux of this consideration is the judgmental expression of therapy. Excessive fundal pressure has the potential to cause trauma, especially if shoulder dystocia is encountered.

# Philosophy of Labor Management

Once it has been established that labor is under way, the goal of the health care professionals managing the labor is to have labor and delivery proceed as normally as possible with regard to duration, intensity, maternal and fetal responsiveness, and outcome. As long as all aspects of the labor process are normal, the perinatal team managing labor simply observes and waits for delivery to occur. The health care professionals managing labor and delivery must constantly evaluate and observe the process for abnormalities.

**Table 16–1**
LOW-RISK PATIENT CARE SUMMARY FOR LABOR*

| | First Stage | Second Stage | Third Stage | Fourth Stage (Postpartum) |
|---|---|---|---|---|
| Patients Not at Risk BP,P,R | On admission; then q 1 h | q 30 min | q 15 min | On admission; then q 15 min × 4; then q 30 min × 2; then q 1 h until stable; then on discharge to postpartum floor; then every shift |
| T | On admission; then q 4 h | q 4 | | On admission; then q 4 h, then on discharge to postpartum floor; then every shift |
| Urinalysis for protein | On admission; then with each void | | | |
| Fetal heart rate | EFM continuous or intermittent during labor | EFM continuous or intermittent during labor | | |
| | Initial 20–30 min strip demonstrating acc. Without monitor, listen through at least 1, but preferably 2–3 contractions. With or without EFM, assess and record q 30 min | With or without EFM assess and record q 5–10 min | | |
| Contractions Frequency Duration Quality Resting Tone | Continuous during labor, with or without EFM, assess and record q 1 h | With or without EFM assess and record q 15 min | | |
| I & O | Each shift | Each shift | Each shift | While in recovery, note first void |
| Lochia | | | | On admission; then q 15 min × 4; then q 30 min × 2; then q 1 h until stable; on discharge to postpartum floor; then q 4–8 h |
| Fundus | | | | |
| H & H | On admission or normal within 1 week before delivery | | | Morning following delivery |

* Nurse-patient ratio = 1 : 2. or 2 : 3

This requires analysis, measurement, timing, and emotional and psychologic support of the parents. To provide this supervision, the nurse–patient ratio should be 1 : 2 or 2 : 3 to allow for adequate labor and delivery management. In high-risk labor and delivery situations, the nurse-patient ratio may need to be 1 : 1.

Unfortunately, not all labor processes are normal, and it is the responsibility of the health care professional to recognize when an abnormality is present and to take the appropriate medical, psychologic, pharmacologic, and, if necessary, surgical measures to ensure that a healthy mother and a healthy neonate emerge from the labor process. In the past 2 to 3 decades, the significant advances made in maternal and fetal surveillance, blood banking, pharmacology (particularly antibiotic administration), and labor management have resulted in a significant decline in both maternal and fetal and neonatal morbidity and mortality (Shamsi et al, 1979). There remains room for significant additional reductions in morbidity and mortality rates; however, these reductions will be achieved only through hard work, evaluation, and critical analysis in order to promote further refinements of management protocol that will result in improved care. As the population at large becomes more educated about health care, health professionals must perform even more teaching, including educating patients as much as possible in areas involving their own health care. Only by so doing can we hope to achieve the highest quality of medical care. Table 16–1 summarizes the management of the labor patient.

# References

ACOG: Obstetric forceps. ACOG Committee Opinion 71. Washington, DC, ACOG, 1989.

ACOG Technical Bulletin: Operative Vaginal Delivery. Number 152. Washington, DC, February 1991.

Arey LB: Developmental Anatomy, 7th ed. Philadelphia, WB Saunders Co, 1965.

Beall M, Eglinton GS, Clark SL, Phelan JP: Vaginal delivery after cesarean section in women with unknown types of uterine scar. J Reprod Med 29(1):31–35, 1984.

Burnhill MS, Danezis JD, Cohen J: Uterine contractility during labor studies by intraamniotic fluid pressure recordings. Am J Obstet Gynecol 83:561, 1962.

Farmakides G, Duvievier R, Schulman H, Schneider EP: Vaginal birth after two or more previous cesarean sections. Am J Obstet Gynecol 156(3):565–566, 1987.

Flamm BL, Dunnett C, Fischermann E, Quilligan EJ: Vaginal delivery following cesarean section: use of oxytocin augmentation and epidural anesthesia with internal tocodynamic and internal fetal monitoring. Am J Obstet Gynecol 148(6):759–763, 1984.

Flamm BL, Goings JR: Vaginal birth after cesarean section: is suspected macrosomia a contraindication? Obstet Gynecol 74(5):694–697, 1989.

Friedman EA: The graphic analyses of labor. Am J Obstet Gynecol 68:1568, 1954

Friedman EA: Effects of labor and delivery procedures on the fetus. In Cohen WR, Friedman EA (eds): Management of Labor. Baltimore, University Park Press, 1983.

Fuchs AR, Fuchs F, Husslein P, et al: Oxytocin receptors in human parturition. Scientific Abstract #231, 28th Annual Meeting of Society for Gynecologic Investigation, San Antonio, 1981.

Gai MY, Zhao SF: Use of an insufflatable abdominal girdle to shorten the second stage of labor. AJOG 1966(2):338, 1992.

Garfield RE, Hayashi RH: A review of formation and regulation of gap junctions of myometrium during labor. Scientific Abstract #10, Society of Perinatal Obstetricians, San Antonio, 1981.

Gimovsky ML, Petrie RH: The neonatal performance of the low birth weight vaginal breech delivery. J Reprod Med 27:45, 1982.

Gimovsky ML, Petrie RH, Todd WD: The neonatal performance of the term vaginal breech delivery. Obstet Gynecol 56:687, 1981.

Hall DG: Serum magnesium in pregnancy. Obstet Gynecol 9:158, 1957.

Hartelendy F, Linter F: Myometrial $F_{2a}$ receptors during pregnancy and parturition. Scientific Abstract #293, 29th Annual Meeting of Society for Gynecologic Investigation, Denver, 1982.

Horenstein JM, Phelan JP: Previous cesarean section: Risks and benefits of oxytocin use in trial of labor. Am J Obstet Gynecol 151:564–569, 1985.

Huey JR Jr, Al-Hadjiev A, Paul RH: Uterine activity in the multiparous patient. Am J Obstet Gynecol 126:682, 1976.

Lavin JP, Stephens RJ, Miodovnik M, Barden TP: Vaginal delivery in patients with a prior cesarean section. Obstet Gynecol 59(2):135–148, 1982.

Lawson GW: Vaginal delivery after 3 previous cesarean sections. Aust N Z J Obstet Gynecol 27(2):115–167, 1987.

Lederman RP, McCann DS, Work B Jr, et al: Endogenous plasma epinephrine and norepinephrine in last trimester pregnancy and labor. Am J Obstet Gynecol 129:5, 1977.

Leppert PC, Keller S, Cerreta J, et al: Elastin in the uterine cervix, its role in dilation. Dallas, Society of Gynecologic Investigation, Scientific Abstract #104, 1982.

Meyers RE, Meyers SE: Use of sedative, analgesic, and anesthetic drugs during labor and delivery: bane or boon? Am J Obstet Gynecol 133:83, 1979.

Miller FC, Yeh S-Y, Schifrin BS, et al: Quantitation of uterine activity in 100 primiparous patients. Am J Obstet Gynecol 124:398, 1976.

Mitchell MD, Strickland DM, Brennecke SP, et al: New aspects of arachidonic acid metabolism and human parturition in initiation of parturition: prevention of prematurity. Report of the Fourth Ross Conference on Obstetric Research, Columbus, OH, 1983, p 145.

Moore, ML: Realities in Childbearing, 2nd ed. Philadelphia, WB Saunders Co, 1980.

Morishima HO, Pederson H, Fenster M: The influence of maternal psychological stress on the fetus. Am J Obstet Gynecol 131:899, 1978.

Murphy H: Delivery following cesarean section. Ten years' experience at the Rotunda Hospital, Dublin. Ir Med J 69(20):533–534, 1976.

Nochimson DJ, Petrie RH, Shah BL, et al: Comparison of conservative and dynamic management of premature rupture of membranes/premature labor syndrome. Clin Perinatol 7:17, 1980.

Petrie RH: The pharmacology and use of oxytocin. Clin Perinatol 8:35, 1981.

Rosengren WR: Some social psychological aspects of delivery room difficulties. J Nerv Ment Dis 132:515, 1961.

Rusu O, Lupan C, Baltescu V, et al: Magneziul seric in sarcina normala la termen si nasterea permatura: rolul magneziterapiei in combatera nasterii permature. Obstetrica Si Ginecologia 14:215, 1966.

Saldana R, Schulman H, Reuss L: Management of pregnancy after cesarean section. Am J Obstet Gynecol 135(5):555–561, 1979.

Shamsi HH, Petrie RH, Steer CM: Changing obstetrical practices and amelioration of perinatal outcome in a university hospital. Am J Obstet Gynecol 133:855, 1979.

Soloff MS, Swartz TL: Characterization of a proposed oxytocin receptor in rat mammary gland. J Biol Chem 248:6471, 1973.

Soloff MS, Schroeder J, Chakraborty J, et al: Characterization of oxytocin receptors in the uterus and mammary gland. Federation Proceedings 36:1861, 1977.

Yeh S-Y, Read JA: Management of post-term pregnancy in a large obstetric population. Obstet Gynecol 60:282, 1982.

# CHAPTER 17

# Induction of Labor

## Roy H. Petrie and Athanasia M. Williams

Early in this century, an impure biologic preparation containing oxytocin was made available. In the 1950s, a synthetically derived, pure preparation of oxytocin, devoid of the side effects secondary to the impurities of the biologic preparation, became commercially available. Until these preparatons became available, there was no satisfactory manner of influencing the onset, the stimulation, or the suppression of labor; therefore, all gestations continued until spontaneous labor occurred and the fetus was delivered. Maternal morbidity and mortality was commonplace, and perinatal morbidity and mortality rates, even in the most advanced countries, were unacceptably high. Presently, maternal mortality has become rare, and perinatal morbidity and mortality generally has been restricted to the very low-birth-weight infant. Perinatal morbidity and mortality rates have improved because of a few philosophic, diagnostic, and therapeutic innovations. One innovation is the ability to medically control uterine activity to cause the uterus either to contract and expel the fetus and the products of conception or to suppress uterine contractions in order to achieve an improved outcome. Although there a number of nonpharmacologic approaches to the control of labor, pharmacologic methods are used most often.

## Definitions

**Induction of labor** is the nonspontaneous initiation of uterine activity to provoke the onset of uterine contractions that result in progressive cervical effacement and dilatation with descent of the presenting part. Generally, induction of labor is carried out near term and when there is a medical indication for the termination of a particular gestation.

**Augmentation of labor** is the medical stimulation, once labor has begun, of additional uterine activity to bring about more progressive cervical dilatation and effacement and descent of the presenting part. Presently, most augmentation is performed through pharmacologic methods. Generally, augmentation is required when there is a dysfunctional (nonprogressive) form of labor or when there is less than the normal amount of uterine activity required to promote progressive cervical effacement and dilatation and descent of the presenting part.

## The Physiology of Labor

A number of outstanding investigators, including Csapo, Liggins, Turnbull, Mac-Donald, du Vigneaud, and Karim, have advanced the study of the physiology and origin of labor. A great body of research has been collected; nevertheless, the origin of the onset of spontaneous labor and its physiology are as yet unknown. In Chapter 16, an analogy was drawn between the starting of an automobile engine and the initiation of labor. Analogies of this sort serve the purpose of clinical consideration and thinking only; however, clinical expression must be buttressed by biologic facts and concepts.

There are a number of theories concerning

the onset and control of labor. For example, it is known that prior to the onset of labor, the maternal estrogen-to-progesterone ratio shifts in favor of estrogen. The predominance of estrogen and the formation of the prostaglandins from arachidonic acid result in an inflammatory reaction similar to that seen with an infection (Mitchell et al, 1983). This inflammatory environment provides a biochemical-biophysical stimulus that provokes and alters action potentials that may be required to initiate the contraction of individual muscle cells.

It has been known for some time that the posterior pituitary octapeptide oxytocin causes the term or near-term uterus to respond with contractions; however, the nongravid uterus or the uterus early in gestation does not respond well to oxytocin administration (Petrie, 1981). The uterus growing near to term, and especially after the onset of uterine activity, becomes sensitive to oxytocin. Oxytocin receptors in the myometrium have been identified (Soloff and Swartz, 1973; Soloff et al, 1977), and more functional oxytocin receptors are available as pregnancy and labor progress (Fuchs et al, 1981). Concomitant with the rise in the number of oxytocin receptor sites that become available is the formation of apparent cellular communication routes or myometrial gap junctions. Garfield and Hayashi (1981) have demonstrated specialized cell-to-cell contacts that are thought to lower the impedance of current flow between cells. Gap junctions are present in increased number as parturition approaches and as labor ensues. The release of arachidonic acid from the fetal membranes and the formation of the prostaglandins, particularly the $F_{2a}$ and the $E_2$ fractions, establishes that these compounds are intimately involved as uterine stimuli in the initiation of uterine activity and the continuation of labor. Unfortunately, the information dealing with the relationship of the prostaglandins and oxytocin in the initiation, maintenance, and regulation of labor is as yet unclear. Myometrial prostaglandin $F_{2a}$ receptors have been identified and have been demonstrated to increase with impending parturition and with the duration of labor (Hartelendy and Linter, 1982).

As pregnancy progresses, serum magnesium levels fall (Hall, 1957; Rusu et al, 1966). With the onset of either preterm or term labor, a further fall in serum magnesium can be identified. Considering that the combination of actin, myosin, ATP, and calcium yields an actin-myosin-ATP-calcium complex, or a myometrial contraction response, it is obvious that controlling calcium flow enables the obstetrician to control labor. The $\beta_2$-sympathomimetic agents are thought to regulate calcium by altering cyclic AMP control, and magnesium probably acts by displacing calcium.

It appears that the uterus approaching term is being prepared biochemically and physiologically to perform its contractile function. Hormone levels shift, microscopic anatomic changes occur, hormones are released, hormones are formed, the myometrium is prepared to act independently from a cellular level, and as labor ensues, the various elements of the myometrium function in unison to produce a singular muscular effort. The exact etiology of the onset of spontaneous labor is as yet unknown; however, it is clear that there may be multiple physiologic, biochemical, and pharmacologic avenues by which labor may ensue, and accordingly, there may be multiple avenues by which the onset of uterine activity leading to labor may be blocked.

Compared with the changes required to achieve active labor, much less uterine activity is required to bring about progress of labor (see Figs. 16–11 and 16–12). The same applies to the oxytocin augmentation and induction schedules, which use a reduction in dosage and a lengthening in the interval between the increases in doses that are subsequently recommended in this chapter. To summarize, it requires lesser amounts of uterine activity and, therefore, lesser amounts of pharmacologic stimulation to achieve the amount of cervical dilatation between 7 and 8 cm than it requires to achieve the same amount at the earlier stage between 2 and 3 cm of cervical dilatation.

To what degree does the clinician need to alter or control uterine activity or labor? Obviously, the ability to induce normal labor may be desirable in certain clinical situations. Likewise, the inhibition of labor is also desirable in some circumstances, although the true indications for this practice may be far fewer than initially suspected. An overall risk-benefit analysis of the control of labor is needed each time its use is entertained.

# Methods and Techniques of Labor Induction and Augmentation

Four medical techniques have been used to induce or augment labor: (1) electrical stimulation, (2) surgical intervention, (3) mechanical intervention, and (4) pharmacologic administration. Although electrical stimulation of the uterus has been used in the past to stimulate uterine activity (Waltman and Hassimi, 1966), it is seldom used in the United States, and thus, we limit our discussion to the three methods currently in common use: surgical, mechanical, and pharmacologic.

## SURGICAL METHODS

Surgical induction of labor is the easiest to perform of all the artificial forms of induction. When it has been established in the term gestation that there is pulmonary maturity or that the gestation should be medically terminated, the surgical rupture of membranes is performed. In the majority of instances, rupture of the chorioamnion is followed by spontaneous uterine activity that leads to productive labor within the first 12 to 24 hours. It is uncommon in the multiparous patient at term that this form of induction is unsuccessful; however, this form of labor induction may require the addition of pharmacologic agents. With a favorable (ripe) cervix, the membranes are ruptured by inserting an instrument through the cervix or through an endoscope placed through the cervix. Care must be taken that a prolapsed cord does not occur; for this reason, many clinicians will not rupture membranes in the presence of an unengaged presenting part. Although the success rate of surgical induction in the nulliparous patient is less than that for the multiparous patient, it is frequently used because the labor that results from the procedure is spontaneous in nature and type (Turnbull and Anderson, 1967). The underlying theory is that, with rupture of the membranes, arachidonic acid is converted into prostaglandins, which then initiate uterine activity. Once the uterine activity is initiated, it is further regulated and augmented with the release of endogenous oxytocin. Once labor is initiated, no further stimulation is required. Because surgical induction of labor is an irreversible process and mandates the delivery of the fetus, many clinicians are afraid to take this step, although it is a very legitimate form of labor induction.

## MECHANICAL METHODS

Mechanical induction of uterine activity and labor can be achieved in several ways: (1) by mechanical stimulation of the uterus by manual palpation; (2) by artificial dilatation of the cervix with the use of laminaria or a cervical vibrator (Beard et al, 1973); and (3) by the digital separation of the membranes overlying the lower uterine segment through a process known as digital stripping of the membranes (Swann, 1958). Mechanical measures to induce labor have not been used extensively in the United States because of the risk of damaging the cervix or introducing an infectious agent.

Most likely, the digital separation of the membranes from the underlying cervix and uterus works in a manner similar to that of surgical induction of labor. It is also less successful than other forms of induction, and it has the potential of introducing an infection at a time when it is not desirable or in the best interest of the patient; therefore, experienced clinicians tend to use stripping of the membranes only in those instances in which the cervix is very ripe and a short induction is anticipated (Muldoon, 1968).

The insertion of a cervical dilator into the cervical canal is gaining favor in this country after reports of successful outcomes with this method from around the world (Darney, 1983). The desiccated material is packed into the cervical canal, where it absorbs fluid and slowly and progressively dilates the cervix, promoting uterine activity over several hours. The cervical dilator is thought to work through the same mechanism as stripping of the membranes and the surgical induction of labor. Three forms of cervical dilators are available: *Laminaria japonicum,* a desiccated seaweed; Lamicel (magnesium sulfate); and Dilapam, a synthetic hygroscopic material (polyacrylate hydrogel). Many clinicians insert laminaria the evening before an anticipated induction, in order to prime the cervix for rupture of the membranes and the infusion of a pharmacologic uterine stimulant. There is a very small but real potential for the introduction of an unwanted infection with this method, especially when using the biologic preparation of desiccated seaweed.

## PHARMACOLOGIC METHODS

Before one decides which technique should be used to alter or control labor, it is important that the condition of both the mother and the fetus be known and that both the mother and the fetus be able to safely undergo the proposed therapy to control labor. For every agent used, there are maternal and fetal complications and side effects; for example, the chief side effects for both mother and fetus with the use of oxytocin are listed in Table 17–1.

Pharmacologic uterine stimulants include the estrogens, the $F_{2a}$ fraction of prostaglandins, the $E_2$ fraction of prostaglandins, and oxytocin. The ergot alkaloids and the alkaloid tocosamine (Sparteine) are such potent stimulants of the uterus that they are no longer used if a living fetus and neonate is the expected product from the labor. Intravenous infusion of large doses of estrogen to simulate the fall of progesterone will induce some uterine activity and contractions, but this infrequently induces labor unless the cervix is very ripe, and for this reason estrogen infusions are rarely used. Other agents, such as quinine, that promote uterine activity by stimulating surrounding organs are no longer in the medical arsenal.

The $F_{2a}$ fraction of prostaglandins has been used intravenously to promote uterine activity and labor; however, it has not received approval by the Food and Drug Administration for use for this purpose at term

because of associated side effects including nausea, vomiting, hyperthermia, and an elevated baseline uterine pressure tone. Some investigators have found a low-dose intravenous transfusion of $F_{2a}$ (Baxi et al, 1980) to be most effective. The $E_2$ fraction of prostaglandins has been used in a number of clinics, either administered orally (Yip et al, 1973) or applied as a local, extra-amniotic cervical vaginal gel, used to prime or pretreat the woman for a routine induction process (Calder et al, 1974; Clarke et al, 1980).

The only agent currently approved for the induction of term labor is oxytocin. It has been known since the first decade of this century that extracts of the posterior pituitary gland had properties that could be used as a uterine stimulant. By the 1930s, it was confirmed that there were two substances in the posterior pituitary extract, and subsequently, these were separated. In the 1950s, both vasopressin (also called antidiuretic hormone, or ADH) and oxytocin were synthesized de novo in the laboratory (du Vigneaud et al, 1953; du Vigneaud, 1956). For this work, the Nobel Prize was awarded to du Vigneaud. A pure preparation of oxytocin enabled the obstetrician to use oxytocin for the augmentation or induction of uterine activity without the side effects that the original Pitressin injection carried as an extract of the posterior pituitary. Oxytocin is destroyed in the stomach by trypsin, and accordingly, it is given as a nasal spray, a buccal tablet (Chalmers and Prakash, 1971), or an intramuscular (Rysso and Kosar, 1967) or intravenous injection. Because of its uptake and an erratic absorption, only the intravenous infusion of oxytocin is considered to be appropriate for the induction of term labor. The half-life of synthetic oxytocin has been determined to be between 1 and 6 minutes in early pregnancy and between 1 and 3 minutes in late pregnancy and during lactation. The liver, kidneys, and functional mammary glands remove oxytocin from the plasma. Oxytocinase has been found in plasma, and it inactivates oxytocin by breaking the cystine-tyrosine bond in oxytocin (Petrie, 1981).

Based on the work of a number of investigators (Baxi et al, 1980; Seitchik and Castillo, 1983), a schedule of increasing the dose of oxytocin delivered that employs an interval of between 45 minutes and 1 hour is provided. Most patients undergoing oxytocin induction or augmentation of labor generate

**Table 17–1**
SIDE EFFECTS OF OXYTOCIN

| Fetal Effects | Maternal Effects |
|---|---|
| Hyperbilirubinemia | Allergy |
| Hypoxia | Uterine hypertonus |
| Asphyxia | Uterine rupture |
| Death | Water intoxication |
| | Hypertension |
| | Hypotension |

sufficient uterine activity to bring about progress of labor with use of a mean dose of 4 to 5 $\mu$U/min, and the majority of patients will respond appropriately to doses of 8 $\mu$U/min or less. Using this slower temporal and low-dose approach for augmentation and induction of labor, minimal cervical change may be noted during the first few hours of induction; however, the active phase of labor frequently is reached after a few hours and then proceeds at a normal to slightly accelerated pace. During an induction of labor, once the patient has reached 4 to 5 cm of cervical dilatation, the oxytocin infusion can be reduced or eliminated, and labor proceeds without further pharmacologic stimulation. Augmentation of labor with oxytocin proceeds well with the use of very minimal (less than 8 $\mu$U/min) doses of oxytocin. Frequently, when an adequate labor has been established, an augmentation infusion can be discontinued altogether. It should be noted that, in some cases, when the uterus is not properly prepared for labor by whatever unknown mechanisms may be involved, doses of oxytocin of 10 to 20 $\mu$U/min (or even higher) may be required to effectively stimulate adequate labor. Using an infrequently increased, low-dose administration of oxytocin for the induction of labor with a favorable Bishop score (Table 17–2) (Blakemore et al, 1990), it has been demonstrated that such a low-dose protocol is as effective as a more frequent higher dose protocol that obstetricians have been using in the past. Using an hourly increase rather than the more traditional quarter-hourly increase in oxytocin, these investigators demonstrated that for an induction with a Bishop score of 5 or greater, there was no statistically significant difference in the duration of labor or subdivisions of labor except for a considerably lower dose of oxytocin, which necessitates the discontin-uation or reduction in dose of oxytocin for potential fetal compromise secondary to excessive uterine activity.

In an attempt to extend the pharmacophysiologic principles involved in low dose and hourly incremental increases in the induction of labor with a favorable Bishop score as described earlier, patients with an unfavorable Bishop score (less than or equal to 4) have undergone preinduction cervical ripening with oxytocin (Blakemore and Petrie, 1988). When the clinician believes that a given patient may require a longer preparatory interval to perform an amniotomy and a standard low-dose induction protocol, an overnight preinduction ripening is carried out with oxytocin. With very low Bishop scores, artificial laminaria may be used. The patient is admitted in the midafternoon and started on intravenous oxytocin at 0.5 $\mu$U. The dose is increased hourly to 1.0, 2.0, and finally 4.0 $\mu$U/min. The patient is monitored externally, and the oxytocin is not increased further. The patient is fed supper, and she takes nothing by mouth after 10 PM. At bedtime, around 11 PM, the patient is sedated with 15 mg morphine and 150 mg Seconal intramuscularly. At approximately 6 AM, an amniotomy usually can be performed, and an internal scalp electrode and an intrauterine pressure catheter are placed. The oxytocin level is reduced to 0.5 $\mu$U/min, and the oxytocin is increased for an induction of labor with a favorable Bishop score. The use of such a preinduction cervical ripening protocol has been successful for completing an induction that would otherwise be believed to be too difficult, and many clinicians would resort to delivery by cesarean section.

It should be noted that any time a labor is being induced or augmented by any means, including pharmacologic uterine stimulants

---

**Table 17–2**

BISHOP SCORE

| Component | Points* | | | |
|---|---|---|---|---|
| | 0 | 1 | 2 | 3 |
| Cervical dilatation (cm) | 0 | 1–2 | 3–4 | 5–6 |
| Cervical effacement (%) | 0–30 | 31–50 | 51–70 | >70 |
| Cervical consistency | Firm | Medium | Soft | — |
| Cervical position | Posterior | Mid | Anterior | — |
| Station | −5/−3 | −2 | −1 | +1/+2 |

* Total score of 0–5 points = difficult induction; 6–13 = easy induction. Adapted from Bishop EH: Pelvic scoring for elective induction. Obstet Gynecol 24:266, 1964.

such as oxytocin, attention must be paid to how well the fetus is tolerating the stresses of labor. Primarily, this is accomplished by external or preferably internal fetal heart rate and uterine activity monitoring and by appropriate backup fetal surveillance based on acid-base commentary whenever fetal heart rate data do not completely reassure the obstetrician of fetal well-being.

When a pharmacologic preparation for the induction or augmentation of labor is used, it is necessary that a careful administrative or delivery system is employed. This requires use of primary intravenous infusion, with all pharmacologic preparations administered as a secondary intravenous system into the first, using the piggyback method. This secondary intravenous infusion should be inserted as close to the needle site as possible, using a short Y-site adaptor. The Y-type insertion above the needle site should not be used, because the fluid between the Y and the needle site contains oxytocin and would give the patient a bolus of fluid if the patient's primary intravenous infusion is increased, as in the case of fetal distress. It is important to administer the oxytocin by secondary infusion, so that if there is a hypertonic response of the uterus or if fetal bradycardia or decelerations occur, the infusion can very simply and quickly be discontinued. Most institutions now consider that the technique of administration of these pharmacologic preparations is of such importance that a regulated infusion system is necessary. Two types of regulated infusion systems are available: (1) a regulated drip system and (2) a constant infusion system. The two systems are similar, but their implementation requires the use of different administrative protocols. Many of the new pumps allow the practitioner to keep track of the amount of milliliters infused, which aids in the observation of the amount of fluid the patient receives. Also, some new IV tubing will automatically discontinue the piggyback infusion if it free flows.

An easy formula to use is to add 15 U of oxytocin to 250 ml of stock solution. This preparation will allow 60 m$\mu$/ml; therefore 1 ml/h equals 1 $\mu$U/min of oxytocin solution. This preparation provides the practitioner with a simple calculation that can be easily converted without a chart. It also allows flexibility of dose and minimizes the amount of fluid the patient receives.

Table 17–3 provides an oxytocin infusion schedule for augmentation and induction of labor. For convenience, the infusion rates using milliunits per minute and the approximate equivalent number of drops per minute and milliliters per hour are included. Note that two different standard solutions— 15 U/250 ml of IV solution and 10 U/1000 ml of IV solution—are used; this is to obtain flexibility of doses delivered at the greater dosage schedule. The clinical goal with oxytocin induction and augmentation is to stimulate a normal labor pattern—i.e., contractions every 2 to 3 minutes, lasting 40 to 90 seconds at an intensity of 40 to 90 mm Hg— and provide adequate progress of labor. It is relatively easy to exceed the optimal oxytocin dose range. A summary of the factors involved in oxytocin administration is given in Table 17–4.

Before the induction of labor is begun, it is essential to check the working condition of the infusion pump. Once this is done, the induction may proceed by slowly increasing the amount of medication administered. Careful observation of the patient is necessary to ascertain whether the medication should be increased or kept at the present dosage. Because responses to a particular drug may vary from one individual to an-

**Table 17–3**
ADMINISTRATION OF OXYTOCIN FOR AUGMENTATION AND INDUCTION

| 15 U Oxytocin/250 ml IV Solution | | | 10 U/1000 ml IV Solution | | |
|---|---|---|---|---|---|
| Milliunits/Min | Approximate Equivalent Drops/Min | ml/h | Milliunits/Min | Approximate Equivalent Drops/Min | ml/h |
| 0.35 $\mu$U/min | | 0.35 | 1.0 $\mu$U/min | 2 gtt/min | 1 |
| 0.75 $\mu$U/min | 1.5 gtt/min | 0.75 | 2.0 $\mu$U/min | 4 gtt/min | 2 |
| 1.50 $\mu$U/min | 3.0 gtt/min | 1.50 | 3.0 $\mu$U/min | 6 gtt/min | 3 |
| 3.50 $\mu$U/min | 6.0 gtt/min | 3.50 | 5.0 $\mu$U/min | 8 gtt/min | 5 |
| 7.50 $\mu$U/min | 12.0 gtt/min | 7.50 | 7.0 $\mu$U/min | 12 gtt/min | 7 |

other, no fixed dose of medication can be given. One should always have magnesium sulfate and other tocolytic agents readily available during an induction of labor in case hypertonicity occurs.

Oxytocin has a weak antidiuretic effect. This could cause water intoxication in the mother if a large volume of fluid is given during oxytocin administration. Therefore, unnecessary fluids should not be given, and a careful intake and output assessment should be made. The patient's fluid intake should be kept to 1000 ml per 8-hour shift, unless the patient is dehydrated.

Until recently, once a patient had undergone a cesarean section, term induction of labor was contraindicated. Recently, it has been demonstrated that, with a horizontal lower uterine segment cesarean delivery, a vaginal delivery following cesarean delivery can be safely attempted. Initially, vaginal delivery following cesarean delivery was performed with spontaneous labor only. More recently, the judicious use of low-dose oxytocin to both augment and induce labor when labor induction or augmentation is medically warranted has been reported to be appropriate and safe (Flamm et al, 1989; Horenstein and Phelan, 1985). As in spontaneous labor, the patient should be prepared for a cesarean delivery, with blood readily available and the patient's informed consent for a cesarean delivery. The judicious use of oxytocin for augmentation and labor induction with the appropriate indications appears to be a safe and logical procedure. The health care professionals who administer oxytocin should be experienced with its use and completely familiar with the potential problems and management alterations that may be required. With complicated high-risk patients undergoing induction of labor or augmentation of labor in the presence of a prior cesarean birth, the nurse-to-patient ratio may reach 1 : 1.

The necessity for the medical induction or augmentation of labor does not terminate with the delivery of the neonate. During the fourth stage of labor, which includes the 1 or 2 hours following delivery, the use of pharmacologic preparations to bring about sufficient uterine contractions to close the uterine sinuses and inhibit excessive blood loss from the uterus is almost essential for the proper management of some patients. Almost routinely, in order to promote effective uterine contractions, intramuscular or intravenous oxytocin is administered just as the fetus is delivered or immediately following the delivery of the placenta. When the intravenous form of oxytocin is administered, great care must be taken to avoid the direct administration of large doses of oxytocin, because of the potential for hypotension and shock (Hendricks and Brenner, 1970). Generally 10 to 30 IU of oxytocin are added to 1000 ml of an electrolyte-containing solution, and the infusion is administered at 100 to 150 ml/h. More oxytocins may be added to the intravenous solution as needed, or it may be given intramuscularly.

In cases in which the uterus does not contract appropriately (atony), more potent uterine stimulants may be required. Ergonovine and methylergonovine maleate may be administered intramuscularly. When bleeding is heavy and unresponsive to oxytocin or intramuscular ergot alkaloids, these agents may be administered slowly intravenously when there are no contraindications such as hypertension or cardiovascular problems. The dosage is generally 0.2 mg, and this dosage may be repeated one or two times as necessary. Because of the potential of these alkaloids to provoke hypertensive states, they are not commonly used in patients with elevated blood pressure. In extreme instances of postpartum hemorrhage, the use of a prostaglandin preparation for injection directly into the myometrium is suggested by some authors (Tropper and Petrie, 1983). A summary of patient treatment is given in Table 17–5.

## Failure of a Pharmacologic Agent to Induce or Augment Labor

When oxytocin fails to adequately induce or augment labor, several questions must be addressed. If the induction has not involved rupture of the membranes, is it wise to wait and attempt the induction the following day, or is it better to proceed with surgical rupture of the membranes to determine whether or not this will augment the induction efforts? With ruptured membranes and an attempt to induce labor, most obstetricians consider the presence of good contractions (i.e., 40 to 80 mm Hg in intensity, lasting 40 to 90 seconds every 2 to 3 minutes) for a period of 8 to 12 hours as an adequate trial of labor before resorting to cesarean birth.

Attempting to shorten the latent phase of labor by either amniotomy or the use of oxy-

**Table 17–4**

MEDICATION SUMMARY FOR INDUCTION OF LABOR*

| Medication | Action | Route | Dose | Pregnancy Precautions |
|---|---|---|---|---|
| Oxytocin | Appears to act primarily on uterine myofibril activity by increasing the permeability of the cell membranes to sodium ions, therefore increasing uterine contractility | Intravenous with constant infusion pump | 0.25 $\mu$U/min double dose/min (after 8 $\mu$U, increase at 1 $\mu$U q 45 min) until adequate contraction pattern is established (q 2–3 min lasting 45–90 sec with 50–80 mm Hg amplitude and $\leq$ 20 mm Hg resting tone) Be prepared to reduce dosage or discontinue in active phase labor Discontinue with fetal distress or hyperstimulation | Contraindications: 1. Significant cephalopelvic disproportion 2. Unfavorable fetal positions or presentations that are undeliverable without conversion prior to delivery 3. When the benefit-risk ratio for either the fetus or mother favors surgical intervention 4. Fetal distress when delivery not imminent 5. Hypertonic uterine patterns |

* Nurse-patient ratio = 1:2

tocin is controversial; however, some authorities believe that neither may be very effective, whereas others believe that oxytocin is of some benefit. Once the latent phase of labor has reached approximately 20 hours, many clinicians believe that an attempt should be made to achieve the active phase of labor by means of intravenous oxytocin augmentation. Although opinions regarding the latent phase of labor may vary from physician to physician, from institution to institution, and from patient to patients, most clinicians believe that an attempt to augment uterine activity is needed before resorting to delivery by cesarean birth.

Most clinicians believe that arrest of labor of 4 hours' duration in the midst of the active phase of labor, with the membranes ruptured and adequate uterine activity that would normally bring about progress of labor, is sufficient indication for a cesarean birth to be performed. Some variation is allowed with regard to the patient's parity, with 3 to 4 hours of lack of progress in the active phase considered an indication for cesarean delivery in the multipara, whereas 4 to 5 hours may be allowed in the nullipara before proceeding to cesarean birth. Figure 17–1 shows the labor curve of a multipara who has experienced an arrest of labor in the active phase. The patient's membranes are intact, and evaluation of uterine activity demonstrates that a subnormal amount of uterine activity has been generated. After appropriate evaluation, augmentation of the labor was begun with intravenous oxytocin. Figure 17–2 is the labor curve of the multipara undergoing induction of labor for prolonged rupture of the membranes. Although a normal amount of uterine activity has been generated, there is an arrest of labor in the active phase, and delivery will be accomplished by cesarean birth in this patient, for whom a clinical diagnosis of cephalopelvic disproportion has been made.

## Effects of Other Pharmacologic Agents on Uterine Activity and Labor

The principles of the primary pharmacologic agents that are currently used to control uterine activity have been discussed; however, almost any pharmacologic agent used in labor has the potential for affecting uter-

**Table 17–4**
MEDICATION SUMMARY FOR INDUCTION OF LABOR*

| Maternal Side Effects | Nursing Considerations | Fetal and Neonatal Considerations | Breastfeeding |
|---|---|---|---|
| Uterine hyperstimulation Uterine rupture Water intoxication | Oxytocin should not be given simultaneously by more than one route<br>Incompatible with: fibrolysis; levarterenol bitartrate; prochlorperazine edisylate; protein hydrolysate; warfarin sodium<br>Compatibility with other intravenous fluids may be influenced by drug concentration, pH, and other factors<br>Monitor maternal vital signs every 15 to 30 min; monitor fetal heart rate and uterine activity q 15 min, preferably with internal monitoring<br>Do not freeze<br>Hourly I & O<br>Discontinue if contractions (1) occur less than 2 minutes apart, or (2) last longer than 90 seconds<br>May cause severe hypertension if given within 3 to 4 hours of vasoconstriction in patients receiving caudal anesthetic | Prematurity Fetal distress | No known contraindications |

ine activity and labor. Some agents, such as the local anesthetics, may either increase or decrease uterine activity, depending on the patient's gravidity, the dosage and mode of administration of the agent, and the timing of its administration within labor itself.

Many drugs given as an intravenous bolus provoke a temporary increase in uterine activity. Some drugs, such as alphaprodine hydrochloride (Nisentil), may initially increase uterine activity, only to decrease it later from the same injection (Petrie et al, 1976); thus, whenever one is managing or controlling labor, great care must be exercised in

**Table 17–5**
PATIENT CARE SUMMARY FOR INDUCTION OF LABOR*

| | Intrapartum | Postpartum |
|---|---|---|
| BP,P,R | On admission; then q 15 min while increasing dose q 30 min on maintenance dose | On admission to RR; then q 15 min × 4; then q 30 min × 2; ten q 1 h until stable; on discharge to PP floor; then follow normal PP routine |
| T | On admission; then q 4 h; q h with ROM | On admission to RR; then q 4 h; then on discharge to PP floor q 8 h on PP floor. |
| Fetal monitoring | Continuous during labor, preferably internal<br>Without monitor, q 10 to 15 min, listening through 2 to 3 contractions | — |
| Contractions Duration Frequency Quality Resting tone | Continuous during labor, preferably internal monitoring<br>Without monitoring, q 10 to 15 min | — |
| I & O | q 8 h (observed for water intoxication) | Total on admission to RR. |

* Nurse-patient ratio = 1:2 may necessitate 1:1 for high-risk patients or VBAC.

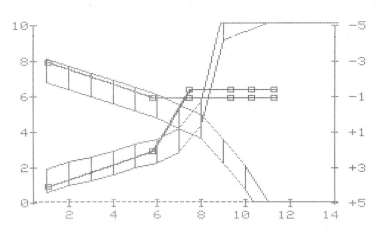

**Figure 17–1.** Labor curve for a multipara with inadequate uterine activity to effect progress of labor. If an evaluation of the patient warrants it, oxytocin will be used to achieve sufficient uterine activity to produce progress of labor. Should an amniotomy be performed or oxytocin be used, the computer will then select a different projected labor curve for the expected progress of labor. The lines connecting the boxes represent the patient's actual dilatation and station changes. The wide bands are the new projected labor and station curves using standard deviation. (Courtesy of Henry R Rey and Dr Roy H Petrie, Columbia University, New York.)

administering pharmacologic agents, so that undesirable results are avoided.

In some instances, depending on the pharmacologic agent used and the timing of its administration, one may effectively control uterine activity and yet promote the progress of labor. For example, studies measuring uterine activity have shown that although meperidine (Demerol) may decrease uterine activity, when the agent is administered in the early to mid-active phase of labor, sufficient relaxation, through the relief of pain and perhaps the diminution of the release of catecholamines, may actually result in greater effectiveness of the uterine activity

that is generated, thus providing greater progress in labor as measured by the degree of cervical dilatation and effacement with descent of the presenting part. Recall from Chapter 16 that less uterine activity is required to achieve 1 cm of cervical dilatation later in labor than in the early stages. Generally, tranquilizing agents suppress uterine activity, perhaps by mechanisms that are the same as or similar to alcohol—that is, by decreasing the outflow of oxytocin as well as by having a general sedative effect. However, Shepard and coworkers have demonstrated an agent such as dimenhydrinate (Dramamine) has oxytocin-like uterine stim-

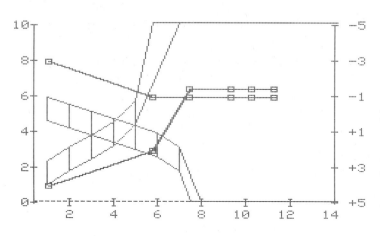

**Figure 17–2.** Labor curve for a multipara with adequate uterine activity to effect progress of labor, which has been stimulated with oxytocin. There has been an arrest of labor in the active phase for 4 hours. Delivery will be accomplished by cesarean delivery. The lines connecting the boxes represent the patient's actual dilatation and station changes. The wide bands indicate standard deviation for dilatation and station. (Courtesy of Henry R Rey and Dr Roy H Petrie, Columbia University, New York.)

ulant properties, especially when given as an intravenous bolus (Shepard et al, 1976). Similarly, some agents that have a tendency to decrease uterine activity when given alone, may actually increase uterine activity when administered in combination, particularly as an intravenous bolus injection (Riffel et al, 1973). Meperidine and promethazine hydrochloride (Phenergan) has been used as a combination intravenous injection. Patients who are being treated for preeclampsia with an anticonvulsant such as magnesium sulfate have been noted to have longer labors and require augmentation of labor in a greater than normal percentage of cases (Hall et al, 1959). Patients with asthma who are using a $\beta_2$-sympathomimetic agent may also require the use of oxytocin augmentation to bring about effective labor, because the $\beta_2$ agent may be acting on uterine smooth muscle as well as on the bronchial smooth muscle.

## EMOTIONAL ASPECTS

When labor is induced, it is of utmost importance to allay the fears of the patient. Many patients feel that induced labor is not natural and have been told by other women that induction causes a much more severe labor than that which occurs naturally. It should be explained to any patient who expresses these fears that induced labor is not really stronger than natural labor; it is only the way in which labor progresses that is different. In spontaneous labor, the uterus slowly contracts in an irregular mild pattern, increasing to strong regular contractions, and allows the patient to gradually get used to and cope with the intensity and duration of the contractions. In induced labor, this prodromal, early form of labor does not exist with many induction techniques, and the patient may progress from complete absence of discomfort to strong active labor. This sudden sensation of pain tends to frighten a patient and cause her a great deal of difficulty in managing to control herself during the labor process. If a patient knows that this will occur, she can better prepare herself for the onset of the active phase of labor.

It is important to keep the patient informed of all progress being made during labor, so that she will be encouraged to cope with the continuing contractions, thereby facilitating the advancement of the fetus. The patient should be made aware that natural childbirth is still possible in induced labor; however, as in spontaneous labor, once a regular active pattern of contractions is achieved, the option of analgesia or anesthesia should be offered.

# Evaluation of the Patient

The obstetrician who is considering using labor control or manipulation must take into account one factor above all others: a detailed risk-benefit analysis must indicate that the patient and her fetus are more likely to benefit from than be harmed by artificial control of labor. In other words, before attempting to control uterine activity and labor, there should be a good medical indication for inducing labor. It has been advised by ACOG (1991) and mandated by the Food and Drug Administration (Postotnik, 1978) that oxytocin should be used for the induction of labor only when there is a medical indication to induce labor; the same can be said for the use of oxytocin to augment labor.

The practice of obstetrics has seen more changes in the past two decades than in the previous few centuries. The indications for the induction and augmentation of labor are not static but dynamic, and they are usually relative; nevertheless, there do exist uniformly accepted indications for the induction of labor. Generally, situations in which the mother and fetus would be best served from a medical standpoint by accomplishing delivery warrant the induction of labor, provided the uterus is sufficiently receptive to the induction technique to be used and the fetus is sufficiently able to tolerate labor. It must be emphasized that this indication does not include the elective induction of labor for the convenience of the patient or her physician. A judicious weighing of the risks and benefits is necessary in situations that do not represent either an absolute medical indication or an absolute nonindication. For example, the induction of labor in a multiparous patient who has a history of short labors with well-controlled hypertension and who lives 2 hours from the hospital may appear to be a convenient type of induction of labor, whereas actually, there may be reasonable justification to induce labor, particularly in the presence of favorable physical (cervical) findings indicating that a labor could be accomplished easily.

Using the same philosophical approach as in determining whether or not to induce labor, the decision to augment labor should not be undertaken without a good indication. The medical indication for the augmentation of labor is based on lack of progress in labor in the presence of subnormal amounts of uterine activity. Whenever labor is induced or augmented, careful attention must be paid to the fetal response to the additional potential insult of increased uterine activity.

Once the decision has been reached to induce labor, certain criteria should be met before the actual induction is carried out, in order to ensure that everything possible has been done to anticipate and, where possible, avoid problems that may be encountered during the induction of labor. These considerations may vary from one institution to another, but for the most part the following criteria must be met:

- Data supporting fetal pulmonary maturity, a medical indication that the benefit of a premature delivery outweighs the possible risk associated with prematurity, or both
- Absence of fetal distress
- Absence of absolute cephalopelvic disproportion
- Absence of overdistention of the uterus with a multiple gestation or hydramnios
- Absence of vaginal bleeding from placenta praevia, abruptio placentae, or vasa praevia
- Absence of a vertical uterine scar
- Absence of an unfavorable presentation or position of the fetus
- Absence of grand multiparity
- Absence of major uterine trauma, significant postcesarean section myometrial infection, or both
- A fetal weight that is not estimated to be excessive for the maternal pelvis
- An evaluation of the cervix (Bishop's score) (see Table 17–2) that is diagnostic of a successful outcome.

Many of the considerations to be met for the induction of labor also apply to the augmentation of labor. The primary consideration for any patient in whom progress is not being made in the active phase of labor is to determine whether or not cephalopelvic disproportion is the cause of the lack of progress. Those obstetricians who manage the labor of the nullipara patient by the protocol known as active management of labor may use oxytocin augmentation earlier; however, the principle of avoiding excess uterine activity in relation to fetal tolerance remains a most important goal.

A major issue to include in considering the induction or augmentation of labor is cervical ripeness or maturity. Although biologic and biochemical considerations are the basic criteria used in determining uterine preparation for labor, clinical evaluation of the cervix causes considerable weight in the determination of whether or not to use labor control, as does any history of the prior performance of a patient in labor. A careful evaluation of the cervix for its general position in relation to the long axis of the vagina—its dilation, its effacement, its consistency, and the station and position of the presenting parts—is important in making an accurate assessment for the induction and augmentation of labor. A system that evaluates cervical ripeness has been developed by Bishop (1964) and is shown in Table 17–2.

## PHILOSOPHICAL CONSIDERATIONS IN THE CONTROL OF LABOR

The techniques to induce or augment uterine activity are tools available to the obstetrician to attempt to improve outcome in terms of morbidity and mortality for both the fetus and neonate and the mother. The old adage of "for every advantage there is a disadvantage" applies to the control of labor. The techniques and pharmacologic agents used to achieve desired results are often potent and have potential side effects. The obstetrician and other team members involved must be completely familiar with these risks, in order to anticipate and avoid problems.

Our current approach to the control of labor leaves much room for improvement, and current protocol concepts and techniques need to be altered as we become more knowledgeable about the labor process itself and as additional pharmacologic agents become available. An analysis of this medical endeavor indicates that considerable research from both a basic and a clinical standpoint is needed before the clinician who is involved in controlling labor can be completely comfortable.

## References

ACOG: Induction and Augmentation of Labor. Technical Bulletin #157, July 1991.

Baxi LV, Petrie RH, Caritis SH: Induction of labor with low dose $PFG_{2a}$ and oxytocin. Am J Obstet Gynecol 136:28, 1980.

Beard R, Boyd I, Hold E: A study of cervical vibration in induced labor. J Obstet Gynaecol Br Commonw 80:9, 1973.

Bishop EH: Pelvic scoring for elective induction. Obstet Gynecol 24:266, 1964.

Blakemore K, Petrie RH: Oxytocin for the induction of labor. Obstet Gynecol Clin North Am 15:339–353, 1988.

Blakemore K, Qin N, Petrie RH, Paine LL: A prospective comparison of hourly and quarterly-hourly oxytocin dose increase interval for the induction of labor at term. Obstet Gynecol 75:757–761, 1990.

Calder AA, Embray MP, Hillier K: Extraamniotic $PGE_2$ for the induction of labour at term. J Obstet Gynaecol Br Commonw 81:39, 1974.

Chalmers JA, Prakash A: Optimal dosage of buccal oxytocin for the induction of labor. Am J Obstet Gynecol 111:227, 1971.

Clarke GA, Letchworth AT, Noble AD: Comparative trial of extraamniotic and vaginal prostaglandin $E_2$ in tylogel for induction of labor. J Perin Med 8:23, 1980.

du Vigneaud V: The isolation and proof of structure of the vasopressins and the synthesis of octapeptide amides with pressor-antidiuretic activity. In Liebiecq C (ed): Proceedings of the Third International Congress on Biochemistry, New York, Academic Press, 1956.

du Vigneaud V, Ressler C, Swan JM, et al: The synthesis of an octapeptide amide with the hormonal activity of oxytocin: enzymatic cleavage of glycinamide from vasopressin and a proposed structure for the pressor-antidiuretic hormone of the posterior pituitary. J Am Chem Soc 75:4879, 1953.

Flamm BL, Goings JR: Vaginal birth after cesarean section: is suspected macrosomia a contraindication? Obstet Gynecol 74(5):694–7, 1989.

Fuchs A-R, Fuchs R, Husslein P, et al: Oxytocin receptors in human parturition. Scientific Abstract #231, 28th Annual Meeting of Society for Gynecologic Investigation, San Antionio, 1981.

Garfield RE, Hayashi RH: A review of formation and regulation of gap junctions of myometrium during labor. Scientific Abstract #10, Society of Perinatal Obstetricians, San Antonio, 1981.

Hall DG: Serum magnesium in pregnancy. Obstet Gynecol 9:158, 1957.

Hall DG, McGaughey HS, Corey EL, et al: The effects of magnesium sulfate therapy on the duration of labor. Am J Obstet Gynecol 78:27, 1959.

Hartelendy F, Linter F: Myometrial $F_{2a}$ receptors during pregnancy and parturition. Scientific Abstract #293, 29th Annual Meeting of Society of Gynecologic Investigation, Denver, 1982.

Hendricks CH, Brenner WE: Cardiovascular effects of oxytocic drugs used postpartum. Am J Obstet Gynecol 108:751, 1970.

Horenstein JM, Phelan JP: Previous cesarean section: risks and benefits of oxytocin use in a trial of labor. Am J Obstet Gynecol 151:564–569, 1985.

Mitchell MD, Strickland DM, Brennecke SP, et al: New aspects of arachidonic acid metabolism and human parturition in initiation of parturition: Prevention of prematurity. Report of the Fourth Ross Conference on Obstetric Research, Columbus, OH, 1983, p 145.

Muldoon MJ: A prospective study of intrauterine infection following surgical induction of labor. J Obstet Gynaecol Br Commonw 75:1144, 1968.

Petrie RH: The pharmacology and use of oxytocin. Clin Perinatol 8:35, 1981.

Petrie RH, Wu R, Miller FC, et al: Effects of drugs on uterine activity. Obstet Gynecol 48:431, 1976.

Postotnik P: Drugs and pregnancy. FDA Consumer 12:7, 1978.

Riffel HD, Nochimson DJ, Paul RH, et al: Effects of meperidine and promethazine during labor. Obstet Gynecol 42:738, 1973.

Rusu O, Lupan C, Baltescu V, et al: Magneziul seric in sarcina normala la termen si nasterea premature: rolul magneziterapiei in combatera nasterii prematura. Obstetrica Si Ginecologia 14:215, 1966.

Rysso JN, Kosar WP: The use of intramuscular oxytocin for the elective induction of labor. Am J Obstet Bynecol 97:203, 1967.

Seitchik J, Castillo M: Oxytocin augmentation of dysfunctional labor. II. Uterine data. Am J Obstet Gynecol 145:526, 1983.

Shepard B, Cruz A, Spellacy N: The acute effects of dramamine on uterine contractility during labor. J Reprod Med 16:27, 1976.

Soloff MS, Swartz TL: Characterization of a proposed oxytocin receptor in rat mammary gland. J Biol Chem 248:6471, 1973.

Soloff MS, Schroeder J, Chakraborty J, et al: Characterization of oxytocin receptors in the uterus and mammary gland. Fed Proc 36:1861, 1977.

Swann R: Induction of labor by stripping membranes. Obstet Gynecol 11:74, 1958.

Tropper PJ, Petrie RH: Current management of postpartum hemorrhage. In Quilligan EJ (ed): Current Therapy in Obstetrics and Gynecology, 2nd ed. Philadelphia, WB Saunders Co, 1983, pp 87–89.

Turnbull AC, Anderson ABM: Induction of labour. I. Amniotomy. J Obstet Gynaecol Br Commonw 74:849, 1967.

Waltman R, Hassimi M: Electrical current for induction of augmentation of labor. Am J Obstet Gynecol 105:220, 1966.

Yip SK, Ma HK, Ng KH: Induction of labor with oral prostaglandin $E_2$. J Obstet Gynaecol Br Commonw 80:442, 1973.

· · · · · · · · · · · · · · · · · · · · · · · · · ·

# CHAPTER 18

# Fetal Heart Rate

Julie West, Bonnie Flood Chez, and Frank C. Miller

It is a challenge to predict accurately the condition of the fetus through fetal heart rate information. A goal in labor is to detect early signs of fetal compromise so that intervention can prevent adverse neonatal outcomes. However, neither electronic fetal heart monitoring nor auscultation has proved effective in predicting the degree of fetal stress in the intrauterine environment, in differentiating fetal stress from fetal distress, or in predicting neonatal outcomes. Rather, direct tests such as fetal blood sampling, fetal stimulation, or umbilical cord blood analyses are used to diagnose and guide patient management.

In contrast, when reassuring characteristics are present, both electronic fetal heart monitoring and auscultation have proved effective predictors of fetal well-being.

The primary task of fetal monitoring techniques, to assess fetal well-being, is to differentiate accurately reassuring from nonreassuring fetal heart rate changes.

## Fetal Heart Rate Physiology and Pathophysiology

To assess fetal heart rate changes, it is necessary to understand the basis of reassuring and nonreassuring fetal heart rate responses to the labor process.

The electrical conduction system of the fetal heart is similar to that of the adult. The intrinsic control of the fetal heart rate originates in the sinus node, which is found in the wall of the right atrium. This autorhythmic pacemaker provides the electric stimulus to begin cardiac contraction. The impulse travels to the atrioventricular node, to the bundle of His and on to the Purkinje's fibers. These events are represented by the P waves and QRS complexes on the electrocardiogram.

Each cardiac cycle ejects a volume of blood into the fetal circulation. This process is referred to as stroke volume. Stroke volume and the heart rate are the two determinants of cardiac output. Cardiac output in the fetus primarily is dependent on the heart rate, because the fetus has a limited ability to modify stroke volume. Therefore, the fetus must rely on the heart rate to maintain or change cardiac output.

In addition to intrinsic properties of the fetal conduction system, the heart rate is varied by input from extrinsic sources; these include baroreceptors, chemoreceptors, and the autonomic nervous system.

Baroreceptors are pressure receptors that are located in the carotid sinus and the aortic arch, in the area of bifurcation of the internal and external carotid arteries. These stretch receptors are sensitive to blood pressure changes in the fetus. For example, when the fetal blood pressure rises, such as in cord compression, impulses are sent from the baroreceptors through the glossopharyngeal or vagus nerve to the midbrain. Additional impulses are sent via the vagus nerve to the heart, resulting in slowing of the heart rate. This normal physiologic response is a protective mechanism that attempts to lower the blood pressure by decreasing the heart rate and, therefore, lowering the cardiac output.

Chemoreceptors are chemical receptors located both near the baroreceptors and in the brain stem. These receptors are sensitive to alterations in $O_2$, $CO_2$, and $H+$ in blood or cerebrospinal fluid and are responsible for changes observed in the fetal heart rate. For example, a decrease in fetal arterial $O_2$ perfusion or an increase in fetal $CO_2$, such as occurs in umbilical cord compression, stimulates the chemoreceptors to produce a reflex tachycardia that increases cardiac output.

The autonomic division of the central nervous system has two components—(1) the sympathetic and (2) the parasympathetic branches. The sympathetic branch arises out of the brainstem through central cervical ganglia. Its neurotransmitters, epinephrine and norepinephrine, cause an increase of the fetal heart rate. The parasympathetic branch also originates in the brainstem, specifically from the medulla oblongata. This branch causes a decrease in the fetal heart rate through the vagus nerve. The parasympathetic branch begins to exert its influence on the fetal heart between 28 and 32 weeks of gestation. Its effect is to lower the baseline fetal heart rate as the fetus matures.

These two branches of the autonomic nervous system produce a constant push-and-pull effect on the fetal heart rate; the sympathetic division of the autonomic nervous system constantly stimulates an increase in the heart rate, and the parasympathetic division stimulates a decrease. In the well-oxygenated, nonmedicated human, this competition occurs with every beat, causing slight changes in rate that cannot be detected by palpation or auscultation but may be recorded electronically. The result is a visible beat-to-beat variation. These beat-to-beat changes are termed short-term variability.

Short-term variability is an important component of fetal heart rate assessment because it is dominated by the parasympathetic branch of the autonomic nervous system. This branch is more sensitive to hypoxic insults than the sympathetic branch; therefore, short-term variability is a more precise indicator of acute fetal oxygen status or fetal oxygen reserve than other characteristics of the fetal heart rate. It is this correlation between a decrease in oxygen reserve and a loss of variability that has led researchers to determine that fetal stress responses are measured more reliably by changes in the baseline rate and variability than in non-

reassuring patterns alone on electronic fetal heart rate monitors.

# Methods of Intrapartum Fetal Monitoring

The two methods used for intrapartum fetal monitoring are (1) auscultation of the fetal heart, with a stethoscope or a Doppler ultrasound device, and (2) continuous electronic monitoring of the fetal heart rate. Several recent studies have suggested that these two approaches are equally effective in predicting outcome (Luthy et al, 1987; Shy et al, 1990, 1987). It is not possible to determine the specific frequency or duration of monitoring that ensures an optimum perinatal outcome (ACOG Technical Bulletin, September 1989).

## AUSCULTATION

Baseline fetal heart rate, rhythm, and the presence or absence of changes in these characteristics is detected by auscultating between uterine contractions. The presence or absence of fetal heart rate changes associated with contractions is best detected by auscultation both during and immediately following uterine contractions.

Both the technique for and timing of fetal heart rate assessment by auscultation vary according to the individual practitioner's preference, institutional policy, and the clinical circumstances. An NAACOG Practice Resource (March, 1990) offers recommendations on how to auscultate the fetal heart rate. These recommendations are presented in Table 18–1; the frequency for assessment is illustrated in Table 18–2.

Auscultation is an effective technique for intrapartum fetal heart rate assessment if certain criteria are met. These criteria include

- Once the fetal heart tones are required every 15 minutes, the nurse-to-fetus ratio is 1 : 1;
- The presence of practitioners experienced in the technique of auscultation, the palpation of contractions, and the auditory recognition of pertinent fetal heart rate changes;

**Table 18–1**
HOW TO AUSCULTATE FETAL HEART RATE

- Palpate the maternal abdomen to identify fetal presentation and position (Leopold's maneuvers).
- Place the bell of fetoscope or Doppler over the area of maximum intensity of fetal heart sounds (usually over the fetal back).
- Place a finger on mother's radial pulse to differentiate maternal from fetal heart rate.
- Palpate for uterine contractions during period of fetal heart rate auscultation in order to clarify relationship between fetal heart rate and uterine contraction.
- Count fetal heart rate during a uterine contraction and for 30 seconds thereafter to identify fetal response.
- Count fetal heart rate between uterine contractions for at least 30 to 60 seconds to identify average baseline rate.
- If distinct differences are noted between counts, recounts for longer periods are appropriate to clarify the presence and possible nature of periodic fetal heart rate changes, such as abrupt versus gradual changes.
- In clarifying accelerations, recounts for multiple brief periods of 5 to 10 seconds may be particularly helpful.

From NAACOG: Fetal heart rate auscultation. NAACOG Practice Resource, #35, March, 1990.

**Table 18–2**
FREQUENCY OF AUSCULTATION: ASSESSMENT AND DOCUMENTATION

| Low-Risk Patients<br>*First Stage of Labor:* | High-Risk Patients<br>*First Stage of Labor:* |
| --- | --- |
| —q 1 h in latent phase | —q 30 min in latent phase |
| —q 30 min in active phase | —q 15 min in active phase |
| *Second Stage of Labor:* | *Second Stage of Labor:* |
| —q 15 min | —q 5 min |

***Labor Events***
***Assess Fetal Heart Rate Prior to***
—initiation of labor-enhancing procedures (e.g., artificial rupture of membranes);
—periods of ambulation;
—administration of medications; and
—administration or initiation of analgesia/ anesthesia.
***Assess Fetal Heart Rate Following***
—rupture of membranes;
—recognition of abnormal uterine activity patterns, such as increased basal tone or tachysystole;
—evaluation of oxytocin (maintenance, increase, or decrease of dosage);
—administration of medications (at time of peak action);
—expulsion of enema;
—urinary catheterization;
—vaginal examination;
—periods of ambulation; and
—evaluation of analgesia and/or anesthesia (maintenance, increase, or decrease of dosage).

From NAACOG: Fetal heart rate auscultation. NAACOG Practice Resource, #35, March, 1990.

- Institutional policy and procedure addressing the technique and frequency of assessment;
- Defined clinical interventions when non-reassuring findings are present.

## ELECTRONIC FETAL MONITORING

In contrast to auscultation, electronic fetal monitoring is both an auditory and visual assessment technique that provides continuous data for evaluation of uterine activity and fetal heart responses. The heart rate components include baseline heart rate, baseline variability, and periodic and nonperiodic fetal heart rate changes over time. The uterine components include frequency, duration, quality (intensity), and resting tone.

### Fetal Heart Rate Patterns

Fetal heart rate patterns are divided into two major categories: (1) baseline heart rate and (2) periodic and nonperiodic changes.

#### Baseline Heart Rate

*Baseline heart rate* (Table 18–3) is determined by assessing a tracing for a minimum of 10 minutes. Changes in rate that occur

**Table 18–3**
BASELINE HEART RATE*

| Categories | |
| --- | --- |
| *Tachycardia* | *Bradycardia* |
| A rate greater than 150 to 160 beats/min or a sustained rise in rate 30 beats/min above the previous baseline rate | A rate less than 110 to 120 beats/min or a sustained drop in rate 20 beats/min from the previous baseline rate |
| **Differential Diagnosis** | |
| Hypoxemia | Hypoxia |
| Maternal dehydration | Reflex |
| Maternal or fetal infection | Hypothermia |
| | Bradyarrhythmias |
| Maternal anxiety | Postdates |
| Fetal arrhythmias | Medications |
| Fetal hypovolemia | Maternal connective |
| Medications | tissue disease |

* *Definition:* The heart rate between contractions or between periodic changes in heart rate. "Normal" is considered to be in the range of 120 to 160 beats/min.
*Note:* Many normal fetuses have a heart rate below 120 or above 160 beats/min.

between contractions or between periodic changes are considered baseline changes. After the contraction has concluded, it is determined whether the rate is the same, greater, or less than it was following each and every contraction during that period of time. If the rate is persistently 160 beats/min or more, it is defined as a *tachycardia*. If the baseline rate is persistently below 120 beats/min, it is defined as a *bradycardia*.

Three factors must be kept in mind when assessing the baseline fetal heart rate. First, although studies define normal fetal heart rate as being between 110 to 120 and 150 to 160 beats/min, each fetus must be assessed individually, as the following examples illustrate. If, on admission, the fetal hart rate is 130 beats/min, and then 2 hours later the rate is 150 beats/min, this change represents a relative tachycardia for this particular fetus, even though the two rates are within the normal range. Investigation into the cause of the tachycardia should follow, along with appropriate treatment. Another example is a postdates pregnancy in which the woman may present in labor with a baseline fetal heart rate of 112 to 115 beats/min with average variability. If this rate remains stable and nonreassuring patterns are absent, this may be considered normal for this fetus, reflecting increasing maturity of the parasympathetic nervous system. Conversely, a premature fetus is likely to have a baseline rate in the high normal range owing to the relative immaturity of the parasympathetic system. Second, it should be noted that if periodic or nonperiodic decelerations are occurring, the assessment of the baseline rate must be made after the *recovery* of the heart rate following the deceleration pattern. Finally, the assessment of variability is made during this same recovery baseline period, not during the deceleration itself.

**Baseline Changes.** The causes of baseline changes are many; some are potentially harmful to the fetus, others are not. A tachycardia or bradycardia alone, however, does not necessarily indicate fetal distress. Many normal fetuses have heart rates greater than 160 beats/min and less than 120 beats/min.

Known causes of fetal tachycardia are maternal fever, maternal dehydration, fetal or maternal infection, maternal anxiety, stimulation of the fetus, fetal cardiac arrhythmias (e.g., supraventricular tachycardia and paroxysmal atrial tachycardia), fetal bleeding with hypovolemia, and hypoxemia. During recovery from a hypoxemic episode, tachycardia is seen as a compensatory sympathetic response to stress. Drugs such as the betamimetics (e.g., Yutopar) and the parasympathetic blockers (e.g., atropine, scopolamine) cause fetal tachycardia when administered to the mother.

Fetal bradycardias may be caused by medications, such as those drugs used for paracervical blocks ("caine" drugs) or beta blockers (propranolol). Bradyarrhythmias such as complete heart block are another cause of fetal bradycardia. When a bradyarrhythmia persists, it is associated with a 20 percent incidence of congenital cardiac structural anomalies (Parer, 1983). Fetal bradycardia is also associated with maternal connective tissue disease (e.g., lupus) and hypothermia.

The initial response of the normal fetus to acute hypoxia is always a reflex-mediated bradycardia (Parer, 1983). When the bradycardia is accompanied by average variability, it represents only a stressful incident that is usually well tolerated by the fetus. However, bradycardia accompanied by absent variability represents direct myocardial depression and is a nonreassuring pattern requiring immediate intervention.

**Baseline Variability.** Although the physiologic origin of variability is not completely clear, there is evidence to show that its presence indicates an intact nervous system. It originates either from the interplay of the sympathetic and parasympathetic divisions or from numerous, sporadic inputs traveling from various areas of the cerebral cortex to the cardiac integratory centers in the medulla oblongata and then transmitted down the vagus nerve (Parer, 1983). This interplay of these impulses cause a variation in rate between successive pairs of beats. (If all of these beat-to-beat intervals were the same, the heart rate pattern would be smooth.) This variability is assessed accurately only with internal methods of heart rate monitoring and is evaluated during the baseline heart rate. If there is a discrepancy in the variability during decelerations and the baseline, the correct assessment is made in the baseline period only.

The variability is described as increased, average, decreased, or absent. The presence of average variability is a reassuring sign that represents normal neurologic modulation and cardiac responsiveness in the fetus. Although specific deceleration patterns indicate the mechanism of the insult, variability indicates the ability of the fetus to tolerate that stress; thus, it is a most useful indicator in assessing fetal status.

An increase in the baseline variability usually results from some event that has stimulated the fetal central nervous system. A loose or defective fetal heart rate electrode may simulate increased variability. Variability may also be falsely exaggerated with the external mode of monitoring.

A decrease in or loss of variability can result from many factors, but the factors that most concern the perinatal team are hypoxia and acidosis. With fetal hypoxia, central nervous system and heart function continue, but variability may be decreased or absent. In addition, other factors such as the administration of medications (including narcotics, alcohol, tranquilizers, barbiturates, and anesthetics) or fetal congenital anomalies can cause a possible loss of or decrease in variability. Premature fetuses have less variability than term fetuses because of immaturity of the parasympathetic nervous system. In addition, when tachycardia is present at rates greater than 180 beats/min, variability decreases, because there is less time between each beat, causing fewer fluctuations and there is a predominance of sympathetic input over parasympathetic input (Table 18–4).

Figure 18–1 shows a tracing indicating decreased variability secondary to narcotic administration. Note that the last 3 minutes of the tracing show a return of the variability as the medication loses its effectiveness. Fig. 18–2 is a nonreassuring tracing that shows a

**Table 18–4**
FACTORS AFFECTING VARIABILITY

| Decreased Variability | Increased Variability |
|---|---|
| Hypoxia and acidosis | Contractions |
| Drugs | Second stage of labor |
| Prematurity | Application of direct |
| Tachycardia | electrode |
| Dysrhythmias | Vaginal exams |
| Fetal sleep | pH sampling |
| Anesthesia | Fetal movement |
| Cardiac and CNS | Fetal breathing movement |
| anomalies | |

loss of variability and an absence of spontaneous accelerations.

### Periodic and Nonperiodic Heart Rate Changes

The second category of fetal heart rate changes comprises periodic and nonperiodic deviations above or below the baseline. Periodic heart rate changes are those deviations in rate occurring in response or in relation to contractions. Periodic changes include uniform accelerations and early, late, and variable decelerations. Nonperiodic heart rate changes are also divided into two subgroups: nonuniform (1) accelerations and (2) decelerations. These accelerations and decelerations do not occur repetitively with contractions and, therefore, do not meet the criteria of periodic changes.

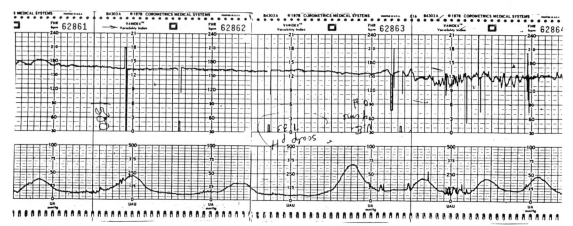

**Figure 18–1.** Mode: Direct electrode, intrauterine catheter. Baseline stable, periodic changes absent, variability decreased but increasing at end of tracing. Demerol 50 mg IV push 1 hour prior to this portion of tracing. (Courtesy of Joan Drukker Dauphinee, RNC, MS.)

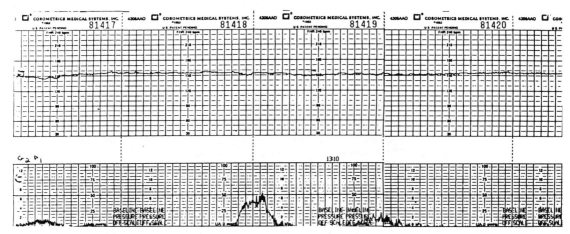

**Figure 18–2.** Mode: External, nonreassuring tracing: No accelerations and absent variability. No medications given. (Courtesy of Joan Drukker Dauphinee, RNC, MS.)

**Periodic Accelerations.** *Uniform accelerations* begin with the onset of the contractions and end with the termination of contractions. The shape of the acceleration is smooth; it gently rises as the contraction builds and decreases as the contraction subsides. The acceleration usually mirrors the size of the contraction; the stronger the contraction, the greater the acceleration. Uniform accelerations are believed to be benign and are *not* associated with fetal compromise. They may be caused by partial umbilical cord compression or tactile stimulation of the fetus during a contraction. They also may be associated with breech presentation (Table 18–5).

**Periodic Decelerations.** Periodic decelerations are classified as early, late, or variable according to their shape and timing in relation to uterine activity. The characteristics of each deceleration pattern should be committed to memory so that error is

### Table 18–5
PERIODIC CHANGES IN HEART RATE:
ACCELERATIONS

| Designation: | Uniform | Nonuniform |
|---|---|---|
| Character: | Mirrors uterine contraction | Abrupt rise and fall |
| Mechanism: | Nonvertex presentations | Response to fetal movement |
| | Umbilical vein compression | Precedes and follows variable decelerations |
| | Stimulation | Stimulation |

avoided when making the interpretation (Table 18–6).

*Early decelerations* begin with the onset of a contraction and return to the baseline with the end of the contraction. The nadir of the deceleration occurs with the peak of the contraction, rarely falling more than 20 beats/min below the baseline rate. These decelerations mirror the contraction, so that the stronger and longer the contractions, the longer and deeper the decelerations. They tend to occur repetitively with each contraction. Early decelerations occur more commonly in the early active phase of labor and after rupture of the membranes. Regardless of cervical dilatation or stage of labor, the decelerations remain smooth in shape and do not drop abruptly. Early decelerations are the result of head compression and are not associated with hypoxia or acidosis; therefore, no treatment is necessary (see Table 18–6).

*Late decelerations* have the same smooth, uniform shape as early decelerations. However, the onset of the deceleration occurs *after* the onset of the contraction (frequently at the peak of the contraction). The nadir of the deceleration occurs after the peak of the contraction, and the recovery of the heart rate to the baseline occurs after the contraction has ended. Therefore, late decelerations have a late onset and offset. The size and depth of the deceleration do not relate to the clinical significance. That is, nonreassuring patterns can be depicted by very shallow late decelerations. However, late decelerations

**Table 18–6**
PERIODIC CHANGES IN HEART RATE: DECELERATIONS

|  | Early | Late | Variable |
|---|---|---|---|
| Definition: | Vagally mediated response to fetal head compression | Response to impaired uterine blood flow | Response to umbilical cord compression |
| Characteristics: | Uniform shape | Uniform shape | Variable shape (abrupt drop) |
|  | Begins at beginning of contraction | Begins at approximately the peak of the contraction | Occurs at any time |
|  | Repetitive | Repetitive | May be repetitive |
|  | Reflects amplitude and duration of contractions | Reflects amplitude and duration of contractions | Variable shape |
|  | Ends with the end of the contractions | Ends after the end of the contraction | Variable duration |
|  | Benign | May be associated with acidosis | May be associated with acidosis |

are of critical significance when they are repetitive. The deceleration pattern indicates the mechanism of the insult, whereas the variability indicates fetal reserve. The underlying mechanism of late decelerations is uteroplacental insufficiency. As the contraction builds, the blood flow through the intervillous space is diminished, leaving the fetus to rely on reserve oxygen. Without adequate reserve, for example, in chronic placental insufficiency, the fetal heart rate begins to slow after the oxygen in the blood of the intervillous space is depleted and the $Po_2$ drops below a critical level. After the contraction has ended, maternal blood flow resumes and the fetus generally recovers. However, this repeated insult can lead to fetal hypoxia and acidosis, followed by permanent organ damage and, eventually, death (see Table 18–6).

Uteroplacental insufficiency results from chronic insults to the placenta and its vasculature. Such conditions usually are not correctable and may result in a chronically hypoxemic fetus with little reserve. In these situations, late decelerations appear early in labor and are often seen with other nonreassuring signs such as decreased variability or loss of spontaneous accelerations (Fig. 18–3).

Late decelerations may also reflect acute uteroplacental insufficiency seen with excessive uterine activity or maternal hypotension. In a normal pregnancy, the fetus initially has adequate reserve, and the late decelerations are seen with average variability. If the underlying situation is corrected,

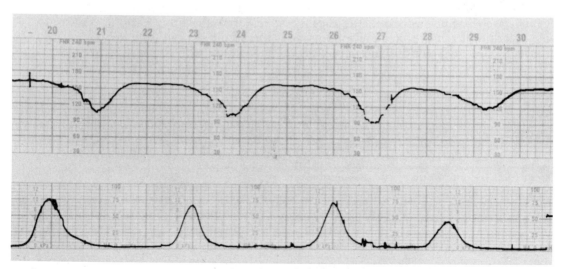

**Figure 18–3.** Mode: Direct electrode, intrauterine catheter. Baseline rate stable, late decelerations, absent variability. (From Schifrin BS: Exercises in Fetal Monitoring, Mosby Year Book, St. Louis, 1990.)

the fetus usually recovers promptly (Fig. 18–4). These *iatrogenic* late decelerations usually are avoided by the judicious use of oxytocin and the careful administration and monitoring of regional anesthesia.

*Variable decelerations*, the most common type of periodic deceleration, may occur before, during, or after the contraction or when no contractions are present. (Variable decelerations also are considered nonperiodic if they do not occur with contractions.) The key characteristic of variable decelerations is the abrupt drop in heart rate, followed by an equally abrupt return to the baseline (see Table 18–6). Variable decelerations vary in size, timing, duration, and depth (Fig. 18–5). They are commonly caused by cord compression and acute cessation of umbilical blood flow. *Shoulder accelerations* precede or follow variable decelerations (Fig. 18–5); the mechanisms of these accelerations is believed to be the result of umbilical vein compression. Occasionally, cord compression develops slowly and only the vein is compressed (as opposed to compression of both the vein and arteries). Blood flow to the fetus is impaired, causing a drop in fetal blood pressure. This stimulates the baroreceptors to increase the heart rate as a compensatory mechanism, causing a primary acceleration. As the contraction continues, the arteries are also compressed, causing fetal hypertension, with a resultant drop in fetal heart rate and a variable deceleration. The same process occurs during the recovery stage: As the compression is alleviated, first the arteries open, allowing the fetal heart rate to begin to return to the baseline, but the continuation of

umbilical vein compression again creates fetal hypotension and the resultant secondary acceleration. Finally, compression ceases totally and the heart rate returns to the baseline. These particular accelerations do not require treatment, but treatment for the variable *decelerations* may be instituted.

The presence of overshoot accelerations, also called prolonged secondary accelerations or rebound accelerations, may be an indication of worsening fetal stress. They are defined as accelerations following variable decelerations, which rise at least 20 beats/min above the baseline rate and persist for more than 20 to 30 seconds before returning to baseline. They always occur with miminal or absent baseline variability (Fig. 18–6). Krebs and associates (1983) hypothesized that these accelerations are a compensatory response to significant fetal hypoxia that occurs during the preceding contraction.

Variable decelerations may last any length of time, from a few seconds, when the cord is briefly compressed, to a prolonged period of time, if the cord is trapped. When the cord is trapped, variable decelerations are seen with every contraction for as long as the cord remains compressed. If the fetus accidentally kicks or squeezes the cord, the variable deceleration may be a solitary event. Variable decelerations seen during antepartum assessment testing, although not usually associated with contractions, also indicate umbilical cord compression. When these decelerations are present, an assessment of amniotic fluid volume is indicated to rule out oligohydramnios and a vulnerable cord (Anyaegbunam et al, 1986).

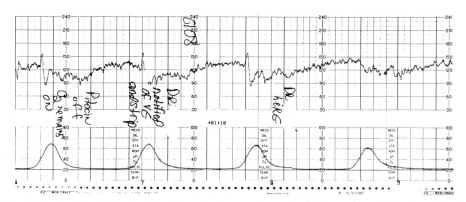

**Figure 18–4.** Mode: Direct electrode, intrauterine catheter. Baseline rate stable, late decelerations, average variability. Oxytocin turned off. Late decelerations resolving, iatrogenic fetal distress. (Courtesy of Linda Bertucci, RNC, MS.)

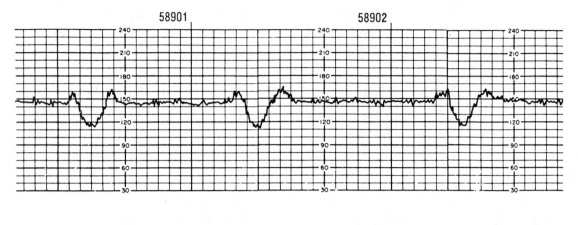

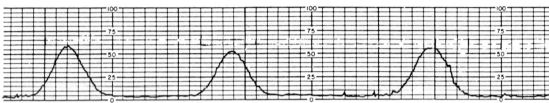

**Figure 18–5.** Mode: Direct electrode, intrauterine catheter. Baseline stable variable decelerations with shoulders, average variability. (From Atterbury JA: Perinatal Educational Resource and Learning System. Department of OB & GYN, University of Arkansas for Medical Sciences, 1992.)

Although variable decelerations indicate that the fetus is under stress (cord compression), the presence of a normal baseline rate and average variability is reassuring (see Fig. 18–5). The pattern of variable deceleration seen with tachycardia, bradycardia, or decreased variability is nonreassuring, indicating a need for intrauterine resuscitation or intervention (see Fig. 18–6).

The goal in treating variable decelerations

is to alleviate the cord compression. To accomplish this goal, a variety of maternal position changes may be initiated, such as turning from side to side or assuming the knee-chest position. Another possible measure is elevation of the presenting part; however, this may cause a prolapsed cord and should be performed only in an emergency situation. Amnioinfusion has also been used successfully in certain situations

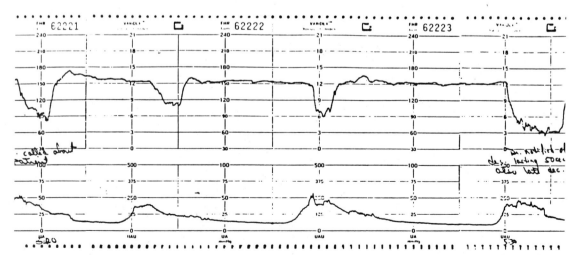

**Figure 18–6.** Mode: Direct electrode, external tocodynomometer. Baseline rate stable, variable decelerations with overshoots and absent variability. (Courtesy of Joan Drukker Dauphinee, RNC, MS.)

to restore a normal amount of fluid in the amniotic cavity, thus alleviating the cord compression (Miyazaki & Nevarez, 1985).

**Nonperiodic Accelerations.** Nonperiodic accelerations that occur are nonuniform accelerations in response to fetal movement or stimulation (see Table 18–5). The basis for the antepartum nonstress test is observation for fetal heart rate acceleration in response to fetal movement or stimulation. These accelerations are irregular in shape and amplitude, and they usually are not associated with contractions. The presence of these accelerations is considered to be reassuring and is generally indicative of an intact, nonacidotic cardioregulatory system (Fig. 18–7).

**Nonperiodic Decelerations.** Nonperiodic (prolonged or undefined) decelerations are most often caused by either cord compression or uteroplacental insufficiency with prolonged contractions (Fig. 18–8). Prolonged decelerations are also associated with significant hypotension seen in a minority of patients following epidural anesthesia. The heart rate drops and stays down for several minutes; if the heart rate recovers to the predeceleration baseline rate with average variability, then it is assumed that the fetus has fully recovered. If the heart rate recovers to a tachycardic or bradycardic baseline or the variability is decreased, intrauterine resuscitation measures should be initiated and further assessment of the fetal status should be performed.

An isolated small deceleration may occur that appears to be unrelated to any of the characteristics described thus far. Generally, such decelerations are intermittent and do not produce any recognizable pattern.

### Pattern Interpretation

Assessment of fetal heart rate patterns should be performed in an organized, systematic fashion, beginning with the determination of the mode of monitoring. Because the ability to accurately assess variability is limited to tracings obtained with the direct fetal scalp electrode, the precise mode of monitoring is taken into consideration. With the external ultrasound transducer, information on variability may not be reliable. However, if the fetal heart rate variability appears decreased or absent with the external ultrasound transducer, this information is most likely correct. Uterine activity is evaluated by determining frequency, duration, and the intensity of the contractions as well as the tone of the uterus at rest (resting tone). Precise determination of uterine baseline tone and the intensity of contractions is obtained only with the intrauterine pressure catheter. After defining the mode of monitoring, the baseline rate is determined as well as any changes in this rate. The baseline variability is assessed as being increased, average, decreased, or absent. Next, the presence or absence of periodic changes (ac-

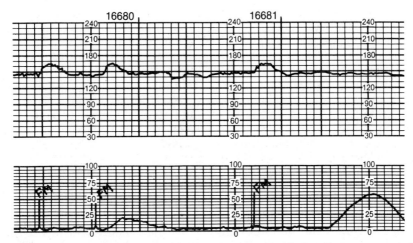

**Figure 18–7.** Mode: external ultrasound and tocodynamometer. Stable baseline rate, nonuniform accelerations in response to fetal movement—reactive nonstress test. (Redrawn From Atterbury JA, West JW, Quirk JG, et al.: Electronic fetal monitoring. In Quirk JG (ed): Perinatal Educational Resource and Learning System. Department of Obstetrics and Gynecology, University of Arkansas for Medical Sciences, Little Rock, AR, 1992.)

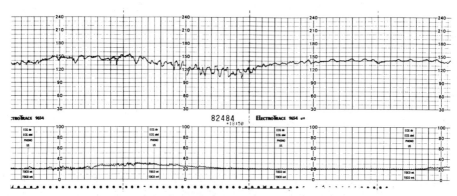

**Figure 18–8.** Mode: Direct electrode, external tocodynamometer. Baseline rate stable. Nonperiodic (prolonged) deceleration with tetanic contraction. (Courtesy of Linda Bertucci, RNC, MS.)

celerations or decelerations) is noted. The patient's medical and obstetric history is considered, as well as the patient's current clinical condition, to look for potential causative or contributory factors. Once these facts have been collected, the differential diagnosis is made and specific treatment of the possible causes of the problem can be carried out.

The interpretation of a fetal heart rate pattern falls into one of two categories: (1) reassuring and (2) nonreassuring.

Examples of reassuring patterns include a normal baseline rate with average variability and spontaneous accelerations, baseline bradycardia between 100 to 120 beats/min with average variability, no decelerations, and accelerations. These patterns are associated with a metabolically normal neonate 95 to 99 percent of the time (Hon, 1969).

Not all nonreassuring patterns are indicative of what has commonly been called fetal distress. Some nonreassuring patterns indicate a fetus that is under a degree of stress but has enough oxygen and metabolic reserve to compensate. This fetal status is evidenced by the presence of such reassuring features as average variability, spontaneous accelerations, or both. Examples of these stress patterns include variable decelerations with a normal baseline rate and average variability, late decelerations with average variability, and prolonged decelerations that recover to a normal baseline rate with average variability.

Other nonreassuring patterns are those without reassuring features and may be associated with acid-base disturbances. Examples of nonreassuring distress patterns include

variable decelerations with a tachycardic baseline rate, decreased or absent variability or overshoots following the variable deceleration, baseline bradycardia with decreased variability, loss of spontaneous accelerations, and late decelerations with decreased variability, baseline tachycardia, or both.

Shields and Schifrin (1988) have described a pattern of chronic distress (Fig. 18–9). Their descriptive study reviewed fetal monitoring patterns of 75 infants with cerebral palsy. Twenty-five of these fetuses had this pattern of chronic distress, and 20 others had a combination of the chronic distress pattern and an acute pattern. The authors postulated that intermittent cord compression may cause "repetitive, transient ischemic episodes in the fetal brain" that may not cause asphyxia or fetal death. However, this cord compression may interfere with the fetal developing brain, resulting in neurologic handicap. This pattern also can be seen with immaturity, transient tachycardia, and the administration of atropine. Several of these fetuses demonstrated normal Apgar scores and uncomplicated neonatal courses; however, some eventually manifested cerebral palsy.

### Intervention for Nonreassuring Fetal Heart Rate Patterns

Not all nonreassuring fetal heart rate patterns indicate worsening fetal stress, but all deserve continued monitoring and careful assessment. The fetal heart rate pattern may be more accurately assessed with the placement of a scalp electrode. Also, the fetus can

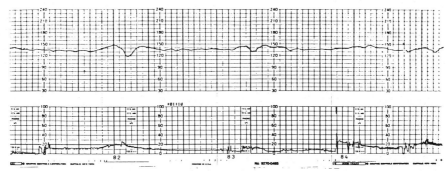

**Figure 18–9.** Mode: Direct electrode, tocotransducer. Pattern of chronic distress. (Courtesy of Joan Drukker Dauphinee, RNC, MS.)

be stimulated by tactile or acoustic means to assess the fetus' ability to produce spontaneous accelerations of the heart rate. If the fetal status remains in doubt, a scalp blood sample can be obtained and the fetal acid-base status can be analyzed.

Interventions to improve uteroplacental blood flow and, thus, fetal oxygenation are called intrauterine resuscitation. Such measures include lateral positioning of the mother to improve blood flow to the uterus. Changes in the maternal position also may be used to alleviate cord compression. Discontinuation of oxytocin or the administration of tocolytic agents to reduce uterine activity also may improve blood flow. The administration of oxygen to the mother may be of limited benefit because it does not remove the mechanism of the insult, and maternal oxygenation is usually normal. The type of intrauterine resuscitation technique that is employed is dictated by the specific fetal heart rate pattern observed, along with other clinical factors (Table 18–7).

Miyazaki and Nevarez (1985) found amnioinfusion to be a simple and safe treatment for the relief of repetitive variable decelerations that lowered the incidence of cesarean delivery for fetal distress in nulliparous patients.

The possible causes of tachycardia were cited earlier. To properly evaluate and treat tachycardia, the maternal temperature is taken. If the patient is afebrile, infection and dehydration are ruled out. In the event that she is febrile, an intravenous line should be placed and fluids infused. Further investigation may be necessary to determine the origin of the infection, and appropriate treatment is given.

It should also be noted that premature fetuses have an inherently higher heart rate than that of full-term infants. Therefore, knowledge of gestational age is necessary. In the event that the fetus is at full term, shows no periodic changes, and has average variability, the final possible cause of the tachycardia may be a dysrhythmia (Table 18–8). If

**Table 18–7**
PRINCIPLES OF INTRAUTERINE RESUSCITATION

| Objective: To improve blood flow to the fetus and to increase oxygen transfer | | |
| --- | --- | --- |
| | **Fetal Heart Rate Pattern** | |
| | *Variable Decelerations* | *Late Decelerations* |
| Change position: | To alleviate cause of cord compression | To improve maternal venous return; correct hypotension |
| Increase intravenous fluids: | — | To increase effective maternal volume |
| Turn off oxytocin: | To improve uterine blood flow; eliminate potentiating factors | To improve uterine blood flow; eliminate potentiating factors |
| Avoid medications: | To avoid other causes of fetal depression | To avoid other causes of fetal depression |
| Oxygen: | To increase oxygen flow across placenta (questionable effect) | To increase oxygen flow across placenta |
| Amnioinfusion: | To cushion the cord in the face of oligohydramnios | Not indicated |

**Table 18–8**
MANAGEMENT OF BASELINE CHANGES IN FETAL HEART RATE

| Tachycardia | Bradycardia | Decreased Variability |
| --- | --- | --- |
| Take maternal temperature | Rule out fetal death (counting maternal heart rate) | Check for possible drug effect (including analgesics and anesthetics) |
| Rule out fetal dysrhythmia | Rule out fetal arrhythmia (fetal echocardiogram) | Stimulate fetus (abdominal palpation, scalp stimulation test) |
| Average variability and no decelerations, observe | Average variability and no decelerations, observe | Change maternal position |
| Decreased variability and/or decelerations, see treatment of nonreassuring patterns | Decreased variability and/or decelerations, see treatment of nonreassuring patterns | No decelerations and accelerations present, observe |
| | | With decelerations; see treatment of nonreassuring patterns |
| pH sampling (?) | pH sampling (?) | pH sampling (?) |

decelerations are present, the onset of tachycardia may indicate that the fetus is not tolerating the cause of the deceleration pattern.

Fetal bradycardia alone with average variability and a stable baseline rate warrants observation but not necessarily intervention. Of primary importance is the need to rule out fetal demise. In the event of a fetal death, the maternal heart rate may be conducted through the dead fetal tissue and fetal electrode and may trigger the machine so that the maternal heart rate is counted in the absence of the fetal heart rate. Emergency cesarean deliveries have been performed for fetal bradycardia when, in fact, the fetus had been dead for several hours or days. This situation is easy to avoid either by taking the mother's pulse and comparing the rates or by obtaining a real-time ultrasound scan to observe fetal heart motion.

Bradycardias are most often observed during the second stage of labor. A distinction must be made between end-stage bradycardia and terminal bradycardia. When there has been a normal tracing and the bradycardia is accompanied by average variability, the condition is characterized as end-stage bradycardia and usually reflects prolonged cord compression or uteroplacental insufficiency due to excessive uterine activity. In most cases, vaginal delivery is anticipated. It is suggested, however, that oxygen be given to the mother and that the woman be encouraged to push in the lateral position, use open glottal pushing, or push with every other contraction to allow for maximum placental blood flow. It may be helpful to discontinue pushing for a short time altogether to allow fetal recovery (see Table 18–8). However, if

variability is absent with bradycardia, it is called terminal bradycardia and may be cause for immediate abdominal delivery (unless vaginal delivery would be faster), because the fetus may be acidotic. This pattern usually is preceded by other nonreassuring patterns.

Other causes of fetal bradycardia are reflex action, vagal stimulation, drugs (primarily associated with paracervical blocks), a postdates pregnancy, cardiac and central nervous system anomalies, and hypoxia or acidosis. In the event of a bradycardia, each possible cause is ruled out systematically. Fetal blood pH sampling may be used to diagnose acidosis (see Table 18–8).

The presence of variable decelerations with a normal baseline rate and average variability constitutes a pattern of stress that should be observed. Signs of worsening of this pattern include a rise or fall in the baseline rate, a decrease in variability, and the presence of overshoot accelerations following the deceleration. Treatment begins with altering maternal position to alleviate the cord compression. Oxygen may be given at 7 to 10 liters/min by face mask, and an intravenous infusion should be started in preparation for possible surgical intervention. If oxytocin is being infused and either the uterine activity is excessive or the fetal heart rate pattern is nonreassuring, the oxytocin should be discontinued. However, if the variability remains average and the variable decelerations are not severe, the administration of oxytocin may continue if the presence of stronger contractions does not increase the fetal stress. This procedure, of course, should always be implemented under careful observation, with a nurse-patient ratio of 1:1. A vaginal examination should be performed to palpate for a prolapsed cord. In some institutions, amnioinfusion is used to treat the patient with severe variable decelerations (see Table 18–7).

In selected patients with variable or prolonged decelerations, amnioinfusion may be used to alleviate cord compression (Miyazaki and Nevarez, 1985). This procedure is reserved for those cases in which conventional therapy, primarily maternal position change, has proved ineffective. Prior to the infusion, a vaginal examination is performed to rule out cord prolapse, to establish cervical dilatation and fetal presentation, and to place a fetal scalp electrode and intrauterine pressure catheter, if not previously done. Normal saline is then infused through the pressure catheter via extension tubing placed between the transducer and the catheter. The saline is infused at a rate of 15 to 20 ml/min until the decelerations are resolved. Then an additional 250 ml is infused. If the decelerations do not resolve after a single infusion of 800 ml, the procedure is considered a failure. If the decelerations recur after gross leakage of fluid from the vagina, the infusion is repeated as needed. Dual lumen intrauterine catheters are available to continue measurement of intrauterine pressure while infusing the saline for amnioinfusion (Fig. 18–10.)

Late decelerations indicate decreased blood flow through the placenta and resultant hypoxia. If the baseline rate remains unchanged and the variability remains average, this indicator reflects a fetus that has adequate metabolic reserves and still is able to compensate for the hypoxemia. Nonreas-

suring changes in the presence of late decelerations include a rise or fall in baseline rate and a decrease in variability. These changes indicate that the fetal reserve is decreasing and intervention is warranted. The initial treatment of late decelerations is to turn the woman to her side to correct supine hypotension and improve uteroplacental perfusion. Intravenous fluids are increased at a rapid rate to expand maternal blood volume and alleviate dehydration. If epidural anesthesia is used, maternal hypotension may cause uteroplacental insufficiency, and intravenous fluids or pressor agents may be used to improve blood pressure. Oxygen may be given by mask. Oxytocin, if it is being infused, should be discontinued (see Table 18–7).

All patients with nonreassuring patterns deserve continued monitoring and careful assessment. Most require other interventions to alleviate the stress or improve uteroplacental blood flow and oxygenation. Since it takes time to prepare for a cesarean delivery, these preparations should be initiated early in case an immediate delivery is needed if the pattern suddenly deteriorates.

## Acid-Base Assessment

A review of the fetal and neonatal acid-base regulatory mechanisms and response to hypoxic stress assist the doctor or nurse in interpreting blood gas parameters.

The pH of blood is directly related to the bicarbonate buffer level (metabolic com-

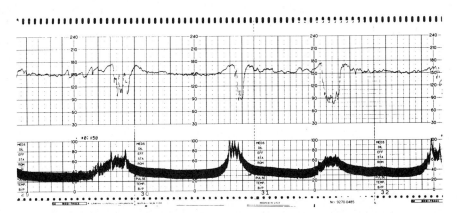

**Figure 18–10.** Internal scalp electrode and intrauterine pressure catheter (IUPC). Amnioinfusion is being administered for variable decelerations. Amnioinfusion fluids may interfere with the IUPC single lumen catheter as it does here, creating the wide recording in the contraction channel. (Courtesy of Joan Drukker Dauphinee, RNC, MS.)

ponent) and is inversely related to $CO_2$ levels (respiratory component). The Henderson-Hasselbalch equation demonstrates the metabolic and respiratory components of pH:

$$pH = pK + \log \frac{[Base][HCO_3^-]}{[Acid][CO_2]}$$

In patients with umbilical cord compression, $CO_2$ retention causes a reduction in pH (respiratory acidosis). Fortunately, $CO_2$ diffuses across the placenta very rapidly with its rate of elimination being directly related to blood flow rates on both sides of the placenta. If, however, the cord compression is persistent and perfusion is impaired for a prolonged period, hypoxia and acidosis may result.

Decreased uteroplacental perfusion and hypoxemia (low blood oxygen content) may lead to tissue hypoxia, anaerobic metabolism, metabolic acidosis, and asphyxia. In the acute clinical situation, decreased uteroplacental perfusion and the resultant hypoxemia may be caused by a hypertonic contraction pattern or maternal hypotension noted with epidural anesthesia or the supine position. Chronic uteroplacental insufficiency is noted in patients with hypertension or other vascular disease, intrauterine growth retardation, and a host of other conditions. If these conditions are not corrected or ameliorated, the reduction in oxygen delivery may interfere with normal aerobic metabolism, and the fetus converts to anaerobic metabolism. Several organic acids, including lactic acid, are products of anaerobic metabolism. These acids diffuse across the placenta much more slowly than $CO_2$. Consequently, fetal metabolic acidosis takes longer to correct than does respiratory acidosis. With the accumulation of these acids, the fetus may suffer end-organ damage with sequelae, such as seizures, necrotizing enterocolitis, or death.

The pH is also related to the ratio of buffer base to acid. The buffer base may be depleted from buffering a fixed acid, and the pH remains unchanged because of compensatory changes in $CO_2$. When this occurs, a base deficit exists. The terms *base deficit* and *base excess* refer to the amount of buffer below or above the normal levels. Base deficit or excess is not measured directly but can be calculated from a nomogram when two of the three following components are known: pH, $HCO_3^-$, and $CO_2$.

In general, fetal or newborn acidosis is classified as either respiratory, metabolic, or mixed. The relationship of $CO_2$, $HCO_3^-$, and base deficit to each type of acidosis is summarized in Table 18–9.

## FETAL BLOOD GAS ANALYSIS

The investigation of fetal acid-base balance was pioneered by Yippö (1916), who reported that, by adult standards, the cord blood of the fetus is acidotic. The current techniques of fetal blood sampling were introduced by Saling (1964). Fetal capillary blood pH is of clinical interest because it is directly related to tissue oxygenation. The pH is used more frequently than $Po_2$, because $Po_2$ is more difficult to measure, is more often subject to technical error, and fluctuates more rapidly. The $Po_2$ reflects the status of the fetus only at the time of sampling and gives no indication of what the preceding levels may have been. The pH of blood is influenced by both respiratory and metabolic factors and, therefore, reflects rapid (respiratory) and prolonged (metabolic) changes.

However, respiratory and metabolic acidosis cannot be differentiated by pH alone. It is important to perform a complete blood gas assessment, including pH, $Po_2$, $HCO_3^-$, and base deficit/excess, to establish the presence of respiratory or metabolic acidosis (see Table 18–9). This assessment is important be-

**Table 18–9**
CLASSIFICATION OF ACIDOSIS

| Type of Acidosis | Pco₂ (mm Hg) | Po₂ (mm Hg) | HCO₃⁻ (mEq/L) | Base Deficit (mEq/L) |
|---|---|---|---|---|
| Respiratory | High (> 65) | Normal (≥ 18) | Normal (≥ 22) | Normal (−6.4 ± 1.9) |
| Metabolic | Normal (< 65) | Low (≤ 18) | Low (≤ 17) | High (−15.9 ± 2.8) |
| Mixed | High (≥ 65) | Low (≤ 18) | Low (≤ 17) | High (−9.6 ± 2.5) |

From The American College of Obstetricians and Gynecologists: Assessment of Fetal and Newborn Acid–Base Status. ACOG Technical Bulletin #127. Washington, DC © April, 1989.

cause respiratory acidosis is rapidly correctable, whereas metabolic acidosis can cause end-organ damage or death.

## Technique

Fetal heart rate monitoring is used as a screening tool to detect nonreassuring heart rate patterns, and fetal blood gases are obtained after the failure of *in utero* treatment to correct such patterns. Indications for fetal blood sampling for measurement of pH are listed in Table 18–10. Withdrawal of blood for a pH should be obtained over the scalp or buttocks, not over the face, brow, or genitals, Other relative contraindications to be considered before performing this procedure are: (1) when the fetus has a known or suspected blood dyscrasia, hemophilia, or von Willebrand's disease; (2) when the procedure might require undesirable rupture of the membranes; (3) when there is vaginal bleeding; (4) when several previous scalp punctures have been made; (5) when the mother has either herpes simplex or human immunodeficiency virus; and (6) when the mother has a genital tract infection such as gonorrhea or $\beta$-hemolytic streptococcus.

To obtain a fetal blood sample for pH, the patient is placed in the Sims' or lithotomy position at the end of her bed or delivery table. Birthing beds providing leg support in the Sims' position are helpful in positioning the labor patient for this procedure. The presenting part is visualized through an endoscope, and debris are removed with long cotton-tipped applicators. Silicone cream is placed over the anticipated site to help contain the blood droplet. Increased blood perfusion of the fetal skin may be produced by spraying it with ethyl chloride. However, this method is not generally recommended, because it may alter the results of the blood tests. Once the skin is prepared, a single incision is made with a $2 \times 1.5$ mm blade. The sample of blood should be collected from free-flowing blood into a capillary tube. It is best to collect the sample between contractions, because values from samples obtained during decelerations may be falsely low.

After the sample has been collected, pressure should be applied to the incision site to prevent further bleeding. Other potential complications include (1) bleeding from sites during vacuum extraction; (2) scalp infections (usually fewer than 1 percent, which require only local treatment); (3) lacerations, which occasionally require suturing; and, (4) fetal death caused by exsanguination (rare). If a sinusoidal pattern is identified on the fetal monitor after a fetal blood sample, the fetus is assessed for excessive bleeding from the sampling site.

In current practice, pH determination is used primarily in a supportive or complementary role to electronic fetal heart rate monitoring. Academic institutions use pH determination more frequently than community hospitals, because many physicians have not been trained in the technique, and few hospitals have a micro–blood gas analyzer available 24 hours a day. Fetal heart rate monitoring has the advantage of providing a record that immediately reflects changes in the fetal condition, and it can be applied almost universally. During situations in which there is some question about the significance of a fetal heart rate pattern, a pH determination may help to clarify the problem.

## Interpretation

When the fetal heart patterns and blood gas tests agree, confidence in the diagnosis is increased whether they are both normal or abnormal.

It is difficult to establish exact limits of pH that would indicate when intervention is required. The range for normal fetal pH values is considerable. Table 18–11 is a summary of pH values from 14 different studies. Therefore, assessment of all parameters of blood gas sampling are helpful in patient management.

**Table 18–10**
INDICATIONS FOR FETAL BLOOD SAMPLING FOR pH

- Absent variability on initiation of monitoring without known cause
- Absent variability in the case of potential fetal hypoxia
- Late decelerations with decreasing variability when the problem is not resolved in a reasonable time (30 minutes)
- Unusual tracings, i.e., sinusoidal, arrhythmias
- Variable decelerations with baseline tachycardia and/or decreased variability

*Lesser Considerations for pH*
- Late decelerations with good variability that cannot be resolved
- Severe variable decelerations with good variability that cannot be resolved

**Table 18–11**
NORMAL FETAL ACID–BASE RANGE

|  | Lower Limits | Upper Limits |
|---|---|---|
| pH | 7.15 to 7.30 | 7.33 to 7.47 |
| $P_{CO_2}$ (mm Hg) | 22 to 34 | 50 to 67 |
| $P_{O_2}$ (mm Hg) | 7 to 17 | 23 to 36 |
| Base excess | −14.1 to 5.3 | −4.3 to +3.0 |

Modanlou and associates (1973) have clearly shown that the fetal pH decreases as labor progresses. There is also a correlation between fetal acidosis and progressively severe fetal heart rate patterns, as reported by Kubli and coworkers (1969) and by Renou and Wood (1974). Apgar scores correlate with fetal pH values in late labor, although there is considerable overlap. Hon and colleagues (1969) reported a false-normal rate of 20.1 percent and a false-abnormal rate of 57.7 percent. Bowe and coworkers (1969) reported a false-normal rate of 10.4 percent and a false-abnormal rate of 7.5 percent.

Conditions that may result in a false-normal pH (normal pH, low Apgar) include the following:

1. Maternal hyperventilation
2. Drugs
3. Airway obstruction (newborn)
4. Prematurity
5. Infection
6. Congenital anomalies
7. Asphyxia between sampling and delivery
8. Air contamination
9. Delivery trauma

Some causes of false-abnormal pH (low pH, normal Apgar) are

1. Contraction during sampling
2. Stage of labor when sampling was performed
3. Maternal acidosis
4. Anesthesia and analgesia
5. Small amount of bleeding from scalp, causing slow collection
6. Delay in analyzing the sample
7. Caput succedaneum

There is evidence that the fetal scalp blood is a reliable index of fetal central circulation. Bowe and coworkers (1969) reported a positive correlation between the pH of the scalp blood just prior to delivery and the pH of blood from the umbilical artery and vein.

Adamsons and coworkers, working with the rhesus monkey fetus, compared the pH of blood taken simultaneously from the fetal scalp and that from the carotid artery and jugular vein. They reported that capillary blood remained representative even under conditions of extreme asphyxia (Adamsons et al, 1975). The capillary blood more closely resembled the jugular venous blood.

Fetal blood pH values above 7.25 are considered normal, and the values should be measured again as indicated by the fetal heart rate pattern, labor progress, or other clinical parameters. Values between 7.20 and 7.25 are considered borderline, or *preacidotic,* and the values generally should be measured again within 15 to 30 minutes to detect the possibility of a downward trend in pH. A fetal blood pH below 7.20 is considered to be indicative of significant acidosis. An abnormally low pH (< 7.20) and a downward trend in pH values not associated with a correctable condition are indications for intervention.

# Fetal Evoked Response

## SCALP STIMULATION

Fetal scalp stimulation with associated fetal heart rate acceleration can reduce the need for scalp blood sampling. One hundred fetuses with tracings judged to be suggestive of fetal asphyxia were studied prospectively (Clark et al, 1984). Each fetus was stimulated by firm digital pressure on the scalp followed by a pinch with an atraumatic clamp, after which a scalp blood sampling was performed in the usual manner. If the fetal heart rate demonstrated an acceleration of 15 beats/min lasting 15 seconds, the pH was uniformly found to be greater than or equal to 7.20. Fifty-one of the fetuses responded with acceleration to the stimulation. Thirty-nine percent of those fetuses not responding with an acceleration of fetal heart rate were acidotic (pH < 7.20). Clinical application of scalp stimulation could reduce the necessity for scalp pH determination. It may also be useful when a vaginal examination may not permit a scalp blood sample or if scalp blood sampling is not available to the patient.

## ACOUSTIC STIMULATION

Use of fetal acoustic stimulation as a test of fetal well-being was first described by Read and Miller in 1977. Since that time, several investigations have confirmed the findings that fetal heart rate acceleration in response to acoustic stimulation is a sensitive test of fetal well-being. The correlation of fetal heart rate acceleration in response to vibroacoustic stimulation and fetal scalp blood pH was reported by Smith and co-workers (1986). As with direct fetal scalp stimulation, no fetus had an acceleration of fetal heart rate greater than or equal to 15 beats/min and lasting 15 seconds if the pH was less than 7.20.

# Umbilical Cord Blood Analysis

Analysis of venous and arterial cord blood samples provides an objective assessment of acid-base status at the time of birth. It is a useful adjunct to the Apgar score when assessing the newborn condition.

In the past, a low Apgar score often was considered to be synonymous with perinatal asphyxia. However, because asphyxia implies the presence of hypoxia with metabolic acidosis, the Apgar score alone cannot be used to indicate its existence. Also, low Apgar scores have been associated with congenital anomalies, sepsis, maternal drug administration, and other causes. Clearly, cord blood gas analysis is a more appropriate tool for use in assessing newborn acid-base status.

Even when acidosis is present, cord blood gas analysis can quantify the degree of acidosis and can determine whether the acidosis is metabolic or respiratory in nature. In the absence of metabolic acidosis, it is unlikely that a low Apgar score is due to intrapartum asphyxia.

The situations where one might benefit from cord blood acid-base analysis include

1. Nonreassuring fetal heart rate patterns
2. Meconium-stained amniotic fluid
3. Prematurity
4. Postdates
5. Intrauterine growth retardation
6. Infection
7. Abruptio placentae
8. Low Apgar score
9. Traumatic delivery

## TECHNIQUE

Because cord blood gas values can change rapidly after only 5 to 10 seconds of neonatal breathing, the cord must be double clamped immediately after delivery and preferably before the first breath (Lievaart and deJong, 1984). Two clamps should be placed close together several inches from the navel. With the clamping of the cord, umbilical circulation stops and gas values change very slowly, obviating any urgency to collect samples (Strickland, 1984). The cord may then be cut between the clamps and the infant handed to the nurse or the mother if the infant is stable. The second set of clamps is then placed approximately 8 to 10 inches from the first set. Then the cord is cut again between the second pair of clamps, providing a segment from which the samples are collected. Optimally, the blood is immediately drawn, placed on ice, then analyzed. However, if a delay is unavoidable, it is reassuring to note that leaving the cord segment at room temperature for up to 20 minutes creates only minimal changes in blood gas values (Strickland, 1984). The sample also can be maintained for up to 60 minutes in capped syringes.

Specimens are drawn into a 1-cc or 3-cc syringe with an 18- to 22-gauge needle that has been heparinized with a 1000 U/ml heparin solution. Excess air and heparin should be expelled prior to drawing the sample, because these elements may affect the results. The blood is removed first from the artery, because the larger distended vein adds turgor to the cord. It is advisable to insert the needle with the bevel facing upward to avoid insertion through the back wall of the artery into the vein. Next, the venous sample is collected from the prominent, single vein. If circumstances dictate that only one sample can be obtained, the artery should be chosen because arterial blood provides the most reliable indication of fetal acid-base status. However, if only venous blood is available, it can be analyzed. A mixed sample is least desirable; but if it is the only blood available, use it and mark it clearly as a venous and arterial blood sample. Note that most micro-analyzers require a minimum of 0.2 to 0.6 ml of blood. After the blood has been successfully obtained, the needles are plugged with clay or the caps are replaced and tightened.

Normal values for arterial and venous cord blood gases are listed in Table 18–12. These values were obtained from patients with uncomplicated labors at term that ended in spontaneous vaginal deliveries. Ramin and associates (1989), found that normal values for preterm infants born following uncomplicated pregnancies are similar to those of term infants.

Traditionally, neonatal acidosis has been defined as an umbilical artery pH of less than 7.2 (Gilstrap, 1987). However, values below 7.15 may be more important in terms of clinical significance. Table 18–12 offers further information to aid in the interpretation of cord blood gases with the assessment of $Pco_2$, $HCO_3$, and base deficit.

## Patient Education and the Team Approach

As is true with all types of medical and nursing care, thorough explanation of the procedure (in this case, fetal heart rate monitoring and fetal blood sampling) and its benefits and risks should be provided to the patient prior to the procedure. Because labor itself can be a stressful period for the patient, this information should be given prior to the onset of labor, preferably during the antepartum period. This ensures that parents will have time to digest the information, have their questions answered, and investigate the procedure more thoroughly, if desired. This encourages the woman (and her partner) to participate more fully in her plan of care.

Literature is an important supplementary source of information for the patient. Many doctors and hospitals provide a booklet explaining electronic fetal monitoring along with the hospital policy and procedure. Other information frequently is provided in childbirth education classes or during hospital tours.

After all the information is given and all questions are answered, the parents must decide whether or not they wish to have the monitor applied. In a normal (low-risk) pregnancy, there is little evidence that continuous fetal heart rate monitoring reduces perinatal mortality. Intermittent auscultation, according to ACOG guidelines (1989), is an acceptable method of intrapartum monitoring. Most practitioners agree that electronic fetal heart rate monitoring is beneficial in high-risk patients, although information in the literature is mixed regarding the reductions in perinatal morbidity and mortality.

Open communication benefits all health care practitioners. However, communication does not stop after the patient has consented to be monitored. In the event of nonreassuring fetal monitoring patterns, in which many manipulations and treatments may be carried out in a very hurried fashion, one member of the team must take responsibility for explaining what is being done *as* it is being done. Reassurance and comfort must be given to the patient continually. The entire perinatal team must work together in support of this mother, father, and fetus. Although many of these events are daily occurrences for the nurses and clinicians, they constitute a new experience for this family. When a decision is made to perform an emergency cesarean delivery, the health care practitioner must remember that the par-

**Table 18–12**
CORD BLOOD GASES

| | Normal Values | | | | | |
|---|---|---|---|---|---|---|
| | Arterial | | | Venous | | |
| | Mean | SD | Range | Mean | SD | Range |
| pH | 7.28 | 0.05 | 7.15 to 7.35 | 7.35 | 0.05 | 7.24 to 7.49 |
| $Pco_2$ (mm Hg) | 49.20 | 8.40 | 31.10 to 74.30 | 38.20 | 5.60 | 23.20 to 49.20 |
| $Po_2$ (mm Hg) | 18.00 | 6.20 | 3.30 to 33.80 | 29.20 | 5.90 | 15.40 to 48.20 |
| Bicarbonate (mEq/L) | 22.30 | 2.50 | 13.30 to 27.50 | 22.40 | 2.10 | 15.90 to 24.70 |

From Yoemans ER, Hauth JC, Gilstrap LC III, et al: Umbilical cord pH, $Pco_2$, $Po_2$, and bicarbonate following uncomplicated term vaginal deliveries. Am J Obstet Gynecol, 151(6):798, 1985.

ents are suffering tremendous anxiety. The parents should be given as much information and support at this time as the situation allows. After delivery, further explanation and support can be provided to help decrease anxiety. We, as professionals, often lose sight of this level of anxiety, which may remain with families for many years following this type of event.

Technology in obstetrics has advanced rapidly during the last 30 years and will continue to do so in the future. Obstetricians, nurse midwives, obstetric nurses, and all other members of the health care team have a responsibility to provide optimum care for the pregnant woman, her baby, and her family. Because diagnosis of fetal distress based on information provided by electronic fetal monitoring and fetal blood gas analysis is relatively new, these techniques and the possibilities they offer for optimum treatment of the fetus and newborn must be kept in perspective and be open to careful scrutiny and improvement. Advances are being made, and new equipment is being introduced, but there is still a great deal to be learned.

The current state of technology suggests that, in combination, fetal response to stimulation, electronic fetal monitoring, and fetal blood gas trends improve our ability to assess fetal status and predict fetal or neonatal distress. Other alternatives may yet be developed. While we try to absorb and at the same time perfect and improve on all this, it should be kept in mind that we are using high level technology to assist in one of the most human experiences life holds.

---

### Acknowledgment

Acknowledgment is given to Cydney I. Afriat, BSN, CNM, MSN, for her contribution to the first edition.

# References

ACOG: Assessment of fetal and newborn acid–base status. ACOG Technical Bulletin #127, April, 1989.

ACOG: Intrapartum fetal heart rate monitoring. ACOG Technical Bulletin #132, September, 1989.

Adamsons K, Beard RW, Myers RE: Comparison of the composition of arterial, venous, and capillary blood of the fetal monkey during labor. Am J Obstet Gynecol 107:435, 1975.

Afriat CI: The nurse's role in fetal heart rate monitoring. J Perinatol Neonatol 3:29, 1983.

Afriat CI, Schifrin BS: Sources of error in fetal heart rate monitoring. J Obstet Gynecol Neonatal Nurs 5(Suppl):5, 1976.

Anyaegbunam A, Brustman L, Divon M, et al: The significance of antepartum variable decelerations. Am J Obstet Gynecol 155:707, 1986.

Atterbury, JA, West, JW, Quirk JG, et al: Electronic fetal monitoring. In Quirk, JG (ed): Perinatal Educational Resource and Learning System. University of Arkansas for Medical Sciences, Little Rock, AR, 1992.

Beall RC, Paul RH: Artifacts, blocks and arrhythmias. Clin Obstet Gyn 29:84, 1987.

Bowe ET, Beard RW, Finster M, et al: Reliability of fetal blood sampling. Am J Obstet Gynecol 107:237, 1969.

Campbell WA, Vintzileos AM, Nochimson DJ: Intrauterine versus extrauterine management/resuscitation of the fetus/neonate. Clin Obstet Gynecol 29:33, 1986.

Clark S, Gimovsky M, Miller F: The scalp stimulation test: a clinical alternative to fetal scalp blood sampling. Am J Obstet Gynecol 148:274, 1984.

Cohen WR, Yeh SY: The abnormal fetal heart rate baseline. Clin Obstet Gynecol 29:73, 1986.

Fields LM: Electronic fetal monitoring: practices and protocols for the intrapartum patient. J Perinat Neonat Nurs 1:5, 1987.

Freeman RK, Garite TJ, Nageotte MP: Fetal Heart Rate Monitoring, 2nd ed. Baltimore, Williams & Wilkins, 1991.

Gilstrap LC, Hauth JC, Hankins GDV, et al: Second-stage fetal heart rate abnormalities and type of neonatal acidemia. Obstet Gynecol 70(2):191–195, 1987.

Hon, E: Detection of fetal distress. In C. Wood (ed): Fifth World Congress of Gynecology and Obstetrics. Sydney, Australia, 1967.

Hon EH, Khazin AF, Paul RH: Biochemical studies of the fetus. Obstet Gynecol 33:237, 1969.

Krebs HB, Peters RE, Dunn LJ: Intrapartum fetal heart rate monitoring. VIII. Atypical variable decelerations. Am J Obstet Gynecol 145:297, 1983.

Kubli FW, Hon EH, Khazin AF, et al: Observations on fetal heart rate and pH in the human fetus during labor. Am J Obstet Gynecol 104:1190, 1969.

Lievaart M, deJong PA: Acid-base equilibrium in umbilical cord blood and time of cord clamping. Obstet Gynecol 63:44, 1984.

Luthy DA, Shy KK, Van Belle A: Randomized trial of electronic fetal monitoring in preterm labor. Obstet Gynecol 69:687, 1987.

Miyazaki FS, Nevarez F: Saline amnioinfusion for relief of repetitive variable decelerations: A prospective randomized study. Am J Obstet Gynecol 153:301, 1985.

Modanlou HD, Yeh SY, Hon EH, et al: Clinical fetal monitoring. III. The evaluation and significance of intrapartum baseline fetal heart variability. Am J Obstet Gynecol 117:942, 1973.

NAACOG: Fetal heart rate auscultation. NAACOG Practice Resource #35, March, 1990.

Parer JT: Handbook of Fetal Heart Rate Monitoring. Philadelphia, WB Saunders Co, 1983.

Paul RH, Suidan AK, Yeh SY, et al: Clinical fetal monitoring. III. The evaluation and significance of intrapartum baseline fetal heart variability. Am J Obstet Gynecol 123:206, 1975.

Ramin SM, Gilstrap LC III, Leveno KJ, et al: Umbilical artery acid-base status in the preterm infant. Obstet Gynecol 74:256, 1989.

Read JA, Miller FC: Fetal heart rate acceleration in response to acoustic stimulation as a measure of fetal well-being. Am J Obstet Gynecol 129:512, 1977.

Reece EA, Antoine C, Montgomery J: The fetus as the final arbitrator of intrauterine stress/distress. Clin Obstet Gynecol 29:23, 1986.

Renou P, Wood C: Interpretation of the continuous fetal heart rate record. Clin Obstet Gynecol 1:191, 1974.

Saling EZ: Die Blutgasverhaltnisse und der sauve Basen-Haushalt der Feten bei ungerstörtem geburtsablauf. Z Geburtsh Gynaekol 161:262, 1964.

Schifrin BS: Exercises in Fetal Monitoring. St. Louis, Mosby Year Book, 1990.

Schneider EP, Topper P: The variable deceleration, prolonged deceleration, and sinusoidal fetal heart rate. Clin Obstet Gynecol 29:64, 1986.

Shields JR, Schifrin BS: Perinatal antecedents of cerebral palsy. Obstet Gynecol 71(6):899, 1988.

Shy KK, Larson EB, Luthy DA: Evaluating a new technology. Ann Rev Pub Health 8:165, 1989.

Shy KK, Luthy DA, Bennett FC, et al: Effects of electronic fetal heart rate monitoring as compared with periodic auscultation on the neurologic development of premature infants. N Engl J Med 322(9):588, 1990.

Smith CV, Mguyan HN, Phelan JP, Paul RH: Intrapartum assessment of fetal well-being: a comparison of fetal acoustic stimulation with acid–base determinations. Am J Obstet Gynecol 155:726, 1986.

Strickland DM, Gilstrap LC III, Hauth JC, et al: Umbilical cord pH and $pCO_2$: Effect of interval from delivery to determination. Am J Obstet Gynecol 148(2):191–193, 1984.

Tucker SM: Pocket Guide—Fetal Monitoring, 2nd ed. St. Louis, Mosby Year Book, 1992.

Yippö, A: Ueber Magenalmung beim Menschen. München Med Wchnschr 63:1650, 1916.

Yoemans ER, Hauth JC, Gilstrap LC, Strickland DM: Umbilical cord pH, $P_{CO_2}$, $P_{O_2}$, and bicarbonate following uncomplicated term vaginal deliveries. Am J Obstet Gynecol 151(6):798, 1985.

# CHAPTER 19

# Cesarean Birth

Jeffrey P. Phelan, Abbe Bendell, and Vicki G. Colburn

Twentieth century technology has produced many changes, with some of the most dramatic having occurred in medicine. In obstetrics, in particular, management of the pregnant mother and her fetus and neonate have undergone overwhelming changes.

Prior to the availability of anesthesia, suture material, antibiotics, and blood, the incidence of recorded cesarean births was low. Because the risks were excessive, with a maternal death rate of almost 100 percent, it is doubtful that the physician would have attempted such a risky procedure. Even at the beginning of this century, when suture material and chloroform were available, cesarean birth was extremely rare.

Edith Potter's studies early in this century indicated that intracranial bleeding was the leading cause of perinatal mortality (Hoffman, 1982). Later, Friedman's work showed the relationship of prolonged labor and forceps delivery to poor perinatal outcome (Friedman, 1989). As a result of these and other studies, there has been a progressive decrease in the incidence of operative vaginal deliveries and a concomitant increase in the cesarean birth rate. This is not a direct cause and effect relationship, because many other factors have contributed to these changes. Most of all, there has been a shift in focus from the mother to the fetus (Phelan, 1990). For example, changing attitudes toward infant survival, quality of life, and limited family size have resulted in continued changes in obstetric management. Neonatal intensive care units and the development of the subspecialty areas of neonatology and maternal-fetal medicine have also contributed considerably to these changing attitudes and improved survival rates.

What is not known is whether long-term infant morbidity is affected by the increased cesarean birth rate. By morbidity, we refer to mental retardation, cerebral palsy, and birth trauma, which may or may not be directly labor related. Not to be ignored is the legal climate and the attitude of families toward complications during the course of pregnancy, labor, and delivery that may ultimately affect the outcome of the pregnancy. To reduce the morbidity rates, hospital committees have been formed to review cesarean deliveries. It should be noted that although abnormal outcomes are often attributed to events surrounding labor and delivery, the damage may, in fact, have occurred prior to labor.

## Maternal Mortality and Morbidity

In the United States, maternal mortality associated with cesarean birth was 2 percent for the period from 1933 to 1939 and decreased to 0.2 percent for the period from 1949 to 1956 (Cohen, 1982). This decline appears to be associated with (1) improved blood bank facilities, (2) antibiotics, (3) improved anesthesia, (4) change in surgical technique from the classic cesarean birth to the low segment transverse procedure, and (5) improved maternal status prior to surgery. A study by Sachs and associates (1990) reported a maternal mortality rate from 1976 to 1984 of 0.06 percent from cesarean birth as compared with an overall maternal mortality of 0.027 percent (Slee, 1976). Hemorrhage; hypertensive disorders, with their associated cardiovascular complications; and infection account for the majority of the deaths. Interestingly, the classic cesarean birth, which accounted for 4 percent of all cesarean births, was performed in 13 percent of the patients who subsequently died. The Report of Confidential Enquiries into Maternal Deaths in England and Wales from 1982 to 1984 quotes a mortality rate of 0.037 in cesarean births.

Although mortality rates have been reduced, morbidity rates with cesarean birth remains high (20 to 80 percent). In the majority of instances, this morbidity is relatively benign (e.g., endomyometritis, urinary tract infection, anemia, wound infection, atelectasis); however, a small percentage of patients develop major complications, such as wound dehiscence, evisceration, pneumonia, thrombophlebitis, pulmonary embolus, and pelvic or abdominal abscesses. Some of these complications can be prevented by the routine use of prophylactic antibiotics. On the other hand, their use can be limited to specific instances that predispose to maternal morbidity, such as prolonged labor with ruptured membranes, in which the risk of infection is higher than it is in the routine elective repeat cesarean birth. More recently, irrigation of operative wounds, including the uterine wound and uterine cavity, has been suggested as an alternative to the administration of prophylactic antibiotics. This is performed using saline or antibiotics.

# Definition and Incidence of Cesarean Birth

Cesarean birth is the transabdominal delivery of an intrauterine fetus or fetuses weighing 500 g or more through a uterine or cervical incision. To quote Webster, it is "the operation of taking a child from the uterus by cutting through the walls of the abdomen and the uterus."

The incidence of cesarean birth has changed considerably over the last decades. In the 1930s and early 1940s, the cesarean birth rate was 2.6 to 3.0 percent. Following World War II and throughout the 1950s, the rate increased to 4 percent. However, since 1960s, the increase has been more precipitous, so that at the present time, the rate varies somewhere between 12 and 50 percent.

## TYPES OF CESAREAN BIRTH

Cesarean births are categorized by the type of uterine incision, as follows (Fig. 19–1):

I.  **Low Segment**—an incision in the isthmic or cervical portion of the uterus
    A. Transverse (Munro Kerr)
    B. Vertical (Beck or Krönig)
II. **Classic**—an incision in the fundus of the uterus
    A. Longitudinal
    B. Transverse (rare)
III. **Extraperitoneal**—a low-segment incision without entering the intra-abdominal cavity
    A. Transverse (Waters)
    B. Vertical (Latzko)
IV. **Postmortem**—uterine incision, generally fundal, performed shortly after maternal death

**Low Segment.** The lower uterine segment incision may be difficult technically, compared with the classic incision (discussed later). Nonetheless, in experienced hands, delivery occurs within a few minutes, in the absence of complications. There is less bleeding intraoperatively, because the blood supply and muscle thickness are less than those in the fundus. The major advantage is that the uterine incision is retroperitoneal. This approach protects the peritoneal cavity from infection and decreases the incidence of adhesions forming postoperatively. Moreover, a patient with an incision in the lower uterine segment can have an attempted vaginal delivery in a subsequent pregnancy. For these reasons, this is the procedure of choice. A technical disadvantage of the low-segment incision is the risk of extension into the broad ligament, resulting in laceration of the uterine arteries. This risk can be minimized by using scissors to cut the lower segment rather than separating it with the fingers. The advantage of finger separation is decreased blood loss. The low vertical incision is often indicated for the delivery of the premature breech, transverse lie, and fundally

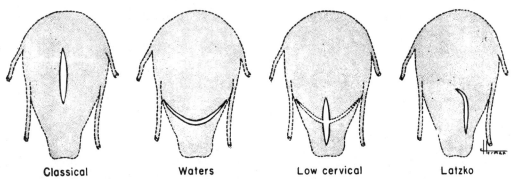

Classical        Waters        Low cervical        Latzko

**Figure 19–1.** Uterine incisions for cesarean sections. (From Quilligan E, Zuspan F, Douglas-Stromme Operative Obstetrics, 4th ed. New York, Appleton-Century-Crofts. 1982.)

located anterior placenta praevia. It has, however, the disadvantage of a risk of extension toward the vagina. Often, because of poor development of the lower uterine segment, the incision must be extended into the upper segment of the uterus and becomes a classic incision.

**Classic.** The classic cesarean operation was the standard procedure in the early part of the 20th century. By the late 1930s and mid 1940s, the classic cesarean was being replaced by the low-segment technique. At the present time, the classic procedure is seldom performed. The low-segment operation is preferred because of improved maternal results. The postoperative course is less morbid, and the chance of rupture of the lower segment is far less than that of rupture of the classic incision. Twenty-five percent of classic scar ruptures occur prior to the onset of labor.

The advantage of the classic incision is rapid delivery of the infant. Disadvantages include a higher risk of infection, greater blood loss, a potentially more morbid postoperative course, and a greater long-term risk of rupture.

Although the classic procedure is seldom performed today, it still has several possible indications. Among these are (1) a back down transverse lie, especially in patients in whom development of the lower uterine segment is poor; (2) an anterior low-lying placenta; (3) extensive lower uterine segment varicosities or myomas; (4) adhesions as a result of previous surgery, which makes exposure difficult; and (5) the rare situation in which the uterus is adherent to the anterior abdominal wall, making identification of the lower uterine segment impossible.

**Extraperitoneal.** The extraperitoneal section is rarely performed in modern obstetrics, because, even in the presence of overt infection, the use of antibiotics appears to provide sufficient protection for the patient. The theoretical advantage of this procedure is protection of the intra-abdominal cavity from exposure to contaminated or infected intrauterine contents. Its disadvantages include technical difficulty performing the operation, which involves staying outside the abdominal cavity and at the same time not entering the bladder. The procedure takes longer because of these difficulties. In spite of this, and even in the most careful hands, the peritoneum may be inadvertently entered. Few obstetricians are trained to perform the procedure.

**Postmortem.** The postmortem cesarean is also rarely performed. It is performed within moments of maternal death to avoid fetal death or injury. Anesthesia and sterile technique are unnecessary. Any scalpel or knife that can cut through the abdominal and uterine cavities can be used. The purpose is to deliver a live infant who has a reasonable chance of survival. Often, however, the decision is made too late to affect survival. Whenever there is a critically ill pregnant patient, preparations should be made for a postmortem section if there is any possibility the mother might die. Of course, whenever possible, the procedure should be discussed with the family. Attempts at resuscitation of the mother precede attempts at delivery of the infant. However, unless an endotracheal tube is in place with adequate oxygenation of the mother, a period of greater than 15 minutes of resuscitation decreases the chances of delivering a liveborn normal infant.

## INDICATIONS FOR CESAREAN BIRTH

The standard indications for abdominal delivery are listed in Table 19–1. Because of the potential risk of uterine scar rupture, previous cesarean birth or any other operative procedure that involved entry into the uterine cavity through the myometrium (e.g., myomectomy, Strassman's procedure, or hysterotomy) historically has been considered an indication for a repeat cesarean delivery.

Among the indications listed under dystocia in Table 19–1, absolute cephalopelvic disproportion is rare but may be recognizable at initial clinical pelvimetry. In most if not all of the patients, a trial of labor is necessary to fully determine the adequacy of the maternal pelvis. Other conditions listed under this heading often are not discovered until after the onset of labor. Some may be obvious in early labor, including malpresentations such as a transverse lie, and a tumor obstructing the birth canal. Others may not be diagnosed until the later stages of labor, such as relative cephalopelvic disproportion. As previously mentioned, the presence of borderline clinical pelvimetry demands a trial of labor to determine whether or not the fetus will negotiate the maternal pelvis. Arrest of progress for 2 hours in active labor, in the presence of ruptured membranes, with no evidence of disproportion, and good uterine contractions with oxytocin stimulation, may be the result of uterine dysfunction, cervical dystocia, or even unrecognized positional cephalopelvic disproportion. Cervical dystocia usually is preceded by a history of cervical surgery, such as cone biopsy, encirclage, or surgical repair of previous cervical trauma, that has resulted in cervical fibrosis or scarring, which prevents progressive cervical dilatation despite good uterine activity in the absence of disproportion.

Malpresentations include transverse lie, brow, and persistent mentum posterior. A floating brow presentation in early labor, in the presence of intact membranes, may, with continued contractions, flex to a vertex or further deflex to a face presentation. Once the membranes are ruptured, the aforementioned event is unlikely. In a brow presentation, the diameter presenting to the pelvis is the occipitomental, which, at term, is approximately 13 cm. A fetus with a persistent brow presentation is unlikely to get through the pelvis. For a persistent mentum posterior, there is no way to deliver the fetus vaginally without inducing an injury. Therefore, the fetus must be delivered abdominally. However, this diagnosis cannot be established until late in labor, because the mentum does not rotate until it reaches the pelvic floor. Fortunately, about two thirds of all fetuses presenting as a mentum posterior rotate and deliver vaginally. In present-day obstetrics, however, there are some who believe that all primigravidas with a face presentation (mentum) in labor should be delivered abdominally, especially if the fetus is in the mentum posterior position, regardless of the station.

Placenta praevia is usually diagnosed either as an incidental finding on routine sonography or when painless vaginal bleeding is a presenting symptom. These patients generally are managed conservatively, because marginal or low-lying placentas seldom present a problem as gestation progresses. With progressive uterine growth, the placental location appears to rise as the lower uterine segment undergoes continued development. If bleeding is excessive, the pregnancy lasts longer than 37 weeks or more, or both, there is little room for procrastination, and one may proceed to double set-up (vaginal examination in the operating room with a team scrubbed for immediate cesarean delivery) or proceed directly to cesarean deliv-

### Table 19–1
STANDARD INDICATIONS FOR CESAREAN BIRTH

**Previous Cesarean Birth or Uterine Surgery**
**Dystocia**
    Cephalopelvic disproportion
    Pelvic contraction
    Malpresentation
    Uterine dysfunction
    Cervical dystocia
    Tumor obstructing birth canal
**Hemorrhage**
    Placenta praevia
    Abruptio placentae
    Vasa previa
**Fetal Distress**
    Prolapsed cord
**Failed Induction**
**Miscellaneous**
    Premature rupture of membranes
    Hypertensive disorders of pregnancy
    Elderly primigravida
    Rh incompatibility
    Previous successful vaginal plastic surgery
    Invasive cervical cancer

ery without a double set-up based on an ultrasound diagnosis alone. An obvious abruptio placentae, without labor or in the presence of fetal distress, requires delivery by the most expeditious route, which is likely to be a cesarean birth. A very rare cause of vaginal bleeding is vasa praevia. This condition presents as fetal distress after amniotomy (spontaneous or artificial), associated with vaginal bleeding with no apparent evidence of abruption. The bleeding in such cases is fetal. Because the term infant's circulating blood volume is only 350 to 375 ml, a significant loss is 80 to 100 ml. The diagnosis should be suspected when bleeding occurs at amniotomy and can be confirmed by an Apt test.

Prior to the era of electronic monitoring, fetal distress was usually diagnosed on the basis of bradycardia, and irregular fetal heart rate, or both, especially if associated with meconium. This condition was a rare indication for a cesarean birth. In fact, prolapsed cord was more commonly the cause of fetal distress and, therefore, a more common indication for cesarean birth. With the advent of electronic fetal monitoring, however, there has been a whole new approach to this area. The diagnosis of fetal distress is now frequently based on fetal heart rate patterns. Some contend this approach has resulted in an increase in the number of abdominal deliveries performed for fetal distress.

Little has changed over the years with regard to the remaining indications listed in Table 19–1, and all are still acceptable reasons for performing a cesarean delivery.

Table 19–2, listing newer indications for cesarean delivery, reflects an increased awareness of the fetus and its chances of survival because of the development of the fields of maternal fetal medicine and neonatology. Experience indicates that the better the condition of the neonate at delivery, the better its chances of survival without long-term handicaps. It is now generally accepted that the small premature breech is best delivered abdominally, although some controversy still exists because of the absence of well-controlled studies. One major reason for abdominal delivery is the hypoxia that might occur during vaginal delivery as a result of cord compression as the small body is delivered through the incompletely dilated cervix, which then results in further hypoxia and trauma as the head is trapped behind the cervix. Premature neonates of less than 33

**Table 19–2**
NEWER INDICATIONS FOR
CESAREAN BIRTH

**Breech presentation**
  In primigravida
  With premature infant
  All breeches
**Macrosomia (fetus greater than 4000 g)**
**Herpes genitalis**
**Placental insufficiency**
**Severe preeclampsia or eclampsia with an unripe cervix**
**Multiple gestation**
**Failed progress in labor**
  Failure to descend
  Failure to dilate
**Fetal distress, as indicated by:**
  Fetal heart rate patterns
  Acid-base balance
**Fetal anomalies diagnosed by ultrasound**
  Meningomyelocele
  Severe prune-belly syndrome
  Hydrocephaly
  Encephalocele
  Conjoined twins
  Gastroschisis/omphalocele
**Maternal cerebral aneurysm**

weeks' gestation have a higher incidence of intracerebral bleeding, probably because of immaturity of the subependymal vessels. Trauma, hypoxia, and changes in cerebral blood flow increase these risks. The most commonly associated factor with intracerebral bleeding is young gestational age; however, hyaline membrane disease is also an associated factor, as are intubation and the administration of bolus fluids. There are some who believe that all small premature infants should be delivered by cesarean birth to prevent intracerebral bleeding; however, this subject generates even more controversy than abdominal delivery of the breech. The best candidate for vaginal breech delivery is the term fetus with a frank breech presentation, a well-flexed head, no evidence of nuchal arms, and weight of less than 4000 g and whose mother is a multipara with normal gynecoid pelvic measurements. Finally, the most important factor is that a vaginal breech delivery be conducted by an experienced obstetrician.

As the weight of the term infant increases, the risks of trauma during vaginal delivery increase; therefore, it is recommended that macrosomic infants (birth weight >4000 g) be considered for cesarean delivery. Macrosomia is associated with an increased incidence of shoulder dystocia, fractures of the clavicle or humerus, Erb-Duchenne paralysis (brachial plexus palsy), hypoxia, anoxia, and maternal trauma.

Herpes genitalis that is active at the time of delivery is associated with an increased risk of neonatal herpes, which has high rates of infant morbidity and mortality; thus, active herpes is now an accepted indication for cesarean birth regardless of the duration of ruptured membranes. Patients with previously active disease and asymptomatic carriers may deliver vaginally provided they have no lesion present at the time of delivery.

Abdominal delivery of the fetus may be indicated when biochemical or biophysical tests indicate placental insufficiency, which may cause deterioration of fetal well-being in the intrapartum period. However, in the presence of a nonreactive nonstress test and a positive contraction stress test or a nonreassuring biophysical profile, a trial of labor is reasonable with a ripe cervix and a normal presentation, because these tests have a high false-positive rate. It is important to point out that fetal well-being must be established prior to aggressive use of oxytocin. If evidence of fetal distress is found in labor, expeditious delivery is desirable.

In the presence of an acute severe hypertensive disorder of pregnancy, eclampsia, or both, in the interests of both mother and infant, rapid stabilization and control are essential, followed by delivery by the most expeditious route. If the cervix is inducible, then attempted vaginal delivery is preferable; otherwise, cesarean delivery may be the procedure of choice.

There are some who believe that all multiple gestations should be delivered abdominally. Certainly, when there is malpresentation of the first infant, or if there are more than two infants, there is general agreement that cesarean delivery is the procedure of choice. If twin A is a vertex, regardless of the presentation of twin B, and labor progresses normally, twin A should be allowed to deliver vaginally. The management of twin B depends on the presentation, fetal condition, and experience of the delivering physician.

Failed progress or secondary arrest, one of the most common indications listed for cesarean birth (in contrast to 15 to 20 years ago), appears to include the older standard indications of uterine dysfunction, cervical dystocia, and positional dystocia, which at the present time are almost never listed as indications. Failed progress is described as failure to dilate, failure to descend, or both. It is diagnosed in a laboring patient with ruptured membranes and no evidence of cephalopelvic disproportion who is having good uterine contractions but who has not progressed after a reasonable period of time despite oxytocin augmentation. Some physicians use a 2-hour limit; however, each patient must be evaluated individually and consulted. Depending on her birth plans, given a reassuring fetal heart rate pattern, the time frame should remain flexible. Because current obstetric practice favors the active management of labor, there is a reluctance to implement the older practice of resting such a patient with sedation for a few hours and then allowing her to resume labor to determine whether or not she will deliver vaginally.

Since the advent of electronic fetal monitoring, there has been an increase in the incidence of cesarean birth for fetal distress. This development is related to changes in the definition of fetal distress and to our overall attitude toward the quality of the neonate. Unfortunately, abnormalities detected on electronic heart rate monitoring alone may not be sufficient to make the diagnosis of fetal distress. They do alert the obstetrician to those infants who are likely to have acidosis and, therefore, should be used wherever possible, in combination with fetal pH determinations. This approach results in a more accurate diagnosis and should decrease the incidence of overdiagnosis of fetal distress. Once the diagnosis of fetal distress is made, delivery should be undertaken in a timely manner.

When a fetus is diagnosed with an anomaly, the route of delivery must be considered. Often, cesarean delivery is preferred over the vaginal route. These instances include meningomyelocele, gastroschisis, and omphalocele. Also, cesarean delivery should be considered for any fetal anomaly that is likely to obstruct vaginal delivery. These include prune-belly syndrome, conjoined twins, and omphalocele.

# Choice of Skin Incision

The choice of abdominal incision depends on many factors. The easier incisions are vertical, midline, and paramedian. The advantages of the vertical incision include decreased blood loss and operating time. The disadvantages are the cosmetic location of the scar and the minimal postoperative risk of decreased healing, resulting in dehiscence, evisceration, or both. Over the last few decades, probably as a result of the popularity of bikini swimsuits, the transverse abdominal incision has gained increasing popularity. This incision is technically more difficult. There are two types of transverse incisions used obstetrically. One is the Pfannenstiel, which involves incising the skin and fascia transversely. The fascia is then dissected off the underlying rectus muscle. The muscle is separated in the midline, and the peritoneum is opened longitudinally. The other is the Joel-Cohen incision, in which the abdomen also is entered through a transverse incision in the skin and fascia. However, the fascia is not separated from the muscle, and the peritoneum is incised transversely. The latter is associated with a lower incidence of seromas and less blood loss than with the Pfannenstiel incision.

## Physical and Psychologic Preparation of the Patient

Because 12 to 50 percent of pregnant women are delivered by cesarean means, all patients should be prepared for this possibility. At times, the obstetrician can predict a cesarean delivery based on the medical problems of the patient, her past obstetric performance, the size of her pelvis and her infant, and fetal anomalies. Once it becomes apparent during the course of pregnancy that cesarean delivery is likely, this should be expressed to the patient and her family. The patient and physician then have time to discuss the procedure, the possible presence of family members in the operating room, anesthesia choices, and operative risks. The patient may be given the opportunity to meet the anesthesiologist in order to discuss various anesthetic choices and their risks. Finally, she should have an opportunity to meet the nurses on the labor floor and become familiar with those who will be providing direct care for her. Many childbirth education courses include cesarean delivery in their format, which is helpful for those patients who may come to abdominal delivery unexpectedly. Additionally, there are childbirth education classes specifically for the cesarean birth or vaginal birth after cesarean.

Some women perceive cesarean childbirth as a failure of their reproductive performance and, as a result may become hostile and depressed. Physicians and nurses must be aware of this, provide adequate explanations, and be understanding. There is even the rare patient who refuses surgery under any circumstances so that a court order may become necessary. Although this behavior may incite anger on the part of the staff dealing with her, one must accept the fact that understanding is far more important than anger, and gentle urging is far more successful than force.

The type of anesthesia to be selected depends on the indication for surgery, the expertise of the anesthesiologist, and the preferences of the patient and her obstetrician. In cases of bleeding, such as in placenta praevia or abruptio placentae, or when there is acute fetal distress, the choice of anesthesia is usually general. Regional block is contraindicated because of the associated sympathetic blockade, which reduces the patient's ability to vasoconstrict her splanchnic vessels to compensate for blood loss.

Prior to any elective cesarean delivery, it is essential that fetal maturity be established. This can be based on the last menstrual period, uterine size at the first prenatal visit, fetal heart tones at 20 weeks with a DeLee stethoscope, and an early ultrasound before 24 weeks. If these are compatible in an otherwise uncomplicated pregnancy, amniocentesis for fetal lung maturity is not essential. Also, if there is sonographic evidence of fetal lung maturity, such as biparietal diameter (BPD) greater than or equal to 9.2 cm, femur length (FL) greater than or equal to 7.3 cm, or grade III placenta in a patient with a negative diabetes screen, elective cesarean delivery can be undertaken. If this is not the case, or if the pregnancy is complicated by a maternal medical condition such as diabetes, then amniotic fluid studies for fetal lung maturity are considered. Awaiting the spontaneous onset of labor usually provides assurance that the fetus is as mature as possible. However, this approach may result in a cesarean birth, which may come at an inconvenient time and may increase the risk of maternal morbidity such as aspiration during anesthesia if the mother recently has eaten.

The physician and the nurse begin the education and preparation of the patient during her prenatal course, especially when elective cesarean has been chosen. Because of third party reimbursement policies, many elective cesarean births are performed as same day admissions to decrease the length of hospital stay. Therefore, the preadmission and ambulatory work-up is scheduled and completed while the patient is receiving out-patient care. Autologous blood donation programs offered by hospitals give the patient the ability to bank her own blood in the antepartal period for her own use (Tighe and Sweezy, 1990). For those patients undergoing morning surgeries, innovative methods to provide preoperative orientation and teaching need to be considered (e.g., sessions in physicians' offices and appointments at the hospital for teaching prior to the day of surgery). The amount of ongoing information, its level of detail, and its necessity increase the nurse's essential role after hospital admission in preparing the patient for her hospital stay.

On admission, a thorough history is taken, and a physical assessment is performed, including fetal heart rate and fetal position. This is a good time to assess the patient's understanding of her need for surgery, her expectations, and her overall attitude toward the procedure. The admission laboratory studies include a complete blood count; a serology, if not performed during the last 6 weeks of gestation, and blood type; Rh; antibodies, where necessary; and a urinalysis. In some hospitals, a crossmatch is routine, whereas in others, type and screening are sufficient but only in the absence of specific antibodies. If unusual antibodies are present, then crossmatched blood is necessary. In areas where HIV infection and hepatitis are epidemic, many doctors are screening for these communicable diseases, either during prenatal care or prior to surgery. When there has been no prenatal care, these tests should be encouraged.

The patient who is admitted the day before surgery should be oriented to her new environment in the hospital. She is taught how to work the call light and the mechanics of her electric bed and where the bathroom, shower, and lounge are located; and, finally, she is encouraged to visit the newborn nursery. Many hospitals provide a tour of the labor and delivery suite or operating room, so that the parturient can see where her surgery will be performed. A preoperative educational checklist (Table 19–3) is helpful to make certain that patient education is completed.

**Table 19–3**
PREOPERATIVE TEACHING LIST

Preparation for O.R.
  Removal of cosmetics, glasses, contact lenses, jewelry
  Catheter
  Preoperative medications
  Role of care givers
Location of delivery and transportation to and from
  Stretcher/wheelchair
  Waiting on call in operating and delivery area
Anesthesia—type and procedure
  General
  Regional
Involvement in birth process
  Patient
  Family and significant other
Recovery room procedures
  Intravenous fluids
  Oxygen mask/inspirometer
  Transfer to postpartum area
Postpartum and operative care and expectations
  Respiratory assistance
  Ambulation
  Pain relief
  Engorgement and postpartum blues
Involvement in newborn care
  Bonding
  Feeding—breast/bottle
  Newborn care

Time is set aside to prepare the patient psychologically for surgery, to ascertain her past surgical experience, and to start her preoperative teaching. Some hospitals have slide and tape presentations that give a step-by-step account of the cesarean birth as experienced from the patient's viewpoint (Alley, 1981). If such a presentation is not available, a detailed description should be given regarding the transport to the operating room, the intravenous infusion, the abdominal preparation, and the Foley catheter. The procedure for anesthesia should be described.

Preparation of the abdomen prior to surgery is a source of controversy among surgeons. There are several divergent opionions relative to scrubbing and shaving that need to be acknowledged. Some believe that an abdominal preparation includes washing and shaving the abdomen. An antibacterial soap is commonly used, and in some hospitals, a 20-minute scrub or an antiseptic shower the night before surgery is routine. Some shave the entire abdomen, whereas others shave only the area of the expected incision. Some shave the night before surgery, others just before surgery. The patient should be educated in the timing of these preparations, because she may be awake in the operating room during these preparatory procedures and have concern that she will not be asleep before the incision is made.

Preparing the patient for postoperative care before surgery and telling her of the necessity for deep breathing and use of an incentive spirometer or balloons are helpful.

It is important to encourage the parturient to express her feelings about the upcoming surgical birth experience. Patients express a variety of feelings such as fear of pain and disfigurement and fear of being unable to mother their babies. Others express a sense of relief that the pregnancy is finally coming to an end so that motherhood can begin. It is safe to assume that patients will experience some preoperative anxiety; therefore, enough time should be provided to reassure the patient and to allow her to voice her concerns (Affonso and Stickler, 1978).

Often, a father or a significant other expresses concern for the safety of the mother and child. Some fathers experience guilt or disappointment that childbirth cannot be achieved in the conventional manner (Clark and Affonso, 1979). Many couples express concern over the increased financial burden of a surgical delivery. Once again, parent education may help to allay these fears.

The birth experience should be as close to normal as possible. Most hospitals provide family-centered surgical births, allowing the father to be present during the surgery to support the mother and to hold their newborn baby. Mothers are also encouraged to hold their babies shortly after delivery, to facilitate bonding. When this process occurs, couples have described the experience positively and demonstrated a genuine enjoyment of the birth process (Gawse, 1982).

If this is the patient's first experience with surgery, it could be beneficial to introduce her to a woman who has undergone surgery 4 or 5 days previously or to call a volunteer representative from the local chapter of the Cesarean Section Support Group or the Childbirth Education Association. Interaction with someone who has experienced surgical birth and perceives it in a positive fashion helps to set a favorable emotional climate (Conklin, 1977).

Ultimately, emphasis should be placed on a healthy, positive outcome for mother and baby. Because abdominal delivery has become so common for a large percentage of the population, it should be viewed simply as an alternative to vaginal birth. It is hoped that the emergence of this attitude continues to open surgical birth experiences to those who desire a family-centered birth. More hospitals, physicians, and nurses now recognize that couples should not be excluded from the shared fulfillment of childbirth, wherever and whenever possible (Donovan and Allen, 1977).

# Intraoperative Care

Most hospitals use a preoperative checklist to ensure thorough preparation for surgery. All requirements must be fulfilled, including consent forms, history, and physical and laboratory work. Preparation of the patient for surgery often includes removal of dentures, contact lenses, jewelry, hairpins, and hairpieces or wigs. No nail polish or cosmetics should be worn, because these may give a false appearance of color to the lips, face, and nail beds. The patient should be wearing a hospital gown, and all underwear should have been removed. She should be *nulla per os* (NPO). The patient should either void on call or have the Foley catheter inserted. Some surgeons may prefer the Foley catheter to be inserted after the epidural anesthesia has been initiated. Although this saves the patient from experiencing any physical pain, some have expressed embarrassment at having such an intrusive procedure performed in an operating room with so many people present. Blood administration tubing should be used for the intravenous in case the need for blood arises.

Some of these preoperative procedures may be perceived as a threat to a young mother who is particular about her grooming and appearance. Simple explanations about what to expect are helpful before and during the procedures. Insertion of the Foley catheter and the intravenous line are sometimes described by patients as traumatic events. Many patients better express their worries and fears during these procedures; therefore, it is advisable to encourage discussion during preparation.

The patient's identification plate should be sent to the operating and delivery suite with the chart so that intraoperative financial charges and labels can be facilitated. In some hospitals, the intraoperative records are generated and sent to the operating room along with baby bracelets and footprint sheets.

These may be filled out in advance (except for the time of delivery and sex of the baby), thus reducing the amount of paperwork at the time of delivery. On arrival at the operating area, the preoperative checklist is again reviewed by the circulating nurse.

Many anesthesiologists order an antacid, such as cimetidine (Tagamet) or ranitidine (Zantac), prior to surgery. Cimetidine is given orally, whereas ranitidine may be given intravenously 30 minutes prior to surgery. Both drugs reduce the acidity of the stomach contents, thereby decreasing the risk of Mendelson's syndrome (aspiration pneumonitis). In addition, a nonparticulate antacid such as sodium citrate is preferable to the colloidal antacids because aspiration of the colloidal antacids may contribute to the syndrome.

Before the patient enters the operating room, a preoperative inspection of the room is important. The delivery table should be checked to make sure that the Trendelenburg and lateral tilt positions work (Fig. 19–2). A safety strap and armrests should be available. The supply cupboard should have adequate quantities of intravenous and irrigating fluids, as well as a proper supply of sutures and other necessary surgical supplies. Irrigation solutions should be prewarmed. A blood warmer and a rapid infusion pump are available and functioning, and suction equipment is functional.

The anesthesia cart and equipment should be inspected. Usually, this is performed by the anesthesia staff. Adequate supplies of drugs should be on hand. A separate compartment may be used to keep controlled drugs; these must be checked priodically for expiration dates, and replacements are made as necessary.

The infant laryngoscope, ambu bag, face mask, airways, and intubation equipment should be present and functioning. If the laryngoscope shows a dull yellow light, the batteries, the bulb, or both should be replaced. The necessary pediatric drugs and dosages should be available in case the need for them arises for emergency resuscitation. An umbilical vessel catheter and introducer kit should be on hand (American Heart Association, 1990). It is important to check the heating element in the infant warmer. The temperature should range from 36.6° to 37.2°C (96° to 99°F). A supply of prewarmed blankets should be available to dry the baby. The necessary equipment for infant identification procedures must be available.

Finally, surgical lamps should be functioning, and the thermostat should be set at 22.2°C (72°F) so that the patient and infant will not suffer from environmental hypothermia (Bacon et al, 1981). A preoperative room inspection checklist is shown in Table 19–4.

Once the room has passed scrutiny, the scrub technician sets up a sterile field and prepares the instruments and drapes for surgery (Fig. 19–3). The first count of sponges, instruments, and needles is accomplished and recorded at this time (AORN, 1991).

When the patient is brought into the room, she is assisted onto the table. If already in place, the Foley catheter is placed under the

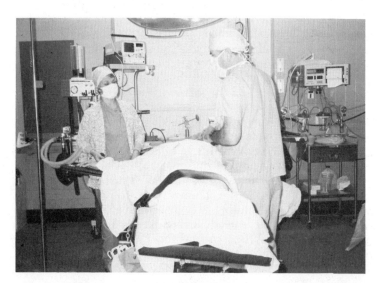

**Figure 19–2.** The patient is positioned in a lateral tilt to the left.

**Table 19–4**
PREOPERATIVE ROOM INSPECTION

| | Yes | No |
|---|---|---|
| 1. Suction equipment functional | ☐ | ☐ |
| 2. Delivery table functional | | |
|   a. Trendelenburg | ☐ | ☐ |
|   b. Lateral tilt | ☐ | ☐ |
|   c. Foot of bed | ☐ | ☐ |
|   d. Arm rests | ☐ | ☐ |
| 3. Safety strap present | ☐ | ☐ |
| 4. Intravenous fluid stock level adequate | ☐ | ☐ |
| 5. Irrigating fluid level adequate | ☐ | ☐ |
|   a. Normal saline prewarmed | ☐ | ☐ |
|   b. Sterile water | ☐ | ☐ |
| 6. Suture stock level adequate | ☐ | ☐ |
| 7. Blood warmer functional | ☐ | ☐ |
| 8. Anesthesia cart properly stocked | ☐ | ☐ |
| 9. Stock drugs not expired | ☐ | ☐ |
| 10. Infant laryngoscope functional | ☐ | ☐ |
| 11. Infant ambu bag—no holes or leaks | ☐ | ☐ |
| 12. Face mask for a premature infant | ☐ | ☐ |
|      Face mask for a term infant | ☐ | ☐ |
| 13. Umbilical catheter and insertion kit | ☐ | ☐ |
| 14. Pediatric emergency drugs in date | | |
|   a. Bicarbonate | ☐ | ☐ |
|   b. Epinephrine | ☐ | ☐ |
|   c. Dextrose | ☐ | ☐ |
|   d. Narcan | ☐ | ☐ |
|   e. Plasma expanders | ☐ | ☐ |
| 15. Infant endotracheal tubes in date | | |
|   a. 4.0 | ☐ | ☐ |
|   b. 3.5 | ☐ | ☐ |
|   c. 3.0 | ☐ | ☐ |
|   d. 2.5 | ☐ | ☐ |
|   e. 2.0 | ☐ | ☐ |
| 16. Infant heater at 96° to 99°F | ☐ | ☐ |
| 17. Infant blankets | ☐ | ☐ |
| 18. Infant identification apparatus | ☐ | ☐ |
| 19. Surgical lamps functional | ☐ | ☐ |
| 20. Room temperature 70° to 76°F | ☐ | ☐ |

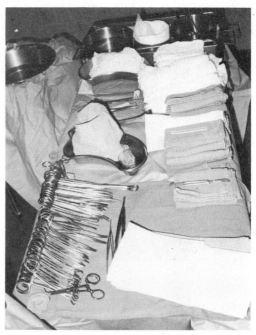

**Figure 19–3.** The back field.

leg. This decreases the chance of urine flowing back into the bladder. The bag is hung at the head of the table, which allows the anesthesiologist to monitor urinary output and report direct observations to the obstetric team.

An epidural injection requires proper positioning and emotional support. Usually, the procedure is performed with the patient in the sitting position. A footrest is provided so that the patient's spine and upper legs form a 90° angle. Placing a pillow across the patient's abdomen and instructing her to sit without leaning to either side, putting her arms around the pillow, relaxes her shoulders and allows her to push out or round out her back. Many patients have great difficulty getting into this position because of tenseness due to anxiety, and subsequently they tighten their muscles. Additional support is

provided by having the patient put her chin against her chest as the nurse puts her hands on the patient's shoulders and instructs the patient to lean against her. This is described as a therapeutic embrace (Fig. 19–4). The assistant then offers words of instruction or encouragement during the procedure.

If the patient is placed in the lateral position for spinal anesthesia, the spine should be horizontal to the table, and the patient is instructed to put her chin and knees to her chest. Again, this is an extremely difficult position for a patient to achieve at term. The patient is assisted by placing one hand against the back of the patient's neck and the other behind her knees. Gentle pressure behind the knees and neck helps the patient to flex the spine and open the intervertebral spaces. Because this position places the assistant in very close proximity to the patient, verbal as well as physical reassurance is facilitated.

Once either of these procedures is completed, the patient is returned to the supine position, a safety strap is applied, and the fetal heart is checked. The operating table is placed in a lateral tilt toward the left or a small towel is placed under the mother's right hip to encourage blood flow to the uterus and to avoid aortocaval syndrome.

If general anesthesia is used, someone may

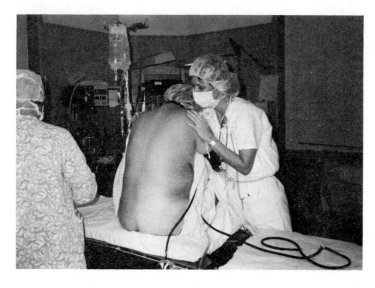

**Figure 19–4.** The therapeutic embrace—positioning for epidural anesthesia.

be required to assist the anesthesiologist during induction and intubation. Prior to beginning the procedure, the safety strap is placed securely over the patient's thighs. The patient's abdomen is prepped, drapes are placed, and the entire surgical team is dressed and ready to begin surgery. Ideally, someone should remain in physical contact with the patient until she is asleep, assisting the anesthesiologist by handing him or her drugs, the endotracheal tube, and applying cricoid pressure according to the anesthesiologist's instructions. Once the tube is secure and assistance is no longer necessary, surgery should commence.

The timing of induction of general anesthesia varies. In the United States, most patients are draped prior to induction, whereas in Great Britain, it is not unusual to induce anesthesia first and then drape the patient.

Either the doctor or the circulating nurse scrubs and paints the abdomen. The Association of Operating Room Nurses (AORN, 1992) standards advise a 5-minute scrub with an antibacterial agent, such as povidone-iodine. The scrub begins along the suture line and proceeds in gradually larger circles. The abdomen is dried with sterile towels, and the antimicrobial paint is applied in the same fashion.

## DUTIES OF THE SCRUB NURSE

The duties of the scrub nurse or technician during a cesarean birth are much the same as for any abdominal surgery. The nurse,

however, must give special consideration to the fact that the fetus is totally dependent on its mother for ventilation, nutrition, excretion, and other vital functions, and therefore, time is of the essence. Valuable time is saved by anticipating the surgeon's needs during the procedure. For the most part, the surgery follows certain predictable patterns.

In general, the scrub nurse is relied on to furnish the appropriate instruments, sutures, and sponges and to monitor the sterile field and technique of all participants. The scrub nurse assists in gowning and gloving the physicians and in draping the patient. As a rule, all laparotomy sponges should be moistened with warm normal saline. Commonly, two of these sponges are kept on the surgical field at all times. The scrub nurse must keep track of any instruments, suture needles, and lap sponges placed on the field, and the fetal scalp electrode, if it is placed on the field. Only items in use should be on the field. Instruments likely to be used are kept on the Mayo stand. A list of instruments and what is necessary on the Mayo stand is given in Table 19–5. Those items least likely to be used should be accessible on the back table. Occasionally, a hysterectomy is performed, and the additional instruments required for this procedure are listed in Table 19–6. Any laparotomy sponges that enter the abdominal cavity should be tagged or attached to a hemostat so that they can be identified and accounted for easily. A sterile bag is used for discarded suture materials, which is disposed of at the end of the case. A complete sponge and instrument count is performed before surgery begins, and the scrub nurse

## Table 19–5
### CESAREAN BIRTH INSTRUMENTS

#### Mayo Stand—Emergency Tray

| | |
|---|---|
| 1 Tissue forceps—smooth | 1 #4 Scalpel handle |
| 1 Tissue forceps—toothed | 1 Bandage scissors |
| | 1 Straight Mayo scissors |
| 1 Short Russian forceps (5″) | 1 Curved Mayo scissors |
| 1 #3 scalpel handle | 4 Curved Kelly's scissors |
| 2 Allis's forceps | 3 Péan's forceps—straight |
| 2 Adson-Brown forceps—toothed | 2 Péan's forceps—curved |
| | 2 Right angle retractors |

#### Back Table

| | |
|---|---|
| 4 Towel clips | 2 Straight Kocher's forceps |
| 4 Pennington's clamps | |
| 2 Babcock's clamps | 1 Singley's forceps |
| 3 Needle holders | 1 Bladder blade retractor |
| 4 Sponge sticks | 1 Large Richardson retractor |

should be certain that a radiopaque tag is attached to each counted sponge (AORN, 1992). Once the patient is draped, the scrub nurse drops the distal end of the suction tubing out of the sterile field, and the circulating nurse attaches it. The suction tube is then tested for proficiency. The Mayo stand and back table are moved into place, and surgery may begin.

For the skin incision, the surgeon needs a #21 blade. Once used, this is considered contaminated and is placed in a receptacle on the back table. Next, a #10 blade is used to incise the fat and nick a small hole in the fascia. The surgeon then needs a forceps with

## Table 19–6
### EXTRA SUPPLIES FOR HYSTERECTOMY

6 Ballantine or heavy clamps
4 Straight Kocher's long forceps
2 Curved Kocher's long forceps
2 Péan's forceps
4 Carmalt clamp
4 Curved Criles
6 Long right-angled clamps
4 Long tonsil clamps (Schnidt angled)
3 Long Babcock's clamps
1 Single-toothed tenaculum
2 Long dissecting scissors (Mayo)
1 Long dissecting scissors (Metzenbaum's)
2 10″ Mayo-Hegar needle holders
1 Bozeman's vaginal packing forcep
1 Singley's forcep
2 Long Russian forceps
2 Tissue forceps (smooth)
2 Tissue forceps (toothed)
1 Long #3 scalpel handle
1 Skin hook
1 Myoma screw
2 Sponge sticks
1 Balfour's retractor

teeth and curved Mayo scissors to open the remaining fascia. The instruments used to grasp the peritoneum prior to incising it may vary. Some surgeons use two Péan forceps, whereas others use Kelly or toothed forceps. Once grasped, the peritoneum is usually incised with a knife, and the incision is extended with Metzenbaum scissors. Next, the bladder is dissected off the uterus. For this procedure, the surgeon needs a smooth forceps and Metzenbaum scissors. The bladder blade is positioned to keep the bladder out of the way. To enter the uterus, the surgeon incises the myometrium with a #10 blade and either spreads the muscles manually or cuts them with a bandage scissors. It is very important that suction and lap sponges be available at this time. When the amniotic sac is ruptured, approximately 700 to 1000 ml of fluid flows out of the uterus. For this reason, sterile towels may be draped around the wound for absorption. There are drapes with a pouch around the incisional opening available to catch the amniotic fluid and blood to prevent it from running on the floor or contaminating the surgical team. Sometimes, the surgeon requires an Allis clamp to rupture membranes. The bladder blade is removed just before starting the delivery of the baby.

Once the baby's head is delivered, the physician needs a bulb syringe to suction the baby's mouth and nose. If meconium is noted in the amniotic fluid, a sterile suction catheter is used to suction the baby. For universal precautions OSHA's guidelines recommend the use of suction rather than a DeLee catheter.

Following delivery, two straight Péan forceps are used to clamp the cord, and bandage scissors are used to sever the cord between the clamps. The baby is then handed to the circulating nurse or pediatrician, with care taken to maintain sterility. Often, before the placenta is delivered, the physician collects cord blood to be sent for analysis. If cord gases are requested, a double-clamped section of umbilical cord will be handed to the circulating nurse so that he or she can obtain the blood sample. (In multiple deliveries, each umbilical cord is identified so that one knows with delivery of the placenta which cord belongs to which baby. Obviously, all tubes of cord blood should be properly identified.) Then the placenta is delivered into a basin and set on the back table. At this time, the surgeon will need sponge sticks or Pennington clamps for removal of the membranes and to identify the uterine wound angles and the upper and lower portions of the uterine incision. The surgical field should be kept clear of excess blood, amniotic fluid, unused lap pads, and towels. Dry sterile towels can be placed around the opening to help maintain a dry sterile field when a pouch drape is not used.

Next, the bladder blade is repositioned, and the uterine closure is begun. Usually, #0 or #1 atraumatic chromic sutures are used to suture the uterus. Uterine closure may be performed in one or two layers. If a two-layer closure is elected, the surgeon also needs a toothed forceps for this step, and two hemostats are needed to tag these sutures until muscle closure is completed. After uterine closure, a count is needed to ensure that no lap pads or needles are left behind. Next, the bladder flap is reapposed. The surgeon generally uses smooth forceps and a 2-0 chromic atraumatic suture. The bladder blade is now removed, and the tagged sutures are cut with a suture scissors.

A second sponge, needle, and instrument count is necessary before closing the parietal peritoneum. All lap sponges must be removed from the abdominal cavity. Some surgeons also remove blood clots and amniotic fluid from the abdomen. The abdomen then is explored, and the fallopian tubes and ovaries are inspected. The peritoneum usually is identified with three Péan forceps, and is sutured with a #0 chromic atraumatic suture. To appose the fascia, the surgeon needs a forceps with teeth and a #0 Vicryl or chromic absorbable suture. If interrupted stitches are used, approximately 16 sutures are needed. They are available with pull-off needles as a convenience. If a running stitch is used, two sutures on general closure needles are required. Every time a surgeon uses sutures or ties, the suture scissors are required to cut the excess material.

The fat is approximated using a toothed forceps and a 3-0 chromic or a plain catgut suture. This may not be a necessary step. Often, it depends on the abdominal wall thickness and the surgeon's preference .

Skin closure may be accomplished by any of several different methods, such as staples, suture, or butterfly dressing (Steri-Strips). If staples are chosen, the skin edges usually are held together during stapling with Adson-Brown forceps. A subcuticular suture of absorbable or nonabsorbable suture material may be used. The skin may also be closed using skin suture of nonabsorbable material, usually 3-0 or 4-0. Once the skin is closed, the nurse should provide a nonadhesive dressing, 4 × 4 gauze pads, and tape to dress the wound. A final sponge and instrument count is performed following closure of the parietal peritoneum (AORN, 1992).

## DUTIES OF THE CIRCULATING NURSE

The circulating nurse must record the times when the patient entered the operating room, anesthesia was started, surgery was started, delivery occurred, surgery and anesthesia were completed, and the patient left the room. This information becomes a permanent part of the patient's record and should be accurate.

If the patient is receiving general anesthesia, the circulating nurse may be asked by the anesthesiologist or anesthetist to apply pressure over the cricoid cartilage. Enough pressure should be applied to prevent passive regurgitation. This procedure is helpful in preventing aspiration, especially if the patient has eaten recently. However, it usually is recommended in all pregnant patients, because they have a slower rate of digestion.

Once surgery has begun, the circulating nurse should take a moment to scrutinize the environment, keeping the room neat. The laparotomy bucket should be placed so that the technician can easily dispose of used lap sponges for later counting and evaluation of blood loss. The AORN recommends that used laps be counted and placed in plastic bags as they accumulate (AORN, 1992). This helps to reduce splattering of blood and simplifies the counting process. Many hospitals require the bagging of laps by fives or tens. The circulating nurse should alert the anesthesiologist prior to bagging the blood-soaked laps so that blood loss can be accurately measured.

The nurse should make herself available for the care of the newborn before the uterine incision is made. In some hospitals, the infant warmer is covered with sterile drapes and the baby is placed directly into the warmer by the physician. In others, either the nurse or a pediatrician is covered with sterile drapes and the baby is handed directly to that person.

Resuscitation of the newborn proceeds as it would with a vaginal delivery. If the mother has received a general anesthetic, the baby may be lethargic and may have to be ventilated and stimulated until the ability to breathe spontaneously is demonstrated. The nurse should be able to respond quickly should the baby need to be intubated, in which case she must provide the doctor with the necessary equipment and assistance.

Once the baby has been stabilized, he or she should be presented to the mother, if she is awake (Harmon et al, 1982) (Fig. 19–5). Eyecare and identification can be delayed until eye-to-eye contact has been accomplished. The mother should have her arms released so that she can hold and examine her infant. Bonding can proceed as it would with a vaginal delivery, provided the integrity of the sterile field is not violated. Breastfeeding can be initiated at this time.

Once bonding is facilitated and eye care and identification are completed, the baby is sent to the nursery according to the usual hospital routine.

Lap pads, instruments, and needles are counted by the scrub nurse as previously mentioned. The circulating nurse observes sterile technique and adherence to universal precautions and reports any breaches. The circulating nurse may insist on a change of gloves, gowns, instruments, or drapes without fear of recrimination. He or she serves as a patient advocate and recognizes his or her role in reinforcing quality assurance in the operating room.

On completion of the surgery, the patient's abdomen is cleansed before the dressings are applied. Because the patient may be lying in a pool of amniotic fluid and blood, the nurse will want to make sure that the patient is thoroughly bathed before moving her to a clean stretcher with a clean gown and perineal pad. Many anesthesiologists agree that, regardless of the type of anesthesia, the patient should be moved gently, preferably using a roller. Sudden changes in position or rough handling may result in hypotension.

In a family-centered birth experience, coordination among the anesthesiologist, the surgeon, and support person is important. Some physicians prefer that the significant other wait until the patient has been anesthetized and draped. Others prefer that the visitor be ushered in earlier to give support throughout the entire procedure.

Obviously, the support person should be in scrub attire with cap and mask. He or she is seated at the head of the table, close to the patient, so that physical contact and verbal intimacy can be enjoyed. If the father and mother wish to see the delivery, mirrors can be strategically placed. Frequently, the surgeon instructs the father to stand up and watch as his baby is being delivered.

If the father has been excluded from the birth process, a message should be sent to him in the waiting room announcing the time of birth and the sex of the infant. The father also will appreciate reassurance that the surgery is proceeding as expected and that the mother and child are doing well. He should be given a realistic idea as to when he, the baby, and the mother will be reunited. If the baby is taken to the NICU, the father should be advised and allowed to visit as appropriate.

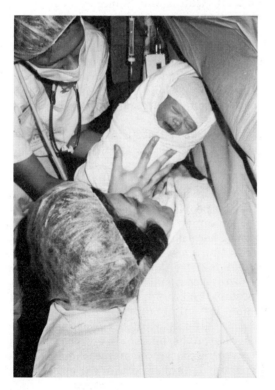

**Figure 19–5.** Bonding in the *en face* position can be accomplished even during surgery.

## Emergency Cesarean Birth

Normal labor can suddenly and unpredictably become an obstetric emergency necessitating cesarean birth. Some are true emergencies in which the surgery must be performed immediately, to avoid serious risk to the mother or the fetus, or both. Other situations are characterized as semi-emergencies: secondary arrest, cephalopelvic disproportion, and determination of the need for a repeat section in early labor. The emergency cesarean delivery is surgical removal of the fetus from the womb specifically aimed at saving the baby or mother from life-threatening complications.

Indications for emergency cesarean delivery are fetal distress, prolapsed cord, abruptio placentae with fetal distress, placenta praevia accompanied by vaginal hemorrhage, ruptured uterus, and a transverse lie in active labor. Occasionally, a multiple gestation requires an emergency cesarean birth.

Because time is of the essence, it is obvious that neither the physician, the nurse, nor the patient will have time to make elaborate plans. Thus, the emotional and educational preparation described previously will largely be eliminated. It is important to emphasize that *although physiologic needs must take priority during the emergency, psychologic needs must not be neglected.* Unfortunately, in the rush to get the infant delivered the patient's questions may go unasked and unanswered. Therefore, especially in a life-threatening crisis, any education and support to the patient and her family will be appreciated.

The labor room nurse is expected to demonstrate considerable expertise in the interpretation and treatment of fetal distress. Since the advent of fetal monitoring, the nurse's role and responsibilities have increased. Once fetal distress or any other acute situation is detected, and the necessity for cesarean birth is established, the preparatory tasks must be performed expeditiously. Emergency cesarean delivery equipment should be conveniently located in every operating and delivery suite.

Although the patient may not have been prepared for a cesarean birth, as mentioned earlier, information about cesarean delivery should have been included as part of her routine prenatal care and education. Again, during the preparation and catheterization of the patient, an explanation of the problem should be given, along with supportive reassurance that under the circumstances, this is the best possible delivery choice.

Everyone's anxiety level is increased during an emergency. Aimless rushing about serves only to increase confusion and results in unnecessary mistakes. Thus, it is necessary to minimize chaos and organize priorities of care to meet the life-threatening crisis.

Preparation for an emergency or semi-emergency cesarean birth should be a consideration for every patient admitted to the labor and delivery department. As a result, many obstetric services on admission routinely request permission for cesarean delivery, fetal blood sampling, and blood administration. When consent for these procedures is requested, the patient is advised that this is in order to save precious time later, in the event that surgical intervention becomes necessary. Permissions signed on admission, when stress is less than during an acute emergency and when the patient is not receiving any drugs, are more valid. Again, prenatal courses provide a good opportunity to inform the patient and her family about these forms; this is best included in the discussion on hospital admission procedures. The consent forms should be discussed clearly and in language the patient can comprehend (Quinn and Sommers, 1974). She should be reassured, however, that operative intervention will be undertaken *only* if absolutely necessary. If the patient is actively bleeding or is anemic, or if excessive blood loss is expected, then blood should be crossmatched. While preparing for the emergency or semi-emergency cesarean, all personnel perform the same tasks practiced at a more leisurely pace during the planned cesarean. The difference is the time element and its impact on the emotions of all involved.

During a medical crisis, there is a tendency for people to congregate. All nonessential personnel should be told to leave the room. There is *no need* for more than two circulating nurses during an emergency cesarean delivery. Ideally, all members of the operating room staff clearly understand the procedure and their responsibilities. It is advisable for only one person to give instructions; traditionally, this is done by the surgeon, but if he or she is preoccupied, the assertive, experienced nurse should be the organizer. Talking is kept at a minimum and limited to necessary instructions.

The circulating nurse must prioritize her

activities, starting by opening items that are needed initially, such as gloves, gowns, drapes, and blades. Nonessential items clutter the operating table, confuse the scrub nurse, and waste time. Ideally, the operating room will have been scrutinized at shift change, and all equipment is present and functional. Some hospitals have an emergency Mayo tray already prepared with everything needed to reach the baby (even the blades having been previously placed on the scalpel or disposable scapels can be used). Then, when time permits, another tray, with the remaining instruments needed, is opened for the back table.

It is imperative to realize that any emergency situation will have some traumatic effect on the patient (Hillan, 1991). Some patients express anger at the medical staff for neglecting labor pains during the preparations for emergency surgery. Others report they felt embarrassed by being stripped naked and "crucified." Fortunately, the majority are grateful and express genuine admiration for the staff as they adeptly move through their paces. Finally, some patients express a sense of unreality described as a feeling of having their hands disengaged from their bodies!

It is important to remember that the patient will be watching the team spring into action. She is frightened and sensitive to facial expressions, tone of voice, and all movement going on in the room. By minimizing confusion and providing support, the staff can prevent her from becoming panicky. Patients frequently remember that they were treated well during the crisis or that they were emotionally abandoned. They respond very favorably to physical reassurance, such as holding of a hand or stroking of the face. Ideally, a specific person should have responsibility for maintaining emotional contact with the patient; the importance of this support should not be underestimated.

Another emotion that a mother experiences is fear for the welfare of her baby and/or herself. As soon as the patient emerges from anesthesia, she should be apprised of the status of the baby, and if the father or a significant other is not in the operating room, he or she should be sent word as to the baby's and mother's well-being at the earliest possible time.

Some mothers go through a grief reaction because of what they perceive as reproductive failure and will need substantial emotional support later on. However, most accept that the cesarean birth was the best choice.

## The Postanesthetic Period: The Fourth Stage of Labor

Once the patient has been moved to the postanesthesia and recovery room, she is placed on an ECG monitor, or a pulse oximeter, or both, and vital signs are taken; breath sounds are checked; the intravenous line, dressings, fundus, and lochia are inspected; and the Foley catheter is checked to make sure that it is draining. The patient's skin color and level of consciousness is also noted. Return to normothermia is an essential component of postanesthesia care; therefore, prewarmed blankets should be placed next to her skin to accelerate this process. If she has received general anesthesia or breathing is labored, she should receive 35 percent oxygen by face mask or nasal cannula. If the patient is recovering from regional anesthesia, she is asked to move her legs, and her level of activity is noted. While the patient is in the recovery room, her I & O should be recorded at a minimum of every hour.

Vital signs should be taken about every 15 minutes for 1 or 2 hours or until the patient is stable. The patient should be fully alert and oriented (in the case of general anesthesia) or able to lift her knees against gravity (in the case of regional anesthesia) before discharge to floor care.

According to the *Joint Commission Accreditation Manual for Hospitals* (1992), recovery room standards should be the same whether the patient is in the main hospital recovery room or the obstetric recovery room.

Postanesthesia care includes careful gentle assessment of uterine contractility and lochia flow. Should the uterus become boggy, resulting in excessive bleeding or accumulation of clots, gentle fundal massage and oxytocics should be instituted. Fundal massage is painful, so caution is exercised, and a sympathetic explanation is given as to its necessity. Postcesarean care combines postanesthetic and mother-infant nursing skills.

Breastfeeding may be initiated in the operating room with assistance from the circulating nurse or the significant other, if present. If the mother is unable to initiate breastfeeding in the operating room, it may be initiated in the recovery room if the mother is feeling up to it. Assistance and reassurance that cesarean birth does not interfere with breastfeeding is important.

# Postoperative Care

Just as preoperative care and understanding of the procedure of cesarean delivery are important to the patient, so is postoperative care. Usually, management is conservative. Patients are kept in bed approximately 6 to 8 hours following surgery.

On transfer to the postpartum area, an overall physical, psychologic, and social assessment of the patient is made, and the information is entered on a form such as the one shown in Figure 19–6. It is important to know the location and status of the neonate, because a sick neonate is a signal that the patient may need even more emotional support. Based on the aforementioned factors, a nursing care plan is outlined. Because the mother may not be able to visit the intensive care nursery, a photograph of her baby will help her to initiate bonding. However, if possible, the mother should be encouraged to visit the baby in the nursery, even if it is by wheelchair or stretcher. This is particularly true if there is a chance that the baby may die. If the baby must be transported to another hospital, every effort should be made for the mother to view the baby before transport. The father or support person may want to go with the baby to the other hospital, stay during stabilization, and then bring a report back to the mother.

Among the postpartum clinical problems is the potential for increased blood loss or hemorrhage. Vital signs should be taken at least every 4 hours for the first 48 to 72 hours. Any significant changes in the patient's pulse (rhythm and character) and blood pressure necessitate further investigation to determine what, if any, hemodynamic changes are occurring. Other measures include observation of the lochia, the number of pads used, fundal height and firmness, and the dressing for evidence of increased bleeding. Oxytocin may be added to the intrave-

## Cesarean Birth—Patient Assessment

Name
Age
Religion/culture
General practitioner
Allergies
Language
Cesarean birth
  Planned
  Unplanned
  Emergency
Patient's perception of the procedure (before and/or after)
Significant medical obstetric history and complications
  Past
  Present
Present medications
Physical assessment
  Vital signs
    Temperature
    Pulse
    Respirations
    Blood pressure

Breath sounds
  Present
  Absent
Elimination
  Bladder
    Foley
    Voiding
    Color
    Consistency
Incision site
  Dressing intact
  Bloody
  Drainage
Additional drainage in place?
Other pertinent observations
Lochia
  Profuse
  Moderate
  Scanty
  Rubra
  Serosa
  Alba

Signature

**Figure 19–6.** Patient assessment form for cesarean section.

nous line in an effort to control uterine bleeding, and manual pressure may be applied to the fundus to express blood clots from the uterus and vagina. Breastfeeding also can be initiated to increase oxytocin release to decrease bleeding. If bleeding from the incision is noted, the wound should be inspected for defects and to determine the bleeding site. Postoperatively, there are usually orders for two blood counts, one within several hours of surgery and one for the next day. These results should be reviewed to determine whether or not there has been a drop in hematocrit, which would indicate continued blood loss.

The patient's respiratory status is an important key to her recovery. Breath sounds should be checked at least once every 8 hours to make sure that they are clear and that there is no congestion. Generally, respiratory care is preventive. Volume inspirometers encourage deep breathing, helping to prevent postoperative atelectasis. Pillows may be used for splinting the incision site should coughing occur. Other respiratory treatments (e.g., jet nebulizers, intermittent positive-pressure breathing, and antibiotics) may be ordered depending on whether respiratory complications, such as pneumonia, develop.

Alimentation generally progresses gradually: The patient may be kept NPO on the day of surgery or clear liquids may be given the following day; the patient gradually progresses to full liquids and then to a regular diet by the second or third postoperative day. This approach gives the intestinal tract the chance to recover from major abdominal surgery. Intravenous therapy provides nutritional support and hydration during this time. When bowel sounds are present, a regular diet can be given.

A more aggressive approach may be taken, which includes feeding patients clear hot liquids in the recovery room postoperatively as early as 1 1/2 hour after general anesthesia or immediately following the operation if only a regional block was used (Thomas et al, 1990). If the patient tolerates fluids without difficulty, and the vast majority of patients do, she can be started on a regular diet for the next feeding, if desired. Ambulating patients as early as 6 hours postoperatively, together with early feeding, stimulates gastrointestinal motility, is effective in the relief of gas pain, and decreases the need for narcotics. An antiflatulent or a Harris flush is also helpful in relieving discomfort from gas. Early ambulation may be even more important for those mothers whose babies are in the intensive care unit, because visits to the intensive care unit facilitate bonding and involvement in the infant's care. All patients should have had a bowel movement prior to discharge.

Urinary output should be monitored frequently and recorded at least every 4 hours; it should average 30 ml per hour. The catheter is often left in place for 6 to 12 hours postoperatively. After it has been discontinued, the patient's output should continue to be monitored for at least 8 hours, to verify that normal bladder and urinary tract function has returned.

Patients experience two different types of pain: incisional site and afterbirth pains. Pain perception is highly individualized because of vast differences in pain threshold. Patients may be medicated intramuscularly or orally. Pain relief is generally in the form of narcotics for the first 24 to 48 hours and in some cases even as long as 72 hours. Many facilities are using patient-controlled analgesic (PCA) pumps for intravenous and intrathecal pain management (Tighe, 1990). Use of these devices for postoperative pain control is becoming increasingly popular and has been shown to reduce the amount of narcotic needed to produce relief. Positioning, early ambulation, and general comfort measures can also help to relieve pain. Patients on pain medication can provide care to their newborns, provided they have proper supervision. In some areas of the country, a device called a transcutaneous nerve stimulator (TENS) is used to decrease the degree of postoperative pain felt by the patients.

Sutures or staples are removed on the fourth postoperative day, and a patient with an uncomplicated, uneventful course may be sent home on that day. Some patients who are fully ambulatory, able to care for themselves, and have help at home may be discharged as early as the third postoperative day. Of course, this also depends on the psychologic makeup of the patient—her initiative and drive—and on the absence of postoperative complications.

Infection is another concern in the postpartum period. An increasing temperature, pulse rate, or both are signs that an infectious process may be present.

The most common cause of postoperative infection is endomyometritis, which usually is a result of prolonged labor, multiple pelvic examinations, or prolonged rupture of the membranes. Because postoperative infection most commonly results from a combination of aerobic and anaerobic bacteria, it is very difficult—even with good culturing techniques—to identify the offending organisms. Most of these infections respond to broad-spectrum intravenous antibiotics (e.g., penicillin and gentamicin) within 24 to 36 hours, but if they do not, they will generally respond to the addition of clindamycin (Cleocin) or chloramphenicol (Chloromycetin), which covers *Bacteroides* organisms. In cases in which infection is resistant to antibiotic treatment, hyperbaric therapy for open wounds should be considered. Hyperbaric treatment has been found to be particularly successful when healing by second intention is necessary (Glowacki and Chew, 1988). The presence of infection, however, is not a reason to limit ambulation. Methylergonovine maleate (Methergine), administered intramuscularly or orally, augments treatment of uterine infection by stimulating contractions and encouraging involution. Breastfeeding accomplishes the same purpose, but one must be concerned about the possibility of neonatal sepsis if the mother is infected. As long as the patient does not have an open draining wound or a known bacteremia, and once she is sufficiently covered by antibiotics, there is no contraindication to her breastfeeding unless certain antibiotics are used (see Chapter 9).

Other causes of postoperative fever include wound infections and urinary tract infections. Patients who are exposed to anesthesia, specifically general anesthesia, may develop atelectasis or pneumonia. Finally, although rare, pelvic thrombophlebitis may also be a source of fever and may result in pulmonary emboli. Any patient who postoperatively has a persistent fever that does not respond to triple antibiotic therapy and who has no other source of infection seriously should be considered as having a suppurative venous thrombophlebitis (septic pelvic vein thrombosis) must be treated with heparin. Of course, intra-abdominal abscesses also must be ruled out. If she develops chest pain, shortness of breath, or both, in the postoperative period, pulmonary embolus is a distinct possibility. Patients diagnosed as having deep thrombophlebitis or pulmonary emboli should be treated with intravenous heparin. If the diagnosis is deep phlebitis without an embolus, heparin is continued for 7 to 10 days. If pulmonary embolus is diagnosed based on chest pain, dyspnea, and arterial blood gases, and is confirmed by ventilation perfusion lung scans, then treatment will also include warfarin (Coumadin) for 3 to 6 months. Patients receiving anticoagulants require multiple laboratory tests to follow the coagulation studies. The Lee-White or activated PTT is kept at $1\frac{1}{2}$ to $2\frac{1}{2}$ times normal to follow heparin, and the Pro-Time is kept at $1\frac{1}{2}$ to $2\frac{1}{2}$ times normal to follow Coumadin for anticoagulation effect.

Continued family-centered maternity care can be fostered by allowing a significant other to participate in those activities that the patient would normally perform, for example, feeding the baby or changing its diapers. Rooming-in during the first 48 hours, when the mother is the most uncomfortable, can be accomplished by means of surrogate care given in the patient's room. Bonding between mother and baby may be impeded as a result of the mother's immobility from pain and the effects of narcotics. In such cases, bonding should be assisted by the nursing staff via frequent contacts with the baby and properly timed pain medication. When a patient who has undergone a cesarean birth desires to breastfeed, assistance should be given in determining the easiest position for her. For those mothers whose infants are in the intensive care unit, assistance in using the breast pump, manual or electric, is necessary as soon as possible. This is also a good time to offer emotional support to the mother with a sick neonate.

For those mothers not breastfeeding, suppressive therapy may or may not be used. If it is not used, the patient should be instructed to wear a well-fitting bra. If engorgement occurs, she should apply cold packs to the breasts to relieve pain. If the pressure is great, small amounts of milk can be expressed just to relieve pressure.

Acetaminophen, given every 3 hours, is most helpful for pain relief and has decreased the incidence of postoperative thrombophlebitis as well.

Psychologic support for the mother is a continuing aspect of care. Encouraging the patient to express her feelings regarding the surgery is important to her psychologic well-being in the future. This is especially true if she has undergone an emergency cesarean delivery and therefore had little or no time to mentally prepare herself. Women who have had cesarean births under emergency circumstances have reported feelings that range from fear to sensations of having been attacked. Women whose infants are in the intensive care unit are also in need of special support.

It has been found that holding postpartum support groups, either in the hospital or later in the postpartum period, has been beneficial in reducing fears for future pregnancies and in explaining the circumstances surrounding the actual delivery.

Postpartum blues may occur about the third day or later. During this period, she may be minimally depressed or, in rare cases, severely depressed. If she is made aware that this occurs and is normal, she probably will react much better. Making the family aware that the patient may be upset for approximately 24 hours certainly helps them to cope with the situation as well. One has to remember that these patients, in addition to their physical discomfort, are now learning to cope with a new infant and wondering how they will interrelate with their infant and husband or significant other. Their physical limitations at this time may not be recognized as temporary; therefore, feelings of inadequacy may surface.

Patient education should be an ongoing process during the hospital stay and should include both maternal and newborn care. Additionally, special guidelines for the cesarean birth patient to follow after discharge should be provided. These should include:

- A list of warning signs to alert them when to see their physician or go to the emergency room (e.g., if they develop a fever, chills, increased bleeding, problems with the incision site)
- A list of contraindications to performing certain activities; this should limit driving, lifting, housework, and exercises.
- Instructions to take showers instead of baths for a week, until external incisional healing has taken place.
- Information about changes to expect in the lochia, which will change in color from red to brown to white.

Many cesarean birth patients feel ready to return to work by 4 weeks postpartum, and as long as all is well, they may do so. Certainly, from a medical point of view, there is no question that most mothers should be able to return to work by 6 weeks postpartum.

## Cesarean Hysterectomy

Rarely, a patient undergoes a cesarean hysterectomy, for example, either as a preplanned procedure or as an emergency procedure at the time of cesarean birth for uncontrollable bleeding, infection, or the inability to close the uterus because of fibroids. Such a patient loses her reproductive function. The patient who has an emergency procedure is totally unprepared for this loss. It is essential that physicians and nurses spend enough time with the patient and her family to ensure that they fully understand the need for the procedure and what its results will be. Although it is not necessarily the case for all patients, the loss of reproductive function may result in a grieving process. Should this loss also be combined with the loss of a child, the situation becomes extremely difficult for the patient and her family to handle. The patient needs counseling over the next several days, whether it be by a nurse, a bereavement counselor, a social worker, or a psychiatrist. This support may need to be extended after discharge. These patients may be especially difficult to treat because of their anger and sense of loss. It is the responsibility of all health care providers to try and understand the patient's anger and not to overreact to what they may perceive as a lack of cooperation on her part. Such patients are extremely challenging to deal with, but if one takes the time and effort, the majority will respond.

## Vaginal Birth After Cesarean Birth

One of the major contributing factors to the increased cesarean birth rate has been the elective repeat procedure, which accounts for 25 to 30 percent of the increase in rates from 1970 to 1978 (NICHD, 1980).

In the first part of this century, the majority of abdominal deliveries were carried out through an incision in the fundal portion of the uterus. In a subsequent pregnancy, rupture was a real risk. Therefore, it became standard procedure to do elective repeat cesarean deliveries.

The risk of rupture of a classic scar is approximately 15 to 30 percent, which is 4 to 5 times greater than the risk of rupture with a lower-uterine-segment scar (0.5 percent). Rupture of either scar most commonly occurs following vaginal delivery. The classic scar is 12 times more likely to rupture during labor and delivery than is the lower-segment scar (25 versus 2 percent). Maternal mortality from a fundal scar rupture is 5 percent, with a fetal mortality of 73 percent, as compared with the lower-segment situation, in which maternal mortality is almost nonexistent and fetal mortality is approximately 8 percent (Rodriguez et al, 1989). Therefore, in terms of future obstetric performance, the lower-segment transverse incision offers a better opportunity for a safe trial of labor, because the risk of rupture is considerably lower than that associated with a classic incision.

Numerous publications show that from 33 to 75 percent of all patients previously delivered abdominally can subsequently deliver vaginally, depending on selection criteria. Because more primary cesarean deliveries are being performed at the present time as a result of a more liberal attitude toward positive fetal and maternal outcome, it only stands to reason that if the risks are acceptable, more consideration should be given to allowing a subsequent trial of labor under carefully set criteria.

Repeat cesarean births increase the risk of maternal mortality to at least twice that for vaginal delivery. Health care costs also are considerably more. The National Institutes of Health (NIH) therefore has recommended that serious consideration be given to attempted vaginal delivery following a low-segment transverse operation for a previous cesarean birth. Selection criteria vary somewhat from hospital to hospital, as do exclusion criteria. However, one essential criterion is that facilities and staff be available for prompt emergency cesarean delivery. Other criteria for vaginal delivery in women with previous cesarean delivery may include the following:

1. One or more prior low-segment incisions, as documented by hospital records and operative note.

2. Previous indication for the initial cesarean delivery no longer exists.

3. Patient acceptance after an explanation of the risks of delivery vaginally versus abdominally.

4. No medical or obstetric contraindication to labor.

5. No previous uterine rupture.

In view of these criteria, *excluded* from a trial of labor would be patients for whom any of the following apply:

1. Any patient whose uterine incision was in the upper segment of the uterus.

2. Inadequate facilities for a prompt emergency cesarean birth.

3. Patient refusal.

4. Medical or obstetric complications that contraindicate labor.

Ideally, when conducting a trial of labor, the onset of labor is spontaneous. The patient is instructed to report to the hospital as soon as she suspects that labor has begun. Once admitted to the hospital, blood is drawn for routine studies and crossmatching, and intravenous fluids are initiated. Continuous external monitoring is instituted. Once membranes are ruptured or labor is active, a scalp electrode can be used. Uterine contractions can be monitored with or without an intrauterine pressure catheter (Rodriguez et al, 1989). If a tocotransducer is used, it should be remembered that it does not assess contraction intensity and, therefore, requires manual palpation. The patient should be closely observed, with a nurse-to-patient ratio of no less than 1:2.

Labor should progress normally. This can be assessed through the use of a labor graph. Vital signs must be carefully monitored. Many physicians use oxytocin for induction and or stimulation of labor in these cases. However, improper use of this drug has been associated with rupture of a previously nonscarred uterus; therefore, extreme caution should be exercised when using oxytocin in patients with a uterine scar.

The patient should be very carefully watched for the signs and symptoms of scar rupture listed in Table 19–7.

Analgesia is selected, keeping the signs and symptoms of rupture in mind as well as the effects of analgesia on uterine contractility, pelvic floor relaxation, and the possibility of a subsequent need for instrument

**Table 19–7**
SIGNS AND SYMPTOMS OF RUPTURED
CESAREAN SCAR

| | Classic | Low Segment |
|---|---|---|
| Pain | Continuous | + |
| | Tearing, then relief | ± |
| Scar | Tenderness | +, suprapubic |
| Fetus | Extruded into abdomen | Rarely |
| | | Irregularity or swelling suprapubically |
| | Fetal distress | Occasionally |
| | Fetal death | Rarely |
| Contractions | Frequently cease | Continue |
| Abdomen | Distention | Rarely |
| | Tenderness | ± |
| Pulse | Tachycardia | + |
| Restlessness | + | ± |
| Collapse | + | Rare |
| Cervical dilatation | Arrested | ± |
| Vaginal bleeding | ± | ±/L late, first stage, postpartum |
| Hematuria | – | ± |

From O'Sullivan MJ, Fumia F, Holsinger KK, et al: Vaginal delivery after cesarean section. Clin Perinatol 8:138, 1981.

assistance in delivery, such as forceps or vacuum extractor.

Once the infant is delivered, the lower uterine segment is carefully examined to determine the presence or absence of a defect. Of course, the cervix and vagina also are evaluated and checked for possible lacerations, regardless of whether delivery was assisted or spontaneous. Should a defect be palpable, indicating that the abdominal cavity or broad ligaments have been entered, then a laparotomy must be performed. A defect in which the abdominal cavity or broad ligaments have *not* been entered and that is not bleeding can be closely observed to determine whether or not there is concealed bleeding. The development of tachycardia, restlessness, hypotension, thirst, tachypnea, air hunger, and abdominal pain is highly suggestive of concealed bleeding. If the fundus rises and is pushed to one side in the presence of an empty bladder, a broad ligament hematoma must be ruled out. On vaginal examination, fullness anteriorly (after bladder evacuation) or in either parametrial region also suggests bleeding and warrants further evaluation. Any abnormal bleeding, either associated with a defect or that is not easily

explained or controlled, warrants laparotomy.

Before a trial of labor, all patients are told that if a scar rupture occurs they may require a hysterectomy, although this procedure is not usually necessary. Neither the postpartum hospital stay nor febrile morbidity is affected by a patient who underwent a previous cesarean delivery and who is allowed a trial of labor that failed, compared with patients having primary cesarean births for secondary arrest, cephalopelvic disproportion, and other complications. (O'Sullivan et al, 1981). The cost of care for patients who deliver vaginally following a trial of labor is considerably reduced, as is the number of postpartum hospital days. A patient who successfully delivers vaginally is not by any means immune from scar rupture in her next pregnancy. Each subsequent labor should be conducted as carefully as the first one following cesarean delivery. If a defect is palpable after delivery but is asymptomatic, the woman's next delivery is better conducted abdominally.

Following a primary cesarean delivery, discussion is held with the patient concerning her future method of delivery. If she is a candidate for vaginal delivery in the future she can be reassured this is the case, but if the physician believes she is not a candidate, he or she should tell her so. It is important that she know the type and location of her uterine incision; extensions, if any; and the indication for her primary cesarean delivery. Careful documentation on the hospital chart is very important and helpful in future management. Also, a surgery summary may be given to the patient for her own records (Hemminki, 1990).

Obstetrics has changed radically over this century and will continue to change. As providers of health care, we must be informed, sensitive to our patients, and adaptable to changes that are beneficial and important but not too eager to jump on bandwagons.

The greatest gains in perinatal outcome have been made in cases of premature infants. Some of these gains are the result of an increase in abdominal deliveries for these infants, but the greatest increase in cesarean births has actually been in term pregnancies—without a concomitantly increased improvement in perinatal outcome. It is the responsibility of the medical profession to provide good health care to the maternal-fetal unit at minimal risk.

## Acknowledgment

Acknowledgment is given to Mary Jo O'Sullivan, MD, for her contribution to the first edition.

## References

Affonso D, Stickler J: Women's reactions to their cesarean births. Birth Family Journal 5:1, 1978.

Alley A: Pre-operative teaching for cesarean birth. AORN J 34:846, 1981.

American Heart Association: Textbook of Neonatal Resuscitation. American Academy of Pediatrics, 1990.

Anderson B, Camacho M, Stark J: Interruptions in family health during pregnancy. *In* The Childbearing Family, Vol II. New York, McGraw-Hill, 1975.

AORN Standards of Practice. Association of Operating Room Nurses, Inc. Denver, CO, 1992.

Bacon K, Louch G, Louch K, et al: Care of the neonate after cesarean section. AORN J 34:860, 1981.

Choate JW, Lund CJ: Emergency cesarean section. Am J Obstet Gynecol 100:703, 1968.

Clark A, Affonso D: Childbearing: A Nursing Perspective, 2nd ed. Philadelphia, FA Davis, 1979.

Cohen SA: The aspiration syndrome. Clin Obstet Gynaecol 9:235, 1982.

Conklin M: Discussion groups as preparation for cesarean section. JOGN Nurs 6 (4):52, 1977.

Cox B, Smith E: The mother's self-esteem after a cesarean delivery. MCN 7:309, 1982.

Dewhurst CJ: The ruptured cesarean section scar. J Obstet Gynaecol Br Commonw 74:113, 1957.

Donovan B, Allen R: The cesarean birth method. JOGN Nurs 6:37, 1977.

Friedman E: Labor: Clinical Evaluation and Management, 3rd ed. New York, Appleton-Century-Crofts, 1989.

Gawse R: Fathers at the cesarean delivery. American Baby 44:32, 1982.

Gibb D: Confidential enquiry into maternal death. Br J Obstet Gynaecol 97:97, 1990.

Glowacki M, Chew N: Hyperbaric oxygen therapy. AORN J 47:1370–1378, 1988.

Greer K: RT's play increasingly important role in use of hyperbaric chambers. Advance for Respiratory Therapists 2(48):1989.

Harmon R, Glicken A, Good W: A new look at maternal-infant bonding. Perinatol Neonatol 6:27, 1982.

Hemminki E: Comparability of reasons for cesarean sections in patient records and mother interviews. Birth 17(4):207, 1990.

Hillan E: Cesarean section: psychosocial effects. Nurs Stand 5(50):30, 1991.

Hoffman N: Edith Potter, MD, PhD: Pioneering infant pathology. JAMA 248:1551–1553, 1982.

Integration of the cesarean birth experience—the various adjustment cycles. Perinatal Press, 4:136, 1980.

Joint Commission Accreditation Manual for Hospitals. Oakbrook, IL, 1992.

Mann LI, Galant JM: Modern indications for cesarean section. Am J Obstet Gynecol 135:437, 1979.

NICHD: Consensus Report by the Task Force on Cesarean Childbirth. Bethesda, MD, NICHD, 1980.

O'Sullivan MJ, Fumia F, Holsinger KK, et al: Vaginal delivery after cesarean section. Clin Perinatol 8:131, 1981.

Quilligan E, Zuspan F: Douglas-Stromme Operative Obstetrics, 4th ed. New York, Appleton-Century-Crofts, 1982.

Quinn N, Sommers A: The Patient's Bill of Rights. Nurs Outlook 22:240, 1974.

Phelan JP: Uterine rupture. Clin Obstet Gynecol 33(3):432–437, 1990.

Rodriguez MH, Masaki D, Phelan JP, Diaz F: Uterine rupture: are intrauterine pressure catheters useful in the diagnosis? Am J Obstet Gynecol 161:666–669, 1989.

Sachs BP, Brown DA, Driscoll SG, et al: Maternal morbidity in Massachusetts. Trends and prevention. N Engl J Med 316(11):667–772, 1987.

Schlosser S: The emergency C-section patient. Why she needs help . . . what you can do. RN 41:53, 1978.

Slee VN (ed): Cesarean sections in US. Ann Arbor, MI, PAS Reporter CPHA, 1976, p 15.

Thomas, et al: The effects of rocking, diet modifications and antiflatulent medication on post cesarean gas pain. Perinat Neonatal Nurse 4(3):12, 1990.

Tighe D, Sweezy S: The perioperative experience of cesarean birth: preparation, considerations, and complications. Perinatal Neonatal Nurs 3:14–30, 1990.

# CHAPTER 20

# Anesthesia Principles for Labor and Delivery

John S. McDonald

At the present time, in most labor and delivery areas, close cooperation exists among obstetricians, pediatricians, anesthesiologists, prenatal nurses, labor nurses, nurse midwives, and Certified Registered Nurse Anesthetists. The subspecialty of perinatal medicine has advanced over the last decade, pointing to the intense interest in and sophistication of obstetrics. Teamwork is essential at all times. This chapter introduces the many methods currently used in relief of pain during the labor process. The labor and delivery process can be one of the most beautiful times that a couple will share, and the more we can do to make this process an enjoyable one, the more we do to further the science of medicine. The protection of the mother and baby is a priority regardless of the method of analgesia chosen.

This chapter discusses various aspects of analgesia currently available to the mother. The difference between analgesia and anesthesia is an important one; for the most part, we are discussing analgesia in reference to obstetrics. The modern mother wants to be in touch with herself, her environment, and most of all, her baby. Above all, she wants to maintain safety for her unborn baby.

The first part of this chapter discusses pain relief methods for labor, and the second part covers pain relief methods for delivery and the postoperative period. It is important that the anesthesiologist, obstetrician, Certified Registered Nurse Anesthetist, and labor nurse work together to provide the best care possible for the laboring mother and her unborn infant. The mother and her unborn infant are considered together, because it is impossible to separate them when considering the effects of analgesic and anesthetic techniques and agents.

## Analgesia for Uncomplicated Labor

In centers where anesthesia coverage is available, regional analgesia is preferred over any other technique offered today. In the past two decades, there have been questions concerning the safest technique for pain relief for the first stage of labor. Regional analgesia by lumbar epidural method has been scrutinized by every possible investigative test. The lumbar epidural method clearly has withstood the test of time. There is no one standard of anesthesia in the country, and other methods are more common in centers where full-time anesthesia coverage is not available. A discussion of many of the methods of analgesia available to the mother in modern centers around the country follows. Some are administered by anesthesiologists or Certified Registered Nurse Anesthetists, but most are administered by obstetricians as ancillary backup methods to the technique of lumbar epidural, which is generally administered by the anesthesiologist or Certified Registered Nurse Anesthetist.

**Table 20–1**
PATIENT CARE SUMMARY FOR ANESTHESIA*

| | Intrapartum | Postpartum |
|---|---|---|
| **Regional Anesthesia** | | |
| BP, P, R | q 5 min × 20 min initially and after each reinjection. (q 5 min should be continued longer if patient is not stabilized in 20 min) After stabilization, q 15 min | q 15 min × 4 q 30 min × 2 then q 1 hr, then on discharge to PP |
| T | q 4 hr | On admission, then q 4 hr, then on discharge to PP |
| Position | Alternate side lying (right & left) initially. Once anesthetic effective, lateral preferred | — |
| Fetal monitoring | Continuous FM during anesthesia, preferably with internal; without monitor, q 10 to 15 min | — |
| Contractions Frequency Duration Quality Resting tone | Continuous FM during anesthesia q 30 min | |
| I & O | q shift (if patient has no other complications) | |
| **General Anesthesia (for cesarean section)** | | |
| BP, P, R | By anesthesia standards | q 15 min × 4; if stable, then q 30 min × 2: if stable, then q 1 hr until stable; then q 4 hr |
| T | By anesthesia standards | On admission to RR, then q 4 hr, then on discharge to PP |
| I & O | | q shift in RR |
| **Inhalants** | Same as routine labor, 1:1 supervision | |
| **Scopolamine** | Not recommended for use in labor | |

* Nurse–patient ratio = 1:1 until stabilization; 1:2 after stabilization.

## PSYCHOLOGIC METHODS

At the present time, three psychologic methods of analgesia are used in modern centers. Each demands close understanding and cooperation of the nurse in the labor area and, in fact, all personnel in the area. The obstetrician and the nurse are the key individuals here and must encourage the patient to participate in one of these three methods. In some instances, the obstetrician is the one who teaches hypnosis, but generally, the obstetrician's support staff members are the responsible teachers and motivators of these methods.

*Natural childbirth* has been used with great success for relief of labor pain, which has never been well understood. In some instances, poor understanding of the effects of the emotional and psychologic aspects of labor and delivery has blocked the use of this method of pain relief by obstetricians. On the other hand, overzealous insistence on the tenet that pain can be entirely eradicated by natural childbirth has also blocked the ancillary use of other methods of pain relief such as regional analgesic methods combined in late labor for beneficial effect.

Dick-Read (1933) popularized natural childbirth at a time when little else could be offered for pain relief, and for that contribution, he should be appreciated. The primary emphasis of his method was on the physical condition of the mother. It was paramount that she be in excellent physical condition so that she could endure the challenge of labor; therefore, conditioning became very important in the early phases of the development of the technique, and later on the psychologic aspects were added. Dick-Read also stressed the need for the patient to have control over the process of labor. This method was enhanced greatly by the cooperation of a friendly and helpful nurse who would act as a coach and facilitator for the patient during stressful times.

The *psychoprophylactic method* of analgesia modified the Dick-Read method with another method of analgesia that was popularized in Russia. These techniques were used for many years and soon were accepted elsewhere in Europe with success. By the middle of the century, the psychologic methods were known by many different names, but the most popular names were Psychoprophylaxis and Childbirth Without Pain, as Dick-Read originally described it. The method was popularized by Lamaze (1954) of France, who successfully introduced it to the United States around the same time that regional anesthesia was being reintroduced, thanks to pioneers such as Bonica (1967), Cleland (1949), and Edwards and Hingson (1942). Various exercises in ventilation were added, and it was understood that control of this aspect of breathing could have a salutary effect on the pain experience. In the mid 1970s there were still not many physicians involved in obstetric anesthesia. All of these methods demanded the close communication and coordination of the teachers, the nurses, the patient, and the obstetrician. The health care team helped to foster confidence and optimism in the parturient, which was very important in developing a pleasing, fulfilling experience at childbirth.

The *hypnotic method* demands complete cooperation between the obstetric patient and the obstetrician. As previously mentioned, the obstetrician may act as the teacher for the hypnosis sessions. I had the distinct pleasure of observing a group of patients during intense hypnotic lessons with their obstetrician a few years ago, and I was impressed by the interviews of the patients, who were genuinely enthusiastic about the method. The relationship between the patient and her obstetrician is usually a very strong and positive one that makes the physician's lessons in hypnosis effective. A patient's enthusiasm for this method demands time, concentration, dedication to learning a new technique, and the patient's belief in her own inner self and strength.

In all of the above-mentioned methods, the nurse's role in the success of the patient is vital. The patients need, seek, and appreciate understanding and kindness during their first encounter with the labor process. Here is a wonderful example of an area in which there is still much to be accomplished in cooperation and coordination of these patients and in the fulfillment of the goals set forth by

the obstetrician early in the pregnancy. It emphasizes the importance of the fact that obstetrics is a team effort among many individuals including the patient, the nurse, the obstetrician, the anesthesiologist, and the pediatrician. Cooperation, communication, coordination, and mutual respect and admiration are essential for the success and enjoyment of the entire process.

## SYSTEMIC METHODS

In past years, the primary responsibility for pain relief of labor rested primarily on use of systemic administered drugs. As mentioned earlier, when we treat the mother, we also treat the baby. Figure 20–1 demonstrates the fate of maternally administered drugs as they move between the maternal and fetal compartments and are distributed to fetal tissues. It was common to give narcotics alone with various potentiating drugs such as hydroxyzine hydrochloride (Vistaril) or promethazine hydrochloride (Phenergan).

*Sedatives* also were used frequently to help allay anxiety and to encourage sleep in patients who were not in labor but were experiencing Braxton Hicks'–type contractions. The most popular sedatives were the hypnotic barbiturates, especially secobarbital and pentobarbital. The phenothiazine sedatives, such as hydroxyzine hydrochloride and promethazine hydrochloride, also were used, both as potentiating drugs and primary sedatives. Less frequently, the benzodiazepine group of drugs, especially diazepam, was used.

*Narcotics* are the primary agents administered for pain relief in labor not managed by regional analgesic methods. These agents were easy to use and required only a verbal order from the obstetrician, who would be contacted by the labor nurse, the primary health care person responsible for decision making in regard to comfort of the patient and the timing of the medication for pain relief. The nurse would establish a relationship with the patient, make regular rounds on her during labor, and contact the patient's physician when deemed necessary. Usually, an order for meperidine (Demerol) would be given when the patient was in active labor with regular contractions. Other narcotic drugs include butorphanol (Stadol), pentazocine (Talwin), alphaprodine (Nisentil), fentanyl, or nalbuphine (Nubain Injection). These narcotics initially were administered

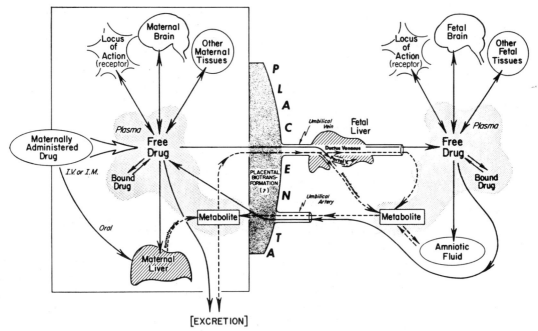

**Figure 20–1.** Distribution of drugs administered to the parturient during pregnancy. Note that once in the fetal compartment, all the principles of drug dynamics come into play to determine the level of drugs in specific fetal tissues. (From Mirkin BL: Drug distribution in pregnancy. In Boreus L [ed]: Fetal Pharmacology. New York, Raven Press, 1973.)

intramuscularly, but at the present time they are given in small intravenous doses to decrease the total amount needed for labor pain and, thus, decrease the amount available for effect on the fetus by placental transmission.

The fact that labor pain is not well appreciated and understood is one of the major problems today regarding the control of this pain. In modern centers, progress is being made through classes for the patients that help to eradicate many of the superstitions surrounding labor pain. It is important to attend these classes, because they help to allay the patients' fears and encourage them that they will be cared for with the utmost consideration for their comfort and the baby's safety. Patients fear that they will be unable to handle the degree of pain that is associated with labor. Some patients are terrified by various stories they have heard from other people or read in popular magazines. They need special handling and reassurance that all resources are available to relieve their pain. Such discussion emphasizes the importance of the nurse member of the team, who can plan for and help the physicians in both obstetrics and anesthesiology by offering a logical plan of care to the patient.

## REGIONAL METHODS

This section discusses the paracervical block and the lumbar epidural block for pain relief during the labor period. Figure 20–2 shows labor and delivery pain pathways and regional techniques used to block them.

The *paracervical block* (Figure 20–3) is used in some centers as a dilute concentration only. Generally, this method has been abandoned because of the problems of bradycardia in the fetus after administration of the drug to the mother. It had been a very popular method of pain relief and was extremely effective for many years. It was administered by the obstetrician, took effect immediately, and provided excellent analgesia, but unless the technique can be rejuvenated by discovery of some agent other than local anesthetic, it is probably not a method that will be used with any frequency.

The *lumbar epidural block* became popular in the late 1960s and early 1970s, although it was a method used by pioneers in the field of anesthesia for many years before that. In the late 1950s, medical literature reported that babies born of mothers who received regional anesthesia were more active and vigorous at delivery than babies born of mothers

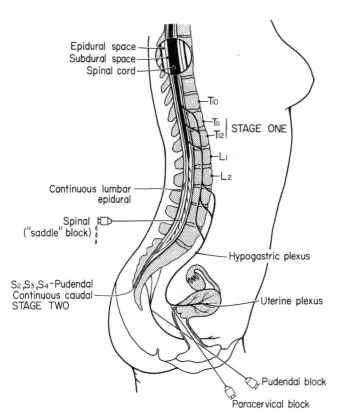

Epidural space
Subdural space
Spinal cord

—T₁₀

—T₁₁
—T₁₂ | STAGE ONE

—L₁

—L₂

Continuous lumbar
epidural

Spinal
("saddle" block)

Hypogastric plexus

S₂,S₃,S₄–Pudendal
Continuous caudal
STAGE TWO

Uterine plexus

Pudendal block

Paracervical block

**Figure 20–2.** Obstetric pain pathways and anesthetic techniques used for blocking them. (Modified from Bonica JJ: An Atlas on Mechanisms and Pathways of Pain in Labor. Abbott Laboratories, 1960.)

who received general anesthesia. At that time, general anesthesia often meant deep anesthesia, which caused significant placental transfer and depression of the fetus also caused by agents like cyclopropane and ether. Initially, epidural analgesia was continued by injecting medication intermittently through the epidual catheter. Shortly thereafter, the use of epidural analgesia rather than narcotics and other systemic drugs was found to decrease maternal work, oxygen consumption, and maternal and fetal metabolic acidosis (Jouppilla and Hollmen, 1976; Pearson and Davies, 1974a,b; Sangoul et al, 1975; Thalme et al, 1974a,b; Zador and Nilsson, 1974; Zador et al, 1974). Another advantage discovered was the continuous technique, which allowed the mother to receive uninterrupted pain relief throughout the first stage of labor and to enjoy the benefits of continued pain relief during the second and third stages.

In the early 1970s, modified techniques frequently were used to try to decrease the amount of drug the fetus would be exposed to. Initially, smaller volumes of 8 to 10 ml of local anesthetic were used to get only a T-10 to T-12 block for early labor and to increase it

slightly to a T-10 to L-2 block for later labor. At the present time, many patients receive a very small injection of 8 to 10 ml of 0.25 percent bupivacaine followed by a continuous dosage throughout their labor. The continuous dosage includes a dilute local anesthetic, 0.625 percent bupivacaine and epinephrine, and a dilute concentration of sufentanil. The combination is administered via a continuous pump throughout labor until the patient is ready for delivery. For those who desire a more detailed account of the various aspects of this method, please see the articles by Albright (1986b), Bonica (1967), Ramanathan (1988), and Shnider and associates (1987).

The *caudal epidural block* was popularized before lumbar epidural block as a method of pain relief for labor. It was championed by Cleland and Hingson, who were strong advocates of regional methods of pain relief for mothers as early as the late 1930s and early 1940s. Regional methods were gaining popularity at that time, and they would have undoubtedly provided for a much earlier acceptance of regional analgesia for labor and delivery had not neurologic complications occurred that were secondary to resteriliza-

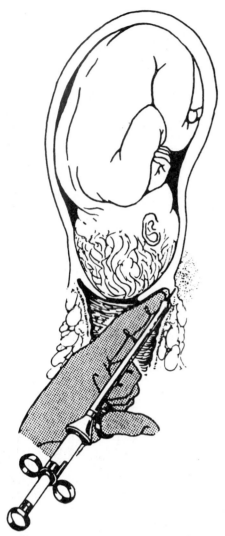

**Figure 20–3.** Paracervical block. (From McDonald JS: Obstetric analgesia and anesthesia. *In* Pernoll MC, Benson RC [eds]. Current Obstetric and Gynecologic Diagnosis and Treatment. 6th ed. Norwalk, CT, Appleton & Lange, 1987.)

tion of equipment and contamination with cleansing solutions. These problems caused many spinal complications between the middle 1940s and early 1950s, and these complications retarded the popularity of regional analgesia significantly. At the present time, with our readily disposable needles and catheters, the problem is nonexistent provided that proper preparations and precautions are taken. The caudal epidural block, although ideal for second stage analgesia, is not suited for first-stage pain relief because of the fact that a generous amount of local anesthetic must be used to obtain analgesia at the T-10 level from the point where the catheter tip

resides, which is in S-4 or S-2. In some instances, as much as 20 to 25 ml has been used to effect first-stage pain relief. All the intermediary segments are also blocked so that the patient has a resultant large degree sympathetic block with all the attendant complications. Nevertheless, the caudal epidural block is mentioned because it is such an effective method of pain relief for labor and was the mainstay for so many years earlier in the history of obstetric anesthesia. More detailed information on performing caudal analgesia is available in the writings of Albright (1986a), Bonica (1967), Ramanathan (1988), and Shnider and associates (1987).

# Analgesia for Uncomplicated Delivery

## LOCAL METHODS

The *pudendal block* has been a mainstay of obstetric analgesia since the beginning of this century. It is a method that the obstetrician can administer and have under his or her control, and it is a method that every young physician trained in obstetrics learns and employs. The obstetrician is comfortable and adroit at administration of both this technique and the method of local infiltration block of the perineum, which is mentioned in the following section. An understanding of the anatomy of the pudendal nerve and its course around the ischial spine is essential to completion of this technique. The success of this method is closely linked to the expertise of the administrator and the timing of the block, but usually, it can produce an intense or near complete block for pain relief for the delivery. Drugs used include either a stronger concentration of 10 ml of 2 percent lidocaine or 10 ml of 0.25 percent or even 0.50 percent bupivacaine. It is unusual to have serious or even mild side effects from the pudendal block, but as in all cases in which local anesthetics are administered, there may be toxic maternal side effects. Delivery usually is accomplished in the most comfortable fashion possible, either with spontaneous pushing or assisted by other means such as forceps application and traction, if necessary. The perineum is richly innervated and receives at least three or four other nerve supplies, such as the ilioinguinal, the genital branch of the genitofemoral, and the perineal branch of the posterior femoral cutaneous nerve, but usually only the bilateral blockade of the pudendal nerve is needed to provide adequate perineal denervation for delivery.

Both maternal and fetal complications have been reported after pudendal block, but generally, these complications are secondary to misplacement of the drug or the result of a technical error in needle placement. Maternal complications include (1) nerve damage, (2) toxic reaction, (3) hematoma in the vagina, and (4) an infectious process of the pelvis. Fetal complications include fetal seizures in utero; depression after delivery due to possible direct fetal injection; and one tragic case in which a mistaken epinephrine injection caused both a maternal and fetal death (Stevenson, 1954).

Pudendal nerve block is easy to perform, as it is facilitated by an instrument referred to as the Iowa trumpet, which helps to guide the needle paravaginally into the vicinity of the ischial spine, where the pudendal nerve courses posteriorly on its way to innervate the vagina laterally on both sides. Usually, 10 ml of drug is injected on each side for a total drug volume of 20 ml. Once the obstetrician feels the ischial spine, he or she must insert the needle deeply to inject the local anesthetic in close proximity to the pudendal nerve itself.

The *local infiltration block* of the perineum is a method of analgesia for delivery that also is under the control and administration of the obstetrician. The procedure involves a subcutaneous injection of a local anesthetic at the site of planned operation, which in the case of delivery is the episiotomy. The optimum timing is just prior to perineal distension by the fetal head. At this point, the perineum is stretched, and the pain from injection is usually not even noted by the patient. The usual injection is 10 ml of 1 percent lidocaine or other similar small amounts of local anesthetics. The dilute concentrations suffice in this case, because the nerves to be affected are the small subcutaneous projective endings that innervate the periphery.

The objective of local infiltration block is to relieve pain of episiotomy and not that of perineal distension, which is the objective of the pudendal block. Neither the pudendal block nor the local infiltration block have any deleterious effects on labor or the mother's ability to push to effect delivery. In cases of a generous perineal body, in which a generous episiotomy is planned, one can infiltrate deeply by use of a 3 1/2 inch spinal needle, which can be bent to slide under the subcutaneous tissues about 3 inches during an episode of perineal distension.

## REGIONAL METHODS

The *subarachnoid block* is another method originally used by the obstetrician for the delivery stage when there was not adequate coverage in obstetrics by anesthesiologists. The method may have been designed initially for the primiparous patient who, after laboring for hours, could expect an assisted comfortable delivery by the obstetrician giving a saddle block in the sitting position. The primary goal is to effect second-stage pain relief and to do it in a safe manner; thus, it is necessary to monitor blood pressure carefully so that hypotension can be detected early. Management of this type of hypotension is simple and effective; it is usually accomplished by position alone or by intravenous injection of a mild vasopressor such as 10 mg of ephedrine.

In some centers lacking anesthesiologists, the obstetrician performs saddle block for delivery with close monitoring performed by Certified Registered Nurse Anesthetists or by Registered Nurses, who are specially trained by Certified Registered Nurse Anesthetists or anesthesiologists to attend, to assess, and to report important changes immediately. Again, the nurse has a very important and appreciated role in the framework of the team effort. The obstetrician *must not* perform this method of analgesia if adequately trained assistance is not available; there were many examples of serious complications in the 1940s and 1950s because of just such a scenario.

The *lumbar epidural block* for labor is the result of the eloquent pioneer work of one man who dedicated a portion of his life to identification of the pain pathways of labor. This man is Dr. John G. P. Cleland, who single-handedly worked out the pathways during his surgical training in Canada in the 1930s. He published his findings in 1933 and used his work to develop a method of pain relief for labor based on introduction of a catheter into the peridural space. His work has gone unchallenged even today, and this author had the distinct pleasure of knowing him personally and having him teach the caudal method. Dr. Cleland was truly an unselfish man who had the best interest of womankind at heart when he did his pioneer work and for many years after that. He never lost an opportunity to talk about the importance of better care and better pain relief for mothers who suffered from labor pain.

The *lumbar epidural* method for obstetrics underwent many changes over the years, including both technical and drug modifications. This method is currently the most popular technique used for labor, vaginal delivery, and cesarean section. The doubts about the methods resulting from the occurrence of the complications of earlier years have given way to full acceptance by both obstetricians and pediatricians because of the dilute concentrations and minimal amounts used currently. The incidence and severity of hypotension with the lumbar epidural method compared with the subarachnoid block are minimal, and this has helped to entrench this method as the most sought after pain relief technique available today.

This method often is adequate for delivery as well as labor because the larger sacral fibers have been saturated long enough to be denervated. When this situation is not the case, one can use various supplements such as the pudendal block, local infiltration block of the perineum, or even inhalation analgesia, which is covered in the next section.

*Caudal epidural block* is the ideal regional analgesic block method for delivery, because it is placed in the sacral area where the sacral fibers exit on their way to innervate the perineum. Thus, the drugs injected can have maximum effect on pain relief by concentrating the drug effect on the associated nerves of the perineum innervated by the S-2 to S-4 fibers. The caudal block technique has experienced great swings in popularity since its introduction in this country in 1923. Its early impact was less than impressive until the 1940s, when Cleland and Hingson and colleagues emphasized the single-dose caudal technique for labor. Other reports confirmed the usefulness of this technique for vaginal delivery (Baptisti, 1939; Lahmann and Mietus, 1942; Pickles and Jones, 1928). The popularization of the continuous technique was reported by Edwards and Hingson (1942), and this method soon became one of the most important regional advances in obstetrics. Since then, hundreds of articles have described over 2 million applications and attested to its popularity (Auad and Castro, 1977; Bush, 1959; Chen et al, 1987; Eastman and Hellman, 1961; Fox et al, 1974; Green-

hill, 1965; Hansen and Ueland, 1966; Hingson and Cull, 1961; Hingson and Hellman, 1956; Lull and Hingson, 1944; Reid, 1962; Roberman, 1974). Through the 1960s, caudal block was considered one of the best methods of providing anesthesia for obstetrics; this popularity was due to the fact that obstetricians learned the technique themselves and taught other colleagues. Obstetricians were motivated to learn another method of pain relief for labor, because their analgesic techniques were so limited. Anesthesiologists were less motivated to learn the more difficult caudal technique, because they already were comfortable with the lumbar epidural technique. Currently, lumbar epidural block is the preferred technique and completely overshadows caudal block. This development mirrors both a larger involvement of the anesthesiologist in obstetrics and a coincidental tendency to limit the obstetrician as candidate to perform his own labor analgesia.

Today, the greatest usefulness of caudal block is in combination with lumbar epidural block in primiparas and in second-stage management of certain high-risk pregnancies. The combined use of these two techniques offers ultimate control of the pain of the first and second stages of labor. This combined technique was popularized by Cleland (1949). Caudal block can be used in several forms:

1. As a continuous technique combined with lumbar epidural for blockade of segments T-10 through L-2, to control pain during the active phase of labor, and later caudal injection with blockade of S-2 through S-5, to produce analgesia for delivery;

2. As a low caudal technique with blockade of segments S-1 through S-5 only for perineal analgesia for delivery; and

3. As a high caudal technique with blockade of T-4 through S-5 for cesarean section in certain instances in which lumbar epidural is contraindicated or unsuccessful (this is exceptionally rare).

*Inhalation analgesia* is effective during expulsion of the baby. It was made available at a time when no other alternative was available. This method of gas analgesia has been practiced since the days of ether anesthesia. It was administered by whoever happened to be at the call of the obstetrician in the labor and delivery suite; sometimes it was a nurse who had been schooled for a few hours in the technique of ether pouring; other times it was by a Certified Registered Nurse Anesthetist or by medical students who were working part-time to pay their way through medical school. Shortly thereafter, nitrous oxide became the choice for labor analgesia, and later, some of the newer drugs such as methoxyflurane were used. Generally, the administration of potent anesthetics has been restricted these days, and the practice of inhalation analgesia is not nearly as popular. However, the technique is still very effective in the right circumstances and, in some cases of multiparous pain, may be preferred for a few moments during pushing to relieve the intense discomfort of perineal distension. If inhalation analgesia is administered, the patient must be kept in the first stage of anesthesia, by definition analgesic, not anesthetic, i.e., not subject to deeper planes of anesthesia in which all sorts of problems can occur. This is easily achieved by those who are schooled in the technique, and no one except those trained in anesthesia should have such a responsibility.

## MANAGEMENT OF PATIENT WITH EPIDURALS

Epidural anesthesia underwent dramatic changes in the 1970s and 1980s, with a tendency toward smaller dosages being used at the present time for pain relief in the first stage of labor. Today, it is fairly standard practice to use only 6 to 8 ml of medication to reach a T-10 to L-2 block. The continuous technique has, in many institutions, superseded the use of even the repeated "minidose" epidural technique. Often, epidural anesthesia is administered by a continuous pumping arrangement with dilute local anesthetics such as 0.0625 to 0.125 percent bupivacaine, some very dilute mixtures of opioids, and epinephrine to reduce vascular uptake. A typical administrative dose might be between 8 to 10 ml/h, or it may be adjusted to the patient's pain relief status. This type of continuous dose follows the single bolus dose of 6 to 8 ml of a stronger 0.25 percent bupivacaine, and periodic small rescue doses for analgesia purposes may be administered as needed. The latter are not usually necessary, because the added dilute narcotics such as fentanyl and sufentanil greatly support the analgesic potency of these very dilute, continuous concentrations of drugs. One of the obvious advantages of a continuously administered technique for primiparous patients is that the drug's effect may last for a longer period of time. Because the effect of the drug may last for 4 to 6 hours, there may be some tendency for full sensory blockade of the sacral fibers so that, for second stage, minimal or no local analgesia is needed for the perineum for purposes of episiotomy.

The ability to select the appropriate dose and concentration of local anesthetics makes these blocks even more desirable. Bupivacaine, 0.25 percent, 2-chloroprocaine, 2 percent, and lidocaine, 1 percent, block pain fibers but leave motor fibers relatively intact. Thus, the patient has no pain but does not feel paralyzed and can move about in bed. Both bupivacaine and chloroprocaine minimally transfer across the placenta, because bupivacaine is highly protein-bound, and 2-chloroprocaine, an ester, is broken down rapidly by cholinesterases (Ralston and Shnider, 1978; Tucker et al, 1970; Finster, 1976).

Unfortunately, the reputations of chloroprocaine and bupivacaine have been tarnished in the recent past, because both have been associated with serious complications in the mother. Chloroprocaine may produce severe and prolonged nerve damage (Covino et al, 1980; Moore et al, 1982), whereas high concentrations (0.75 percent) of bupivacaine injected intravascularly may cause arrhythmias and cardiovascular depression (Albright, 1979). Although the scope of these problems is too great for adequate discussion in this chapter, in the case of chloroprocaine, final conclusions regarding complications are not available. Some experts have chosen to avoid one or both drugs, whereas others still use both. Most authorities believe that chloroprocaine is no more dangerous than any other local anesthetic. However, some still believe the question has not been settled conclusively (Barsa, 1982; deJong, 1981; Gibbs and Munson, 1980; Moore et al, 1982; Ravindran, 1980; Reisner, 1980; Rosen, 1983). Some have chosen to use lidocaine, a drug tainted only by early reports indicating neonatal neurobehavioral depression (Scanlon et al, 1974). In a well-controlled study, Abboud and colleagues reported that neurobehavioral depression of newborns whose mothers had received epidural analgesia with lidocaine was no greater than that of newborns whose mothers had received bupivacaine or no local anesthetic (Abboud et al, 1982).

The problems associated with epidural analgesia in general include its effects on labor and blood pressure, production of total spinal anesthesia in rare cases, and anesthetic toxicity or overdose. Normally, unless the block is administered before a good labor pattern is established or the pattern is irregular, the effects of epidural anesthesia on labor are minimal (Ralston and Shnider, 1978). During a normal labor, a transitory decrease in the frequency of contractions may occur immediately after the injection of the local anesthetic, but the original pattern resumes within minutes. An obstetrician who doubts the efficacy of a labor pattern during epidural analgesia can supplement a desultory labor with oxytocin or allow the anesthesia to wear off and then evaluate labor without having to take the effects of the epidural into account. The anesthesia can be reinstituted through the previously placed catheter when the labor pattern is satisfactory or the delivery begins. Although the incidence of forceps deliveries may increase with epidural analgesia (Hoult et al, 1977), this is not necessarily the case (Doughty, 1976). Optimum management of the epidural block and the delivery can result in a low incidence of forceps deliveries. Furthermore, with epidural analgesia, the application of indicated forceps and the delivery are facilitated, resulting in an easy, comfortable, and controlled delivery, thus minimizing risk to the fetus. With some small, premature infants, such a delivery is desirable.

Although it is usually preventable, hypotension, the most common complication or side effect of epidural analgesia, occurs in approximately 4 to 5 percent of epidurals used for labor (McDonald et al, 1974). Hypotension results from sympathetic nerve blockade, which blocks not only pain sensation but also sympathetic control of blood vessels below the level of analgesia. Thus, with sympathetic blockade, there is widespread vasodilatation and subsequent pooling of blood in the lower extremities. These effects cause decreased cardiac return, which, in turn, causes decreased cardiac output and hypotension. Decreased cerebral and uterine blood flow may subsequently occur and jeopardize both mother and fetus. Although systolic blood pressures of 80 mm Hg are usually considered hypotensive, for the mother, a 20 to 30 percent reduction or systolic pressures below 100 mm Hg may threaten the fetus. Because of this complication, electronic fetal monitoring should be employed during this procedure. If external monitoring is used, it is imperative to maintain an adequate tracing. If the side-lying position makes this difficult or the belts interfere with the procedure, an internal monitor should be inserted.

Usually, effective prevention includes left uterine displacement to ensure that cardiac return is not mechanically impeded, together with administration of 1000 ml Ringer's lactate to help fill the enlarged vascular space created by the vasodilatation. Care should be taken to avoid fluid overload, especially in preeclamptic and eclamptic patients, patients with cardiac disease, and any other patients who would be hemodynamically unstable, as well as patients who broke through ritodrine therapy. It should be emphasized that rarely is more than 1000 ml needed, and more fluid may cause fluid overload and pulmonary edema. Uterine displacement is accomplished either manually or by insisting that the patient remain on her left side, a good practice any time during labor. However, alternating sides gives the same effect and may produce a more even pain relief.

Treatment of hypotension consists of administering still more intravenous fluids and exaggerating the uterine displacement. In addition, one should lower the head of the bed to improve cerebral blood flow, and elevate the foot of the bed or legs to facilitate cardiac return of blood pooled in the lower extremities. If these maneuvers do not suffice, administration of ephedrine, 10 to 15 mg intravenously, is indicated. Rarely is this regimen not effective. Ephedrine is an appropriate vasopressor to use, because much of its pressor activity is beta- rather than alpha-adrenergic; thus, the blood pressure increases without the widespread vasoconstriction (including that of uterine arteries) that characterizes many other vasopressor agents (Shnider et al, 1968) Hypotension treated rapidly in the above manner is not likely to harm the fetus (James et al, 1977). However, even brief periods of hypotension may be dangerous to the fetus that is already severely compromised, either acutely or chronically (Datta and Brown, 1977). Datta and associates (1982) have suggested that any fall in blood pressure greater than 10 mm Hg is an indication for ephedrine. In following this guideline, he reported no hypotension in a series of patients receiving spinal analgesia for cesarean section.

Total spinal anesthesia after epidural

anesthesia, meaning anesthesia to the C-5 to C-6 level (affecting the shoulders and hands), occurs rarely; however, when it does occur, it must be treated effectively. A total spinal anesthesia may compromise the patient's breathing by weakening the intercostal muscles and, perhaps, even the diaphragm. The anesthesiologist should reassure the patient and then maintain her airway with a mask and an ambu-type bag or even endotracheal intubation until her muscle control returns. An extremely apprehensive patient may be sedated once her airway is secure. Hypotension in these cases, if present, should be treated as described earlier. Because there may be more tasks to perform than one person can handle, good judgment dictates calling for assistance. When treated appropriately, no serious or permanent damage should occur to the patient. The incidence of total spinal anesthesia after epidural analgesia varies from 0.03 to 0.06 percent (Ralston and Shnider, 1978).

Local anesthetic toxicity, a manifestation of excessively high blood levels of local anesthetic, usually results from intravascular injection or miscalculation of dosage. (Maximum recommended doses are found in all package inserts.) The symptoms range from excitement and mental confusion to convulsions to cardiovascular and respiratory depression. Although the blood levels at which central nervous system symptoms occur are high, they are usually considerably lower than those required to cause cardiovascular depression. Thus, the patient usually manifests the central nervous system symptoms long before any cardiovascular symptoms. The recent controversy surrounding bupivacaine (as discussed earlier) is concerned with precisely this point. There appears to be little distinction between levels required to produce both central nervous system and cardiovascular effects (Albright, 1979; deJong et al, 1983; Morishima et al, 1983). Therefore, once a reaction begins, treatment may be more difficult because of accompanying arrhythmias and cardiovascular depression. Moreover, cardiac resuscitation may prove ineffective. Because of these concerns, several manufacturers have recommended that the 0.75 percent concentration of bupivacaine not be used for obstetrics and that the drug be contraindicated for paracervical block (Abbott Laboratories, Astra Pharmaceutical Products, Inc., Breon Laboratories, 1984).

In the usual case of local anesthetic toxicity, any sort of anxiety or abnormal behavior on the part of a patient should alert the physician to stop administering the drug if possible. If convulsions occur, they will usually subside spontaneously in a short period of time. Even so, it is imperative that oxygen be administered immediately, because these patients soon become severely hypoxic and acidotic. If the convulsions do not subside immediately, small doses of thiopental (25 mg) or diazepam (5 mg) can counteract them. However, the physician administering these drugs must be prepared to deal with a drug-depressed as well as postictally depressed patient. Thus, the ventilatory and circulatory systems may need support. Some authorities recommend avoiding these drugs completely. Instead, they recommend the use of succinylcholine, a muscle relaxant, to stop the convulsions (Moore et al, 1960; Moore and Bonica, 1985). Certainly this admonition seems prudent when bupivacaine has caused the reaction. If succinylcholine is used, endotracheal intubation and manual ventilation are necessary. Also, it is extremely important to remember that during resuscitation of a pregnant patient for whatever reason, the uterus must be kept off the inferior vena cava and aorta. The incidence of local anesthetic overdose with epidural anesthesia varies from 0.03 to 0.5 percent (Ralston and Shnider, 1978).

During any major regional block, equipment in proper working order and drugs to treat complications must be available and should include a bag and mask for ventilation, oral and nasal airways, laryngoscope, endotracheal tubes, vasopressors, anticonvulsant drugs, oxygen, a suction apparatus, and equipment for intravenous therapy.

Another area of concern is the possibility of paralysis or permanent nerve damage after regional techniques. Ralston and Shnider (1978) discussed this problem in an excellent review of regional anesthesia in obstetrics. In over 31,000 epidural and caudal epidurals reviewed in the literature, the authors found no instance of permanent nerve damage. In 29,000 patients in whom spinal anesthetics were used, there were only two instances. Both of these patients experienced footdrop, which could have been of obstetric as well as anesthetic origin. Thus, serious neurologic sequelae are indeed rare.

Firm contraindications to regional analgesia include

1. Hemorrhage or hypovolemia, because the sympathetic blockade may attenuate the patient's compensatory mechanisms.

2. Anticoagulation or inadequate clotting mechanisms, because a punctured vein in the epidural space will not stop bleeding and may form a large hematoma, which could compress and compromise the spinal cord.

3. Infection at the site of puncture.

4. Allergy to the local anesthetic.

5. Patient refusal.

Other instances in which the risks and benefits of regional analgesia should be thoroughly evaluated are:

1. Fetal distress. If acute and severe, it is usually best to avoid regional analgesia.

2. Severe preeclampsia or eclampsia. Regional analgesia can be used safely and effectively in these patients if their condition is optimized before instituting the block. Volume status should be evaluated by means of a central line. Any deficit should then be corrected by appropriate fluid administration. In any patients, use of an arterial line is necessary for accurate continuous monitoring of blood pressure. Finally, clotting studies must be done to rule out a preeclampsia-induced coagulopathy.

3. Some forms of maternal heart disease that cannot tolerate hypotension, e.g., aortic stenosis.

4. Pre-existing neurologic abnormality.

## INTRATHECAL NARCOTICS

The use of a continuous subarachnoid analgesia for labor and delivery has recently been suggested and it also appears to be a viable technique for pain relief in labor. In the past, use of any technique of subarachnoid continuous administration has been limited because of the high incidence of postdural puncture headaches, which were often incapacitating to the mother after delivery. However, use of the recently developed smaller gauged catheters, such as the 32-gauge microcatheter or the 25-gauge catheter has stimulated new interest in consideration of use of the intrathecal technique (Benedetti and Tiengo, 1990; Benedetti et al, 1990).

Patients are evaluated very early in labor, and they are prepped and draped in the fashion usual for an epidural, but a small 26-gauge needle can be used for introduction of the 32-gauge microcatheter, or a standard 22-gauge spinal needle can be used for introduction of the 25-gauge catheter, which is placed and then taped into position for later activation. Small doses of isomeric bupivacaine in the range of 0.5 ml to 1 ml of 0.25 percent solution usually effect adequate pain relief in labor. This continuous intrathecal technique is also advantageous from the standpoint of providing perinatal analgesia for episiotomy and delivery because small doses of 0.5 percent bupivacaine in the range of 0.2 to 0.3 ml can be used to provide adequate pain relief at this time. Of course, one important advantage of this technique is that, if it is decided during labor that emergency cesarean section is required, the same catheter can be used to provide rapid analgesia for surgical anesthesia for cesarean section.

# Postoperative Analgesia

## PATIENT-CONTROLLED ANALGESIA PUMPS FOR POSTOPERATIVE PAIN CONTROL

A revolution has occurred in postoperative pain relief in medicine. It is no longer necessary to suffer from the rigors of the healing process after surgery. Patients can receive either patient-controlled analgesia (PCA) via intravenous opioids for pain relief, over which they have complete control, or they may receive continuously administered opioids via the epidural space, to obtain optimum pain relief in regard to analgesic potency. These methods not only provide the patient with comfort, but it is thought that it is possible that the body heals more rapidly after surgery in such patients, so that they may be discharged to resume their normal activities at an earlier time. These techniques presently are available in many hospitals and offer the patients control over one of the aspects of their medical care that they often feared in the past, namely, pain in the postoperative period. For patients who have regional anesthetics, an epidural may be used for pain relief in labor or for cesarean section; the epidural catheter may be left in place for several days postoperatively and continuous small doses of either pure narcotic or a combination of extremely dilute local anesthetic mixture with narcotic may be used. In those patients who do not have an epidural catheter in place, either one may be placed for patients who have general anesthesia, or a PCA method with administration of the opioid through the intravenous route may be used so that the patient may periodically dial her own effective pain relief dose. The most favored drugs for use in epidural pain relief include morphine and fentanyl. Only preservative-free opioids are used for epidural administration at this hospital.

General epidural dosage guidelines are as follows:

1. Initial epidural bolus
   a. Preferably 1 h before the case is finished or immediately after delivery.
   b. Morphine, 1 to 5 mg (as the bolus dosage of morphine is increased, the incidence of pruritus can be expected to increase; the combination of 1 to 3 mg morphine with 50–100 mcg of fentanyl should result in a low incidence of pruritus and other side effects such as nausea/vomiting or respiratory depression).
   c. Bolus doses should be decreased by 10 to 20 percent for patients over 60 years of age.
2. Continuous infusions
   a. Continuous infusions are used for all patients receiving epidural narcotics.
   b. Typical continuous infusion doses are 200 to 400 mcg/h for morphine, and 50–130 mcg/h fentanyl in a concentration of 10 mcg/ml. Local anesthetics such as bupivacaine have been added to continuous infusion of epidural narcotics with reportedly better pain relief. A concentration of 0.625% bupivacaine can be used. Side effects secondary to this concentration of bupivacaine are rare but can include paresthesias and decreased blood pressure.

Morphine and Dilaudid are the opioids of choice when a patient is using PCA. The use of meperidine (Demerol) is discouraged owing to the risk of seizure activity secondary to meperidine toxicity.

General PCA dosage guidelines are as follows:

1. Morphine dose is 1.2 to 2 mg (0.02 mg/kg) every 10 minutes for patients younger than 60 years of age.
2. The 4-hour limit should be roughly 20 to 30 mg/4 h (0.35 mg/kg).

3. Dilaudid dose is 0.2 to 0.4 mg every 10 minutes (0.004 mg/kg) for patients younger than 60 years of age.
4. The 4 hour limit should be roughly 4 to 8 mg/4 h (0.075 mg/kg).

# Effects of Anesthetic Agents on the Newborn

It is safe to generalize about the placental transfer of anesthetic agents and say that all cross the placenta to the fetus (Moya and Thorndike, 1962). Muscle relaxants, for clinical purposes, are the only important exceptions (Moya and Kvisselgaard, 1961). Despite this ready transfer, anesthesiologists, obstetricians, and physiologists have combined their clinical and experimental efforts to provide anesthesia that does little, if any, harm to the newborn, as evaluated by Apgar scores and acid-base and blood-gas status (Marx et al, 1970; Kosaka et al, 1969; Galbert and Gardner, 1972; James et al, 1977; Magno et al, 1976; Datta and Alper, 1980). These measurements, however, evaluate only brainstem function. They evaluate functions of a newborn necessary for physical well-being and survival but not functions of the higher cortical centers. For several years, psychologists have used tests such as the Brazelton, Prechtal, and Bientema to evaluate the newborn's and older infant's more subtle neurobehavioral activities and, occasionally, to evaluate drug effects. However, these tests, which were long and cumbersome, were not widely used in the early neonatal period. Therefore, Scanlon developed a neurobehavioral examination that included features from the neurologic examinations of Prechtal and Bientema as well as from behavioral testing of the Brazelton examination (Scanlon et al, 1974). The behaviors selected were considered easier to elicit during the first few hours and days of life:

1. Apgar score
2. State
   a. Awake
   b. Asleep
3. Response to pinprick
4. Tone evaluation
   a. Pull to sitting
   b. Arm recoil
   c. Truncal tone
   d. General body tone

5. Rooting
6. Sucking
7. Moro's response
8. Response decrement to light in eyes
9. Response to sound
10. Placing
11. Alertness
12. General assessment

The Apgar score serves as an indicator of vital signs to begin the examination. Next, the general state of the fetus is recorded. This is scored by various states of wake or sleep of the infant. The fetal state is then recorded again before each of the specific tests. Each of these tests is scored from 0 to 3, with the higher number indicating a more alert, responsive newborn. To complete the scoring, general scores for alertness, overall assessment, predominant state, and lability of state are added to all of the above mentioned factors. Scores above 33 to 35 indicate a normal fetal condition, provided that points were not lost in one specific category, such as tone or adaptive capacity (Bonica, 1980).

Since the first appearance of Scanlon's test, many anesthetic agents and techniques have been found to have some effect according to this now widely accepted neurobehavioral scoring system (Hodgkinson et al, 1978a, 1978b; Corke, 1977; Hodgkinson et al, 1977; Scanlon et al, 1976). Although many anesthetic agents alter these tests, the alterations are subtle and transient (Tronick et al, 1976). Infants of mothers who received regional analgesia had higher scores than did those whose mothers received general anesthesia. Ketamine as an induction agent produced better scores than did thiopental (Hodgkinson et al, 1978; McGuinness, 1978).

Infants also responded better when the local anesthetic used was chloroprocaine or bupivacaine as opposed to lidocaine or mepivacaine (Scanlon et al, 1974). However, more recent studies have exonerated lidocaine (Abboud et al, 1982).

Gibbs (1986) and many other obstetric anesthesiologists believe that neuro-behavioral testing can be summarized as follows:

1. Anesthetic agents alter neurobehavioral performance in newborns.
2. There is no evidence to suggest that these alterations have any effect on later development.
3. The results of such tests probably should not significantly influence the anesthesiologist's choice of anesthetic or technique.

# Anesthesia Selection for Cesarean Section

The selection of anesthesia technique and agents for cesarean delivery is an important consideration in obstetrics because both the mother and the life of the baby are affected. For a period of time in the past few decades, regional anesthesia was preferred over general anesthesia because of the safety it provided to the mother, that is, reduction or eradication of the fear of aspiration of gastric contents and death from that disease process that was known in the late 1940s and 1950s as Mendelson's syndrome. However, in the 1970s, a new low-dose analgesic method with continuous controlled relaxation for cesarean section was introduced, and it was shown that the Apgar scores of babies delivered with such regimens were similar at birth regardless of whether regional or general anesthetic techniques were used. It must be noted that, early in the decade, inhalational anesthetics such as cyclopropane and other potent agents were used in cesarean deliveries and crossed the placenta to depress the baby; therefore, the Apgar scores of these babies were much lower than those of babies who were delivered by either spinal or epidural techniques. However, with use of a low-dose barbiturate induction and a 50 percent nitrous oxide concentration with continuous succinylcholine or longer acting muscle relaxants, maternal control during the short induction-to-delivery phase can be managed, and the baby is delivered in excellent condition. Therefore, in the mid 1970s and 1980s, there was a resurgence in the use of the general anesthetic technique for cesarean delivery. In retrospect, this was probably a mistake, because there may have been several lives placed at risk with this procedure. Again, the primary problem has been and continues to be aspiration. If the mother aspirates at the time of cesarean delivery, it is a very serious problem; the surest way to avoid it is the use of a regional technique. Therefore, the the author of this chapter is overwhelmingly in favor of the use of either subarachnoid or epidural techniques for cesarean delivery. Both of these techniques provide excellent analgesia with good relaxation and often excellent conditions for delivery of the baby.

The general anesthetic technique still may be used in some instances, such as those necessitating very rapid delivery of the baby, and in mothers who are deemed to have no contraindications to a rapid-sequence induction, such as no possibility of a difficult intubation. These conditions include placenta praevia, rupture of the uterus, or other life-threatening maternal hemorrhagic conditions in which regional anesthesia may further jeopardize the patient's cardiovascular stability and the safety of both the baby and the mother. The selection of anesthesia for cesarean section should be taken very seriously. At the present time, it is preferable to meet with the patient prior to her admission to the labor and delivery suite and to discuss her preference for anesthesia during cesarean delivery, that is, whether she prefers to be awake and participate in the delivery or prefers to be asleep. The overwhelming choice for most patients is to be awake and participate during this very special moment in life. Therefore, the choice usually is not complicated in most instances. Some patients are fearful of having a needle placed in their back and are concerned about complications of regional anesthesia, but most of these fears are based on horror stories related to them by relatives and friends. There may be instances in which the obstetrician is anxious for a rapid delivery, such as when the life of the fetus is in jeopardy. Naturally, the anesthesiologist wants to comply and, as a member of the health care team, wants to facilitate his or her task so that operative conditions can be met. However, the anesthesiologist must remember that his or her primary responsibility is to maintain the health, safety, and welfare of the patient. In a situation in which the airway may be blocked and in which the anesthesiologist believes that rapid-sequence inductor in an emergency situation, such as with a morbidly obese patient or a patient with a guarded airway, the anesthesiologist may suggest to the obstetrician that he or she consider a subarachnoid or epidural technique to ensure the mother's safety. Sometimes, a rapidly placed subarachnoid block is performed. In many instances, practitioners have suggested that spinal anesthesia can be administered as quickly as general anesthesia. However, this is a very sensitive area, and it is an area in which all the health care team members must work together to come to a rapid and satisfactory solution to the main problem facing them, namely, the necessity for an emergency delivery in conjunction with complications that may be serious or even lethal for the mother. Under intrathecal analgesia, the placement of a catheter in such a patient may be one of the solutions to this problem, because in that instance, rapid analgesia can be obtained because the catheter is already in place.

At the present time, the pregnant woman expects excellent pain relief for labor and delivery, and she expects this to be performed in a setting that protects the health and welfare of her unborn baby. She may want to have her husband participate with her in the delivery, and I would encourage this practice. There may not be a more wonderful time in a woman's life than when she gives life to her baby. It may be the realization of many years of planning. More than ever before, this event is performed through the teamwork and cooperation of health care professionals of many different disciplines. It demands careful attention, planning, discussions, and experience with many different methods of pain relief, some of which were mentioned in this chapter. Many other references are available for the reader for more in-depth coverage of specific areas, and further study is encouraged. Each situation must be treated individually, and the method of analgesia chosen is based on the many years of experience and expertise of the management team. Safe and effective pain relief is a privilege well worth the planning.

**Acknowledgment**

Acknowledgment is given to Charles Gibbs, the author of the first edition.

# References

Abboud TK, Khoo SS, Miller F, et al: Maternal, fetal, and neonatal responses after epidural anesthesia with bupivacaine, 2-chloroprocaine, or lidocaine. Anesth Analg 61:638, 1982.

Albright GA: Cardiac arrest following regional anesthesia with etidocaine or bupivacaine. Anesthesiology 51:285, 1979.

Albright GA: Caudal Epidural Anesthesia. *In* Albright GA, Ferguson JE II, Joyce TH III, Stevenson DK (eds):

Anesthesia in Obstetrics. Maternal, Fetal, and Neonatal Aspects. Boston, Butterworths, 1986a.

Albright GA: Lumbar Epidural Anesthesia. *In* Albright GA, Ferguson JE II, Joyce TH III, Stevenson DK (eds): Anesthesia in Obstetrics. Maternal, Fetal, and Neonatal Aspects. Boston, Butterworths, 1986b.

Auad A, Castro AR: Anestesia caudal: Nuestra experiencia. Rev Esp Anestesiol Reanim 24:459, 1977.

Baptisti A Jr: Caudal anesthesia in obstetrics. Am J Obstet Gynecol 38:642, 1939.

Barsa J, Batra M, Fink BR, et al: A comparative in vivo study of local neurotoxicity of lidocaine, bupivacaine, 2-chloroprocaine, and a mixture of 2-chloroprocaine and bupivacaine. Anesth Analg 61:961, 1982.

Benedetti C, Tiengo M: Continuous subarachnoid block for labor and delivery. Pain Suppl 5:S400, 1990.

Benedetti C, Chadwick HS, Mancuso JJ, et al: Incidence of postspinal headache after continuous subarachnoid analgesia for labor using a 32-gauge microcatheter. Anesthesiology 73(suppl):A922, 1990.

Bonica JJ: Obstetric Analgesia and Anesthesia. Amsterdam, World Federation of Societies of Anaesthesiologists, 1980.

Bonica JJ: Principles and Practice of Obstetric Analgesia and Anesthesia. Philadelphia, FA Davis Co, 1967.

Bush RC: Caudal analgesia for vaginal delivery. Anesthesiology 20(31):186, 1959.

Chen JS, Lau HP, Chao CC: Caudal block in vaginal delivery. Ma Tsui Hsueh Tsa Chi (Taiwan) 25:145, 1987.

Cleland JGP: Continuous peridural and caudal analgesia in obstetrics. Curr Res Anesth Analg 28:61, 1949.

Corke BC: Neurobehavioral responses of the newborn: the effect of different forms of maternal analgesia. Anaesthesia 32:539, 1977.

Datta S, and Alper MH: Anesthesia for cesarean section. Anesthesiology 53:142, 1980.

Datta S, and Brown WU: Acid-base status in diabetic mothers and their infants following general or spinal anesthesia for cesarean section. Anesthesiology 47:272, 1977.

Datta S, Kitzmiller JL, Naulty JS, et al: Acid-base status of diabetic mothers and their infants following spinal anesthesia for cesarean section. Anesth Analg 61:662, 1982.

deJong RH: The chloroprocaine controversy. Am J Obstet Gynecol 140:237, 1981.

deJong RH, Gamble CA, and Bonin JD: Bupivacaine-induced cardiac arrhythmias and plasma cation concentrations in normokalemic cats. Regional Anesth 8:104, 1983.

Dick-Read G: Natural Childbirth. London, William Heinemann Ltd, 1933.

Doughty A: Selective epidural analgesia and the forceps rate. Br J Anaesth 41:1058, 1976.

Eastman NJ, Hellman LM: Williams Obstetrics, 12 ed. New York, Appleton-Century-Crofts, 1961.

Edwards WB, Hingson RA: Continuous caudal anesthesia in obstetrics. Am J Surg 57:459, 1942.

Fox LP, Weller WJ, Wilder H: Obstetrical caudal anesthesia in a community hospital: A satisfactory plan. West J Med 120:189, 1974.

Galbert MW, and Gardner AE: Use of halothane in a balanced technic for cesarean section. Anesth Analg 51:701, 1972.

Gibbs CP: Anesthesia in Pregnancy. *In* Knuppel, RA and Drukker JE: High Risk Pregnancy: A Team Approach. Philadelphia, WB Saunders, 1986.

Gibbs CP, Munson ES: Local anesthetic toxicity (letter). Anesthsia Analg 59(12):955, 1980.

Greenhill JP: Obstetrics, 13 ed. Philadelphia, WB Saunders Co, 1965.

Hansen JM, Ueland K: The influence of caudal analgesia on cardiovascular dynamics during normal labor and delivery. Acta Anaesthesiol Scand 23:448(suppl), 1966.

Hingson RA, Cull WA: Conduction anesthesia and analgesia for obstetrics. Clin Obstet Gynecol 4:87, 1961.

Hingson RA, Edwards WB: An analysis of the first ten thousand confinements managed with continuous caudal analgesia with a report of the authors' first one thousand cases. JAMA 123:538, 1943.

Hingson RA, Hellman LM: Anesthesia for Obstetrics. Philadelphia, JB Lippincott Co, 1956.

Hingson RA, Cull WA, Benzinger M: Continuous caudal analgesia in obstetrics. Curr Res Anesth Analg 40:119, 1961.

Hodgkinson R, Bhatt M, Kim SS, et al: Neonatal neurobehavioral tests following cesarean section under general and spinal anesthesia. Am J Obstet Gynecol 132:670, 1978a.

Hodgkinson R, Bhatt M, and Wang CN: Double-blind comparison of the neurobehaviour of neonates following the administration of different doses of meperidine to the mother. Can Anaesth Soc J 25:405, 1978b.

Hodgkinson R, Marx GF, Kim SS, et al: Neonatal neurobehavioral tests following vaginal delivery under ketamine, thiopental, and extradural anesthesia. Anesth Analg 56:548, 1977.

Hoult IJ, MacLennan AH, and Carrie LES: Lumbar epidural analgesia in labour: relation to fetal malposition and instrumental delivery. Br Med J 1:14, 1977.

James FM, Crawford JS, Hopkinson R, et al: A comparison of general anesthesia and lumbar epidural analgesia for elective cesarean secion. Anesth Analg 56:228, 1977.

Jouppila, R, Hollmen A: The effect of segmental epidural analgesia on maternal and foetal acid-base balance, lactate, serum potassium and creatine phosphokinase during labour. Acta Anaesth Scand 20:259, 1976.

Kosaka Y, Takahashl T, and Mark LC: Intravenous thiobarbiturate anesthesia for cesarean section. Anesthesiology 31:489, 1969.

Lamaze F: L'experience francaise de l'accouchement sans douleur. Bull Circle Claude Bernard 8:2, 1954.

Lahmann AH, Mietus AC: Caudal anesthesia: Its use in obstetrics. Surg Gynecol Obstet 74:63, 1942.

Lull CB, Hingson RA: Control of Pain in Childbirth. Philadelphia, JB Lippincott Co, 1944.

Magno R, Kjellmer I, and Karlsson K: Anaesthesia for cesarean section. III. Effects of epidural analgesia on the respiratory adaptation of the newborn in elective cesarean section. Acta Anaesth Scand 20:73, 1976.

Marx GF, Joshi CW, and Orkin LR: Placental transmission of nitrous oxide. Anesthesiology 32:429, 1970.

McDonald JS, Bjorkman LL, and Reed EC: Epidural analgesia for obstetrics. Am J Obstet Gynecol 120:1055, 1974.

McDonald JS, Bjorkman LL, Reed EC: Epidural analgesia for obstetrics. Am J Obstet Gynecol 120:8, 1055, 1975.

McGuinness GA, Merkow AJ, Kennedy RL, et al: Epidural anesthesia with bupivacaine for cesarean section: neonatal blood levels and neurobehavioral response. Anesthesiology 49:270, 1978.

Moore DC, and Bonica JJ: Convulsions and ventricular tachycardia from bupivacaine with epinephrine: successful resuscitation—congratulations! (Letter to the Editor) Anesth Analg 64:843, 1985.

Moore DC, and Bridenbaugh LD: Oxygen: the antidote for systemic toxic reaction from local anesthetic drugs. JAMA 174:842, 1960.

Moore DC, Spierdijk J, van Kleef JD, et al: Chloroprocaine neurotoxicity: four additional cases. Anesth Analg 61:155, 1982.

Morishima HO, Pedersen H, Finster M, et al: Is bupivacaine more cardiotoxic than lidocaine? Anesthesiology 59:A409, 1983.

Moya F, and Kvisselgaard N: The placental transmission of succinylcholine. Anesthesiology 22:1, 1961.

Moya F, and Thorndike V: Passage of drugs across the placenta. Am J Obstet Gynecol 84:1778, 1962.

Pearson JF, Davies P: The effect of continuous lumbar epidural analgesia upon fetal acid-base status during the first stage of labour. J Obstet Gynaecol Br Commonw 81:971, 1974a.

Pearson JF, Davies P: The effect of continuous lumbar epidural analgesia upon fetal acid-base status during the second stage of labour. J Obstet Gynaecol Br Commonw 81:975, 1974b.

Pickles W, Jones SS: Regional anesthesia in obstetrics with a report of twenty-eight deliveries under epidural block. N Engl J Med 199:988, 1928.

Ralston DH, and Shnider SM: The fetal and neonatal effects of regional anesthesia in obstetrics. Anesthesiology 48:34, 1978.

Ramanathan S: Obstetric Anesthesia. Philadelphia, Lea & Febiger, 1988.

Ravindran RS, Bond VK, Tasch MD, et al: Prolonged neural blockade following regional analgesia with 2-chloroprocaine. Anesth Analg 59:447, 1980.

Reid DE: A Textbook of Obstetrics. Philadelphia, WB Saunders Co, 1962.

Reisner LS, Hochman BN, and Plumer MH: Persistent neurologic deficit and adhesive arachnoiditis following intrathecal 2-chloroprocaine injection. Anesth Analg 59:452, 1980.

Roberman B: Single shot caudal epidural anaesthesia in obstetrics. PNG Med J 17:360, 1974.

Rosen MA, Baysinger CL, Shnider SM, et al: Evaluation of neurotoxicity after subarachnoid injection of large volumes of local anesthetic solutions. Anesth Analg 62:802, 1983.

Sangoul F, Fox GS, Houle GL: Effect of regional analgesia on maternal oxygen consumption during the first stage of labor. Am J Obstet Gynecol 121:1080, 1975.

Scanlon JW, Brown WU, Weiss JB, et al: Neurobehavioral responses of newborn infants after maternal epidural anesthesia. Anesthesiology 40:121, 1974.

Scanlon JW, Ostheimer GW, Lurie AO, et al: Neurobehavioral responses and drug concentrations in newborns after maternal epidural anesthesia with bupivacaine. Anesthesiology 45:400, 1976.

Shnider SM, deLorimier AA, Holl JW, et al: Vasopressors in obstetrics. I. Correction of fetal acidosis with ephedrine during spinal hypotension. Am J Obstet Gynecol 102:911, 1968.

Shnider SM, Levinson G, Ralston DH: Regional Anesthesia for Labor and Delivery. In Shnider SM, Levinson G (eds): Anesthesia for Obstetrics, 2 ed. Baltimore, Williams & Wilkins, 1987.

Stevenson CS: Obstetric analgesia and anesthesia—current problems. J Michigan Med Soc 53:857, 1954.

Thalme B, Belfrage P, Raabe N: Lumbar epidural analgesia in labour. I. Acid-base balance and clinical condition of mother, foetus and newborn child. Acta Obstet Gynecol Scand 53:27, 1974a.

Thalme B, Belfrage P, Raabe N: Lumbar epidural analgesia in labour. II. Effects on glucose, lactate, sodium chloride, total protein, haematocrit and haemoglobin. Acta Obstet Gynecol Scand 53:113, 1974b.

Tronick E, Wise S, Als H, et al: Regional obstetric anesthesia and newborn behavior: effect over the first ten days of life. Pediatrics 58:94, 1976.

Zador G, Nilsson BA: Low-dose intermittent epidural anesthesia with lidocaine for vaginal delivery. II. Influence on labour and foetal acid-base status. Acta Obstet Gynecol Scand Suppl 34:17, 1974.

Zador G, Englesson S, Nilsson BA: Low-dose intermittent epidural anaesthesia with lidocaine for vaginal delivery. I. Clinical efficacy and lidocaine concentrations in maternal, foetal, and umbilical cord blood. Acta Obstet Gynecol Scand Suppl 34:3, 1974.

# CHAPTER 21

. . . . . . . . . . . . . . . . . . . . . . . . . . . . . . . . . . . . . . . . .

# Premature Rupture of the Membranes

Kenneth A. Kappy, Mary McTigue, and Edwin R. Guzman

The optimal management of patients with premature rupture of the membranes (PROM) remains unsettled, because of two main complicating factors. The first is infection. Intact membranes act as a formidable barrier to infectious agents, preventing infections from ascending the genital tract. If the bag of waters is no longer intact, normal vaginal flora may become serious pathogens and place both the mother and fetus in jeopardy. Therefore, an aggressive management plan that may involve induction or augmentation of labor is called for to minimize the dangerous risk of infection.

The second complicating factor is prematurity. PROM frequently occurs in patients who are carrying premature infants. A lack of functional maturity in a fetus may cause devastating complications that can easily result in great expenditures of time, money, and energy. To minimize this risk, a conservative management scheme may be appropriate, to allow intrauterine development to progress for as long as possible.

Some of the variables involved in the management of PROM include the use of antepartum steroids, prophylactic antibiotics, and fetal monitoring studies. Despite the amount of research done in these areas, there is still no universally accepted management scheme. In fact, a survey of members of the Society of Perinatal Obstetricians (Capeless and Mead, 1987) showed 97 percent of the respondents favored an expectant management approach. However, there was no consensus in exactly how to best follow and treat patients with PROM (Capeless and Mead, 1987).

Therefore, each patient with PROM presents a dilemma, namely: Which is a more serious complicating factor, the risk of infection or that of prematurity? The optimal managment protocol must take both of these factors, plus others, into consideration and weigh each separately to make a logical decision for each patient.

## Definition and Incidence

A definition of PROM is not universally agreed on. Some authors make the diagnosis whenever the bag of waters ruptures before the onset of true labor. The time interval between rupture and labor is defined as the latent period. Other authors require that a specific minimal latent period elapse before a diagnosis of PROM is made. This period may vary from 1 to 12 hours depending on the study (Burchell, 1964; Taylor et al, 1961).

Latent periods tend to vary with the length of the gestation. The general rule is that the more premature the pregnancy, the longer the latent period. In a study by Kappy and associates (1979), 85 percent of the patients at term had latent periods of less than 24 hours, whereas 57 percent of patients at less than 37 weeks' gestation went more than 24 hours before labor commenced. These values are consistent with those reported in other studies (Gunn et al, 1970).

The exact incidence rate of PROM varies with each study. Most studies report a rate of 7 to 12 percent, but the range can be anywhere from 2.7 to 17 percent (Gunn et al, 1970). This wide range may be due to a number of variables, such as the exact diagnosis and the investigator's definition of the latent period. In our referral center, (Newark Beth Israel Medical Center, Newark, New Jersey), PROM in a premature pregnancy accounts for more than 50 percent of our referred cases. This factor affects the incidence rates in many individual hospitals. The risk of recurrence of PROM also needs to be studied. Many physicians have seen patients who have PROM in subsequent pregnancies even when clear, etiologic factors cannot be identified. Asrat and associates (1991) have reported on preliminary data that show a 32 percent frequency of recurrent PROM in future pregnancies after a single occurrence.

## Etiology

The exact etiology of PROM remains unknown; many causes have been postulated, but a single common denominator has not yet been found. Possible predisposing factors that have been suggested are incompetency of the cervical os; cervicitis; amnionitis; placenta praevia; genetic abnormalities; fetal malpresentation; increased uterine tension, as in multiple pregnancies or hydramnios; trauma; previous induced abortions; abruptio placentae; and vaginal infections (Sweet, 1981).

Others have suggested that the membranes themselves may have an inherent weakness that predisposes to PROM. Sbarra (1978) has been working on a theory that local bacterial action may produce a peroxidase that weakens the membranes and causes PROM. However, other studies have failed to verify such a weakness (Al-zaid et al, 1980; Danforth et al, 1953; Polishuk et al, 1962). Nutritional deficiencies have also been implicated. Wideman and colleagues (1964) have postulated that an ascorbic acid deficiency predisposes the membranes to premature rupture.

Infection has always been a leading contender as a cause of PROM. It has been postulated that the infection may act on the membranes directly, via an ascending route from the vagina or an intra-amniotic fluid infection (Naeye, 1977; Naeye and Peters, 1980). Infection also may be the etiologic factor for labor for these patients. Romero and colleagues (1988) have presented information that suggests the onset of labor in patients with PROM is associated with subclinical intra-amniotic or extra-amniotic infections as well as other noninfectious processes.

## Diagnosis

The correct diagnosis of PROM is of great importance. The false-positive diagnosis threatens the patient with a nonindicated intervention involving a potential early delivery or a surgical delivery. The false-negative diagnosis places the infant and mother at an increased risk of infection that may be life threatening to one or both. Therefore, every attempt should be made to diagnosis this condition as quickly and as accurately as possible. To achieve this, one or all of the following factors may be considered.

**History.** The patient's history is important but may be erroneous. Every patient who presents with a story of "feeling wet," or having a "sudden gush of fluid from the vagina" may be describing ruptured membranes, but frequently it is found not to be so. In many cases, a thorough history of recent sexual intercourse, vaginitis, urinary incontinence, or excessive fetal activity may point to other sources of excessive vaginal moisture. Therefore, all cases require objective documentation of ruptured membranes before a definitive diagnosis can be made.

**Physical Examination.** After a complete history is obtained, the vulva should be examined. Any sample of moisture should be inspected for color, consistency, odor, and pH. The fluid may be urine or vaginal secretions. The pH of the fluid can be evaluated by the use of a nitrazine paper analysis (Abe, 1940). The vaginal secretions of the pregnant female are normally acidic, with a pH of 4 to 5. This pH does not turn nitrazine paper from its normal yellow color. However, amniotic fluid with a pH of 7 to 7.5 changes nitrazine paper to a blue color. If blood is present in the fluid sample, it also may change the nitrazine paper to a blue color because of its higher pH.

Regardless of the results of the vulvar inspection, a sterile speculum examination should also be carried out. This procedure permits inspection of the vaginal canal, the posterior vaginal pool, and the cervix itself.

Direct visualization of fluid leaking from the cervical os is the most reliable diagnosis of PROM. If gross leakage is not seen spontaneously, then fundal pressure is applied or the patient is asked to cough or strain down (Valsalva maneuver) to help demonstrate leakage of fluid. If these maneuvers do not produce leakage of fluid, then further evaluation should be made of the cervix and vagina. A sterile cotton swab can be placed at the external cervical os or the posterior vaginal vault to gather moisture, which is then transferred to nitrazine paper. If the paper turns blue, it is presumptive evidence of PROM; however, on occasion, the secretions within the canal itself may be more basic (alkaline) than those of the vagina, and this can lead to an incorrect diagnosis of PROM. Therefore, the posterior vaginal vault is a better area to sample. If gross fluid is not seen and the nitrazine test is positive, then a fern test should also be performed (Tricomi et al, 1966). This is accomplished by placing a sample of the vaginal secretions onto a glass slide and allowing it to air dry. The slide is then inspected under a low-power microscope to look for crystallization or a ferning pattern. Vaginal secretions do not show the ferning pattern during pregnancy, but if amniotic fluid is present, the fern pattern is seen. This is due to an increased concentration of protein and electrolytes within the fluid. The combination of these two tests should provide a correct diagnosis in over 90 percent of cases.

If the diagnosis of PROM is in question, the patient should be asked to ambulate. This change in position may allow fluid to drain from the cervix, and a repeat examination may confirm the diagnosis. If there is still some question of the diagnosis, amniocentesis with injection of 1 ml of indigo carmine may prove helpful. However, this procedure is invasive and should be used in relatively few cases. To document leakage in these patients, a sterile tampon should be placed in the vagina, and the patient is asked to ambulate. After a few hours, the tampon is removed and the internal end is inspected. If it is blue, the diagnosis is confirmed. However, because the dye is excreted mainly through the maternal urine, one must be careful *not* to make an erroneous diagnosis of PROM when the patient urinates and stains the external end of the tampon. Ultrasound may also assist in making the diagnosis by demonstrating oligohydramnios. However,

it must be kept in mind that oligohydramnios may be caused by conditions other than PROM. Ultrasound is also useful for obtaining information on gestational age and presentation of the infant. These parameters help in making a decision on the timing and route of the delivery.

**Other Diagnostic Measures.** During the sterile speculum examination, it is imperative to take a culture of the cervix if a diagnosis of PROM is made or even if it is suspected. This allows for early identification of potentially serious pathogens such as *Escherichia coli* and group B β-hemolytic streptococci. These pathogens are discussed later in this chapter.

Careful consideration must be given to deciding whether or not a bimanual examination should be carried out in patients with PROM. In the patient who has not reached term and who is not in labor, vaginal examination is usually unnecessary and rarely alters the early management of patients with PROM (Gunn et al, 1970; Kappy et al, 1979). It may even be deleterious in that the examining finger may inoculate the lower uterine segment with the normal vaginal flora. These organisms can quickly and easily become serious pathogens. The digital examination should be performed only in those patients with PROM in whom labor has begun spontaneously or for whom labor induction is to begin. The total number of examinations should be kept to a minimum even in these cases.

Many other tests have been used for the diagnosis of PROM. Smith (1976) has reviewed the use of such tests as the Papanicolaou smear, Nile blue sulfate stain, fluorescein staining test, Sudan stains, and even lanugo hair identification, and has reported varied results. More recently, other diagnostic tests have been used to diagnose PROM. One such diagnostic tool is to determine the presence of α-fetoprotein by a rapid latex agglutination test (Rochelson et al, 1983). Further evaluation, however, is necessary to show its appropriateness.

## Initial Evaluation

When the diagnosis of PROM is made, an initial evaluation is performed to ascertain the status of the patient. Gestational age is very important. To determine this age accurately, a thorough history and chart review is mandatory. Information is obtained concerning last menstrual period, regularity of menstrual cycles, initial pelvic examination, availability of an early pregnancy test, date of quickening, date the fetal heart tones were first heard with a fetoscope, growth of the fundus, abdominal examination, and results of any ultrasound examinations that may have been performed. All of these parameters help identify the gestational age of the fetus.

Gestational age alone may not be a reliable indicator of fetal maturity. For this reason, amniotic fluid can be used for an evaluation of fetal lung maturity. There has been some skepticism of the results of fetal lung maturity studies based on amniotic fluid collected from the vagina. The argument has been that the vaginal and cervical secretions in some way alter the lecithin–sphingomyelin (L/S) ratio, giving erroneous results. However, there are data that show that amniotic fluid collected vaginally is a reliable indicator of fetal lung maturity (Sbarra et al, 1981). The authors have compared vaginally collected amniotic fluid with that collected from transabdominal amniocentesis and found them to have good correlation (Kappy, unpublished data). Investigators have recently evaluated phospholipids such as phosphatidylglycerol to determine fetal lung maturity. There are reports in the literature of phosphatidylglycerol being used in cases of PROM to accurately predict fetal lung maturity, based on an analysis of vaginally collected fluid (Stedman et al, 1981).

Part of the initial examination must be directed toward ruling out chorioamnionitis. Possible indicators of this serious infectious problem are maternal fever, maternal or fetal tachycardia, uterine tenderness to palpation, uterine contractions, odoriferous vaginal discharge, and elevated white blood cell counts with a shift in the differential.

All patients should also have external electronic fetal heart rate monitoring as part of an initial evaluation. This method may show a fetal tachycardia or variable decelerations that may indicate occult cord prolapse or fetal compromise. Early labor also can be diagnosed by using the fetal monitor. A nonstress test should be performed during the initial examination to evaluate fetal wellbeing.

At the time of the sterile speculum examination, attention should be given to the condition of the cervix itself. On visual inspection, the examiner should be able to give a rough estimate of whether the cervix is (1) dilated or tightly closed, (2) anterior or posterior in the vagina, and (3) markedly effaced or very long. In other words, an estimate of inducibility may be obtained by visual inspection. This procedure is not as accurate as a bimanual examination, but it will provide a good estimate without exposing the patient to an added risk of infection. An assessment for a prolapsed cord can also be done at this time.

# Subsequent Management Variables

Once the diagnosis of PROM has been made and an initial evaluation has been carried out, other variables must be considered. These would include such complicating factors as risk of respiratory distress syndrome (RDS), risk of infection, and cervical inducibility. These variables should be considered for each patient before an individualized plan of management is made.

## RISK OF RDS

Aggressive management is ideal if there is some assurance that the infant is mature and that the attempted delivery would not put the infant and mother at an increased risk of morbidity or mortality. Maturity can be estimated with increasing gestational age, but even term newborns may show RDS if complicating factors—such as maternal illnesses (e.g., diabetes), birth trauma, or hypoxia—are present.

With PROM in a preterm gestation, there is always a risk of RDS; in fact, RDS is the major cause of neonatal morbidity and mortality. It is a far greater threat to the newborn than is neonatal sepsis. This risk has been shown to decrease, however, with antepartum exogenous steroid administration to the mother (Liggins and Howie, 1972). Recent use of neonatal surfactant preparations after delivery look promising to reduce RDS. PROM is not a contraindication to the use of these drugs. It is also possible for naturally occurring steroids to be an aid in fetal lung maturation. A stimulus for steroid release is stress. Whether this stress is from the loss of amniotic fluid, subclinical infection, or compression of the fetus in utero, the result is the same. A number of studies have shown an increased level of cortisol in patients with PROM as compared with normal patients. These studies have shown increased cortisol in the maternal serum in as short a time as 16 hours (Bauer et al, 1974) and in amniotic fluid after 24 hours of ruptured membranes (Cohen et al, 1976). Many investigators have demonstrated that this stress accelerates fetal lung maturity (Berkowitz et al, 1978; Richardson et al, 1974; Sell and Harris, 1977; Worthington et al, 1977). The length of the latent period required for this pulmonary maturation ranges from as little as 16 hours to 72 hours. Others have suggested that the pulmonary maturation actually precedes rather than results from the PROM (Worthington et al, 1977). An increased L/S ratio has been observed in patients with PROM for more than 24 hours (Morrison et al, 1977; Richardson et al, 1974; Verder et al, 1978). A study by Yeung (1982), showed a positive effect of PROM on RDS by comparing twins with PROM. In the first twin with PROM, there was a 13.8 percent incidence of RDS compared with an 80 percent incidence in the second twin, who was not stressed with PROM.

There are, however, other studies that have not been able to show an accelerated fetal lung maturation in patients with PROM when compared with matched controls (Barrada et al, 1977; Christensen et al, 1976; Jones et al, 1975). The largest review of cases has been conducted by Jones and coworkers (1975). In their report, a review of 16,458 neonates, weighing more than 500 g and delivered from patients with and without PROM, was carried out to evaluate the effect that PROM for more than 24 hours before delivery had on the eventual development of RDS. There was no significant difference between the two groups when infants of the same gestational age were compared. The different conclusions in these studies may be due to a number of factors. One factor may be that a study with a large number of cases provides for more equal distribution of patients into smaller subgroups, thereby eliminating confounding variables. Another is that none of the studies routinely used the same variables, such as definition of ruptured membranes, length of latent period, and definition of RDS. These variations make it difficult to compare individual results and conclusions. Therefore, at this time, it must be considered that PROM does *not* provide definite protection against RDS.

One must also remember that lung maturity does not mean fetal maturity. A mature L/S ratio with the presence of phosphatidylglycerol indicates lung maturity alone. It does not provide information about the central nervous system, liver function, or other organ systems. Premature infants who do not have problems with RDS may have serious problems, such as necrotizing enterocolitis, hyperbilirubinemia, or intracerebral bleeding. A mature L/S ratio does *not* mean that a 33-week-old fetus should be delivered without concern. Continued intrauterine development in these premature patients may be of considerable importance and benefit.

## INDUCIBILITY

Labor inductions are frequently carried out in patients with PROM who are thought to be at term. Frequently this occurs in a patient whose cervix is not inducible, and thus, attempted inductions may fail, because the cervix may not be ready to respond to oxytocin. This problem has been reported in the past with term patients with PROM (Kappy et al, 1979, 1982). In those patients in whom labor inductions were carried out because of PROM, as compared with those who began labor spontaneously, there was a higher risk of cesarean birth (39 versus 19 percent) owing to lack of progress of labor. In many cases, this complication occurred in patients who had delivered larger infants in prior pregnancies; therefore, bony cephalopelvic disproportion could not be the cause.

It is also well known that patients who undergo cesarean deliveries have higher morbidity and mortality rates than those who deliver vaginally. These statistics may be due to anesthesia, operative complications, or infection. If one adds to this the increased risk of infection from multiple bimanual examinations to evaluate progress during the induction (Burchell, 1964), the total risk may outweigh the benefits of the induction (Duff et al, 1984).

## RISK OF INFECTION

The major maternal complication with PROM is the development of chorioamnionitis, which may progress to general sepsis. The incidence of chorioamnionitis seems to be related to the length of the latent period and the route of delivery. Bryans and associates (1965) reported that 6.4 percent of patients with PROM exhibited clinical infection within 24 hours but that this number increased to 30 percent of patients beyond 24 hours. Others have shown similar data, with chorioamnionitis reported in 26 to 28 percent of patients with a latent period of greater than 24 hours (Lanier et al, 1965, Schreiber and Benedetti, 1980). As already discussed, cesarean deliveries place the mother at increased risk, especially for postpartum endometritis and bacteremia (Bada et al, 1977; Kappy et al, 1979; Mead and Clapp, 1977). These infections are frequently mixed bacterial infections with anaerobic organisms. Maternal outcome, however, tends to be good according to most studies.

Along with RDS, the major *fetal* complication associated with PROM is infection leading to sepsis. The risk of fetal and neonatal infection was investigated by St. Geme and associates (1984), who reviewed 2556 pregnancies complicated by PROM. In this review, infection occurred in 1.3 percent of the births complicated by PROM alone, and in 8.7 percent of births following prolonged rupture with signs of clinical chorioamnionitis. The risk of infection has long been considered to be in direct relationship to the length of the latent period. Gunn and associates (1970) demonstrated an increased perinatal mortality rate after 48 hours of PROM and advocated early delivery. However, the length of the latent period alone may not entirely account for the degree of risk of infection. It is probable that gestational age and maturation also play a role.

What factors influence the risk of infection? Clearly there are at least two: (1) the infectivity of the offending organism and (2) the available host defenses.

The normal bacteria flora of the vagina and cervix consists of many different organisms, both aerobic and anaerobic. Lactoba-

cilli are the most common, but staphylococci, streptococci, *E. coli*, *Klebsiella* spp., clostridia, peptococci, and *Bacteroides* spp. have been identified. As a normal pregnancy progresses through the second and third trimesters, there is a decreasing number of anaerobic bacteria in the cervical flora, followd by an increase during the first week postpartum. The total number of bacteria returns to the level of the first trimester by the sixth postpartum week (Goplerud et al, 1976). The bacteria found in the uterus during labor or postpartum can be any of these normally occurring bacteria.

An organism that is of grave concern is the group B β-hemolytic streptococcus. It has been shown that 80 percent of newborn infants with early-onset group B streptococcus sepsis are of low birth weight and that 62 percent were born after a prolonged latent period following PROM (Baker and Barrett, 1973). Part of the problem with group B streptococci is that they have been found to colonize in 5 to 27 percent of asymptomatic women (Sweet and Ledger, 1973), and these women may be at increased risk of PROM and premature labor (Regan et al, 1981). Rapid treatment with broad-spectrum antibiotics is indicated if group B β-hemolytic streptococci chorioamnionitis is suspected. Many experts recommend initiating intravenous penicillin and inducing labor with PROM if gestational age is greater than 32 weeks.

Amniotic fluid itself may have an antimicrobial property. According to the data of several investigators, there is a phosphate-sensitive bacterial growth inhibitor in amniotic fluid (Larsen, 1980; Schlievert et al, 1977). This substance is inactivated by phosphate and is dependent on zinc for its activity. It is also inactivated by large numbers of bacteria and seems to reach its peak activity in term pregnancies. Amniotic fluid seems to be bacteriostatic near term. This explains why occult bacterial contamination can exist without evidence of sepsis at term. However, if PROM permits further contamination of the amniotic fluid and bacterial numbers reach a critical level, then bacterial growth will not be inhibited and sepsis will develop. Unfortunately, the action of the amniotic fluid's inhibitory substances against anaerobic organisms are only temporary (Thadepalli et al, 1977). This inhibition also may be related to diet and could explain why patients of low socioeconomic class have an increased risk of infection.

Other antimicrobial substances have also been identified in the amniotic fluid. One is a bactericidal protein, a $\beta$ lysin that is believed to be present in pregnancies greater than 14 weeks and that acts against the cytoplasmic membranes of gram-positive bacteria (Ford et al, 1977). Lysozyme, another inhibitory substance that is normally contained in phagocytic leukocytes, may also provide bacteriolytic activity. The function of lysozyme remains unclear, but it may provide nonspecific resistance to bacterial infection. This substance also seems to increase from 25 weeks until term (Bratlid and Linoback, 1978).

## DIAGNOSIS OF CHORIOAMNIONITIS

The diagnosis of chorioamnionitis, once it is fulminant, is not difficult. Clinically, one may observe fetal or maternal tachycardia, maternal fever, uterine tenderness, foul vaginal or cervical discharge, and uterine contractions. A leukocytosis with a shift in the differential also is frequently noted. However, the early signs of chorioamnionitis are not as easily identified. In fact, none of the signs of chorioamnionitis are very reliable indicators of early infection. When these signs are compared with bacteriologic identification of the offending organisms or pathologic evidence of infection on microscopic examination of the placenta, more than 50 percent of the cases are false-positive (Townsend et al, 1966).

In an effort to make a more correct diagnosis in these cases, alternative parameters have been examined. One such parameter is microscopic examination of the amniotic fluid for the presence of leukocytes or bacteria. However, this determination is controversial. Some have reported that the presence of bacteria in an amniotic fluid sample shows an increased risk of infection (Bobitt and Ledger, 1978; Garite et al, 1979; Zlatnick et al, 1984). Some of these amniotic fluid samples, however, were obtained by using an intrauterine pressure catheter or by transcervical amniocentesis, and both of these methods are unreliable for obtaining samples free of cervical contaminants. Similarly, other studies in which fluid was obtained by the same routes have shown that leukocytes are more indicative of risk than are bacteria (Larsen et al, 1974). Another study shows that neither bacteria nor leukocytes correlate with the potential for infection (Listwa et al, 1976). Any study, however, that uses leukocytes in amniotic fluid for predicting infection has a drawback. These white blood cells could be a contaminant from the cervix or blood or may be present as a result of the mechanical effects of labor.

Another potential sign of impending infection is an elevated level of C-reactive protein. In one study based on this indicator, there were no false-positive results and only 10 percent false-negative results (Evans et al, 1980). This test has the obvious advantage of dealing with factors from maternal serum, making it preferable to a more invasive test such as amniocentesis.

Low glucose concentrations seem to be promising as an early prognostic sign of infection, and recent work has shown this study to be of value in predicing early intraamniotic infection (Romero et al, 1990). Some preliminary studies also have been performed to evaluate this test in patients with PROM, but more studies are needed to determine the true value of this test (Dildy et al, 1991).

The biophysical profile also has been used as a predictor of the risk of infectious morbidity. Vintzileos and associates (1985) have shown a close association between a low biophysical profile within 48 hours of delivery and infectious morbidity. These low scores mainly reflected decreased amounts of amniotic fluid and nonreactive nonstress tests. Further studies have shown the closest relationship to be between infectious morbidity and decreased fetal breathing activity on the biophysical profile (Vintzileos et al, 1986). Vintzileos and associates believe that this problem is due to the release of prostaglandins from infected membranes, causing a depression of the fetal respiratory centers.

The correct early diagnosis of fetal maturity and chorioamnionitis is important. If a test is performed to accurately predict which fetuses are mature and which are at increased risk of infection, rapid delivery is accomplished before the morbidity and mortality rates increase. These tests probably involve amniotic fluid, thereby necessitating amniocentesis. Amniocentesis is a relatively simple procedure, but it does carry some risks, even in patients with intact membranes. The procedure carries the risk of trauma, bleeding, initiation of labor, and infection. Once the patient has PROM with leakage of varying amounts of fluid, the risk increases. In the authors' experience and in that of others (Garite et al, 1979), the success rate for obtaining fluid in PROM patients was only 50 percent even with ultrasonic guidance.

## ANTIBIOTIC USE

Antibiotic prophylaxis has been shown to be of value in certain obstetric and gynecologic procedures. In patients with PROM, the benefits have ranged from small to none at all (Bobbitt and Ledger, 1978). The consensus in the past has been that, although there may be a decrease in postpartum fever due to genitourinary infection, perinatal mortality had not decreased (Gordon and Winegold, 1974; Lebherz et al, 1963). Some recent studies have pointed to a benefit of prophylactic antibiotic use. Johnston and associates (1990) have shown a decreased frequency of chorioamnionitis and endometritis when patients were treated with antibiotics. Similarly, Morales and coworkers (1989) have shown a benefit from using antibiotics and steroids in patients with immature lungs and PROM. Further studies are still needed to make a more convincing argument. Prophylaxis may also increase the risk of more serious nosocomial infections and may interfere with culture reliability in the neonate. If chorioamnionitis is present, therapeutic doses of antibiotics are given with delivery, which should be accomplished as soon as possible by the least traumatic route.

## USE OF ANTEPARTUM STEROIDS

The use of antepartum steroids to accelerate fetal lung maturity has become widespread since is was originally described by Liggins and Howie (1972). Although there have been no significant adverse effects reported by these examiners, others have reported neurologic and electroencephalographic abnormalities in the offspring (Fitzharding et al, 1974). The use of steroids in patients with PROM is also controversial because of the potential suppression of the immune system, with possible increased infection risk for mother and fetus (Garite et al, 1981; Collaborative Group on Antenatal Steroid Therapy, 1981). However, in patients with PROM, it appears that the major risk to the fetus is from RDS and prematurity rather than from infection. Therefore, steroids may be of benefit for these patients. Using this logic, Mead administered steroids and then delivered patients after 24 hours. He showed a significant reduction in neonatal morbidity and mortality, mainly as a result of a decreased incidence of RDS without an increase in maternal infectious morbidity (Mead and Clapp, 1977). The authors' studies and those of others support these findings (Kappy et al, 1979; Morales et al, 1986; Quirk et al, 1979). A number of studies now have accumulated suggesting that antenatal glucocorticoid steroids are of no major benefit in patients with PROM. These studies have shown no marked reduction in the incidence of RDS following PROM as compared with patients not receiving the medication (Iams et al, 1985; Nelson et al, 1985; Simpson and Harbert, 1985).

## USE OF TOCOLYTICS

The use of tocolytics in patients with PROM is also controversial. Labor can be one of the signs of chorioamnionitis. Because of this, many feel that if labor occurs, no effort should be made to stop it, because if tocolytics are used, an infection problem may go unrecognized and worsen. Others say that because prematurity is such a serious problem in these patients, steroids should be used for lung maturation with concomitant tocolytics, if needed, to prolong the pregnancy for 24 to 48 hours. This approach allows enough time for the steroids to work (Mead and Clapp, 1977). At the end of that time, either labor can be induced, or tocolytics can be stopped and labor allowed to ensue. Tocolytics are less effective in patients with PROM. However, frequently a delay of only 24 hours can be obtained by using tocolytics in these patients (Christensen et al, 1980; Wesselius deCasparis et al, 1971).

The role of tocolytics in PROM patients was reviewed in a collaborative study on antenatal steroid therapy (Curet et al, 1984). In this study, patients with PROM who were treated with tocolytics in an effort to prolong gestation to prevent RDS *showed no significant benefit* when compared with those with PROM who did not receive tocolytics.

## ROUTE OF DELIVERY

Various opinions are held regarding the route of delivery in patients with PROM. As mentioned previously, patients with PROM who undergo cesarean delivery have an increased risk of infection. These infections not only occur more frequently but are also more serious, with more aggressive bacteria as causative agents. A vaginal delivery diminishes this risk (Ledger, 1979). In contrast, there are those who believe that the route of delivery should be dictated by the risks to the fetus, especially in the premature infant (Quirk et al, 1979). In his study of predominantly lower socioeconomic patients, Quirk and associates made every effort to achieve a nonhypoxic, nonstressful, atraumatic labor and delivery, along with the use of steroids for induction of pulmonary maturity. If an induction was not considered to be easy, or if there were signs of fetal distress, a cesarean delivery was carried out. This very strict surveillance resulted in a cesarean delivery rate of 40 percent. In this study, in which the mean gestational age was 31 weeks, there was a 15 percent incidence of RDS and an 88 percent survival rate.

In a similar study, Nochimson and coworkers (1980), using a middle-class population, showed comparable results. The study group consisted of patients pregnant for less than 34 weeks with PROM who were treated with steroids. If labor began within 24 hours, magnesium sulfate was started as a tocolytic agent until at least a 24-hour delay of labor was obtained after steroid administration. Elective delivery was then carried out by the least traumatic route. The control group was treated conservatively, without steroids, and delivered whenever spontaneous labor began, or when infection was found. In the study group, 11.9 percent of the fetuses developed RDS, and 16.6 percent were delivered by cesarean delivery. In the control group, 31.1 percent developed RDS and 9.8 percent were delivered by cesarean delivery. There was a mortality of 4.8 percent in the study group, compared with a 9.8 percent rate in the control group. The authors concluded that a nonconservative, dynamic management plan, with avoidance of delivery trauma, improved neonatal survival.

The emphasis was on the avoidance of intrapartum stress, hypoxia, and trauma.

## NEONATAL DEFORMITIES

One of the areas that must be considered in treating patients with PROM is the effect of decreased amniotic fluid on the further structural development of the fetus. Graham and associates (1980) believed that limb reduction anomalies can occur from early in utero limb compression as seen in cases of PROM. This may be from the formation of amniotic bands from the amnion to fetal parts, particularly the limbs and digits (Torpin, 1965). These bands may produce amputation defects of limbs and digits. Similarly, band-induced craniofacial defects have also been described (Jones et al, 1974). These defects may be caused not only by bands of adhesions but also by compression of the fetal parts (Fig. 21–1). Kennedy and Persaud (1977) believe that compression may cause a vascular insult within the developing limb, resulting in necrotic absorption and loss of previously normal tissue. These defects would be considered non-band limb reduction defects. Limb–body wall defects have also been described by Miller and colleagues (1981). They postulate that all of these defects fit a spectrum of abnormalities that may occur with PROM, which they have named the amnion rupture sequence. There is a review of this subject by Seeds and associates (1982) that goes into greater detail.

In premature infants younger than 28 weeks' gestation, when PROM was prolonged for greater than 24 hours, a higher incidence of positional foot deformities, congenital dislocations of the hips, and hypoplastic lungs was demonstrated in comparison with other newborns (Kanjanapone et al, 1979). These limb deformities are believed to be related to the lack of adequate amniotic fluid to allow free motion of the fetus in utero.

Another complication noted in patients with PROM is fetal pulmonary hypoplasia. This lack of pulmonary development seems to be related to a deficiency of amniotic fluid necessary to sufficiently bathe the fetal lungs during development. This problem is noted only when PROM occurs early in pregnancy (<20 weeks) and the membranes have been ruptured for a long period of time (>4 weeks) (Nimrod et al, 1984).

Moretti and Sibai (1988) investigated the

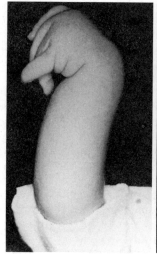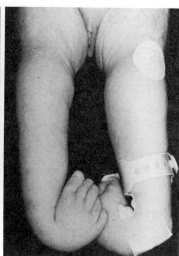

**Figure 21–1.** This neonate presented with arthrogryposis after prolonged rupture of the membranes. (Courtesy of University of South Florida, College of Medicine, Tampa, FL.)

perinatal outcome in mid-trimester pregnancies complicated by PROM. They showed a 13 percent perinatal survival rate in pregnancies in which PROM occurred before 23 weeks. However, this rate climbed to 50 percent survival in the 24-to-26-week group, the developmental abnormality rate in this same group was 33 percent, placing even those patients who survived at substantial risk of further complications.

## A Management Plan

There is no ideal management for *all* patients with PROM. The management varies depending on gestational age, risk of infection, presence of labor contractions, and the specific patient population. For example, a management plan that works in a private institution treating well-educated, well-nourished patients may not be the same one used to manage indigent patients in an inner-city hospital. The well-nourished patients may have a minimal risk of infection, whereas the indigent patients may be at such a high risk for morbidity and mortality due to infection that any attempt at conservative management may be completely out of the question. With these factors in mind, a plan for the *average* patient may be outlined.

Initially, it is of utmost importance that a correct diagnosis of PROM be made. A combination of history, sterile speculum exami-

nation, nitrazine paper test, fern test, and instillation of a dye into the amniotic fluid may be necessary for a truly accurate diagnosis. Reliance on only one of these parameters may easily result in an erroneous diagnosis. Of special note is that only a sterile speculum examination should be performed. The amount of information gained by the digital examination over that gained by the visual inspection of the cervix is not sufficient to add the extra risk of infection that is inherent with this procedure. A bimanual examination should never be performed unless the patient is in labor or thought to be already infected, with an induction of labor forthcoming. Patients with documentation of PROM should then be admitted to the hospital for evaluation.

The initial examination must evaluate the fetal status. Fetal monitoring for signs of occult cord prolapse (variable decelerations) or infection (fetal tachycardia) is mandatory. Also, the presence of accelerations demonstrates fetal well-being. An estimation must be made of gestational age based on information on the last menstrual period, early examination, early pregnancy test, date of quickening, date of first fetal heart tones auscultated with a DeLee fetoscope, ultrasound examinations, and uterine growth rates, all of which should be verified if possible. Despite the sophistication of some of these parameters, a reliable date of the last menstrual period is still the best indicator of gestational age. The presence of infection must also be evaluated on the initial examination. A high white blood cell count with a shift in the differential, maternal fever, maternal or fetal tachycardia, uterine tenderness, a foul vaginal discharge, or labor may indicate infection. A transabdominal amniocentesis with fluid analysis for bacteria or white blood cells may give helpful information as to the risk of infection. An initial cervical bacterial culture and sensitivity test should be obtained at the time of the sterile speculum examination, to obtain information on the cervical flora. Fetal lung maturity should be determined, if feasible; amniotic fluid from an amniocentesis or from the vaginal pool may be used for this purpose.

If there are signs of chorioamnionitis, an aggressive approach with delivery as soon as possible is indicated. In all such cases, broad-spectrum antibiotics in high doses should be started as soon as the initial cultures are obtained. If a cesarean delivery is deemed necessary, it should be carried out after the antibiotics are begun.

For the patient with PROM who shows no signs of infection, labor, or fetal distress, a conservative approach may be followed. This approach should consist of bed rest in the hospital with daily CBCs and differentials; vital signs and temperature every 4 hours while the patient is awake; daily evaluation of uterine tenderness; and weekly antepartum fetal heart rate evaluations (NST/CST/BPP). This approach is followed in the hospital for as long as the patient is leaking fluid. If the leaking stops, even with increased ambulation, the patient may be given discharge instructions, including no sexual intercourse, douching, or tampons, and sent home. She is told to take her temperature three to four times a day and to report if there is any elevation of the temperature or if there is uterine tenderness, decreased fetal movement, or a foul vaginal discharge. Weekly antepartum fetal heart rate assessment should be continued. If at any time an infection is suspected, no matter what the gestational age, an aggressive approach is taken. Antibiotics are given, and the patient should be delivered. Prophylactic antibiotics and tocolytics may have a place in the routine care of patients with PROM. It is our belief that labor may be an initial sign of chorioamnionitis and should not be ignored or suppressed.

This general management scheme, however, is modified depending on the gesta-

tional age of the patient. Patients of less than 20 weeks' gestation may be managed in either of two ways. Because of the risk of infection and the need for intrauterine development to reach a minimal age of viability, the patient may choose to have a termination of pregnancy. This route should be favored if the risk of infection is high. On the other hand, some patients may be treated conservatively even at this early stage of gestation, for the amniotic sac may seal over and the pregnancy may continue. If the patient continues to leak fluid, however, the fetus may be at increased risk of having compression deformities. In general, most of these early pregnancies are interrupted because of these risks.

In PROM patients with a gestational age of 20 to 27 weeks, conservative management is advised. All of these patients should be kept at bed rest and followed closely for as long as they continue to leak fluid.

Patients with a gestational age of 28 to 32 weeks who have PROM may be offered the benefits of antepartum steroid therapy to promote fetal lung maturation. This therapy may consist of betamethasone given in a dose of 12 mg intramuscularly initially with a repeat dose in 24 hours. Further repeat injections are not indicated.

Between 32 and 36 weeks' gestation, the fetus still benefits from continued intrauterine development. Patients at this stage should be followed conservatively in the hospital, and signs of chorioamnionitis should be sought. The use of labor inductions in this group may lead to unnecessary problems with RDS or other prematurity complications. If an analysis of the amniotic fluid has shown fetal lung maturity, then labor induction may be carried out in patients who are at high risk for infection. All others may be allowed to wait for spontaneous labor, so that the fetus may benefit from continued intrauterine development.

Infants delivered at greater than 36 weeks' gestation infrequently have RDS, or if they do, it is usually very mild. Thus, for patients with PROM at this gestational stage, delivery is indicated. The timing of the delivery should be based on an estimate of inducibility of the cervix. If visualization of the cervix at the time of the sterile speculum examination shows an inducible cervix (effaced, anterior, and partially dilated), then an induction can be carried out immediately. If the cervix is not favorable, then observation for 24 to 48 hours should follow. Of the patients at term with PROM, approximately 90 percent begin spontaneous labor during this period. If, at the end of this time, labor has not started, than an induction may be attempted if deemed appropriate.

The use of neonatal support systems is mandatory with all deliveries of premature infants. The possibility of concomitant infection in these infants further increases their risks of morbidity and mortality. Therefore, they should be delivered in a tertiary perinatal center where neonatal support is available in the form of skilled personnel and high-tech equipment.

## PATIENT EDUCATION

The length of the antepartum hospitalization period for the patient with PROM may run from hours to weeks depending on the latency period from rupture to labor. The health care team's major role at this time, along with clinical assessment for symptomatology of labor and infection, is in patient education and psychosocial support.

Patient teaching should be initiated on admission in order to help the patient understand the purpose of procedures and laboratory testing and the need for hospitalization. The patient should be made aware of the purpose of the speculum examination as well as that of the baseline cervical culture and the CBC with differential. If the patient is aware of the importance of such testing, she is more likely to be compliant with the prescribed regime. At this time she should be instructed in the signs and symptoms of chorioamnionitis so that she is able to recognize them as complicating factors. The purpose and need of daily CBCs and the role of the leukocyte in the infectious process should be explained.

Patient education also needs to focus on the physiology of the membranes and the purpose of the amniotic fluid. Explanation of the terms high leak, gross rupture, and seal-over should be explained to the patient. She should be encouraged to express any points of confusion. The membranes may be compared to the skin of the patient, operating as a barrier to bacteria and infection. Frequently, the patient with PROM may ask about dry birth, thinking that the amniotic fluid will not be replaced. It is necessary to explain that fluid will continue to be pro-

duced, although there may be smaller amounts surrounding the baby (Kilbride et al, 1989). Amniotic fluid helps to maintain fetal temperature; it acts as a cushion for the cord; and it allows the baby to grow, move, and develop symmetrically (Gilbert and Harmon, 1986). This explanation helps the patient understand the significance of fetal monitoring and the need for intervention when abnormalities in the fetal heart rate occur. The patient should also be reassured that the amount of amniotic fluid is being determined during the biophysical profile so that early diagnosis of a problem can be made.

The most common complaint of patients with long-term hospitalization due to PROM is "Why can't I go home? I can do this at home." The PROM patient at our institution usually is not discharged until she delivers because of the major risk of infection; the only exception to this is if the membranes seal over. If, however, the physician decides that discharge is appropriate and the patient is deemed reliable, a special emphasis on self-care at home must be communicated to the patient. This approach would also be appropriate for the patient whose membranes have sealed over. Only a patient deemed reliable should be discharged. Reliability may be determined by a history of consistent attendance at scheduled prenatal visits, immediate seeking of medical care on rupture of the membranes, and in-hospital compliance with the PROM regime. Assessment of the home environment is imperative. A social worker or a visiting nurse usually is helpful in this assessment. The assessment should include factors that would affect her compliance at home, such as whether the woman has help at home; whether it is imperative that she return to work once released, owing to financial hardship; and the number and ages of children at home. Prior to discharge, the patient must be able to demonstrate the correct reading of a thermometer, list the symptoms of infection and labor, demonstrate understanding of daily fetal movement counts, and verbalize the conditions that necessitate return to the hospital. She should be instructed to take her temperature every 4 hours and to note any foul-smelling discharge, uterine tenderness, or contractions. These symptoms, as well as a temperature above 37.8°C (100°F) and a decreased frequency in fetal movements, should be reported to the physician. The patient also should be instructed to avoid douching, tampons, sexual intercourse, and tub baths.

Maintaining a supportive environment should be of the utmost concern for the patient who becomes infected. This in fact may be the first time that the complication becomes real for the patient. The patient and her significant other are now faced with the impending delivery of their infant, who may be preterm or previable. They need to be aware of all procedures that are being performed as well as the presence of all available resources to care for the infant. After delivery and stabilization of the infant, the parents should be encouraged to see and touch the baby, to initiate the bonding process.

## PSYCHOSOCIAL CONSIDERATIONS

### Continuity of Care

The patient with PROM frequently poses a special challenge to medical and nursing personnel because she usually feels well and, thus, may have difficulty understanding the implications of this complication. Psychosocial aspects with regard to family and financial responsibilities may be an overwhelming concern during her hospitalization. The high-risk pregnant woman who is hospitalized for any period of time needs a reality-based orientation to the complication as well as education to aid her and her significant other to face the potential outcomes of the pregnancy. This is best accomplished through the development of a trusting relationship with a consistent nurse and physician, in whom the patient feels she can confide the fear, anxiety, and guilt that she may be experiencing. Nursing continuity may best be achieved through a Clinical Nurse Specialist, primary nurse, or case manager who can support, educate, and advocate for the patient (Heaman, 1990). Especially difficult for the patient with PROM is the fact that she often has been transferred from the care of a primary physician near her home to the care of a high-risk team in a tertiary center miles away from her family. In this case, it is important that the patient be informed of the high-risk team's consultation with her physician as well as any collaborative decisions the physician may have been involved in (Johnson and Murphy, 1986).

### Active Participation

The patient should be encouraged to take on an active role in her care, especially after transfer to the antepartum unit. Powerlessness and a lack of control, in addition to fear and eventual boredom, have been expressed as concerns for the hospitalized, high-risk antepartum patient (Loos and Julius, 1989). Knowledge, education, and involvement in decision-making can help to reduce these concerns.

A more active role can be assumed by the patient in many different forms. For those patients who are being routinely monitored with a fetal monitor, the patient may be taught to apply the monitor to herself at the appropriate times with the assistance of the nurse. The patient may also be taught to take her own temperature and to read the thermometer with confirmation by the nurse. This helps the patient to feel more involved in her care. Another aspect of antepartum surveillance that may help the patient feel she is an active participant in her care is daily fetal movement counts. This should be performed for 1 hour after each meal, with the patient lying quietly on her left side. Decreased frequency in movements is considered to be a signal of possible stress to the infant (Cunningham et al, 1989).

### Overcoming Loss of Control

Loss of control over one's life and health is frustrating for any hospitalized patient but particularly for the patient with PROM, because these patients do not feel sick and, therefore, do not perceive themselves as sick or in need of hospitalization. Loss of control, accompanied by the boredom of bed rest and the isolation experienced within a strange environment, can be lessened by a flexible health care team. A more personal atmosphere can be achieved by allowing families to bring food and items such as quilts and pictures from home. Activities such as puzzles, word games, and needlework can help to reduce boredom. Allowing the patient to determine her own schedule of care activities, including hygiene, monitoring, and antepartum testing, helps her feel more in control of her life despite the complications of pregnancy.

Nursing must also support the patient through the normal developmental tasks of pregnancy (Rubin, 1975) as well as help her feel normal despite the high risk of her pregnancy. This goal is achieved by being flexible, especially with regard to visits by the significant other. This person needs to remain involved and supportive, and this need may not be met within the confines of regular visiting hours. Some support persons may even want to spend the night. Supervised child visitation should also be allowed to maintain family integrity as much as possible. If possible, the patient with PROM should be allowed to attend childbirth classes in the hospital setting via individualized teaching, written materials, or videos. Antepartum hospitalization also provides an environment for postpartum education such as baby baths, breastfeeding, car seat safety, and so on.

## Realistic Expectations

The goal of maintaining the pregnancy to allow for maturity as long as the uterine environment is healthy (Gilbert and Harmon, 1986) must be emphasized to the patient and her significant other. The patient's greatest concerns are for the health of her baby, followed by concerns for her own health and the fear of the outcome (Merkatz, 1978). Supportive measures should focus on verbalization of these emotions, allaying anxieties, and emphasizing the availability of skilled health care practitioners and current technology in the tertiary care center. The patient needs a candid, realistic explanation of the benefits of the conservative approach to PROM (Kappy et al, 1979) versus the risk of delivery of a preterm infant by cesarean delivery. Discussing the risks of prematurity, including respiratory distress syndrome, bronchopulmonary dysplasia, intraventricular hemorrhage, and retinopathy (Goldstein et al, 1989), may foster a better understanding of the need to follow the prescribed regimen. A calm, professional manner must be used by the health care professional so as not to create greater anxiety for the patient. This is especially true in light of the fact that the patient may deliver a preterm infant despite strict compliance with the PROM regimen.

It is also important to introduce the patient to the Neonatal Intensive Care Unit. If the patient is unable to tour the unit, a nursing representative from this unit should visit the patient in her room to talk with her about

the facility, usual procedures, and the type of care that her baby will receive. A staff neonatologist should also visit with the patient to answer questions concerning viability and prognosis in anticipation of a preterm delivery.

## Other Concerns

Frequently, the patient with PROM may have other children at home for whom she has been the primary or sole caretaker. Beside the blame and guilt she may be internalizing, thinking that something she did caused her membranes to rupture (Lemons, 1981), she may also exhibit anxiety about the welfare of her other children. Support should be given to the patient regarding her concerns about her children at home. Sometimes it is hard for the perinatal team to understand that the patient may be more concerned about her children at home than the fetus, to whom she is less attached. Health care professionals can help to alleviate this anxiety by encouraging frequent contacts via the telephone or by having the children visit, as long as they are not sick and have not been exposed to infections or childhood diseases. For those patients whose children are temporarily being cared for by neighbors or friends, social work intervention may be necessary in light of a potential prolonged hospitalization. This may also be warranted if the hospitalization is causing financial difficulties through the loss of the patient's job or income, or the lack of health care insurance. The health care team must take a holistic approach to the care of the patient with PROM to influence all aspects of the patient's care positively and to give her resources so that she is able to comply with the proposed regimen.

It must be emphasized that the management critical paths described here are those that work for us in our institution, at the present time, and with our present population. Each physician must be flexible enough to modify this approach to fit his or her patients. (Table 21–1 summarizes the general management for the patient with PROM.) As more information is obtained regarding patients with PROM, our capacity to manage this complication improves. Analysis of infection risks, host resistance factors, and neonatal complications further refine our management to allow a delivery at the most

**Table 21–1**
PATIENT CARE SUMMARY FOR PREMATURE RUPTURE OF THE MEMBRANES*

| | Antepartum | | Intrapartum | Postpartum |
| | *Outpatient* | *Inpatient* | | |
|---|---|---|---|---|
| Blood pressure | Weekly | q shift | q 1 hr | q 15 min × 4; then q 30 min × 2; then q 1 hr until stable; then on discharge to PP; then q shift |
| Pulse, Respiration | Weekly | q shift | q 1 hr | q 15 min × 4; then q 30 min × 2; then q 1 hr until stable; then on discharge to PP; then q shift |
| Temperature | Weekly | q shift | q 2 hr | q 15 min × 4; then q 30 min × 2; then q 1 hr until stable; then on discharge to PP; then q shift |
| Bed rest | Yes | Yes | Yes | |
| Fetal monitoring | NST/CST weekly at onset of PROM. Presence of fetal movement | NST/CST weekly at onset of PROM; FHR q shift | Continuous during labor, preferably internal. Without a monitor, q 15–30 min listening through 2–3 contractions | — |
| Monitoring of contractions Frequency Duration Quality Resting tone | Daily by patient at home | q shift, prn | Continuous during labor, preferably internal. Without monitor, q 1 hr | — |
| I & O | | | q shift | — |
| Sonogram | q 1 week | q 1 week | | — |
| Amniocentesis | May be done for gestational age Depends on availability of fluid | May be done for gestational age Depends on availability of fluid | — | — |
| Chemistry blood count | Weekly | CBC with differential daily | On admission | On admission to PP; then prn per infection |
| Sexual counseling | No intercourse | No intercourse | — | — |
| Check for uterine tenderness, foul vaginal discharge, cervical discharge | Daily | q shift | Continuous assessment for changes | — |
| Amniotic fluid cultures | Depends on protocol | Depends on protocol | — | — |

* Nurse–patient ratio is 1 : 6–8 antepartum; 1 : 2 intrapartum.

appropriate time and by the most appropriate route.

## References

Abe T: The detection of the rupture of fetal membranes with the nitrazine indicator. Am J Obstet Gynecol 39:400, 1940.

Al-zaid NS, Bou-Resli MN, Goldspint G: Bursting pressure and collagen content of fetal membranes and their relation to premature rupture of the membranes. Br J Obstet Gynecol 8:227, 1980.

Asrat T, Lewis DF, Garite TJ, et al: Frequency of recurrence of preterm premature rupture of membranes. Am J Obstet Gynecol 164:374, 1991. Abstract.

Bada HS, Alojipan LC, Andrews BF: Premature rupture of membranes and its effect on the newborn. Pediatr Clin North Am 24:491, 1977.

Baker CJ, Barrett FF: Transmission of group B streptococci among parturient women and their neonates. Pediatrics 83:919, 1973.

Barrada MI, Virnig NL, Edwards LE, et al: Maternal intravenous ethanol in the prevention of respiratory distress syndrome. Am J Obstet Gynecol 128:25, 1977.

Bauer CR, Stern L, Collie E: Prolonged rupture of membranes associated with a decreased incidence of respiratory distress syndrome. Pediatrics 53:7, 1974.

Berkowitz RL, Kantor RD, Beck GJ, et al: The relationship between premature rupture of the membranes and the respiratory distress syndrome: an update and plan of management. Am J Obstet Gynecol 131:503, 1978.

Bobitt JR, Ledger WJ: Amniotic fluid analysis: its role in maternal and neonatal infection. Obstet Gynecol 51:56, 1978.

Bratlid D, Linoback T: Bacteriolytic activity of amniotic fluid. Obstet Gynecol 51:63, 1978.

Bryans CI, in discussion, Lanier LR, et al: Incidence of maternal and fetal complication associated with rupture of the membranes before onset of labor. Am J Obstet Gynecol 93:403, 1965.

Burchell RC: Premature spontaneous rupture of the membranes. Am J Obstet Gynecol 88:251, 1964.

Capeless E, Mead PB: Management of preterm rupture of membranes: lack of a national consensus. Am J Obstet Gynecol 157:11, 1987.

Christensen KK, Christensen P, Ingemarsson I, et al: A study of complications in preterm deliveries after prolonged premature rupture of the membranes. Obstet Gynecol 48:670, 1976.

Christensen KK, Ingemarsson I, Leidenman T, et al: Effect of ritodrine on labor after premature rupture of the membranes. Obstet Gynecol 55:187, 1980.

Cohen W, Fencl MM, Tulchinsky D: Amniotic fluid cortisol after premature rupture of membranes. J Pediatr 88:1007, 1976.

Collaborative Group on Antenatal Steroid Therapy: Effect of antenatal dexamethasone administration on the prevention of respiratory distress syndrome. Am J Obstet Gynecol 141:276, 1981.

Cunningham F, MacDonald P, Gant N (eds): Williams Obstetrics, 18th ed. East Norwalk, CT, Appleton & Lange, 1989, p 290.

Curet CB, Rao V, Zachman RD, et al: Association between ruptured membranes, tocolytic therapy and respiratory distress syndrome. Am J Obstet Gynecol 148:263, 1984.

Danforth ON, McElin TW, States MN: Studies on fetal membranes. Am J Obstet Gynecol 65:480, 1953.

Dildy GA, Pearlman MD, Smith L: Amniotic fluid glucose as a predictor of intraamniotic infection in preterm labor and preterm rupture of membranes. Am J Obstet Gynecol 164:298, 1991. Abstract.

Duff P, Huff RW, Gibbs RS: Management of premature rupture of membranes and unfavorable cervix in term pregnancy. Obstet Gynecol 63:697, 1984.

Evans MI, Hajj SN, Devoe LD, et al: C-reactive protein as a predictor of infectious morbidity with premature rupture of membranes. Am J Obstet Gynecol 138:648, 1980.

Fitzharding PM, Eisen A, Lehtenyi C, et al: Sequela of early steroid administration of the newborn infant. Pediatrics 53:877, 1974.

Ford LC, Delance RJ, Lebherz TB: Identification of a bactericidal factor (B-Lysin) in amniotic fluid at 14 and 40 weeks gestation. Am J Obstet Gynecol 127:788, 1977.

Garite TJ, Freeman RK, Linzey EM, et al: Prospective randomized study of corticosteroids in the management of premature rupture of the membranes and the premature gestation. Am J Obstet Gynecol 141:508, 1981.

Garite TJ, Freeman RK, Linzey EM, et al: The use of amniocentesis in patients with premature rupture of membranes. Obstet Gynecol 54:226, 1979.

Gilbert E, Harmon J: High Risk Pregnancy and Delivery. St Louis, CV Mosby, 1986, pp 347–361.

Goldstein I, Copel J, Hobbins J: Fetal behavior in preterm premature rupture of the membranes. In Manning FA, Smith MK (eds): Clinics in Perinatology, Vol 16:3. Philadelphia, WB Saunders Co, 1989, pp 735–754.

Goplerud CP, Ohm MJ, Galask RP: Aerobic and anaerobic flora of the cervix during pregnancy and puerperium. Am J Obstet Gynecol 126:858, 1976.

Gordon M, Winegold AB: Treatment of patients with premature rupture of the fetal membranes: a) Prior to 32 weeks; b) After 32 weeks. In Reid DE, Christian CD (eds): Controversy in Obstetrics and Gynecology. Philadelphia, WB Saunders Co, 1974.

Graham JM, Miller ME, Stephan MJ, et al: Limb reduction anomalies and early in utero limb compression. J Pediatr 96:1952, 1980.

Gunn GL, Mishell DR, Morton DG: Premature rupture of the membranes: a review. Am J Obstet Gynecol 106:469, 1970.

Heaman M: Psychosocial apsects of antepartum hospitalization. In McCormick A (ed): NAACOG's Clinical Issues in Perinatal and Women's Health Nursing, Vol 1:3. Philadelphia, JB Lippincott, 1990, pp 333–341.

Iams JD, Talbert ML, Barrows H, et al: Management of preterm prematurely ruptured membranes: a prospective randomized comparison of observation versus use of steroids and time delivery. Am J Obstet Gynecol 151:32, 1985.

Johnson T, Murphy J: Psychosocial implications of high-risk pregnancy. In Knuppel R, Drukker J (eds): High-Risk Pregnancy: A Team Approach. Philadelphia, WB Saunders Co, 1986, pp. 173–186.

Johnston MM, Sanchez-Ramos L, Vaughn AJ: Antibiotic therapy in preterm premature rupture of membranes: a randomized, prospective, double-blind trial. Am J Obstet Gynecol 163:743, 1990.

Jones KL, Smith DW, Hall BD, et al: A pattern of cranioacial and limb defects secondary to aberrant tissue bands. J Pediatr 84:90, 1974.

Jones MD, Burd LI, Bowes WA, et al: Failure of association of premature rupture of membranes with respiratory distress syndrome. N Engl J Med 292:1253, 1975.

Kanjanapone V, Kappy KA, Herschel MJ, et al: The influences of prolonged premature rupture of membranes on the fetus. Pediatr Res 12:528, 1979.

Kappy KA: Unpublished data.

Kappy KA, Cetrulo CL, Knuppel RA: Premature rupture of the membranes at term: a comparison of induced and spontaneous labors. J Reprod Med 27:29, 1982.

Kappy KA, Cetrulo CL, Knuppel RA, et al: Premature rupture of the membranes: a conservative approach. Am J Obstet Gynecol 134:655, 1979.

Kennedy LA, Persaud TVN: Pathogenesis of developmental defects induced in the rat by amniotic sac puncture. Acta Anat 97:23, 1977.

Kilbride H, Yeast J, Thibeault D: Intrapartum and delivery room management of PROM complicated by oligohydramnios. In Hageman JR, Smith MK, (eds):

Clinics in Perinatology Vol 16:4. Philadelphia, WB Saunders Co, 1989, pp 863–868.

Lanier RL, Scarbrough RW, Fillingim DW, et al: Incidence of maternal and fetal complication associated with rupture of the membranes before onset of labor. Am J Obstet Gynecol 93:398, 1965.

Larsen B: How does amniotic fluid protect mother and fetus against infection? Contemp Obstet Gynecol 15:127, 1980.

Larsen JW, Goldhrand JW, Hanson TM, et al: Intrauterine infection on an obstetric service. Obstet Gynecol 43:838, 1974.

Lebherz TB, Hallman LP, Madding R, et al: Double-blind study of premature rupture of the membranes. Am J Obstet Gynecol 87:218, 1963.

Ledger WJ: Premature rupture of membranes and maternal-fetal infection. Clin Obstet Gynecol 22:329, 1979.

Lemons P: The family of the high risk newborn. In Perez R (ed): Protocols for Nursing Practice. St Louis, CV Mosby Co, 1981, pp 440–444.

Liggins GC, Howie RN: A controlled trial of antepartum glucocorticoid treatment for prevention of the respiratory distress syndrome in premature infants. Pediatrics 50:515, 1972.

Listwa HM, Dobek AS, Carpenter J, et al: The predictability of intrauterine infection by analysis of amniotic fluid. Obstet Gynecol 48:31, 1976.

Loos C, Julius L: The client's view of hospitalizations during pregnancy. J Obstet Gynecol Neonatal Nurs 18:52, 1989.

Mead PB, Clapp JE: The use of betamethasone and timed delivery in management of premature rupture of the membranes in the preterm pregnancy. J Reprod Med 19:3, 1977.

Merkatz R: Prolonged hospitalization of pregnant women: the effects on the family. Birth 5:204, 1978.

Miller ME, Graham JM, Higginbottom MC, et al: Compression-related defects from early amnion rupture: evidence for mechanical teratogenesis. J Pediatr 98:292, 1981.

Morales WJ, Angel JL, O'Brien WF, et al: Use of ampicillin and cortcosteroids in premature rupture of membranes: a randomized study. Obstet Gynecol 73:721, 1989.

Morales WJ, Diebel ND, Lazar AJ, et al: The effect of antenatal dexamethasone administration on the prevention of respiratory distress syndrome in preterm gestations with premature rupture of membranes. Am J Obstet Gynecol 154:591, 1986.

Moretti M, Sibai B: Maternal and perinatal outcome of expectant management of premature rupture of membranes in the mid-trimester. Am J Obstet Gynecol 159:390, 1988.

Morrison JC, Whybrew WD, Bucovaz ET, et al: The lecithin/sphingomyelin ratio in cases associated with fetomaternal disease. Am J Obstet Gynecol 127:363, 1977.

Naeye RL: Causes of perinatal mortality in the United States: collaborative perinatal project. JAMA 238:229, 1977.

Naeye RL, Peters EC: Amniotic fluid infection with intact membranes leading to prenatal death: a prospective study. Pediatrics 61:171, 1978.

Naeye RL, Peters EC: Causes and consequences of premature rupture of fetal membranes. Lancet 1:192, 1980.

Nelson LH, Meis PJ, Hatjis CG, et al: Premature rupture of membranes: a prospective randomized evaluation of steroids, latent phase, and expectant management. Obstet Gynecol 66:55, 1985.

Nimrod C, Varela-Gittings F, Machin G, et al: The effect of very prolonged membrane rupture on fetal development. Am J Obstet Gynecol 148:540, 1984.

Nochimson DJ, Petrie RH, Shah BL, et al: Comparison of conservative and dynamic management of premature rupture of membranes/premature labor syndrome. Clin Perinatol 7:17, 1980.

Polishuk WZ, Hohane S, Peranio A: The physical properties of the fetal membranes. Obstet Gynecol 20:204, 1962.

Quirk JG, Rake RK, Petrie RH, et al: The role of glucocorticoids, unstressful labor and atraumatic delivery in the prevention of respiratory distress syndrome. Am J Obstet Gynecol 134:768, 1979.

Regan JA, Chao S, James LS: Premature rupture of membranes, preterm delivery and group B streptococcal colonization of mothers. Am J Obstet Gynecol 141:184, 1981.

Richardson CJ, Pomerance JJ, Cunningham MD, et al: Acceleration of fetal lung maturation following prolonged ruptures of the membranes. Am J Obstet Gynecol 118:1115, 1974.

Rochelson BL, Richardson DA, Macri JN: Rapid assay—possible application in the diagnosis of premature rupture of the membranes. Obstet Gynecol 62:414, 1983.

Romero R, Jinemez C, Lohda AK, et al: Amniotic fluid glucose concentration: a rapid and simple method for the detection of intraamniotic infection in preterm labor. Am J Obstet Gynecol 163:968, 1990.

Romero R, Quintero R, Oyarzun E, et al: Intraamniotic infection and the onset of labor in preterm premature rupture of the membranes. Am J Obstet Gynecol 159:661, 1988.

Rubin R: Maternal tasks in nursing. Matern Child Nurs J 4:143, 1975.

Sbarra AJ: Personal communication, 1978.

Sbarra AJ, Blake G, Cetrulo CL, et al: The effect of cervical/vaginal secretions on measurement of lecithin/sphingomyelin ratio and optical density at 650 mm. Am J Obstet Gynecol 140:214, 1981.

Schlievert P, Johnson W, Jalask RP: Bacterial growth inhibition by amniotic fluid. VII. The effect of zinc supplementation on bacterial inhibitory activity of amniotic fluids from gestations of 20 weeks. Am J Obstet Gynecol 127:603, 1977.

Schreiber J, Benedetti T: Conservative management of preterm premature rupture of the fetal membranes in a low socioeconomic population. Am J Obstet Gynecol 136:92, 1980.

Seeds JW, Cefalo RC, Herbert WN: Amniotic band syndrome. Am J Obstet Gynecol 144:243, 1982.

Sell EJ, Harris ZR: Association of premature rupture of membranes with idiopathic respiratory distess syndrome. Obstet Gynecol 49:167, 1977.

Simpson GF, Harbert GM: Use of betamethasone in management of preterm gestation with premature rupture of membranes. Obstet Gynecol 66:168, 1985.

Smith RP: A technic for the detection of rupture of the membranes: a review and preliminary report. Obstet Gynecol 48:172, 1976.

St Geme JW, Murray DL, Carter J, et al: Perinatal bacterial infection after prolonged rupture of amniotic membranes: an analysis of risk and management. J Pediatr 104:608, 1984.

Stedman CM, Crawford S, Staten E, et al: Management of preterm premature rupture of membranes: assessing amniotic fluid in the vagina for phosphatidylglycerol. Am J Obstet Gynecol 140:34, 1981.

Sweet RL: Perinatal infections: bacteriology, diagnosis and management. *In* Iffy L, Kaminetzky H (eds): Principles and Practice of Obstetrics and Perinatology. New York, Wiley Medical Publications, 1981, pp 1035–1071.

Sweet RL, Ledger WJ: Puerperal infectious morbidity: a two year review. Am J Obstet Gynecol 117:1093, 1973.

Taylor ES, Morgan RL, Bruns PD, et al: Spontaneous premature rupture of the fetal membranes. Am J Obstet Gynecol 82:1341, 1961.

Thadepalli H, Appleman MD, Maidman JE, et al: Antimicrobial effect of amniotic fluid against anaerobic bacteria. Am J Obstet Gynecol 127:250, 1977.

Torpin R: Amniochorionic mesoblastic fibrous strings and amniotic bands: associated constricting fetal malformations or fetal death. Am J Obstet Gynecol 91:65, 1965.

Townsend L, Aickin DR, Fraillon J: Spontaneous premature rupture of the membranes. Aust NZ Obstet Gynecol 6:226, 1966.

Tricomi V, Hall JE, Bittar A, et al: Arborization test for the detection of ruptured fetal membranes. Obstet Gynecol 27:275, 1966.

Verder H, Fonseca J, Falck L, et al: Lecithin/sphingomyelin ratio in eight cases of premature rupture of the membranes. Dan Med Bull 25:218, 1978.

Vintzileos AM, Campbell WA, Nochimson DJ, et al: Fetal breathing as a predictor of infection in premature rupture of the membranes. Obstet Gynecol 67:813, 1986.

Vintzileos AM, Campbell WA, Nochimson DJ, et al: The fetal biophysical profile in patients with premature rupture of the membranes—an early predictor of fetal infection. Am J Obstet Gynecol 152:510, 1985.

Wesselius deCasparis A, Thiery M, Yo Le Sian A, et al: Results of a double-blind, multicenter study with ritodrine in premature labor. Br Med J 3:144, 1971.

Wideman GL, Baird GH, Baldin OT: Ascorbic acid deficiency and premature rupture of fetal membranes. Am J Obstet Gynecol 88:592, 1964.

Worthington D, Maloney AHA, Smith BI: Fetal lung maturity. I. Mode of onset of premature labor: influence of premature rupture of the membranes. Obstet Gynecol 49:275, 1977.

Yeung CY: Effects of prolonged rupture of membranes on the development of respiratory distress syndrome in twin pregnancy. Aust Pediatr J 18:197, 1982.

Zlatnick F, Cruikshank D, Petzold C, et al: Amniocentesis in the identification of inapparent infection in preterm patients with premature rupture of the membranes. J Reprod Med 29:656, 1984.

# CHAPTER 22

. . . . . . . . . . . . . . . . . . . . . . . . . . . . . . . . . . .

# Preterm Labor

Jeffrey Lipshitz, Patricia M. Pierce, and Meichelle Arntz

Preterm delivery, which accounts for over 75 percent of all cases of perinatal morbidity and mortality, remains the most important obstetric problem in the world today. Although ritodrine hydrochloride was introduced as the first FDA-approved drug for the treatment of preterm labor in the United States, it is far from a panacea and has resulted in serious iatrogenic problems such as maternal pulmonary edema and death. Part of the problem has been due to a poor understanding of the diverse nature of preterm labor, poor selection of patients for tocolytic therapy, the widespread metabolic and cardiovascular effects of the $\beta$-agonists ($\beta$-stimulators), and a failure to recognize the dangers and pitfalls associated with the use of these drugs in the treatment of preterm labor. This chapter is written with these issues in mind.

## Definition and Incidence

In the past, the term *premature* was used to describe babies born before 37 or 38 weeks' gestation as well as those with a weight of less than 2500 g. This definition is confusing, because approximately 40 percent of these babies, although they weigh less than 2500 g, have a gestational age of greater than 37 weeks. The term premature should no longer be used, and infants should be described in terms of either birth weight or gestational age. The World Health Organization's (WHO) recommendation is that infants delivered at less than 37 completed weeks' (<259 days') gestation from the first day of the last menstrual period be defined as preterm, and infants weighing less than 2500 g be classified as low birth weight (Anderson, 1977). Most statistics, however, refer to birth weight, because gestational age is often difficult to determine.

The incidence of low-birth-weight babies in the United States from 1950 to 1987 is depicted in Figure 22–1. In 1987, the preterm delivery rate was 101 per 1000 live births (Gabbe et al, 1991). The incidence of low-birth-weight babies by race in the United States from 1950 to 1987 is depicted in Figure 22–2.

## Consequences of Preterm Birth

Preterm birth is the leading cause of early neonatal death. This factor is demonstrated in a study from England (Rush et al, 1976). Although the preterm birth rate was only 5.1 percent, 85 percent of early neonatal deaths not due to lethal deformity occurred in these newborns. Preterm newborns born alive had a chance of survival 120 times lower than that of newborns born later in gestation. The introduction of specialized neonatal intensive care units has greatly improved the prognosis for the small newborn from the depressing outcomes of the 1940s and 1950s, when the survival expectation for the neonate under 1500 g was less than 20 percent and up to 70 percent of the survivors had significant developmental handicaps. The incidence of major handicap is still approximately 10 percent (Fitzhardinge, 1975; Sabel

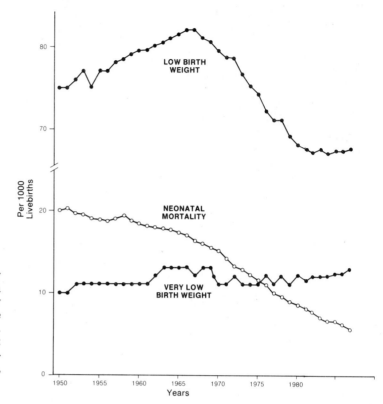

**Figure 22–1.** Incidence of low birth weight, very low birth weight, and neonatal mortality per 1000 live births in the United States for 1950 to 1987. (From Gabbe, et al: Obstetrics: Normal and Problem Pregnancies, 2nd ed. New York, Churchill Livingstone, 1991.)

et al, 1976; Stewart, 1977), but with improvements in neonatal intensive care, survival rates continue to improve for newborns weighing less than 1000 g (Hack and Fanaroff, 1989; Sell, 1986). Because of a decrease in the size of the family unit, there has been a shift of emphasis from mere survival to greater expectations for *quality* of life. Therefore, the goal is not just to ensure survival but also to decrease handicaps.

Data from the National Collaborative Perinatal Study of the National Institute of Neurological and Communicative Disorders and Stroke, in which children were followed to age 7 or 8 years, indicate a relationship between birth weight and gestational age statistics and, later, IQ scores and incidence of neurologic abnormalities (Hardy and Mellits, 1977). Preterm babies and low-birth-weight babies had lower IQ scores and a higher incidence of neurologic abnormalities.

Morrison (1990) stated that neurodevelopmental handicaps, such as cerebral palsy, seizure disorders, and mental retardation, are 22 times more common in infants who weigh less than 1500 g than in those who weighed 2500 g.

Parents are usually emotionally unprepared for the birth of a preterm infant. Anxiety about survival of the infant is accompanied by feelings of guilt, anger, and depression. These usual feelings of parents after the birth of a preterm infant are symptomatic of grief for the expected healthy, full-term infant that they did not have, and of the realistic fear of the loss of the newborn (Taylor and Hall, 1979). The psychologic counseling of the parents is addressed in greater detail later in this chapter. The recognition of the importance of parent-infant bonding has led to parents no longer being excluded from the neonatal intensive care unit.

The financial drain caused by the delivery of a preterm infant is enormous. Average daily neonatal intensive care unit costs keep climbing. Stahlman (1984) found the average daily cost for surviving infants was $902 and for nonsurvivors was $1183. The average cost per normal survivor now likely exceeds $100,000 (Hernandez et al, 1986). In 1990, Morrison stated that the average cost to

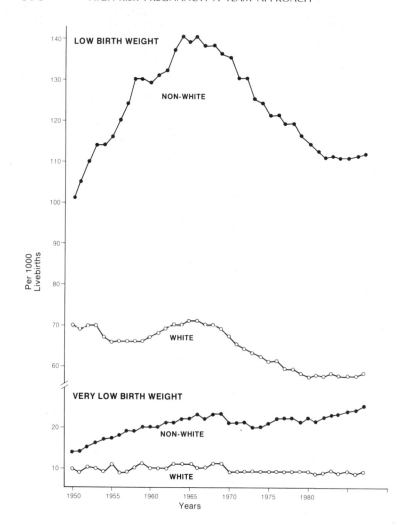

**Figure 22–2.** Incidence of low birth weight and very low birth weight per 1000 live births by race in the United States for 1950 to 1987. (From Gabbe, et al: Obstetrics: Normal and Problem Pregnancies, 2nd ed. New York, Churchill Livingstone, 1991.)

graduate a sick newborn from the NICU was $20,000 to $100,000 per infant and that for newborns weighing less than 1000 g, the average cost was $140,000 per patient. Care for infants with severe neurologic and physical handicaps can cost over $100,000 for special education and long-term care, whereas lifetime custodial care may cost as much as $450,000 (Morrison, 1990).

## Initiation of Labor

The sequence of events leading to the initiation of labor has been well documented in the sheep, in which it is the *fetus* that initiates the onset of parturition through activation of its hypothalamic-pituitary-adrenal axis (Lipshitz, 1980). A prelabor rise in fetal cortisol is the key to the fetal control of the onset of parturition in the sheep. Fetal cortisol, which increases during the last 8 to 10 days of gestation, stimulates a placental enzyme ($17\text{-}\alpha$-hydroxylase) that decreases the level of progesterone and, at the same time, increases the level of estrogen. Estrogens are potent stimulators of prostaglandin production, whereas the fall in progesterone enables the release of prostaglandin to occur. Figure 22–3 details this sequence of events. The cortisol has a dual role in the sheep, in which it not only stimulates the onset of parturition, but also prepares the fetus for extrauterine life, for example, by the induction of fetal lung maturity.

If, as in the sheep, the human fetus initiated labor and simultaneously prepared itself for extrauterine survival, babies born

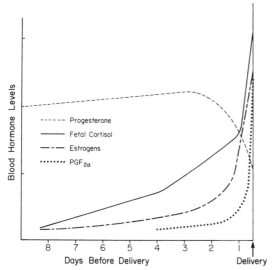

**Figure 22-3.** Sequence of events leading to the initiation of labor in the sheep.

prematurely would rarely get respiratory distress syndrome (RDS), and it would almost never be necessary to use drugs to inhibit preterm labor. However, it is obvious from clinical practice that this is not the case.

Although many studies have reported on maternal and fetal cortisol levels, it has thus far not been shown that a sharp rise in maternal or fetal cortisol precedes the onset of labor in the human. Although an increase in the estrogen-to-progesterone ratio associated with the onset of labor has been described, the data in humans remain contradictory and confusing (Lipshitz, 1980).

The local production of prostaglandins, from precursors located in the fetal membranes and decidua, appears to be the primary mechanism by which labor is initiated in the human. The fetal membranes contain glycerophospholipids highly enriched with arachidonic acid. An enzyme, phospholipase $A_2$, is required to split off the arachidonic acid from the phospholipids. However, this enzyme is contained in the lysosomes, and its activity depends on release from them.

Schwarz and colleagues (1976) described a progesterone-binding substance in fetal membranes near term that competes with lysosomes for progesterone. As a consequence, the lysosomes become more unstable and their contents leak out. Milewich and coworkers (1977) showed that progesterone metabolism was decreased in fetal membranes several weeks before normal labor when compared with the progesterone in midtrimester fetal membranes. Thus, there is a local withdrawal of progesterones in the membranes, independent of maternal plasma levels.

The phopholipase $A_2$, which is released from the lysosomes, strips off arachidonic acid from the phospholipids. This results in an increased local production of prostaglandins, which diffuse to the myometrium and initiate uterine contractions (Fig. 22-4).

# Etiology of Preterm Labor

The etilogy of preterm labor is multifaceted and poorly understood. It can be broadly classified under four headings: Complications of Pregnancy, Epidemiologic Factors, Iatrogenic Factors, and Unknown Causes (Table 22-1).

A retrospective analysis of 486 preterm infants revealed that spontaneous labor of unknown cause accounted for 38 percent of all preterm deliveries and 35 percent of all preterm early neonatal deaths (Rush et al, 1976). Spontaneous labor associated with complications occurred in 24 percent of the preterm deliveries and accounted for 29 percent of the deaths. The most common complication was antepartum hemorrhage, followed by fetal growth retardation, cervical incompetence, and hypertension. Multiple pregnancy accounted for 10 percent of the preterm deliveries and 27 percent of the preterm early neonatal deaths. The final 28 percent of preterm deliveries were accounted for by elective obstetric intervention due to complicating maternal or fetal factors. This group accounted for only 9 percent of the preterm early neonatal deaths. Thus, spontaneous preterm delivery was associated with either no apparent cause or with multiple pregnancy in almost 50 percent of the infants.

## COMPLICATIONS OF PREGNANCY

Although infection undoubtedly plays an important role in the etiology of preterm labor, at present, it is unknown to what extent unrecognized infection contributes to preterm birth when no apparent cause is

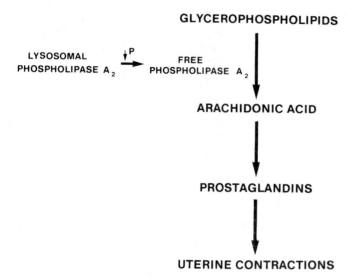

**GLYCEROPHOSPHOLIPIDS**

LYSOSOMAL
PHOSPHOLIPASE A$_2$ →$\downarrow$P FREE
PHOSPHOLIPASE A$_2$

**ARACHIDONIC ACID**

**PROSTAGLANDINS**

**UTERINE CONTRACTIONS**

**Figure 22–4.** Initiation of labor in the human.

found (Lipshitz, 1977). Roos and coworkers (1980) were able to culture bacteria from the intrauterine environment in 72 percent of 56 preterm infants. Several more recent studies (Martius et al, 1988; Gravett et al, 1986) demonstrated a relationship between bacterial vaginosis and prematurity; however, more data are necessary to confirm the relationship of these organisms to prematurity and to resolve the use of antibiotic therapy (Gabbe et al, 1991; Lee, 1988). An understanding of the factors that initiate parturi-

**Table 22–1**
ETIOLOGY OF PRETERM LABOR

**Factors in Pregnancy**
Infection
Uterine bleeding
Multiple pregnancy and hydramnios
Uterine abnormalities
Incompetent cervix
Maternal illness
Premature rupture of the membranes
Fetal growth retardation
Fetal anomalies
**Epidemiologic Factors**
Maternal age
Height and weight
Socioeconomic status
Race
Antenatal care
Smoking
Psychologic factors
Coitus
Previous obstetric history
Unwanted pregnancies
**Iatrogenic Factors**
**Unknown Causes**

tion has clarified the possible mechanism by which bacteria may initiate preterm labor. The bacterial endotoxin itself is unable to stimulate the pregnant rat uterus (Wren, 1970). Bejar and colleagues (1979) have shown that the organisms associated with preterm labor have specific activity of phospholipase A$_2$ higher than that of the intracellular phospholipase A$_2$ of the amnion and chorion. Also, intact gram-positive and gram-negative bacteria were able to release stable prostaglandin E$_2$ and F$_{2\alpha}$ in the presence of arachidonic acid (Gulbis et al, 1979).

An association between pyelonephritis and preterm labor has been described (Sweet, 1985). Although it is not clear whether there is an association between asymptomatic bacteriuria and preterm labor, 70 to 80 percent of acute pyelonephritis could be prevented by screening pregnant patients and treating their asymptomatic bacteriuria (Sweet, 1985).

Placenta praevia and abruptio placentae both commonly result in the delivery of preterm infants (Niswander, 1977). Threatened abortion in early pregnancy, and antepartum uterine bleeding that is *not* due to placenta praevia or abruptio placentae, are both associated with an increased risk of preterm labor (Turnbull, 1977).

Maternal uterine abnormalities increase the risk of both spontaneous abortion and preterm delivery (Craig, 1975; Gibbs, 1973). The chance of a woman with Asherman's syndrome carrying a pregnancy to term is less than 50 percent (Forssman, 1965). Cervical incompetence results in repeated abortions as well as preterm deliveries. Cervical suture is usually successful if used for the correct indication. However, it is a procedure not without risk and is often unsuccessful when used for conditions other than cervical incompetence (Gabbe et al, 1991; Lipshitz, 1975).

Chronic systemic diseases such as diabetes mellitus, hypertension, and chronic renal disease may result in preterm delivery, as a result of either spontaneous labor or obstetric intervention (Rush et al, 1976). Almost any severe maternal illness, as well as endocrine disorders such as untreated hypothyroidism (Mestman et al, 1974) and hyperparathyroidism (Johnstone et al, 1972), is associated with preterm labor.

## EPIDEMIOLOGIC FACTORS

Epidemiologic factors are merely associated with preterm labor, and there is no evidence that they actually *cause* preterm labor. Great care needs to be taken when interpreting specific epidemiologic factors, because the apparent effect may be due to other associated variables. For example, it has been shown that, when analyzed separately, both maternal height and weight influence the weight of the infant (Hardy and Mellits, 1977) as well as the rate of preterm delivery (Fedrick and Anderson, 1976). However, when these two factors were examined simultaneously, it became obvious that maternal weight, but not height, was of importance to the rate of preterm delivery (Fedrick and Anderson, 1976). The preterm birth rate was almost three times as high in mothers who weighed less than 112 pounds at the start of their pregnancies than in mothers who weighed more than 126 pounds.

It has been shown that the younger the mother, the lighter the baby (Hardy and Mellits, 1977), and the higher the rate of preterm delivery (Fedrick and Anderson, 1976).

Women in lower socioeconomic groups have a 50 percent higher rate of spontaneous preterm births than do those in the higher socioeconomic groups. The rate for unmarried mothers is even greater (Fedrick and Anderson, 1976).

In the United States, the preterm birth rate among blacks is twice is high as among whites (Chase, 1977; Garn et al, 1977). This may in part be due to socioeconomic factors. As socioeconomic status increases, the prevalence of low-birth-weight and preterm deliveries markedly decreases (see Fig. 22–2). However, at equivalent socioeconomic levels, the incidence of low-birth-weight black neonates is still twice that of white neonates (Garn et al, 1977).

It has been shown that patients who have poor antenatal care have a higher incidence of preterm deliveries (Fedrick and Anderson, 1976; Schwartz, 1962).

The increased rate of preterm deliveries associated with smoking is directly proportional to the number of cigarettes smoked per day, being much worse in mothers who smoke more than 20 cigarettes per day (Meyer, 1977).

Several retrospective studies have reported that sexual orgasm is more frequent in mothers of preterm infants (Goodlin, 1969; Wagner et al, 1976). The prostaglandins implicated in the mechanism of orgasm, as well as their presence in the seminal fluid, may lead to preterm labor in certain susceptible individuals. A more detailed discussion of this subject is presented in Chapter 15.

Of all the epidemiologic factors, a history of previous preterm delivery correlates the most strongly with spontaneous preterm birth. Patients with one previous spontaneous preterm delivery have a 37 percent risk of having a second, and those with two or more preterm deliveries have a 70 percent risk of again delivering preterm (Keirse et al, 1978).

## PREVENTION

In patients with a high risk of preterm labor, education and home monitoring for uterine contractions may allow preterm labor to be detected early in its course so that successful tocolysis is possible (Blondel et al, 1990; Copper et al, 1990; Iams et al, 1988; Konte et al, 1988; Morrison et al, 1987). Controversy exists over whether it is actually the education and daily contact with a trained nurse rather than the contraction monitor that is the major factor leading to success of such programs (Anderson et al, 1989; The Diagnostic and Therapeutic Technology Assessment, 1989).

# Specific Treatment of Preterm Labor

A significant number of patients in so-called preterm labor respond to placebo treatment. This finding has resulted in claims of success for numerous regimens and therapeutic agents ranging from bed rest, sedatives and analgesics, alcohol, magnesium sulfate, progesterone, calcium inhibitors, aminophylline, diazoxide, anti-prostaglandin drugs, and the β-sympathomimetic agents. Unfortunately, there are very few randomized, placebo-controlled trials with large enough numbers to draw valid conclusions for most of these therapies.

## BED REST AND INTRAVENOUS FLUIDS

It is not known whether patients who respond to bed rest and intravenous fluids were originally in true preterm labor or in false labor. Bed rest increases uterine blood flow and reduces myometrial activity, whereas the infusion of water inhibits the secretion of antidiuretic hormone and may also inhibit the secretion of oxytocin. Bed rest and intravenous fluids may be used in the patient who has no evidence of cervical changes, in order to avoid the unnecessary use of potent drugs. However, once the preterm labor appears to be progressing, as evidenced by cervical change, this regimen cannot be relied on to prevent preterm delivery, as evidenced by the large number of patients who deliver preterm infants while at bed rest.

## ANALGESICS, NARCOTICS, AND SEDATIVES

Because of their effect on the central nervous system, drugs such as meperidine, morphine, promethazine, and phenobarbital have been used in attempts to relax the uterus. However, these agents do not seem to significantly reduce uterine activity (Petrie et al, 1976; Riffel et al, 1973), and they may cause depression and respiratory difficulties in the preterm baby.

## MAGNESIUM SULFATE

The administration of a 2-g intravenous dose of magnesium sulfate to women in labor has been found to decrease uterine activity by approximately 10 percent (Petrie et al, 1976). Steer and Petrie (1977) compared magnesium sulfate and alcohol in the treatment of preterm labor. In patients with a cervical dilatation of 1 cm or less, magnesium sulfate was found to inhibit contractions for 24 hours in 96 percent of the patients, compared with 72 percent for alcohol. However, when the cervix was dilated more than 1 cm; only 25 percent of the patients responded to magnesium sulfate and only 8 percent to alcohol. The dosage of magnesium sulfate used was a 4-g loading dose administered as a slow intravenous infusion, followed by a maintenance dose of 2 g/h. Hollander (1987) reported $MgSO_4$ to be as effective as β-mimetics in stopping premature labor, however, it was found to be slower to take effect.

Following magnesium sulfate administration, the mother may experience a sensation of warmth and flushing owing to peripheral vasodilatation. Transient nausea and headache and palpitations may occur after rapid intravenous injection. Overdosage is followed by disappearance of the knee-jerk reflex, and as the plasma concentration increases, depression of respiration and, eventually, cardiac arrest may occur. McCubbin and coworkers (1981) reported on a patient who inadvertently received a 20-g loading dose of magnesium sulfate with resultant cardiopulmonary arrest. Of interest was the fact that although spontaneous uterine contractions ceased immediately, they resumed spontaneously at a serum magnesium level of 11.6 mg/dl, a level far in excess of that achieved on a normal therapeutic regime.

Because the kidney is the primary route of elimination, caution is required in patients with renal disease. The patellar reflex and urinary output should be checked regularly, at least once every hour.

It is rare for magnesium therapy to depress the fetus, although neonatal depression manifested by decreased muscle tone and cynasosis secondary to hypoventilation due to magnesium has been reported, particularly after prolonged intravenous therapy and in cases in which high doses have been given close to delivery (Lipshitz, 1971; Stone and Pritchard, 1970).

## PROSTAGLANDIN SYNTHETASE INHIBITORS

As already discussed, the prostaglandins play a central role in the initiation of labor, and, thus, it is not unexpected that drugs such as aspirin and indomethacin, which inhibit prostaglandin synthetase, would affect the labor process. These drugs have minimal maternal effects and would be attractive agents in the treatment of preterm labor if not for the possible adverse fetal effects.

Retrospective surveys of patients who had chronically ingested high doses of acetylsalicylic acid during pregnancy revealed that they had a highly significant increase in the average length of gestation, the frequency of pregnancy lasting longer than 37 weeks, and the mean duration of spontaneous labor (Collins and Turner, 1973; Lewis and Schulman, 1973). Maternal ingestion of this drug during pregnancy may interfere with both neonatal and maternal hemostatic mechanisms. Computed tomographic (CT) scanning performed on 108 infants born at 34 weeks' gestation or earlier, and weighing 1500 g or less, revealed a higher incidence of intracranial hemorrhage in the infants whose mothers had ingested aspirin, compared with controls and with infants whose mothers had ingested acetaminophen (Rumack et al, 1981). Stuart and associates (1982) reported that of 10 mothers who ingested acetylsalicylic acid within 5 days of delivery, 6 mothers and 9 infants had bleeding tendencies; the same study found that of 7 maternal-neonatal pairs in which the mothers ingested aspirin 6 to 10 days before delivery, all were free of clinical bleeding. The neonatal hemostatic abnormalities seen in the first group included numerous petechiae over the presenting part, hematuria, cephalhematoma, subconjunctival hemorrhage, and bleeding from a circumcision. The authors concluded that aspirin should be avoided during pregnancy, and that if ingestion has occurred within 5 days of delivery, the neonate should be evaluated for the presence of bleeding (Stuart et al, 1982).

Several clinical studies have described the use of indomethacin to treat preterm labor. Zuckerman and associates (1974) were the first to report on this treatment modality, and in an uncontrolled study they reported an 80 percent success rate in 50 patients. Wiqvist and coworkers (1975) confirmed that indomethacin was useful in the treatment of six patients in preterm labor and showed that the drug produced a reduction in the metabolites of prostaglandin $F_{2\alpha}$. Niebyl and colleagues (1980) showed that indomethacin was signficantly more effective than placebo in the inhibition of preterm labor during a 24-hour course of therapy. They also showed that indomethacin markedly reduced the prostaglandin $F_{2\alpha}$ metabolite. No indomethacin-related adverse neonatal effects were described in any of the aforementioned studies.

Because prostaglandins are important in fetal cardiovascular homeostasis, and because indomethacin crosses the placenta without difficulty, it is not surprising that there have been several cases reported of untoward neonatal cardiovascular effects. These consist mainly of narrowing of the fetal ductus arteriosus and persistent fetal circulation (primary pulmonary hypertension). Most adverse effects of indomethacin have been reported when the drug is given in large doses, for a long period of time, or in mothers past 34 weeks' gestation with fetuses larger than 2000 g (Witter and Niebyl, 1986). Studies on rats have determined that the response of the ductus arteriosus depends on gestational age. It was shown that a large dose of indomethacin given to the mother within 18 hours of term delivery resulted in intrauterine narrowing of the fetal ductus arteriosus (Sharpe et al, 1974), whereas this did not occur when the drug was administered several days prior to term (Sharpe et al, 1975). Indomethacin has been shown to decrease amniotic fluid volume via a decrease in fetal urine output (Kirshon et al, 1988), although the exact mechanism is unclear (Mari et al, 1990). Thus, indomethacin may be useful in cases in which preterm labor is initiated or aggravated by hydramnios. The dosage is 50 mg orally or (if not tolerated orally) 50 to 100 mg by rectal suppository (if not tolerated orally) every 8 hours for 24 hours, then 25 mg orally every 6 hours. The amniotic fluid volume should be checked by ultrasound twice weekly to ensure that it does not diminish excessively. The renal changes are reversible once the indomethacin is stopped.

Although these drugs cannot be recommended for general use in preventing preterm labor, in the early third trimester, in selected patients in whom conventional agents are contraindicated, a short course of antiprostaglandin drugs may have a favorable benefit-to-risk ratio. To be safe, it is best not to use indomethicin beyond 32 weeks' gestation.

## β-ADRENERGIC AGONISTS

During the first half of this century, studies with epinephrine, the parent compound of the β-adrenergic agonists, produced perplexing and contradictory results. In certain animal species, epinephrine produced relaxation of the uterus; whereas in other species, it produced contraction. In some animals, it produced relaxation in the pregnant as well as nonpregnant uterus; whereas in others, it produced contractions in both the gravid and nongravid uterus. It was left to Ahlquist (1948) to clarify these seemingly contradictory effects of epinephrine on the uterus. He showed that the adrenergic agonists produced their effects through two receptors, which he called α-adrenergic and β-adrenergic. Depending on dose, species, and hormonal status, epinephrine could stimulate either the α-receptors, which produced stimulation of the uterus, or the β-receptors, which produced uterine relaxation. In 1967, Lands and associates (1967) further subdivided the β-receptors into $\beta_1$ and $\beta_2$. The $\beta_1$-receptors mediate the increase in rate and force of the heart and produce lipolysis. The $\beta_2$-receptors cause relaxation of the smooth muscles of the bronchi, uterus, and arterioles (Fig. 22–5). There are, however, no pure $\beta_1$ or $\beta_2$ stimulants. Although a particular drug may affect mainly one type of receptor, there is usually some degree of overlap. Thus, when comparing the different drugs, the most $\beta_2$-selective agonists tend to have the least $\beta_1$ effects.

Isoxsuprine was the first β-sympathomimetic drug to be widely used as a tocolytic agent in the treatment of preterm labor (Hendricks, 1964). Baillie and coworkers (1970) showed that metaproterenol (Orciprenaline) was also an effective tocolytic agent. The therapeutic usefulness of these

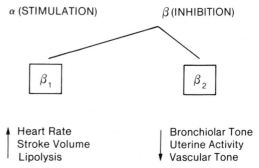

Figure 22–5. Physiologic effects of the adrenergic receptors.

drugs was somewhat compromised by their significant degree of cardiovascular $\beta_1$ effects. They have been replaced by a second generation of selective $\beta_2$-sympathomimetic drugs that have fewer $\beta_1$ effects, a listing of which follows:

1. Fenoterol (Th 1165, Berotec, Partusisten)
2. Hexoprenaline (Ipradol, Delaprem)
3. Ritodrine (Du 21220, Yutopar)
4. Salbutamol (albuterol, Ventolin)
5. Terbutaline (Brethine, Bricanyl)

## Comparison of $\beta_2$-Sympathomimetic Drugs

To determine if any of the $\beta_2$-sympathomimetic drugs exhibit increased uterine selectivity (increased $\beta_2$-selectivity), fenoterol, hexoprenaline, ritodrine, and salbutamol were compared in dosages having equivalent uterine effects in pregnant patients at term who were undergoing oxytocin-induced labor (Lipshitz et al, 1976; Lipshitz and Baillie, 1976). For an equivalent uterine response, hexoprenaline had significantly less effect ($p < 0.001$) on the maternal rate heart than the other three drugs.

Hexoprenaline and fenoterol were compared in prostaglandin $F_{2\alpha}$–induced labor, and once again, hexoprenaline was shown to produce significantly less effect on the maternal heart rate than fenoterol ($p = 0.005$). The tocolytic effects of the drugs were just as good in the prostaglandin $F_{2\alpha}$–induced as in the oxytocin-induced uterine contractions (Lipshitz and Lipshitz, 1984).

Preliminary data from the United States Multicenter Study comparing hexoprenaline and ritodrine in the treatment of preterm labor reveal the following: (1) hexoprenaline had significantly less effect on the maternal heart rate and blood pressure than did ritodrine; (2) untoward effects of the drugs, such as nausea and palpitations, occurred significantly less with hexoprenaline than with ritodrine; and (3) the drugs had to be discontinued owing to cardiovascular manifestations in 4.5 percent of the hexoprenaline patients, as compared with 15.4 percent of the ritodrine patients (p < 0.01) (Lipshitz et al, 1983). Because it is mainly the maternal cardiovascular effects of these drugs that limit their therapeutic application, hexoprenaline appears to be the safest and best tolerated of the $\beta_2$-sympathomimetic drugs. Hexoprenaline is not commercially available in the United States at this time; therefore, ritodrine and terbutaline are the drugs most often used.

## Mechanism of Action

A detailed review of this subject was published by Huszar and Roberts (1982). Uterine contractions occur when actin-myosin interaction takes place. This interaction is regulated through enzymatic phosphorylation or dephosphorylation of the myosin light chain. Myosin light chain phosphorylation depends on the activity of an enzyme, myosin light chain kinase. Relaxation of the uterine smooth muscle occurs when another enzyme, myosin light chain phosphatase, removes the phosphate group from the myosin light chains. Thus, uterine activity depends on the ratio of myosin light chain kinase and myosin light chain phosphatase (Fig. 22–6). Myosin light chain kinase, the key regulator of uterine contractility, depends on an adequate supply of free intracellular calcium, which binds with a protein, calmodulin.

The $\beta$-adrenergic agonists interact with $\beta$-adrenergic receptors located on the outer surface of the cell membrane. This interaction then activates adenyl cyclase, an enzyme located on the internal surface of the plasma membrane of the cell. This stimulates the conversion of adenosine triphosphate to cyclic AMP (cAMP), which increases in concentration. The increase in cAMP stimulates a protein kinase, which results in phosphorylation of specific membrane proteins. This process produces uterine relaxation via two mechanisms:

1. A decrease in free intracellular calcium ions. The activation of cAMP-dependent protein kinases results in the phosphorylation of a protein associated with the sodium pump. Thus, $Na^+$ is pumped out of the cell in exchange for $K^+$, which enters the cell. This may partially explain the mechanism for the decrease in serum potassium that occurs with the use of the $\beta_2$-agonists. The increased $Na^+$ gradient also accelerates the

THE SMOOTH MUSCLE CELL

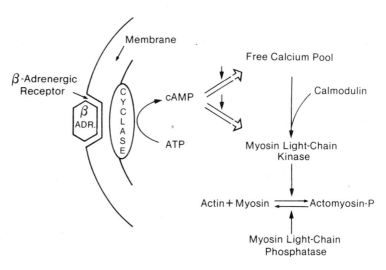

**Figure 22–6.** Mechanism of action of the $\beta$-adrenergic drugs.

rate of $Na^+/Ca^{2+}$ exchange, resulting in increased calcium efflux from the cytoplasm and sequestration of calcium by the sarcoplasmic reticulum.

2. Direct inhibition of the activity of myosin light chain kinase as a result of the cAMP-mediated phosphorylation (Fig. 22–6).

## Cardiovascular Effects

Administration of the $\beta$-adrenergic agonists produces a consistent, dose-related increase in maternal heart rate. These drugs relax the smooth muscle in the vascular wall of resistant vessels, resulting in lowered peripheral vascular resistance. A decrease in diastolic pressure occurs that facilitates venous return and results in an increased stroke volume and a rise in systolic and pulse pressures (Bieniarz, 1977) (Table 22–2). Bieniarz (1977) described a consistent increase in maternal cardiac output in five patients receiving ritodrine for the treatment of preterm labor. As diastolic blood pressure tends to decrease more than the systolic pressure increases, the mean blood pressure tends to decrease slightly (Lipshitz and Baillie, 1976; Miller et al, 1976).

Direct measurement of uteroplacental blood flow in the human is not possible, but indirect evidence suggests that it is favorably influenced by these drugs, especially when vasospasm has resulted in a decrease in perfusion (Lippert et al, 1976; Brettes et al, 1976). Data from studies in sheep are conflicting, which may be because, in the sheep, the vessels may already be fully dilated. Hexoprenaline increases placental blood flow on day 14 of gestation in the rat (Lipshitz et al, 1982).

## Metabolic Effects

The metabolic effects produced by the administration of $\beta$-adrenergic agonists are due, in part, to the increase in cAMP (see Table 22–3). Maternal hyperglycemia results mainly from hepatic glycogenolysis. Because muscle does not contain glucose-6-phosphatase, an end product of glycogenolysis in muscle is lactate, which causes hyperlactacidemia. Lipolysis results in the outpouring of free fatty acids and glycerol into the bloodstream. In a study of the metabolic changes that occur in response to an intravenous bolus of hexoprenaline, it was found that the maximum increase in insulin and glucagon concentrations occurred before the peak in glucose and free fatty acid levels, which suggests a direct action on the $\alpha$- and $\beta$-cells of the maternal pancreas (Lipshitz and Vinik, 1978).

Although plasma potassium concentration is reduced, urinary potassium and excretion is unchanged (Smith and Thompson, 1977), which is compatible with redistribution from the extracellular to the intracellular compartment. Electrocardiograms performed in a few patients showed no evidence of hypokalemia or disturbances in rhythm (Thomas et al, 1977). Potassium supplementation is not recommended, because no adverse effects have been reported, and the change is of a temporary nature, with a return to normal within 24 hours.

**Table 22–2**

CARDIOVASCULAR EFFECTS OF
$\beta$-SYMPATHOMIMETIC DRUGS

| |
|---|
| **Decreased** |
| Vascular resistance |
| **Increased** |
| Heart rate |
| Stroke volume |
| Pulse pressure |
| Venous return |
| Cardiac output |
| ? Uteroplacental blood flow |

**Table 22–3**

METABOLIC EFFECTS OF THE
$\beta$-ADRENERGIC AGONISTS

| Increased | Unchanged | Decreased |
|---|---|---|
| cAMP | Pituitary hormones | Serum iron |
| Glucose | Calcium | Transferrin |
| Insulin | Phosphorus | TIBC |
| C-peptide | Cortisol | Potassium |
| Glucagon | Bilirubin | Cholesterol |
| Free fatty acids | Haptoglobin | Alanine |
| Triglycerides | Creatinine | Estriol |
| Lactate | Uric acid | Bicarbonate |
| Pyruvate | Sodium | |
| Glycerol | Chloride | |
| $\beta$- | HPL | |
| Hydroxybutylate | pH | |
| Acetoacetic acid | | |
| Renin | | |

## Adverse Reactions

In the United States trials, intravenous ritodrine was associated with palpitations in one third of the patients (New Drug Application No. 18280). Tremor, nausea, vomiting, headache, and erythema was observed in 10 to 15 percent of patients. Nervousness, jitteriness, restlessness, emotional upset, or anxiety was reported in 5 to 6 percent of patients. Cardiac symptoms, including chest pain or tightness (rarely associated with abnormalities in the echocardiogram) and arrhythmia, were reported in 1 to 2 percent of patients. Other infrequently reported maternal effects included anaphylactic shock, rash, epigastric distress, ileus, bloating, constipation, diarrhea, dyspnea, hypoventilation, sweating, and weakness.

A rare but serious complication of β-agonist therapy is *pulmonary edema*. The widespread use of ritodrine in the United States has resulted in several maternal deaths due to pulmonary edema associated with this therapy in the treatment of preterm labor. Although the exact mechanism for the occurrence of pulmonary edema is unknown, several high-risk factors have become apparent:

1. Fluid overload, which may be due to iatrogenic overvigorous hydration during therapy as well as to the antidiuretic effect of the β-agonists, which results in gradual water retention with prolonged intravenous therapy.
2. Patients with a multiple gestation, in whom there is a natural volume overload, are at increased risk of developing pulmonary edema.
3. Corticosteroids used in combination with the β-agonists have been implicated in the development of pulmonary edema, but convincing evidence is lacking.
4. The maintenance of maternal tachycardia for prolonged periods of time. Pulmonary edema does not usually develop within the first 24 hours of intravenous therapy. Maternal tachycardia results in a shortening of the diastolic filling time of the heart, which over a prolonged period of time may result in the slow accumulation of fluid in the lungs.
5. The patient with unrecognized subclinical amniotic fluid infection may be at particular risk for the development of pulmonary edema (Benedetti, et al, 1982).

Acute cerebral ischemic episodes during terbutaline therapy have been reported in two patients with a history of migraine headaches (Rosen et al, 1982). Thus, these drugs probably should not be used in patients with a history of migraine headaches.

Because of the metabolic effects of these drugs, the patient with diabetes requires careful blood glucose monitoring and usually needs increased insulin administration during treatment of preterm labor. We have found that a continuous intravenous infusion of insulin, adjusted to the patient's blood glucose level, gives the most satisfactory results. Use of the β-agonists may result in ketoacidosis in the unrecognized diabetic patient.

## Fetal and Neonatal Effects

Possible fetal effects of β-agonists can occur via two mechanisms: (1) direct action of the active drug on the fetus, and (2) indirect effects secondary to maternal changes, such as an eleviated plasma glucose or alterations in uteroplacental blood perfusion. Differences in the physical properties of the various β-adrenergic agonists may account for the differences in placental transfer of these drugs. Ritodrine has been shown to cross to the fetus in both sheep (Kleinhout et al, 1974) and humans (Gandar et al, 1980), although fetal levels are usually less than maternal levels. The fetus seems to be protected from the direct effect of fenoterol because of two mechanisms: first, placental transfer of the active substance is minimal (Meissner and Klostermann, 1976), and second, the small amount that is transferred to the fetus is further inactivated by conjugation at the time of passage (Kords, 1977). In animal experiments on $^{14}$C-hexoprenaline, it was found that none of this drug crossed the placenta to the fetus, perhaps because hexoprenaline is not fat soluble (Lipshitz et al, 1982). No adverse effects of ritodrine have been described either in the newborn (Blouin et al, 1976; Freysz et al, 1973) or in follow-up studies on infants between 1 and 3 years of age (Freysz et al, 1977). Most infants tolerate β-mimetic drugs; however, there is a potential, although small, for cardiotoxicity (Givens, 1988).

In a retrospective study, isoxsuprine was associated with neonatal hypoglycemia, hypocalcemia, ileus, hypotension, and death (Brazy and Pupkin, 1979). However, the isoxsuprine was administered as an intravenous bolus and produced hypotension or marked tachycardia in 58 percent of the mothers. Hypotension and death occurred mainly in those infants who were in the 26- to 31-week gestational age group and whose mothers had only a short interval from loading dose to delivery, developed hypotension or tachycardia, or both. Maternal hypotension and resultant decreased uteroplacental blood flow is a serious risk with bolus injection of isoxsuprine because of its poor $\beta_2$-selectivity.

## Patient Management

(Tables 22–4 and 22–5)

## ANTEPARTUM OUTPATIENT MANAGEMENT

Many preterm births occur not because of the lack of effective tocolytic agents or maternal contraindications to the use of these drugs, but because by the time the mother arrives at the hospital, her labor has progressed to a stage (cervix dilated greater than 4 cm) at which it is too late to treat the preterm labor. This happens when the patient either ignores or does not recognize the early warning signs of preterm labor. At the E.H. Crump Women's Hospital and Perinatal Center in Memphis, approximately 25 percent of preterm deliveries occur solely because the patient has arrived too late for treatment. Thus, an extremely important part of the treatment of preterm labor should

**Table 22–4**
PATIENT CARE SUMMARY FOR PRETERM LABOR

| | Antepartum | |
| --- | --- | --- |
| | *Outpatient Stable* | *Inpatient Stable* |
| Blood pressure, pulse and respirations | At each office visit. Woman should monitor pulse before taking tocolytics. | Oral meds q 2 to 6 h (maternal pulse 120 fetal pulse < 180) |
| Temperature | If elevated > 100° F, call office/clinic | q shift |
| Nursing assessment | Prn depending on uterine contractions and cervical change | q shift and prn |
| Bed rest | | Bed rest with bathroom privileges |
| I&O | | q shift |
| Fetal monitoring and ultrasound | While on oral medications, weekly NST, AFI. Kick count every day.<br>Ultrasound for:<br>  Size and dates<br>  R/O polyhydramnios<br>  R/O oligohydramnios<br>  R/O abruption<br>  R/O IUGR | < 26 weeks–fetal heart rate q shift<br>Biophysical profile biweekly<br>> 26 weeks—nonstress test, biophysical profile, kick count bid<br>> 4 in 1 h |
| Contractions | Baseline set for each patient. Generally < 5 per hour ok ≥ 5 h—increase rest, adjust tocolysis, or report to Labor and Delivery Department | Educate patient to palpate uterus and recognize uterine activity. Notify nurses if ≥ in 1 h |
| Laboratory Studies | | prn |
| Echocardiogram | No | No |
| Amniocentesis | prn | prn<br>Tocolysis versus delivery |
| Vaginal examinations | As indicated | As indicated |
| Sexual counseling | No intercourse<br>No orgasm<br>No breast stimulation | No intercourse<br>No orgasm<br>No breast stimulation |

begin before the patient is actually in labor. This involves education of the patients, the nurses, and medical staff dealing with these patients. The early signs of preterm labor are as follows:

- Change of Braxton Hicks contractions from an irregular pattern to a regular pattern. Medical attention should be sought whenever contractions are gradually increasing in intensity, duration, and frequency and are occurring 10 minutes apart or closer.
- Abdominal cramping, sometimes associated with diarrhea.
- Menstrual-like cramps.
- Low backache, often of a different character than that previously felt. This may come and go or be constant.
- Intermittent pressure in the pelvis.
- Change in the character or amount of vaginal discharge. This is especially ominous when the discharge becomes bloody.

Because many of these symptoms frequently occur throughout gestation, the importance of any change or increase is stressed.

It is important to teach patients at risk how to palpate for uterine contractions. The patient should be taught how to feel the contractions with her fingertips placed on the fundus of her uterus. She should be taught to recognize a contraction as a tightening or hardening of the uterus, which then relaxes.

| Active Preterm Labor | Intrapartum | Postpartum |
|---|---|---|
| Intravenous or subcutaneous medications q 15 min while stabilizing q 30 min maintenance dose (maternal pulse should be < 140—fetal heart rate < 180) | q 1 h | On admission to RR or continue in LDRP; then q 15 min × 4; then q 30 min × 2; then q 1 h until stable; then on discharge to PP; then q shift |
| q 4 h If elevated > 100° F, q 1 h Head to toe assessment on admission q shift and prn (pay special attention to pulse and lung sounds) | q 4 h prn | On admission; then q 4 h; then on discharge to PP; then q shift prn |
| Strict bed rest | Prn depending on uterine contractions and cervical change | |
| q 1 h Continuously during tocolysis, chart q 15 min Without monitor, q 15 min listening through 2-3 contractions | q shift Continuously during labor, preferably internal Without monitor, q 30 min listening through 2 to 3 contractions | While in RR |
| Monitor continuously by tocolysis and palpation of uterus by nurse | Continuously during labor, preferably internal Without monitor, 1 h 30 min | |

A. Blood sugars (R/O) diabetes)
B. Electrolytes (obtain baseline)
C. Hematocrit (R/O anemia)
D. CBC, differential (R/O infection)
E. Urinalysis (R/O urinary tract infection)
F. Vaginal cultures

Baseline echocardiogram if possible

Often used to check fetal lung maturity

Tocolysis versus delivery
As indicated
Limit if possible (may cause uterine contractions)
No intercourse
No orgasm
No breast stimulation

**Table 22–5**

MEDICATION SUMMARY FOR PRETERM LABOR

| Medication | Action | Route | Dose | Pregnancy Precautions |
|---|---|---|---|---|
| $\beta$-Adrenergic agonists | Prevents smooth muscle contractions by inhibiting actin and myosin interaction through two mechanisms: (1) decrease of free calcium pool, (2) inhibition of myosin light-chain kinase (see Fig. 22–4) | IV & PO | Start infusion at recommended initial dose and increase every 10–20 min<br>Titrate against contractions, pulse, and side effects; keep maternal pulse less than 140 beats/min<br>Generally continued for 6–12 h after cessation of contractions<br>Give first PO tablet, then discontinue IV medication 30 min later<br>Usual PO dose is 1 tab every 2 h for 24 h, followed by 1–2 tabs every 3–6 h depending on contractions, pulse, and side effects<br>Continue until fetal maturity | Not indicated in the first half of pregnancy |
| Magnesium sulfate | Central nervous system depressant<br>Diminishes excitability of muscle fibers and relaxes the uterus | IV | Loading dose 4–6 g<br>Titration dose 2 g/hr<br>Maintenance dose 1 g/h<br>Continue 24 to 72 hr after cessation of contractions | None |

If these contractions are recognized at home, the patient should be encouraged to lie in the partial left lateral position, and to time the contractions from the beginning of one contraction to the beginning of the next. She should time the contractions for 1 hour. If the contractions occur at a frequency of 10 minutes or less for a period of 1 hour, she should seek medical attention and *not* wait for them to disappear, because cervical dilatation may become advanced, which jeopardizes her chances of successful treatment. Education programs and in-home uterine contraction monitoring can allow many patients to detect preterm labor at an early enough stage for successful treatment to be implemented (Blondel et al, 1990; Copper et al, 1990; Iams et al, 1988; Konte et al, 1988; Morrison et al,

**Table 22–5** *Continued*

| Side Effects | Nursing Considerations | Fetal/ Neonatal | Breast- Feeding |
|---|---|---|---|
| Tachycardia, nervousness, anxiety, tremor, palpitations, nausea, vomiting, sweating, headache, chest pain, dyspnea, pulmonary edema, widened pulse pressure, metabolic effects, water retention | *DO NOT* fluid overload these patients, because of cardiovascular changes and water retention<br>Strict I & O<br>Contraindicated: before 20 weeks, antepartum hemorrhage, eclampsia, fetal death, IUGR, chorioamnionitis, maternal cardiac disease, pulmonary hypertension, maternal hyperthyroidism, uncontrolled diabetes<br>Maternal and fetal vital signs every 15-30 min on IV dose<br>Observe for maternal pulse > 140<br>Do not use if solution is discolored or has a precipitate<br>Keep patient in left lateral position<br>If stable, other positions can be tried | Observe for hypoglycemia, fetal tachycardia ≥ 180 | No information is available about excretion in breast milk<br>These agents not indicated after delivery<br>The half-life is short and, therefore, should not cause problems for nursing mothers. |
| Sweating, drowsiness, depressed reflexes, flaccid paralysis, hypothermia, hypotension, depressed cardiac function, heart block, respiratory paralysis, hypocalcemia | Use cautiously in patients with impaired renal function, myocardial damage, heart block; have IV calcium gluconate (1 g) available to reverse MgSO$_4$<br>Monitor maternal vital signs q 1 h; FHR q 15 min; I & O q 1 h; urinary output should be over 30 cc/h<br>Reflexes q 1 h | Crosses placenta, producing hypotonia, lethargy, weakness, and low Apgar scores | Not indicated after delivery |

1987). Recent studies demonstrated that home monitoring by itself is probably not the answer to the problem of preterm labor. However, it should be considered one of the components of a preterm pregnancy program, which should also include patient education of the early signs and symptoms of preterm labor and daily contact with trained nurses (Creasy, 1990).

During the antepartum period, it is extremely important to obtain an accurate assessment of gestational age. If there is any discrepancy between dates and size, an ultrasonic examination should be obtained. It is important that the patient's weight gain be checked at each visit and that she be adequately informed about correct nutrition. If she smokes, the risks of preterm birth should be explained to her and she should be strongly encouraged to stop smoking.

## ANTEPARTUM INPATIENT MANAGEMENT

The patient who presents with a diagnosis of possible preterm labor should receive prompt evaluation and treatment, because any delay may result in the progression of labor to a stage at which any attempted treatment is doomed to fail. It is tragic enough when the patient at risk delays seeking treatment for preterm labor because she ignores the signs of early labor that appear weeks before she expects them, but it is even worse when the delay is due to negligence by the perinatal team.

### Requirements to Treat Preterm Labor

For a physician to undertake the treatment of a patient in preterm labor, the following should be present:

1. The personnel and equipment necessary to assess the mother.
2. The personnel and equipment necessary to assess the fetus.
3. The facilities to perform an amniocentesis and to do fetal lung maturity studies on the amniotic fluid. The introduction of the Lumadex-foam stability index test makes this possible even in the smallest hospital (Lipshitz et al, 1984).
4. Close access to a neonatal intensive care unit.

Because the treatment of preterm labor is not always successful, and because the resultant degree of infant morbidity and mortality is directly related to the quality of subsequent neonatal care and expertise, if a neonatal intensive care unit is not available, it is better to transfer the infant in utero than after delivery.

### Selection of Patients for Tocolytic Therapy

It is often extremely difficult to distinguish between true preterm labor and so-called false labor. Often, the diagnosis of preterm labor can be made only in retrospect. No more than 50 percent of patients with regular painful contractions proceed to preterm delivery (Anderson, 1977). Thus, if all patients presenting with regular uterine contractions are treated, many will receive unnecessary pharmacologic treatment, the side effects of which may be life threatening. With false labor, there is often no progressive cervical change, and the contractions cease spontaneously. However, the frequency, regularity, or pain of the contractions may not necessarily distinguish true labor from false labor.

Patients admitted without any evidence of cervical changes, that is, whose cervix is found to be posterior, long, and closed, can safely be observed with regular pelvic assessments by the same examiner. During this interval, the patient should be placed at bed rest in the partial left lateral position, and an intravenous crystalloid infusion is begun. In many such cases, the contractions stop before any changes in the cervix occur. This is especially important in research trials on new modalities of therapy. If patients are selected for therapy on the basis of contractions alone, a high success rate is achieved no matter which therapy is employed.

Many of the epidemiologic factors associated with preterm labor are also found in patients who have growth-retarded fetuses. Thus, it is often in the case of the low-socioeconomic, high-risk, indigent patient, who may have unreliable dates, that a decision has to be made as to whether she is in preterm labor or whether the small fetus is mature but growth retarded. A single ultrasound examination at this stage is of very little value. The intrauterine growth-retarded fetus has an increased risk of asphyxia and stillbirth. It is, thus, unwise to use tocolytic drugs to maintain these fetuses in an unfavorable intrauterine environment. An excellent way to distinguish the mature growth-retarded fetus from the small preterm fetus is by performing an amniocentesis and analyzing the fluid for fetal lung maturity. The potential complications of amniocentesis are minimal compared with the benefits gained (Dancis, 1979). In the presence of frequent contractions, tocolytic agents are used to inhibit the contractions until the results of pulmonary maturity studies are known. Another important reason to perform an amniocentesis is the fact that unrecognized chorioamnionitis may lead to preterm labor, and if β-adrenergic agonists are used in these patients, pulmonary edema is more likely to occur (Benedetti et al, 1982). Caution must also be used if the patient is to receive corticosteroids for lung maturity.

Figure 22–7 summarizes the selection of patients for tocolytic therapy developed for our hospital and used in the United States Multicenter Trial comparing hexoprenaline to ritodrine in the treatment of preterm labor. We have since found that the Lumadex-foam stability index test is more accurate than the L/S ratio in diagnosing the very small growth-retarded fetus (Lipshitz et al, 1983).

## Patient Assessment

A complete history and physical examination should be performed to evaluate the patient's suitability for receiving β-adrenergic drugs. The history should include details of the patient's past reproductive performance. Details should be sought regarding previous episodes of preterm labor, premature rupture of the membranes, number of preterm, low-birth-weight and stillborn infants delivered, and previous infants with RDS or other problems. A history of allergies, long-standing medical diseases, and any relative or absolute contraindications to tocolytic therapy should be listed. Special attention should be paid to symptoms of cardiac disease, which should be outlined for the patient. A social history should include the consumption of alcohol, drugs, and tobacco, and other factors epidemiologically associated with the onset of preterm labor.

A detailed physical examination should be performed to recognize any possible contraindication to the use of β-sympathomimetic drugs (Table 22–6). It is especially important to examine the cardiovascular system very carefully to exclude any heart disease. If membranes are intact, a pelvic examination should be performed. The cervix should be examined for any evidence of effective uterine action. These changes are (1) *position*—the cervix moves from a posterior to an anterior position during early labor; (2) *effacement*—the cervix becomes shorter before significant dilatation occurs; and (3) *dilatation* of the cervix, which usually follows effacement. Effacement of the

**Table 22–6**
RECOMMENDED CONTRAINDICATIONS FOR THE ADMINISTRATION OF THE β-ADRENERGIC AGONISTS

Gestation < 20 weeks
Maternal cardiac disease
Eclampsia or preeclampsia
Significant hypertension of any etiology
Abruptio placentae, severe bleeding with placenta praevia, or significant vaginal bleeding of unknown cause
Intrauterine infection and probably fever of unknown origin
Fetal mortality or significant abnormality
Significant fetal growth retardation
Maternal hyperthyroidism
Uncontrolled maternal diabetes mellitus
Maternal medical conditions that would be seriously affected by the pharmacologic properties of the β-adrenergic agonists
Any obstetric or medical condition that contraindicates prolongation of pregnancy
Known hypersensitivity to any component of the product
Possibly migraine headache

cervix associated with uterine contractions usually indicates the onset of preterm labor, and treatment should be instituted before any significant dilatation of the cervix. Assessment by the same perinatal team member is useful in detecting early changes of the cervix.

If the patient presents a history of having ruptured her membranes, no pelvic examination should be performed. Instead, a sterile speculum examination should be carried out to confirm whether or not the membranes are ruptured and to assess the state of the cervix. Although it is a controversial practice, the authors use tocolytic drugs in the patient with ruptured membranes if the following criteria are met: (1) regular uterine contractions are present, (2) there is no evidence of infection, and (3) fetal lung immaturity is documented.

## Criteria for the Use of Tocolytic Drugs

1. Gestational age is between 20 and 36 weeks.

2. At least two uterine contractions have occurred in a 15-minute period of time.

3. Cervical effects of contractions are present.

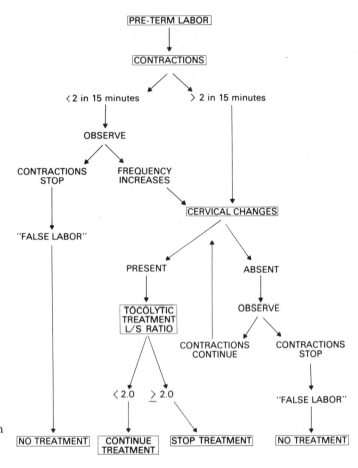

**Figure 22–7.** Protocol for the selection of patients for tocolytic therapy.

4. The cervix is dilated less than 5 cm.

5. If there is any doubt about gestational age, or if there is a possibility of fetal growth retardation or unrecognized chorioamnionitis, an amniocentesis should be performed.

6. There should be no contraindications to the use of β-adrenergic agonists (see Table 22–6).

7. The patient should be fully informed about the plan of action as well as the possible side effects of the drugs.

## Special Investigations

1. A clean-catch specimen of urine should be examined for bacteriuria. This test is mandatory in all patients, because there is an association between asymptomatic bacteriuria and preterm labor. When appropriate antimicrobial therapy is instituted at the time of treating the preterm labor, excellent results usually follow. However, if a urinary tract infection is missed, the patient may continue having episodes of preterm labor that will require prolonged tocolytic therapy, with the concomitant increased risk of untoward effects.

2. Blood sugars should be checked to exclude unrecognized diabetes.

3. It is recommended that baseline electrolytes be obtained.

4. If possible, an echocardiogram should be obtained before starting therapy.

5. Hematocrit.

6. A full blood count to exclude unrecognized infection.

## Administration of Drugs

### Intravenous Administration

The authors' protocol for the administration of hexoprenaline sulfate and ritodrine hydrochloride is as follows:

1. Dilute 150 mg ritodrine hydrochloride (3 ampules) in a 500-ml solution of 5 percent w/v dextrose, which yields a final concentration of 0.3 mg/ml. To administer, hexoprenaline, 150 $\mu$g (6 ampules) is added to 500 ml of fluid, which yields a final concentration of 0.3 $\mu$g/hml. An intravenous microdrip chamber (1 ml = 60 drops) provides a convenient range of infusion rates within the recommended dosages of these drugs.
2. The patient is kept in the partial left lateral recumbent position, and a large-bore indwelling catheter is kept open by a slow intravenous infusion.
3. Baseline values for maternal heart rate, respirations, blood pressure, uterine contractions, and fetal heart rate are determined.
4. The drug infusion is piggybacked onto the main intravenous line, using a controlled infusion device to adjust the rate of flow in drops per minute (60 microdrops = 1 ml).
5. The drug infusion is started at 20 microdrops/min (ritodrine, 0.1 mg/min; hexoprenaline, 0.1 $\mu$g/min) and increased usually by increments of 10 microdrops (ritodrine, 0.05 mg/min; hexoprenaline, 0.05 $\mu$g/min) every 10 to 15 minutes.
6. Maternal heart rate, blood pressure, respirations, and uterine contractions, as well as fetal heart rate, should be recorded immediately before the rate of the infusion is increased. These vital signs should be recorded every 15 minutes until the correct dose of the intravenous infusion is achieved, and then every 30 minutes throughout the intravenous infusion.
7. A strict intake and output chart should be maintained throughout the intravenous infusion. The total amount of intravenous fluid should not exceed 100 ml/hour.
8. The rate of the infusion is increased until one of the following occurs:
   a. Uterine contractions have stopped completely, or are reduced to less than one contraction/15-min period. If contractions occur less frequently than one /15-min period, it is advisable not to increase the dose of the drug further in an attempt to totally inhibit all uterine contractions.
   b. Maternal heart rate reaches 140 beats/minute. If the heart rate increases beyond this, the dosage of the drug should be reduced.
   c. Unacceptable side effects develop. The drug infusion may have to be reduced or discontinued.
9. We do not use an arbitrary maximum dosage of a particular drug, because the patient's sensitivity to the drugs may vary widely. Instead, once the maternal heart rate reaches 140 beats/minute, this is regarded as the maximum dosage for that particular patient, and the rate of the infusion is not increased any further. It is rare for a patient to require more than 350 $\mu$g/min (0.35 mg/min) of ritodrine or more than 0.5 $\mu$g/min of hexoprenaline.
10. We have found that the mean maximum dosage required to treat preterm labor is approximately 0.32 $\mu$g/min for hexoprenaline and 270 $\mu$g/min (0.27 mg/min) for ritodrine. However, dosages may vary widely among individual patients.
11. If a patient is sensitive to the drug and exhibits a rapid increase in heart rate, or experiences undesirable side effects, the dosage should be increased more slowly.
12. On effective inhibition of uterine contractions (or the reduction to less than one contraction/15-min period), the infusion should be continued at the same flow rate for 6 hours.
13. At the end of the 6-hour period, weaning should be commenced by reducing the infusion rate in decrements of 10 microdrops/min at half-hour intervals. When the maternal heart rate decreases to 100 beats/min, 1 tablet of hexoprenaline or ritodrine should be administered by mouth, and the infusion is stopped 30 minutes later.
14. The intravenous infusion may be repeated, if necessary, as long as the patient still meets the selection criteria.

### Oral Administration

Following the initial administration of 1 tablet of ritodrine or hexoprenaline, further oral therapy consists of the administration of 1 to 2 tablets every 2 to 6 hours until it is decided to let the patient deliver. Tablet dosage must be tailored to individual patient needs, based on maternal heart rate, uterine activity, and undesirable subjective effects. Ideally, resting maternal heart rate should be maintained between 100 and 110 beats per minute. If the uterus remains relaxed, it may become unnecessary to disturb the patient during the night, and drug administration may be limited to her waking hours. Undesirable effects may be reduced, both in occurrence and intensity, by administering the tablets with meals.

Administration of the β-agonists, whether by intravenous infusion or by mouth, should be discontinued in any patient presenting with chest pain or dyspnea. An echocardiogram should be recorded immediately and a chest x-ray taken. The patient should be evaluated for the presence of pulmonary rales or other pertinent clinical manifestations of incipient pulmonary edema.

### Terbutaline Sulfate

Terbutaline sulfate, although not approved by the FDA in the treatment of labor, is used to arrest contractions. Subcutaneous injections of 0.25 mg may be given 20 minutes apart up to a total of three injections. Then oral administration of terbutaline is begun with 2.5 mg to 5.0 mg orally every 2 to 6 hours. More recently, terbutaline has been given subcutaneously via a continuous pump device similar to that used for insulin infusions (Lam, 1989). A baseline dose of terbutaine is continuously infused and boluses can be added if required. Overall, this method allows use of the lowest daily dose of terbutaline (Lam et al, 1988). It is especially useful in patients who are difficult to control with oral medication and is used in conjunction with home uterine monitoring.

### Clinical Significance of the Maternal Pulse Rate

Whether or not the β-adrenegic agonists are administered as an intravenous bolus (Lipshitz et al, 1976), intravenous infusion (Lipshitz and Baillie, 1976a), oral tablet (Lipshitz, 1977b), or aerosol (Lipshitz and Baillie, 1976b), there is a close correlation between the time of onset of the uterine inhibitory effect and the time of increase in the maternal pulse rate. The same correlation holds true for the time taken for uterine activity to return to normal after stopping the

drugs, and the time taken for the heart rate to return to normal. Thus, the maternal pulse rate is an important clinical parameter during the administration of the β-agonists. The drug infusion is titrated against the patient's contractions as well as against the rise in maternal pulse rate. Conversely, if contractions recur during intravenous administration at close to maximum dosages, then, provided the maternal pulse rate is slow, the dose usually can be increased further. The maternal pulse rate also should be used to adjust the oral dosage of the β-agonists.

## Psychologic Aspects of Treatment

The psychologic effects of prolonged hospitalization and the emotional needs of the patient are often overlooked by the health care team. In addition to suffering the untoward effects of the drugs, the patient seldom has an undisturbed night's sleep, often resulting in chronic fatigue. Scheduling of medications, vital signs, fetal surveillance, and other procedures should, whenever possible, be tailored to meet the maternal patient's needs. A collaborative approach should be taken by nurses, physicians, and other health care providers to meet this goal. The patient often has feelings of guilt that the preterm labor is due to something that she has done or failed to do during the pregnancy. It is important that she be reassured that the preterm labor is not her fault. Although many pregnant women fear that their baby will not be normal, this is of even greater concern to many patients in preterm labor.

Health care providers are occasionally faced with the patient who refuses further treatment and expresses the desire to end the pregnancy, even though it has been explained to her that this may result in the loss of her baby. This ambivalence toward her pregnancy is normal for a woman who has been hospitalized for a long period of time. Some patients blame the baby for their confinement, the separation from the rest of the family, and their inability to conduct a normal life. It should be explained to the patient that these are normal emotions faced by many women in preterm labor and that these emotions do not make them an uncaring or unloving mother. Some patients have great difficulty confining themselves to bed when they do not feel ill. These patients may be encouraged to develop activities that can be done in bed, such as reading, writing, and crafts.

It is not uncommon for a patient confined to bed to experience periods of depression. Correct counseling and emotional support, including a liberal visitation policy, play a very important part in the patient's treatment for preterm labor (see Chapter 14).

## Postpartum Management

The patient who has delivered a preterm baby requires intensive emotional support during the postpartum period. The preterm birth cuts short a normal developmental process of adjustment and attachment to the fetus. By the time the pregnancy has progressed to the stage of viability, the parents have made a significant psychologic and emotional investment in the fetus.

Preterm delivery presents a family crisis. Grief, guilt, and anxiety are the primary emotional responses to the preterm birth. The parents experience all the elements of grief, first, because they did not have the baby that they expected. Anticipatory grief for the potential threats to their vulnerable newborn may follow. At the same time, they are attempting to bond with their baby. It is important to allow and encourage them to see their newborn as soon as possible. The sooner they see their baby, the sooner they can work through their feelings and begin the process of bonding with the baby. If visiting is impossible because of transport of the baby or the mother's condition, it is a good idea to provide the parents with a picture of their baby, which can help them deal with the real baby. The father and grandparents should be encouraged to visit the baby if the mother is unable to do so. They can give support to the mother as well. To help reduce anxiety, it is essential that the medical staff communicate with the family about the baby's condition. The elements of grief are essentially the same, regardless of the cause. They have been described as shock, denial, anger, bargaining, and acceptance. Parents of preterm babies exhibit varying degrees of these emotions at one time or another.

The initial emotion exhibited by the mother and family of the preterm baby is usually *shock*. The patient can expect to have periods of crying and silence and at times, to experience emotional numbness. The patient should be allowed to express her feelings, and sedation should not be prescribed in order to help her deal with the seemingly negative emotions that will need to be dealt with eventually.

The *denial* phase is generally the longest and is probably the most troublesome response for the nursing and medical staff to handle. During this phase, the family apparently refuses to grasp and understand what is told to them about the baby's condition. Denial is a normal self-defense mechanism that the family uses to cope during such a crisis. This enables the family to feel that they are maintaining control and also enables them to cushion themselves against the pain of the reality of the circumstances. Denial does not necessarily mean that the family refuses to hear what they are told by the staff. During this time, the staff is called on to give repeated explanations regarding the condition of the baby. During each meeting with the family, the staff should provide accurate information and prevent confrontation.

*Anger* is another common response to the birth of a preterm baby. The anger and hostility of the family is often directed at the physicians and hospital staff, especially the nurses who care for the baby. The mother may be jealous of the nurses who are caring for her baby while she cannot. To alleviate this situation, the nurses should allow the mother to participate in as much of the infant's care as possible.

The mother may experience a period of *bargaining*, which is usually done in a religious context. The staff should withhold their personal feelings during this time and continue to provide emotional support without setting unrealistic expectations for the patient regarding the baby's condition. The easiest phase of grief for the nursing and medical staff to deal with is when the family members begin to *accept* the circumstances and ask pertinent questions on how to handle their situation.

Each of these responses is a phase. The phases may not occur in any particular order, and families may have different responses at different times. It is important that the staff be supportive and allow family members to express their feelings and ask questions, while at the same time correcting the parents in areas in which they are misguided with regard to their child's condition.

The mother of the preterm infant may feel guilty that she has failed to produce a healthy, full-term infant. She may ask the staff repeated questions in her search for something that she possibly did wrong and that may have resulted in her preterm delivery. The father may also have guilt feelings with regard to whether something he did, or failed to do, contributed toward the preterm delivery. Siblings may worry that their jealousy or fantasies were what caused the problem. The entire family needs to be listened to and reassured that they were not responsible for the preterm delivery.

The postpartum nursing staff and the neonatal intensive care unit staff should expect the family to experience episodes of severe anxiety in response to the daily fluctuations in the infant's condition. It is imperative for the postpartum nursing staff to have good communication with the neonatal staff to give the parents current information on the status of their baby. The family may experience fear and anxiety about their infant's prognosis; in addition to this, there may be a great concern about the financial consequences of the neonate's prolonged hospitalization. The mother may feel inadequate and lack confidence in her ability to care for the baby in the neonatal intensive care unit. These feelings of inadequacy may be intensified by her lack of understanding of the medical terminology being used in reference to her baby's condition, as well as the various life support systems and monitors in the intensive care unit. Antepartum visits to the intensive care unit may help to decrease the mother's anxiety.

When the parents are ready to take their infant home, "nesting" rooms can be made available so that the parents can spend a few days and nights caring for their baby alone within the hospital with help readily available. This type of safe environment increases the parents' confidence in caring for their child.

The medical and nursing staff can be invaluable when they provide for both the emotional and physical well-being of the mother during the postpartum period. Explanations regarding the infant's condition should be given in simple terms to the patient and her family. Responses to the grief, guilt, and anxiety of the family should be expected, perceived as normal by the nurses, and dealt with in a professional manner. Without disregarding the physical condition of the patient, it is imperative that staff members exhibit an empathetic and nonjudgmental attitude as well as pay close personal attention to the emotional well-being of the patient in this situation (see Chapters 33 and 34).

Finally, when a mother has had preterm labor, she should be counseled that she is at risk for another preterm labor. She should be advised that, with subsequent pregnancies, she should seek medical care as soon as she knows that she is pregnant and advise the practitioners that she has had a previous preterm labor. She should also be told that she should seek prenatal care at a center in which comprehensive services are available.

### Acknowledgment

Acknowledgment is given to Rebecca L. Brown, RN, for her contribution to the first edition.

## References

Ahlquist RP: A study of the adrenotropic receptors. Am J Physiol 153:586, 1948.

Anderson ABM: Pre-term labour: definition. In Anderson ABM, et al. (eds): Proceedings of the Fifth Study Group of the Royal College of Obstetricians and Gynaecologists. London, Royal College of Obstetricians and Gynaecologists, 1977.

Anderson HF, Freda MC, Damus K, Brustman L, Merkatz IR: Effectiveness of patient education to reduce preterm delivery among ordinary risk patients. Am J Perinatol 6(2):214, 1989.

Baillie P, Meehan PP, Tyack AJ: Treatment of premature labour with orciprenaline. Br Med J 4:154, 1970.

Bejar R, Cuberlo V, Davis C, et al: Premature labor: infections as possible triggers. Twenty-sixth Annual Meeting of the Society for Gynecologic Investigation. San Diego, March 1979, Abstract No. 285.

Benedetti TJ, Hargrove J, Rosene KA: Maternal pulmonary edema during premature labor inhibition. Obstet Gynecol 59(Suppl.)33, 1982.

Bentley DL, Bentley JL, Watson DL, et al: Relationship of uterine contractility to preterm labor. Obstet Gynecol 76(suppl):1, 1990.

Bernbaum J, Hoffman-Williamson M: Following the NICU graduate. Contemp Pediatr 3:22, 1986.

Bieniarz J: Cardiovascular effects of beta-adrenergic agonists. In Anderson ABM, et al (eds): Proceedings of the Fifth Study Group of the Royal College of Obstetricians and Gynaecologists. London, Royal College of Obstetricians and Gynaecologists, 1977.

Bishop EH, Woutersz TB: Arrest of premature labor. JAMA 178:116, 1961.

Blondel B, Breart G, Llado J, Chartier M: Evaluation of the home-visiting system for women with threatened preterm labor: results of a randomized controlled trial. Eur J Obstet Gynecol Reprod Biol 34(1–2):47, 1990.

Blouin D, Murray MAF, Beard RW: The effect of oral

ritodrine on maternal and fetal carbohydrate metabolism. Br J Obstet Gynaecol 83:711, 1976.

Brazy JF, Pupkin MG: Effects of maternal isoxsuprine administration on preterm infants. J Pediatr 94:444, 1979.

Brettes JP, Renaud R, Gandar R: A double-blind investigation into the effects of ritodrine on uterine blood flow during the third trimester of pregnancy. Am J Obstet Gynecol 124:164, 1976.

Brustman LE, Langer O, Anyaegbunam A, Belle C, Merkatz IR: Education does not improve patient perception of preterm uterine contractility. Obstet Gynecol 76(suppl):1, 1990.

Chase HC: Time trends in low birth weight in the United States, 1950–1974. In Reed DM, et al (eds): The Epidemiology of Prematurity. Baltimore, Urban and Schwarzenberg, 1977, pp 17–34.

Chibber G, Cohen AW, Lindenbaum CR, Teplick F: Patient attitude toward home uterine activity monitoring. Obstet Gynecol 76(suppl):1, 1990.

Collins E, Turner G: Salicylates and pregnancy. Lancet 2:1494, 1973.

Copper RL, Goldenberg RL, Davis RD, et al: Warning symptoms, uterine contractions and cervical examination findings in women at risk of preterm delivery. Am J Obstet Gynecol 162(3):748, 1990.

Craig CJT: Congenital abnormalities of the uterus and foetal wastage. S Afr Med J 49:2013, 1975.

Creasy RK, Merkatz IR: Prevention of preterm birth: clinical opinion. Obstet Gynecol 76(suppl):1, 1990.

Dancis J: Task force of predictors of fetal maturity. Washington, DC, United States Department of Health, Education, and Welfare, Public Health Service, National Institutes of Health, 1979.

Diagnostic and Therapeutic Technology Assessment (DATTA): Home monitoring of uterine activity. JAMA 261:3027, 1989.

Fedrick J: Anderson ABM: Factors associated with spontaneous preterm birth. Br J Obstet Gynaecol 83:342, 1976.

Fisher Lee ML: Infections and prematurity: is there a relationship? J Perinat Neonatal Nurs 2(1):10, 1988.

Fitzhardinge PM: Early growth and development in low birth weight infants following treatment in an intensive care nursery. Pediatrics 56:162, 1975.

Forssman L: Posttraumatic intrauterine synechiae and pregnancy. Obstet Gynecol 26:710, 1965.

Freda MC, Damus K, Andersen, HF, et al: A "PROPP" for the Bronx: preterm birth prevention education in the inner city. Obstet Gynecol 76(suppl):1, 1990.

Freysz, H, Willard D, Berland H, et al: Effets lointains de la thérapeutique sur le foetus: répercussions sur le métabolisme hydrocarbone et les fonctions hépatiques du nouveau-né d'un traitement beta-mimique (ritodrine ou PrePar) administré au cours de la gestation. J Gynecol Biol Repr 2:987, 1973.

Freysz H, Willard D, Lehr A, et al: A long term evaluation of infants who received a beta-mimetic drug while in utero. J Perinat Med 5:94, 1977.

Gandar R, de Zoeten LW, van der Schoot JB: Serum level of ritodrine in man. Eur J Clin Pharmacol 17:117, 1980.

Garite TJ, Bentley DL, Hamer CA, Porto ML: Uterine activity characteristics in multiple gestations. Obstet Gynecol 76(suppl):1, 1990.

Garn SM, Shaw HA, McCabe KD: Effects of socioeconomic status and race on weight-defined and gestational prematurity in the United States. In Reed DM, et al (eds): The Epidemiology of Prematurity. Baltimore, Urban and Schwarzenberg, 1977, pp 127–140.

Gibbs CE: Diagnosis and treatment of uterine conditions that may cause prematurity. Clin Obstet Gynecol 16:159, 1973.

Givens SR: Update on tocolytic therapy in the management of preterm labor. J Perinat Neonatal Nurs 2(1):21, 1988.

Goodlin RC: Orgasm and premature labor. Lancet 2:646, 1969.

Gravett MD, Nelson HP, DeRouen T, et al: Independent association of bacterial vaginosis and Chlamydia trachomatis infection with adverse pregnancy outcome. JAMA 256:189, 1986.

Gulbis E, Marion AM, Dumont JE, et al: Prostaglandin formation in bacteria. Prostaglandins 18:397, 1979.

Hack M, Fanaroff AA: Outcomes of extremely low-birth-weight infants between 1982 and 1988. N Engl J Med 321:1642, 1989.

Hardy JB, Mellits ED: Relationship of low birth weight to maternal characteristics of age, parity, education and body size. In Reed DM, et al (eds): The Epidemiology of Prematurity. Baltimore, Urban and Schwarzenberg, 1977, pp. 105–117.

Hendricks CH: The use of isoxsuprine for the arrest of premature labor. Clin Obstet Gynecol 7:687, 1964.

Hernandez JA, Offutt J, Butterfield LJ: The cost of care of the less-than-1000-gram infant. The Tiny Baby. Clin Perinatol 13(2):461–476, 1986.

Herron MA: One approach to preventing preterm birth. J Perinat Neonatal Nurs 2(1):33, 1988.

Hess LW, McCaul JF, Perry KG, et al: Correlation of uterine activity using the term guard monitor versus standard external tocodynamometry compared with the intrauterine pressure catheter. Obstet Gynecol 76(suppl):1, 1990.

Hill WC, Fleming AD, Martin RW, et al: Home uterine activity monitoring is associated with a reduction in preterm birth. Obstet Gynecol 76(suppl): 1, July 1990.

Hollander DI, Nagey DA, Pupkin MJ: Magnesium sulfate and ritodrine hydrochloride: a randomized comparison. Am J Obstet Gynecol 156:631, 1987.

Huszar G, Roberts JM: Biochemistry and pharmacology of the myometrium and labor: regulation at the cellular and molecular levels. Am J Obstet Gynecol 142:225, 1982.

Iams JD: Johnson FF, Hamer C: Uterine activity and symptoms as predictors of preterm labor. Obstet Gynecol 76(suppl):1, 1990.

Iams JD, Johnson FF, O'Shaughnessy RW: A prospective random trial of home uterine activity monitoring in pregnancies at increased risk of preterm labor. Am J Obstet Gynecol 159(3):595, 1988.

Johnstone RE II, Kreindler T, Johnstone RE: Hyperparathyroidism during pregnancy. Obstet Gynecol 40:580, 1972.

Katz M, Newman RB, Gill PJ: Assessment of uterine activity in ambulatory patients at high risk of preterm labor and delivery. Paper presented at Annual Meeting of Society of Perinatal Obstetricians, Las Vegas, Nevada, February, 1985.

Keirse MJNC, Rush RW, Anderson ABM, et al: Risk of preterm delivery in patients with previous preterm delivery and/or abortion. Br J Obstet Gynaecol 85:81, 1978.

Kirshon B, Moise KJ Jr, Wasserstrum N, Ching-Nan, O, Huhta JC: Influence of short term indomethacin therapy on fetal urine output. Obstet Gynecol 72:51, 1988.

Kleinhout J, Stolte LAM, Veth AFL: Passeert ritodrine de placenta? Med T Geneesk 118:1248, 1974.

Knuppel RA, Lake MF, Watson DL, et al: Preventing preterm birth in twin gestation: home uterine activity monitoring and perinatal nursing support. Obstet Gynecol 76(suppl):1, 1990.

Knuppel RA, Lake MF, Watson DL, et al: The contribution of symptomatology and/or uterine activity to the incidence of unscheduled visits. Obstet Gynecol 76(Suppl):1, 1990.

Konte JM, Creasy RK, Laros RK Jr: California North Coast Preterm Birth Prevention Project. Obstet Gynecol 71:727, 1988.

Kords H: Pharmacology and pharmacokinetics of Partusisten (fenoterol). In Weidinger H (ed): Labour Inhibition Betamimetic Drugs in Obstetrics. New York, Gustav Fischer Verlag, 1977, pp 41–46.

Kosasa TS, Abou-Sayf FK, Li-Ma G, Hale RW: Evaluation of the cost-effectiveness of home uterine activity monitoring in Medicaid population. Obstet Gynecol 76(suppl):1, 1990.

Lam F: Miniature pump infusion of terbutaline—an option in preterm labor. Contemp Ob/Gyn 31:52, 1989.

Lam F, Giu P, Smith M, Kitzmiller JL, Katz M: Use of the subcutaneous terbutaline pump for long-term tocolysis. Obstet Gynecol 72:810, 1988.

Lands AM, Arnold A, McAuliff JP, et al: Differentiation of receptor systems activated by sympathomimetic amines. Nature 214:597, 1967.

Lawhon G, Melzar A: Developmental care of the very low birth weight infant. J Perinat Neonatal Nurs 2(1):56, 1988.

Lefrak-Okikawa L: Nutritional management of the very low birth weight infant. J Perinat Neonatal Nurs 2(1):66, 1988.

Lewis RB, Schulman JD: Influence of acetylsalicylic acid, an inhibitor of prostaglandin synthesis, on the duration of human gestation and labour. Lancet 2:1159, 1973.

Lippert TH, De Grandi PB, Fridrich R: Actions of the uterine relaxant fenoterol on uteroplacental hemodynamics in human subjects. Am J Obstet Gynecol 125:1093, 1976.

Lipshitz J: Initiation of labor. In Givens JR (ed): Endocrinology of Pregnancy. Chicago & London, Year Book Medical Publishers, Inc, 1980, pp 133–151.

Lipshitz J: Preventing premature delivery. S Afr Med J 52:1110, 1977a.

Lipshitz J: The uterine and cardiovascular effects of oral fenoterol hydrobromide. Br J Obstet Gynaecol 84:737, 1977b.

Lipshitz J: Cerclage in the treatment of incompetent cervix. S Afr Med J 49:2013, 1975.

Lipshitz J, Baillie P: The uterine and cardiovascular effects of beta$_2$-selective sympathomimetic drugs administered as an intravenous infusion. S Afr Med J 50:1973, 1976a.

Lipshitz J, Baillie P: The effects of fenoterol hydrobromide (Partusisten) aerosol on uterine activity and the cardiovascular system. Br J Obstet Gynaecol 83:864, 1976b.

Lipshitz J, Lipshitz EM: Uterine and cardiovascular effects of fenoterol and hexoprenaline in prostaglandin F$_{2\alpha}$ induced-labor in the human. Obstet Gynecol 63:396, 1984.

Lipshitz J, Vinik AI: The effects of hexoprenaline, a $\beta_2$-sympathomimetic drug, on maternal glucose, insulin, glucagon and free fatty acid levels. Am J Obstet Gynecol 130:761, 1978.

Lipshitz J, Ahokas RA, Broyles K: Effect of hexoprenaline on utero-placental blood flow. Proceedings of the Second Annual Scientific Meeting of the Society of Perinatal Obstetricians. San Antonio, TX, 1982.

Lipshitz J, Anderson GD, Whybrew WD: Accelerated pulmonary maturity as measured by the Lumadex-foam stability index test. Obstet Gynecol 62:31, 1983.

Lipshitz J, Baillie P, Davey DA: A comparison of the uterine beta$_2$-adrenoreceptor selectivity of fenoterol, hexoprenaline, ritodrine and salbutamol. S Afr Med J 50:1969, 1976.

Lipshitz J, Broyles K, Whybrew WD: Placental transfer of 14C-hexoprenaline. Am J Obstet Gynecol 142:313, 1982.

Lipshitz J, Depp R, Hauth J, et al: Comparison of the cardiovascular effects of hexoprenaline and ritodrine in the treatment of preterm labor. Proceedings of the Third Annual Scientific Meeting of the Society of Perinatal Obstetricians. San Antonio, TX, 1983.

Lipshitz J, Whybrew MS, Anderson GD: Comparison of the Lumadex-foam stability index test, lecithin:sphingomyelin ratio, and simple shake test for fetal lung maturity. Obstet Gynecol 63:349, 1984.

Lipsitz PJ: The clinical and biochemical effects of excess magnesium in the newborn. Pediatrics 47:501, 1971.

Mari G, Moise KJ Jr, Deter RL, Kirshon B, Carpenter RJ: Doppler assessment of renal blood flow velocity waveform during indomethacin therapy for preterm labor and polyhydramnios. Obstet Gynecol 75(2):199, 1990.

Martin JN Jr, McColgin SW, Martin RW, et al: Uterine activity among a diverse group of patients at high risk for preterm delivery. Obstet Gynecol 76(suppl):1, 1990.

Martin RW, Gookin KS, Hill WC, et al: Uterine activity compared with symptomatology in the detection of preterm labor. Obstet Gynecol 76(suppl):1, 1990.

Martius J, Krohn MS, Hillier SL, et al: Relationships of vaginal Lactobacillus species, cervical Chlamydia trachomatis, and bacterial vaginosis to preterm birth. Obstet Gynecol 71:89, 1988.

McCoy R, Kadowaki C, Wilks S, Engstrom J, Meier P: Nursing management of breast feeding for preterm infants. J Perinat Neonatal Nurs 2(1):42, 1988.

McCubbin JH, Sibai GM, Abdella TM, et al: Cardiopulmonary arrest due to acute maternal hypermagnesaemia [letter]. Lancet 1:1058, 1981.

McLendon MS: Home ambulatory uterine activity monitoring: a new tool in the management of women at risk for preterm bith. J Perinat Neonatal Nurs 2(1):1, 1988.

Meissner J, Klostermann H: Distribution and diaplacental passage of infused $^3$H-fenoterol hydrobromide (Partusisten) in the gravid rabbit. Int J Clin Pharmacol Biopharm 13:27, 1976.

Mestman JH, Manning PR, Hodgman J: Hyperthyroidism and pregnancy. Arch Intern Med 134:434, 1974.

Meyer MB: Effects of maternal smoking and altitude on birth weight and gestation. In Reed DM, Stanley FJ (eds): The Epidemiology of Prematurity. Baltimore, Urban and Schwarzenberg, 1977, pp 81–101.

Milewich L, Gant NF, Schwarz BE, et al: Initiation of human parturition. VIII. Metabolism of progesterone by fetal membranes of early and late human gestation. Obstet Gynecol 50:45, 1977.

Miller FC, Nochimson DJ, Paul RH, et al: Effects of ritodrine hydrochloride on uterine activity and the cardiovascular system in toxemic patients. Obstet Gynecol 47:50, 1976.

Morrison JC: Preterm birth: a puzzle worth solving. Obstet Gynecol 76(suppl):1, 1990.

Morrison JC: Introduction: home uterine activity monitoring and other initiatives in preterm birth prevention. Obstet Gynecol 76(suppl):1, 1990.

Morrison JC, Martin RW, Johnson C, Hess LW: Characteristics of uterine activity in gestations less than 20 weeks. Obstet Gynecol 76(suppl):1, July 1990.

Morrison JC, Pittman KP, Martin RW, McLaughlin BN: Cost/health effectiveness of home uterine activity monitoring in a Medicaid population. Obstet Gynecol 76(suppl):1, 1990.

Morrison JC, Martin JN Jr, Martin RW, et al: Prevention of preterm birth by ambulatory assessment of uterine activity: a randomized study. Am J Obstet Gynecol 156(3):536, 1987.

New Drug Application No. 18280, for ritodrine hydrochloride, submitted to the FDA on March 8, 1979, by Mid-West Medical Research, Inc, Columbus, Ohio, on behalf of Philips-Duphar, BV, Weesp, The Netherlands.

Newman RB, Richmond GS, Winston YE, et al: Antepartum uterine activity characteristics differentiating true from threatened preterm labor. Obstet Gynecol 76(suppl):1, 1990.

Niebyl JR, Blake DA, White RD, et al: The inhibition of premature labor with indomethacin. Am J Obstet Gynecol 136:1014, 1980.

Niswander KR: Obstetric factors related to prematurity. In Reed DM, Stanley FJ (eds): The Epidemiology of Prematurity. Baltimore, Urban and Schwarzenberg, 1977, pp 249–264.

Petrie RH, Wu R, Miller FC, et al: The effects of drugs on uterine activity. Obstet Gynecol 48:431, 1976.

Richardson C: Hyaline membrane disease: future treatment modalities. J Perinat Neonatal Nurs 2(1):78, 1988.

Riffel HD, Nochimson DJ, Paul RH, et al: Effects of meperidine and promethazine during labor. Obstet Gynecol 42:738, 1973.

Roberts WE, Morrison JC, Hamer C, Wiser WL: The incidence of preterm labor and specific risk factors. Obstet Gynecol 76(suppl):1, 1990.

Robichaux AG III, Stedman CM, Hamer C: Uterine activity in patients with cervical cerclage. Obstet Gynecol 76(suppl):1, 1990.

Roos RJ, Malan AF, Woods DL, et al: The bacteriological environment of preterm infants. S Afr Med J 57:347, 1980.

Rosen KA, Featherstone HJ, Benedetti TJ: Cerebral ischemia associated with parenteral terbutaline use in pregnant migraine patients. Am J Obstet Gynecol 143:405, 1982.

Rumack CM, Guggenheim MA, Rumack VH, et al: Neonatal intracranial hemorrhage and maternal use of aspirin. Obstet Gynecol 58:52S, 1981.

Rush RW, Keirse MJN, Howat P, et al: Contribution of preterm delivery to perinatal mortality. Br Med J 2:965, 1976.

Sabel KG, Olegard R, Victorin L: Remaining sequelae with modern perinatal care. Pediatrics 57:652, 1976.

Scheerer LJ, Campion S, Katz M: Ambulatory tocodynamometry data interpretation: evaluating variability and reliability. Obstet Gynecol 76(suppl):1, 1990.

Schwartz S: Prenatal care, prematurity and neonatal mortality. Am J Obstet Gynecol 83:591, 1962.

Schwarz BE, Milewich L, Johnston JM, et al: Initiation of human parturition. V. Progesterone binding substance in fetal membranes. Obstet Gynecol 48:685, 1976.

Sell EJ: Outcome of very very low birth weight infants. The Tiny Baby. Clin Perinatol 13(2):1986.

Sharpe GL, Larsson KS, Thalme B: Studies on closure of the ductus arteriosus. XII. In utero effect of indomethacin and sodium salicylate in rats and rabbits. Prostaglandins 9:585, 1975.

Sharpe GL, Thalme B, Larsson KS: Studies on closure of the ductus arteriosus. XI. Ductal closure in utero by a prostaglandin synthetase inhibitor. Prostaglandins 8:363, 1974.

Smith SK, Thompson D: The effect of intravenous salbutamol upon plasma and urinary potassium during premature labour. Br J Obstet Gynaecol 84:344, 1977.

Stahlman MT: Newborn intensive care: success or failure? J Pediatr 105:162, 1984.

Steer CM, Petrie RJ: A comparison of magnesium sulfate and alcohol for the prevention of premature labor. Am J Obstet Gynecol 129:1, 1977.

Stewart A: Follow-up of pre-term infants. In Anderson ABM, et al (eds): Proceedings of the Fifth Study Group of the Royal College of Obstetricians and Gynaecologists. London, Royal College of Obstetricians and Gynaecologists, 1977, pp 372–384.

Stone SR, Pritchard JA: Effect of maternally administered magnesium sulfate on the neonate. Obstet Gynecol 35:574, 1970.

Stuart MJ, Gross SJ, Elrad H, et al: Effects of acetylsalicylic-acid ingestion on maternal and neonatal homeostasis. N Engl J Med 307:909, 1982.

Sweet RL, Gibbs RS: Urinary tract infection. In Infectious Diseases of the Female Genital Tract. Baltimore, Williams & Wilkins, 1985.

Taylor PM, Hall BL: Parent-infant bonding: problems and opportunities in a perinatal center. Semin Perinatol 3:73, 1979.

Thomas DJB, Dove AF, Alberti KGMM: Metabolic effects of salbutamol infusion during premature labour. Br J Obstet Gynaecol 84:497, 1977.

Turnbull AC: Aetiology of pre-term labour. In Anderson ABM, et al (eds): Proceedings of the Fifth Study Group of the Royal College of Obstetricians and Gynaecologists. London, Royal College of Obstetricians and Gynaecologists, 1977, pp 56–78.

Vital Statistics of the United States: Natality. Rockville, Maryland: United States Department of Health, Education, and Welfare, 1987, p. 255.

Vital Statistics of the United States: Natality. Rockville, Maryland: United States Department of Health, Education, and Welfare, 1977, p 1.

Vrbicky K, Hill WC, Lambertz EL, Jurgensen WW: Home uterine activity monitoring in a rural setting. Obstet Gynecol 76(suppl):1, 1990.

Wagner NN, Butler JC, Sanders JP: Prematurity and orgasmic coitus during pregnancy: data on a small sample. Fertil Steril 27:911, 1976.

Watson DL, Welch RA, Mariona FG, et al: Management of preterm labor patients at home: does daily uterine activity monitoring and nursing support make a difference? Obstet Gynecol 76(suppl):1, 1990.

Wiqvist N, Lundstrom V, Green K: Premature labor and indomethacin. Prostaglandins 10:515, 1975.

Witter FR, Niebyl JR: Inhibition of arachidonic acid metabolism in the perinatal period: pharmacology, clinical application, and potential adverse effects. Semin Perinatol 10:316, 1986.

Wren BG: Premature labor with renal infections: the action of coliform endotoxin on the pregnant rat uterus. Aust NZ J Obstet Gynaecol 10:211, 1970.

Zuckerman H, Reiss U, Rubinstein I: Inhibition of human premature labor by indomethacin. Obstet Gynecol 44:787, 1974.

# CHAPTER 23

. . . . . . . . . . . . . . . . . . . . . . . . . . . . . . . . . .

# Prolonged Pregnancy

Winston A. Campbell, David J. Nochimson, and Anthony M. Vintzileos

## Definition

The gestational period for a developing embryo varies depending on the species. In humans, the expected date of confinement (EDC) is usually calculated from the first day of the last menstrual period. The average EDC is 280 ± 14 days (40 ± 2 weeks); an alternative calculation is based on the day of ovulation and is 266 ± 14 days (38 ± 2 weeks). A pregnancy is considered prolonged when it has exceeded 294 days from the last menstrual period (42 weeks) or 280 days from the time of ovulation. The majority of pregnant patients (80 percent) deliver within ± 2 weeks of their EDC. Eight percent of pregnant women deliver preterm (before 36 weeks' gestation), and the remaining 12 percent continue the pregnancy to or beyond 42 weeks. Beyond 42 weeks, there are fewer patients (1 to 4 percent) who remain pregnant (Lagrew and Freeman, 1986).

A weakness in the definition is that it is based on the clinical last menstrual period. This is a variable parameter and assumes that each patient has a 28-day menstrual cycle and that ovulation occurs on day 14 of the cycle. Those patients who have longer or shorter menstrual cycles, as well as patients who have irregular menses or who have vague recall of the last menstrual period, can account for a significant number of pregnancies that are incorrectly classified as a prolonged pregnancy (postdates). It has been estimated that approximately 15 to 30 percent of incorrect EDCs are based on some of these factors. A more precise method to determine the duration of gestation would be to use the time of conception, as reflected by the day of ovulation. This information can be obtained from basal body temperature charts; however, since a majority of pregnancies are not so well planned, the obstetrician usually does not have this information available. The usefulness of this technique was indicated by a study of pregnancies in which temperature charts had been kept as an aid to conception. This study showed that pregnancies classified as prolonged by the usual clinical means were erroneously classified 70 percent of the time (Boyce et al, 1976). In a review of prolonged pregnancies, it was observed that 7.5 percent of pregnancies continued to 42 weeks' gestation when menstrual dating was used. However, when gestational age was calculated on the basis of a second trimester ultrasound, only 2.6 percent of pregnancies continued to 42 weeks (Boyd et al, 1988). These investigators reported an even lower incidence of postdates pregnancies (1.1 percent) when menstrual dates confirmed by a second trimester ultrasound were used to define gestational age.

Although there are a number of clinical parameters that can be used to establish gestational age, the most useful, easily available, and informative method uses the last menstrual period, which is confirmed by a second trimester (16 to 20 weeks) ultrasound. This ultrasound examination is very beneficial for two reasons: (1) it serves to confirm or correct menstrual dates early in the pregnancy when the error of the examination is less than it would be in the third trimester (7 to 10 days versus 14 to 21 days), and (2) it can identify other obstetric conditions (congenital anomalies, multiple fetuses, oligohydramnios, fetal demise) that could alter management.

## Significance and Risks

It is realized that a significant number of pregnancies classified as prolonged are the result of errors in dating. In such cases, provided there are no other medical or obstetric complications, there should be no increased risk to the fetus. The risk arises when the pregnancy is not only prolonged but when there is placental dysfunction as well. Placental dysfunction (placental insufficiency) places the fetus at risk of developing dysmaturity (postmaturity). The posmaturity syndrome reflects the detrimental effects on the fetus of diminished placental function. Clifford (1957; 1954) and Vorherr (1975) have written extensively about placental dysfunction and the postmaturity syndrome. There is also risk to the fetus in prolonged pregnancies when macrosomia (trauma), oligohydramnios (cord accidents), and meconium (meconium aspiration) are present (Bochner et al, 1987; Chervenak et al, 1989; Usher et al, 1988).

Extensive study of placental development and physiology indicates that placental development is complete by the fifth month of gestation. From this point on, there are minor modifications to ensure adequate nutritional and oxygen supply to the growing fetus. It appears that peak placental function is achieved at approximately 36 weeks of gestation, after which diminishing function is normal. Although peak function is reached at 36 weeks gestation, there is still fetal and placental growth, but at a slower rate. As depicted in Figure 23–1, an actual plateau of fetal growth and then a decrease would not be seen until after 42 weeks of gestation. However, the presence of predisposing factors that can alter placental function may cause abnormalities in fetal growth to appear at an earlier time (Fig. 23–2). This is an important concept, because the postmaturity syndrome has been observed prior to 42 weeks' gestation (Fig. 23–3). The difference is that there are fewer cases that occur prior to 42 weeks' gestation. The overall incidence of postmaturity syndrome is estimated at 2 to 6 percent, with an incidence of 3 percent at term compared with 20 to 40 percent when

the pregnancy is prolonged. The risk to the fetus is increased perinatal mortality (Fig. 23–4) and morbidity, with rates varying with different reports. At term, the average perinatal mortality rate (PMR)* is from 1 to 2 percent compared with 5 to 7 percent in cases of prolonged pregnancy. The PMR also varies with maternal age, parity, and sex of the fetus (Vorherr, 1975). The PMR is higher with increasing maternal age, in primigravidas (Fig. 23–4), and in male infants. Compared with term pregnancies, there is about a two- to fivefold increase in PMR at 43 weeks' gestation; and at 44 weeks' gestation, a three-, to sevenfold increase.

Placental dysfunction is a factor that complicates a prolonged pregnancy and increases the risk to the fetus. Placental dysfunction occurs in approximately 5 to 12 percent of all pregnancies, and placental pathology is observed in 20 to 40 percent of all perinatal fetal deaths. Depending on the cause of placental insufficiency and the rate at which it develops, one may see a different effect on the fetus. If placental dysfunction initially involves a small part of the placenta and then gradually progresses to further placental involvement, chronic placental insufficiency can occur. This can cause nutritional deficiency, as reflected by underweight infants. This form of insufficiency can also cause chronic hypoxia, which can be a significant risk. Chronic hypoxia has been found in some studies to be the cause of 60 to 70 percent of antepartum fetal deaths (Manning et al, 1982). In cases of acute placental dysfunction (e.g., due to abruptio placentae or cord complications), the effect on the fetus is reflected as poor fetal oxygenation manifested as either hypoxia (decreased oxygen concentration) or asphyxia (decreased oxygen and increased carbon dioxide concentration). The placental insufficiency involved in prolonged pregnancy is of the chronic type; however, this condition can also be complicated by superimposed acute insufficiency. Clifford (1954) has described the clinical findings of infants who are affected by the dysmaturity syndrome. These infants show evidence of growth retardation and have different stages of skin maceration secondary to loss of the vernix caseosa, which functions to protect the skin. In addition, these infants

---

$$* \text{ PMR} = \frac{No.\ of\ Stillbirths + No.\ of\ Neonatal\ Deaths}{1000\ Births}$$

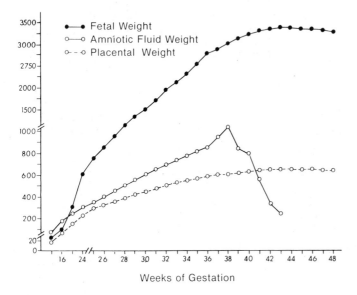

**Figure 23–1.** Average weights of fetus, placenta, and amniotic fluid throughout human gestation. (From Vorherr H: Placental insufficiency in relation to postterm pregnancy and fetal postmaturity. Am J Obstet Gynecol 123:67, 1975.)

have an alert appearance, long nails, and staining of the body, umbilical cord, and placenta from meconium. Clifford (1957; 1954) has classified the disorder into stages of severity as follows:

*Stage I*—Dry and cracking skin that is parchmentlike, wrinkled (owing to loss of subcutaneous fat), and peeling. Infant appears malnourished but alert or apprehensive. Absence of meconium staining.

*Stage II*—All of the findings of stage I plus presence of meconium-colored amniotic fluid and meconium covering the skin. Also, green meconium staining of the

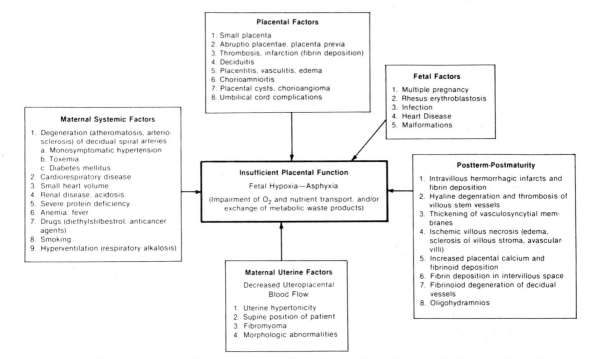

**Figure 23–2.** Abnormal maternal, placental, or fetal conditions. (From Vorherr H: Placental insufficiency in relation to postterm pregnancy and fetal postmaturity. Am J Obstet Gynecol 123:67, 1975.)

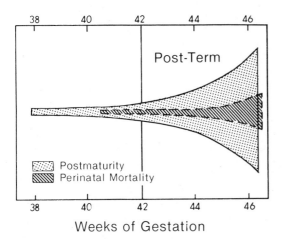

**Figure 23–3.** Relative incidence of fetal postmaturity syndrome and perinatal mortality. (From Vorherr H: Placental insufficiency in relation to postterm pregnancy and fetal postmaturity. Am J Obstet Gynecol 123:67, 1975.)

placental membranes and the umbilical cord.

*Stage III*—All of the findings of stages I and II, in addition to which there is bright yellow staining of nails and skin and a conversion to yellow-green staining of umbilical cord, membranes, and placenta.

It is believed that the severity of placental dysfunction in stage II is such that sufficient fetal anoxia exists to cause the passage of meconium. Meconium is a normal product of

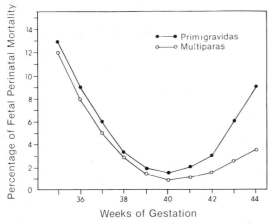

**Figure 23–4.** Preterm, term, and postterm perinatal fetal mortalities in primigravidas and multiparas. (From Vorherr, H.: Placental insufficiency in relation to postterm pregnancy and fetal postmaturity. Am J Obstet Gynecol 123:67, 1975.)

fetal gastrointestinal function. Its passage in utero is believed to occur when oxygen delivery to the smooth muscle of the gastrointestinal tract is inadequate. This results in relaxation of the anal sphincter and meconium passage. The finding of meconium in stage II is significant; it represents a severe level of anoxia. According to Clifford (1957), infants in this stage have the highest rates of morbidity and mortality. The overall mortality rates for infants with dysmaturity syndrome is 36 percent; of those delivered during stage II, however, two thirds have significant clinical problems and respiratory complications from meconium aspiration, and about 50 percent die. A smaller number may develop intracranial bleeding.

For clinical, medical, and legal purposes, it is important to keep in mind that meconium staining occurs over time and that meconium aspiration can occur in utero. The time required for meconium staining varies depending on whether the focus of attention is the fetus or the placenta. Desmond and associates (1956) demonstrated that 4 to 6 hours of exposure to meconium is needed to yield staining of a newborn's toenails. Twelve to 14 hours of exposure are needed to cause staining of the vernix caseosa. Similar information regarding placental staining was determined from in vitro studies by Miller and associates (1985). Using increasing concentrations of a meconium bath solution, they determined that gross meconium staining of the placental membranes and the umbilical cord is a surface phenomenon. They concluded that gross superficial staining begins within an hour of meconium passage. However, maximal staining time varies depending on the concentration of meconium; the time in this particular study varied from 3 to 6 hours. Similar observations are noted for the umbilical cord. Microscopic examination of the placenta yielded a more reliable index of time for meconium staining; the findings were independent of the concentration of meconium. Meconium-laden macrophages were identified in the amnion layer (the innermost layer of the placental membranes in direct contact with the amniotic fluid) after 1 hour of exposure to meconium. It required 3 hours of exposure to demonstrate meconium-laden macrophages in the chorion layer. The implication of these findings is that meconium passage and its complications can occur prior to labor; thus, some of the complications may not be preventable.

Such an event has been described for meconium aspiration (Manning et al, 1978; Paul et al, 1986)

Those infants who have survived stage II and reach stage III have a lower mortality rate. The major clinical problems in stage III are respiratory distress syndrome (which results from meconium aspiration) and anoxic injury to the central nervous system. The mortality rate for infants delivered during stage III is about 15 percent.

Placental dysfunction is not the only cause of mortality and morbidity in prolonged pregnancies. Leveno (1986) noted that if placental dysfunction was the most significant feature of prolonged pregnancies, then we should expect to see fetal heart rate patterns that are characteristic for uteroplacental insufficiency—late decelerations. The most frequent cause of fetal distress requiring cesarean delivery was variable decelerations (Leveno, 1986). This is a pattern suggestive of umbilical cord compression, a condition that can be caused by decreased amniotic fluid (Leveno, 1986).

The major risks to the fetus in prolonged pregnancy have been summarized by Vorherr (1975) as follows: (1) lack of adequate fetal and placental growth after 41 weeks' gestation, (2) progressive degenerative placental changes, (3) increased incidence of meconium staining, (4) decreased amniotic fluid, (5) inadequate fetal oxygen and nutrition, (6) increased pathologic function of the fetoplacental unit, and (7) increased rates of fetal distress and consequent perinatal deaths.

Other features of a prolonged pregnancy that may increase the risk to the fetus are (1) macrosomia—birth weight greater than 4000 g (Chervenak et al, 1989); this condition can increase the risk of shoulder dystocia and birth trauma, (2) congenital anomalies (2.5 percent), especially central nervous system malformations (Ahn and Phelan, 1989), and (3) meconium aspiration (Usher et al, 1988).

# Diagnosis

The key to diagnosing prolonged pregnancy lies in recognizing that it is a potential complication of any pregnancy. With this in mind, the obstetric care providers can look for clues to indicate which patients are at risk. A number of clinical factors seem to be associated with an increased risk of prolonged pregnancy; these factors are listed in Table 23–1.

The number of pregnancies that are prolonged as a result of the factors cited in Table 23–1 varies with different reports. Also, not all of these factors have a known associated risk for the pregnancy to be prolonged. Disorders of the menstrual cycle, for example, often result in a pregnancy being diagnosed as prolonged because of difficulty in determining the correct gestational age. In all likelihood, the majority of these cases are term, and even preterm, pregnancies and are probably not associated with placental insufficiency if there are no complicating medical or obstetric problems.

Although the overall incidence of prolonged pregnancy in multigravidas and primigravidas is essentially the same for the entire reproductive age group (about 20 percent), it varies among specific age groups. There is a tendency for multigravidas to have a lower incidence of prolonged pregnancy. The age groups with the highest incidence for both multigravidas and primigravidas are 21 to 25 years old and 26 to 30 years old. For multigravidas, the incidence is 31 percent and 30 percent for the respective age groups. For primigravidas, it is 44 percent and 18 percent, respectively. Over the age of 30, there is a reversal in the incidence for multigravidas versus primigravidas; by age

**Table 23–1**
CONTRIBUTING FACTORS IN
PROLONGED PREGNANCY

**Disorder of Menstrual Cycle**
  Irregular menses
  Conception during lactation
  Conception with use of oral contraceptives
  Delayed ovulation
**Social***
  Parity and age
  Multigravidas—21 to 30 years old
  Primigravidas–21 to 30 years old
**Race**
  Whites more frequently than blacks
**Obstetric**
  Late registration for prenatal care
  Inadequate prenatal care
  Previous prolonged pregnancy
  First-trimester bleeding
  Sex of fetus (more common with males than with
    females)
  Congenital anomalies

* See text for details.

35 or more, the incidence for multigravidas is 15 percent versus 4 percent for primigravidas (Vorherr, 1975).

The obstetric factors listed in Table 23–1 (late registration, inadequate prenatal care, disorders of the menstrual cycle) can be a source of gestational dating error. In these instances, it is more likely that the gestational dating error would lead to a diagnosis of prolonged pregnancy. A previous history of a prolonged pregnancy carries a 50 percent chance for a repeat occurrence. Some studies have indicated that women pregnant with a male fetus have a higher risk of a prolonged pregnancy than if the fetus were female—8.5 percent versus 4 percent (Vorherr, 1975). This increased incidence with a male fetus is not appreciably changed with parity. Various congenital anomalies (especially anencephaly) have been associated with prolonged pregnancy (about 9 percent of cases).

These epidemiologic factors provide guidance in identifying pregnancies at risk. Some are more helpful than others. However, these guidelines do not provide the criteria to make a definitive diagnosis of prolonged pregnancy. The correct diagnosis for true prolonged pregnancy is based on having an accurate gestational age and knowing that the pregnancy has gone beyond 42 weeks from the last menstrual period. There are clinical milestones and diagnostic tests that can help to establish clinical dates. The simplest method is early prenatal care. If a patient seeks prenatal care within 2 weeks after her first missed menses and has a positive urine pregnancy test, this is indicative of a pregnancy of 6 weeks' duration. Alternatively, dating conception by means of a basal body temperature chart with serum testing for human chorionic gonadotropin (hCG) confirmation is also highly accurate. Another clinical milestone is quickening (maternal perception of the first episode of fetal movement), but this is known to vary with maternal parity and placental location. In general, quickening occurs between 18 and 20 weeks of gestation; it may occur earlier, and this may be related to placental location. When the placenta is located on the anterior uterine wall, quickening occurs at a mean gestational age of 19 weeks in primigravidas and 17.5 weeks in multiparas. When the placenta is located on the posterior uterine wall, quickening occurs at a mean gestational age of 18 weeks in primigravidas and 16.1 weeks in multiparas (Gillieson et al, 1984). In order

to determine the EDC based on quickening, add 22 weeks for primiparas and 24 weeks for multiparas to the date of quickening. The ability to auscultate fetal heart tones using an unamplified stethoscope occurs at 20 weeks' gestation; this tends to correlate with the size of the uterus being enlarged to the level of the umbilicus. Beyond 20 weeks, the height of the fundus in centimeters above the symphysis pubis roughly correlates with gestational age. This commonly accepted measurement is termed McDonald's rule and is, in fact, a modification of the rule. McDonald's rule states that the height of the fundus in centimeters should be multiplied by a factor of 8/7 to give the gestational age in weeks.*

These clinical milestones, although useful, are not very accurate. In order to be 90 percent certain that a pregnancy has lasted 38 weeks or more, one needs to be sure that there have been 42 weeks of amenorrhea, unamplified fetal heart tones for 21 weeks, and quickening for 25 weeks (Hertz et al, 1978). A more accurate method for confirming or establishing gestational age is diagnostic ultrasound. Many studies have confirmed that the accuracy of ultrasound for dating is most precise in the early part of pregnancy. In the first trimester, crown-rump lengths (in millimeters) are within ± 4 days of the EDC; from 16 weeks to 26 weeks, measurement of the fetal biparietal diameter (in centimeters) and fetal femur length (in millimeters) is accurate to within ± 1 week of the EDC. After this time, the accuracy of ultrasound measurements decreases and predicts the EDC to within only ± 2 to 3 weeks. This must be taken into consideration when a patient registers late for prenatal care and an ultrasound examination is obtained to determine gestational age, or when the initial ultrasound examination is obtained late in pregnancy for patients who started early prenatal care.

## Management

There is no consensus about the correct management of prolonged pregnancy. Management plans reported in the literature ei-

---

* However, the modified method is clinically accepted and used.

ther support routine induction at 42 weeks' gestation (Dyson et al, 1987; Witter and Weitz, 1987) or find no benefit over expectant management with antepartum testing until labor ensues or fetal indications for delivery develop (Augensen et al, 1987; Cardozo et al, 1986). It is important to state that any pregnancy with a specific complication that, in itself, carries an increased risk for the fetus (e.g., insulin-dependent diabetes, Rh or other isoimmunization, preeclampsia, chronic hypertension) should not be allowed to progress beyond 40 weeks' gestation. Such pregnancies have a higher incidence of poor outcome (Eden et al, 1982).

The management for prolonged pregnancy is classified for two groups of patients: those with a *favorable cervix* for induction and those with an *unfavorable cervix*. Because of the increased morbidity and mortality rates that can accompany complications of prolonged pregnancy (placental insufficiency, oligohydramnios, meconium, fetal growth abnormalities), labor induction, if the cervix is favorable (Bishop score of 5 to 8) (Friedman and Niswander, 1966), is the best choice. Even when fetal assessment is normal, it is safer to deliver the infant rather than incur the increased risk should placental dysfunction develop. This approach pertains only to the well-established diagnosis of prolonged pregnancy. If the gestational age is questionably prolonged* (> 42 weeks) but the cervix is inducible, pulmonary maturity must be established by amniocentesis prior to initiating induction of labor.

Those patients who do not have a favorable cervix should be entered into a fetal surveillance testing protocol. Current protocol varies depending on the institution, but there seems to be some uniformity in that there is assessment of the fetus (nonstress test, biophysical profile) as well as its environment (amniotic fluid volume) (Bochner et al, 1988; Guidetti et al, 1989; Johnson et al, 1986; Silver et al, 1987).

In view of the risks of fetal growth abnormalities and oligohydramnios, ultrasound evaluation of the fetus provides more direct information about these risks than does biochemical monitoring (i.e., serum estriol); thus, it is not necessary to include a biochemical

assessment. A new diagnostic modality (umbilical Doppler velocimetry), which is believed to reflect placental vascular resistance, also has not been of any benefit in fetal assessment of this condition (Brar et al, 1989; Farmakides et al, 1988; Guidetti et al, 1987).

Some protocols follow a nonreactive nonstress test by performance of a contraction stress test. However, this method does not offer as much information as the ultrasound examination. Ultrasound evaluation allows one to gain more information: Fetal activity, which is governed by levels of oxygenation, can be directly assessed; amniotic fluid volume can be evaluated, with diminished or absent fluid levels being associated with an increased risk of umbilical cord complications (Moya et al, 1985; Phelan et al, 1985); and lastly, one might identify a congenital anomaly that could alter the obstetric management (Thornton et al, 1982). A clinical evaluation of different protocols for management of prolonged pregnancy (Eden et al, 1982) demonstrated that the best outcome was achieved when both antepartum fetal heart rate testing (AFHRT) and ultrasonic evaluation (biophysical profile) were used.

Observations regarding the nonstress test warrant mention at this time. Although the nonstress test may be reactive, if there are variable decelerations present on the tracing, the test should not be considered normal (Myasaki and Myasaki, 1981; Phelan et al, 1982; Phelan and Lewis, 1981). Such findings have been associated with umbilical cord complications (e.g., cord compression associated with oligohydramnios, occult prolapse, and entanglement) in 50 to 95 percent of cases (O'Leary et al, 1980; Phelan and Lewis, 1981). Umbilical cord compression (reflected as variable decelerations on AFHRT) has been associated with antepartum deaths within 1 week after the test. In our management protocol for the postdate pregnancy, we use the presence of variable declerations or diminished amniotic fluid as an indication for delivery (Fig. 23–5). Leveno and coworkers (1984) have described the importance of oligohydramnios and cord compression as a cause of fetal distress in prolonged pregnancy.

Regardless of which testing protocol is employed, it is important to realize that oligohydramnios can develop within 24 hours of a normal evaluation (Clement et al, 1987);

---

* A pregnancy is questionably prolonged when the EDC was calculated by uncertain clinical milestones or by an initial third trimester (≥ 28 weeks) ultrasound.

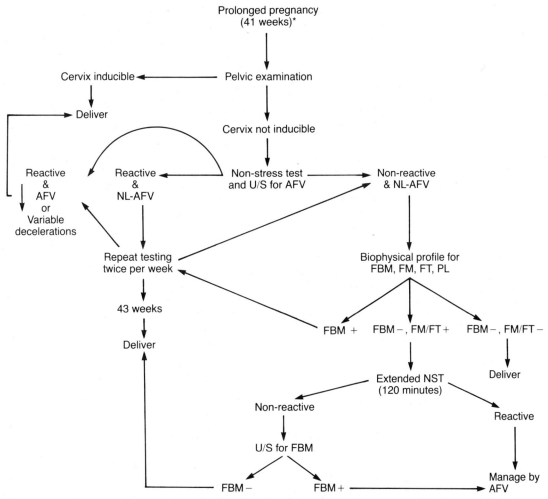

**Figure 23–5.** Protocol of antepartum fetal evaluation for prolonged pregnancy. Testing is initiated at 41 weeks. NST = non-stress test, AFV = amniotic fluid volume, FBM = fetal breathing movement, FM = fetal movement, FT = fetal tone, NL = normal, + = present / normal, − = absent / abnormal

thus, particular attention should be paid to any changes in the amniotic fluid status. There are differences of opinion in the literature regarding what constitutes an abnormal amount of amniotic fluid by ultrasound measurement (Manning et al, 1982; Vintzileos et al, 1983). Clinical protocols in prolonged pregnancies have found that amniotic fluid pockets less than 3 cm in vertical dimension have been associated with an increased incidence of fetal distress and necessitate cesarean section for delivery (Bochner et al, 1987). When one evaluates the amniotic fluid volume by ultrasound examination, one should measure the vertical depth of the fluid pockets that do not contain any segment of umbilical cord (cord-free vertical pocket). Although we consider an umbilical

cord–free vertical pocket measurement of greater than 2 cm as normal, delivery still may be indicated. If there is only one adequate fluid pocket and, overall, the fluid volume is diminished, then delivery is prudent. Also, if the twice-weekly testing and amniotic fluid assessment show that the fluid pocket dimensions are decreasing dramatically, then delivery also is prudent. In this setting, oligohydramnios (and a cord accident) could occur prior to a repeat assessment of the fluid status.

Most protocols recommend that testing be initiated at 42 weeks. Because we are aware that some cases of placental insufficiency exist prior to this time (see Fig. 23–3) and in order to obtain baseline information, we initiate our testing at 41 weeks' gestation (see

Fig. 23–5); this approach is supported by the observations of others (Bochner et al, 1988; Guidetti et al, 1989). Abnormalities of the biophysical profile (see Fig 23–5) (Vintzileos et al, 1987; 1983) or evidence of poor fetal growth are also indications for delivery. We also use a gestational age of 43 weeks as a limit, and we induce labor at this point. Although the presence of meconium in the amniotic fluid carries an increased risk for the infant, studies show that use of amniocentesis to detect meconium has not been helpful (Green and Paul, 1978; Knox et al, 1979). In such situations, when the nonstress test has been normal, intervention based on the finding of meconium did not improve the outcome.

The intrapartum management of prolonged pregnancy should not differ from that for any other complicated pregnancy. Internal monitoring of the fetal heart rate should be achieved at the earliest possible time. A normal fetal heart rate provides assurance that the infant is not hypoxic. Because the membranes need to be ruptured for this monitoring technique, one can also evaluate the fluid for meconium. The presence of meconium should serve as a reason for closer surveillance of the fetal heart rate tracing, because there may be an increased tendency for these infants to be acidotic if thick meconium is found (Miller and Read, 1981). Because in utero meconium aspiration has been reported (Manning et al, 1978, Paul et al, 1986), the clinician should be aware of the triad of findings, which includes (1) elevated baseline fetal heart rate, (2) decreased variability, and (3) meconium-stained amniotic fluid, that have been reported for fetuses at risk for this complication. In cases in which a patient is undergoing oxytocin induction or there is evidence of abnormal fetal heart rate patterns, intrauterine pressures should also be monitored by an intrauterine pressure catheter. This procedure ensures that uterine stimulation is adequate (not too excessive or insufficient) and allows better classification of the fetal heart rate patterns. Fetal scalp blood sampling to assess the fetal acid-base status is performed when there are abnormal findings in the fetal heart rate tracing. This technique allows one to detect fetuses that may be acidotic and may require immediate delivery, as compared with those with an abnormal fetal heart rate pattern but without acidosis. In fetuses with a normal fetal heart rate and no acidosis, labor may continue with vigilant monitoring. If meconium is present, the fetal oropharynx and nasopharynx should be suctioned with a DeLee suction as the head is delivered, prior to the delivery of the chest. In view of the recommendation of universal precautions and OSHA standards as of March, 1992, to avoid human immunodeficiency virus (HIV) infection, the operator should not use his or her mouth when using the DeLee suction trap. Instead, the suction trap should be connected to a wall suction device at a low setting. Prolonged pregnancy in itself is not an indication for cesarean delivery; this should be performed only when there are appropriate obstetric indications for doing so (see Chapter 19).

## Emotional Aspects

The mother and her family may become very anxious when pregnancy continues past the expected date of confinement. This date is anticipated with great excitement, and when it passes without delivery of the baby, everyone becomes frustrated. Also, for mothers who are physically uncomfortable, extension of the pregnancy can seem unbearable.

These women and their families need emotional support and recommendations to try to make them more comfortable. These suggestions could include placing a pillow under her abdomen while resting or sleeping to decrease the pull on her ligaments; raising the head of her bed to aid in breathing and to decrease indigestion; placing a heating pad or hot water bottle on her abdomen while she is awake to soothe sore ligaments; elevating her legs to increase circulation; and eating small, frequent meals to aid digestion. If she is physically comfortable, she should be better able to tolerate waiting for delivery.

Maternal anxiety or physical discomfort may not be recognized as a medical indication for delivery. However, even though the patient's cervix may not be suitable for induction of labor, there may be some situations in which the physician may decide that induction is the best course of action. After a thorough discussion with the couple about the risks and benefits involved, one can consider labor induction with the use of prostaglandin for cervical ripening. Its use has been reported to improve the success rate of labor induction in prolonged pregnancies (Rayburn et al, 1988).

The family should be given as much information as possible regarding the timing of delivery, because they will probably be anxious about the fetus not being delivered. A full explanation of the tests to be performed and the circumstances that necessitate delivery is helpful. The mother should also be educated about fetal movements; she can be instructed to count fetal movements for 1 hour, once or twice a day. If there are less than three movements in an hour, she should be instructed to come to the hospital (Rayburn, 1982).

Reassurance during this extended waiting period is very important to the mother and her family. This reassurance should include information that the baby is well (this can be given during testing) and that she *will* eventually deliver.

## Overview

Prolonged pregnancy presents a risk to the fetus when there is associated placental insufficiency, oligohydramnios, meconium-stained amniotic fluid, or macrosomia. These problems can lead to fetal growth retardation, umbilical cord compression, meconium aspiration, or birth trauma. These complications can increase morbidity and mortality rates for the fetus and neonate depending on the severity of the complication. The increased morbidity and mortality rates associated with this condition can be avoided by (1) paying attention to clinical history and clues that may identify patients with prolonged pregnancy, (2) inducing labor in prolonged pregnancies when the cervix is favorable, (3) using an antepartum fetal testing protocol to assess the fetus in cases of prolonged pregnancy with an unfavorable cervix, (4) delivering the patient when the antepartum fetal testing is abnormal, and (5) admitting the patient to the hospital at the earliest sign of spontaneous labor.

## References

Ahn MO, Phelan JP: Epidemiologic aspects of the postdate pregnancy. Clin Obstet Gynecol 32(2):228, 1989.

Augensen K, Bergsjo P, Eikeland T, et al: Randomised comparison of early versus late induction of labour in post-term pregnancy. Brit Med J 294:1192, 1987.

Bochner C, Medearis A, Davis J, et al: Antepartum predictors of fetal distress in postterm pregnancy. Am J Obstet Gynecol 157:353, 1987.

Bochner C, Williams J, Castro L, et al: The efficacy of starting postterm antenatal testing at 41 weeks as compared with 42 weeks of gestational age. Am J Obstet Gynecol 159:550, 1988.

Boyce A, Mayaux MJ, Schwarts D: Classical and "true" gestational postmaturity. Am J Obstet Gynecol 125:911, 1976.

Boyd M, Usher R, McLean F, et al: Obstetric consequences of postmaturity. Am J Obstet Gynecol 158:334, 1988.

Brar H, Horenstein J, Medearis A, et al: Cerebral, umbilical, and uterine resistance using Doppler velocimetry in postterm pregnancy. J Ultrasound Med 8:187, 1989.

Cardozo L, Fysh J, Pearce M: Prolonged pregnancy: the management debate. Brit Med J 293:1059, 1986.

Chervenak J, Divon M, Hirsch J, et al: Macrosomia in the postdate pregnancy: Is routine ultrasonagraphic screening indicated? Am J Obstet Gynecol 161:753, 1989.

Clement D, Schifrin B, Kates R: Acute oligohydramnios in postdate pregnancy. Am J Obstet Gynecol 157:884, 1987.

Clifford SH: Postmaturity. Adv Pediatr 9:13, 1957.

Clifford SH: Postmaturity—with placental dysfunction. J Pediatr 44:1, 1954.

Desmond MM, Lindley JE, Moore, J, et al: Meconium staining in newborn infants. J Pediatr 49:540, 1956.

Dyson D, Miller P, Armstrong M: Management of prolonged pregnancy: induction of labor versus antepartum fetal testing. Am J Obstet Gynecol 156:928, 1987.

Eden RD, Gergely RZ, Schifrin BS, et al: Comparison of antepartum testing schemes for the management of the postdate pregnancy. Am J Obstet Gynecol 144(6):683, 1982.

Farmakides G, Schulman H, Ducey J, et al: Uterine and umibilical artery Doppler velocimetry in postterm pregnancy. J Reprod Med 33:261, 1988.

Friedman EA, Niswander KR, Bayonet-Rivera NP, et al: Relation of prelabor evaluation to inducibility and the course of labor. Obstet Gynecol 28:495, 1966.

Gauthier RJ, Griego BD, Goebelsmann U: Estriol in pregnancy. VII. Unconjugated plasma estriol in prolonged gestation. Am J Obstet Gynecol 139:382, 1981.

Gillieson M, Dunlap H, Nair R, et al: Placental site, parity and date of quickening. Obstet Gynecol 64:44, 1984.

Green JN, Paul RH: The value of amniocentesis in prolonged pregnancy. Obstet Gynecol 51:293, 1978.

Guidetti D, Divon M, Langer O: Postdate fetal surveillance: is 41 weeks too early? Am J Obstet Gynecol 161:91, 1989.

Guidetti D, Divon M, Cavalieri R, et al: Fetal umbilical artery flow velocimetry in postdate pregnancies. Am J Obstet Gynecol 157:1521, 1987.

Hertz RH, Sokol RJ, Knoke JD, et al: Clinical estimation of gestational age: rules for avoiding preterm delivery. Am J Obstet Gynecol 131:395, 1978.

Johnson J, Harman C, Lange I, et al: Biophysical profile scoring the management of the postterm pregnancy: an analysis of 307 patients. Am J Obstet Gynecol 154:269, 1986.

Knox GE, Huddleston JF, Flowers CE: Management of prolonged pregnancy: results of a prospective randomized trial. Am J Obstet Gynecol 134:376, 1979.

Lagrew D, Freeman R: Management of postdate pregnancy. Am J Obstet Gynecol 154:8, 1986.

Leveno K: Amniotic fluid volume in prolonged pregnancy. Semin Perinatol 10:154, 1986.

Leveno KJ, Quirk JG, Cunningham FG, et al: Prolonged pregnancy. I. Observations concerning the causes of fetal distress. Am J Obstet Gynecol 150:465, 1984.

Manning FA, Schreiber J, Turkel SB: Fatal meconium aspiration "in utero": a case report. Am J Obstet Gynecol 132:111, 1978.

Manning FA, Morrison I, Lange IR, et al: Antepartum determination of fetal health: composite biophysical profile scoring. Clin Perinatol 9:285, 1982.

Miller FC, Read JA: Intrapaturm assessment of the postdate fetus. Am J Obstet Gynecol 141:516, 1981.

Miller PW, Coen RW, Benirschke K: Dating the time interval from meconium passage to birth. Obstet Gynecol 66:459, 1985.

Mittendorf R, Williams MA, Berkey CS, et al: The length of uncomplicated human gestation. Obstet Gynecol 75:929, 1990.

Moya F, Grannum P, Pinto K, et al: Ultrasound assessment of the postmature pregnancy. Obstet Gynecol 65:319, 1985.

O'Leary JA, Andrinopoulous GC, Giordano PC: Variable decelerations and the nonstress test: an indication of cord compression. Am J Obstet Gynecol 137:704, 1980.

Paul RH, Yonekura ML, Cantrell CJ, et al: Fetal injury prior to labor: does it happen? Am J Obstet Gynecol 154:1187, 1986.

Phelan JP, Lewis PE: Fetal heart rate decelerations during a nonstress test. Obstet Gynecol 57:288, 1981.

Phelan JP, Cromartie AD, Smith CV: The nonstress test: the false negative test. Am J Obstet Gynecol 142:293, 1982.

Phelan JP, Platt LD, Sze-Ya Y, et al: The role of ultrasound assessment of amniotic fluid volume in the management of the postdate pregnancy. Am J Obstet Gynecol 151:304, 1985.

Rayburn WF: Antepartum fetal assessment. Monitoring fetal activity. Clin Perinatol 9:231, 1982.

Rayburn W, Gosen R, Ramadei C, et al: Outpatient cervical ripening with prostaglandin $E_2$ gel in uncomplicated postdate pregnancies. Am J Obstet Gynecol 158:1417, 1988.

Silver R, Dooley S, Tamura R, et al: Umbilical cord size and amniotic fluid volume in prolonged pregnancy. Am J Obstet Gynecol 157:716, 1987.

Thornton YS, Yeh SY, Petrie RH: Antepartum fetal heart rate testing and the post-term gestation. J Perinat Med 10:196, 1982.

Usher R, Boyd M, McLean F, et al: Assessment of fetal risk in postdate pregnancies. Am J Obstet Gynecol 158:259, 1988.

Vintzileos AM, Campbell WA, Ingardia CJ, et al: The fetal biophysical profile and its predictive value. Obstet Gynecol 62:271, 1983.

Vintzileos AM, Campbell WA, Nochimson DJ, et al: The use and misuse of the fetal biophysical profile. Am J Obstet Gynecol 156:527, 1987a.

Vintzileos A, Gaffney S, Salinger L, et al: The relationship between fetal biophysical profile and cord pH in patients undergoing cesarean section before the onset of labor. Obstet Gynecol 70:196, 1987b.

Vorherr H: Placental insufficiency in relation to postterm pregnancy and fetal postmaturity. Evaluation of fetoplacental function; management of the postterm gravida. Am J Obstet Gynecol 123(1):67, 1975.

Witter F, Weitz C: A randomized trial of induction at 42 weeks' gestation versus expectant management for postdates pregnancies. Am J Perinatol 4:206, 1987.

# CHAPTER 24

# Twins and Other Multiple Gestations

Robert A. Knuppel and Joan Drukker

Twinning occurs in approximately 1 of every 80 pregnancies, constituting an important biologic event. Although it has long been known that two types of twins exist, identical (monozygotic) and fraternal (dizygotic), it was Sir Francis Galton (Charles Darwin's first cousin), who first proposed using twins as a model for the understanding of disease and, by doing so, made twin research an active field. Other multiple gestations are not as frequent; spontaneous triplets occur in 1 of 8000 births, quadruplets in 1 of 700,000 (Sheppard, 1992), and quintuplets in 1 of 65,610,000 (Crane, 1984).

## Predisposing Factors

### DIZYGOTIC TWINS

Dizygotic twins make up two thirds of all the twins born in the United States. This type of twinning involves the independent release and subsequent fertilization of two ova. Dizygotic twins, genetically, are as similar as any other siblings, except that they are the same age and are *in utero* at the same time. The sex of the fetuses can be the same or different. They might have different fathers if coitus occurs with two different men within a relatively short period.

### Familial Inheritance

Dizygotic twinning has a hereditary basis; that is, there is a familial tendency toward multiple ovulation. This phenomenon may be partly due to increased levels of pituitary gonadotropins, which predispose a woman to double ovulations. If such traits are partly inherited (carried and transmitted by both females and males), they are expressed only in women, because they act through the ovaries exclusively. Women who have given birth to spontaneous dizygotic twins probably have a twofold increased likelihood, as compared with the general population, of having dizygotic twins in each succeeding pregnancy, although the precise nature of the inheritance remains to be established.

### Race

There is a high incidence among blacks in Nigeria, where 1 of every 25 births involves twins. At the other extreme, there is a very low incidence among Asians; in Japan, for example, twinning occurs in 1 of every 150 births.

### Age and Parity

For reasons that are poorly understood, the twinning rate correlates with maternal age, steadily rising from 20 and reaching a maximum between ages 35 and 39, after which the rate falls abruptly (Fig. 24–1). It has been postulated that this increase may be partly due to increasing levels of gonadotropins and a higher incidence of double ovulation. There is also a high correlation between increased number of pregnancies and multiple births (Fig. 24–2).

**433**

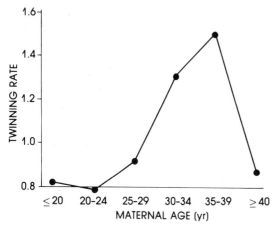

**Figure 24–1.** Rate of twinning in relation to maternal age, expressed as the ratio of twin births to all births per thousand for comparable ages (at MacDonald House). (From Hendricks CH: Twinning in relation to birth rate, mortality and congenital anomalies. Obstet Gynecol 27:48, 1966. Reprinted with permission from The American College of Obstetricians and Gynecologists.)

## Medications

**Clomiphene Citrate.** The induction of ovulation with clomiphene citrate (Clomid) has been associated with a high incidence of multiple gestation (mostly twins), and national statistics show an 8 percent rate of multiple births among women who have taken this drug. Kistner (1968) reports a rate of 6 percent, and Hack and coworkers (1972) report a rate of 8.4 percent. Speroff and col-

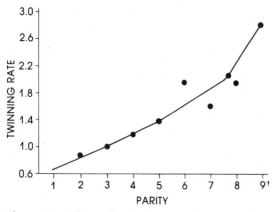

**Figure 24–2.** Rate of twinning at various parities, expressed as a fraction of the rate in each parity group. (From Hendricks CH: Twinning in relation to birth rate, mortality and congenital anomalies. Obstet Gynecol 27:48, 1966. Reprinted with permission from The American College of Obstetricians and Gynecologists.)

leagues (1981) state that in recent years, with a standardization of therapy and doses of about 50 mg/day or less, fewer cases of ovarian hyperstimulation syndrome have been reported, and the incidence of twins has approached that of the normal population.

**Gonadotropins.** Human menopausal gonadotropin, or hMG (Pergonal: one vial contains 75 U of follicle-stimulating hormone and 75 U of luteinizing hormone), in combination with human chorionic gonadotropins, or hCG (one vial contains 10,000 U of luteinizing hormone), is being used at the present time for induction of ovulation in patients with hypothalamic hypogonadotropic hypogonadism (primary or secondary amenorrhea and anovulation), and in patients with oligomenorrhea or amenorrhea and anovulation secondary to hypothalamic pituitary dysfunction (e.g., polycystic ovarian syndrome). Gonadotropins also are used to induce hyperstimulation in preparation for *in vitro* fertilization, gamete intrafallopian transfer, and zygote intrafallopian transfer.

The most common complication is multiple pregnancy in the range of 20 to 40 percent, owing to the fact that there is a very narrow margin between dose-related pregnancy rates and ovarian hyperstimulation with multiple gestation (Hollenbach and Hickok, 1990). This incidence may be decreased by several factors, such as (1) proper selection of patients; (2) choice of suitable treatment; and (3) careful monitoring of follicular growth, using serial ultrasound and daily estradiol determinations.

**Oral Contraceptives.** It has been speculated that after cessation of oral contraceptive therapy, pituitary gonadotropin release is increased, possibly leading to an increase in twin conception (Benirschke and Kim, 1973).

## Miscellaneous Factors

The twinning pregnancy rate appears to be greater when a woman conceives during the first 3 months after marriage, which may be related to coital frequency.

In some areas of northern Finland, there is a strong seasonal frequency for multiple gestation (peak twin conception is in July); this frequency may be explained by the continuous exposure to light during the summer months, which might result in hypothalamic pituitary stimulation and, consequently, multiple ovulation.

## MONOZYGOTIC TWINS

One third of all twins born in the United States are monozygotic. These twins are derived from a single fertilized ovum that duplicates at any of the preimplantation stages, before the embryo has been formed. There is no valid hypothesis that explains monozygotic twinning; this form of twinning should probably be considered a teratogenic phenomenon. The frequency is constant around the world, being roughly 1 in 250 pregnancies, and it is not influenced by race, maternal age, drugs, or any other known factors. The concept that monozygotic twins occur with greater frequency with advancing maternal age, that malformations often occur, that conjoined twins develop, and that monozygotic twins can be induced by teratogens have led to the hypothesis that monozygotic twins may result from a teratologic event.

## DIZYGOTIC TWINS

Dizygotic twins are the result of fertilization of more than one egg by separate spermatozoa. Two thirds of all twins are dizygotic and genetically, are as similar as any two siblings (Hollenbach and Hickok, 1990). Dizygotic twins are thought to be the result of multiple ovulations, which may be related to "increased levels of follicle-stimulating hormone or luteinizing hormone surges." Their placentas are usually diamniotic-dichorionic and can be fused or separate. The sex of the fetuses can be the same or different.

---

# Placentation
(Figs. 24–3 and 24–4)

## MONOZYGOTIC TWINS

There are basically two types of placentas in monozygotic twins. The first type is monochorionic, with a single placental disk that might or might not have developed two separate amnions. Monochorionic-monoamniotic and monochorionic-diamniotic twin placen-

tas exist only in monozygotic twins; therefore, the twins are the same sex (Fig. 24–5). The diagnosis can be made readily by examination of the placenta of twins who are born with the same sex.

The second type of placenta in monozygotic twins is dichorionic-diamniotic. About 20 to 30 percent of all monozygotic twins have dichorionic-diamniotic placentas with infants of the same sex, and therefore, the zygosity in such a circumstance should be assessed genotypically. This type of placenta can be either fused or separated. Dichorionic-diamniotic placentation is accomplished when splitting of the inner cell mass from the blastocyst occurs before cells appear that eventually will make up the chorion. This phenomenon occurs very early after fertilization, perhaps in the first 60 hours. In the other extreme, if separation occurs very late after fertilization, conjoined twins will develop as a last possible twinning phenomenon (Fig. 24–6).

Vascular anastomoses between the two fetal circulations in monochorionic placentas are common and are of two types: artery-to-artery and arteriovenous. Artery-to-artery anastomoses are rare, but when they occur, they represent an acute emergency during the delivery because of shifting of blood from one twin to the other. More common are the arteriovenous shunts between the two fetal circulations, which are believed to be the basis of what is known as the twin-to-twin transfusion syndrome. The placental vascular anastomosis is more often an artery-to-artery anastomosis than a vein-to-vein communication, and sometimes, both types are present and multiple. An interfetal anastomosis of large caliber may lead to significant shifts of blood between fetuses. The most important anastomosis, the arteriovenous shunt, is also the most difficult to diagnose. It is not a direct communication but occurs when one cotyledon is fed by an artery from one twin and is drained by a vein into the other twin. Arteriovenous shunts may occur singly or in combination with other arteriovenous shunts and may be in opposing directions.

## DIZYGOTIC TWINS

The number and size of follicles can now be determined readily by serial sonographic examination of the ovaries during the proliferative phase of the menstrual cycle. There-

## Monochorionic Twin Placentation

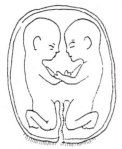

Monoamnionic, Monochorionic
(conjoined twins)

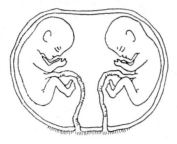

Monoamnionic, Monochorionic

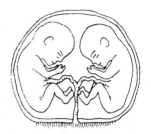

Monoamnionic, Monochorionic
(forked cord)

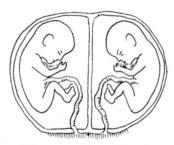

Diamnionic, Monochorionic

## Dichorionic Twin Placentation

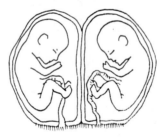

Diamnionic, Dichorionic (fused)

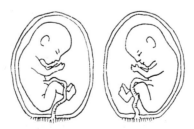

Diamnionic, Dichorionic (separated)

**Figure 24–3.** Monochorionic and dichorionic twin placentation.

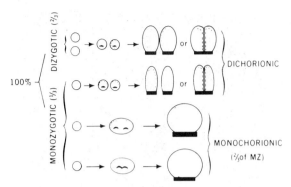

**Figure 24–4.** Incidence and placental development of MZ and DZ twins. (From Iffy L, Kaminetzky H: Principles and Practice of Obstetrics in Perinatology, Vol 2. © 1981, John Wiley & Sons, Inc. Reprinted by permission of John Wiley & Sons, Inc.)

fore, zygosity of twins can be determined at or before the time of ovulation. All dizygotic twins are derived from two follicles containing two separate ova and fertilized by two separate spermatozoa.

All dizygotic twins have dichorionic-diamniotic placentas. They might appear as entirely separated organs, or they may be fused if implantation occurred side-by-side. If the infants differ in sex and if pathologic examination of the divided membrane shows four layers (amnion/chorion/chorion/amnion), the diagnosis of zygosity readily is established. This situation accounts for about 35 percent of all twins born in the United States (see Fig. 24–3). Placen-

tal relationships of triplets, quadruplets, and so on follow the same principles and, in some monochorionic and dichorionic placentations, may coexist. With an increased number of placentas, there are an increased number of placental anomalies, including marginal and velamentous cord insertions and single umbilical arteries (D'Alton et al, 1990).

## DETERMINATION OF ZYGOSITY

In the United States, about 80 percent of twins are dichorionic and about 20 percent are monochorionic. Through pathologic examination of the placenta, 20 percent of the monozygotic twins who have monochorionic placentas (same sex) are detected. Another 30 percent are detected who have dichorionic placentas, fused or separated, and who are of different sexes. These twins will be diagnosed as dizygotic. In the remaining 45 percent of the cases, the zygosity must be established genotypically through blood grouping, enzymatic determinations, and human leucocyte antigen typing.

## TWIN-TO-TWIN TRANSFUSION SYNDROME

There are no vascular connections in dichorionic placentas. On the other hand, monochorionic placentas may have a vascu-

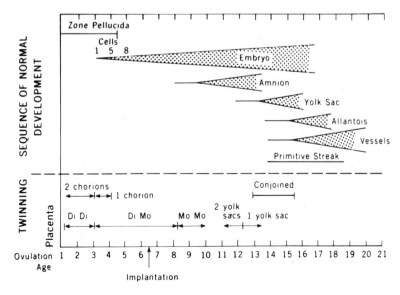

**Figure 24–5.** Hypothetical scheme of timing of monozygotic placental development. (From Benirschke K, Kim CK: Multiple pregnancy. N Engl J Med 288:1276, 1973. Reprinted by permission of the New England Journal of Medicine.)

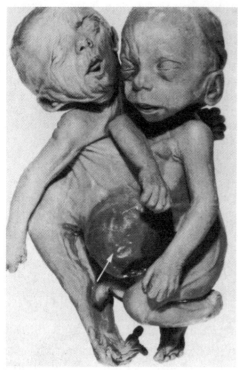

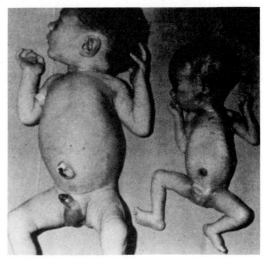

**Figure 24–8.** Discordant twins caused by twin transfusion syndrome. (From Lubchenco LO: The High Risk Infant. Philadelphia, WB Saunders Co, 1976.)

**Figure 24–6.** Thoraco-omphalopagus twins with omphalocele (*arrow*)—postmortem appearance. (From Moore KL: The Developing Human: Clinically Oriented Embryology, 3rd ed. Philadelphia, WB Saunders Co, 1982.)

as outlined in Table 24–1. Twin transfusion syndrome, if diagnosed before 32 weeks of gestation, has a low survival rate of approximately 17 percent.

lar connection between the two fetal circulations (Fig. 24–7). This can be an artery-to-artery connection or, more commonly, an arteriovenous anastomosis within the placental bed. The latter can result in the twin-to-twin transfusion syndrome (Fig. 24–8), which can cause discordance in twins,

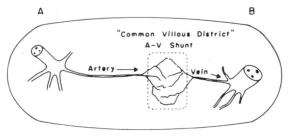

**Figure 24–7.** Vascular arrangement of the transfusion syndrome. (From Benirschke K, Kim CK: N Engl J Med 288:1276, 1973. Reprinted by permission of the New England Journal of Medicine.)

**Table 24–1**
CHARACTERISTICS OF DISCORDANT TWINS

| Twin Recipient | Twin Donor |
| --- | --- |
| Twin is usually larger; up to 1000-g disparity | Twin is usually smaller |
| Polycythemia with hemoconcentration thrombosis and disseminated intravascular coagulation (DIC) in the newborn | Anemia that can be rather severe |
| | Hypoglycemia |
| | Cardiac atrophy |
| | Decreased muscle mass |
| | Oligohydramnios |
| | Small pale placenta |
| Jaundice secondary to hemolysis, occasionally causing kernicterus | Retarded growth and retarded mental development postnatally |
| Cardiac hypertrophy | ***Treatment*** |
| Increased muscular mass | Blood transfusion |
| Polyhydramnios secondary to increased glomerular size and polyuria | |
| Large congested placenta | |
| ***Treatment*** | |
| Exchange transfusion with phlebotomy | |

## PERINATAL MORBIDITY AND MORTALITY

Several factors are thought to be of relevance for increased perinatal mortality and morbidity in cases of multiple gestation as compared with singleton pregnancies. Naeye and coworkers (1978) found a perinatal mortality of 13.9 percent for twins as compared with 3.3 percent for singletons. In most cases, the reason for this excess in perinatal mortality is prematurity secondary to preterm labor, with the second most important factor being intrauterine growth retardation (IUGR), especially after 30 weeks' gestation (Figs. 24–9 and 24–10).

Hypertension, anemia, and birth trauma also are mentioned as possible factors for increased perinatal morbidity and mortality in twin gestations. It has been reported that 70 percent of the perinatal mortalities occur before the 30th week of gestation, which is also the period of greatest neonatal morbidity. As the number of fetuses *in utero* increases, both the mean birth weight and the duration of pregnancy decrease.

The multiple pregnancy mortality rate, which rises progressively as the number of fetuses increases, was demonstrated by Botting and associates (1987). The mortality rates were 6.3 percent, 16.4 percent, 20.0 percent, 21.4 percent, and 41.6 percent, respectively, among twins, triplets, quadruplets, quintuplets, and sextuplets.

Although prematurity of multiple fetal gestations has not decreased over the past 20 to 30 years, perinatal mortality has decreased, probably owing to improved neonatal care. The long-term morbidity of these infants has not been assessed. Seventy-five percent of triplets deliver prematurely, many before 32 weeks' gestation. The statistics on morbidity for four or more fetuses are too small to analyze; however, it can be surmised that they are only as good as triplet outcomes and probably worse (Alvarez and Berkowitz, 1990).

## Diagnosis

In cases of multiple gestation, as with any other condition in obstetrics that can cause complications or harm to the mother and her fetus, early diagnosis is paramount if a good outcome is to be achieved.

A study by Barter and associates (1965) revealed that up to 50 percent of twin pregnancies were undiagnosed at the time of labor. Farooqui and coworkers (1973) found that the diagnosis of twins was missed before labor in 58 percent of the cases; in about 30 percent of the cases, the diagnosis was made only after delivery of the first twin. Today, if patients have access to care and ultrasound imaging, the diagnosis should be 99 percent accurate.

### HISTORY

As mentioned earlier, there is a hereditary tendency to multiple ovulation. Therefore, a family history of twins should alert the physician to the possibility of multiple gestations.

Women who have been treated with fertility drugs (clomiphene citrate or gonadotropins) or who become pregnant after cessation of oral contraceptive therapy also should be screened for multiple gestation.

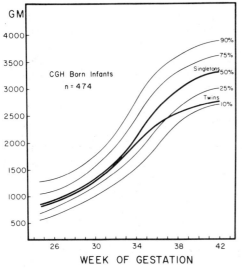

**Figure 24–9.** Intrauterine growth of twin pregnancies compared with singletons: Weight curve is parallel until approximately 35 weeks, at which time the rate of growth in twin pregnancies slows. (From Lubchenco LO: The High Risk Infant. Philadelphia, WB Saunders Co, 1976.)

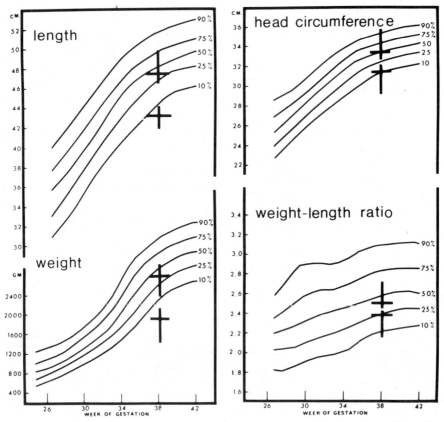

**Figure 24–10.** Discordant twins with intrauterine growth retardation: comparison of length and weight, head circumference, and weight-length ratio after 35 weeks' gestation. (From Lubchenco LO: The High Risk Infant. Philadelphia, WB Saunders Co, 1976.)

## CLINICAL EXAMINATION

If the fetus gestational age is considered accurate, the McDonald measurements of the abdomen may be helpful in diagnosing multiple gestation. The height of the uterus can be measured with a measuring tape from the symphysis pubis to the fundus. Between 22 and 34 weeks' gestation, the fundal height should equal gestational age in centimeters. Jarvis (1979) reported that in 66 of 94 sets of twins, the initial suspicion of multiple pregnancy arose from finding a uterus larger than would be expected at that gestation age. A discrepancy of 4 cm or more suggests multiple gestation (Fig. 24–11). Ultrasound should be used to confirm the diagnosis of multiple gestation. Ultrasound also can be used to rule out other causes of an enlarged uterus, such as polyhydramnios, dating errors, uterine leiomyomata, and ovarian tumors (D'Alton and Mercer, 1990). Palpation of multiple fetal parts through the Leopold maneuver, with the presence of more than two fetal poles, should alert the clinician to the possibility of multiple gestation.

The auscultation of more than one fetal heart sound, particularly with a difference of 10 beats/min, may be another important finding during the physical examination for twin gestation.

Anemia that may not respond to the usual treatment with iron and folic acid (multiple fetuses require extra iron and folic acid) and hypertension, especially in a multiparous patient, also should raise the suspicion of multiple gestation.

## ULTRASOUND EXAMINATION

Ultrasound is probably the most important technologic contribution to obstetrics, equal to what computed tomography (CT) scanning and magnetic resonance imaging (MRI) have contributed to radiology. At the

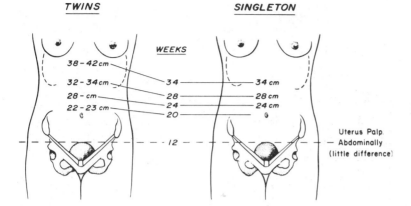

**Figure 24–11.** Uterine fundal height in twins versus singletons. (From Cetrulo CL, Ingardia CJ, Sbarra SJ: Management of multiple gestation. Clin Obstet Gynecol 23:536, 1980.)

present time, the most important reasons for increased perinatal morbidity and mortality are prematurity and congenital anomalies. Hawrylyshyn and coworkers (1982) found that 70 percent of the perinatal mortality in twin pregnancies occurred when delivery took place before the 30th week of gestation.

In 1973, routine screening with ultrasound of the entire pregnant population of Malmo, Sweden was instituted (Persson et al, 1979). The purpose of the study was to improve early diagnosis and, therefore, prevent preterm labor and allow early diagnosis of complications, such as hypertension, anemia, and IUGR in multiple gestation. Studied in the 17th week of gestation, 98 percent of the twins were diagnosed during the first sonographic examination, with no false-positive results. In contrast, before routine ultrasound was instituted, the mean gestational age at the time the diagnosis of twin gestation was made was 35 weeks. When sonographic examination was performed routinely in 1983, the mean gestational age at the time of diagnosis was reduced to 30 weeks; by 1987, it was down to 20 weeks. The diagnosis can be made as early as 6 to 8 weeks by identifying two separate sacs within the uterus (Fig. 24–12). Cardiac activity usually can be identified during the next 2 weeks with abdominal ultrasound. Identification of the sacs and cardiac activity can be detected earlier with vaginal ultrasound (D'Alton and Mercer, 1990). Between 8 and 13 weeks' gestation, separate sacs and two fetal poles with separate cardiac activity and fetal movements can be identified clearly (Figs. 24–13, 24–14 and 24–15).

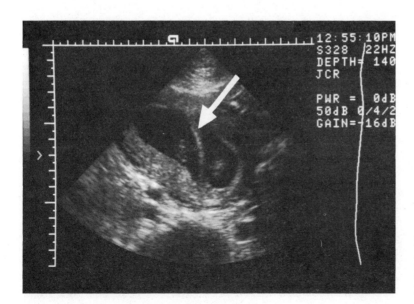

**Figure 24–12.** A longitudinal ultrasound through an 8-week twin pregnancy. The *arrow* demonstrates the membrane separating the twins. Fetal poles are noted in each echolucent sac. (Courtesy of Robert A. Knuppel.)

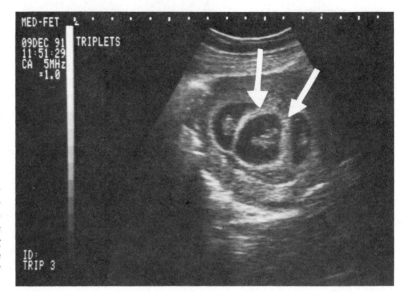

**Figure 24–13.** A longitudinal section through a 9-week pergonal-induced triplet pregnancy. Both *arrows* point to the thick separating membranes. Fetal parts are noted in each sac. (Courtesy of Robert A. Knuppel.)

From 16 weeks' gestation on, different fetal parts can readily be observed, and the measurement of biparietal diameter (BPD), femoral length, and abdominal circumference should be attempted serially to assess fetal growth (Figs. 24–16). In an effort to reduce maternal and fetal complications frequently seen in association with multiple gestation, a strong argument can be made for routine screening with ultrasound of all pregnant patients for early diagnosis of this condition. Misdiagnosis of twins by ultrasound can occur because of (1) refraction errors, (2) a bicornuate uterus with a decidual pseudosac within the contralateral horn, or (3) spontaneous abortion of the twin (D'Alton and Mercer, 1990). When structures examined by ultrasound are small, refraction may cause an apparent duplication of the image (Buttery and Davison, 1984). By altering the incident angles, the duplication will change or disappear (D'Alton and Mercer, 1990). A pseudosac may develop in the adjacent horn of a bicornuate uterus. This occurs because of the thickening of the decidua and glandular secretions into this uterine cavity, which are stimulated by ovarian and placental hormones. This pseudosac can be confused with an additional gestation (D'Alton and Mercer, 1990).

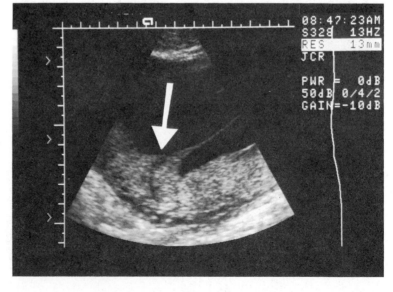

**Figure 24–14.** Transverse section through a twin pregnancy demonstrating 2 separate but adjacent posterior wall placentas. *Arrow* shows the echolucent line of demarcation. A thin membrane is also noted separating the sacs. (Courtesy of Robert A. Knuppel.)

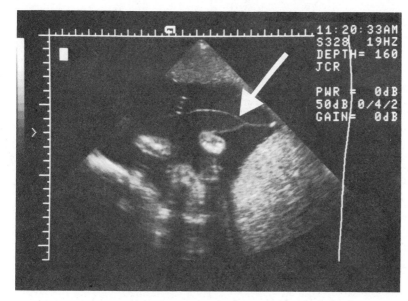

**Figure 24–15.** *Arrow* indicates the thin membrane separating second trimester triplet pregnancy. (Courtesy of Robert A. Knuppel.)

Early identification of pregnancy through the use of ultrasound has demonstrated pregnancy loss of not only singletons but also multiple gestations. Approximately 20 percent (Jones et al, 1990) to 50 percent (D'Alton and Mercer, 1990) are lost *in utero*. A spontaneous abortion of one member of a multiple gestation may be asymptomatic or may be associated with vaginal bleeding early in pregnancy (D'Alton and Mercer, 1990). The vanishing twin phenomenon has been described when one fetus completely disappears by the time of delivery (Benirschke, 1990). This phenomenon also can happen with more than two fetuses (Fig. 24–17). Larger fetuses that have developed bone ossification become progressively compressed, a phenomenon known as fetus papyraceus (Fig. 24–18). Occasionally, large fetus papyracei may cause dystocia, and some are masses of fetal-compressed bone seen in the placenta at delivery and, therefore, often are overlooked. Frequently, anomalies are present in the surviving twin (Benirschke, 1990).

The prognosis for a surviving twin is good. However, although rare, fetal death of one twin may stimulate premature labor or labor

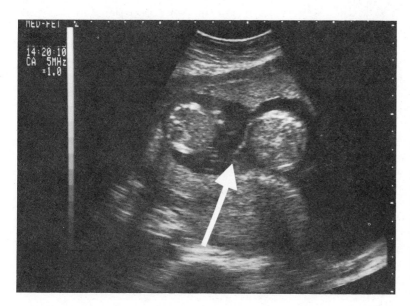

**Figure 24–16.** Transverse section through a 17-week twin pregnancy. The *arrow* demonstrates the separating membrane. Transverse sections of both fetal abdomens at approximately the same level are demonstrated. The growth of the twin to the right of the membrane is appropriate for 17.6 weeks; whereas the growth of the twin on the left is lagging and has a composite age of 15.4 weeks. (Courtesy of Robert A. Knuppel.)

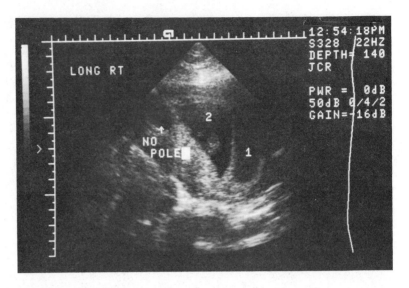

**Figure 24–17.** This demonstrates a longitudinal ultrasound through an 8-week multiple gestation. Three distinct sacs are noted. Sacs 1 and 2 have positive fetal cardiac activity. The third sac is empty and eventually would be reabsorbed; this was not detectable in the 2nd trimester. (Courtesy of Robert A. Knuppel.)

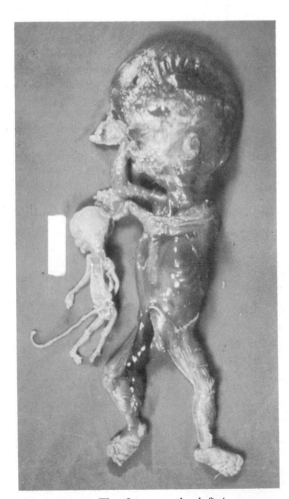

**Figure 24–18.** The fetus on the left is a papyraceous twin. (Courtesy of Trevor MacPherson, Magee-Womens Hospital, Pittsburgh, PA.)

may be obstructed by the macerated fetus (Dudley and D'Alton, 1986). Twin embolization syndrome can occur in monochorionic gestations in which vascular injuries occur in the surviving twin owing to thrombotic emboli or disseminated intravascular coagulation (DIC). However, the risk is minimal (Benirschke and Kim, 1973; Dudley and D'Alton, 1986; Enbom, 1985; Patten et al, 1989; Samuels, 1988; Winter et al, 1988). Since the risk for the surviving twin is small, conservative management, including continued assessment of maternal-fetal well-being and aggressive intervention when necessary, may be used until 37 weeks' gestation (Burke, 1990; Cattanach et al, 1990; D'Alton et al, 1984; Van Den Veyver et al, 1990).

Doppler flow studies should be used in cases of discordancy and IUGR (Fig. 24–19). However, the value of velocimetry data in cost–benefit analyses has yet to be realized. It may be that we are dealing with a different placental pathophysiology in many multiple gestations than we see in singleton cases of IUGR.

Antepartum surveillance for multiple gestations is critical because of increased complications in twin gestations (Table 24–2). The rate of undiagnosed twins before labor and delivery is approximately 20 to 40 percent (Jones et al, 1990). Early detection of twins is critical to prepare for premature labor and other complications as well as to prepare the parents for more than 1 newborn.

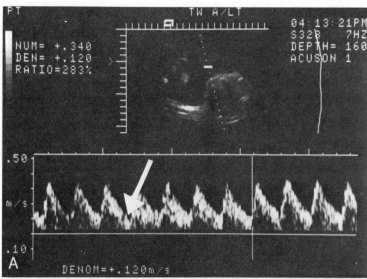

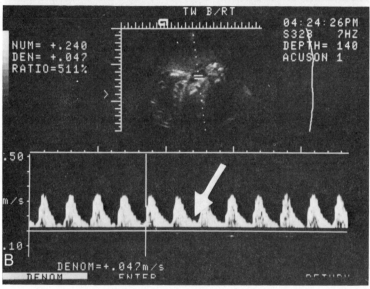

**Figure 24–19.** Doppler flow studies were performed on this third-trimester discordant twin pregnancy. Twin A birthweight was <10 percent, whereas twin B remained in the 32 percentile. *A,* the umbilical artery blood flow of twin A. The systolic/diastolic ratio was calculated, measuring 2.8, which is normal. The *arrow* demonstrates the normal amount of diastolic flow present. *B,* an umbilical artery waveform from the growth retarded twin. The systolic/diastolic ratio was increased to 5.1, which indicates increased resistance in the umbilical circulation. The *arrow* shows the decreased amount of diastolic flow as compared to the normal twin (*A*). (Courtesy of Robert A. Knuppel.)

Table 24–2

RISKS AND COMPLICATIONS
OF TWIN GESTATION

Anemia
Preeclampsia
Polyhydramnios
Fetal malformations
Intrauterine growth retardation
Vanishing twin
Premature rupture of membranes
Preterm delivery
Intrauterine fetal demise
Malpresentations, malpositions, and cord prolapse
Increased perinatal mortality and morbidity
Psychologic problems

From Jones JM, Sbarra AJ, Cetrulo CL: Antepartum Management of twin gestation. Clin Obstet Gynecol 33(1): March, 1990.

## BIOCHEMICAL TESTS

Indirect biochemical methods are based on the fact that total placental mass and fetal mass are greater in multiple gestations than in singleton pregnancies.

Estriol, hCG, and alpha$_1$-fetoprotein (AFP) levels were measured in an attempt to establish the normal range for twin gestation. The results in the literature are conflicting. AFP, hCG, and human placental lactogen (hPL) were reported in a number of studies to be higher in twin than in singleton pregnancies, with an accuracy rate of 80 to 95 percent (Garoff and Seppala, 1973).

However, levels of hPL in twin gestations were reported to be similar to those in singleton pregnancies (Garoff and Seppala, 1973). Persson and associates (1979) measured hPL levels in an entire population of pregnant women in Malmo, Sweden; 16 percent had levels high enough to indicate twin pregnancy, but this was not the case, suggesting that other measures, mainly ultrasound, should be used to make a definitive diagnosis.

## RADIOGRAPHIC EXAMINATION

Radiography should be used as a last resort for the exceptional situation in which the sonogram is doubtful, especially if more than two fetuses are suspected to be *in utero*. Another unusual circumstance in which radiographic examination might be used is for the diagnosis of presentation when the patient arrives in active labor. It must be emphasized, however, that in general, the availability of ultrasound equipment and skillful personnel on a 24-hour basis in the labor and delivery area should obviate the need to expose the fetus to unnecessary radiation.

# Antepartum Management

## DIET

Increased placental and fetal mass in multiple gestation dictate the need for increased caloric intake as well as increased intake of proteins, minerals (iron), vitamins, and folic acid. Dietary intake should be increased to at least 2400 calories/day, with additional milk intake. Maternal weight gain during a multiple pregnancy frequently ranges from 35 to 45 lbs.

## THE BED REST CONTROVERSY

There are few studies examining the management of multiple gestation, and bed rest remains a controversial issue. Nevertheless, the majority of the reports appear to support the view that it has a beneficial effect (Table 24–3).

Power (1973) stated that in England, over 88 years of bed rest have been expended on healthy mothers to prolong their twin pregnancies, although the efficacy of bed rest remained unproved.

O'Connor and colleagues (1979) reported on 101 twin pregnancies in which routine bed rest in the hospital was replaced by intensified antenatal care in special twin clinics. This group of patients clearly benefitted from the special care, as evidenced by the fact that there was no increase in the prematurity rate, IUGR rate and perinatal mortality. The possibility of psychologic benefit (placebo effect) to the women, who were managed carefully and evaluated frequently, was mentioned as one of the contributing factors.

The study by Persson and colleagues (1979) is probably the most widely quoted. Their approach was as follows: bed rest at home and discontinuance of work as soon as the diagnosis of multiple gestation is made, followed by bed rest in the hospital from 28 to

Table 24–3
TWIN PERINATAL MORTALITY AND THE EFFECTIVENESS OF BED REST

| Author | Place | Years | No. of Twins | | PND*/1000 Live Births | | Labor < 36 wk (%) | |
|--------|-------|-------|------|--------|-----|--------|-----|--------|
| | | | *Bed†* | *Active‡* | *Bed* | *Active* | *Bed* | *Active* |
| Barter et al | Washington, DC | 1954–64 | 25 | 225 | 80 | 217 | 35 | 25 |
| Robertson | Scotland | 1956–62 | 152 | 237 | 75 | 206 | ? | ? |
| Laursen | Denmark | 1958–70 | 79 | 107 | 32 | 85 | 13 | 45 |
| Misenhimer et al | Baltimore | 1964–75 | 70 | 161 | 7 | 55 | 57 | 48 |
| Jeffrey et al | Denver | 1968–73 | 41 | 31 | 61 | 229 | | |
| Jouppila et al | Finland | 1971–73 | 117 | 161 | 31 | 78 | | |
| Weekes et al | England | 1973–77 | 60 | 36 | 66 | 55 | 23 | 22 |
| Perrson et al | Sweden | 1973–77 | 86 | 24 | 6 | 105 | | |

* PND = perinatal deaths
† Bed = patient treated with bedrest
‡ Active = bedrest not instituted
From Hawrylyshyn PA, Barkin M, Bernstein A, et al: Twin pregnancies—a continuing perinatal challenge. Obstet Gynecol 59:65, 1982.

36 weeks' gestation. The results were impressive.

1. The mean duration of pregnancy was 255 days, without the use of tocolytic agents.
2. There was a decreased incidence of twins born with weights below 1500 g, although no increase in the mean gestational age was found.
3. Decreased incidence of small-for-gestational-age neonates, with all of the twins born after 35 weeks' gestation.
4. The incidence of preterm labor as compared with the control group decreased from 33 percent to 30 percent (P < 0.01).
5. No twins were born before 33 weeks' gestation.
6. Eighty-five percent of the patients were induced at 38 weeks' gestation, because in Sweden, this has been determined to be the time in pregnancy when twins have the lowest perinatal mortality rate; the incidence of cesarean delivery in this group was 17 percent.
7. The perinatal mortality rate in the group on bed rest was 0.6 percent, equal to that of a singleton pregnancy in Sweden. More recent data suggest no benefit to hospitalized bed rest between 26 and 32 weeks' gestation (Table 24–4).

Appropriate management of the patient includes bed rest at home. Home uterine activity monitoring and evaluation by home health care nurses should result in appropriate evaluations between obligatory office visits for fetal surveillance.

## PROGESTERONE

Johnson and coworkers (1975) reported that hydroxyprogesterone caproate administered intramuscularly at a dosage of 250 mg weekly, beginning at 16 to 20 weeks' gestation, may be efficacious in the prevention of premature labor. Although it is recommended by some, this hormonal treatment has not achieved a national consensus.

**Table 24–4**
PREGNANCY OUTCOME BY TREATMENT ALLOCATION—NO BENEFIT TO BED REST
IN HOSPITAL

| | Mean (SD) or no (%) of infants | |
| --- | --- | --- |
| | Inpatients (n = 138) | Outpatients (n = 144) |
| Gestation at birth (wk) | 35-1 (3-2) | 35-7 (2-7) |
| Birth weight (g) | | |
| Twin I | 2309 (667) | 2399 (598) |
| Twin II | 2268 (727) | 2348 (560) |
| No. delivered before 32 wk | 22 (16%) | 10 (7%) |
| No. with birthweight | | |
| < 1500 g | 20 (14%) | 12 (8%) |
| Days in nursery | | |
| Total in level 3 | 390 | 234 |
| Mean in all nurseries | 11-2 (8-2) | 9-0 (7-9) |
| No. of perinatal deaths | 8 (6%) | 2 (1%) |
| No. with early major neurologic handicap | 3 (2%) | 0 |
| No. with 1-min Apgar score < 7 | | |
| Twin I | 17 (36%) | 18 (25%) |
| Twin II | 25 (36%) | 32 (44%) |
| No. with 5-min Apgar score < 7 | | |
| Twin I | 3 (4%) | 1 (1%) |
| Twin II | 4 (%) | 2 (3%) |

From MacLennan AH, Green RC, O'Shea R, Brooks C, Morris D: Routine Hospital Admission in twin pregnancy between 26 and 30 weeks' gestation. Lancet 335:268, 1990.

## CERVICAL CERCLAGE

The placement of a prophylactic cervical cerclage in patients with multiple gestation has been suggested. We, in agreement with Dor and colleagues (1982), believe that this technique has not proved to be beneficial when it is performed only because of the presence of multiple gestation.

If the diagnosis of incompetent cervix is made on the basis of past obstetric history, or if the cervix is found to be effaced or dilated prior to 20 weeks' gestation, the suture should be placed around the internal cervical os. Again, ultrasound imaging may provide a more specific and sensitive indicator of cervical change at the internal os (Michaels et al, 1991).

## TOCOLYTIC AGENTS

O'Connor and coworkers (1979) conducted a double-blind study using ritodrine, 40 mg daily, and showed that prophylactic tocolytic therapy in multiple gestation did not increase birth weight; they also were unable to show any decreased incidence of preterm labor. Cetrulo and colleagues (1980), in a randomized double-blind study at the University of Southern California, showed that the oral administration of ritodrine in a prophylactic fashion was ineffective.

Preterm labor in the presence of multiple gestation should be treated according to established protocols, using either intravenous magnesium sulfate, ritodrine hydrochloride, or other tocolytic. In addition, betamethasone is being used at the present time to enhance pulmonary maturity between 28 and 34 weeks' gestation. If intravenous treatment with the tocolytic agent is successful, the patient is placed on bed rest on the antepartum floor and given either terbutaline or ritodrine by mouth until 34 completed weeks. If there are no further cervical changes or added complications, she is discharged home.

# Antepartum Assessment

## NONSTRESS TEST AND OXYTOCIN CHALLENGE TEST

In multiple gestations, antepartum electronic fetal monitoring is performed on a weekly basis, starting at 32 or 30 weeks if there is evidence of discordant twins or if any other complications, such as diabetes mellitus, hypertension, and anemia, are present. Nonstress tests can be used as the primary approach in antepartum fetal heart rate evaluation of twin gestation. The biophysical profile is becoming the primary source of surveillance if the technology and fiscal support are available. The criteria for a reactive nonstress test at the Robert Wood Johnson Medical School are as follows: two accelerations with an amplitude of 20 beats/min and a duration of 15 seconds occurring within any 10-min interval.

If after 20 min the fetus has not achieved a reactive test, attempts are made to arouse the fetus by abdominal manipulation, maternal position change, or acoustic stimulation. The tracing is continued after 20 min. If the nonstress test remains nonreactive at the end of 40 min, it is repeated later in the day, because most of the fetuses become reactive by that time. A nonreactive nonstress test does not imply immediate fetal jeopardy; rather, it should be viewed as an indication for further evaluation (i.e., biophysical profile).

Some controversy exists as to whether an oxytocin challenge test should be performed in cases of twin gestation, because these patients are prone to preterm labor. A report from Braly and Freeman (1977), however, failed to demonstrate an increased incidence of premature labor before 38 weeks' gestation in patients who underwent nonstress tests prior to that time. Our data from the University of South Florida support their results: Of 14,215 deliveries between January 1, 1980 and July 1, 1982, a total of 160 sets of twins was delivered. Ninety of these were managed under the protocol. Six patients carrying twins received an oxytocin challenge test. The incidence of premature labor was not increased for this group. However, patients with nonreactive nonstress tests are routinely followed up with a biophysical profile.

The position of the patient and monitoring techniques are similar to those used on patients with singleton pregnancies. However, in twin gestations, two fetal monitors and, often, two operators are needed to perform simultaneous nonstress tests, although with two distinctive fetal heart rates, the tests may be performed separately, which makes them easier for one operator to perform. New electronic fetal monitors with external twin capabilities have simplified nonstress testing of multiple gestations. One company even provides external triplet capabilities with two heart rate tracings and a digital read-out of the third fetus.

One major unresolved clinical problem is deciding on the proper management when one fetus shows a persistent abnormal pattern, the other one being normal. The decision about timing of delivery in such cases requires careful clinical judgment. Under these circumstances, our recommendation is, first, to make a careful evaluation of other underlying complications, including sensitization, hypertension, diabetes mellitus, vaginal bleeding, premature rupture of membranes, and IUGR; and then to proceed as follows.

1. If one of the fetuses is nonreactive but shows no late decelerations with uterine contractions, a biophysical profile is performed. Pregnancy should be allowed to continue if the biophysical profile demonstrates fetal well-being.

2. If one fetus has a persistent nonreacting pattern followed by late decelerations or a low biophysical profile score, an amniocentesis should be performed. If pulmonary maturity has been achieved, delivery should be accomplished by an expeditious and safe method. If the lecithin-sphingomyelin (L/S)

ratio is below 2, our approach is to administer betamethasone (12 mg intramuscularly in two doses over 24 h) and then proceed with the delivery. This is a difficult decision, because the normal fetus is delivered electively and might suffer the consequences and complications of prematurity, whereas the fetus with the abnormal fetal heart rate might demonstrate this pattern because of multiple congenital anomalies incompatible with extrauterine life. The parents as well as the health care team should be actively involved in the decision-making process when confronted with this clinical dilemma, but it is obvious that the optimal management of a nonreactive fetus that has not achieved pulmonary maturity remains unresolved.

## BIOPHYSICAL PROFILE

The continuing search for a more specific and sensitive test that would reduce antepartum stillbirth and neonatal losses led Manning and associates (1982) to develop the composite biophysical profile scoring technique (Table 24–5), which they proposed as a primary method of fetal surveillance.

There is speculation that fetal biophysical activities are not random events but rather are initiated and regulated by a complex in-

**Table 24–5**
TECHNIQUE OF BIOPHYSICAL PROFILE SCORING

| Biophysical Variable | Normal (score = 2) | Abnormal (score = 0) |
| --- | --- | --- |
| Fetal breathing movements | One or more episodes of ≥ 30 sec in 30 min | Absent or no episode of ≥30 sec in 30 min |
| Gross body movements | Three or more discrete body/limb movements in 30 min (episodes of active continuous movements considered as single movement) | Two or less episodes of body/limb movements in 30 min |
| Fetal tone | One or more episodes of active extension with return to flexion of fetal limb(s) or trunk; opening and closing of hand considered normal tone | Either slow extension with return to partial flexion or movement of limb in full extension or absent fetal movement |
| Reactive fetal heart rate | Two or more episodes of acceleration of ≥15 bpm and of ≥15 sec associated with fetal movement in 20 min | Less than 2 episodes of acceleration of fetal heart rate or acceleration of <15 bpm in 40 min |
| Qualitative amniotic fluid | One or more pockets of fluid measuring ≥1 cm in two perpendicular planes | Either no pockets or a pocket <1 cm in two perpendicular planes |

From Manning FA, Morrison I, Lange IR, Harman CR, Chamberlain PPC: Fetal biophysical scoring: selective use of the nonstress test. Am J Obstet Gynecol 156:709, 1987.

tegrated mechanism of the central nervous system. The presence of a normal response, therefore, indicates that that portion of the central nervous system is intact and functioning. A multivariant assessment, such as the biophysical profile, appears to be effective in differentiating the normal sleeping fetus from the asphyxiated fetus, and therefore, its use may result in an even greater decrease in the antepartum stillbirth rate.

## ASSESSMENT OF FETAL LUNG MATURATION

There are several clinical situations in which amniotic fluid may need to be obtained from each separate sac. These include genetic studies and Rh-sensitized patients.

Spellacy and colleagues (1977) found no significant difference in the L/S ratios obtained from separate sacs in 14 sets of twins. Sims and associates (1976), testing 20 sets of twins, found that the L/S ratio in each pair of sacs was closely related and suggested using L/S ratios of 2.5 or greater to predict functional pulmonary maturity if only one sac is available. Verduzco and associates (1976) reviewed 294 pairs of twins and concluded that the second twin's increased risk of hyaline membrane disease was due to birth asphyxia and not lung immaturity at birth. Thus, the data available to us indicate that in the majority of cases, the information obtained in one sac is probably a reliable estimate of functional pulmonary maturity for both twins and is even more so if one uses an L/S ratio of 2.5 or greater as a lower limit for lung maturation.

An amniocentesis in twin gestation should be performed under careful sonographic examination of the fetuses. The position of the twins, the location of the placenta, and if possible, the location of the divided membranes should be established. Then, the site for a safe tap should be chosen, always starting with the easier sac. A 22-gauge needle is introduced and fluid aspirated. After the fluid is withdrawn, 0.5 ml of indigo carmine (blue dye) is instilled into the sac, the needle is removed, and the patient is rescanned to select the site for the second tap. If the fluid on the second tap is clear, the procedure has been successful; if it is blue-stained, how-

ever, the amniocentesis for the second twin must be repeated. Indigo carmine should be used, because Cowett and associates (1974) reported hemolysis of fetal red blood cells with methylene blue, which may lead to fetal anemia.

## ULTRASOUND SURVEILLANCE

### Normal Fetal Growth

Early diagnosis of twins and other multiple gestations in the first and second trimesters has been difficult. Sonography has made a significant impact on the early detection of the multifetal pregnancy. The routine use of ultrasound in obstetrics is now associated with the reduction of the mean gestational age of twin diagnosis from 35 to 20 weeks. Early diagnosis is crucial in order to prevent approximately 70 percent of perinatal deaths that occur prior to 30 weeks of gestational age. High resolution real-time equipment and the advent of ultrasonography have allowed the diagnosis of multifetal gestation to be consistently accomplished shortly after 6 to 7 weeks of menstrual age. The identification of the amnion is now common, allowing for the reliable determination of amnionicity and chorionicity in multifetal pregnancy. Cervical length can be readily measured and may lead to methods of treatment for cervical incompetence (Michaels et al, 1991).

Using transvesical sonography, twin sacs should be identifiable within the uterus by 6 weeks' menstrual age. At this stage, one would expect to see two distinct chorionic sacs as two echogenic rings within the endometrium. The yolk sacs can be observed at 38 to 40 days (5.5 to 6 weeks' menstrual age), with a mean sac diameter of 8 mm. In the first trimester, the chorion is a thick hyperechoic ring, whereas the amnion is a thin filament. The amnion, however, is not normally identified until the visualization of the yolk sac and fetus, which occurs by 6 to 6.5 weeks' menstrual age.

The true breakthroughs in sonographic evaluation of twin gestations have been in the early detection of fetal membranes and fetal anomalies. It is critical to visualize the amniotic membrane because of the poor prognosis, higher incidence of congenital anomalies, and fetal wastage in monoamniotic twins. It is important to perform early serial studies until the amnionicity can be determined sonographically (see Figs 24–12 to 24–15).

In the second trimester, documentation of two placentacal sites are indicative of a dichorionic pregnancy. It is not, however, always easy to identify the presence of two separate placentas when they are fused. It is important to remember that generally it is not possible after fusion of the amniotic chorion at 16 weeks' gestation to differentiate between monochorionic and dichorionic twins.

Although there is some controversy, the growth pattern in the first and second trimesters appears to be the same for twins when compared with singletons. The reduction in growth curves in twins as compared with singletons usually begins at 27 to 35 weeks' menstrual age (see Fig. 24–9). A decrease in weight of fetal organs may be demonstrated for twins by about 30 weeks' gestation through term. The importance of serial measurement of growth parameters in twins in the second and third trimester is to enable the early identification of IUGR. Normative data are essential to the successful evaluation of this pathologic entity. Without normative data, there will continue to be unacceptably high numbers of false-positive and false-negative diagnoses.

Studies of normal fetal growth in multiple gestations have been conflicting in their results. Most of the studies focused on the BPD of the fetal head. Crane and associates (1980) demonstrated BPD growth in normal twins to be similar to that of a singleton. Other authors have suggested a relative decrease in BPD growth in twin gestations (Benson and Doubilet, 1991).

It is recognized that measurement of the BPD technically is more difficult in multiple gestations. Difficulties in visualization of the BPD and in obtaining measurements deep within the pelvis or under the costal margins as well as difficulties in maternal intolerance of the supine position during scanning are the predominate reasons for lack of success in obtaining an appropriate BPD. Others recognize that dolichocephaly (head shaped like a banana, therefore, shortening the BPD), which is attributable to intrauterine crowding or the breech position, is more common in twin gestations. A dolichocephalic head generally requires the presence of a cephalic index (CI = BPD/occipitofrontal

diameter × 100) less than 75 percent. The head circumference or the BPD should be used. When comparing twin with singleton fetuses, Socol and associates (1984) demonstrated a slowing of growth for the BPD and abdominal circumference (AC) at 32 to 34 weeks' gestation in the twin fetuses. Newborn measurements, when contrasted with standard singleton curves, indicated that birth weight and abdominal circumference lagged in the twin infants, whereas head circumference and body lengths were comparable to those of singletons. These neonatal data suggest an asymmetric retardation of fetal growth in twin pregnancy and are consistent with ultrasound data. The association of dolichocephaly in multiple gestations leads to a relative decrease in BPD (D'Alton and Mercer, 1990). Therefore, in the third trimester, it is best to use twin-specific BPD tables or femur lengths to determine gestational age (Benson and Doubilet, 1990).

## Abnormal Fetal Growth

Discordant fetal growth is described as an intrapair birth weight discrepancy of greater than 20 percent. Although twins are already in a high-risk group, this discrepancy predisposes them to increased IUGR. If discordant growth is present, the risk of perinatal death (usually of the smaller twin) is 20 percent, which is 6.5 times greater than in twins with concordant growth. Leveno and associates (1979, 1980) stated that differences between twins in BPD of 5 mm or greater after 28 weeks' gestation are suggestive of discordant fetal growth; if greater than 7 mm, the differences are associated with fetal death in 20 percent of cases. As highlighted earlier, more recent studies have shown that the BPD is an insensitive and nonspecific indicator of discordancy in twin gestations. O'Brien and associates (1986) suggest that if the intrapair birth weight difference is less than 20 percent, there is less than a 10 percent probability of a small-for-gestational-age neonate.

Criteria for diagnosis of discordant twin growth include (1) a 5 mm difference in BPD measurements, (2) a 5 percent difference in head circumference, (3) a BPD of the small twin below 2 standard deviations of the normal curve, and (4) a 20 mm difference in AC between the twins (D'Alton and Mercer, 1990). IUGR, therefore, is a relatively common finding in multiple gestations. It needs to be confirmed with very strict criteria. When discussing the issue with the parents, recognize that the term IUGR is synonymous with mental retardation to most patients. Although this may clearly distinguish between small for gestational age and IUGR, it is recommended to use the term small for gestational age in order to relieve any questions the patient may have regarding neurologic impairment. Furthermore, abnormal growth in one twin may be associated with the twin-to-twin transfusion syndrome. It is our impression that the twin-to-twin transfusion syndrome has been overdiagnosed in cases of chronic hypoxia, IUGR, and an elevated hematocrit in the smaller fetus. These two distinct entities, IUGR and twin-to-twin transfusion syndrome, will require definitive management schemes that are different.

Although IUGR usually affects one twin, IUGR in both fetuses (concordant IUGR) does occur. Concordant IUGR highlights the need for an early ultrasound evaluation, which can be used as a baseline indicator of gestational age. As with IUGR in singletons, biophysical profiles are more reliable indicators of outcome than is fetal measurement. As a result, it is important to monitor fetal growth in the second and third trimesters through assessment of the biophysical profiles.

# Antepartum Complications

## SPONTANEOUS ABORTIONS

Spontaneous abortions are more common in twin gestations than in singleton pregnancies. Hellman and coworkers (1973) and Robinson and Caines (1977) reported cases in which there was sonographic evidence of two sacs early in pregnancy, with disappearance and reabsorption of one embryo later. Schenker and colleagues (1981) reported that monozygotic twins are more likely to abort in the first trimester than singleton pregnancies. They also found an increased incidence of second trimester spontaneous abortion in cases of multiple gestation, with the risk increasing according to the number of fetuses. Finally, in cases in which drugs were used to induce ovulation, a lower incidence of

spontaneous abortion was noted with clomiphene than with hMG and hCG.

Schenker and associates (1981) speculate that several factors may account for increased abortion rates (between 20 and 30 percent) in drug-induced pregnancies: (1) faulty ovum as a result of exogenous stimulation with different drugs; (2) a very high level of estradiol, which may increase tubal motility, resulting in early arrival of the conceptus to a very poorly prepared endometrium and, therefore, poor implantation with subsequent abortion; (3) luteal phase deficiency; and (4) earlier diagnostic rate in this special group of patients on fertility drugs.

## ANEMIA

As reported by Pritchard and MacDonald (1980), the mean increment of blood volume in twin gestation is about 50 to 60 percent. As mentioned earlier, multiple gestation causes increased placental as well as fetal mass. These factors predispose the mother to a greater prevalence of maternal anemia. Good nutrition with an increased iron intake as well as supplementation of iron and vitamins with folic acid is recommended.

## HYPERTENSIVE DISORDERS

Hypertensive disorders in pregnancy are more common in women with multiple gestation. The development of hypertension in a multiparous patient who had previous, otherwise uncomplicated pregnancies should alert the obstetrician to the possibility of twin gestation.

The incidence is recognized to be two to three times higher than in singleton pregnancies. This complication not only is more common in twin pregnancies but also tends to develop earlier and to be more severe than in patients with a singleton pregnancy (Cunningham et al, 1989).

## HYDRAMNIOS

The uterus with multiple fetuses may have a volume of 10 liters and weigh over 20 lbs. Rapid accumulation of excessive amounts of amniotic fluid is common, especially in monozygotic twin pregnancies. Approximately 12 percent of all multiple gestations are complicated with this disorder (Cetrulo et al, 1980). The overdistention of the uterus by excessive amounts of amniotic fluid, in addition to the burden of carrying two or more fetuses, increases the likelihood of premature labor, premature rupture or both, of the membranes. Hydramnios also has been associated with increased incidence of gastrointestinal and central nervous system abnormalities in the fetus; therefore, perinatal mortality rates might be as high as 41 percent when this condition is present in multiple gestation.

## ANTEPARTUM HEMORRHAGE

The condition of large placental mass combined with overdistention of the uterus might lead one to believe that multiple gestations commonly are more complicated with placenta praevia and abruptio placentae. Several authors (Cetrulo et al, 1980; Farooqui et al, 1973; O'Connor et al, 1981) have listed antepartum hemorrhage as a complication observed in multiple gestations; however, it is difficult to assess whether this phenomenon is more common in these cases than in singleton pregnancies.

## PREMATURE RUPTURE OF THE MEMBRANES

Premature rupture of the chorioamniotic membranes occurs more frequently in multiple gestation and can lead to premature labor. It also may be associated with increased incidence of cord prolapse.

## CONGENITAL ANOMALIES

The incidence of certain congenital anomalies is higher in twin gestations than in singleton pregnancies. In 1195 twins studied in the Collaborative Perinatal Project (Iffy and Kaminetzky, 1981), the incidence of cardiovascular and gastrointestinal tract anomalies in twin gestation was more than twice that for singleton pregnancies. The incidence of central nervous system and skeletal abnormalities was also much higher in multiple gestation. Another study of 2000 twins resulted in a higher incidence of anencephaly, hydrocephaly, and congenital heart disease in twins of the same sex, suggesting that placental anastomosis may play a role in the etiology of these manifestations (Iffy and Kaminetzky, 1981). No increase in overall prevalance of malformations has been reported (Neilson, 1992).

Monozygotic twins have a higher incidence of congenital anomalies than do dizygotic twins, and as previously mentioned, the former type of twinning should be considered a teratologic process. Acardia (absence of the heart) is a malformation confined to only monozygotic twins and occurs in 1 in every 100 cases. Fetuses affected by acardia may differ greatly in appearance and may have different degrees of organogenesis. They probably represent the ultimate discordance in the development of genetically identical individuals (Benirschke and Kim, 1973).

The anomaly of conjoined twins is also more common in monozygotic twins. Most of them are female (70 percent) and are fused by the chest (thoracopagus) (70 percent). The incidence is between 1 in 33,000 and 1 in 165,000 births, and the condition is believed to result from separation of the inner cell mass, occurring very late on the time scale (13 to 15 days after implantation).

Selective termination may be a consideration for pregnancies in which one twin has an anomaly or when the number of fetuses may jeopardize the survival of any of the fetuses. Malgar and associates (1991) suggest that there is improved gestational age at delivery and outcome when quadruplet pregnancies are reduced to twins; the situation is less clear with triplets. Although the technology is available, the ethics of such management are debatable (Laube, 1990). Evans and colleagues (1988) presented the use of ethical decision-making for selective termination for each individual case, with careful attention given to the parent's choice. Berkowitz and colleagues (1988) argue that because abortion is available on demand, the parents' choice is the only criteria for selective termination.

# Intrapartum Management

Common intrapartum complications are abnormal presentation, dysfunctional labor, cord prolapse, fetal distress, and abruptio placentae. At the time of labor, several important measures should be implemented to ensure a good outcome in cases of multiple gestation.

## VAGINAL DELIVERY FOR VERTEX-TO-VERTEX PRESENTATION

Electronic fetal monitoring has been used successfully to monitor both fetuses simultaneously at the time of labor. During premature labor or until the membranes are ruptured, twin monitoring can pick up simultaneous external fetal heart rate using the same monitor. One monitor even allows external triplet monitoring. When a vaginal delivery is planned and a twin monitor is not available, artificial rupture of the membranes should be performed, after which the scalp electrode is applied to the first twin. An intrauterine pressure catheter is then introduced into the uterus for accurate monitoring of the uterine activity. The internal elec-

trode on the first twin and the intrauterine pressure catheter are attached to a first monitor. The fetal heart tones of the second twin are recorded on a second monitor externally, by ultrasound (Fig. 24–20). A second catheter filled with sterile water is then run between the strain gauges of the first and second monitors (Fig. 24–21). In this way, the tracing from the second twin also will show uterine activity being recorded internally. Several monitor companies now offer an electronic monitor that simultaneously monitors both twins (Figs. 24–22 and 24–23). In some cases, if the same pen on the monitor traces both fetal heart rates, an accurate assessment of variability is lost. This problem can be overcome by intermittently allowing only the internal lead to pick up the signal. However, some brands have dual channels, so that variability can be assessed from the internal electrode.

As soon as the first twin is delivered, the vertex of the second twin should be guided gently into the pelvis. This can be observed by using ultrasound equipment if it is available in the labor and delivery area. As soon as this procedure has been accomplished, the fetal scalp electrode should be applied immediately to the head of the second fetus. As long as no complications develop, there is no time limit for the delivery of the second twin, provided that there is a normal pattern of

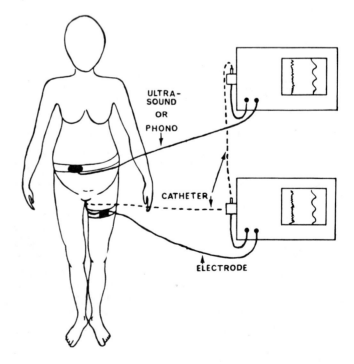

Figure 24–20. Twin gestation—simultaneous monitoring of intrapartum fetal heart rate and uterine activity. Fetal heart rate on Twin A monitored with internal scalp electrode. Twin B monitored by Doppler ultrasound or phonocardiogram through maternal abdominal wall. Intrauterine pressure catheter is used for uterine activity. (From Cetrulo CL, Ingardia CJ, Sbarra AJ: Management of multiple gestation. Clin Obstet Gynecol 23:536, 1980.)

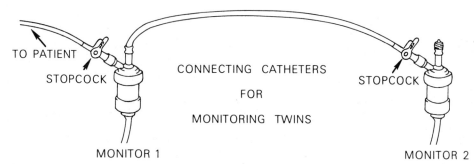

**Figure 24–21.** Connecting catheters for monitoring twins using two monitors. (From Paul RH, et al: Fetal Intensive Care. Wallingford, CT, Corometrics Medical Systems, Inc, 1979.)

fetal heart rate. We have found few contraindications to the use of oxytocin for augmentation of labor, provided that both fetuses are properly monitored.

### Additional Guidelines for Vertex-to-Vertex Delivery

On admission to the labor floor, blood should be drawn from the mother, and two units of cross-matched whole blood should be readily available.

An intravenous infusion system with a large bore catheter is mandatory. The delivery area should be immediately operational for emergency surgery.

An appropriately trained obstetrician and an assistant should be available to follow the mother in labor.

Epidural anesthesia is probably the best choice for a vaginal delivery.

An anesthesiologist or nurse anesthetist capable of administering general anesthesia is available in case the need for cesarean delivery or intrauterine manipulations arises.

A neonatal team comprised of two neonatologists with assistants should be alerted and present at delivery, because infant resuscitation may be needed.

With this team approach, every patient with a twin gestation and a vertex-to-vertex presentation should be allowed to progress into labor spontaneously.

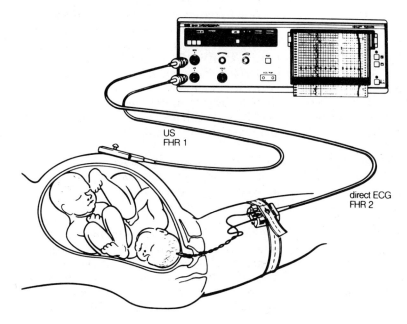

**Figure 24–22.** The attachment of a single fetal monitor to monitor both twins simultaneously with ultrasound and the internal electrode. (Courtesy of Hewlett-Packard.)

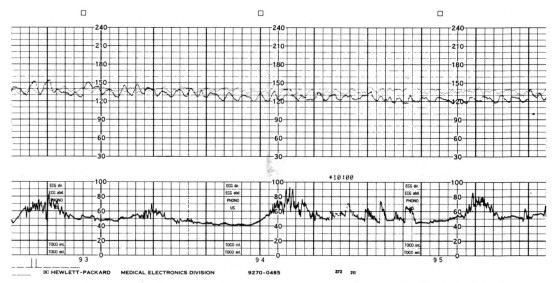

**Figure 24–23.** Tracing from the monitor that monitors twins simultaneously. The light fetal heart rate line is the internal tracing, and the dark line is the ultrasound tracing. (Courtesy of the Division of Maternal-Fetal Medicine, University of South Florida, College of Medicine, Tampa, FL.)

If, at the onset of labor, there is a question about the presentation of one or both fetuses, an ultrasound examination of the uterus (or an x-ray study of the abdomen) is performed immediately to accurately assess fetal position.

## VAGINAL DELIVERY FOR PRESENTATIONS OTHER THAN VERTEX-TO-VERTEX

Much controversy exists in the literature about vaginal delivery of twin fetuses with other than vertex-to-vertex presentations. With fetuses in a breech-to-vertex presentation, cesarean delivery should be performed because of the possibility, although rare (1 in 1000), of interlocking twins.

The risks of a breech infant in a vaginal delivery are meticulously described by Seeds and Cefalo (1982).

- Intrapartum death is 16 times higher.
- Intrapartum asphyxia is 3 to 8 times higher.
- Cord prolapse is 5 to 20 times higher.
- Trauma is 13 times higher.
- Incidence of spinal cord injury is 21 percent.

- Incidence of hyperextended head is 5 percent.
- Arrest of the aftercoming head is 8 percent.
- Congenital anomalies are in the range of 6 to 18 percent.

Kelsik and Minkoff (1982) suggest that the perinatal mortality is higher for a breech first or second twin in a vaginal delivery (5 percent) than with cesarean delivery (2.5 percent). The outcome for the first breech twin is not better than that for the second breech twin, and cesarean deliveries should be performed as frequently for breech second twins as for breech first twins. The indications for cesarean delivery for breech twins are (1) prematurity, with an estimated fetal weight between 800 and 2500 g; (2) footling breech; (3) evidence of contracted pelvis; (4) hyperextension of the fetal head; (5) lack of expertise of the medical staff in vaginal deliveries; (6) fetal distress; and (7) abnormal labor patterns.

It is well known that twin B may be heavier than twin A (Friedman et al, 1977). In a situation in which twin B is breech and larger than vertex twin A, labor management should be altered (Roberts, 1976) and cesarean delivery should be considered to prevent potential birth trauma.

# CESAREAN DELIVERY

Numerous reports in the literature have exposed a recent trend to routinely deliver multiple fetuses by cesarean delivery. Cunningham and associates (1989) reported that 47 percent of the twins followed at the High-Risk Pregnancy Clinic at Parkland Memorial Hospital were delivered by cesarean section. After evaluation of several studies conducted by Ware (1971), Cetrulo and associates (1980), and Barter and associates (1965), it seems reasonable to conclude that cesarean delivery probably should be performed for multiple pregnancies of larger fetal numbers (three or more) or for twins other than those with vertex-to-vertex presentation. A vertical incision in the lower uterine segment may be indicated if a fetus lies transversely or when a very thick lower uterine segment is encountered. Indications for cesarean delivery are fetal distress; abruptio placentae; prolapsed umbilical cord; coexistence of twin gestation with other complications of pregnancy, such as hypertension, diabetes mellitus, and Rh sensitization; evidence of discordant twins with IUGR; and perhaps, any presentations other than vertex-to-vertex, in order to avoid birth trauma, the most important labor complication leading to perinatal mortality.

# DELIVERY OF THE SECOND TWIN

It has been said that the main problem in delivering twins is the delivery of the second twin. Many authors have stressed that the second twin is at a greater risk of mortality and morbidity than the first-born. Early reports of cesarean deliveries performed for second twins after vaginal delivery of the first twin, were mainly in the form of case reports. Evrard and Gold (1981) reviewed four such cases presented over 4 years and added five cases from the literature. If one follows the advice of typical textbooks, maternal and perinatal mortality and morbidity undoubtedly would be higher with this mode of delivery. However, when the management protocol includes cesarean delivery for all twins other than those with vertex-to-vertex presentation, this complication cannot be avoided.

In an attempt to define the risks of cesarean delivery for twin B after a vaginal delivery of twin A, we undertook a review of our experience from 1973 to 1982. As shown in Table 24–6, the indications for cesarean delivery for the second twin are prolapse of the cord, abruptio placentae, fetal distress, failed forceps, failed internal podalic version, and probably any presentation other than vertex. One of the concerns regarding cesarean delivery for the second twin is the risk of infection to the mother when cesarean delivery is undertaken in these circumstances. Because there is a paucity of literature regarding this subject, some physicians might be reluctant to perform a cesarean delivery for twin B when twin A has been delivered vaginally. On the other hand, some physicians, in order to avoid this possibility altogether, might use cesarean delivery for all twins.

In our review, we found that 21 of the 352 twin deliveries (6 percent) required cesarean delivery of twin B after vaginal delivery of twin A. This group of 21 cesarean deliveries made up 15 percent of all cesarean deliveries that were performed throughout the study for twin gestations. Even with the liberal use of cesarean delivery in 1979, 11 of the 85 cesarean deliveries of twins were performed for twin B after a vaginal delivery of twin A, and they made up 13 percent of the total number of cesarean deliveries performed in twin pregnancies in this latter period. This compares with 10 cesarean deliveries for twin B after vaginal delivery of twin A performed out of a total of 50 cesarean deliveries (20 percent) between 1973 and 1978. Despite the antepartum use of ultrasound imaging, the failure to diagnose twins continues to be a major factor in the management of twins and often accounts for the need to perform a cesarean delivery for twin B after vaginal delivery of twin A. This factor accounted for about 35 percent of all such cases.

**Table 24–6**

PRIMARY INDICATIONS FOR CESAREAN IN TWIN B AT TAMPA GENERAL HOSPITAL DELIVERY (UNIVERSITY OF SOUTH FLORIDA), 1973–1982

| Indication | Number of Cases (%) |
|---|---|
| Transverse lie | 8 (33%) |
| Fetal distress | 5 (24%) |
| Contracted cervix | 3 (20%) |
| Prolapsed cord | 2 (9%) |
| Premature breech | 2 (9%) |
| Failed extraction | 1 (5%) |
| Total | 21 (100%) |

In our experience, the time interval between vaginally and abdominally delivered twins was not associated with an increase in low Apgar scores for the second twin at 5 min, even when delivered after the usual time interval of 15 to 20 min which is considered safe (Table 24–7). Many reports have appeared in the literature regarding postcesarean delivery morbidity, with infection being the most important complication in the postpartum period. In our review of cases, 3 mothers in 21 (14 percent) experienced extensive febrile morbidity, and all had significant predisposing factors. This review, which covers the largest number of such cases reported, was prepared to address the safety of cesarean delivery for twin B only. It supports the view that, whenever indications exist, cesarean delivery can be performed safely for the delivery of twin B after vaginal delivery of twin A. We recognize that indications for cesarean delivery in twin pregnancy sometimes are controversial; however, in this small number of patients, there was no increase in maternal morbidity when pregnancy was not complicated. There was no increase in neonatal mortality or morbidity resulting from cesarean delivery for twin B. The success of this management scheme reemphasizes the need for anesthesia availability at every twin delivery and continued fetal monitoring for twin B in the operating room.

## MULTIFETAL GESTATIONS GREATER THAN TWO

Multifetal gestations of more than two intrauterine fetuses require even more enhanced surveillance and prevention of prematurity than do twins. These are highly unusual cases, except after the use of artificial reproductive technology, with a very low prevalance in the overall population.

**Table 24–7**
DELIVERY INTERVAL AND APGAR SCORES OF SECOND TWINS

| Time Interval (min) | Number of Twins | Apgar Scores (below 7 at 5 min) |
| --- | --- | --- |
| 0–10 min | 0 | — |
| 10–20 min | 7 | 2 |
| 21–60 min | 9 | 0 |
| 61–120 min | 5 | 1 |
| Total | 21 | 3 |

These mothers must be encouraged to improve uterine perfusion, decrease activity, and maintain a well-balanced diet. Prophylactic measures to reduce premature labor have not been successful.

More than two intrauterine fetuses are difficult cases to manage, because the perinatal team frequently has to allow one or two distressed, hypoxemic fetuses to die *in utero* in order to maintain one or two healthy, live newborns. Serial biophysical profile scoring, interaction with social workers and geneticists, and close communication with the family reduces the tensions associated with these extremely high-risk cases.

The method of delivery generally accepted is cesarean delivery. The prevalence (frequency) of these gestations is so low that a prospective study is unlikely to occur. Perhaps a multicenter study with meta-analysis may develop some data for us to acknowledge the safety of a vaginal delivery. At the present time, a cesarean delivery is the method of choice, with all of the support team available for at least three neonates at the time of delivery.

## Conclusions Regarding Management

1. The treatment of infertility by the use of drugs for induction of ovulation has increased the overall incidence of multiple gestation.

2. Ultrasound is the most accurate method of diagnosis. However, whether or not a sonogram should be performed in every pregnancy remains controversial. The accuracy is about 98 percent. If the diagnosis is still in doubt after ultrasound, or if ultrasound equipment is unavailable, a flat plate of the abdomen is not contraindicated.

3. Because the most common problem in multiple gestations is prematurity, every attempt should be made to diagnose twin gestations early (between 16 and 20 weeks). Early diagnosis, prolonged bed rest between 26 and 34 weeks' gestation, and the use of tocolytic agents might prolong the pregnancy; maternal administration of glucocorticoids for enhancement of fetal lung maturation also may improve the perinatal outcome. Early diagnosis allows prompt detection and treatment of other complications

that are encountered frequently in this clinical situation, such as anemia, hypertension, polyhydramnios, IUGR, and discordance.

4. The patient's diet should be well balanced, with supplements of iron and folic acid.

5. Malpresentation is a common finding. Cesarean delivery is preferable in these cases to avoid potential complications. In cases of fetal distress, prolapse of the umbilical cord, and abruptio placentae, the fetuses probably are best served by an abdominal delivery. Avoid birth trauma. Optimal neonatal care requires a team effort.

6. Malformations are more common in monozygotic twins. These anomalies usually affect only one twin. These defects include anencephaly; hydrocephalus; holoprosencephaly; cloacal exstrophy; vertebral defects, imperforate anus, tracheoesophageal fistula, and radial and renal dyplasia (VATER) syndrome; and sacrococcygeal teratoma. These defects occur three to seven times more frequently in monozygotic twins than in dizygotic twins or singletons (Benirschke and Kim, 1973; Coleman et al, 1987; Crane, 1984; Winter et al, 1988).

7. In a review of 59 triplet deliveries, the mortality rate was 23 percent. The most important factors relating to neonatal death were prematurity and birth order. The mortality rate for those infants born last was double that for first-borns (Itzkowicz, 1979). Holeberg and colleagues (1982) demonstrated that the neonatal mortality rate was 53 percent for the third-born infant compared with 27 percent for the first-born infant and 30 percent for the second-born infant during vaginal delivery. Although there were no neonatal deaths in the cesarean delivery group, the gestational age was significantly higher. Although prematurity of multiple fetal gestations has not decreased over the past 20 to 30 years, perinatal mortality has decreased, probably owing to improved neonatal care. The long-term morbidity of these infants has not been assessed. Seventy-five percent of triplets deliver prematurely, many before 32 weeks. The statistics on the morbidity for four or more fetuses are too small to analyze; however, it can be surmised that they are only as good as triplet outcomes and probably worse (Alvarez and Berkowitz, 1990).

8. Labor and delivery of twins with a vertex-to-vertex presentation require intensive electronic fetal monitoring, including the internal pressure catheter. Oxytocin is not contraindicated. An epidural is probably the preferred method of anesthesia. If nuchal cord is encountered, do not cut the cord to deliver twin A.

9. As soon as the first twin is born, guide the head of the second twin into the pelvis, proceed to rupture the membrane, and apply the scalp electrode. Allow labor under very close surveillance. Oxytocin is not contraindicated. Time between deliveries is not as relevant as it once was, provided that the second twin is monitored properly and labor is well tolerated by the fetus.

10. If delivery is anticipated before 36 weeks' gestation, with a birth weight below 2500 g, the patient is best served by an early transfer *in utero* to a level III hospital.

A summary of the management for multiple gestations is presented in Table 24–8 and Figure 24–24.

# Psychosocial Considerations

When the diagnosis of a multiple gestation is made, the parents may have many fears concerning the addition of more than one baby to the family. These concerns may include fears of being unable physically and emotionally to care for more than one infant; financial concerns for the cost of caring for more than one baby, which involves doubling items such as clothing, cribs, and strollers; and increased hospitalization costs for the mother and her infants. Broadbent (1985) found that women had three major concerns when expecting twins: (1) worries about the birth itself; (2) concern for one or both of the babies; and (3) apprehension over her and her partner's ability to cope with two babies practically, emotionally, and financially. She also found that these fears were exacerbated by a lack of information and counseling and a lack of continuity of care. These fears may be overwhelming to the new parents, and psychologic and financial counseling should be available to decrease parental anxiety by continuous and personalized care during and after pregnancy (Hunter, 1989).

The parents probably recognize that there is a higher risk for prematurity and other maternal and fetal complications, such as anemia, hypertension, increased incidence of congenital anomalies, IUGR, abruptio pla-

**Table 24–8**
PATIENT CARE SUMMARY FOR MULTIPLE GESTATION*

| | Antepartum | | Intrapartum | Postpartum |
|---|---|---|---|---|
| | *Outpatient* | *Inpatient* | | |
| BP, P, R | Each visit | Every 8 h (more frequently if hypertensive) | Every 1 h | On admission; then every 15 min × 4; then every 30 min × 2; then every 1 h until stable; then every 8 h on PP (unless also hypertensive, then more frequent BP indicated) |
| T | Each visit | Every 8 h | Every 4 h | On admission to RR; then every 8 h |
| FHR | Weekly NST/ CST starting 30–32 weeks' gestation | Weekly NST/ CST starting at 30–32 weeks' gestation | Continuously with electronic fetal monitor (both internal and external). If monitor not available, every 15 min first stage; then every 5 min second stage | |
| Contractions | Weekly, (daily home monitoring may be used) | Every 8 h | Continuously with electronic fetal monitor, preferably internal. If monitor not available, every 1 h by palpation | Fundal checks: every 15 min × 4; then every 30 min × 2; then every 1 h until stable; then every 8 h on PP floor |
| Lochia | — | — | — | Lochia checks: every 15 min × 4; then every 30 min × 2; then every 1 h until stable; then every 8 h on PP floor |
| Laboratory studies: | | | | |
| Hemoglobin | Each visit | Weekly | Admission | First day PP |
| Hematocrit | Each visit | Weekly | Admission | First day PP |
| GTT (2-h postprandial) | At 20, 24, 28, 32, and 36 weeks | Same as under outpatient | Admission | PP |
| Sonogram | At least one level II sonogram before 24 weeks to R/O major congenital anomalies. Serial sonograms for EFW q 3 weeks. Biophysical profile weekly from 30 weeks. | Serial sonogram 2–3 weeks from 28 weeks to R/O discordance; on admission, to check fetal presentations | | |
| Assess fundal heights | Each visit | Each visit | | |

* Nurse–patient ratio as follows: antepartum, 1 : 6–8; intrapartum, 1 : 1; at delivery, 1 : 1; postpartum, 1 : 6–8.

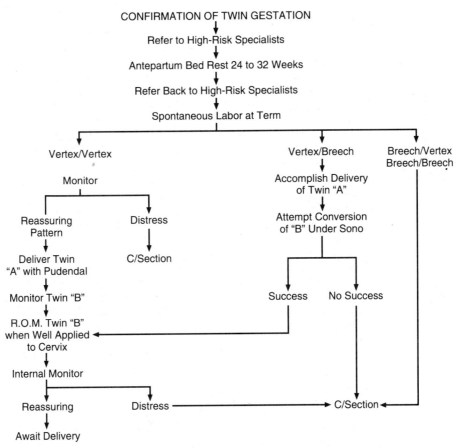

**Figure 24–24.** Management flow chart for multiple gestations.

centae, prolapse of the cord, placenta praevia, and postpartum hemorrhage. The parents should have a clear understanding of these potential complications, which will help them to deal with the stresses that may occur. In some situations, the parents may want to tour the neonatal intensive care nursery in order to prepare for their babies' admittance. They may want to take prepared childbirth classes earlier than they would if they were expecting a singleton birth, in anticipation of premature labor and restricted activity later in the pregnancy.

Some of the minor discomforts of pregnancy become exaggerated with a large uterus. Small meals can help to decrease the heartburn caused by the enlargement of the uterus pressing on the stomach. The woman may feel awkward with the size of her uterus. This awkwardness and discomfort may lead to difficulty sleeping. A pillow can be used under her side to support the uterus when she sleeps. A heating pad or hot water bottle can be used while she is awake to soothe aching ligaments. (One of our patients, pregnant with triplets, was so uncomfortable that the physical therapy department devised a harness to help support her uterus.)

These women also may be depressed by their large size and may be anxious over their weight gain; nevertheless, they should be encouraged to maintain their increased caloric intake. Psychologic support is important.

Home visits to these families can be helpful in the antepartum period to help the family prepare for the arrival of more than one baby. Discussions for delivery options help the family prepare for delivery. The parents should be encouraged to verbalize their concerns to the health care team and to work on solutions for the demands of increased caretaking. Other family members, hired help, or family aides may facilitate the caretaking, at least until schedules can be devised in the postpartum period.

Information on multiple gestation support

groups should be provided so that the parents can have contact with other families with more than one baby. These families can provide emotional support and helpful hints to problems, such as attaching two umbrella strollers rather than using the larger twin strollers available and, initially, allowing the babies to sleep in the same crib.

Fathers should be included in these preparatory plans and should be encouraged to help with the caretaking. Some fathers may find this difficult because of their work schedules and demands. The parents also should be counseled that these increased caretaking jobs will decrease their time together. They should be encouraged to try to find some time to spend together.

Once the babies have been delivered, the family should be given continued support. This is especially true because abuse of twins occurs nine times more often than in singletons (Theroux, 1989). Home visits should be maintained and care plans continued and modified as needed in the postpartum period. If the multiple gestation was not identified until the time of delivery, these parents will need additional support and planning in the postpartum period. The late discovery of twins may even delay bonding.

Goshen-Gottstein (1980) observed how mothers coped with twins and other multiple gestations. The frequently expressed ambivalence sometimes is manifested pathologically "by projecting negative qualities onto one twin and positive attributes onto the other" (Neifert and Thorpe, 1990). Goshen-Gottstein (1980) concluded that parents should be supported and allowed to express these negative feelings to help them cope with these feelings. Fathers as well as mothers can experience this ambivalence. Older children who normally may experience jealousy may have even stronger feelings about multiple siblings because of the increased attention that the newborns require. Special time alone with the older siblings can help to alleviate some of these anxieties. However, exhausted parents may not be able to meet everyone's needs (Neifert and Thorpe, 1990).

Making a specific schedule for the care for more than one infant may be helpful, at least initially, in getting the family organized. However, the family also should try to remain flexible, because the schedule probably will be interrupted. Keeping records of when each baby was fed, bathed, and so on may be

helpful, because fatigue may cause the parents to forget whose turn it is. It should be reinforced that as long as the babies are cleaned well with each diaper change, daily bathing is not necessary. The parents may find it helpful to bathe the babies on the same day or, perhaps, to bathe each baby on alternating days.

Initially, the sounds the babies make may disturb others in the family, but the family will quickly become accustomed to these sounds. Some parents have suggested having the babies share a crib, because the babies may enjoy the closeness and may rest better.

Breastfeeding should be encouraged and supported if the mother desires. Addy (1975) questioned 173 mothers of twins and found that 23.7 percent breastfed the infants from birth, even though 30 percent of those babies were premature. Several mothers did not breastfeed because of erroneous information. Nine percent were discouraged by their physician, 11 percent did not think they had enough milk, and 11 percent did not think it was possible to breastfeed twins. Rooming-in in the hospital can give the mother a chance to feed the babies while help and instruction are available. It should be explained to the mother that she will have enough milk to feed more than one baby; supply will equal demand. Establishing regular breastfeeding during the first week after delivery is important in establishing a sufficient supply of breast milk. If the babies are unable to empty the mother's breasts regularly, she should be encouraged to pump her breasts until they are empty. This helps establish an adequate milk supply (Neifert and Thorpe, 1990). The family should be encouraged to be supportive, so that the mother will continue to have caretaking help at home. Additional support can be provided by home visits from the visiting nurses or lactation consultants and by contact with other mothers who have breastfed more than one infant. This advice and support is important, because the mother's milk supply can be diminished if she becomes fatigued or does not get enough nourishment. More calories are needed to produce milk to feed additional babies. She also needs to increase her fluid intake and continue taking her vitamin and mineral supplements.

Additional support from the perinatal team will be necessary for those mothers who want to breastfeed their babies who are premature or have complications.

The mother may want to feed the infants separately, at first, until she becomes more comfortable with the babies. Later, with more practice, she may be able to feed both babies simultaneously (Fig. 24–25). It takes less time to feed both babies simultaneously. Simultaneous feeding also has the advantage of allowing the more vigorous infant to initiate the milk let down reflex for a smaller twin (Neifert and Thorpe, 1990). It has been suggested that because simultaneous nursing may generate higher prolactin levels, it also may increase milk production (Neifert and Seacat, 1985; Tyson et al, 1976). The mother also may want to express milk so that another family member can feed one of the babies. A combination of feeding the babies separately and together may save time and offer individual attention for each baby.

Mothers also should be prepared for the increased demand of breastfeeding when the babies have growth spurts, at about 6 weeks and 3 months. This increased demand from the babies will increase the milk supply for these growth spurts. If sore nipples develop, the babies should be assessed to determine whether or not they have latched on cor-rectly and that the baby's mouth covers the areolar area, not just the nipple. Changing the position of the babies when they feed will change the areas of pressure on the nipples. The less hungry baby should be fed from the sorer breast and the hungrier baby fed from the fuller breast. The mother also may find that a baby may prefer one breast over the other. If the babies have different appetites, the breast will become fuller on the side that supports the hungrier baby; therefore, the babies should alternate breasts.

Mothers may not realize how time-con-suming breastfeeding twins can be in the early postpartum period. Some mothers think the long-term rewards of breastfeeding are worthwhile, whereas others, who have less support may not choose to continue breastfeeding. Some mothers may choose to combine breast-feeding and bottle-feeding (Neifert and Thorpe, 1990). To maintain a sufficient milk supply, adequate nursing must take place and may need to be supple-mented by pumping.

Some mothers may choose to bottle-feed owing to a variety of reasons, including the availability of more people to feed the babies.

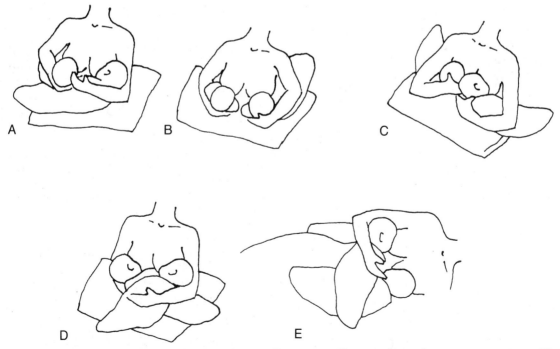

**Figure 24–25.** Positions for breastfeeding twins. All positions illustrated permit eye-to-eye contact with both infants. For women who have incisional pain from cesarean delivery, position B and a modification of C are comfortable. In C, the infants can be placed on a padded table at the correct height with the mother moving in close to feed them.

If the mother is bottle-feeding both twins at the same time, several positions can be used; usually, the mother holds one infant and supports the other or uses an infant seat (Fig. 24–26). The baby that is held for feedings should be alternated with his or her sibling. Bottle propping is not recommended, especially in the supine position, and should only occur when the parents can observe the infant (Neifert and Thorpe, 1990).

Attachment and grieving can be much more difficult when dealing with more than one baby. Klaus and Kennell (1982) have described principles that guide human bonding (Table 24–9). The fact that the mother and father can bond optimally to only one infant at a time has special implications for multiple gestations. Bowlby (1958) used the term monotropy to describe a "tendency for instinctual responses to be directed toward a particular individual or group of individuals and not promiscuously toward many." Although this was described as the response of the child toward the mother, it also has significance in the bonding process of parent to child in multiple gestations. Klaus and Kennell (1982) have described nursery settings in which nurses never have more than one special infant at a time. They like the other infants, but one is special. This may be why mothers often dress their babies alike, because this enables them to see the babies as one unit.

Because bonding may be more difficult for the parents in cases of multiple gestation, they should be encouraged to work with each

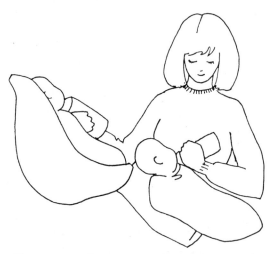

**Figure 24–26.** Positioning for bottlefed twins.

**Table 24–9**
CRUCIAL COMPONENTS IN THE PROCESS
OF ATTACHMENT

For later development to be optimal, there is a sensitive period in the first minutes and hours of life during which it is necessary that the mother and father have close contact with their neonate.

There appear to be species-specific responses to the infant in the human mother and father that are exhibited when they are first given their infant.

The process of the attachment is structured so that the father and mother become attached optimally to only one infant at a time. Bowlby (1958) earlier presented this principle of the attachment process and termed it *monotropy.*

During the process of the mother's attachment to her infant, it is necessary that the infant respond to the mother by some signal such as body or eye movements. We have sometimes described this as "You can't love a dishrag."

People who witness the birth process become strongly attached to the infant.

For some adults, it is difficult simultaneously to go through the processes of attachment and detachment, that is, to develop an attachment to one person while mourning the loss or threatened loss of the same or another person.

Some early events have long-lasting effects. Anxieties about the well-being of a baby with a temporary disorder in the first day may result in long-lasting concerns that may cast long shadows and adversely shape the development of the child.

From Klaus MH, Kennell JH: Parent-Infant Bonding, 2nd ed. St. Louis, CV Mosby Co, 1982.

child individually, especially in the initial "getting acquainted" period. The nurse can help the parents to relate to each child as an individual, not as a unit, and to identify the unique physical and behavioral characteristics of each child. The individual reactions of each baby to the parents should be pointed out. Early contact with the babies, together and separately, which might include rooming-in, helps the mother gain confidence in caretaking and gets her acquainted with her babies. Antepartum ultrasound also can help the parents to recognize more than one baby and start the bonding process even before delivery. There are usually differences in the fetuses, even at this early age, in activity level and positioning that should be pointed out to the parents (Neifert and Thorpe, 1990).

Evans and associates (1972) further investigated the problems of this difficult simultaneous bonding and found that not only the process of attachment but also that of detachment cannot easily occur simultaneously (Evans et al, 1972). They found that if one baby dies, it is difficult to completely mourn that child while at the same time trying to attach to the survivor. (This same phenomenon can be observed if a mother quickly becomes pregnant after the loss of a neonate.) Evans and associates (1972) also found that one third of infants with failure-to-thrive that was not organic had parents who had recently suffered the loss of a close family member. He concluded that while they were grieving the loss, the parents could not adequately care for their newborns.

The nurse can care for the parents by encouraging the grieving process while helping the parents establish a relationship with their new baby. Kollantai and Fleischer (1989) have stated that mementos, including a picture of the parents that also includes both the twins, are very important to the parents. These photographs also may be used to help the sibling understand the loss. Parents should be encouraged to verbalize their feelings regarding the loss of one of their newborns. The grieving process will probably take longer, and it may take 3 to 5 years to incorporate the loss of this infant into the parents' lives (Sainsbury, 1987).

This grieving process has implications when one of the babies is sick or has congenital anomalies and the other is well. The parents do not have enough energy to mourn for the less-than-perfect child. Klaus and Kennell (1982) found that when one twin was sent home and the other was left to grow in the nursery, more mothering disorders were observed with the latter twin. Therefore, if possible, twins should be discharged together, either back to the referring hospital or to the home.

Singleton newborns develop one primary attachment to their mother, whereas twins form two early attachments—one to the mother and one to the other twin. Therefore, ongoing parenting should include assisting the children in separation from their sibling as well as their mother. It also should include assisting the children in perceiving themselves as separate and distinct. Siblings of the twins should be encouraged to interact with them as individuals (Neifert and Thorpe, 1990). To assist in this process, "parents should be discouraged from giving their babies rhyming names, dressing them alike, referring to them as the twins, and otherwise encouraging the blending of their identities" (Neifert and Thorpe, 1990).

There is a great need for support and education for parents in cases of multiple gestation. This process should start as soon as the diagnosis is made and continue well into the postpartum period.

## References

Addy HA: The breastfeeding of twins. Environ Child Health 21:231, 1975.

Alvarez M, Berkowitz R: Multifetal gestation. Clin Obstet Gynecol 33(1):79, 1990.

Barter RH, Hsu I, Ekkenbech RV, et al: The prevention of prematurity in multiple pregnancy. Am J Obstet Gynecol 91:787, 1965.

Benirschke K: The placenta in twin gestation. Clin Obstet Gynecol 33(1):18, 1990.

Benirschke K, Kim J: Multiple pregnancy. N Engl J Med 288:1276, 1973.

Benson CB, Doubilet PM: Sonography of multiple gestations. Radiol Clin North Am 286(1):149, 1990.

Benson CB, Doubilet PM: Ultrasound of multiple gestations. Semin Roentgenol 1:50, 1991.

Berkowitz RL, Lynch L, Chitkara U, et al: Selective reduction of multifetal pregnancies in the first trimester. N Engl J Med 318:1043, 1988.

Botting BP, McDonald-Davies I, McFarlane HA: Recent trends in the incidence of multiple births and associated mortality. Arch Dis Child 62:941, 1987.

Bowlby J: The nature of the child's tie to his mother. Int J Psychoanal 39:350, 1958.

Braly P, Freeman RK: The significance of fetal heart rate reactivity with a positive oxytocin challenge test. Obstet Gynecol 50:669, 1977.

Broadbent B: Multiple births: women's needs. Midwife Health Visitor Community Nurse 21:425–430, 1985.

Burke MS: Single fetal demise in twin gestation. Clin Obstet Gynecol 33(1):69, 1990.

Buttery B, Davison G: The ghost artifact. J Ultrasound Med 3:49, 1984.

Cattanach SA, Wedel M, White S, Young MB: Single intrauterine fetal death in a suspected monozagotic twin pregnancy. Aust NZ J Obstet Gynaecol 30:137, 1990.

Cetrulo CL, Ingardia CJ, Sbarra AJ: Management of multiple gestation. Clin Obstet Gynecol 23:536, 1980.

Coleman BG, Grumbach K, Arger P, et al: Twin gestation: monitoring of complications and anomalies by ultrasound. Radiology 165:449, 1987.

Cowett RM, Hakanson DO, Kocon RW: Untoward neonatal effect of intra-amniotic administration of methylene blue. Obstet Gynecol 43(suppl):74, 1974.

Crane JP: Sonographic evaluation of multiple pregnancy. Semin Ultrasound CT MR 5:144, 1984.

Crane JP, Tomich PG, Kopta M: Ultrasonic growth patterns in normal and discordant twins. Obstet Gynecol 55:678, 1980.

Cunningham FG, MacDonald PC, Gant NF: Williams Obstetrics, 18th ed. East Norwalk, CT, Appleton & Lange, 1989.

D'Alton ME, Mercer BM: Antepartum management of twin gestation: ultrasound. Clin Obstet Gynecol 33(1):42, 1990.

D'Alton ME, Newton Er, Cetrulo CL: Intrauterine fetal demise in multiple gestation. Acta Genet Med Gemellol, 33:43, 1984.

Dor J, Shalev S, Mashiach J, et al: Elective cervical

suture of twin pregnancies diagnosed ultrasonically in the first trimester following induced ovulation. Gynecol Obstet Invest 13:55, 1982.

Dudley DKL, D'Alton ME: Single fetal death in twin gestation. Semin Perinatol 10:65, 1986.

Eganhouse BJ: Fetal monitoring of twins. J Obstet Gynecol Neonatal Nurs 21(1):17, 1992.

Enbom JA: Twin pregnancy with intrauterine death of one twin. Am J Obstet Gynecol 152(4):424, 1985.

Evans MI, Fletcher JC, Zandor IE, Newton BW, Quigg MH, Struyk CD: Selective first-trimester termination in octuplet and quadruplet pregnancies: clinical and ethical issues. Obstet Gynecol 71:289, 1988.

Evans S, Reinhart JB, Succop RA: A study of 45 children and their families. J Am Acad Child Adolesc Psychiatry 11:440, 1972.

Evrard JR, Gold EM: Cesarean section for the delivery of the second twin. Obstet Gynecol 57:581, 1981.

Farooqui MO, Grossman JH III, Shannon RA: A review of twin pregnancies. Obstet Gynecol Surv 28:144, 1973.

Friedman EA, Sachtleben MR: Relative birth weights of twins. Obstet Gynecol 49:717, 1977.

Garoff L, Seppala M: Alpha fetoprotein and human placental lactogen levels in maternal serum in multiple pregnancies. J Obstet Gynaecol Br Commonw 80:695, 1973.

Goshen-Gottstein E: The mothering of twins, triplets, and quadruplets. Psychiatry 43:189, 1980.

Hack M, Brish M, Serr DM, et al: Outcome of pregnancy after induced ovulation. Follow-up of pregnancies and children after clomiphene therapy. JAMA 220:1329, 1972.

Hawrylyshyn PA, Barkin M, Bernstein A, et al: Twin pregnancies—a continuing perinatal challenge. Obstet Gynecol 59:463, 1982.

Hellman LM, Koboyashi M, Cromb E: Ultrasonic diagnosis of embryonic malformations. Am J Obstet Gynecol 115:615, 1973.

Holeberg G, Biale Y, Lewenthal H, et al: Outcome of pregnancy in 31 triplet gestations. Obstet Gynecol 59:472, 1982.

Hollenbach KA, Hickok DE: Epidemiology and diagnosis of twin gestation. Clin Obstet Gynecol 33(1):3, 1990.

Hunter LP: Twin gestation: antepartum management. J Perinat Neonatal Nurs 3(1):1, 1989.

Iffy L, Kaminetzky H: Principles and Practice of Obstetrics and Perinatology, vol 2. New York, John Wiley & Sons, 1981, p 1172.

Itzkowicz D: A survey of 59 triplet pregnancies. Br J Obstet Gynaecol 86:23, 1979.

Jarvis GJ: Diagnosis of multiple pregnancy. Br Med J 2:593, 1979.

Jeffrey RL, Bowes WA, DeLaney JJ: Role of bedrest in twin gestation. Obstet Gynecol 43:822, 1974.

Johnson JWC, Hustink L, Jones GS, et al: Efficacy of 17-alphahydroxyprogesterone caproate in the prevention of premature labor. N Engl J Med 293:675, 1975.

Jones JM, Sbarra AJ, Cetrulo CL: Antepartum management of twin gestation. Clin Obstet Gynecol 33(1):32, 1990.

Jouppila P, Kauppila A, Kovisto M, et al: Twin pregnancy—the role of active management during pregnancy and delivery. Acta Obstet Gynecol Scand 44:13, 1975.

Kelsik F, Minkoff H: Management of breech second twin. Am J Obstet Gynecol 144:783, 1982.

Kistner KW: Induction of ovulation with clomiphene citrate. In Bertram SJ, Kistner KW (eds): Progress in Infertility. Boston, Little, Brown & Co, 1968, p 407.

Klaus MH, Kennell JH: Parent-Infant Bonding, 2nd ed. St Louis, CV Mosby Co, 1982.

Kollantai J, Fleischer L: Parents who have lost one twin respond (Letter to the Editor). J Perinat Neonatal Nurs 3:1, 1989.

Laube DW: Multiple pregnancy, operative delivery, anesthesia, and analgesia. Curr Opin Obstet Gynecol 2:40, 1990.

Laursen B: Twin pregnancy. Acta Obstet Gynecol Scand 52:367, 1973.

Leveno K, Santos-Ramos R, Duen Hoelter J, et al: Sonar cephalometery in twins: a table of biparietal diameters for normal twin fetuses and a comparison with singletons. Am J Obstet Gynecol 135:727, 1979.

Leveno K, Santos-Ramos R, Duen Hoelter J, et al: Sonar cephalometery in twins: discordancy of the biparietal diameter after twenty-eight weeks of gestation. Am J Obstet Gynecol 138:615, 1980.

MacLennan AH, Green RC, O'Shea R, et al: Routine hospital admission in twin pregnancy between 26 and 30 weeks' gestation. Lancet 335:268, 1990.

Malgar CA, Rosenfeld DL, Rawlinson K, Greenberg M: Perinatal outcome after multifetal reduction to twins compared with nonreduced mutiple gestations. Obstet Gynecol 78:763, 1991.

Manning FA, Morrison I, Lange IR, et al: Fetal Biophysical Scoring: Selective use of the nonstress test. Am J Obstet Gynecol 156:709, 1987.

Michaels WH, Schrieber FR, Padgett RJ, Ager J, Pieper D: Ultrasound surveillance of the cervix in twin gestations: management of cervical incompetency. Obstet Gynecol 78:739, 1991.

Misenhimer HR, Kaltreider DF: Effects of decreased prenatal activity in patients with twin pregnancy. Obstet Gynecol 51:692, 1978.

Naeye RL, Tafari N, Judge D, et al: Twins: causes of perinatal death in 12 United States cities and one African city. Am J Obstet Gynecol 31:267, 1978.

Neifert M, Seacat J: Milk yield and prolactin rise with simultaneous breast pumping. Presented at the annual meeting of the Ambulatory Pediatric Association. Washington, DC, May, 1985.

Neifert M, Thorpe J: Twins: family adjustment, parenting, and infant feeding in the fourth trimester. Clin Obstet Gynecol 33(1):102, 1990.

Neilson P: Prenatal diagnosis in twins. Curr Opin Obstet Gynecol 4:280, 1992.

O'Brien WF, Knuppel RA, Scerbo J, Rattan PK: Birth weight in twins: an analysis of discordancy and growth retardation. Obstet Gynecol 67:483, 1986.

O'Connor MC, Murphy H, Dalrymple IJ: Double blind trial of ritodrine and placebo in twin pregnancy. Br J Obstet Gynaecol 86:706, 1979.

O'Connor MC, Arias E, Royston JP: The merits of special antenatal care for twin pregnancies. Br J Obstet Gynecol 88:222, 1981.

Patten RM, Mack LA, Harvey D, Cyr DR, Pretorius DH: Disparity of amniotic fluid volume and fetal size: problem of the stuck twin—US studies. Radiology 172(1):153, 1989.

Persson PH, Grennert L, Gennser G, et al: An improved outcome of twin pregnancies. Acta Obstet Gynecol Scand 58:3, 1979.

Power WF: Bedrest in twin pregnancy: identification of a critical period. Obstet Gynecol 42:795, 1973.

Pritchard JA, MacDonald PC (eds): Multifetal pregnancy. In Williams Obstetrics, 16th ed. New York, Appleton-Century-Crofts, 1980, p 639.

Roberts RB: Infant weights in multiple births. Obstet Gynecol 47:382, 1976.

Robertson JG: Twin pregnancies. Obstet Gynecol 91:787, 1965.

Robinson HP, Caines JS: Sonar evidence of early pregnancy and failure in patients with twin conceptions. Br J Obstet Gynecol 84:22, 1977.

Sainsbury M: Unique aspects of grief in multifetal demise. Read before the National Mothers of Twins Convention, Anaheim, CA, July 29, 1987.

Samuels P: Ultrasound in the management of the twin gestation. Clin Obstet Gynecol 31(1):110, 1988.

Schenker JG, Yarkoni S, Gronat M: Multiple pregnancy following induction of ovulation. Fertil Steril 35:105, 1981.

Seeds JW, Cefalo RC: Malpresentations. Clin Obstet Gynecol 25:145, 1982.

Sims CD, Cowan DB, Parkinson CE: The lecithin/sphingomyelin (L/S) ratio in twin pregnancies. Br J Obstet Gynaecol 83:447, 1976.

Socol ML, Tamura RK, Sabbagha RE, et al: Diminished biparietal diameter and abdominal circumference growth in twins. Obstet Gynecol 64:235, 1984.

Spellacy WH, Cruz AC, Buhi WC, et al: Amniotic fluid L/S ratio in twin gestation. Obstet Gynecol 50:68, 1977.

Speroff L, Glass RH, Kaso NG: Clinical Gynecological Endocrinology and Infertility, 2nd ed. Baltimore, Williams & Wilkins, 1981.

Theroux R: Multiple birth: a unique parenting experience. J Perinat Neonatal Nurs 3(1):35, 1989.

Tyson J, Freedman R, Perez A, Zacurit, Zanartu J: Breastfeeding and the mother. In CIBA Foundation Symposium No 45. London, CIBA Foundation, 1976.

Van den Veyver E, Schatteman E, Vanderheyden JS, Van Wiemeersch J, Meulyzer P: Antenatal fetal death in twin pregnancies: a dangerous condition mainly for the surviving co-twin; a report of four cases. European J Obstet Gynecol Reprod Biol 38:69, 1990.

Verduzco R, Rosario R, Rigatto H: Hyaline membrane disease in twins. Am J Obstet Gynecol 125:668, 1976.

Ware HH: The second twin. Am J Obstet Gynecol 110:865, 1971.

Weekes AR, Menzies DN, DeBoer CH: The relative efficacy of bedrest, cervical suture and no management of twin pregnancy. Br J Obstet Gynaecol 84:161, 1977.

Winter RM, Knowles SAS, Bieber FR, et al: Biology and Pathology of Twinning in the Malformed Fetus and Stillbirth. Chichester, John Wiley & Sons, 1988 p 219.

# CHAPTER 25

. . . . . . . . . . . . . . . . . . . . . . . . . . . . . . . . . . . . . . . . .

# Hypertension in Pregnancy

Robert A. Knuppel and Joan Drukker

The term toxemia of pregnancy was formerly applied to a number of conditions manifesting vascular derangements that arise either during pregnancy or during the early peurperal period. These conditions were characterized by hypertension and other signs. Unfortunately, the term toxemia was all-inclusive; thus, discrepancies in statistical reporting occurred, making it extremely difficult to evaluate the results obtained with different treatment programs. These problems highlight only a few of the controversies surrounding the data supporting the empirical management of preeclampsia-eclampsia and chronic hypertension. Despite 40 years of intensive research, the etiology of preeclampsia-eclampsia is still unknown, and epidemiologic surveys remain clouded in the shroud of confounding variables (Chesley, 1978; Friedman, 1976). This chapter discusses preeclampsia, eclampsia, chronic hypertension, and chronic hypertension with superimposed preeclampsia.

## Terminology

In 1972, the Committee on Terminology of the American College of Obstetricians and Gynecologists, after careful consideration and consultation with authorities in the field, suggested a classification for the group of conditions hitherto loosely referred to as toxemias of pregnancy; this is shown in Table 25–1 (Page and Christianson, 1976).

The term toxemia has been in widespread use for so long that probably the best we can

hope for is the adoption of one inclusive term, with preeclampsia and eclampsia used to designate the two clinical phases of the same disorder. A recent modification in terminology suggests the overall designation gestational edema–proteinuria–hypertensive disorders (GEPH), with the recommendation that no preeclampsia be considered mild. Hypertension complicated by pregnancy is synonymous with the chronic hypertensive state, which is different from the elevated blood pressure in GEPH.

This chapter uses the terms preeclampsia, eclampsia, chronic hypertension, and superimposed preeclampsia, as referred to in the 1972 terminology report mentioned above and defined in Table 25–1.

## Preeclampsia-Eclampsia

### THE CLASSIC TRIAD: HYPERTENSION, EDEMA, AND PROTEINURIA

#### Hypertension

Hypertension is a measurable sign of preeclampsia. Hypertension is a rise in the systolic pressure (SP) of at least 30 mm Hg, a rise in the diastolic pressure (DP) of at least 15 mm Hg, or a diastolic pressure of at least 90 mm Hg. A blood pressure of 140/90 mm Hg represents a mean arterial pressure (MAP) of 107 mm Hg. The MAP is an indicator of cardiac work, for it measures the resistance against which the heart works. The

**Table 25–1**
CLASSIFICATION OF "TOXEMIAS OF PREGNANCY"

| | |
|---|---|
| **Gestational Edema** | The occurrence of a general and excessive accumulation of fluid in the tissues of greater than 1+ pitting edema after 12 hours in bed, or of a weight gain of 5 lb or more in 1 week due to the influence of pregnancy. |
| **Gestational Proteinuria** | The presence of proteinuria during or under the influence of pregnancy, in the absence of hypertension, edema, renal infection, or known intrinsic renovascular disease. |
| **Gestational Hypertension** | The development of hypertension during pregnancy or within the first 24 hours postpartum, in a previously normotensive woman. No other evidence of preeclampsia or hypertensive vascular disease is present. The blood pressure returns to normotensive levels within 10 days following parturition. Some patients with gestational hypertension may in fact have preeclampsia or hypertensive vascular disease, but they do not satisfy the criteria for either of these diagnoses. |
| **Preeclampsia** | The development of hypertension with proteinuria, edema, or both, due to pregnancy or the influence of a recent pregnancy. It occurs after the 20th week of gestation, but it may develop before this time in the presence of trophoblastic disease or isoimmunization. Preeclampsia is predominantly a disorder of primigravidas. |
| **Eclampsia** | The occurrence of one or more convulsions, not attributable to other cerebral conditions such as epilepsy or cerebral hemorrhage, in a patient with preeclampsia. |
| **Superimposed Preeclampsia or Eclampsia** | The development of preeclampsia or eclampsia in a patient with chronic hypertensive vascular or renal disease. Occurs when the hypertension antedates the pregnancy, as established by previous blood pressure readings, or when there is a rise in the systolic pressure of 30 mm Hg and/or a rise in the diastolic pressure of 15 mm Hg, and the development of proteinuria or edema, or both. |
| **Chronic Hypertensive Disease** | The presence of persistent hypertension, from whatever cause, before pregnancy or before the 20th week of gestation, or persistent hypertension beyond the 42nd postpartum day. |
| **Unclassified Hypertensive Disorders** | Those in which information is insufficient for classification. They should compose a minority of the hypertensive disorders of pregnancy. |

MAP is calculated by adding the DP to one third of the pulse pressure:

$$MAP = DP + \left[ \frac{(SP - DP)}{3} \right].$$

Page and Christianson (1976) believe that a rise of 20 mm Hg in the MAP is ominous and that MAP of 100 is abnormal. MAP of 105 indicates hypertension. The blood pressures cited above must be manifested on two occasions at least 6 hours apart and should be judged on the basis of *previously known blood pressure levels*. Ideally, baseline blood pressures should be established early in the first trimester.

Attempts to standardize techniques for obtaining blood pressure levels have been unsuccessful. Patients in a supine position can develop the supine hypotensive syndrome, resulting in falsely low values. Even in the lateral position, when the blood pressure is taken in the upper arm, the systolic and diastolic measurements are usually falsely low (10 to 20 mm Hg) owing to hydrostatic pressure (Fleming et al, 1983; Gallery et al, 1977; Redman et al, 1977; Reiss et al, 1987; Sibai, 1988; Wichman et al, 1984). When standing, the systolic and diastolic pressures are significantly higher than when sitting (Wichman et al, 1984). There is an increase of systolic and diastolic pressures when the arm is held in a dependent position rather than at heart level (Webster et al, 1984). Sibai (1988) recommends the blood pressure be taken in a sitting position with the arm supported in a horizontal position at heart level. Standardization of position for recording a blood pressure should be maintained from the outpatient to the inpatient departments. Ideally, patients who have hypertension as outpatients should have their blood pressures checked in the hospital in a similar standardized fashion.

There continues to be a controversy about whether Korotkoff's fifth phase (the disappearance of sound) correlates better with the true diastolic pressure than does the fourth phase (muffling). Most American authorities use the fifth phase, whereas many investigators and some clinicians use the fourth phase, because the complete disappearance of sound fails to occur in many pregnant women. Korotkoff's fourth phase is approximately 5 to 10 mm Hg higher than the fifth phase (Sibai, 1988). However, it is much more difficult to educate observers to record the fourth phase, and this difficulty is reflected in a large variance of fourth phase pressure readings; thus, this chapter refers to the fifth phase method. Furthermore, the physiologic reduction in the mean arterial pressure during weeks 8 to 30 of gestation underlines the importance of having an accurate record of first trimester blood pressure evaluations.

The cuff of the sphygmomanometer can be another confounding variable in epidemiologic evaluation. The cuff must be wide enough and long enough for the blood pressure to be assessed accurately. A small cuff gives a falsely high reading, and a cuff that is too large gives a falsely low reading (Sibai, 1988; Wheeler and Jones, 1981). Many other studies have called into question the sensitivity and specificity of single measurements and recommend that two blood pressure measurements be obtained 6 hours apart to ensure that the abnormal reading is accurate. Other factors also may influence blood pressure readings (Table 25–2).

Data from over 50,000 pregnancies have shown that a maternal blood pressure as low as 125/75 mm Hg is ominous if it occurs before the 32nd week of gestation or exceeds 84 mm Hg thereafter (Friedman, 1976). However, each case must be treated individually, because a blood pressure level of 140/90 mm Hg in a patient whose pressure is usually 134/84 is less significant than is a pressure of 140/90 mm Hg in a patient whose usual level is 110/70 mm Hg. The *degree of elevation* is more important than the absolute value.

An important feature of preeclampsia is the variance of *nocturnal hypertension* (Redman et al, 1976). During pregnancy, there appears to be a reversal of the nor-

**Table 25–2**
FACTORS THAT MAY INFLUENCE BLOOD PRESSURE READINGS

Type of equipment
Faulty equipment
  Not calibrated
  Leaks
  Faulty control valves
Size of cuff
Exercise
Duration of rest period before assessment
Pain
Posture of patient
Position of arm
Korotkoff phase used—4 or 5
Environmental factors
  Noise in the room
Tight clothing
Anxiety
Smoking (wait at least 10 minutes after smoking to measure blood pressure)

Adapted from Sibai BM: Pitfalls in diagnosis and management of preeclampsia. Am J Obstet Gynecol 159:1, 1988.

mal diurnal-nocturnal pattern. Normally, in the nonpregnant state, the lowest blood pressures are found during sleep; however, because in pregnancy the reverse is true, any regimen of hypotensive therapy in preeclampsia should be scheduled to have the maximum effect during the nocturnal hours of sleep, when the blood pressure is higher.

The critical blood pressure at which an individual will develop permanent vascular damage is unknown. Although direct evidence is lacking, it has been found experimentally that arterial damage can occur rapidly. In women with severe preeclampsia, examination of the optic fundi reveals segmental arteriolar constriction and dilatation that are indistinguishable from the changes observed in experimental hypertensive encephalopathy. Preeclampsia does not cause chronic arteriolar changes; thus, the presence of arteriolar sclerosis detected by increased light reflex, copper wiring, or arteriovenous nicking indicates pre-existing vascular disease (Creasy and Resnik, 1989). Hypotensive agents may prevent this damage. Blood pressure levels of 170 to 180 over 110 to 120 mm Hg (MAP of 130 to 140 mm Hg) are similar to those at which acute vascular damage occurs experimentally. A blood pressure of 160/110 is the critical level at which antihypertensive agents are needed for the urgent reduction of the blood pressure.

Unfortunately, at the present time, it is

not known whether or not suppression of hypertension ameliorates the underlying disorder; thus, the disease may progress despite antihypertensive treatment and bed rest. Therefore, even if apparent control of blood pressure has been achieved, the fetus must be monitored for uteroplacental insufficiency and the mother must continually be observed for disseminated intravascular coagulation, excessive weight gain, renal failure, and central nervous system irritability.

## Edema

Edema has traditionally been described as the earliest sign of developing preeclampsia. However, edema by itself is a common symptom of pregnancy. Edema is a general and excessive accumulation of fluid in the tissues, generally demonstrated by the swelling of the extremities and face. Edema of the face and hands may be a better indicator of preeclampsia because it is associated with sodium retention rather than dependent edema, which is caused by hydrostatic mechanisms (Creasy and Resnick, 1989). The fluid may be intracellular or extracellular, and edema usually is not demonstrated until there is a weight gain of 10 percent from the prepregnancy weight. Edema is usually physiologic, but when it occurs in association with hypertension and proteinuria, the perinatal mortality rate is increased. When vasoconstriction occurs, it can cause a decrease of oxygen and glucose to the body tissues. When this occurs, there is a shift of fluid, especially blood plasma, from the circulation to the body tissues. As the intravascular volume shifts, edema can be seen and there is a rise in hemoconcentration demonstrated by an increased hematocrit.

Edema might be a protective mechanism against the development of preeclampsia. Approximately 85 percent of patients who develop generalized edema have normal pregnancies; only about 15 percent develop preeclampsia. Edema is, thus, a very rough clinical parameter and can reflect changes that are nonpathologic. The Perinatal Task Force on Preeclampsia demonstrated a relatively greater incidence of edema among white (39.8 percent) than among black gravidas (23.3 percent). The perinatal mortality rate of 25.4:1000 for offspring of mothers who manifested edema alone was significantly lower than the rate of 32.8:1000 among those without edema. This relationship was observed both in white and in black gravidas. Moreover, edema and high blood pressure were unrelated in white nulliparas (Fig. 25–1). In light of these considerations, we should reassess our previous commitment to the traditional but purely arbitrary standards. Perhaps edema should be deleted from the clinical triad of preeclampsia. It is important, however, not to confuse edema with excessive weight gain (Fig. 25–2). Sibai (1988) reported that 40 percent of patients with eclampsia at the University of Tennessee did not demonstrate edema before the onset of seizures. He, therefore, recommends that presence of edema should not be used as an indication in the diagnosis of preeclampsia.

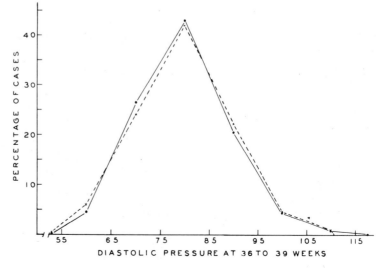

Figure 25–1. Frequency distribution of diastolic blood pressures recorded between 36 and 39 weeks in white nulliparas without proteinuria. Continuous line indicates women with edema, and broken line women without edema. (From Chesley LC: Classification. *In* Friedman EA [ed]: Blood Pressure, Edema and Proteinuria in Pregnancy. New York, Alan R Liss, 1976. Copyright © 1976. Reprinted by permission of Wiley-Liss, A Division of John Wiley and Sons, Inc.)

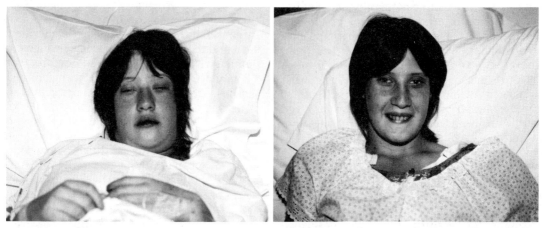

**Figure 25–2.** The patient (*left*) developed severe preeclampsia at 34 weeks' gestation. She gained 10 pounds during the week previous to her admission. She developed central edema, and shortly after this photograph was taken had a respiratory arrest. Her appearance changed markedly by her fourth day postpartum (*right*). (Photographs courtesy of Dr. Gary Cohen, University of South Florida College of Medicine, Tampa, FL.)

The belief that treating edema will prevent toxemia is invalid. In fact, the use of diuretics may be harmful. They reduce the metabolic clearance rate of dehydroisoandrosterone sulfate in relation to maternal weight loss. Because diuretics decrease plasma volume, the decrease in the metabolic clearance rate of dehydroisoandrosterone sulfate probably reflects reduced placental perfusion (Gant et al, 1975). Both of these factors (i.e., decreased plasma volume and reduced uteroplacental perfusion) are believed to be important in the pathogenesis of preeclampsia-eclampsia, so that administration of diuretics actually may predispose the patients to the disease. These considerations and others generally contraindicate the use of diuretics in pregnancy unless there are other compelling reasons for their use or if future research suggests benefit.

## Proteinuria

Proteinuria is usually the last of the triad to appear. Proteinuria is the presence of urinary protein in concentrations greater than 300 mg/liter in a 24-hour collection or in a concentration greater than 1 + or 2 + by standard turbidimetric methods (dipstick) on two or more occasions at least 6 hours apart. The urine must be a clean-voided midstream specimen or one obtained by catheterization. Proteinuria may be the most ominous sign of preeclampsia. A combination of 2 + proteinuria (1 g/liter) and hypertension at least doubles the perinatal mortality rate (deAlvarez, 1976). Edema with proteinuria also increases perinatal risks (Vosburgh, 1976). If the specimen is not contaminated, 1 + proteinuria (300 mg/liter) should be considered significant, particularly with a diastolic blood pressure of 85 mm Hg or higher.

The finding of proteinuria may help to differentiate preeclampsia from other disorders of pregnancy. Also, quantitative and qualitative urinalyses may help to differentiate preeclampsia and eclampsia from other disorders in which proteinuria may occur. In orthostatic proteinuria, the commonly used 24-hour sample demonstrates 1 or 2 g per 24-hour collection, whereas the nephrotic syndrome is indicated by a loss of 10 to 15 g/day. The usual protein content in a 24-hour specimen is 0.3 to 2 g in mild preeclampsia. Proteinuria is greatest during the most severe episodes of the process. The standard definition, in the United States, for diagnosing severe preeclampsia is protein content greater than 5 g/day. However, the standard is much lower in studies from outside the United States, ranging from 0.5 to 5 g/day (Sibai, 1988). Proteinuria reduces the concentrations of the various serum proteins. In fractionation of the proteinuria in severe toxemia, albumin accounts for 50 to 60 percent of the total protein excreted. This may also account for hypoalbuminemia consistently below the level for a normal pregnancy of the same duration. Because of the increased loss of $\alpha_2$-globulin in the urine at the height of preeclampsia, angiotensinase is lost at a greater rate than with a normal pregnancy (deAlvarez, 1976), thus supporting the vasospastic influence of angiotensin II. Chesley (1978) reported that 26 of 199 eclamptic patients had either a trace of or no proteinuria prior to seizures.

## INCIDENCE AND IMPORTANCE

Approximately 10 percent of Americans have hypertension. Approximately 20 to 40 percent of women with chronic renal or vascular disease, such as essential hypertension, diabetes mellitus, and lupus erythematosus, develop preeclampsia (Scott et al, 1990). In the United States, preeclampsia complicates about 1.5 percent of pregnancies among women receiving care from private physicians. However, there is a 15 percent incidence among patients of low socioeconomic status giving birth in public and teaching hospitals. Thus, the overall rate of occurrence in the United States is approximately 5 to 7 percent (Creasy and Resnik, 1989). In general, preeclampsia is a disease of the first pregnancy and tends to beset women who are pregnant for the first time after the age of 25.

Chesley and Cooper (1986) and Sutherland and associates (1981) have established that preeclampsia is a recessive single gene trait. Preeclampsia is demonstrated in 5 percent of the general population during the first viable pregnancy. It is seen in 22 percent of daughters of preeclamptic women and in 35 percent of sisters of preeclamptic women.

Sutherland and associates (1981) also reported that 15 percent of mothers of preeclamptic women had preeclampsia, whereas only 4 percent of their mother-in-laws had preeclampsia. Adams and Finlayson (1961) reported a four times higher incidence of preeclampsia in sisters of women who had the disease. O'Brien (1990) stated that "a nullipara whose sister demonstrated preeclampsia has about a one-hundredfold higher risk of preeclampsia than a multipara whose mother and sister have remained normotensive."

The diagnosis may be complicated by the fact that the mean blood pressure tends to rise with increasing age. If the prepregnancy blood pressure is unknown, the differential diagnosis between preeclampsia and preeclampsia superimposed on chronic hypertension cannot be made with certainty. Preeclampsia-eclampsia has its highest incidence among groups of women who have a high predilection for hypertension. Thus, the incidence of preeclampsia and eclampsia is always higher among blacks than among whites. Few studies, however, have corrected for the higher prevalence of essential hypertension in the black population.

The incidence of preeclampsia is higher in women who have received little or no prenatal care (Sachs et al, 1987). Therefore, more accessible prenatal care would increase early detection of this disease and decrease maternal and fetal morbidity and mortality.

Preeclampsia-eclampsia is an important entity for several reasons:

1. It is a major cause of perinatal mortality.
2. It is the second leading cause of maternal deaths in the United States.
3. It is often associated with intrauterine fetal growth retardation.
4. It is associated with an increased tendency toward mental retardation in surviving offspring.

## ETIOLOGY AND PATHOGENESIS

Study of the etiology and pathogenesis of preeclampsia-eclampsia has focused on six major factors:

1. *Immunologic phenomena:* Interest in this aspect has been lacking until recently, when immunofluorescent studies identified immunoglobulins in the tissues of women with preeclampsia-eclampsia. This is the most promising research frontier for finding the etiology of preeclampsia.

2. *Dietary factors:* The geographic distribution of eclampsia suggests that diet plays an important part in the etiology. Various dietary factors have been incriminated, including deficiencies of protein, thiamine, calcium, iron, and vitamins, and excesses of carbohydrate and sodium.

3. *Endocrine dysfunction:* During normal pregnancy, enlargement of the anterior pituitary, adrenal, thyroid, and parathyroid glands occurs. Interference with hormonal activity or metabolism by the developing placenta has also been noted.

4. *Toxic manifestations:* Water intoxication and other miscellaneous agents have been incriminated.

5. *Hemodynamic hypotheses:* Preeclampsia and placenta praevia rarely coexist. It has been suggested that when the placenta is implanted in the upper uterine segment, much of the venous blood returns to the heart via the ovarian veins. In traversing this route, the additional blood volume encourages congestion of the renal, hepatic, and cerebral venous systems, resulting in hypoxic changes. Another hemodynamic theory is that the cause of toxemia is hypovolemia, which leads to a hypoperfusion syndrome.

In normal pregnancy, the spiral arteries are eroded by the invading trophoblast as uteroplacental circulation is established. This process decreases the content of neurotransmitters, causing a functional degeneration that decreases uterine vascular tone and maximum dilatation. In preeclampsia, there is less erosion and, therefore, the spiral arteries are thicker and narrower with higher vascular tone. This decreases blood flow through the intervillous space and can cause intrauterine growth retardation (IUGR) and hypoxia (Walsh, 1990).

The weight of evidence suggests that hypovolemia, like disseminated intravascular coagulation, plays an important part in pathogenesis but is not the primary cause of preeclampsia-eclampsia.

6. *Uterine stretch reflex:* It has been suggested that the resistance of the myometrium to stretching initiates a uterorenal reflex and results in renal cortical ischemia. This, in turn, has been said to result in generalized vasoconstriction, with hypertension, proteinuria, and edema as the major clinical manifestations. Although this theory is appealing, because of the association between toxemia and such factors as multiple pregnancy, the weight of experimental evidence of pathogenesis is against it.

Preeclampsia has a geographic distribution that is not entirely related to the quality of obstetric care and is sometimes seen *de novo* in the immediate postpartum period. Misenhimer and associates (1970) reported on an experimental model of chronically impaired uterine artery flow in the rhesus monkey. These workers did not measure blood pressure, but angiographic studies showed a marked reduction in intervillous space in-

flow in some animals; the fetal mortality rate was 60 percent, with all deaths occurring near the beginning of the third trimester of pregnancy.

If the uteroplacental blood flow is decreased, the uterine renin-angiotensin system is activated. There is some evidence that plasma-renin levels are higher in the uterine vein than in the peripheral circulation in preeclampsia. Thus, the release of angiotensin II from the uterus, stimulated by a decrease in uteroplacental blood flow, may explain the apparent paradox of low renin-angiotensin levels in this condition.

Cavanagh and associates (1974; 1977) conducted a multidisciplinary program with the aim of developing a toxemia model in a subhuman primate. The baboon was used in these studies because the reproductive physiology of baboons is remarkably similar to that of human subjects. When the ovarian arteries were transected in pregnant animals, hypertension, proteinuria, and reduced renal artery flow followed. The same sequelae were observed in those animals whose uterine arteries had been partially occluded by metal clips prior to conception. Subsequently, 50 percent occlusion of aortic blood flow produced the same changes. In addition, fibrin-fibrinogen deposits were detected in pregnant study animals by immunofluorescence, although no evidence of disseminated intravascular coagulation could be found in those baboons whose coagulation profiles were studied. Investigations by light microscopy, electron microscopy, and immunofluorescence revealed the renal lesions in the toxemic baboon to be indistinguishable from those in women with preeclampsia-eclampsia.

At present, it appears that uteroplacental ischemia is the trigger mechanism for initiating toxemia, not only in the rabbit and dog but also in the primate experimental model. Immunologic mechanisms may play a critical role. If blocking antibodies develop against antigenic sites on the placenta, the risk of pregnancy-induced hypertension is increased. Present evidence suggests that a different mate may make a multigravid patient react as a primigravida in regard to the risk of preeclampsia (Scott and Freeney, 1980).

Some important features in the pathogenesis of preeclampsia are presented in Figure 25–3 and Table 25–3.

Walsh (1985) described an imbalance in pros-

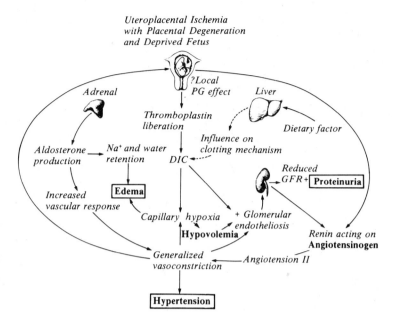

Figure 25–3. The presumed pathologic mechanism of eclamptogenic toxemia. (From Cavanagh D, Woods RE, O'Connor LCF, Knuppel RA: Obstetric Emergencies, 3rd ed. New York, Harper & Row, 1982.)

tacyclin and thromboxane in preeclamptic women. Prostacyclin decreases blood pressure, prevents platelet aggregation, and promotes uterine blood flow because it is a potent vasodilator, inhibitor of platelet aggregation, and inhibitor of uterine contractility (Walsh, 1990). It has been well documented that prostacyclin is decreased in preeclampsia (Bussolino et al, 1980; Downing et al, 1980; Friedman, 1988; Remuzzi et al, 1980; Romero, 1988; Walsh, 1986; Walsh, 1987). A deficiency would contribute to the symptoms of preeclampsia. Prostacyclin probably acts locally through the "paracrine mechanism between endothelial cells and the vascular smooth muscle to relax the blood vessels in which it is produced" (Walsh, 1990). It may not be a circulating hormone.

Thromboxane, on the other hand, is a potent vasoconstrictor, stimulator of platelet aggregation, and stimulator of uterine activity that opposes the action of prostacyclin. Thromboxane, if unopposed, may increase

**Table 25–3**

IMPORTANT OBSERVATIONS
IN PREECLAMPSIA

The trophoblast plays a role. When abundant trophoblast is present (mole, twins), there is an increased incidence of preeclampsia.
When the placenta is removed, the disease abates.
There is an increased risk in preexisting vascular disease.
There is a genetic or familial predisposition.

blood pressure and platelet aggregation and decrease uteroplacental blood flow. Therefore, an imbalance of these hormones, found in the placenta, favoring thromboxane leads to symptoms of preeclampsia. Walsh (1985) found that there were approximately equal amounts of prostacyclin and thromboxane in placentas from normal, uncomplicated pregnancies. Because these hormones are partially produced by the placenta, this would also help to explain the withdrawal of symptoms when the placenta is delivered.

Low doses of aspirin (baby aspirin), 60 to 81 mg/day, which inhibit thromboxane, are being used to treat preeclampsia. The low-dose aspirin acts on the maternal vasculature by making it less sensitive to vasopressors. This decreases systolic, diastolic, and mean blood pressure, as well as reduces proteinuria. Inhibiting thromboxane has been preferential over increasing prostacyclin, because prostacyclin has a potent systemic vasodilator effect and outcomes have not been as successful with this treatment.

Thromboxane therapy should be started at about 30 to 36 weeks' gestation or when tests such as the roll-over test indicate a tendency for preeclampsia. Women whose mothers or sisters had preeclampsia or eclampsia could also benefit from this treatment. This may be before preeclampsia symptoms are present (O'Brien, 1990). Schiff (1989) found that when 791 women were screened for preeclampsia with the roll-over test, 69 had a positive test. During the third trimester, 34 women were treated with low-dose aspirin and 31 with a placebo. Four developed preeclampsia with protein on low-dose aspirin and 11 developed it with the placebo. An additional advantage of thromboxane therapy is that it ameliorates or corrects decreased growth in fetuses suffering from intrauterine growth retardation. This has been demonstrated by increased fetal, neonatal, and placental growth as well as increased umbilical-placental blood flow and perfusion. There has also been an increase of pregnancies that advance to term and, therefore, a decreased need for neonatal intensive care (Ballerini et al, 1989; Benigni et al, 1989; Elder et al, 1988; Frusca et al, 1989; Gastaldi et al, 1988; Kopernick et al, 1988; Schiff et al, 1989; Trudinger et al, 1988a; Trudinger et al, 1988b; Wallenburg, 1988; Wallenburg and Rotmans, 1987).

Although higher doses of aspirin have been associated with closure of the ductus arteriosus, low-dose aspirin therapy does not appear to cause this neonatal problem. There are no neonatal bleeding problems nor have there been any fetal or neonatal deaths. Several authors have reported that there are no adverse affects on the fetus or neonate (Ballerini et al, 1989; Benigni et al, 1989; Gastaldi et al, 1988; Giannatlasio et al, 1988; Louden et al, 1988; Schiff et al, 1989; Sibai et al, 1989; Wallenburg, 1986; Wallenburg et al, 1987).

Calcium may also play a role in preeclampsia, because decreased urinary calcium occurs in women who are otherwise asymptomatic and who will later develop preeclampsia (Sanchez-Ramos et al, 1991a; Sanchez-Ramos, et al, 1991b). This is probably due to tubular reabsorption of calcium in those women who become preeclamptic (Taufield et al, 1987).

## PATHOLOGY

Donnelly and Lock (1954) investigated the cause of death in 533 women with toxemia of pregnancy and found that death was directly attributable to the disease in 393 cases. The most common causes of death were cerebral vascular accidents, cardiopulmonary insufficiency, and acute renal failure.

The characteristic lesion in preeclampsia-eclampsia is a renal glomerular endotheliosis. The endothelial cells are swollen, and the amorphous material deposited in the cytoplasm causes enlargement of the capillary tufts. The lumens of the glomerular capillaries become narrow so that ischemia is the result of organic narrowing as well as vasospasm. These changes presumably reduce the glomerular blood flow and the glomerular filtration rate (GFR). This can be a decrease of 25 percent in mild disease to 50 percent in severe cases (Gabbe et al, 1986). Immunofluorescent techniques have been used to demonstrate the presence of fibrin-fibrinogen immunoglobulins and complement in the glomerular mesangium of the capillary vessel walls. Renal tubules usually show abnormalities consistent with ischemia, and proteinaceous material often is noted within the tubular lumens. In women who survive, complete repair of the glomerular lesion following pregnancy is the rule. However, some patients show evidence of glomerular damage months or even years after delivery. Severe renal involvement may produce extensive arterial thrombosis resulting in bilateral renal cortical necrosis. This is especially likely to occur in patients with preeclampsia-eclampsia complicated by abruptio placentae. Serum creatine rarely is elevated; however, uric acid commonly is increased (Gabbe, 1986).

Significant liver damage may occur in pregnancy-induced hypertension. In eclampsia, about 75 percent of the patients show some evidence of hepatic dysfunction, but permanent damage is rare. The most common hepatic lesion in the eclamptic patient is periportal hemorrhagic necrosis; this lesion may extend toward the center of the hepatic lobule. The surrounding blood sinuses may be compressed. In some areas, extravasation may occur and fibrin clots may form, especially at the bases of the liver cell columns. These changes are believed to result from thrombosis in the hepatic arterioles. Hemorrhage under the capsule of the liver may occur in severe preeclampsia-eclampsia, and the associated intra-abdominal bleeding presents an acute surgical emergency. Another serious complication is hepatic rupture, which has a 70 percent maternal mortality rate (Bis and Waxman, 1976; Nelson, 1977; Severino et al, 1970).

Arias and Mancilla-Jimenez (1976) reported immunofluorescent evidence of fibrin-fibrinogen, immunoglobulins, and complement in the livers of patients with preeclampsia-eclampsia. Fibrin-fibrinogen deposits of immunoglobulins G and M (IgG, IgM) and of the heat-stable component of complement (C3) are found in areas of necrosis. These investigators postulated that changes in the liver and kidneys in patients with toxemia are due to generalized vasospasm. They pointed out that the increased vasospasm, in the presence of systemic blood hypercoagulability, creates adequate local conditions for the precipitation of fibrin-fibrinogen.

In patients who die of eclampsia, there is almost always evidence of pulmonary edema and diffuse hemorrhagic bronchopneumonia. In the mycoardium, subendothelial hemorrhages, fibrin thrombi, and focal necroses may be found. These changes are sometimes so severe as to cause discoloration in the heart. This damage helps to explain the related pathophysiologic changes, such as impaired cardiac reserve, arrhythmias, and rapid pulse.

Histologic changes in the placenta reveal signs of advanced villous maturation, increase in syncytial knots, villous crowding, and infarction. Decidual vessel changes include acute atheromas, hyperplastic arteriosclerosis, and necrotizing arterioles. Infarction is a typical gross lesion in the placenta; it is present in up to 60 percent of cases.

In preeclampsia, the intramyometrial cytotrophoblast invasion may be defective and may demonstrate "acute atheromatosis (fibrinoid necrosis and lipid deposition), hyperplastic atherosclerosis, and necrotizing arteriolitis of maternal spiral arteries" (Macpherson, 1991). These changes can be assessed only by placental site biopsy. These changes reduce profusion to the intervillous space and may cause adverse outcomes, such as fetal IUGR, fetal hypoxia, and perinatal death (MacPherson, 1991).

## MANAGEMENT

The obstetric team always treats two patients: the mother and the fetus. The most definitive treatment for preeclampsia-eclampsia is termination of the pregnancy. All other treatment is supportive, the main objective being to ensure maternal and fetal well-being.

The rate of maternal mortality in preeclampsia is low. However, the risks of maternal death from eclampsia are appreciable, especially when cerebral hemorrhage, pulmonary edema, or repeated seizures occur, or syndrome of hemolysis, elevated liver enzymes, and low platelets (HELLP) is present. Long-term follow-up studies have failed to implicate preeclampsia and eclampsia as significant factors in the development of subsequent cardiovascular or renal disease.

Naeye and Friedman (1979), reviewing information from the Collaborative Perinatal Project, found a twofold increase in perinatal mortality rates among women with hypertension and proteinuria (diastolic blood pressure higher than 85 mm Hg and proteinuria of 1 + or more) as compared with normotensive patients without proteinuria. The excessive perinatal mortality rate was due to placental infarcts, placental growth retardation, and abruption of the placenta.

Often, preeclampsia cannot be prevented, but it is possible to select groups of patients who are particularly prone to develop it and to monitor those patients carefully for predisposing factors and early signs of the disease. Table 25–4 lists those conditions that predispose a woman to preeclampsia.

## OUTPATIENT ANTEPARTUM CARE

The blood pressure should be checked at each prenatal visit, with the patient in the sitting position. The systolic pressure fourth and fifth phases of Korotkoff should be recorded. A significant rise in blood pressure usually indicates developing preeclampsia. A MAP in excess of 92 mm Hg during the second trimester is a good indicator that the patient will subsequently develop pre-

**Table 25–4**
CONDITIONS THAT PREDISPOSE
TO PREECLAMPSIA*

| |
|---|
| Nulliparity |
| Multiple pregnancy |
| Hydatidiform mole |
| Chronic hypertension |
| Chronic renal disease |
| Diabetes mellitus |
| Hydrops fetalis |
| Malnutrition |
| Age <18 |
| >35 |

* The first three factors are beyond the control of the obstetrician, but meticulous control of the remaining ones, with frequent hospitalization when necessary, helps to decrease the adverse effects of this disease.

eclampsia. However, in many patients, the MAP does not attain this level in the second trimester, and hypertension may develop rapidly without premonitory symptoms. The need for a test to detect patients who will develop preeclampsia is obvious, especially if patients are to be treated with low doses of aspirin. The roll-over test, or a modification of the same, may serve this need (Table 25–5). The roll-over test has not met with universal application, primarily because of its difficult requisites.

Gant and coworkers (1974) found that patients in whom the roll-over test was positive were very sensitive to angiotensin infusion. They also found that 98 percent of these patients subsequently developed preeclampsia, whereas 91 percent of the patients in whom the test was negative did not become hypertensive. Gusdon and colleagues (1977), however, were more conservative in their assessment of the test. They found that only a negative test was accurate in predicting the failure to develop preeclampsia. Pregnancy-induced hypertension is insidious, and its subtle changes are often missed. However, progression to the severe forms of the disease should be preventable. Good prenatal observation is necessary for the success of the treatment of pregnancy-induced hypertension. It is important for the nurse and physician to observe subtle changes and to screen for patients with a potential for this disease. Any patient with a pregnancy of 20 weeks or more with the predisposing criteria should be seen once or twice a week, and a roll-over test should be performed between the 28th and 32nd week of gestation (O'Shaughnessy and Zuspan, 1981; Zuspan, 1980).

Angiotensin II testing in the antepartum period, which is used to predict pregnancy-induced hypertension, has also had conflicting successful results and may not be helpful

in predicting this complication (O'Brien, 1990; Sibai, 1988). A combination of predictive tests, such as the roll-over test and the MAP determination, is used to increase reliability (O'Brien, 1990; Phelan et al, 1977). Family history and parity should also be assessed for the most effective prediction of preeclampsia (O'Brien, 1990).

Some authors have suggested that once the diagnosis of preeclampsia has been made, the patient should be hospitalized (Cavanagh and Knuppel, 1982; Zuspan, 1980). Others have suggested that *selected* patients could be managed on an outpatient basis (Pritchard, 1980; Zuspan, 1980). Patients managed on an outpatient basis must maintain a diastolic blood pressure no greater than 85 mm Hg and have a good knowledge of the signs and symptoms of their disease, a home environment conducive to bed rest, and provide the opportunity to be examined twice a week. Patients can be taught to take their own blood pressure, measure their urinary output, and use a dipstick to test for protein. However, hospitalization is recommended for most of these patients.

If the patient can be examined only once a week, a visiting nurse could observe the patient at home during the week. These patients should follow a good diet with increased protein and no added salt (salt restriction is not necessary [Zuspan, 1980]) and should rest at mid-day for 1 1/2 hours. If the roll-over test is positive, the bed rest should be increased, even if the patient is asymptomatic. Once the diagnosis of pregnancy-induced hypertension has been made, the patient should be examined weekly or twice a week for signs of the following:

1. Increased blood pressure (when increased, the blood pressure should be taken again in 15 minutes and both the high and low readings should be recorded).
2. Proteinuria.
3. Increased deep tendon reflexes.
4. Increased weight.
5. Increased edema.
6. Increased hematocrit and hemoglobin.
7. Visual changes.
8. Reduced fundal growth.
9. Thrombocytopenia.
10. Epigastric pain.

Weekly nonstress testing (contraction

**Table 25–5**
ROLL-OVER TEST

**Procedure**
1. Measure blood pressure in the lateral recumbent position until stable
2. Roll patient to supine position
3. Measure blood pressure immediately
4. Repeat blood pressure in 5 minutes

**Positive test**—An increase of 20 mmHg or more in the diastolic pressure at the 5-minute reading
**Negative test**—Less than a 20 mmHg rise in diastolic blood pressure at the 5-minute reading

stress testing, when indicated), biophysical profile and Doppler testing should be started at 30 to 32 weeks of pregnancy to observe for fetal compromise. A sonogram should be performed every 3 to 4 weeks to serially measure fetal growth, and an amniocentesis should be carried out at 33 weeks for an L/S ratio to assess fetal maturity in case delivery is indicated. An oral glucose tolerance test should be performed, because diabetic patients have a higher incidence of preeclampsia than does the normal population.

Because decreased peripheral resistance during pregnancy lowers the blood pressure, it is important that serial blood pressure with baseline values be established. Also, it is imperative to have good gestational dating through the use of early pregnancy testing, early ultrasound, auscultation of the fetal heart sounds with a DeLee stethoscope at 18 to 20 weeks, documentation of quickening, and a good menstrual history. The patient must also realize that although she may feel better, the disease is only controlled, not cured. The regimen should be continued despite abatement of symptoms. Strict bed rest in the left lateral position and good nutrition are necessary for outpatient management. However, with clinical improvement, allowance of some patient activity to encourage compliance has been suggested.

The patient who remains at home must have a very good understanding of signs and symptoms of worsening disease and should observe for increasing edema, especially in the face and hands and, if at bed rest, over the sacrum; severe or persistent headache; epigastric or upper right quadrant pain; visual disturbances; decreased urinary outputs; increased proteinuria; severe nausea and vomiting; bleeding gums; and disorientation. If any of these signs and symptoms persist, she should contact her physician.

Decreasing fetal movement also should alert the patient to contact her physician. Family members should be included in the teaching of these signs and symptoms so that they can detect them, especially disorientation, because the patient may not be able to understand the change in her condition.

If the patient is noncompliant, is not stable on the home management program, or if a proper surveillance program does not exist, she should be hospitalized. We recommend hospitalization for the vast majority of our patients.

## INPATIENT ANTEPARTUM CARE

The patient should be hospitalized if she demonstrates *any* of the following signs or symptoms:

1. A blood pressure of 140/90 mm Hg on two readings, 6 hours apart (home blood pressure monitoring can help).
2. A systolic increase of 30 mm Hg on two readings, 6 hours apart at bed rest.
3. A diastolic increase of 15 mm Hg on two readings, 6 hours apart at bed rest.
4. Proteinuria of 3 g/liter in a 24-hour urine collection, or 1 g/liter in at least two random samples, 6 hours apart (5 g of protein demonstrates severe preeclampsia, or 3 + or 4 + proteinuria on a dipstick).
5. Thrombocytopenia—elevated liver enzymes.

Expectant management is appropriate in mild cases of preeclampsia when it may permit further fetal development. Most obstetric centers in the United States prefer to hospitalize all patients with diagnosed preeclampsia. Immediate evaluation for assessment of fetal maturity is performed on admission if the patient's pregnancy is over 33 weeks' gestational age. If the mother is stable, delivery can be delayed, provided that the fetus does not demonstrate lung maturity and demonstrates fetal well-being during antepartum testing. However, if the maternal or fetal condition deteriorates, delivery is initiated (Gabbe et al, 1986).

Once hospitalized, the patient is put on bed rest with bathroom privileges. The lateral recumbent position is advisable because it avoids compression of the vena cava and aorta and improves renal function by increasing cardiac output. This increases the glomerular filtration rate and should increase urinary output. Bed rest is also beneficial to the fetus by increasing uterine profusion. The patient's room should be arranged to enhance maintenance of this positioning. For example, facing the wall could become boring, whereas facing the television or visitors results in better patient compliance. The patient should be kept in a quiet, dimly lit private room or a well-selected semiprivate room. A semiprivate room allows availability of another person to call for a nurse if the patient should have a seizure.

Blood pressure should be taken at least twice during an 8-hour shift. However, if the blood pressure is stable late in the evening, measurement of the blood pressure in the middle of the night can be eliminated to allow the patient to rest. To be most effective, the width of the blood pressure cuff should be 20 percent greater than the diameter of the limb, and the length of the cuff should be 1.2 times the limb diameter. Because there are standard cuff sizes, choose the one closest to the above-mentioned dimensions (Wheeler and Jones, 1981).

The patient's weight should be measured daily in the hospital, because this is a good indicator of fluid retention. An increase of 1 to 1 1/2 lb/day may indicate fluid retention. For a more accurate measurement, the patient should be weighed at the same time daily, using the same scale. The patient usually will have physiologic diuresis within 36 to 48 hours following hospitalization with bed rest. The weight can decrease as much as 4 to 9 lb during the next 3- to 5-day period.

Serial weekly hematocrits should be obtained and compared with any hematocrits obtained early in pregnancy. An increase in the hematocrit indicates that more fluid has moved from the blood vessels to the interstitial tissue as edema (indicating worsening of the disease). A decrease in the hematocrit shows fluid moving from the tissues back into the bloodstream, thereby diluting the red blood cells, which indicates an improvement in the disease. A complete blood chemistry should be done for proper assessment, including a disseminated intravascular coagulation screen and liver enzyme evaluations.

Intake and output should be measured every 8 hours. Oliguria occurs as pregnancy-induced hypertension worsens. The excess fluid is not excreted. This overloads the vascular system and further stresses the heart. The fluid may move from the circulation into the interstitial space (Wheeler and Jones, 1981).

A urine specimen should be tested daily for protein, and if it is greater than 1 + with a dipstick, a 24-hour collection should be obtained. If the 24-hour urine collection shows more than 300 mg of protein, it should be repeated within the next 24 hours. Contamination of the urine with amniotic fluid and blood increases the protein content. If this presents a problem, a catheterized specimen is recommended. No casts or cells should be seen on microscopic examination of the urine. The normal plasma uric acid should be within normal limits (3.5 to 7 mg/100 ml).

A 24-hour urine collection for creatinine clearance, to test renal function, should be performed weekly (normal = 150 ml/min). However, a serum creatinine may be a more sensitive test and is more easily obtained. Serial measurements of creatine clearance, blood urea nitrogen, and serum creatinine are more helpful so that trends of elevation can be assessed, because there is a wide range of normal for a single value. A 24-hour urine collection should begin at a specific time and continue to that same time the following day (e.g., 6 AM to 6 AM). The first void at 6 AM should be discarded, and the last void at 6 AM the following day should be collected. The urine for a creatinine clearance must be refrigerated or cooled on ice during the collection.

Deep tendon reflexes and vital signs should be checked every 4 to 8 hours while the patient is in the hospital. If the patient is stable, the midnight to early morning vital signs can be eliminated, to allow the patient more rest. When the nurse checks the patient's vital signs, assessment should be made for the patient's general appearance, alertness, condition of skin, edema (especially of the face, hands, and feet), presence of epigastric pain or upper right quadrant pain, headache, visual disturbances, level of consciousness, chest sounds, bleeding from gums or other areas, and increased reflexes. Labor assessment should also be made.

The patient is kept on a regular diet with good protein and caloric intake. (This factor may be a definite improvement from outpatient care.) Salt and fluids should neither be encouraged nor restricted.

Brewer (1970; 1975; 1976) has written extensively on the importance of good nutrition in reducing the tendency to hypovolemia and a hypoperfusion state. In a group of 7000 underprivileged patients in whom particular attention was paid to nutrition, he reported a toxemia rate of 0.55 percent, with no cases of eclampsia. A nutritionist is an integral part of the perinatal team for the preeclamptic mother.

Patients are *not* kept on large doses of sedatives, because it is hard to evaluate the patient's condition when she is heavily sedated. Moreover, sedatives do not adequately prevent seizure activity. The oversedated patient may not be able to control her bodily functions, clear her airway, or verbalize pain, visual disturbances, contractions, and so forth. Because the sedatives cross the placenta, the fetus, which might already be stressed, may also be oversedated. If sedation is used, a nonreactive nonstress test may result from the medication and may be misleading.

Because strict bed rest may improve urine output and decrease the edema, the blood pressure may decline and the patient's general condition and circulatory status may improve. It is a widely accepted policy, therefore, to avoid induction of labor during the first 24 to 36 hours, even in relatively severe cases, if fetal immaturity exists. This time frame also may allow administration of glucocorticoids to improve fetal lung maturity. When the preeclampsia is mild and the improvement is sustained, it is reasonable to postpone induction of labor until fetal lung maturity has occurred. In such cases, amniocentesis may need to be performed to determine fetal lung maturity, as measured by an L/S ratio greater than 2.0.

Under these conditions, the pregnancy may be continued if the maternal status remains improved, the fetoplacental function is stable, and the fetus has not reached the stage of lung maturity. However, worsening of the clinical signs (Table 25–6) warrants intervention irrespective of the stage of fetal maturity.

Bioelectric monitoring of the fetal reserve is accomplished with a nonstress test. Any change in maternal status requires prompt re-evaluation of the fetus. If the maternal status is satisfactory and there is evidence of fetal reactivity, the test may be repeated once a week. However, if the nonstress test is not reassuring, a contraction stress test or biophysical profile is indicated. If the nonstress test is nonreactive and the contraction stress test is positive or if there is a score of less than or equal to 6 on the biophysical profile, induction still may be attempted if the condition of the cervix and the station of the vertex permit rupturing of the membranes and the application of a scalp electrode without difficulty. In the presence of a nonreactive nonstress test and a positive contraction stress test or a low-scoring biophysical profile, in cases in which it is not possible to evaluate the fetus by direct bioelectric monitoring, cesarean delivery should be strongly considered.

Prior to the days of cost-containment, the experience of academic and public institutions, as well as that of Armed Forces units, supported without question the use of hospitalization with limited activity as the primary component of the care of the preeclamptic patient. These experiences raise doubts as to the validity and effectiveness of using sophisticated techniques for evaluating fetal or placental reserve. The data of Parkland Hospital (Hauth et al, 1976) confirm the value of hospitalization among their 346 hypertensive gravidas, 50 percent of whom showed edema, with only 14 percent demonstrating proteinuria. These patients received a normal diet without sedation, antihypertensive therapy, or the use of diuretics. They were allowed free ambulation. Eighty-one percent of these patients became normotensive before delivery.

The perinatal mortality rate was 9 : 1000, as compared with 129 : 1000 for those who left the hospital against medical advice. No patient with any of the following symptoms was ever admitted directly to this unit: diastolic blood pressure of 110 mm Hg or greater, significant proteinuria (2 + or more), headaches, scotomas, and epigastric pain. These patients were managed as severe preeclamptics (discussed later in this chapter).

The same group (Gilstrap et al, 1978) reported equally satisfactory results among 576 nulliparous gestational hypertensive patients with single pregnancies. The blood pressure was taken four times daily, urine dipsticks and weight were checked three times weekly, and creatinine clearance and

**Table 25–6**

SIGNS AND SYMPTOMS OF WORSENING
PREGNANCY-INDUCED HYPERTENSION

Increased edema (weight gain)
Severe headache
Disorientation
Liver tenderness
Epigastric pain
Hepatic distention
Visual disturbance
Increased hematocrit
Decreased urinary output (less than 100 ml/4h)
Increased blood pressure
Increased proteinuria
Decreased creatinine clearance
Increased serum creatinine
Hyperreflexia, especially with clonus
Severe nausea and vomiting
Thrombocytopenia
Elevated liver enzymes

fetal growth (sonography) were monitored weekly. The investigators measured the L/S ratio of the amniotic fluid but performed no bioelectric fetal assessment. Spontaneous labor and delivery at term were permitted unless there was evidence of deterioration of the patient's condition at bed rest. These reports (Fleigner, 1976) raise serious questions as to whether prompt delivery of the mild preeclamptic patient offers the best solution for the mother and the fetus. The conservative management described earlier reduces the rate of prematurity and its associated high incidence of neonatal mortality (Table 25-7).

Severe preeclampsia should not be managed expectantly. These patients should be placed at bed rest and given hydralazine intravenously to maintain the diastolic pressure at approximately 100 mm Hg, but note that the antihypertensive may be masking the disease. Magnesium sulfate should be used liberally. While the preeclamptic patient is being observed closely for signs of neuromuscular hyperexcitability, the fetus should also be evaluated for loss of fetal reserve with antepartum testing (nonstress test, contraction stress test, or biophysical profile). After the condition of the severe preeclamptic patient has been stabilized in the hospital, termination of pregnancy is indicated in the interest of both the mother and the fetus. In Catanzarite and associates' (1991) survey of perinatologists, 71 percent agreed that patients with severe preeclampsia should be delivered after stabilization, whereas 29 percent said they would delay delivery in selective cases. Some even said they would delay delivery in patients with thrombocytopenia.

## INTRAPARTUM CARE

When fetal maturity has been reached, further procrastination serves no useful purpose (Knuppel and Montenegro, 1985). The mode of delivery is established by the condition of the patient, her cervix, and the fetoplacental unit. If the cervix is favorable for induction and the mother and fetus are stable, induction is preferable, with use of oxytocin and (circumstances permitting) artificial rupture of the membranes. Creasy and Resnik (1989) suggest that some preeclamptic women respond well to induction and, therefore, even a woman with an un-

inducible cervix should have a trial of induction (Zuspan and Talledo, 1968). If delivery does not occur in a predetermined amount of time, a cesarean delivery should be performed. Mandatory, adequate fetal monitoring, preferably with internal electrode, is needed to assess this fetus at high risk for compromise during induction. With an uninducible cervix, or with a very premature or distressed fetus, a cesarean section is advisable. This approach is particularly desirable when the estimated fetal weight is less than 1500 g. When the blood pressure cannot be controlled, the weight gain continues at bed rest, or proteinuria increases, the patient is delivered regardless of fetal age or lung maturity (Table 25-8). This approach is justifiable even when the gravida is less than 30 weeks' pregnant, because it is in this group of patients that ominous maternal sequelae are particularly prone to occur.

## MEDICATIONS

The medications that may be used for treatment of preeclampsia-eclampsia are summarized in Table 25-9. The most frequently used medications are highlighted here.

Hydralazine (Apresoline) acts by causing arteriolar vasodilatation. It also increases cardiac output and renal blood flow; appreciable blood pressure reduction usually occurs with an oral dose of 100 mg/day in four divided doses. A recent observation suggests that the administration of the same daily dose in two doses is equally effective for blood pressure control in many patients. Hydralazine is completely absorbed after oral administration; peak serum concentrations are obtained within 1 to 2 hours. Intravenous injections reach a peak effectiveness in 15 to 20 minutes; therefore, adequate reduction of high diastolic blood pressures should be achieved by repeating the appropriate dose every 10 to 15 minutes. One may prefer to administer a 5-mg initial intravenous bolus and to repeat it in 15 to 20 minutes if there is no response. Alternatively, hydralazine may be given slowly by continuous intravenous infusion: 20 to 40 mg in 1000 ml 5 percent dextrose with 0.45 percent saline. The rate of infusion of the intravenous fluid should be titrated to the patient's blood pressure (100 to 110 mm Hg diastolic), which should be stabilized at a level consistent with an ade-

**Table 25–7**
SEVERE PREECLAMPSIA

One or more of the following symptoms indicate severe preeclampsia.
1. BP greater than or equal to 160 systolic
   BP greater than or equal to 110 diastolic;     2 readings, 6 hours apart
   MAP of 127 or more
2. Proteinuria greater than or equal to 5 g/24 h
3. Oliguria less than or equal to 400 ml/24 h
         less than or equal to 30 ml/h
4. Cerebral or visual disturbances
5. Pulmonary edema or cyanosis

From Weinstein L: Preeclampsia/eclampsia with hemolysis, elevated liver enzymes, and thrombocytopenia. Obstet Gynecol 66:5, 1985.

quate urinary output. The fetal heart rate should be monitored carefully during administration of hydralazine because of the patient's depleted blood volume; a sudden fall in blood pressure may cause severe fetal hypoxia. The most common side effect is tachycardia, which may be severe and may occasionally progress to arrhythmias; this effect may be abolished by the intravenous administration of propranolol. Hydralazine is a very valuable drug for the treatment of hypertension associated with toxemia, but chronic administration in doses exceeding 200 mg/day can lead to an acute rheumatoid state, which, when fully developed, gives rise to a syndrome resembling disseminated lupus erythematosus.

**Table 25–8**
HOSPITALIZED PATIENTS: INDICATIONS FOR DELIVERY DESPITE FETAL PREMATURITY

Rapid weight gain at bed rest
Blood pressure progressively elevates at bed rest
Premonitory symptoms of eclampsia
Increasing proteinuria
IUGR diagnosed with lung maturity
Impaired liver function
Thrombocytopenia

**Management Schema**

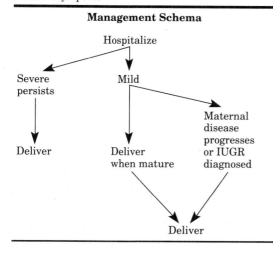

Diazoxide (Hyperstat), administered intravenously as a 300-mg dose, is effective in treating acute hypertensive states. However, because it may cause sudden and irreversible hypotension, which can produce severe fetal hypoxia, it is not the treatment of choice (Neuman et al, 1979). Maternal death has occurred from the administration of 5 mg/kg of body weight.

Magnesium sulfate ($MgSO_4$) has been the cornerstone of treatment for severe preeclampsia for over 50 years. Its main effect is at the neuromuscular junction. It is administered when preeclampsia displays a progressive tendency.

To prevent seizures, $MgSO_4$ can be administered intravenously or intramuscularly. Intravenous administration is preferable because of the rapid achievement of appropriate magnesium levels in the blood and for patient comfort. When $MgSO_4$ is given intravenously, usually a 4-g loading dose is administered over 15 minutes, followed by 1 to 2 g/h (Gant, 1980) administered by a constant infusion pump in a piggyback fashion. Usually, 1 g is given per 50 or 100 ml of D5W. If the dose is increased to a constant level, the concentration of $MgSO_4$ should be increased, not the fluid volume. If the nursing staff is unable to monitor the patient and the intravenous infusion adequately, it is beneficial to give the $MgSO_4$ intramuscularly.

Deep intramuscular injection of $MgSO_4$ is given Z-track in the upper outer quadrant of the buttocks with a 3-inch, 20-gauge needle. It is very painful, and 1 ml of lidocaine may be added to the syringe after the $MgSO_4$ (Gant and Worley, 1980). One-half cc of air should be at the end of the plunger to ensure that the needle is cleared of all medication when injected. The patient should be alerted to the pain of the injection so that she is not startled, which could lead to seizure activity. The intramuscular loading dose is 10 g; 5 g

*Text continued on page 498*

**Table 25–9**

MEDICATION SUMMARY FOR PREECLAMPSIA-ECLAMPSIA

| Medication | Action | Route | Dose | Pregnancy Precautions |
|---|---|---|---|---|
| | | *Anticonvulsants* | | |
| Magnesium sulfate | To control CNS irritability through action at the neuromuscular junction | IV with constant infusion pump | *Loading dose:* 4 g over 15 min<br>*Maintenance dose:* 1–2 g/h to be continued 12–72 hours after delivery<br>*For seizures:* 4 g over 5 min | None |
| | | IM | *Loading dose:* 10 g; 5 g into each buttock<br>*Maintenance dose:* 5 g/4 h alternating hips, to be continued 12–72 hours after delivery (if more than 6 hours elapse between doses, the loading dose should be repeated) | |
| Diazepam (Valium) | Anticonvulsant | IV | 5 mg over 60 sec; may repeat (20 mg or more may be required) | Not recommended for obstetric use<br>Associated with congenital malformations when taken during the first trimester<br>Fetal toxicity |
| | | *Magnesium Antagonist* | | |
| Calcium gluconate | Reverses magnesium intoxication | IV only | 1 g over 3 min (10 ml of a 10 percent solution) | |

| Maternal Side Effects | Nursing Considerations | Fetal and Neonatal Considerations | Breastfeeding |
|---|---|---|---|
| *Anticonvulsants* | | | |
| Hypotension, flushing, circulatory collapse, depressed cardiac function, heart block, respiratory paralysis, hypocalcemia Should not be used on digitalis patients because of danger of arrhythmias | Keep IV calcium gluconate available to reverse MgSO₄ Monitor vital signs q 15 min when administered IV in a specialized care setting I&O IM Z-track Add 1 cc lidocaine to 5-g dose Allow 1/2 cc of air to clear 3″ needle | Occasional hypermagnesemia | Excreted in breast milk but not absolute contraindication to breastfeeding |
| Fatigue, drowsiness, ataxia, dizziness, headache, dysarthria, slurred speech, tremor, hypotension, bradycardia, cardiovascular collapse, blurred vision, nausea | Vital signs q 5 min Do not mix with other IV drugs Do not infuse through plastic tubing or store in plastic syringe Do not inject into small veins | Crosses placenta and is not excreted well by fetus Toxic levels have been detected 3 weeks after maternal administration in the neonate Hypothermia | Excreted in breast milk; because of long-acting metabolites, diazepam should be avoided during breastfeeding |
| *Magnesium Antagonist* | | | |
| Tingling sensation, sense of oppression or heat waves, mild decrease in blood pressure, hypercalcemia, polyuria with rapid administration, syncope, vasodilation, bradycardia, cardiac arrhythmias, and cardiac arrest | Continue to monitor for vital signs closely | No data available | No data available |

*Table continued on following page*

**Table 25-9**
MEDICATION SUMMARY FOR PREECLAMPSIA-ECLAMPSIA *Continued*

| Medication | Action | Route | Dose | Pregnancy Precautions |
|---|---|---|---|---|
| | | ***Barbiturates*** | | |
| Barbiturates | Sedative | Dependent on medication | | Not helpful in preventing eclampsia, but IV amylbarbital useful in eclampsia |
| | | ***Antihypertensives*** | | |
| Aldomet (Methyldopa) | Central-acting adrenergic inhibitor | Oral | 500–2000 mg/day, usually given in divided doses twice daily | None |
| Propranolol hydrochloride (Inderal) | $\beta$-adrenergic inhibitor | Oral | 40–480 mg/day, usually given in divided doses twice daily | Drug is associated with IUGR, prolonged bradycardia, and hypoglycemia |

| Maternal Side Effects | Nursing Considerations | Fetal and Neonatal Considerations | Breastfeeding |
|---|---|---|---|
| *Barbiturates* | | | |
| Drowsiness, lethargy, hangover, nausea and vomiting, rash | May mask symptoms of toxemia if patient is too sedated | Crosses placenta rapidly and should not be given if delivery is imminent | Excreted in breast milk (short-acting preferred, as smaller amounts appear in the milk) |
| *Antihypertensives* | | | |
| Hemolytic anemia, reversible granulocytopenia, thrombocytopenia, sedation, headache, asthenia, weakness, dizziness, decreased mental activity, psychic disturbances, depression, bradycardia, orthostatic hypotension, dry mouth, nasal stuffiness, diarrhea | Monitor BP and potassium frequently<br>Daily weight | None reported | Observe carefully; appears to be secreted in significant amounts |
| Fatigue, lethargy, vivid dreams, hallucinations, bradycardia, hypotension, peripheral vascular disease, nausea and vomiting, diarrhea, hypoglylcemia without tachycardia, rash | Check apical heart rate before administration<br>Monitor BP frequently<br>May mask common signs of shock and hypoglycemia<br>Give with meals<br>Exercise and activity must be monitored by physician<br>Use with caution in patients with heart disease | Associated with hypoglycemia, bradycardia, intrauterine growth retardation; these reports may be exaggerated<br>Respiratory depression has been reported in neonates when propranolol has been administered to the mother by IV immediately before cesarean section | Amounts in breast milk too small to produce adverse effects in normal infants; however, caution should be used in premature or sick infants |

*Table continued on following page*

**Table 25–9**
MEDICATION SUMMARY FOR PREECLAMPSIA-ECLAMPSIA *Continued*

| Medication | Action | Route | Dose | Pregnancy Precautions |
|---|---|---|---|---|
| | | ***Adrenergic Receptor Blocking Agent*** | | |
| Normodyne (Labetalol HCl) | Antihypertensive | | Dose must be individualized | |
| | | P.O. | Initial dose 100 mg twice daily. Usual maintenance dose is 200–400 mg twice daily | Research with rats and rabbits has not shown teratogenicity. No studies conducted in humans |
| | | IV injection | 20 mg (corresponds to 0.25 mg/kg for an 80 kg patient) by slow IV infusion over 2 min. Additional injections of 40 mg or 80 mg can be given at 10 min intervals until desired blood pressure is achieved or a total of 300 mg. (The maximum effect usually occurs within 5 min) | "Should only be used in pregnancy if the potential benefit justifies the potential risk to the fetus." (PDR) |
| | | Continuous IV | Add 40 ml to 160 ml of IV fluid. The resultant 200 ml contains 1 mg labetalol/ml. Rate of 2 ml/min to deliver 2 mg/min. The effective dose is usually in the range of 50–200 mg. A dose of 300 mg may be required in some patients. Dose may be adjusted according to blood pressure response, at the discretion of the physician | |

| Maternal Side Effects | Nursing Considerations | Fetal and Neonatal Considerations | Breastfeeding |
|---|---|---|---|
| | *Adrenergic Receptor Blocking Agent* | | |
| | IV patient should be kept in a supine position during IV administration. Patient should be observed closely for significant hypotension on standing | May cause transient hypotension, bradycardia, and hypoglycemia | Small amounts are excreted in human milk. Use caution when administering IV injection to nursing mothers |
| Hypotension, if patient allowed to assume an upright position within 3 hours of receiving injection | Immediately before injection at 5 and 10 min after injection, measure supine blood pressure | | |
| Rare side effects include sweating, flushing, ventricular arrhythmia, dizziness, tingling of scalp and skin, numbness, vertigo, nausea, vomiting, transient increase in BUN and serum creatinine (usually without drops in BP and renal insufficiency), yawning, wheezing, pruritus | Monitor fetal heart tones after administration. Use EFM if maternal hypotension or fetal bradycardia occur | | |

*Table continued on following page*

**Table 25–9**
MEDICATION SUMMARY FOR PREECLAMPSIA-ECLAMPSIA *Continued*

| Medication | Action | Route | Dose | Pregnancy Precautions |
|---|---|---|---|---|
| | | ***Antihypertensives*** *Arteriolar Dilators* | | |
| Hydralazine (Apresoline) | Arteriolar vasodilation | Oral, IV, or IM | 50–300 mg/day, usually given in divided doses twice daily Maximum effect 3–4 h; duration of action 6 h; 5 percent of dose excreted unchanged in urine | |
| Prazosin (Minipress) | Peripheral-acting α-adrenergic blocker | Oral | 1–20 mg/day; peak action in 2 h | |
| Nitroprusside (Nipride) | To lower BP quickly in hypertensive emergencies | IV in D5W Do not inject | 50 mg/liter Start at 0.2–0.5 ml/min Immediate effect; works only during IV infusion, which should be less than 24 h in duration, carefully controlled with an intravenous pump | The safety of nitroprusside in women who are pregnant or who may become pregnant has not been established; hence, the drug should be given only when the potential benefits outweigh the hazards to mother and child |

| Maternal Side Effects | Nursing Considerations | Fetal and Neonatal Considerations | Breastfeeding |
|---|---|---|---|
| **_Antihypertensives_** _Arteriolar Dilators_ | | | |
| Flushing, headache, tachycardia, palpitations, lupus-like syndrome | Vital signs: with IV check q 1 min for 5 min, then q 5 min for 30 min; with IM check q 5 min for 30 min Watch for signs of SLE-like syndrome | None reported with long-term use | Excreted in breast milk. Care should be taken when administered to nursing mothers |
| Tachycardia, palpitations, dizziness, postural hypotension, weakness, headache, syncope | Use cautiously in patients receiving other hypertensive drugs Monitor blood pressure frequently Severe syncope with loss of consciousness may develop with an initial dose greater than 1 mg Exercise and activity should be monitored by physician | No data available | Excreted in small amounts in breast milk. Care should be taken when administered to nursing mothers |
| Nausea, diaphoresis, apprehension, cyanide poisoning | Use cautiously with hypothyroidism or hepatic or renal disease, or if patient is receiving other hypertensives Wrap IV in foil because of light sensitivity; tubing not necessary to cover Fresh solution should have a slight brownish tint; Discard after 4 h | May cause cyanide poisoning | Not recommended |

_Table continued on following page_

**Table 25–9**
MEDICATION SUMMARY FOR PREECLAMPSIA-ECLAMPSIA *Continued*

| Medication | Action | Route | Dose | Pregnancy Precautions |
|---|---|---|---|---|
| Nitroprusside (Nipride) *Continued* | | | | |
| Minoxidil, guancydine (Loniten) | Vasodilator | Oral | 5–100 mg/day Single daily dose is longacting | No adequate controlled studies |
| | | ***Osmotic Diuretics*** | | |
| Mannitol | Increases blood volume and GFR, reduces cerebral edema | IV | 12.5 g | None known |

| Maternal Side Effects | Nursing Considerations | Fetal and Neonatal Considerations | Breastfeeding |
|---|---|---|---|
| Hirsutism, edema, tachycardia, pericardial effusion and tamponade, congestive heart failure, breast tenderness | Check BP q 5 min × 6 at start of infusion, then q 15 min. Needs intrarterial line<br>Use constant infusion pump<br>Best run piggyback with no other medications<br>Check serum thiocyanate levels q 72 hr<br>Contraindicated in patients with pheochromocytoma<br>Use only when other vasodilators have failed<br>Usually prescribed with a beta-blocking drug to control tachycardia | No data available | Not recommended |
| | ***Osmotic Diuretics*** | | |
| May worsen status in circulatory failure, water intoxication, cellular dehydration | Contraindicated in anuria, severe pulmonary congestion, frank pulmonary edema, severe congestive heart disease, severe dehydration, metabolic edema, progressive renal disease or dysfunction<br>Monitor vital signs at least q h<br>If solution crystallizes, warm bottle in hot water bath, shake vigorously<br>Use IV in-line filter<br>Use catheter to measure I & O | Diuretics apparently have no adverse side effects in the neonate | Can cause a decrease in the production of milk |

*Table continued on following page*

**Table 25–9**
MEDICATION SUMMARY FOR PREECLAMPSIA-ECLAMPSIA *Continued*

| Medication | Action | Route | Dose | Pregnancy Precautions |
|---|---|---|---|---|
| *Aldosterone Antagonists* | | | | |
| Spironolactone (Aldactone) | Potassium-sparing diuretic | Oral | 50–100 mg/day | Diuretics can cause a decrease in maternal intramuscular volume and consequently diminish uteroplacental perfusion |
| Triamterene (Dyazide) | Potassium-sparing diuretic | Oral | 50–100 mg/day | These agents *do not prevent development of toxemia* |
| *Miscellaneous Antihypertensives* | | | | |
| Cryptenamine acetate (Unitensen) | Antihypertensive | Oral IM | 0.15–0.5 $\mu$g/min 4–12 mg/day 0.25–0.5 mg Length of action: 12 h | |
| *Diuretics* | | | | |
| Furosemide (Lasix) | For treatment of pulmonary edema | Oral IV | 40–200 mg/day 20–40 mg/day Diuretic response immediately with IV; in 30 min when given orally; bound to plasma proteins; also produces renal vasodilatation | Safety in pregnancy has not been established Diuretics can cause a decrease in maternal intravascular volume and consequently diminish uteroplacental perfusion These agents *do not prevent development of toxemia* |

| Maternal Side Effects | Nursing Considerations | Fetal and Neonatal Considerations | Breastfeeding |
|---|---|---|---|
| | ***Aldosterone Antagonists*** | | |
| Nausea, vomiting, leg cramps, dizziness | Contraindicated in anuria; occasional acute or progressive renal inefficiency, hyperkalemia | None known | Not recommended |
| | Monitor serum potassium levels, electrolytes, I & O, weight, BP <br> Protect drug from light <br> Give with meals to enhance absorption | No data available | |
| | ***Miscellaneous Antihypertensives*** | | |
| Same as above plus cardiac irritability | Contraindicated in patients with pheochromocytoma <br> Use cautiously in patients with angina, cerebrovascular disease, bronchial asthma, renal insufficiency, or those taking other antihypertensives <br> Monitor BP and P closely <br> Range between therapeutic and toxic dose is narrow | No data available | No data available |
| | ***Diuretics*** | | |
| | Hyponatremia, paresthesias, rash, GI irritability, thrombocytopenia, neutropenia, tinnitus, deafness <br> Patients may have allergic reactions <br> Will need increased potassium <br> May cause hyperglycemia in diabetic patients <br> Store tablets in light-resistant container to prevent discoloration (does not affect potency); store in refrigerator | | Diuretics can cause a decrease in milk production and have been known to suppress postpartum lactation |

*Table continued on following page*

**Table 25–9**
MEDICATION SUMMARY FOR PREECLAMPSIA-ECLAMPSIA *Continued*

| Medication | Action | Route | Dose | Pregnancy Precautions |
|---|---|---|---|---|
| Furosemide (Lasix) *Continued* | | | | |
| | | ***Ganglionic Blocking Agents*** | | |
| Trimethaphan (Arfonad ampules) | To decrease BP quickly in hypertensive emergencies | IV titered Oral intake incomplete, erratic, unpredictable Parenteral dose excreted unchanged; tolerance develops | 0.3–6 ml/min | None noted |

**Table 25–9**
MEDICATION SUMMARY FOR PREECLAMPSIA-ECLAMPSIA *Continued*

| Maternal Side Effects | Nursing Considerations | Fetal and Neonatal Considerations | Breastfeeding |
|---|---|---|---|
| | Do not use discolored (yellow) injectable | | |
| | Use prepared solution within 24 h | | |
| | Use cautiously in cardiogenic shock complicated by pulmonary edema, anuria, hepatic coma, or electrolyte imbalance | | |
| | Monitor BP and $P_1$ potassium level | | |
| | Sulfonamide-sensitive | | |
| | ***Ganglionic Blocking Agents*** | | |
| Dilated pupils, extreme weakness, severe orthostatic hypotension, tachycardia, anorexia, nausea, vomiting, dry mouth, urinary retention, respiratory depression | Contraindicated in patients with anemia, respiratory insufficiency | Meconium ileus | No data available |
| | Use cautiously in patients with cardiac, hepatic, or renal disease, and in patients receiving glucocorticoids and other antihypertensives | | |
| | Monitor vital signs frequently | | |
| | Use constant infusion IV pump | | |
| | Use oxygen therapy during administration of this drug | | |

injected into each buttock, then 5 g every 4 hours, alternating hips. If the dose lapses for more than 6 hours, the loading dose should be given again (Gant and Worley, 1980). With the initial loading dose of $MgSO_4$, the patient may experience nausea and vomiting. She may also feel flushed and state that she "feels hot all over."

Chesley (1979) demonstrated that after an initial intravenous dose of 3 mg of magnesium sulfate followed by 10 mg intramuscularly, the average peak serum level at 60 minutes was 4.5 mEq/liter, and that at the end of 4 hours, the accumulative renal excretions ranged from 38 to 53 percent of the injected dose. The conclusion from this study was that the initial dose is safe even in anuric patients. However, repeated doses may not be safe.

Catanzarite and associates (1991) surveyed perinatologists regarding their care of preeclamptic patients. They found that of the 214 respondents, 179 give $MgSO_4$ all the time, 34 answered only for eclampsia, and one answered that he never used it in his practice. Of 214 responding to dose, 208 said they gave $MgSO_4$ intravenously with a 2 to 10 g loading dose and a maintenance dose of 1 to 4 g/h. Three perinatologists said they used only $MgSO_4$ intramuscularly, with a 10 g loading dose and a maintenance dose of 5 g every 4 hours. Three said they used a combination of intravenous and intramuscular administration of $MgSO_4$.

Constant supervision, with a minimum 1:2 nurse-to-patient ratio, should be provided for the preeclamptic patient receiving $MgSO_4$. These patients should be given the same care as patients in any other intensive care unit, because pregnancy-induced hypertension is associated with high maternal and perinatal mortality rates (Wheeler and Jones, 1981). Mild preeclampsia warrants at least a 1:2 nurse–patient ratio; severe preeclampsia or eclampsia requires a 1:1 nurse-to-patient ratio.

The dose of $MgSO_4$ should be withheld if the patient's reflexes are absent, if the respiratory rate is depressed (lower than 10–14/min), or if the urinary output is less than 30 ml/h, or 100 ml in 4 hours (Chesley, 1979). This assessment must be made prior to each dose of $MgSO_4$. Of the 214 perinatologists who responded to Catanzarite and associates' (1991) survey, 190 used deep tendon reflexes as their primary assessment to manage $MgSO_4$, and 21 stated they used serum magnesium levels as their primary manage-ment screen. Three subjects did not respond to this question.

$MgSO_4$ is used to control seizures–it is *not* an antihypertensive. However, there may be a transient decrease in the blood pressure for the first 60 minutes, owing to the vasodilatation and relaxation of the smooth muscle. $MgSO_4$ may increase cerebral blood flow, urinary output, and the uterine blood flow by decreasing the spasms of the vessels to the uterus and intervillous space. $MgSO_4$ may also cause uterine activity to decrease, and labor augmentation may be necessary.

$MgSO_4$ is excreted through the kidneys. If the patient has an increase in output, an increase in the dose of $MgSO_4$ may be necessary. If the output decreases, a lower dose may be necessary. Impaired renal function may also necessitate a lower dose of $MgSO_4$.

Rarely does a patient convulse if she has received therapeutic levels of magnesium sulfate, as described above. Experimental studies have failed to conclusively demonstrate the primary nervous system effect of parenterally administered magnesium. This has resulted in the controversial speculation that the anticonvulsant effect of magnesium is merely masking the clinical convulsions by neuromuscular blockade. Borges and Gucer (1978) determined the effects of intravenously infused magnesium sulfate on the epileptic neuroactivity induced by the topical application of penicillin in anesthetized cats and dogs and in awake, undrugged primates. Magnesium sulfate was able to suppress directly neuronal burst firing and electroencephalographic spike generation at serum levels below those producing paralysis. There was a direct relation between serum-magnesium concentrations and suppression of spike generation. The effect was reversible.

Although newer anticonvulsants have been introduced for the management of convulsive disorders, magnesium sulfate has remained the medication of choice for the prevention and treatment of eclamptic convulsions. As the levels of $MgSO_4$ reach their therapeutic dose of 6 to 7 mEq/liter, the deep tendon reflexes decrease at 4 mEq/liter, and may be absent when levels approach 10 mEq/liter. At 5 mEq/liter, cardiac conduction is prolonged, as measured by the P-R interval and the QRS restoration. Occasional instances of complete heart block have been reported at levels below 10 mEq/liter. Excessive levels of magnesium block muscular transmission by decreasing the amount of acetylcholine released in response to nerve action potential. Calcium antagonizes this effect. At 15 mEq/liter, an additional hazard is respiratory paralysis, and at 25 mEq/liter, cardiac arrest may occur. These side effects can be counterbalanced by the administration of calcium salts. Magnesium poisoning is characterized by a sharp drop in blood pressure and by respiratory paralysis. Artificial respiration should be administered until calcium salts can be injected intravenously.

As an antagonist to $MgSO_4$, 1 g of calcium gluconate is administered intravenously over 3 minutes (10 ml of a 10 percent solution) (Gant and Worley, 1980). There is usually a good response to the calcium unless the reaction is severe enough to cause cardiac arrest.

Hypermagnesemia in the newborn has not been correlated with maternal or fetal magnesium levels. In normal pregnancy, the maternal and cord serum levels of magnesium are identical. Stone and Pritchard (1970) have shown that after parenteral administration of magnesium sulfate to normal and preeclamptic women, there is delayed increase in the concentration of fetal magnesium. Chesley and Tepper (1957) reported that, using usual doses, the fetal level reaches 90 percent of maternal concentrations in 3 hours.

Barbiturates act as sedatives and anticonvulsants. They cross the placenta rapidly and should not be given if delivery is imminent. Phenobarbital does not prevent convulsions. After an isolated seizure, 0.25 to 0.5 g amylbarbitol (sodium amytal) is effective when given by slow intravenous injection; however, $MgSO_4$ may be the drug of choice in the emergency situation, because sodium amytal must be reconstituted to use.

Diazepam (Valium) produces an anticonvulsant effect when given intravenously; it stops convulsions quickly, but its effect may last only 20 minutes. Convulsions in adults usually stop after one or two 5-mg injections, but 20 mg or more may be required. Because the drug crosses the placenta and the neonate cannot excrete the drug readily, toxic levels have been detected in the infant as long as 3 weeks after delivery. Twelve minutes after maternal intravenous injection of diazepam, concentrations of the drug in the umbilical cord and the maternal plasma are equal. Valium is primarily recommended for postpartum eclampsia.

Mannitol may cause a fluid overload. The role of diuretics should be limited to patients with proved pulmonary edema. Acute pulmonary edema is a common cause of death and should be handled as a very serious medical emergency in an intensive care unit. The treatment involves the administration of oxygen, morphine, and digitalis (digoxin).

Furosemide (Lasix) is very useful in treating pulmonary edema; however, objections have been raised to its use in preeclampsia-eclampsia–induced pulmonary edema, because increased peripheral resistance and systemic hypertension may lead to left ventricular failure and pulmonary edema. Therefore, under ideal circumstances, the use of furosemide and the infusion of colloid or crystallized solutions should be governed by the pulmonary artery wedge pressure.

Digitalization should be considered if signs of congestive heart failure develop. Electrocardiography should be performed to determine whether any contraindication to its use exists. Initially, 0.6 mg lanatoside C is given intravenously for tachycardia above 120. Digitalization is maintained with 0.25 to 0.5 mg digoxin daily. Maintenance of a patent airway may require an endotracheal tube. Tracheostomy may be necessary in case of laryngeal obstruction.

## PATIENT MANAGEMENT

Persistently symptomatic patients, particularly those with severe preeclampsia demonstrating a diastolic pressure of 110 mm Hg or greater, severe proteinuria (3 +), oliguria, pulmonary edema, and cyanosis, should be cared for in a quiet, darkened room with a 1:1 nurse-to-patient ratio (Table 25–10). A

**Table 25–10**
PATIENT MANAGEMENT BASICS WHEN MATERNAL DISEASE OR SEVERE PREECLAMPSIA PERSISTS

1. 1:1 nurse-to-patient ratio
2. $MgSO_4$ administered to prevent convulsions
3. Hydralazine given to keep diastolic blood pressure less than 110 mm HG
4. Type and cross-match and CBC
5. DIC profile
6. Fetal monitoring
7. Urimeter
8. CVP line if indicated
9. Intake and output (hourly)
10. Blood pressure every 15 to 30 minutes
11. Liver enzymes
12. Eclampsia tray at bedside

supportive person should attend to the patient; however, visitors should be limited. All observations must be recorded carefully on flow sheets. Observe for signs and symptoms of impending eclampsia (Table 25–11).

Vital signs, including respirations, pulse, blood pressure, and fetal heart rate, should be monitored every 15 minutes while the patient is receiving MgSO$_4$. The fetal heart rate should be monitored closely. Because uterine perfusion is already compromised, persistent late decelerations and fetal acidosis are anticipated. Abrupt changes in the fetal heart rate have been demonstrated during convulsions (Vink et al, 1980). Uterine activity should be documented with an intrauterine pressure catheter and assessed every hour. If oxytocin is administered, assessment should be made every 15 minutes (Butts, 1965; Wheeler and Jones, 1981). Because these patients are NPO and are mouth breathing during labor, they should have good mouth care.

Fetal monitoring should be initiated, preferably with an internal monitor. It should be documented every 15 minutes in the first stage and every 5 minutes in the second stage of labor. If electronic fetal monitoring is not available, the fetal heart rate should be assessed and documented every 15 minutes during the first stage of labor, and every 5 minutes during the second stage. The fetal heart rate should be listened to during several contractions, through the last half of the contraction and for 30 seconds after the end of the contraction (Wheeler and Jones, 1981).

If the patient has severe preeclampsia, a Swan-Ganz pulmonary artery catheter should be used to accurately assess blood pressure, volume, and cardiac output. However, a central venous pressure catheter is most commonly used to assess fluid replacement and intravascular volume. In Catanzarite and associates' (1991) survey of perinatologists, two thirds said they used arterial lines and rarely or never used central venous pressure or Swan-Ganz catheters. Ten percent said they routinely used the catheters; use increased when these were applied by the perinatologist rather than the anesthesiologist or other health care professional. A urinary catheter with a urimeter should be inserted to measure hourly output. Fluid intake should also be monitored hourly. The patient's fluid intake should be limited; however, if hypovolemia occurs, it requires careful correction. Oliguria may be corrected by fluid infusion (fluid challenge). However, if the oliguria is of renal origin, then the patient is at risk for fluid overload. Hypotonic solutions should not be used. "In patients with decreased colloid oncotic pressure due to decreased serum albumin, colloid-containing fluid should be used" (Creasy and Resnick, 1989). If there are no signs of renal complications or congestive heart failure, "1000 ml of isotonic crystalloid, or if appropriate, 500 ml of colloid-containing solution can safely be infused in one hour" (Creasy and Resnick, 1989). If urinary output increases, maintain administration at 100 ml. If urinary output does not improve, assessment should be continued with central venous or pulmonary wedge pressures (Creasy and Resnick, 1989). The fluid intake for 24 hours should not exceed 1000 ml plus the amount of urinary output of the preceding 24 hours. If the patient is severely hypovolemic and in shock, when demonstrated with monitoring of the circulatory pressure by the central venous pressure line or Swan-Ganz catheter, additional fluid is recommended. Blood replacement (packed red blood cells), if required, should be initiated early, when patients are eclamptic. However, precautions should be observed to prevent overloading of the cardiovascular system. Oliguria is a common consequence of eclampsia and indicates the need for prompt termination of pregnancy. Diuretics may mask the intensity of the hypovolemia and oliguria.

The urine should have a specific gravity of at least 1.018 and should be yellow. Zuspan (1980) has noted that "severe preeclampsia occasionally causes hemolysis manifested by either jaundice or dark-colored urine, which probably represents hepatocellular damage and red blood cell destruction." This is usually an ominous sign. Sometimes, hematuria is found with the administration of MgSO$_4$. The etiology is unknown.

An eclampsia tray (Table 25–12) should be

**Table 25–11**
SIGNS AND SYMPTOMS OF
IMPENDING ECLAMPSIA

Scotomata or blurred vision
Epigastric pain
Persistent or severe headache
Vomiting
Neurologic hyperactivity
Pulmonary edema or cyanosis

**Table 25-12**
ITEMS FOR A PREECLAMPSIA TRAY

Needles
Syringes
An airway
Padded tongue blade
Calcium gluconate—two 1-cc vials
Sodium amylbarbital—two 1-cc vials
$MgSO_4$
Suction and $O_2$ should be available

kept at bedside during the antepartum hospitalization, the intrapartum period, and in the recovery room. It should include needles, syringes, an airway, and a padded tongue blade to be carefully inserted between the jaws to protect the tongue. Calcium gluconate should be included in case of $MgSO_4$ overdose. Sodium amylbarbital can be included to stop seizures. Because $MgSO_4$ potentiates it, the dose should be less than 0.25 to 0.5 g (Cavanagh and Knuppel, 1982).

Because of the use of $MgSO_4$, and also depending on the fetal condition, a pediatrician or neonatologist should attend the birth of the baby of a preeclamptic or eclamptic mother.

Gabbe and associates (1986) recommend that epidural anesthesia be used with these patients, and arterial and central lines be used for hemodynamic monitoring because their contracted blood volume places them at high risk for hypotension. This is supported by the Experts Opine (1985) in an article in which obstetric anesthesiologists and obstetricians gave opinions on preferred anesthesia for severe preeclampsia. It was reported that with careful hemodynamic monitoring, these patients could receive fluids to prevent hypotension without overload (Albright, 1978). The use of general anesthesia may raise two concerns: (1) it may cause aspiration or (2) induction may fail owing to unsuspected laryngeal edema.

## ECLAMPSIA

Eclampsia represents the convulsive phase of preeclampsia. Eclampsia is more prevalent among patients who had inadequate antenatal care and in those who have had unsuspected deterioration of the maternal status during the early puerperium. Approximately 5 percent of preeclamptic patients become eclamptic. Early diagnosis, skillful prenatal care, and careful management of preeclampsia are capable of reducing the incidence of eclampsia and, thus, the accompanying maternal and perinatal risks. The worldwide perinatal mortality rate associated with eclampsia may be as high as 30 to 35 percent. Eclampsia is seldom encountered in patients who have received appropriate antenatal care and were hospitalized promptly when preeclampsia first became evident.

Eclampsia is a preventable disease. However, because it is clearly a disease of lower socioeconomic women, access to care has an impact on the occurrence of eclampsia (Creasy and Resnik, 1989).

Deep tendon reflexes should be monitored, because many women experience increased reflexes before seizures. However, Sibai and associates (1981) reported that seizures can occur without hyperreflexia. Assessment should be made when seizures occur, with notation of the onset of the seizure, the progress of the seizure, the body involvement, the duration of the convulsion, incontinence, status of the fetus, and signs of abruption. Usually the convulsion begins with facial twitching, and then the head turns to one side, with the neck tense and the eyes staring. During the seizure, a patent airway should be maintained with adequate oxygen up to 3 liters per minute. The patient should be turned to her side to prevent aspiration. Suctioning may be necessary to clear the glottis or trachea. During the seizure, the patient should be protected from injury. Tongue blades should be used to protect the tongue. Do not insert the tongue blades into the back of the throat, because this may cause a gag reflex. Do not insert fingers into the patient's mouth, because they may be bitten. Because many facilities no longer advocate inserting anything into the mouth, check hospital protocol for tongue blade insertion (Bobak and Jensen, 1991). Padding of the side rails of the bed has also been recommended. To break the seizure, 4 to 6 g of $MgSO_4$ are administered over 5 minutes. Sodium amylbarbital has also been used; however, administration of this drug requires reconstitution, which may be difficult at the time of an emergency.

During a convulsion, there may be fetal bradycardia. If possible, allow the mother and fetus to recover before delivery. The stress of the seizure may decrease the duration of labor and precipitate delivery (Pritchard, 1980). It is important to give a minimum of constant nursing care (1:1 nurse-to-patient ratio) to assess fetal and maternal status and to avoid precipitous delivery, which has a risk of laceration and increased bleeding.

After the seizure, routine observations are imperative. The maternal lungs are checked frequently, because acute pulmonary edema is common in eclamptic patients. A detailed intake and output chart must be available, with the amounts recorded hourly. Blood should be obtained immediately for typing and cross-matching with a baseline hematocrit.

It may be necessary to establish a patent airway and administer oxygen. A nasogastric tube may be used to empty the patient's stomach and instill 30 ml of antacid. After delivery, coughing, turning, deep breathing, and intermittent positive-pressure breathing treatments may be needed to prevent aspiration pneumonia. If the patient's electrolytes are abnormal, the intravenous may have to be changed to a more physiologic solution, perhaps D5/normal saline. The vital signs should be monitored every 5 minutes until the patient is stable, and then every 15 minutes. Continued assessment of laboratory values, including MgSO$_4$ levels, is important. The patient should be encouraged to stay on her side to increase urinary excretion and uterine perfusion and to prevent aspiration of saliva and nasopharyngeal secretions.

To decrease the patient's agitation and confusion, a family member should be at the bedside as she regains consciousness. Continue to avoid bright lights, noises, and numerous people at the bedside. Also try to organize care to avoid frequent disturbances.

The number of convulsions may vary from 1 or 2 to as many as 10 or 20. "The duration of coma after the seizure is variable. When the convulsions are infrequent, the woman usually recovers some degree of consciousness after each seizure. As the woman arouses, a semiconscious combative state may ensue. In severe cases, the coma persists from one convulsion to another, and death may result before the mother awakens" (Pritchard and MacDonald, 1980).

The most dreaded maternal complication is cerebral hemorrhage, which occurs when the blood pressure is not controlled. Loss of vision from edema or hemorrhage may be a sign of impending cerebrovascular accident, although usually this loss of vision is temporary (Zuspan, 1980). To control the blood pressure, hydralazine is given.

Pritchard has reported excellent success in treating 154 consecutive eclamptics over a 20-year period (Pritchard, 1975). Approximately three fourths of the patients in whom eclampsia developed were delivered vaginally. Steps were initiated to effect delivery as soon as the patient regained consciousness.

The latent period between induction of labor and cesarean birth varies. Procrastination is unwise, and the patient should be delivered soon after stabilization is achieved. It is better to deliver a low-birth-weight infant by cesarean delivery if the cervix is not inducible or if the fetus is not in vertex presentation.

Oxytocin is used for induction; however, assessment of the antidiuretic effect in these patients is imperative. At 45 mU/min, the antidiuretic effect is at its maximum (Chesley, 1979), although this dose is rarely necessary for labor and delivery. Any woman on oxytocin is at an increased risk for water intoxication, and thus, fluid intake and output should be monitored closely. The patient with pregnancy-induced hypertension is at an even greater risk, and thus, a continuous infusion pump should be used to control intravenous fluid intake. This risk of water intoxication is the result of a combination of factors: The patient may already have spontaneous oliguria; oxytocin has an antidiuretic effect; the patient may lie on her back, which decreases urinary blood flow; and antihypertensive drugs decrease urinary output. These combined processes inhibit the excretion of water while increasing the patient's circulating volume and diluting the the electrolytes (Chesley, 1979). Thus, keep intake low. If the oxytocin has to be increased, increase the concentration, rather than continuing to increase the total fluid volume.

If the patient has a seizure, it may be due to water intoxication rather than to eclampsia or vasoconstriction alone. In water intoxication seizures, there is muscle weakness and cramping, and a decrease in respiration. However, the best way to diagnose the cause of the seizure is to look at the intake and output. In addition, a decreased sodium level in the plasma, usually 115 to 125 mEq/liter, is found in patients having seizures caused by water intoxication (Chesley, 1979).

The patient with eclampsia may be very sensitive to oxytocin. Be alert for hyperstimulation and precipitous delivery. Use of an intrauterine catheter is advisable to measure uterine tone. Chesley (1979) has reported that most patients with eclampsia can be delivered by oxytocin induction. Zuspan (1980) reports that most eclamptic patients are delivered within 18 hours.

If the eclamptic patient is being transported to a regional center, MgSO$_4$ should be maintained during transport. The patient should be accompanied by a person trained to use a preeclamptic tray and who understands the use and side effects of MgSO$_4$.

Placental abruption is a complication of pregnancy-induced hypertension. As a result of the vasospasm, there is a decrease in the perfusion of the intervillous space, which seems to increase the risk of abruption. Observe for severe sustained pain with a rigid abdomen. The resting tone on the contraction channel of the internal fetal monitor usually increases significantly. There can be vaginal bleeding; however, in some cases, the blood may accumulate behind the placenta during abruption, with no vaginal bleeding.

## POSTPARTUM CARE OF PREECLAMPSIA-ECLAMPSIA

Once the fetus has been delivered, preeclampsia-eclampsia commonly abates within 24 hours. We continue administering MgSO$_4$ for 24 hours after delivery. Of 210 perinatologists surveyed by Catanzarite and associates (1991), 198 indicated that they administered MgSO$_4$ 1 to 48 hours after delivery, with a mean of 23.5 hours. Twelve of the perinatologists said they continued MgSO$_4$ until diuresis occurred (Catanzarite et al, 1991). However, there are some patients who will continue to be preeclamptic for up to 5 weeks after delivery. It is important to recognize that the salutary effects of delivery result from delivery of the *placenta* rather than that of the fetus. Eclampsia has been reported in several instances after intrauterine fetal death. Although most women become normotensive within a day or two after delivery, their blood pressures occasionally remain elevated for a few weeks rather than a few days. In our service, if the hypertension remains severe with a diastolic

pressure of 110 mm Hg or greater, we reassess the patient to be sure that a detectable cause of hypertension has not been overlooked. If the patient does not demonstrate a diastolic blood pressure of greater than 110 mm Hg and there are no complications, we usually discharge the patient without instituting antihypertensive medication. We do so only after arranging for the patient to return weekly to our office, so that we can continue to monitor her blood pressure.

Patients with preeclampsia should be placed under close observation for 24 hours, because about 10 to 25 percent of the patients have seizures during the first 24 hours. Most occur by 24 hours; virtually all will occur by 48 hours. There have been rare exceptions after 48 hours. The patient should be continued on MgSO$_4$ for 24 hours at a minimum, *or until the blood pressure has returned to normal with normal reflexes for two 4-hour consecutive periods with adequate output.* During the administration of MgSO$_4$, either intramuscularly or intravenously, the patient should remain in the recovery room or under close observation in a labor, delivery, recovery (LDR) room or labor, delivery, recovery, postpartum (LDRP) room. Vital signs should be monitored every 15 minutes until the patient is stable. Because of the toxemic state and the administration of MgSO$_4$, vital signs should be continued every 15 to 30 minutes while the patient is on MgSO$_4$. Remember that the patient with preeclampsia-eclampsia is very sensitive to blood loss because of a decreased intravascular compartment. Even a moderate amount of bleeding after delivery may cause serious hypovolemia, with resulting oliguria. Thus, decreased blood pressure may be a sign of hypovolemia, rather than relief of the vasospasm.

Because output is an indicator of blood volume, hourly intake and output should be continued while the patient receives MgSO$_4$. Oliguria of less than 30 ml/h may signify a worsening of the disease; however, if the oliguria is accompanied by normal blood pressure and normal reflexes, it may indicate hypovolemia and a fluid challenge may be successful. Patients with normal output and normal blood pressures may have relief of their vasospasm. The bladder should be kept empty to avoid uterine relaxation. This should be easy to accomplish, because a Foley catheter should already be in place.

During this initial period, as in the antepartum and intrapartum periods, the patient should be observed for signs of pulmonary edema (see Table 25–13), cardiac failure (see Table 25–14), and DIC (Table 25–15).

While the patient is in the recovery room, LDR, or LDRR, she should be allowed visitors for short periods of time. She should be allowed to visit with her new baby as much as her condition allows. Breastfeeding should not be discouraged, even with the MgSO$_4$ therapy. If the fetus has died, grief counseling can be initiated at this time.

Once the MgSO$_4$ has been discontinued, the patient can then be transferred to the postpartum floor. She should have her blood pressure and pulse observed and recorded every 4 hours, and a hematocrit should be obtained daily. The patient usually remains in the hospital for 3 to 5 days after delivery, depending on her clinical course.

After discharge, the patient should be seen in 1 week. If her blood pressure is still elevated, the patient should be seen weekly until the hypertension is resolved (Zuspan, 1980). If the patient's blood pressure is still elevated at the 6-week checkup, she should be sent for a hypertensive workup. The management for these patients is summarized in Table 25–16.

In regard to counseling the patient for further pregnancies, Zuspan has stated that pregnancy-induced hypertension does not increase the incidence of hypertension in later life (Zuspan, 1980). Chesley (1980) followed 270 women for 40 years and found that women with preeclampsia are not at risk for hypertensive disorders in subsequent pregnancies. Preeclampsia does not cause permanent damage or predispose the patient to chronic hypertension (Creasy and Resnick, 1989). Chesley (1978) found no increase in hypertension, cardiovascular mortality, or death rate in women with eclampsia in their first pregnancy who were followed for more than 40 years.

Because the fetus of a mother with preeclampsia-eclampsia is at high risk, a pediatrician should be in attendance at delivery.

**Table 25–13**

SIGNS AND SYMPTOMS OF
PULMONARY EDEMA

Rales
Tachycardia
Increased CVP (normal: 9–11 cm H$_2$O)
Shortness of breath
Distended neck veins

**Table 25–14**

SIGNS AND SYMPTOMS OF
CARDIAC FAILURE

Cyanosis
Increased pulse rate
Decreased blood pressure
Tachypnea and rales
Distended neck veins
Increased central venous pressure

The baby may be growth retarded (Fig. 25–4) and have the problems associated with this condition, such as hypoglycemia, hypocalcemia, asphyxia at birth due to decreased placental function, meconium aspiration, polycythemia, pulmonary hemorrhage, and an increased risk of infection. The baby also may be depressed as a result of hypermagnesemia. If the baby is hypotonic, he or she can be treated with calcium; however, this rarely occurs.

Lloret and Lloret (1990) demonstrated that patients with hypertensive disorders have fetuses with intrauterine growth retardation (IUGR), general morbidity, and perinatal mortality rates 3 to 5 times higher than the control group. In addition, they found that perinatal morbidity and mortality rates increased not only in relation to type and severity of hypertension but also to the severity of proteinuria (Friedman and Neff, 1978; Lloret and Lloret, 1990). They also found an increase in morbidity and mortality rates when the hematocrit was greater than 38, and the hemoglobin was greater than 12.5 (hemoconcentration).

IUGR is associated with preeclampsia. Accelerated aging of the placenta has been documented and can be visualized by the use of ultrasonography. The obstetrician and the pediatrician must work together closely in order to provide optimum care to both the

**Table 25–15**

SIGNS AND SYMPTOMS OF DISSEMINATED
INTRAVASCULAR COAGULATION

Oozing from IV or suture sites and bleeding gums
Clotting studies—While awaiting laboratory results, set aside a tube of blood and determine how long it takes for it to clot; without DIC, blood should clot in 6 to 7 minutes

| | |
|---|---|
| Prolonged PT | (normal: 10.6 to 13.3 sec) |
| Prolonged PTT | (normal: 27.8 to 38 sec) |
| Fibrinogen < 300 mg/dl | (normal: 400 mg/dl) |
| FSP > 40 $\mu$g/ml | (normal: NONE) |
| Platelets < 100,000 | (normal: 200,000–500,000) |

**Table 25–16**
PATIENT CARE SUMMARY FOR PREECLAMPSIA*

| | Antepartum | | Intrapatrum | Postpartum |
|---|---|---|---|---|
| | *Outpatient* | *Inpatient* | | |
| BP | 1–2 × week | q 4 h | q 15 min | q 15 min until stable; then q 15–30 min while on MgSO$_4$, then q 1 h × 2 then q 4 h |
| P, R | Weekly | q 4 h | q 15 min | As above |
| T | Weekly | q shift | q 4 h | q 4 h |
| Bed rest | Yes | Yes | Yes | While on MgSO$_4$ |
| Weight | Weekly | Daily | — | — |
| Edema | Weekly | Daily | On admission | — |
| Urinalysis | | | | |
|   for protein | Weekly | Daily | On admission; then q 4 h | — |
|   24-h collection | Weekly | Weekly | — | — |
| Retinal changes | Weekly | Daily | On admission | — |
| DTR | Weekly | q shift | q 1 h while on MgSO$_4$ | q 1 h while on MgSO$_4$ |
| I & O | — | q shift | q 1 h | q 1 h while on MgSO$_4$ |
| Fetal heart rate | NST-CST weekly, starting at 30–32 weeks' gestation | NST-CST weekly; q shift FHR | Continuous during labor, preferably internal. If no monitor available, q 15 min in first stage and q 5 min in second stage, listening through 2–3 contractions | — |
| Contractions Frequency Duration Quality Resting tone | Weekly | q shift | Continuously with electronic fetal monitor. If no monitor available, q 1 h; induction 15 min in first stage | Fundal checks: q 15 min × 4; then q 30 min × 2; then q 4 h Lochia: Same as above |
| Sonogram | 3–4 weeks | 3–4 weeks | — | — |
| Amniocentesis (for L/S ratio) | Weekly after 33–34 weeks until mature | | — | — |
| Laboratory values; analysis with: DIC screen Liver enzymes Magnesium levels | — | Weekly | On admission | After delivery |
| CBC and platelets | Weekly | Weekly | On admission | On admission to RR; then prn |
| Serum creatinine and BUN creatinine clearance | Weekly | Weekly | — | — |
| Sexual counseling | No restrictions | — | — | — |

* Nurse–patient ratios: *antepartum,* 1:6–8; *intrapartum,* 1:2; *recovery room,* 1:2–4, *postpartum* 1:6–8.
Severe preeclampsia 1:4, *intrapartum,* 1:1–2:1, *recovery room,* 1:1–1:2.

mother and the neonate. A physician skilled in cardiopulmonary resuscitation must be in the delivery room, because premature or growth-retarded newborns often suffer from poor thermal regulation, hyperviscosity, and episodes of hypoglycemia. The IUGR infant is generally asymmetric, its head appears disproportionately large for its height and weight, and the paucity of subcutaneous fat causes it to have the appearance of an old man (Fig. 25–4). Quirk and coworkers (1979) suggest that atraumatic delivery of the low-

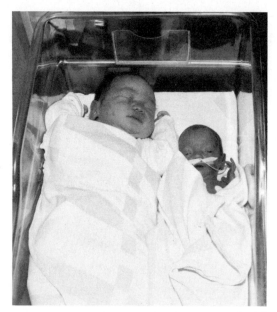

**Figure 25–4.** IUGR infant (*right*) compared with normal newborn (*left*). (Photograph courtesy of Dr Gary Cohen, University of South Florida College of Medicine, Tampa, FL.)

birth-weight infant may reduce the incidence of respiratory distress syndrome. Bowes (1977) has demonstrated that cesarean delivery and atraumatic vaginal delivery may reduce neonatal problems and the probability of respiratory distress syndrome.

## HELLP SYNDROME

Pritchard and associates (1954) reported three cases of preeclampsia complicated by hemolysis, elevated liver enzymes, and low platelets. Goodlin and associates (1978) described the syndrome as EPH (edema, proteinuria, hypertension) gestosis type B. They stated that the condition had been reported in the literature for 100 years. The syndrome is found in older multiparous patients and is associated with abdominal pain, elevated liver function tests, low platelets, and multisystem organ dysfunction. Subsequent cases describing these symptoms were thought to be complications of disseminated intravascular coagulation or acute fatty liver disease (Killam et al, 1975). Weinstein (1982) reported 29 cases of preeclampsia exhibiting HELLP syndrome. Although HELLP syndrome usually is associated with severe preeclampsia, it may occur before the signs of preeclampsia and, therefore, may be diagnosed as gastroenteritis, hepatitis, gallbladder disease, pyelonephritis, chronic renal disease, or idiopathic thrombocytopenic purpura.

Patients with HELLP syndrome usually present with symptoms before term, about 90 percent before 36 weeks' gestation. They have malaise; about 90 percent experience epigastric or upper right quadrant pain, and about 50 percent experience nausea and vomiting. Some have virus-like symptoms as well as symptoms of common anemia, such as fatigue, pallor, anorexia, weakness, lassitude, and dyspnea. Additional symptoms may include significant weight gain and edema. The patient may have slight hypertension or proteinuria or none at all. However, HELLP syndrome usually occurs with symptoms of severe preeclampsia-eclampsia. Regardless of their blood pressure and presence of protein in urine, these patients should have a complete blood cell count with platelets and liver enzymes (Sibai, 1990). Sibai (1990) suggests that LDH and bilirubin values be assessed and added to the criteria to diagnose HELLP syndrome.

Sibai and associates (1986) described an 8-year study of 112 patients with severe preeclampsia-eclampsia and HELLP syndrome. The incidence of HELLP syndrome in this study was 9.7 percent of the severe preeclamptic-eclamptic patients. This is high for the preeclamptic-eclamptic population because 58 percent of the patients with HELLP syndrome were transported from other hospitals. They found that the disease is increased in white, older, multiparous patients. The incidence is higher when the diagnosis of preeclampsia was delayed or if there was a delay in the patient's delivery. In that study, the perinatal mortality rate was 367 per 1000, with significant neonatal morbidity. Maternal morbidity and mortality rates were also high, resulting in two maternal deaths, two patients with ruptured liver hematoma, and nine patients with acute renal failure. Thirty-eight percent had intravascular coagulopathy, and 21.4 percent had prolonged partial prothrombin times. These complications were most often associated with abruption (20 percent) and fetal death (19 percent). Vaginal deliveries were performed in 36.6 percent of the women, and 63.4 percent were delivered by cesarean delivery. Ninety-three percent of the patients received blood or blood products. Of the infants in this study, 26 percent had thrombocytopenia (<150,000); 14 percent had leukopenia and neutropenia; and 11 percent had disseminated intravascular coagulation (DIC). All of the infants with these complications were premature with low APGAR scores or were severely retarded. There was no relationship of maternal and neonatal thrombocytopenia or DIC. Weinstein (1982; 1985) completed two studies that indicated a maternal mortality rate of 3.5 percent. Like Sibai and associates' (1986) study, 24 percent of the infants had thrombocytopenia, and 35 percent had leukopenia.

There is some difference in the definition of the symptoms of the syndrome and, therefore, the true incidence is not known. However, it is believed to occur in about 4 to 12 percent in patients with severe preeclampsia and eclampsia.

## Hemolysis

In preeclampsia, vasospasms occur that damage the endothelial layer of the small vessels, causing lesions that allow platelet aggregation and formation of a fibrin network. As red blood cells flow through the fibrin network, they are damaged, and this process results in hemolysis. Hemolysis is confirmed by the presence of abnormal blood cells, usually schistocytes and echinocytes, on a peripheral blood smear. Echinocytes, also known as burr cells, are caused by increased plasma levels of free fatty acids (increased in HELLP due to hepatic dysfunction) and decreased serum concentration of albumin. This causes contracted red blood cells with spiny projections appearing along the edge of the cell. Sibai (1990) describes criteria for hemolysis:

Abnormal peripheral smear
Increased bilirubin ≥ 1.2 mg/dl

Burrow and Ferris (1986) described an association of increased stillborns and premature infants with a hemoglobin of less than 6 g/100 ml. In preeclampsia, the fetus already may be compromised owing to maternal vasospasm and decreased uteroplacental perfusion. Anemia could further reduce oxygen to the fetus.

## Elevated Liver Enzymes

Increased serum glutamic-oxaloacetic transaminase (SGOT) and serum glutamic-pyruvic transaminase (SGPT) are noted in HELLP syndrome. Liver ischemia and damage occur because of microemboli in the hepatic sinuses, causing local necrosis and subcapsular hemorrhages. Obstruction of blood through the liver probably causes distention resulting in upper right quadrant and epigastric pain and, rarely, hepatic rupture. Sibai (1990) describes the criteria for elevated liver enzymes:

SGOT ≥ 70 U/liter
Increased lactic dehydrogenase (LDH) > 600 U/liter

## Low Platelets

Platelets increase secondary to consumption of circulating platelets that adhere to the damaged endothelium sites caused by vasospasm in preeclampsia. As platelet consumption occurs, thrombocytopenia can be identified. Increased thromboxane also may contribute to this, because it causes not only vasoconstriction but also platelet aggregation. This condition differs from DIC in that the maternal coagulation factors PT and PTT remain normal in HELLP syndrome. Sibai (1990) defines low platelets as less than 100,000 $\mu$l.

## Treatment

The treatment for a patient with HELLP syndrome is similar to that for a patient with severe preeclampsia-eclampsia. Both patients should receive $MgSO_4$. Assessment should be made for worsening preeclampsia (Table 25–6) with continued assessment of platelet counts and liver enzymes as well as other laboratory values. The mother should not take aspirin and should be protected from developing hypoxia and hemorrhage. Clinical signs of thrombocytopenia should be assessed by observing abnormal bleeding such as hematuria, petechiae, ecchymoses, bloody stools or emesis, or oozing from intravenous sites or mucous membranes. Shoulder pain should be noted, because this might be a symptom of massive ascites or pleural effusions. If pain is present, the patient should undergo a computed axial tomography (CT) scan of the liver to rule out hepatic capsular hematoma. If the patient is in shock from subcapsular liver hematoma, the patient should be prepared for transfusions and immediate laparotomy (Sibai, 1990). Hourly intake and output should be precise, to avoid fluid overload and to observe for output that is less than 30 ml/h. Blood replacement is usually necessary for hypovolemia. Platelet transfusion is controversial because the effect is only transient when the platelet count is less than 20,000 $\mu$l. Fresh frozen plasma is recommended to correct coagulopathy. Also, continue to observe for signs of pulmonary edema (Table 25–13) and cardiac failure (Table 25–14).

These maternal changes can affect fetal well-being; therefore, constant assessment of the fetus is imperative. An emotional and psychologic assessment must be made, because the patient and her family are concerned about the status of the fetus as well as the critical state of the mother.

Weinstein (1982; 1985) stated that preeclampsia with HELLP syndrome mandates prompt delivery of the fetus regardless of gestational age, either by induction or cesarean delivery. Killam (1975) and Schwartz (1983) support this practice. MacKenna (1983) has stated that immediate delivery is not always warranted. In his study, patients were at bed rest in the left lateral position receiving MgSO$_4$ intravenously, and delivery was postponed from 24 hours to 24 days. Goodlin (1982) and Thiagarajah (1984) support this more conservative approach. Goodlin (1982) believes that hypovolemia is important in the consideration of the treatment of the disease, and recommends plasma volume expanders with 5 percent albumin; he had a 10 percent success rate in prolonging pregnancy. Thiagarajah (1984) was able to increase the platelet count and improve liver enzymes in five patients by administering prednisone or betamethasone. Two of these patients, however, had abruptio placentae and fetal death. The deliveries of 12 of these patients were delayed and treated with corticosteroids for fetal lung maturity. A review of the overall findings of 231 patients (Goodlin, 1978; MacKenna, 1983; McKay, 1972; Pillay, 1985; Pritchard, 1980; Schwartz, 1983; Thiagarajah, 1984; Weinstein, 1982) demonstrated 7 maternal deaths (corrected 5 in 231), with such high mortality rates delivery should not be delayed, except 48 to 72 hours for corticosteroid therapy to be effective. Serial platelet counts should be assessed closely, and if they drop quickly, intervention should no longer be delayed.

Sibai (1990) recommends administering 10 U of platelets before intubation when a cesarean delivery is indicated. He also advises leaving the bladder flap open with a subfascial drain for 24 to 48 hours and leaving the wound open with sutures in situ from the level of the fascia. The incision can be closed within 72 hours. Closing the wound at the time of surgery caused hematoma in 20 percent of his patients. Although epidural anesthesia with careful hemodynamic monitoring is recommended in severe preeclampsia-eclampsia, it is not recommended in patients with thrombocytopenia or significant coagulopathy. Because of the coagulopathy or thrombocytopenia, these patients may bleed into the epidural space (Experts Opine, 1985). Sibai (1990) recommends epidural anesthesia be used only when it is safer than general anesthesia, such as in patients with marked laryngeal edema, marked obesity with short neck, and pulmonary disease.

In the immediate postpartum period, the patient should be observed closely for blood loss, because the patient may bleed owing to the thrombocytopenia. Also, because of the reduced blood volume, the patient may become hypotensive with very little blood loss. Sibai (1990) reported that 31 percent developed HELLP syndrome during the postpartum period, usually within 48 hours after delivery. Seventy-nine percent of those who developed HELLP syndrome in the postpartum period had symptoms of preeclampsia. McKenna (1983) reported that liver function tests convert to normal within 72 hours postpartum. Sibai (1990) followed 59 patients through 80 subsequent pregnancies, and 3.4 percent (2 patients) had recurrent HELLP syndrome. The two patients that had ruptured subcapsular liver hematoma had no recurrence of the syndrome.

Patients with HELLP syndrome usually need intensive care for at least 48 hours after delivery. It may be longer if DIC also is present. Intensive care is necessary because these patients are at risk for pulmonary edema and compromised renal function (Sibai, 1990).

Infant deaths are related to prematurity, intrauterine asphyxia, and abruptio placentae. About one third of these infants will be growth retarded. Some infants will have thrombocytopenia and leukopenia and must be observed closely, because there is a potential in these infants for central nervous system hemorrhage.

Patients with HELLP syndrome are critically ill and should be rigorously assessed, not only for worsening of their disease, but also for complications such as pulmonary edema, renal shut down, and cardiac failure. Patients should be counseled that although they were very sick, there is only a small chance that HELLP syndrome will recur in future pregnancies.

# Chronic Hypertension

Occasionally, the patient is first seen with symptoms of chronic hypertension. If the patient is seen after the 20th week of gestation, the differential diagnosis may be difficult because of the well-documented decrease in blood pressure that occurs during the second trimester in normotensive as well as in most chronically hypertensive women. It is important to have historical evidence documenting previous hypertension. Typically, as pregnancy progresses, the patient's blood pressure often returns to the previous hypertensive reading, requiring an increase in the antihypertensive medication, or the dilemma of deciding whether the patient has preeclampsia and chronic hypertension. The diagnostic problem for the health care team is to differentiate between the chronic hypertensive state and acute preeclampsia-eclampsia. Chronic hypertensive disease is suggested by the following factors:

1. Hemorrhages and exudates seen in the optic fundi.
2. Plasma creatinine concentrations greater than 1 mg/dl.
3. Plasma urea nitrogen concentrations greater than 20 mg/dl.
4. The presence of chronic diseases, such as diabetes mellitus with nephropathy, and connective tissue disease.

The uric acid level in the maternal serum may also help to differentiate the chronic hypertensive patient from the patient with acute pregnancy-induced hypertension.

The patient with chronic hypertension may have an underlying condition that predisposes her to the hypertension, the two most common being hypertensive disease and renal and urinary tract disease. In addition to these diseases, there are numerous other conditions that may cause or underlie chronic hypertension complicating pregnancy. The obstetric team should search for evidence of such conditions when evaluating

women with pregnancy-associated hypertension. During the physical examination, one can appropriately record blood pressure in both the upper and lower extremities. In addition, the thorax should be auscultated and the femoral pulses palpated to rule out coarctation of the aorta. Auscultation of the flank may identify the bruit of unilateral renovascular stenosis. The urinary metanephrine spot test detects the presence of a pheochromocytoma. A search for antinuclear antibodies or the anti-DNA antibody, a glucose intolerance test, and measurement of the BUN and creatinine, as well as creatinine clearance and quantitative protein excretion determinations, are all part of a reasonable evaluation of the patient.

## MANAGEMENT
(Table 25–17)

### Antepartum Care

The outpatient care for the pregnant patient with chronic hypertension is essentially the same as in a routine case of hypertension, with medications regulated according to the patient's blood pressure response. These patients should be seen weekly for blood pressure checks. Renal function studies should be performed early in pregnancy to establish a baseline to aid in the diagnosis of superimposed preeclampsia. In addition, weekly nonstress contraction stress test biophysical profiles should be performed starting at 30 to 32 weeks, to assess fetal reserve. Observation should be made for IUGR, because these babies are at risk owing to uteroplacental insufficiency. Examinations should include fundal heights and sonograms every 3 weeks.

Antihypertensive medications can be used to decrease maternal risk of severely elevated blood pressure. Use of these medications may decrease fetal morbidity and mortality rates by reducing placental changes.

The patient with chronic hypertension usually can be managed on an outpatient basis as long as her blood pressure remains under control. However, she should be seen every other week at 26 weeks and weekly at 30 weeks to assess her blood pressure and observe for superimposed preeclampsia, because preeclampsia is seen earlier in hypertensive women (Creasy and Resnik, 1989). Occasionally our patients are hospitalized so

**Table 25–17**
PATIENT CARE SUMMARY FOR CHRONIC HYPERTENSION*

| | Antepartum | | Intrapartum | Postpartum |
|---|---|---|---|---|
| | *Outpatient* | *Inpatient* | | |
| BP, P, R | Weekly | q 4 h | q 1 h if normotensive q 15 min with ↑ BP | On admission to RR; then q 15 min × 4; then q 30 min × 2; then q 1 h until stable; then q 4 h on PP floor |
| T | Weekly | q 4 h | q 4 h | On admission to RR; then q 4 h |
| Fetal heart rate | NST-CST weekly starting at 30 to 32 weeks' gestation | NST-CST weekly starting at 30 to 32 weeks' gestation | Continuous electronic fetal monitoring, preferably internal If no monitor available, q 15 min in first stage and q 5 min in second stage, listening through 2–3 contractions | — |
| Contractions Frequency Duration Quality Resting tone | Weekly | q 8 h | Continuous electronic fetal monitoring If no monitor available, q 1 h by palpation | Fundal checks: q 15 min × 4; then q 30 min × 2; then q 1 h until stable; then q 4 h Lochia: Same as above |
| Sonogram Amniocentesis | q 3 weeks Weekly after 33–34 weeks if patient not stable or IUGR is present | q 3 weeks | — — | — — |

* Nurse–patient ratios: *antepartum,* 1:6–8; *intrapartum,* 1:2.

that their medications can be regulated for good blood pressure control. If they are maintained at home, a visiting nurse may be used between weekly visits to take blood pressure measurements and assess the patient. A summary of the medications used for treatment is presented in Table 25–9.

## Intrapartum Care

These patients are managed under normal protocols for labor and delivery, with vital signs taken every hour and intake and output recorded every shift. More frequent monitoring is required if the blood pressure remains high during labor and delivery.

## Postpartum Care

Routine vital signs can be observed in the recovery room. Blood pressure should be monitored twice a shift on the postpartum floor. All other vital signs can be taken per routine. If any of the vital signs are abnormal, they should be assessed more frequently.

The patient may be taking antihypertensive medications to control her blood pressure. Most of these medications are safe to take while the mother is breastfeeding (see Table 25–9).

# Chronic Hypertension with Superimposed Preeclampsia

Approximately 25 percent of patients who have been identified as having chronic hypertension are predisposed to superimposed preeclampsia. It is imperative that the perinatal team identify preexisting chronic hypertension, either historically or before the 20th week of pregnancy. The hypertension of preeclampsia superimposed on chronic hypertension is often severe. In such cases, we maintain the patient on her previous chronic hypertensive medicine and place her in the hospital for observation. If signs of worsening of the hypertension, proteinuria, or weight gain develop while the patient is on bed rest in the hospital, we seriously consider intervention. Management would continue as for the preeclamptic patient (see Table 25–16).

# Patient Education

The patient and her family should be fully informed about her treatment regimen and about the severity of pregnancy-induced hypertension, especially because these patients usually do not feel or appear sick. However, severe facial edema or seizures may cause grave concern. If the patient has a seizure while family members are present, provide dignity and support to the patient and her family. The patient will need a great deal of support in dealing with a disease that may be life-threatening to her and her fetus. Offer information and show the patient the positive results of her being maintained at bed rest, such as decreased blood pressure, weight loss, and decreased facial, hand, and leg edema. Blood pressure and weight charts can be helpful to show the patient her progress or the reason for hospitalization (Fig. 25–5). The patient should be instructed to observe for headaches, visual disturbances, epigastic pain, right upper quadrant pain (liver pain), continued abdominal pain or rigidity, tremors, and increased facial or other edema. If she is at home, she should be instructed to come to the hospital if any of these conditions occur. If she is hospitalized, she should alert the perinatal team.

Long-term hospitalization may be necessary. This would provide a good opportunity for individual or group teaching, because the patient may have had no prenatal classes, or her classes may have been interrupted by her hospitalization. Classes or group sessions can be arranged for all of the antepartum patients to discuss prenatal care; high-risk factors, including equipment to be used and procedures to be completed; and attitude toward hospitalization, including fears, family relationships, and expectations for hospitalization. Our patients are given graphs to chart the progress of their blood pressure.

Blood Pressure Graph

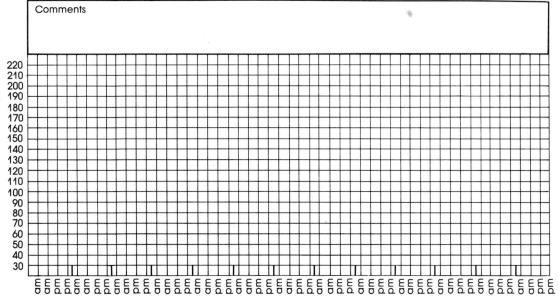

**Figure 25–5.** Blood pressure graph. (Courtesy of Marian Lake and Tom Johnson, University of South Florida College of Medicine, Tampa, FL.)

These charts seem to help the patients better understand their disease (see Fig. 25–5). Information on induction of labor and cesarean delivery should be given, as well as an estimate of when she can expect to deliver. Patients admitted for long-term hospitalization also should be informed that they will stay in the hospital until they deliver, although in some situations in which the patient's condition has stabilized, short out-of-the-hospital passes may be beneficial. Patients who have been transported to the hospital from out of town may have additional needs and fears because of being separated from their families.

The family also may have trouble adjusting to the absence of the mother from the home. Social agencies may be able to provide a homemaker, babysitting services, and other supportive personnel in these cases. Children should be encouraged to visit whenever possible, and family resources such as the church or synagogue should be used.

Maternal-infant attachment should be encouraged. Even if the mother is in an intensive care unit, infant visiting should be encouraged. In very sick patients, we have seen maternal improvement when the infant is brought to the mother. Breastfeeding can be encouraged if the mother is stable, even if she requires a lot of assistance from the staff or her family. This may include positioning or holding the infant for her if she is unable to do that. If the infant is unable to be brought to the mother, photographs should be brought to her. If the mother is planning on breastfeeding, she should be assisted with pumping her breasts so that the milk can be taken to the infant or, at least, to establish her milk so that breastfeeding can occur later. These interactions may help to decrease the stress in these families. If the infant has died, grief support should be provided to the mother and her family.

If the patient convulses, she may not remember coming into the hospital for her delivery. It will be important to go over this information with the patient to help her deal with her delivery and her new infant in the event that this problem occurs.

The patient with pregnancy-induced hypertension has many concerns and physical problems. This potentially serious disease should be controllable by good accessible prenatal care, good nutrition, and good patient education (Zuspan, 1980).

# References

Abitbol MM, Driscoll SG, Ober WB: Placental lesions in experimental toxemia in the rabbit. Am J Obstet Gynecol 125:942, 1976

Abitbol MM, Gallo GR, Pirani CL, et al: Production of experimental toxemia in the pregnant rabbit. Am J Obstet Gynecol 124:460, 1976.

Abitbol MM, Pirani CL, Ober WB, et al: Production of experimental toxemia in the pregnant dog. Obstet Gynecol 48:537, 1976.

ACOG Technical Bulletin 91: Management of preeclampsia. American College of Obstetrics and Gynecology, 1986.

Adams EM, Finlayson A: Familial aspects of preeclampsia and hypertension in pregnancy. Lancet 2:1375, 1961.

Albright GA: Anesthesia in Obstetrics: Maternal, Fetal, and Neonatal Aspects. Menlo Park, CA, Addison-Wesley. 1978, pp 334–335.

Anderson PO: Drugs and pregnancy. Drug Intelligence Clin Pharm 1:208, 1977.

Arias F, Mancilla-Jimenez R: Hepatic fibrinogen deposits in pre-eclampsia: immunofluorescent evidence. N Engl J Med 295:578, 1976.

Assali NS, Vergon JM, Tada Y, et al: Studies on autonomic blockade. VI. The mechanisms regulating the hemodynamic changes in the pregnant woman and their relation to the hypertension of toxemia of pregnancy. Am J Obstet Gynecol 63:978, 1952.

Baca L, Gibbons RB: The HELLP syndrome: a serious complication of pregnancy with hemolysis, elevated levels of liver enzymes, and low platelet count. Am J Med, Volume 85, October 1988.

Ballerini S, Valcamonico A, Gregorini G, et al: Low-dose aspirin (ASA) given to prevent preeclampsia only partially inhibits fetal platelet cyclooxygenase activity. Clin Exp Hypertens [B] B8:219, 1989 (abstr).

Bartholomew RA, Colvin ED, Grimes WH Jr, et al: Facts pertinent to the etiology of eclamptogenic toxemia: a summation of previous observations (1930–1955). Am J Obstet Gynecol 74:64, 1957.

Beecham JB, Watson W, Klapp JF: Eclampsia, preeclampsia and disseminated intravascular coagulation. Obstet Gynecol 18:368, 1929.

Beker JC: The effects of pregnancy on blood circulation in their relation to so-called toxemia. Am J Obstet Gynecol 18:368, 1929.

Benigni A, Gregorini G, Frusca T, et al: Effect of low-dose aspirin on fetal and maternal generation of thromboxane by platelets in women at risk for pregnancy-induced hypertension. N Engl J Med 321:357–362, 1989.

Berger M, Cavanagh D: Toxemia of pregnancy—the hypertensive effect of acute experimental placental ischemia. Am J Obstet Gynecol 87:293, 1963.

Berkowitz RL, Coustan DR, Mockizuki TK: Handbook for Prescribing Medications During Pregnancy. Boston, Little, Brown & Co, 1981.

Bis KA, Waxman B: Rupture of the liver associated with pregnancy: a review of the literature and report of 2 cases. Obstet Gynecol Surv 31:11, 763, 1976.

Bobak IM, Jensen MD: Essentials of Maternity Nursing. 6th ed. St. Louis, Mosby Year Book, 1991.

Bonnar J, McNicol GP, Douglas AS: Coagulation and fibrinolytic systems in pre-eclampsia and eclampsia. Br Med J 2:12, 1971.

Borges LF, Gucer G: Effects of magnesium on epileptic foci. Epilepsia 19:81, 1978.

Bowes W: Results of the intensive perinatal management of very low birth weight infants (150–1500 gms). Proceedings of the Fifth Study Group of Royal College of Obstetricians and Gynaecologists. London, 1977, p 331.

Brewer TH: Letter: role of malnutrition in preeclampsia and eclampsia. Am J Obstet Gynecol 125:281, 1976.

Brewer TH: Consequences of malnutrition in human pregnancy. Ciba Review: Perinatal Medicine, Vol 13, p 175. Basel, Ciba-Geigy, 1975.

Brewer TH: Human pregnancy nutrition: an examination of traditional assumptions. Aust NZJ Obstet Gynaecol 10:87, 1970.

Brosens J, Robertson WB, Dixon HG: The physiological response of the vessels of the placental bed to normal pregnancy. J Pathol Bacteriol 93:569, 1967.

Brown GJ, Curtis JR, Lever AF, et al: Plasma renin concentration at the control of blood pressure in patients on maintenance haemodialysis. Nephron 6:329, 1969.

Browne FJ: Aetiology of pre-eclamptic toxaemia and eclampsia. Lancet 1:115, 1958.

Browne J, Veall N: The maternal placental blood flow in normotensive and hypertensive women. J Obstet Gynecol Br Commonw 60:141, 1953.

Burke TF, Spalding CT, Jones VD: Influence of sodium and potassium content on arterial responsiveness. Circ Res 29:525, 1971.

Burrow W, Ferris T: Medical Complications During Pregnancy, 5th ed. Philadelphia, WB Saunders Co, 1986.

Bussolino F, Benedetto C, Massobrio M, et al: Maternal vascular prostacyclin activity in preeclampsia. Lancet 2:702, 1980.

Butts P: Magnesium sulfate in the treatment of toxemia. Am J Nurs 77:1294, 1977.

Cardwell MS: Maternal death due to the HELLP syndrome. J Tenn Med Assoc 80:8, 1987.

Catanzarite V, Quirk JG, Aisenbrey G: How do perinatologists manage preeclampsia? Am J Perinatol 8:1, 1991.

Cavanagh D, Knuppel RA: Preeclampsia and eclampsia. In Cavanagh D, et al (eds): Obstetric Emergencies. Philadelphia, JB Lippincott, 1982, pp 107–132.

Cavanagh D, Rao PS, O'Connor TCF, et al: Experimental hypertension in the pregnant primate. Am J Obstet Gynecol 128:75, 1977.

Cavanagh D, Rao PS, Tung KSK, et al: Eclamptogenic toxemia: the development of an experimental model in the subhuman primate. Am J Obstet Gynecol 120:183, 1974.

Chesley LC: Hypertension in pregnancy: definitions, familial factor, and remote prognosis. Kidney Int 18:234, 1980.

Chesley LC: Parenteral magnesium sulfate and the distribution, plasma levels, and excretion of magnesium. Am J Obstet Gynecol 133:1, 1979.

Chesley LC: Hypertensive Disorders in Pregnancy. New York, Appleton-Century-Crofts, 1978.

Chesley LC: The renin-angiotensin system in pregnancy. J Reprod Med 15:173, 1975.

Chesley LC, Cooper DW: Genetics of hypertension in pregnancy: possible single gene control of preeclampsia and eclampsia in the descendants of eclamptic women. Br J Obstet Gynaecol 93:898–908, 1986.

Chesley LC, Tepper I: Plasma levels of magnesium attained in magnesium sulfate therapy for preeclampsia and eclampsia. Surg Clin North Am 37:353, 1957.

Common errors in blood pressure measurements. Am J Nurs 65:133, 1965.

Creasy RK, Resnik R: Maternal-Fetal Medicine: Principles and Practice. Philadelphia, WB Saunders Co, 1989.

Cunningham F, Lowe T, Guss S, Mason R: Erythrocyte morphology in women with severe preeclampsia and eclampsia. Am J Obstet Gynecol 153(4):358–62, 1985.

deAlvarez RR: Proteinuria relationships. In Friedman EA (ed): Blood Pressure, Edema and Proteinuria in Pregnancy. New York, AR Liss, 1976.

Demers LM, Gabbe SG: Placental prostaglandin levels in pre-eclampsia. Am J Obstet Gynecol 126:137, 1976.

DeWolf F, Robertson WB, Rosen I: The ultrastructure of acute atherosis in hypertensive pregnancy. Am J Obstet Gynecol 123:164, 1975.

Dieckmann WJ: The Toxemias of Pregnancy. St Louis, CV Mosby Co, 1952.

Doan-Wiggins L: Pregnancy-induced hypertension: combating the dangers. Emerg Med Clin North Am March 30:29–35, 1990.

Donnelly JF, Lock FR: Causes of death in 533 fatal cases of toxemia of pregnancy. Am J Obstet Gynecol 68:184, 1954.

Downing I, Shepherd GL, Lewis PJ: Reduced prostacyclin production in pre-eclampsia. Lancet 2:1374, 1980.

Elder MG, DeSwiet M, Robertson A, et al: Low-dose aspirin in pregnancy. Lancet 1:410, 1988.

Experts Opine. Surv Anesthesiol. 30:306–308, 1986.

Fleming SE, Horvath JS, Korda A: Errors in the measurement of blood pressure. Aust NZJ Obstet Gynaecol 23:136, 1983.

Fliegner JRH: Placental function and renal tract studies in preeclampsia and long term maternal consequences. Am J Obstet Gynecol 126:211, 1976.

Franklin GO, Dowd AJ, Caldwell BV, et al: The effect of angiotensin II intravenous infusion on plasma renin activity and prostaglandins A, E, and F levels in the uterine vein of the pregnant monkey. Prostaglandins 6:271, 1974.

Friedman EA (ed): Blood Pressure, Edema and Proteinuria in Pregnancy. New York, AR Liss, 1976.

Friedman EA, Nelf R: Hypertension in pregnancy: correlation with fetal result. J Am Med Assoc 239:2249, 1978.

Friedman SA: Preeclampsia: a review of the role of prostaglandins. Obstet Gynecol 71:122–137, 1988.

Frusca T, Gregorini G, Ballerini S, et al: Low-dose aspirin in preventing preeclampsia and IUGR. Clin Exp Hypertens [B] B8:218, 1989 (abstr).

Gabbe SG, Neibyle JR, Simpson JL, et al: Normal and Problem Pregnancies, 2nd ed. New York, Churchill Livingstone, 1991.

Gallery EDM, Hunyor SN, Ross M, Gyory AZ: Predicting the development of pregnancy-associated hypertension. The place of standardized blood-pressure measurement. Lancet 1:1274–1275, 1977.

Gant NF, Daley GL, Chand S, et al: A study of angiotensin II pressor response throughout primigravid pregnancy. J Clin Invest 52:2683, 1973.

Gant NF, Chand S, Worley RJ, et al: A clinical test useful for predicting the development of acute hypertension in pregnancy. Am J obstet Gynecol 120:1, 1974.

Gant NF, Madden JD, Siiteri PK, et al: The metabolic clearance rate of dehydroisoandrosterone sulfate. III. The effect of thiazide diuretics in normal and future pre-eclamptic pregnancies. Am J Obstet Gynecol 123:159, 1975.

Gant NF, Worley R: Hypertension in Pregnancy: Concepts and Management. New York, Appleton-Century-Crofts, 1980.

Gastaldi A, Frusca T, Gregorini G: Prevention of preeclampsia and possible correlation with physiopathology. Clin Exp Hypertens [B] B7:139–148, 1988.

Giannattasio M, Coratelli P, Boscia FM, et al: Prevention of pre-eclampsia: Pathophysiological rationale for the use of low-dose aspirin. Clin Exp Hypertens [B] B7:149–158, 1988.

Gilstrap LC, Cunningham FG, Whaley PS: Management of pregnancy-induced hypertension in the nulliparous patient remote from term. Semin Perinatol 2:75, 1978.

Goldblatt H, Kahn JR, Hanzal RF: Studies on experimental hypertension. Effect on blood pressure of constriction of abdominal aorta above and below site of origin of both main renal arteries. J Exp Med 69:649, 1939.

Goldby FS, Beilin LJ: Relationship between arterial pressure and the permeability of arterioles to carbon particles in the rat. Cardiovasc Res 6:384, 1972.

Goldby FS, Beilin LJ: How an acute rise in arterial pressure damages arterioles. Electron microscopic changes during angiotensin infusion. Cardiovasc Res 6:569, 1972.

Goodlin RC: Beware the great imitator—severe preeclampsia. Contemp Obstet Gynecol 20:215, 1982.

Goodlin RC, Cotton DB, Haesslein HC: Severe edema-proteinuria-hypertension gestosis. Am J Obstet Gynecol 132(6):595, 1978.

Grannum PAT, Berkowitz RL, Hobbins JC: The ultrasonic changes in the maturing placenta and their relation to fetal pulmonic maturity. Am J Obstet Gynecol 133:915, 1979.

Greer IA, Cameron AD, Walker JJ: HELLP syndrome: pathologic entity or technical inadequacy? Am J Obstet Gynecol 152:113, 1985.

Gusdon JP, Anderson SG, May WJ: A clinical evaluation of the "roll-over" test for pregnancy-induced hypertension. Am J Obstet Gynecol 127:1, 1977.

Gyongyossy A, Kelentey B: An experimental study of the effect of ischemia of the pregnant uterus on the blood pressure. J Obstet Gynaecol Br Commonw 65:617, 1958.

Hauth JC, Cunningham FG, Whaley PJ: Management of pregnancy-induced hypertension in the nullipara. Obstet Gynecol 48:254, 1976.

Hodgkinson CP, Hodari AA, Bumpus FM: Experimental hypertensive disease of pregnancy. Obstet Gynecol 30:371, 1969.

Hunter CA, Jr, Howard WF: Amelioration of the hypertension of toxemia by post-partum curettage. Am J Obstet Gynecol 81:441, 1961.

Ihle BU, Long P, Oats J: Early onset preeclampsia—recognition of underlying renal disease. Br Med J 294:78–81, 1987.

Ikedif D: Eclampsia in multiparity. Br Med J 280:985, 1980.

Iles A, Collinge DA, McNalty H, et al: Drugs excreted in mother's milk. Patient Care, June, 1980, pp. 2–11.

Kelch BP, Nowak ML: Toward the early diagnosis of the HELLP syndrome in the community hospital. J Am Osteopath Assoc 87:6, 1987.

Killam AP, Dillard SH, Patton RC, Pederson PR: Pregnancy-induced hypertension complicated by acute liver disease and disseminated intravascular coagulation. Am J Obstet Gynecol 123(8):823, 1975.

Kirshon B, Wasserstrum N, Cotton DB: Should continuous hydralazine infusions be utilized in severe pregnancy-induced hypertension? Am J Perinatol 8:3, 1991.

Knuppel RA, Montenegro R: Preeclampsia-eclampsia: an overview. J Fla Med Assoc 70:741, 1983.

Kopernick H, Mest HJ, Schwarz B: Pharmacological management of an impending placental insufficiency. Prostaglandins Leukot Essent Fatty Acids 33:179–183, 1988.

Kumar D: Chronic placental ischemia in relation to toxemia of pregnancy—a preliminary report. Am J Obstet Gynecol 84:1323, 1962.

Letsky E: Coagulaton Problems During Pregnancy. New York, Churchill Livingstone, 1985.

Liaw ST: Pre-eclampsia and the HELLP syndrome. Aust Fam Physician 18:5, 1989.

Lloret P, Lloret M: Perinatal morbidity and mortality in pregnancy hypertensive disorders: prognostic value of the clinical and laboratory findings. Int Fed Obstet Gynecol 32:229, 1990.

Louden KA, Broughton Pipkin F, Heptinstall S, et al: Studies of the effect of low-dose aspirin on thromboxane production and platelet reactivity in normal pregnancy, pregnancy-induced hypertension and neonates. Presented at the First European Congress on Prostaglandins in Reproduction (ECPR), Vienna, July 6–9, 1988 (abstract 30).

MacGillivray I: Some observations in the incidence of preeclampsia. J Obstet Gynaecol Br Emp 65:536–9, 1958.

MacKenna J, Daver N, Brame R: Preeclampsia associated with hemolysis, elevated liver enzymes, and low platelets—an obstetrical emergency? Obstet Gynecol 62:751, 1983.

Macpherson T: Fact and Fancy. Arch Pathol Lab Med 15:672–681, 1991.

Magara M: On the pathogenic power of a placental extract. An experimental and clinical study of the etiology of toxemia of pregnancy. Gynecol Obstet 59:478, 1960.

Martin EJ: Intrapartum Management Modules. Baltimore, Williams & Wilkins, 1990.

Martin JN Jr, Files JC, Blake PG, Norman PH, et al: Plasma exchange for preeclampsia: Postpartum use for persistently severe preeclampsia-eclampsia with HELLP syndrome. Am J Obstet Gynecol 162(1):1, 1990.

McCubbin JH, Siabi BM, Ardella TW, et al: Cardiopulmonary arrest due to acute maternal hypermagnesium. Lancet, 1:1058, 1981.

McKay DG: Hematologic evidence of disseminated intravascular coagulation in eclampsia. Obstet Gynecol Surv 27:399, 1972.

McKay DG: Disseminated Intravascular Coagulation: An Intermediary Mechanism of Disease. New York, Hoeber, 1965.

McKay DG: Cryofibrinogenemia in toxemia of pregnancy. Obstet Gynecol 23:508, 1964.

McKay DG: Clinical significance of the pathology of toxemia of pregnancy. Circulation 30(Suppl II):66, 1964.

McKay DG, Wong TC: Studies of the generalized Shwartzman reaction produced by diet. J Exp Med 115:1117, 1962.

McKay DG, Goldenberg V, Kaunitz H, et al: Experimental eclampsia—an electron microscope study and review. Arch Pathol 84:557, 1967.

McKay DG, Merrill SJ, Weiner AE, et al: The pathologic anatomy of eclampsia, bilateral renal cortical necrosis, pituitary necrosis, and other acute fatal complications of pregnancy, and its possible relationship to the generalized Shwartzman phenomenon. Am J Obstet Gynecol 66:507, 1953.

Misenhimer HR, Ramsey EM, Martin CB, et al: Chronically impaired uterine artery blood flow. Obstet Gynecol 36:415, 1970.

Morris N, Osborn SR, Wright HP, et al: Effective uterine blood flow during exercise in normal and preeclamptic pregnancies. Lancet 2:481, 1956.

Moutquin JM, Rainville C, Giroux L, et al: A prospective study of blood pressure in pregnancy: Prediction of preeclampsia. Am J Obstet Gynecol 151:191–6, 1985.

Nadjii P, Sommers SC: Lesions of toxemia in first trimester pregnancies. Am J Clin Pathol 59:344, 1973.

Naeye RL, Friedman EA: Causes of perinatal death associated with gestational hypertension and proteinuria. Am J Obstet Gynecol 133:8, 1979.

Nelson EW, Archibald L, Albo D: Spontaneous hepatic rupture in pregnancy. Am J Surg 134:817, 1977.

Neuman M, Ron-El R, Langer R, et al: Maternal death caused by HELLP syndrome (with hypoglycemia) complicating mild pregnancy-induced hypertension in a twin gestation. Am J Obstet Gynecol 162:2, 1990.

Newman J, Weiss B, Rabello Y, et al: Diazoxide for the acute control of severe hypertension complicating pregnancy: a pilot study. Obstet Gynecol 53:505, 1979.

Neuweiler W, Berger M, Widmer J: Second World Cong Int Fed Gynecol Obstet Montreal, June, 22–28, 1958. Kongressband: Tendances actuelles en gynécologie et obstétrique, p 398. Montreal, Librairie Beachemin Limitée, 1959.

O'Brien WF: Predicting preeclampsia (review). Obstet Gynecol 75(1):3, 1990.

Ogden E, Hildebrand OJ, Page EW: Rise in blood pressure during ischemia of the gravid uterus. Proc Soc Exp Biol Med 43:49, 1940.

Olds SB: Obstetric Nursing. Reading, MA, Addison-Wesley, 1980, pp 262–267.

O'Shaughnessy R, Zuspan FP: Managing acute pregnancy hypertension. Contemp Ob/Gyn 18:85, 1981.

Page EW: Placental dysfunction in eclamptogenic toxemia. Obstet Gynecol Surv 3:615, 1948.

Page EW, Christianson R: Influence of blood pressure changes with and without proteinuria upon the outcome of pregnancy. Am J Obstet Gynecol 126:821, 1976.

Perez RH: Protocols for Perinatal Nursing Practice. St Louis, CV Mosby Co, 1981, pp 134–148.

Phelan JP, Everidge GJ, Welder TL, Newman C: Is the supine pressor test an adequate means of predicting acute hypertension in pregnancy? Am J Obstet Gynecol 128:173–176, 1977.

Pillay M, Moodley J: The HELLP syndrome in severe hypertensive crises of pregnancy—does it exist? S Afr Med J 67:246, 1985.

Poole JH: Getting Perspective on HELLP Syndrome. MCN, 13:1988.

Pritchard JA: Management of preeclampsia and eclampsia. Kidney Int 18:259, 1980.

Pritchard JA: Standardized treatment of 154 consecutive cases of eclampsia. Am J Obstet Gynecol 123:543, 1975.

Pritchard J, MacDonald PC: Williams Obstetrics, 16th ed. New York, Appleton-Century-Crofts, 1980.

Pritchard JA, Cunningham FG, Mason RA: Coagulation changes in eclampsia: frequency and pathogenesis. Am J Obstet Gynecol 125:855, 1976.

Pritchard JA, Weisman R, Ratnoff O, Vosburgh G: Intravascular hemolysis, thrombocytopenia and other hematologic abnormalities associated with severe toxemia of pregnancy. N Engl J Med 250(3):89–98, 1954.

Quirk JG, Raker RK, Petrie RH, et al: The role of glucocorticoids, unstressful labor, and atraumatic delivery in the prevention of respiratory distress syndrome. Am J Obstet Gynecol 134:768, 1979.

Redman CWG, Beilin LJ, Bonnar J: Treatment of hypertension in pregnancy with methyldopa: blood pressure control and side effects. Br J Obstet Gynaecol 84:419–26, 1977.

Redman WG, Beilin LJ, Bonnar J: Variability of blood pressure in normal and abnormal pregnancy. In Lundheimer MD, Katz AI, Zuspan FP (eds): Hypertension in Pregnancy. New York, John Wiley & Sons, 1976.

Reeder SJ: Maternity Nursing. Philadelphia, JB Lippincott Co, 1980, pp 516–528.

Reiss RE, Tizzano TP, O'Shaughnessy RW: The blood pressure course in primiparous pregnancy. A prospective study of 383 women. J Reprod Med 32:523–6, 1987.

Remuzzi G, Marchesi D, Zoga C, et al: Reduced umbilical and placental vascular prostacyclin in severe preeclampsia. Prostaglandins 20:105–110, 1980.

Roberts JM, May WJ: Consumptive coagulation in severe pre-eclampsia. Obstet Gynecol 48:163, 1976.

Romero R, Lockwood C, Oyarzun E, et al: Toxemia: new concepts in an old disease. Semin Perinatol 12:302–323, 1988.

Rubenstein A: Ueber das toxische Prinsip in der placenta bei schwangerschafts toxaemia. Thesis Berne, 1962.

Sachs BP, Brown DA, Driscoll SG, et al: Maternal mortality in Massachusetts: trends and prevention. N Engl J Med 316(11):667, 1987.

Sanchez-Ramos L, Jones DC, Cullen MT: Urinary calcium as an early marker for preeclampsia. Obstet Gynecol 77:5, 1991a.

Sanchez-Ramos L, Sandroni S, Andres FJ, Kaunitz AM: Calcium excretion in preeclampsia. Obstet Gynecol 77:4, 1991b.

Schiff E, Peleg E, Goldenberg M, et al: The use of aspirin to prevent pregnancy-induced hypertension and lower the ratio of thromboxane $A_2$ to prostacyclin in relatively high risk pregnancies. N Engl J Med 321:351–5, 1989.

Schiff E, Barkai G, Ben-Baruch G, Mashiach S: Low-dose aspirin does not influence the clinical course of women with mild pregnancy-induced hypertension. Obstet Gynecol 76(1):5, 1990.

Schwartz ML, Brenner WE: Pregnancy-induced hypertension presenting with life-threatening thrombocytopenia. Am J Obstet Gynecol 146–756, 1983.

Scott J, Freeney JG: Preeclampsia and eclampsia and change of paternity. Br Med J 281:565, 1980.

Scott JR, and Worley RJ: Hypertensive disorders of pregnancy. In DiSaia PJ, Hammond CB, Spellacy WN (eds): Danforth's Obstetrics and Gynecology. 6th ed. Philadelphia, JB Lippincott Co, 1990.

Severino LJ, Freedman WL, Maheshkumar AP: Spontaneous subcapsular hematoma of liver during pregnancy. NY State J Med 70:2828, 1970.

Sibai BM: The HELLP syndrome (hemolysis, elevated liver enzymes, and low platelets): much ado about nothing? Am J Obstet Gynecol 162:2, 1990.

Sibai BM: Pitfalls in diagnosis and management of pre-eclampsia. Am J Obstet Gynecol 159:1, 1988.

Sibai BM, Mirro R, Chesney CM, et al: Low-dose aspirin in pregnancy. Obstet Gynecol 74:551–557, 1989.

Sibai BM, Abdella TN, Anderson GD: Pregnancy outcome in 211 patients with mild chronic hypertension. Obstet Gynecol 61:571–6, 1983.

Sibai BM, Lipshitz J, Anderson GD, Dilts PV, Jr: Reassessment of intravenous MgSO$_4$ therapy in preeclampsia-eclampsia. Obstet Gynecol 57:199, 1981.

Sibai BM, Taslimi MM, El-Nazer A, et al: Maternal-perinatal outcome associated with the syndrome of hemolysis, elevated liver enzymes, and low platelets in severe preeclampsia-eclampsia. Am J Obstet Gynecol 155:3, 1986.

Sophian J: Correspondence: Hypertension of pregnancy. Br Med J 2:1501, 1961.

Sophian J: Proceedings of the Third World Cong Int Fed Gynecol Obstet, Vienna, September 3–9, 1961.

Sophian J: Correspondence: Toxemia of pregnancy. Am J Obstet Gynecol 78:688, 1959.

Sophian J: Letter to the Editor: Etiology of preeclamptic toxemia and eclampsia. Lancet 1:434, 1958.

Sophian J: Letter to the Editor: Pregnancy toxemia. Lancet 1:48, 1957.

Sophian J: Myometrial resistance to stretch: the cause of preeclampsia. J Obstet Gynaecol Br Commonw 62:37, 1955.

Sophian J: Toxaemias of Pregnancy. London, Butterworths, 1953.

Sophian J: Discussion on the pathological features of cortical necrosis of the kidney and allied conditions associated with pregnancy. Proc R Soc Med 42:387, 1949.

Speroff L: Toxemia of pregnancy. Mechanism and therapeutic management. Am J Cardiol 32:582, 1973.

Spiegelberg O: Lehrbuch der Geburtshilfe fuer Aerzte und Studierende Lahr. Verlage M Schauenburg, 1878.

Stone SR, Pritchard JA: Effect of maternally administered magnesium sulfate on the neonate. Obstet Gynecol 35:574, 1970.

Sutherland A, Cooper DW, Howie PW, et al: The incidence of severe preeclampsia amongst mothers and mothers-in-law of preeclamptics and controls. Br J Obstet Gynecol 88:785, 1981.

Taufield PA, Ales KL, Resnick LM, et al: Hypocalciuria in preeclampsia. N Engl J Med 316:715–8, 1987.

Talledo OE, Chesley LC, Zuspan FP: Renin-angiotensin system in normal and toxemic pregnancies. III. Differential sensitivity to angiotensin II and norepinephrine in toxemia of pregnancy. Am J Obstet Gynecol 100:218, 1968.

Terragno NA, Terragno DA, Pacholczk D, et al: Prostaglandins and the regulation of uterine blood flow in pregnancy. Nature 249:57, 1974.

Thiagarajah S, Bourgeois FJ, Harbert GM, Caudle MR: Thrombocytopenia in preeclampsia: associated abnormalities and management principles. Am J Obstet Gynecol 150:1, 1984.

Thompson RHS, Tickner A: Observations on the monoamine oxidase activity of placenta and uterus. Biochem 45:125, 1949.

Trolle D, Bock JE, Gaeda P: The prognostic and diagnostic value of total estriol in urine and in serum and of human placental lactogen hormone in serum in the last part of pregnancy. Am J Obstet Gynecol 126:834, 1976.

Trudinger BJ, Cook CM, Thompson RS, et al: Low-dose aspirin therapy improves fetal weight in umbilical placental insufficiency. Am J Obstet Gynecol 159:681–685, 1988a.

Trudinger B, Cook CM, Thompson R, et al: Low-dose aspirin improves fetal weight in umbilical placental insufficiency. Lancet 2:214–215, 1988b.

van Bouwdijk Bastiaanse MA: Etiological aspects in the problem of toxemia in pregnancy. Am J Obstet Gynecol 68:515, 1964.

Vane RR: The dynamics of the renin-angiotensin system. Proc R Soc Lond (Biol) 173:339, 1969.

Villar MA, Sibai BM: Clinical significance of elevated mean arterial blood pressure in second trimester and threshold increase in systolic or diastolic blood pressure during third trimester. Am J Obstet Gynecol 160:419–23, 1989.

Vink GJ, Moodley J, Philpott RH: Effect of dihydralazine on the fetus in the treatment of maternal hypertension. Obstet Gynecol 55:519, 1980.

Vosburgh GJ: Edema relationships. In Friedman EA (ed): Blood Pressure. Edema and Proteinuria in Pregnancy. New York, AR Liss, 1976, p 155.

Wallenburg HCS, Rotmans N: Prophylactic low-dose aspirin and dipyridamole in pregnancy. Lancet 1:939, 1988.

Wallenburg HCS, Rotmans N: Prevention of recurrent idiopathic fetal growth retardation by low-dose aspirin and dipyridamole. Am J Obstet Gynecol 157:1230–1235, 1987.

Wallenburg HCS, Dekker GA, Makowitz JW: Reversal of elevated vascular angiotensin II responsiveness in pregnancy by low-dose aspirin. Presented at the 34th Meeting of the Society for Gynecologic Investigation, March 18–21, 1987, Atlanta, GA (abstract 11).

Wallenburg HCS, Makowitz JW, Dekker GA, et al: Low-dose aspirin prevents pregnancy-induced hypertension and preeclampsia in angiotensin-sensitive primigravidae. Lancet 1:1–3, 1986.

Walsh SW: Physiology of low-dose aspirin therapy for the prevention of preeclampsia. Semin Perinatol 14(2):152–70, 1990.

Walsh SW: Low-dose aspirin: treatment for the imbalance of increased thromboxane and decreased prostacyclin in preeclampsia. Am J Perinatol 1989.

Walsh SW: Eicosanoids and pregnancy-related hypertension. In Hillier K (ed): Eicosanoids and Reproduction. Lancaster, England, MTP Press, 1987, pp 128–162.

Walsh SW: Preeclampsia: an imbalance in placental prostacyclin and thromboxane production. Am J Obstet Gynecol 152:335–340, 1985.

Walsh SW, Parisi VM: The role of arachidonic acid metabolites in preeclampsia: Semin Perinatol 10:334–355, 1986.

Webster J, Newnham D, Petric JC, Lovell HG: Influence of arm position on measurement of blood pressure. Br Med J 288:1574–5, 1984.

Weinstein L: Preeclampsia/eclampsia with hemolysis, elevated liver enzymes, and thrombocytopenia. Obstet Gynecol 66:5, 1985.

Weinstein L: Syndrome of hemolysis, elevated liver enzymes, and low platelet count: a severe consequence of hypertension in pregnancy. Am J Obstet Gynecol 142:159, 1982.

Wichman K, Ryden G, Wichman M: The influence of different positions and Korotkoff sounds on the blood pressure measurements in pregnancy. Acta Obstet Gynecol Scand [Suppl] 118:25–8, 1984.

Wheeler L, Jones MB: Pregnancy-induced hypertension. JOGN Nurs 10:212, 1981.

Young J: The aetiology of eclampsia and albuminuria and their relation to accidental hemorrhage: an anatomical and experimental investigation. J Obstet Gynaecol Br Empire 26:1, 1914.

Zuspan FP: Acute hypertension. *In* Queenan JT (ed): Management of High Risk Pregnancy. Oradell, NJ, Medical Economics Co, 1980, p 441.

Zuspan FP: Hypertension: chronic and pregnancy-induced—a symposium. *In* Queenan JT (ed): Management of High Risk Pregnancy. Oradell, NJ, Medical Economics Co, 1980, p 375.

Zuspan FP: Hypertension in pregnancy. *In* Quilligan EJ, Kretchmer N (eds): Fetal and Maternal Medicine. New York, Wiley Medical, 1980, pp 547–568.

Zuspan FP: Problems encountered in the treatment of pregnancy-induced hypertension. Am J Obstet Gynecol 131:591, 1978.

Zuspan FP, Talledo OE: Factors affecting delivery in eclampsia: conditions of the cervix and uterine activity. Am J Obstet Gynecol 100:672, 1968.

Zuspan FP, Zuspan K: Strategies for controlling eclampsia. *In* Queenan JT (eds): Managing Ob/Gyn Emergencies. Oradell, NJ, Medical Economics Co, 1981, pp 99–105.

. . . . . . . . . . . . . . . . . . . . . . . . . . . . . . . . . . . . . . . .

# CHAPTER 26

# Diabetes Mellitus in Pregnancy

Lee Rotondo and Donald R. Coustan

Remarkable improvement has been made in the prognosis for the 2 to 3 percent of pregnancies complicated by diabetes mellitus. Excluding deaths due to major congenital malformations, the perinatal mortality rate of infants of diabetic women receiving optimal care is as low as that observed in normal gestations. Such care demands the collaborative efforts of a health care team that should include a physician expert in the management of both high-risk pregnancy and diabetes, a nurse specialist, a nutritionist, a social worker, and a neonatologist.

This chapter reviews the pathophysiology of diabetes mellitus in pregnancy, emphasizing those changes that lead to perinatal morbidity and mortality. The important objectives of therapy, especially the need to maintain maternal glucose levels within physiologic limits throughout gestation, are outlined.

## Carbohydrate Metabolism In Pregnancy

During gestation, significant metabolic changes occur that must be understood for the successful management of the pregnancy complicated by diabetes (Table 26–1). The fetus depends on the maternal compartment for an uninterrupted supply of fuel. Several maternal adaptations are normally made to meet these fetal needs. Pregnancy is characterized by maternal hyperinsulinemia associated with insulin resistance, changes that

are most marked late in gestation (Kalkhoff et al, 1978). There is also an increased likelihood of ketosis developing during maternal food deprivation, a state of accelerated starvation related to the limited availability of gluconeogenic precursors (Metzger and Freinkel, 1978). Metzger and associates (1982) have observed that normal pregnant women who fast after dinner and skip breakfast demonstrate a significant fall in glucose levels. After meals, a state of facilitated anabolism characterized by greater carbohydrate-induced hypertriglyceridemia and enhanced suppression of glucagon has been described. Placental syncytiotrophoblast is the source of human placental lactogen (HPL), a growth hormone–like glycoprotein that produces insulin resistance and augments maternal lipolysis. With increased maternal use of fats for energy, glucose is spared for fetal consumption. Levels of HPL are directly related to placental mass, increasing as pregnancy progresses and heightening the *diabetogenic stress*. Other hormones that also produce this state of insulin resistance include free cortisol and, possibly, prolactin. Estrogen and progesterone directly alter maternal islet cell function, producing $\beta$-cell hyperplasia and hyperinsulinemia (Kalkhoff et al, 1978).

The diabetogenic stress of pregnancy demands increased insulin production by the maternal pancreas. In most pregnancies, the patient's pancreas can increase insulin secretion severalfold and preserve maternal glucose homeostasis. Glucose crosses the placenta by carrier-mediated diffusion. The rate of glucose transfer from mother to fetus is limited largely by these transport characteris-

**Table 26–1**
METABOLISM IN PREGNANCY

|  | Early | Late |
|---|---|---|
| Fasting glucose | ↓ | ↓ |
| Oral GTT | Normal | Deteriorates |
| Intravenous GTT | Improved | Normal |
| Fasting insulin | ↑ | ↑ ↑ |
| Postprandial insulin | ↑ | ↑ ↑ ↑ |
| Free fatty acids | Normal | ↑ |
| Triglycerides | ↑ | ↑ ↑ ↑ |
| Body fat | ↑ | ↑ |
| Liver glycogen | ↑ | Normal |
| Lean muscle | ? | ? |

Data from Kalkhoff RK, Kissebah AH, Kim HJ: Carbohydrate and lipid metabolism during normal pregnancy: relationship to gestational hormone action. Semin Perinatol 2:291, 1978.

istics as well as by the glucose consumption rate of the placenta (Simmons et al, 1979). Free insulin does not cross the placenta, however, and although the fetus receives a continuous supply of maternal glucose, it is not affected by maternal insulin. Although a recent study has demonstrated the presence of antibody-bound, animal species insulin in the fetal circulation of mothers treated for diabetes, the advent of human insulin renders this observation clinically irrelevant (Menon et al, 1990). During pregnancy, periods of maternal hyperglycemia produce fetal hyperglycemia. Late in pregnancy, elevated levels of glucose in the fetus stimulate the fetal pancreas, resulting in fetal $\beta$-cell hyperplasia and hyperinsulinemia (Van Assche, 1975). This combination of fetal hyperglycemia and hyperinsulinemia contributes to much of the morbidity and mortality observed in the infant of the diabetic mother.

# Maternal Morbidity and Mortality

Patients with vascular and unstable diabetes are at greatest risk for morbidity and mortality during pregnancy. Although there is no evidence that pregnancy shortens the life expectancy of women with diabetes, and maternal mortality is rare, women with diabetes who have coronary artery disease may suffer an increased rate of mortality in pregnancy (Silfen et al, 1980). Pregnancy does not produce a permanent deterioration of renal function in women with diabetic *nephropathy* (Kitzmiller et al, 1981). Carstensen and associates (1982) observed no difference in the prevalence or severity of *retinopathy, nephropathy,* or *neuropathy* in patients who had been pregnant when compared with those who had never been pregnant. Nevertheless, there does remain uncertainty concerning the course of diabetic retinopathy during gestation. Benign retinopathy may worsen as the pregnancy advances, but usually regresses after delivery. Dibble and associates (1982) have reported that women who demonstrate neovascularization that has not been treated with laser therapy before pregnancy may be at great risk for deterioration of their vision.

Much of the maternal morbidity observed in pregnancies complicated by diabetes can be attributed to the changes in maternal metabolism reviewed earlier, which cause deterioration of glycemic control. A review of maternal mortality in diabetic patients showed that 7 of 24 deaths could be directly attributed to the metabolic complications of diabetes (Gabbe et al, 1976). Before the use of home glucose monitoring techniques, severe *hypoglycemic reactions* requiring hospitalization occurred in approximately 10 percent of insulin-dependent patients (Roversi et al, 1979). Early in gestation, estrogen increases the sensitivity of adipose tissue and skeletal muscle to insulin (Kalkhoff et al, 1978). Therefore, deaths due to hypoglycemia were observed in the first trimester. Nausea and vomiting, common problems early in pregnancy, may also necessitate a reduction in insulin dosage. After delivery, the contrainsulin effects of HPL are lost, and hypoglycemia may again result. Insulin-dependent diabetics usually require only a small dose of insulin or no insulin replacement at all during the first days after delivery.

Ketoacidosis most often occurs during the second and third trimesters, when the diabetogenic stress of pregnancy is greatest. The recently diagnosed diabetic who becomes pregnant is most likely to develop ketoacidosis, because she fails to appreciate its causes and symptoms. Ketoacidosis has been associated with a maternal mortality rate of 5 to 15 percent and a perinatal mortality rate as high as 90 percent (Kitzmiller, 1982).

# Perinatal Morbidity and Mortality

Because maternal glucose is readily carried across the placenta to the fetus, maternal diabetes may be associated with fetal hyperinsulinemia. The fetal pancreas responds to hyperglycemia by increasing insulin production and release, leading to fetal hyperinsulinemia, which in turn is probably the cause of many of the cases of morbidity and mortality observed in the fetus of the diabetic mother. For example, Jovanovic and associates (1980) analyzed data from a review of the literature on diabetic pregnancy and found a direct correlation between lower ambient maternal glucose concentrations in the third trimester and perinatal survival (Figure 26–1). Susa and associates (1984) infused insulin directly into fetal rhesus monkeys and reported a stillbirth rate of 20 percent. Similarly, insulin infusion in the sheep fetus increases the oxidative metabolism of glucose and reduces fetal arterial oxygen

content (Carson et al, 1980). Thus, a possible mechanism exists for the increased stillbirth rate in poorly controlled diabetic pregnancies. Other risk factors for perinatal mortality in such pregnancies include nephropathy, hypertension, and poor adherence to the medical regimen.

Fetal hyperinsulinemia is also the most likely explanation for the various forms of morbidity encountered in diabetic pregnancy (Coustan, 1986). Macrosomia can be produced by the infusion of insulin directly into the fetal rhesus monkey (Susa et al, 1979), and problems such as respiratory distress syndrome, neonatal hypoglycemia and plethora also appear to be related to this mechanism. For example, Robert and associates (1976) have demonstrated that at any gestational age, the infant of a diabetic mother is five to six times more likely to develop respiratory distress syndrome.

Historically, the decision as to when to deliver the infant of a diabetic mother has been influenced by the high stillbirth rate near term and moderated by concern about respiratory distress syndrome, even at relatively

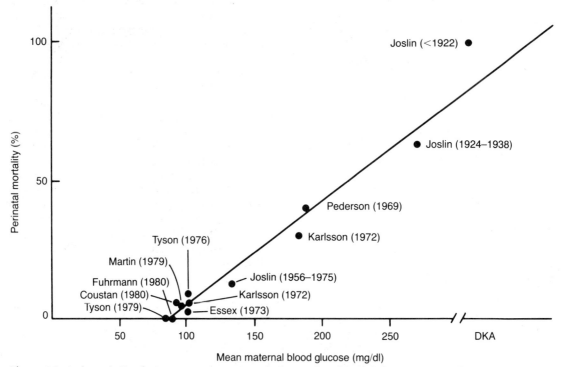

**Figure 26–1.** Association between mean maternal glucose level in third trimester and perinatal mortality rate in diabetic pregnancies. (Adapted from Jovanovic and Peterson: Management of the Pregnant, Insulin Dependent Diabetic Woman. Diabetes Care, 3:64, 1980. (Reproduced with permission of the American Diabetes Association, Inc.)

advanced gestational ages. The ability to measure lung maturity by assessment of amniotic fluid phosphatidylglycerol (PG) determinations or other tests has allowed for individualization of such delivery decisions, and improvements in glucose control have lowered the incidence of fetal death as well as respiratory distress syndrome. A recent study demonstrated that approximately 20 percent of fetuses of diabetic mothers did not have PG as late as 39 weeks (Ojomo and Coustan, 1990). Because the babies were not delivered without PG, it is impossible to say whether or not they would have developed respiratory distress syndrome had they been born. Nevertheless, in many centers, the patient with documented well-controlled diabetes who has no complicating factors is allowed to proceed to term or until pulmonary maturity is documented before elective delivery.

Because fetal macrosomia may be associated with shoulder dystocia and birth injury, particularly in the broad-shouldered infant of a diabetic mother (Acker et al, 1985; Modanlou et al, 1982), cesarean delivery without a trial of labor has been advocated in cases in which macrosomia is evident. Unfortunately, current methods for estimating fetal weight, such as ultrasound, are not accurate, and clinicians are likely to be faced with vaginal deliveries of babies who are much bigger than anticipated or cesarean deliveries of babies much smaller than predicted. The prediction of shoulder dystocia is not always possible, so it is important to be well versed in the management of this potential hazard.

Improved understanding of maternal metabolism and of the need to carefully regulate maternal glycemia, together with the development of reliable techniques for fetal surveillance and improved neonatal care, have markedly reduced perinatal mortality arising from intrauterine deaths, trauma, and respiratory distress syndrome. At the present time, the most frequent cause of perinatal loss in pregnancies complicated by insulin-dependent diabetes is the fatal *congenital malformation*. Infants of diabetic mothers have a two- to threefold greater frequency of severe malformations involving many organ systems (Gabbe, 1977). Whereas the incidence of major malformations in normal pregnancies may be 2 to 3 percent, the frequency observed in the offspring of

insulin-dependent diabetic patients is 6 to 8 percent (Mills, 1982). The caudal regression syndrome and cardiac, renal, and central nervous system anomalies are the most common defects. Such anomalies must occur during the first 7 weeks of development, long before most diabetic patients seek prenatal care (Mills et al, 1979).

There is increasing evidence that these malformations, which today account for 30 to 50 percent of all deaths in infants of diabetic mothers, may be attributed to poor metabolic control during the early weeks of pregnancy. Hemoglobin $A_{1c}$ levels reflect glycemic control in previous weeks and months. The incidence of major anomalies is significantly higher in pregnancies of diabetic mothers who have elevated hemoglobin $A_{1c}$ concentrations during the first trimester (Greene et al, 1989; Miller et al, 1981). Baker and associates (1981) have demonstrated that the increased incidence of lumbosacral skeletal defects observed in fetuses of diabetic rat mothers can be reduced to control levels by aggressive insulin treatment. Eriksson and associates (1982) have confirmed these findings in a similar study.

The possible role of maternal hypoglycemia during critical periods of organogenesis has been suggested by studies using animal models (Ellington, 1987; Sadler and Hunter, 1987), but the timing of such an aberration is apparently critical (Buchanan and Sipos, 1989); applicability to the human embryo has yet to be established. It is not clear how intensive preconception and early pregnancy metabolic control must be in order to avoid an increased likelihood of congenital anomalies (Mills et al, 1988). What is clear, however, is that preconception counseling and attention to metabolic control is associated with a significant reduction in the malformation rate (Fuhrmann et al, 1984; Mills et al, 1988).

After delivery, considerable neonatal morbidity has been reported in the offspring of diabetic women. The characteristic triad of hypoglycemia, hypocalcemia, and hyperbilirubinemia may be seen in as many as 25 percent of these offspring (Soler et al, 1978). The incidence of macrosomia and hypoglycemia can be related to cord blood C-peptide levels (Sosenko et al, 1979). Infants of diabetic mothers have been observed to demonstrate a cardiomyopathy associated with septal hypertrophy, polycythemia with hyperviscosity, and the small left colon syndrome. The long-term prognosis for infants of diabetic mothers remains to be determined. The incidence of subsequent insulin-dependent diabetes in the infants of those women who themselves have insulin-dependent diabetes is approximately 1.5 percent (Kobberling and Bruggeboes, 1980).

# Detection of Diabetes in Pregnancy

*Gestational diabetes* constitutes 90 percent of all diabetes in pregnancy, occurring in approximately 30,000 to 90,000 women in the United States each year (Freinkel, 1980). Using a rat model, Aerts and Van Assche (1979) have observed that the female offspring of rats who are made mildly diabetic during pregnancy are at an increased risk to develop gestational diabetes when they become pregnant. This suggests that the propensity for gestational diabetes may be acquired during *in utero* exposure to hyperglycemia.

Gestational diabetes is defined as "carbohydrate intolerance of varying severity with onset or first recognition during the present pregnancy" (Second International Workshop-Conference on Gestational Diabetes, 1985). These patients are diagnosed by means of a 100-g oral glucose tolerance test (Table 26–2). A well-organized *screening program* must be established to detect this abnormality. In the past, screening was based on recognized historical or clinical clues, including a family history of diabetes; delivery of a macrosomic infant, an infant with a malformation, or an unexplained

stillborn; and maternal obesity, hypertension, and glycosuria (Gabbe et al, 1977). A number of studies have shown that screening patients by such means is inadequate, because approximately 50 percent of women with gestational diabetes fail to develop these clues (Coustan et al, 1989; O'Sullivan et al, 1973). The American Diabetes Association (ADA) (1990) has recommended that all pregnant women be screened at 24 to 28 weeks, using a 50-g glucose load followed by a 1-hour plasma glucose determination, given without regard to the time of the last meal or the time of day. A result of greater than or equal to 140 mg/dl indicates the need for a full, 100-g 3-hour oral glucose tolerance test. The American College of Obstetricians and Gynecologists (ACOG) (1986), on the other hand, has suggested that this screening test be used on all women aged 30 and older, and younger women who have historic risk factors for diabetes. Using the ACOG approach, one population-based study (Coustan et al, 1989) demonstrated that 65 percent of cases of gestational diabetes will be diagnosed at a cost of $190 per case. The ADA recommendation, on the other hand, would lead to the diagnosis of 90 percent of the cases at a cost of $222 per case. The same study demonstrated that 10 percent of women with gestational diabetes have 1-hour screening test values between 130 and 139 mg/dl.

Approximately 10 to 15 percent of all gestational diabetics demonstrate significant fasting or postprandial hyperglycemia and require a program of care identical to that used for the pregestational diabetic (Gabbe et al, 1977). As many as 35 to 50 percent of patients who exhibit gestational diabetes show further deterioration of carbohydrate metabolism during the next 15 years of life (O'Sullivan, 1975). Diabetes is most likely to occur in the obese woman who has carbohydrate intolerance during pregnancy (O'Sullivan, 1982). Patients who have been diagnosed as gestational diabetics should not subsequently take high-dose combined oral contraceptive agents, because these hormones may produce the derangements in carbohydrate metabolism observed during pregnancy (Kalkhoff, 1975). Skouby and associates (1982) observed no significant changes in glucose tolerance in women with a history of gestational diabetes treated with a low-dose (30 $\mu$g ethinyl estradiol) combination oral contraceptive.

**Table 26–2**
DETECTION OF DIABETES IN PREGNANCY
(UPPER LIMITS OF NORMAL)

|  | Plasma[1] (mg/dl) |
| --- | --- |
| Oral GTT* | |
| Fasting | 105 |
| 1 h | 190 |
| 2 h | 165 |
| 3 h | 145 |

[1] National Diabetes Data Group, 1979.
* Diagnosis of gestational diabetes is made when any two values are exceeded.

# Management of the Diabetic Pregnant Patient

(Table 26–3)

## RISK ASSESSMENT

A program of patient care may be best developed when the risks to the patient and her infant are first considered. Pregnancies complicated by diabetes mellitus may be divided into two groups: (1) those women with pregestational diabetes, including patients with vascular complications, and (2) those women with gestational diabetes.

The most widely applied risk assessment system has been that of Dr. Priscilla White. She observed that the age of onset of diabetes, its duration, and the presence of maternal vascular disease, factors that could be determined in the prepregnant state, would all have an important impact on pregnancy outcome (White, 1949) (Table 26–4). In general, the earlier the onset of diabetes, the longer its duration; and the greater the degree of vasculopathy, the worse the prognosis

**Table 26–3**
PATIENT CARE SUMMARY FOR DIABETES*

| | Antepartum | | Intrapartum | Postpartum |
|---|---|---|---|---|
| | *Outpatient* | *Inpatient* | | |
| BP, P, R | Weekly | q shift except while sleeping (if stable); may be more frequent | q 15 min | On admission; then q 15 min × 4; then q 30 min × 2; then on discharge to PP floor; then q 8 hr |
| T | Weekly (optional per discretion of physician) | q shift; more frequently if infection present | q 1 h | On admission; then q 4 h; then on discharge to PP floor; then q 8 h |
| Bed rest | No (May be indicated with vasculopathy) | No | Yes | — |
| Fetal monitor | Class A patients begin at 36–40 weeks. All Class B, C, D, and R patients, and Class A patients with a previous stillbirth, PIH, chronic hypertension, or fetal growth retardation are given weekly (or twice weekly) NSTs beginning as early as 28 weeks; OCT only if NST is nonreactive. Diabetics with vascular disease (e.g., Class F) are tested more frequently (even daily), at discretion of physician | | Continuously during labor, preferably with internal monitor | |
| Contractions | — | — | Continuously during labor, preferably with internal monitor | — |
| I & O | | q shift | q 1 h | While in RR note first void |
| Amniocentesis | 37–38 weeks (or as clinically indicated) | 37–38 weeks (or as clinically indicated) | | |
| Sonogram | q 4–6 weeks | q 4–6 weeks | — | — |
| Blood sugar | Glucose oxidase strips or glucose meter daily, fasting and before or after each meal, and prn | Same as for outpatient | On admission; then q 1–2 h | In RR, q 10, then fasting, and before each meal and PRN |
| Ophthalmologic examination | At first visit; with return visits based on initial findings and with any visual changes | | | |

* Nurse–patient ratio equals 1 : 2; with intravenous insulin (intrapartum), 1 : 1.

BP, Blood pressure; I & O, intake and output; NST, nonstress test; OCT, oxytocin challenge test; P, pulse; PIH, pregnancy-induced hypertension; R, respiration; RR, recovery room; T, temperature.

**Table 26–4**
WHITE CLASSIFICATION OF DIABETES IN PREGNANCY

| Class | Age of Onset (yr) | | Duration (yr) | Vascular Disease | Insulin |
|---|---|---|---|---|---|
| A | Any | | Any | 0 | Diet only |
| B | >20 | | <10 | 0 | + |
| C | 10–19 | or | 10–19 | 0 | + |
| D | <10 | or | >20 | Benign retinopathy | + |
| F | Any | | Any | Nephropathy | + |
| R | Any | | Any | Proliferative retinopathy | + |
| H | Any | | Any | Heart disease | + |

in pregnancy. Although maternal vascular disease is a risk factor, most current experts believe that the most important prognosticator for pregnancy outcome is the metabolic control of the diabetes (Karlson and Kjellmer, 1972).

Pedersen and associates (1974) noted that *prognostically bad signs of pregnancy*, specifically ketoacidosis, pyelonephritis, pregnancy-induced hypertension, poor clinic attendance, and self-neglect, were associated with an unfavorable outcome.

## PRE-EXISTING DIABETES

Care of the patient with pre-existing diabetes should begin prior to gestation (Table 26–5) (Graber et al, 1978; Steel et al, 1982). The patient must be assessed as to her suitability for pregnancy. Does she have active and untreated proliferative retinopathy or significant nephropathy and hypertension? The patient and her family should be advised of the financial demands of pregnancy. In addition, a program of contraception must be established (Table 26–6) (Steel and Duncan, 1980). The increased risk of thromboembolic disease precludes the use of high-dose combined estrogen and progestogen oral contraceptive preparations, and the efficacy of copper-containing intrauterine devices has been questioned (Gosden et al, 1982). Therefore, patients may choose a low-dose combined pill or a progestogen-only pill or a mechanical method. In theory, Norplant should be an effective birth control option without side effects, with the benefit of long-term conception regulation. Sterilization should be discussed after the diabetic woman has completed her family.

With increasing evidence indicating that congenital malformations are related to hyperglycemia during early embryogenesis, insulin-dependent patients should be in optimum control at the time of conception and throughout the first trimester of pregnancy. In normal pregnancies, maternal plasma glucose levels rarely exceed 100 mg/dl, with excursions between fasting levels of 60 mg/dl and postprandial levels of 120 mg/dl (Lewis et al, 1976b). Mean plasma glucose concentrations during the third trimester are

**Table 26–5**
PREPREGNANCY CARE FOR THE DIABETIC PATIENT

1. Assess patient's fitness for pregnancy, especially vasculopathy
2. Establish contraceptive program
3. Identify and treat infertility and gynecologic problems
4. Emphasize need for cooperation of patient and her partner
5. Educate both the patient and her partner
6. Obtain optimum glycemic control before conception
7. Check immune status against rubella

Adapted from Steel JM, Johnstone FD, Smith AF, et al: Five years' experience of a prepregnancy clinic for insulin-dependent diabetes. Br Med J 285:353, 1982.

**Table 26–6**
CONTRACEPTION FOR THE DIABETIC PATIENT

**Combination Oral Contraceptives (High Dose)**
Increased risk of vascular complications in insulin-dependent patients
Deterioration of carbohydrate tolerance in gestational diabetics
**Progestogen-only Pills**
Acceptable for insulin-dependent patients
**Intrauterine Device (IUD)**
Possibly less effective in pre-existing diabetic patients
**Mechanical or Barrier Methods**
Less effective than oral contraceptives or IUD
**Sterilization**
When family has been completed
Especially for patients with serious vasculopathy

86 mg/dl (Cousins et al, 1980; Gillmer et al, 1975).

The benefits of careful regulation have been recognized for many years. Nearly 20 years have passed since Karlsson and Kjellmer (1972) observed a perinatal mortality of 38/1000 when mean maternal blood glucose levels were maintained below 100 mg/dl during the third trimester. If mean glucose levels exceeded 150 mg/dl, perinatal mortality rose almost sixfold. In another study (Gabbe et al, 1977), in which the goal was to maintain fasting serum glucose at 100 to 110 mg/dl and postprandial levels at 140 mg/dl, the perinatal mortality rate was 46/1000, and macrosomia occurred in 22 percent of the infants. Twenty-one percent of infants were delivered because of evidence of fetoplacental compromise. A third series (Coustan et al, 1980) reported a perinatal mortality rate of 40/1000 and a macrosomia rate of 11 percent when mean plasma glucose levels averaging 108 mg/dl were maintained. Only 3 percent of these patients were delivered early because of evidence of compromise. In a treatment program in which physiologic glucose levels were achieved, Jovanovic and colleagues (1981) have essentially eliminated macrosomia and neonatal morbidity. The perinatal risks associated with maternal hypoglycemia have not been well documented.

Maintenance of physiologic glucose levels in the pregnant insulin-dependent diabetic usually requires two to three injections of insulin daily as well as careful adjustment of dietary intake. Most patients require a mixture of intermediate acting (NPH) and rapid acting (regular) insulin in the morning. As a general guideline, the amount of NPH exceeds that of regular insulin by a 2-to-1 ratio (Lewis et al, 1976a). In the evening, equal amounts of NPH and regular insulin are employed. Patients usually receive two thirds of their total insulin dose at breakfast and the remaining third at dinnertime. Circulating glucose measurements are made daily by the patient before breakfast, and 2 hours after each of the three main meals. If glucose levels are elevated, the corresponding insulin dose is increased by 10 to 20 percent the next day. An alternative approach is the measurement of preprandial and bedtime glucose levels. Jovanovic and Peterson (1982) have found that the administration of separate injections of regular insulin at dinnertime and NPH at bedtime may reduce the occurrence

of nocturnal hypoglycemia. The latter is likely to occur during the night when the patient is in a relative fasting state and placental and fetal glucose consumption continue (Table 26–7).

The continuous subcutaneous insulin infusion pump has been developed in an attempt to more closely mimic normal pancreatic function, because it allows for a basal dosage plus additional preprandial boluses. Although initial uncontrolled trials (Cohen et al, 1982; Rudolf et al, 1981) appeared to demonstrate advantages to using the pump in diabetic pregnancy, a randomized prospective trial (Coustan et al, 1986) found no intrinsic advantage to pump use compared to intensive conventional insulin therapy in pregnancy. The decision to employ an insulin pump or not should be based on the cost, the patient's degree of enthusiasm and commitment, and an assessment of the risks, such as that of ketoacidosis in the event of unrecognized pump failure.

Diabetic control must be assessed regularly. This surveillance should be achieved at home, with the use of glucose oxidase reagent strips (Schneider et al, 1980; Tattersal and Gale, 1981) and a glucose reflectance meter. In this way, patients may assess their control four to six times each day while following their usual diet and program of exercise. Advances in meter technology have produced models that employ the most simplified user technique. Memory meters with recall features provide the health care practitioner with a more accurate assessment of the glycemic state.

*Hemoglobin $A_{1c}$* determinations may be made at the patient's first visit to provide rapid assessment of the patient's prior diabetic regulation (Schwartz et al, 1976). Along with frequent blood glucose monitoring, hemoglobin $A_{1c}$ determinations may be repeated during pregnancy as an early warning system for unreported problems with glucose control.

Early in gestation, hospitalization may be required to assess diabetic management and educate the patient. The initial hospitalization also provides an opportunity to assess the patient's vascular status with an ophthalmologic consultation, to determine baseline creatinine clearance and protein excretion, and to take an electrocardiogram. Screening for fetal neural tube defects by maternal serum $\alpha$-fetoprotein assessment is appropriate at 16 weeks' gestation

**Table 26–7**
MEDICATION SUMMARY FOR DIABETES

| Medication | Action | Route | Dose* (Individualized per Patient) |
|---|---|---|---|
| **Note:** Insulin is necessary for the efficient transport of glucose to tissues other than those of the central nervous system, renal medulla, pancreatic beta cells, and gut epithelium. It also favors hepatic glycogen synthesis and storage of glucose in adipose tissue as triglycerides. Insulin facilitates the transport of ingested amino acids into cells, thus increasing protein synthesis. It inhibits lipolysis and is, therefore, antiketogenic. Exogenous insulin can reverse the symptoms of diabetes. | | | |
| Regular insulin<br>　Beef<br>　Pork<br>　Concentrated | Peaks in 1–2 h with a duration of 5–6 h | Subcutaneous; may be given intravenously for control, especially during labor<br>Subcutaneous; do not give intravenously | Dose to try to keep the patient euglycemic<br>Fasting values of 60–100 mg/dl and below 120 mg/dl the rest of the day<br>If a combination of an intermediate and short-acting insulin is given, it is usually in a ratio of 2 : 1 in AM and 1 : 1 before dinner; AM dose is twice the evening dose |
| Prompt insulin zinc suspension (Semilente) | Peaks at 2–8 h with a duration of 12–16 h | Subcutaneous; do not give intravenously | |
| NPH (Isophane insulin suspension) | Peaks at 6–12 h with a duration of 24–48 h | Subcutaneous; do not give intravenously | |
| Insulin zinc suspension (Lente) | Peaks at 6–12 h with a duration of 24–28 h | Subcutaneous in a ratio of 2 : 1 in the AM and 1 : 1 prior to dinner<br>The AM dose is twice the PM dose | |
| Globin zinc | Same as for insulin zinc | Same as for insulin zinc | |
| Protamine zinc insulin suspension (PZI) | Same as for insulin zinc | Same as for insulin zinc | |
| Extended insulin zinc suspension | Same as for insulin zinc | Same as for insulin zinc | |
| **_Human Insulins_** | | | |
| Novolin R<br>Humulin Reg | Effect begins in approximately 1/2 h; peaks between 2 1/2 and 5 h; terminates after 8 h | Subcutaneous | U-100 |
| Velosulin | Effect begins in approximately 1/2 h; peaks between first and third hour; terminates after 8 h | Subcutaneous | U-100 |
| Novolin L<br>Novolin N<br>Humulin L<br>Humulin NPH | Effect begins after 2 1/2 h; peaks between 7 and 15 h; terminates at approximately 24 h | Subcutaneous | U-100 |
| Insulatard (NPH) | Effect begins at 1 1/2 h; peaks between 4 and 12 h; terminates at approximately 24 h | Subcutaneous | U-100 |

* During pregnancy, dose is based on careful blood glucose monitoring. Patients may respond to a change in type of insulin (e.g., beef versus pork versus human) with changing dosage requirements.
Patients may react differently to the human insulins than to the beef and pork varieties and must be observed carefully.

| Pregnancy Precautions | Maternal Side Effects | Nursing Considerations | Fetal and Neonatal Considerations | Breastfeeding |
|---|---|---|---|---|
| Insulin requirements may decrease slightly during the first third to half of pregnancy During second half of pregnancy, requirements may increase to 2–3 times that of the prepregnancy dose Immediately postpartum, insulin requirements drop drastically, sometimes to below the prepregnancy dose (insulin may not even be needed the first 24–48 h after delivery) | Overdose may cause hypoglycemia Allergic reactions to *beef* are commonly reported | With regular insulin, a deep secondary hypoglycemic reaction may occur 18–24 h after injection Dosage is expressed in USP units. Strength is U-100 (for very large dose U-500 is available; store in separate area) Regular, intermediate, and long-acting insulins may be mixed; all insulins should be in the same concentration | The use of low doses of NPH and regular insulin in mild gestational diabetics has been found effective in reducing macrosomia in the fetus (even though the mother may not require the insulin to remain euglycemic) Neonates should be observed for hypoglycemia, especially if the mothers have had high blood sugars | Patients may breastfeed their infants while on insulin |
| All suspensions: same as for regular insulin (above) | All suspensions: same as for regular insulin (above) | With all suspensions, gently agitate so that the contents are mixed uniformly; suspension should appear white and cloudy after mixture | | |
| | | Store in a cool area; refrigeration is desirable but not essential except for regular insulin concentrated Do not use insulin that has changed color Check expiration date before administration Press, do not rub injection site. Rotate injection sites. Have patient chart sites to avoid overuse of one area. *However,* unstable patients may achieve better control if injection site is rotated within the same anatomic region | Does not cross the placenta | |
| Same as for regular insulin (above) | Same as for regular insulin (above) | Same as for regular insulin (above) | Same as for regular insulin (above) | Same as for regular insulin (above) |
| Same as for regular insulin (above) | Same as for regular insulin (above) | Store in refrigerator | Same as for regular insulin (above) | Same as for regular insulin (above) |
| Same as for regular insulin (above) | Same as for regular insulin (above) | See notes for suspensions, above (Prompt insulin zinc suspension) | Same as for regular insulin (above) | Same as for regular insulin (above) |
| Same as for regular insulin (above) | Same as for regular insulin (above) | See notes for suspensions, above (Prompt insulin zinc suspension) Avoid heavy foam Do not use if contents remain clear after shaking Do not use if you see lumps that float or stick to the sides | Same as for regular insulin (above) | Same as for regular insulin (above) |

(Milunsky et al, 1982). An initial urine culture is also obtained and then repeated every 4 to 6 weeks.

## Antepartum Management

Ideally, the diabetic gravida should be followed in an outpatient setting. Frequent communication with a member of the health care team ensures continuous counseling and assessment of the glycemic state. The home environment usually provides a more realistic setting for the patient to follow her diabetic regimen. If diabetes cannot be controlled in an outpatient setting, then hospitalization may be necessary. Several factors may enter into such a decision. For example, poor diabetes control or a lack of documentation of diabetes control at the onset of pregnancy requires intensive management, especially during the first 8 weeks of gestation, which is the time of organogenesis. Another factor requiring hospitalization might be unexplained severe hypoglycemia. Nausea and vomiting during the early months of pregnancy, particularly with ketonuria, may require intravenous fluid administration and stabilization of blood glucose. Hyperglycemia that cannot be resolved may require more aggressive insulin therapy to avoid diabetic ketoacidosis. Patients who do not adhere to their regimen or who lack self-management skills also may be admitted to the hospital during their pregnancies. Finally, obstetric complications such as pregnancy-induced hypertension and preterm labor may necessitate hospitalization.

Self-monitoring of blood glucose is an important aspect of the outpatient antepartum self-care regimen. As noted earlier, the pregnant woman with diabetes should monitor her blood glucose at least four to six times per day. The patient may experience difficulty in adapting to lower blood glucose levels and frequent adjustments in insulin dosage. Patience and understanding on the part of the nursing staff assists the patient in coping with these stress factors.

The signs, symptoms, and treatment of hypoglycemia should be part of patient teaching. The methods of treatment including the use of subcutaneous glucagon should also be reviewed with family members or other support persons. During pregnancy, it is important to keep in mind the need to avoid overtreatment that might result in unstable blood glucose levels.

A nutritionist should be scheduled to meet with the patient on the day she presents for care. At this time, a careful dietary history is obtained, caloric requirements are determined, and a modified carbohydrate diet is prescribed.

In a common diet for a pregnant insulin-dependent diabetic patient, 20 percent of the calories are derived from protein, 35 percent from fats, and 45 percent from carbohydrates (Ney and Hollingsworth, 1981). In terms of caloric distribution, 25 percent of the calories are provided with breakfast, 30 percent with lunch, 30 percent with dinner, and 15 percent with a bedtime snack. An alternative diet, used at our center, is based on 30 to 35 kcal/kg of ideal body weight. It is higher in protein content, which is intended to help smooth out the peaks and valleys of glycemia throughout the day. The distribution of calories allows for 45 to 50 percent carbohydrate, 20 to 25 percent protein, and 30 percent fat, divided into 3 meals and 3 snacks. It must be taken into account that many patients are prone to hypoglycemia and may require snacks in mid-morning, mid-afternoon, or both. In such cases, 5 percent of the calories are subtracted from breakfast and lunch, respectively. The average daily caloric intake for the pregnant diabetic woman ranges from 2200 to 2400 calories. Those patients who are restricted in activity or who demonstrate early excessive weight gain may require a lower caloric prescription. Obese patients are not encouraged to lose weight during pregnancy; however, they should be counseled not to overeat. Ideally, all patients should be provided with an exchange list and meal pattern. The nutritionist will then assess their knowledge base and level of understanding on a regular basis. Caloric adjustments are made as needed, varying from one patient to another.

The patient should continue to consult with the nutritionist at the time of each prenatal visit in order to discuss any changes in her dietary regimen. In the event that a nutritionist is not available for routine follow-up, the role of nutrition consultant is, in all probability, taken on by the perinatal nurse.

## Subsequent Antepartum Outpatient Care

A record should be kept of all test results and reviewed by the health care team at each office visit. The patient should also be instructed to inform the physician about glucose levels that are too high or too low. At these visits, the patient may be asked to perform a glucose measurement so that her technique can be evaluated.

Prior to 28 weeks, the patient is assessed at 1- to 2-week intervals, depending on the complexity of the diabetes. However, after 28 weeks, weekly appointments are the rule. At this time, further tests to evaluate fetal well-being may be initiated. The patient requires instruction regarding antepartum heart rate testing and fetal activity assessment.

The stable and cooperative diabetic patient may continue as an outpatient until spontaneous labor occurs. However, factors such as infection, changes in activity, emotional stress, hypertension, and other complications of pregnancy may alter the control, thereby necessitating frequent or long-term hospitalization. If benign retinopathy has been detected early in gestation, repeat ophthalmologic examinations should be obtained in the second and third trimesters. Proliferative retinopathy requires more intensive follow-up.

In mothers with poorly controlled diabetes, and perhaps even in some with apparently well-controlled glucose metabolism, sudden intrauterine fetal death may occur with increased frequency compared with the general population. A number of tests of fetoplacental function have been devised in an attempt to identify those fetuses at greatest risk for this tragedy, so that early delivery may be accomplished and the neonates' survival chances enhanced by management in modern neonatal units. Because preterm delivery carries with it an increased risk of adverse outcomes, including neonatal death, clinicians must always balance the chance of stillbirth if the pregnancy is left undisturbed against the chance of major morbidity if early delivery is accomplished. An important principle is that all tests of fetoplacental function yield some *false-positive* results, meaning that the test suggests a compromised fetus when no problem actually exists. If a group of patients with a low *a priori* risk of compromise is tested, most of the abnormal tests will be false positives. On the other hand, if a group of fetuses at high *a priori* risk is tested, a much higher proportion of the positive results will be true positives, indicating a real problem. The consequences of acting on the result of a false positive test at term may be a long induction, and perhaps a cesarean delivery that might

have been otherwise avoided. However, a delivery at 26 weeks' gestation prompted by a false-positive test result has much more serious implications. Thus, the earlier in pregnancy that a test is administered, the greater is the risk of a false-positive result causing harm by unnecessary early delivery. For this reason, the appropriate time to begin testing fetal well-being is best individualized, with the degree of risk of fetal compromise being assessed for each patient. For example, when the mother is in poor diabetic control, has diabetic nephropathy and hypertension, and her fetus is believed to be growth retarded, it may be perfectly appropriate to begin intensive testing of fetal well-being as early as 24 to 26 weeks, because there is a high likelihood of intrauterine fetal death in such cases, and because some neonates survive even at such an early gestational age. On the other hand, if the mother's diabetes is well controlled and she has no adverse risk factors in her past history or present condition, it makes more sense to begin testing as late as 34 to 36 weeks.

There is no single test of fetal well-being that is unanimously considered the ideal approach to diabetic pregnancy. Each center uses a test or combination of tests that is most familiar to its caregivers. Although in the past, daily urinary or serum estriol determinations were standard in the management of diabetic pregnancies, such testing has now been abandoned throughout the country because of the high rate of false-positive and false-negative results, the inconvenience, and the availability of better biophysical tests.

The *oxytocin challenge test,* popularized by Ray and associates (1972) and applied to a series of diabetic pregnancies by Gabbe and associates (1977), has proved to be an extremely valuable tool for fetal evaluation. In recognition of the fact that some gravidas are already contracting at a rate of 3 in 10 minutes without use of oxytocin, even though they are not in labor, the test is often referred to as the *contraction stress test* (CST). When the CST is negative, indicating the absence of persistent fetal heart rate late decelerations in response to contractions, fetal death within 1 week is extremely unlikely in the metabolically stable diabetic patient. A positive CST appears to be a relatively early sign of decreased placental reserve (Freeman et al, 1982b), and the false-positive rate with the CST has been reported as high as 60 percent. The CST usually requires a longer time to complete than other tests of fetal well-being, and in many cases, an intravenous line must be inserted in order to administer oxytocin. More recently, in some centers, the use of nipple stimulation has been used to obviate the requirement for exogenous oxytocin (Lenke and Nemes, 1984). The CST is usually performed at intervals of no greater than one week in the assessment of fetal well-being in diabetic pregnancies.

The nonstress test (NST) was introduced after the observation was made that if the fetal heart rate accelerated in connection with fetal movements during the CST, then a positive CST was highly unlikely (Rochard et al, 1976). The NST is usually performed weekly. The presence of a nonreactive NST (fewer than two accelerations of 15 beats/minute; duration $\geq 15$ seconds during a 10-minute period) generally dictates that a CST or biophysical profile be performed. The NST is simple to perform, requires no intravenous line, and usually takes 20 minutes or less. In a prospective but nonrandomized comparison of 1542 patients in whom NSTs were used for antepartum testing with 4626 in whom CSTs were used, Freeman and associates (1982a) found a significantly higher antenatal death rate with NSTs than with CSTs (3.2/1000 versus 0.4/1000). On the other hand, the intervention rate for abnormal testing results in patients followed with CSTs was approximately double that for NSTs (45/1000 versus 29/1000). Given the increased expense, patient discomfort, and time consumed with CSTs, many centers continue to opt for NST as the primary means of surveillance in diabetic pregnancies. Golde and associates (1984) have reported excellent results in diabetic pregnancies with a program of *twice-weekly* NSTs as the primary mode of surveillance. Boehm and associates (1986) also have suggested that NSTs be performed twice weekly and reported that the antenatal fetal death rate in their institution decreased from 6/1000 to 2/1000 when twice-weekly testing was introduced. Because of the sample size, this difference was not statistically significant. In our unit, we continue to use weekly NSTs as our primary mode of surveillance in otherwise uncomplicated diabetic pregnancies, but the presence of other risk factors, such as maternal hypertension, fetal growth retardation, or inadequate diabetic control, may dictate that the frequency of surveillance be increased, other fetal tests be administered, or both.

A third commonly used approach to assessment of fetal well-being is the *biophysical profile* (Manning et al, 1980). In addition to the nonstress test, ultrasound examination is used to assess fetal tone, breathing, body movements, and amniotic fluid volume; a biophysical profile score of 0 to 10 is assigned. A randomized prospective trial (Platt et al, 1985) comparing the biophysical profile with the NST alone suggested that weekly biophysical profile testing might be a better predictor of fetal outcome, although statistical significance was not reached. Fewer than 70 of the 652 subjects studied had diabetes, however.

A simple and practical approach to the evaluation of fetal condition is maternal assessment of *fetal activity* (Liston et al, 1982). A number of methods have been described, including one in which the patient is instructed to count movements every morning until 10 are perceived. If that number is not reached within 12 hours, a nonstress test is performed. Although this method has not been reported in a large population of diabetic gravidas, it is inexpensive and is often suggested *in addition* to scheduled antepartum testing, as described earlier.

In summary, no single method has been proved to be the ideal antepartum assessment approach in management of the diabetic pregnancy. Each center uses its own version of the above-mentioned primary screening protocols, with other modalities as backup systems. It is important to point out that no method of fetal assessment can predict fetal deaths due to maternal diabetic ketoacidosis, cord accidents, or other events that may occur in an apparently random manner.

Ultrasound studies have permitted the assessment of fetal growth as well as the detection of hydramnios. After early ultrasound for pregnancy dating and midtrimester observation for fetal anomalies, when appropriate, sonography may be performed at 1- or 2-month intervals, beginning at 22 to 26 weeks, in order to assess growth and fluid volume.

## Hospitalization versus Outpatient Care in Late Pregnancy

As the diabetic gravida approaches the final month of gestation, hospitalization may be required. Such a policy was considered an important part of successful treatment programs established in the past. Many of the centers following this regimen dealt with large indigent populations containing patients who were unable to maintain good diabetic control at home and who could not come to the hospital for antepartum testing. For these reasons, a liberal policy of hospitalization was employed. Physicians have now become more comfortable in treating selected diabetic gravidas as outpatients. At-home assessment of maternal glycemia by means of a glucose reflectance meter and the use of outpatient antepartum testing have reduced the need for hospitalization. Many centers are now reporting comparable reductions in perinatal mortality with such an outpatient approach. However, for the patient who has had poor diabetic control throughout pregnancy or who has been unable to make adequate arrangements for daily antepartum surveillance, hospitalization still remains an important part of the treatment program.

## ANTEPARTUM HOSPITALIZATION FOR FINAL EVALUATION AND MANAGEMENT

As the time of delivery approaches, the patient's anxiety level increases. Frequently, there is uncertainty regarding the method of delivery. The primigravida, as well as those patients who have experienced previous fetal losses, may require extra attention and support. Because diabetic patients are more likely to require an operative delivery, information on cesarean delivery should be included in their childbirth classes.

It is often reassuring for the patient and her support person to visit the labor and delivery suite and nursery facilities prior to delivery. This process may alleviate anxiety and allow the patient the opportunity to orient herself to these unfamiliar environments. Infants of diabetic mothers are frequently admitted to the intensive care nursery for observation. Although the majority of infants require only regular assessment of glucose levels and prompt treatment of hypoglycemia, some may require respiratory assistance and cardiac monitoring. The mother will be less likely to panic if she is familiar with the monitors and ventilators used in her infant's care.

The patient also benefits from a visit by the obstetric anesthesiologist, neonatologist, and primary nursery nurse prior to delivery. Her questions can be answered and she will be further reassured.

## Intrapartum Management

### Timing of Delivery

If the patient has been maintained in excellent glycemic control and all parameters of antepartum surveillance have remained normal, delivery should be safely delayed until fetal maturation has been achieved. Elective delivery may be planned at a gestational age of 38 weeks or later if amniotic fluid analysis reveals evidence of completed *pulmonary maturation,* as documented by the presence of the acidic phospholipid PG (Cunningham et al, 1982). A previously well-controlled and stable diabetic individual might conceivably develop ketoacidosis or an intercurrent illness after full fetal maturation has been attained, a possibility that suggests the advisability of induction of labor near term. On the other hand, induction of labor in the presence of an unripe cervix increases the likelihood of a long induction period and, ultimately, cesarean delivery. A good compromise, then, is to induce labor at 38 weeks or later if the fetal lungs are mature and the cervix feels favorable (Coustan, 1988). Delivery may be considered even without documented lung maturity if maternal or fetal compromise puts the life of either individual at significant risk, as occurs in eclampsia. On the other hand, evidence of fetal pulmonic maturity should be sought earlier than 38 weeks in the presence of such problems as poor or undocumented metabolic control or pregnancy-induced hypertensive disorders. In such cases, if documentation of pulmonic maturity has not been noted before 34 weeks, the use of corticosteroids to induce fetal pulmonic maturation should be undertaken with considerable caution because of the possibility of inducing diabetic ketoacidosis.

When fetal compromise is suggested by antepartum testing, the gestational age of the fetus as well as the type and degree of abnormality determined by the test should determine whether immediate delivery is undertaken without attempts to document fetal lung maturity or whether amniocentesis should be performed. When an elective delivery is contemplated, it is usual to await the presence of PG because of the occasional false-positive L/S ratio; nevertheless, only a few neonates develop severe respiratory distress syndrome in the presence of an L/S ratio greater than 2 (Cunningham et al, 1982). If the lungs are clearly immature, clinical management must be individualized.

Premature labor may occur in pregnancies complicated by diabetes, especially when hydramnios is present. Combined therapy with corticosteroids and tocolytic drugs has been used to accelerate fetal lung maturation and halt uterine contractions. However, such treatment may lead to rapid decompensation of diabetic control and requires intensive glucose monitoring (Schilthuis and Aarnoudse, 1980).

## Selection of the Route of Delivery

Diabetes is not an indication for cesarean delivery, but its complications may be. In a review of 17 published series (Coustan, 1988), an overall cesarean delivery rate of 47 percent was found among 2138 overt diabetic women. Hypertensive disorders of pregnancy may require induction of labor before term in the presence of an unripe cervix, thus increasing the likelihood of cesarean delivery. Macrosomic babies are more likely to require cesarean delivery because of the maternal problem of dystocia. Concern about shoulder dystocia may indicate cesarean delivery when marked macrosomia is suspected. Intrauterine fetal distress during labor often requires cesarean delivery. The history of a previous low transverse cesarean delivery does not preclude vaginal delivery in a woman with diabetes any more than it does so for other gravidas.

During the induction of labor in a diabetic pregnancy, electronic fetal heart rate and contraction monitoring are appropriate. The use of a labor graph is helpful in the early recognition of labor abnormalities. The combination of a prolonged second stage of labor and midpelvic instrumental delivery of a macrosomic infant is associated with a high risk of shoulder dystocia (Benedetti and Gabbe, 1978); therefore, caution should be exercised in such situations. Individuals with expertise in the care of the neonate should be available when diabetic mothers deliver.

## Intrapartum Glucose Control

Delivery produces a rapid change in the hormonal milieu that causes the diabetogenic stress of pregnancy. The fall in HPL levels after the placenta has been removed causes a marked decrease in the insulin replacement required to maintain glycemic control. Thus, management of the patient's blood sugars during labor, delivery, and postpartum is a most challenging and important clinical problem (Cohen and Gabbe, 1981). The incidence of neonatal hypoglycemia can be related to the level of maternal glycemia maintained during labor as well as to the degree of antepartum control. If the mean maternal blood sugar exceeds 90 mg/dl, the frequency of neonatal hypoglycemia in infants of diabetic mothers increases significantly (Soler et al, 1978).

A useful approach to maintaining normal maternal blood glucose levels during labor involves the administration of a constant glucose and insulin infusion with frequent glucose monitoring (West and Lowy, 1977). This method is based on the assumption that the patient has good metabolic control during the third trimester and usually exhibits a normal fasting glucose level. The usual subcutaneous insulin dose is taken on the day and evening (if applicable) before induction, which is begun early the morning after an overnight fast. No subcutaneous insulin is administered on the morning of induction. Rather, an intravenous infusion is begun and 5 percent dextrose in half normal saline is infused at a constant rate; we use 125 ml/h (Coustan, 1988). The maternal circulating glucose level is measured hourly, and regular insulin (10 U/liter) is added to the fluid if maternal glycemia exceeds 120 mg/dl. The concentration can be doubled or halved, depending on the maternal glycemic response. To decrease the insulin-binding capacity of insulin to plastic surfaces, the intravenous tubing should be flushed with the insulin-containing fluid before the fluid is administered to the patient. Another alternative is to use two separate infusion pumps, one for the dextrose solution and the other for insulin in normal saline, so that their infusion rates can be varied independently. Using the artificial pancreas, Jovanovic and Peterson (1980) and Golde and associates (1982) have demonstrated that a significant proportion of diabetic mothers require no insulin at all during the first stage of labor. Thus, it is important to individualize the dosage of insulin depending on frequently measured maternal glucose levels. With the constant glucose and insulin infusion in a nonambulatory patient in labor, who is on *nulla per os* (NPO) stable circulating glucose levels are usually reached in 4 to 6 hours. However, abrupt increases in glucose may be observed during the second stage of labor, and insulin infusion is often begun or increased at this time. If induction is unsuccessful and an overnight rest is planned, it is important to remember to administer the evening subcutaneous insulin dose before the patient eats dinner, because overnight insulinopenia results in ketoacidosis.

If an elective cesarean delivery is performed, the patient is maintained NPO the night before delivery, and her morning insulin dose is withheld. The cesarean delivery should be scheduled in the early morning. Epidural or spinal anesthesia allows the anesthesiologist to continually evaluate the mental status of the patient and detect early signs of hypoglycemia. However, regional anesthesia must be carefully administered, because maternal hypotension has been associated with more profound fetal acidosis in pregnancies complicated by diabetes (Datta and Kitzmiller, 1982). To avoid maternal hyperglycemia with resultant fetal hyperglycemia, dextrose infusions should be limited to no more than 6 g/h (Kenepp et al, 1982). After the operation has been completed, blood sugars should be monitored every 2 to 4 hours and an intravenous solution containing 5 percent dextrose continued, at a rate of 100 to 125 ml/h. No insulin may be required for the remainder of the operative day. Cesarean delivery also may be required if the elective induction of labor is unsuccessful.

## Intrapartum Emotional Support

Emotional support for the patient and her family is essential during the intrapartum period, because fears regarding the condition of the infant are heightened prior to delivery. If possible, a member of the antepartum nursing team should visit the patient during labor and be present at delivery, thereby providing support and continuity of care for the patient and family. The mother should be permitted to see and touch her infant as soon as possible after delivery. This measure will reassure the mother as to the infant's well-being. On the other hand, if there are complications such as respiratory distress syndrome or unexpected congenital anomalies, additional support and encouragement are required. The antepartum, intrapartum, and postpartum nursing teams must work together to meet these needs.

## Postpartum Management

In the postpartum period, the patient's insulin requirements are usually significantly lower than were her prepregnancy requirements (Lev-Ran, 1974). The antepartum objective of physiologic glycemic control is relaxed during this period, and blood sugars of 150 to 200 mg/dl are satisfactory. The patient who has delivered vaginally and is able to eat can be given one half of her prepregnancy dosage of insulin as a 2:1 mixture of NPH and regular insulin on the first postpartum day. Glucose levels should be monitored at least four times daily and regular insulin given for glucose levels greater than 200 mg/dl. The following day, additional insulin is given in the morning based on the previous day's blood glucose values and supplemental insulin needs. Using this method, one can stabilize the patient within several days after delivery.

In addition to the usual postpartum measures of assessing fundal tone, evaluating fluid balance, and providing for comfort, close monitoring of blood glucose levels is necessary. Following a vaginal delivery, hourly glucose evaluations are obtained in the recovery room using a glucose meter. Once the patient has been transferred to the postpartum unit, a fasting glucose as well as measurements 1 to 2 hours after meals and at bedtime are usually needed. If the patient remains NPO the glucose levels should be ascertained every 2 hours. Intravenous fluids are maintained, and regular insulin is prescribed as needed. When glucose levels are stabilized, the frequency of assessment may be decreased to once every 4 hours until a regular meal pattern is resumed.

After delivery, the insulin dose required is usually less than that needed prepregnancy. The safety of insulin for breastfeeding mothers should be emphasized. *Lactation* or *infection* may increase insulin requirements, and this should be explained to the patient, to reassure her that fluctuations in glucose levels are expected and, thus, avoid any unnecessary concern. The postpartum nurse must be particularly observant for the sudden onset of hypoglycemic reactions, which may occur despite reductions of the insulin dose.

The patient who has been delivered by cesarean delivery often requires no additional insulin on the day of delivery. During the first several postoperative days, while her diet is being adjusted, the patient should be given one third of her prepregnancy dosage of insulin. More insulin is required each day as her diet is advanced. Patients should be encouraged to breastfeed, working closely with a nutritionist and with close observation of blood glucose levels.

Prior to discharge, an assessment should be made concerning the need for family planning and further nutritional counseling. It is also important to arrange for a follow-up appointment with the physician for diabetes management.

## THE PATIENT WITH GESTATIONAL DIABETES

Women with gestational diabetes are usually identified late in pregnancy. Once this diagnosis has been established by glucose tolerance testing, these patients are started on a dietary program of approximately 2000 to 2500 calories daily, with the exclusion of simple sugars (Gabbe et al, 1977). Their fasting and postprandial glucose levels should be evaluated at least weekly and more often if values are outside the 60 to 120 mg/dl range. If fasting plasma glucose levels reach 105 mg/dl and/or postprandial glucose values exceed 120 mg/dl, insulin treatment should be instituted in order to reduce the perinatal mortality risk, as in the overt diabetic individual. Once maternal hyperglycemia has necessitated the use of insulin, the patient's treatment should be similar to that of the overt diabetic individual. A number of approaches have been evaluated in order to lower the morbidity, particularly macrosomia, associated with gestational diabetes. The use of prophylactic insulin (Coustan and Imarah, 1982) and daily self-glucose monitoring (Goldberg et al, 1986; Langer et al, 1988) have both been shown to reduce macro-

somia in the offspring of gestational diabetic mothers; either or both may be offered to patients as options for reducing morbidity.

Gabbe and associates (1977) and Landon and Gabbe (1985) have published data showing that women with well-controlled gestational diabetes can safely be followed using only daily fetal movement determinations from 28 until 40 weeks' gestation, providing that no other problems arise. The presence of problems such as previous fetal death, hypertension, and postdatism are indications for earlier testing. If the pregnancy reaches 40 weeks, these authors advocate more intensive fetal surveillance. Another common approach is the initiation of weekly nonstress testing at 36 weeks in women with gestational diabetes and no other risk factors.

# Psychosocial Considerations

## ANXIETY AND CONFLICT

It is conceivable for the diabetic patient to have been told that with careful control of diet and blood glucose levels, a normal life is possible. Nevertheless, the diabetic woman also may have been advised against becoming pregnant because of the potential risk for both her and the fetus. For most women, pregnancy and childbirth is considered to be a natural and normal part of life. Thus, to be denied this experience is to give up that right to be a "whole" woman. Consequently, when the diabetic woman does become pregnant, the customary anxieties are exacerbated by the conflict concerning her own health versus her desire for motherhood. It is not uncommon for the patient to experience deep concern regarding possible congenital anomalies in the infant. Others are apprehensive because of previous fetal loss. Although these fears are often justified, recent advances in patient management have significantly improved the chances for a successful outcome. Taking these facts into consideration helps the health care providers to more appropriately assess the patient's emotional needs and to initiate an individualized plan of care.

It is essential to recognize that despite similarities in diagnosis and history, *no two patients have the same needs.* Consequently, the importance of *individualized care* cannot be overemphasized. Single mothers and patients whose homes are far from the referral center are but two examples of patients facing particular hardship when hospitalization is required. Concern over family welfare, financial status, or the lack of support systems often leads to conflict regarding the need for hospitalization. Women with these concerns are literally torn between acknowledging their need to remain in the hospital for their own well-being and that of the fetus and agonizing over the problems that this separation from their family will cause.

Additional stress factors also must be considered in the management of the pregnant diabetic. The unpredictable fluctuations in glucose levels and the frequent readjustments in insulin dosages are often sources of frustration for the patient. Also, stress may make physiologic glucose control more difficult to achieve. Constant reassurance by the perinatal team that such control can be attained assists the patient in coping with the situation. Superimposed complications, such as hypertension, premature labor, proliferative retinopathy, and nephropathy, increase anxiety. Because the treatment for such conditions frequently involves prolonged periods of hospitalization, restrictions in activity, and early delivery, these patients require consistent therapeutic intervention and emotional support (Barglow et al, 1981).

Regularly scheduled rounds for the entire high-risk team may be established to provide more effective and holistic implementation of the care plan. Often the patient benefits from sharing her experiences with other diabetic patients, either on a one-to-one basis or in an organized group. If such is the case, interaction on this level should be encouraged and provided for whenever possible. For example, women with diabetes who have delivered can be asked to return to the unit for a luncheon with antepartum patients.

## UNMET EXPECTATIONS

Unfortunately, not all diabetic pregnancies will have a successful outcome. Fetal loss may occur, or the infant may be born with congenital anomalies. The parent's hopes are dashed and their worst fears are realized.

Regardless of the circumstances, the grief process is experienced to one degree or another. The shock, suffering, and recovery phases may vary for each individual. Nevertheless, each stage is essential and must be dealt with before resolution occurs and plans for the future can begin. There is usually an element of guilt interspersed with feelings of grief and anger. This, too, must be understood and worked through by the patient and her partner.

During the initial crisis period, the physicians and nursing staff, in collaboration with the social worker, psychiatric liaison service, and the clergy, can provide valuable support to the patient and her family. Prior to discharge, information should be provided regarding available support groups in the community (e.g., *Compassionate Friends, Unite, Share, Resolve*) that can assist her with the long-term process of resolution and adaptation.

Pregnancy presents a special health care opportunity in the life of a woman with diabetes mellitus. The patient is highly motivated to do whatever may be necessary to ensure a good perinatal outcome. The perinatal team must work with the patient, stressing that the knowledge gained and the habits developed during pregnancy be maintained in years to come.

**Acknowledgment**

Acknowledgment is given to Jane L. Berry, RNC, MSN, and Steven G. Gabbe, MD, for their contributions to the first edition.

## References and Recommended Reading

Acker D, Sachs B, Friedman E: Risk factors for shoulder dystocia. Obstet Gynecol 66:762–768, 1985.

Aerts L, Van Assche FA: Is gestational diabetes an acquired condition? J Dev Physiol 1:219, 1979.

American College of Obstetricians and Gynecologists: Management of diabetes mellitus during pregnancy. ACOG Technical Bulletin No 92, 1–2, May, 1986.

American Diabetes Association: Position statement on gestational diabetes mellitus. Diabetes Care 13:5–6, 1990.

Baker L, Egler JM, Klein SH, et al: Meticulous control of diabetes during organogenesis prevents congenital lumbosacral defects in rats. Diabetes 30:955, 1981.

Barglow P, Hatcher R, Wolston J, et al: Psychiatric risk

factors in the pregnant diabetic patient. Am J Obstet Gynecol 140:46, 1981.

Benedetti TJ, Gabbe, SG: Shoulder dystocia: a complication of fetal macrosomia and prolonged second stage of labor with midpelvic delivery. Obstet Gynecol 52:526, 1978.

Borg S, Lasker J: When Pregnancy Fails. Boston, Beacon Press, 1981.

Buchanan TA, Sipos GF: Lack of teratogenic effect of brief maternal insulin-induced hypoglycemia in rats during late neurulation. Diabetes 38:1063–1066, 1989.

Carson BS, Philipps AF, Simmons MA, et al: Effects of a sustained insulin infusion upon glucose uptake and oxygenation of the ovine fetus. Pediatr Res 14:147, 1980.

Carstensen LL, Frost-Larsen K, Fugleberg S, et al: Does pregnancy influence the prognosis of uncomplicated insulin-dependent diabetes mellitus? Diabetes Care 5:1, 1982.

Cohen AW, Gabbe SG: Intrapartum management of the diabetic patient. Clin Perinatol 8:165, 1981.

Cohen AW, Liston RM, Mennuti MT, Gabbe SG: Glycemic control in pregnant diabetic women using a continuous subcutaneous insulin infusion pump. J Reprod Med 27:651, 1982.

Cousins L, Rigg L, Hollingsworth D, et al: The 24 hour excursion and diurnal rhythm of glucose, insulin, and C-peptide in normal pregnancy. Am J Obstet Gynecol 136:483, 1980.

Coustan DR: Delivery: timing, mode and management. In Reece EA, Coustan DR (eds): Diabetes Mellitus in Pregnancy: Principles and Practice. New York, Churchill Livingstone, 1988, pp 525–533.

Coustan DR: Hyperglycemia-hyperinsulinemia: effect on the infant of the diabetic mother. In Jovanovic L, Peterson CM, Fuhrmann K (eds): Diabetes and Pregnancy: Teratology, Toxicology and Treatment. New York, Praeger Publishers, 1986, pp 131–156.

Coustan DR, Imarah JE: Insulin treatment of class A diabetes can reduce operative deliveries and birth trauma. Diabetes 30(Suppl 1):78A, 1982.

Coustan DR, Berkowitz RL, Hobbins JC: Tight metabolic control of overt diabetes in pregnancy. Am J Med 68:845–852, 1980.

Coustan DR, Nelson C, Carpenter MW, et al: Maternal age and screening for gestational diabetes: a population-based study. Obstet Gynecol 73:557–561, 1989.

Coustan DR, Reece EA, Sherwin RS, et al: A randomized clinical trial of the insulin pump vs intensive conventional therapy in diabetic pregnancies. JAMA 255:631–663, 1980.

Cunningham MD, McKean HE, Gillispie DH, et al: Improved prediction of fetal lung maturity in diabetic pregnancies: a comparison of chromatographic methods. Am J Obstet Gynecol 142:197, 1982.

Datta S, Kitzmiller JL: Anesthetic and obstetric management of diabetic pregnant women. Clin Perinatol 9:153, 1982.

Dibble CM, Kochenour NK, Worley RJ, et al: Effect of pregnancy on diabetic retinopathy. Obstet Gynecol 59:699, 1982.

Distler W, Gabbe SG, Freeman RK, et al: Estriol in pregnancy. V. Unconjugated and total plasma estriol in the management of diabetic pregnancies. Am J Obstet Gynecol 130:424, 1978.

Ellington SK: Development of rat embryos cultured in glucose-deficient media. Diabetes 36:1372–1378, 1987.

Elliott JP, Garite TJ, Freeman RK, et al: Ultrasonic prediction of fetal macrosomia in diabetic patients. Obstet Gynecol 60:159, 1982.

Eriksson U, Dahlstrom E, Larsson KS, et al: Increased incidence of congenital malformations in the offspring of diabetic rats and their prevention by maternal insulin therapy. Diabetes 30:1, 1982.

Evertson LR, Gauthier RJ, Collea JV: Fetal demise following negative contraction stress tests. Obstet Gynecol 51:671, 1978.

Freeman RK, Anderson G, Dorchester W: A prospective multi-institutional study of antepartum fetal heart rate monitoring. II. Contraction stress test versus nonstress test for primary surveillance. Am J Obstet Gynecol 143:778–781, 1982a.

Freeman RK, Anderson G, Dorchester W: A prospective multi-institutional study of antepartum fetal heart rate monitoring. I. Risk of perinatal mortality and morbidity according to antepartum fetal heart rate test results. Am J Obstet Gynecol 143:771–777, 1982b.

Freinkel N: Gestational diabetes 1979: philosophical and practical aspects of a major health problem. Diabetes Care 3:399, 1980.

Fuhrmann K, Reiher H, Semmler K, Glückner E: The effect of intensified conventional insulin therapy before and during pregnancy on the malformation rate in offspring of diabetic mothers. Exp Clin Endocrinol 83:173–177, 1984.

Gabbe SG: Congenital malformations in infants of diabetic mothers. Obstet Gynecol Surv 32:125, 1977.

Gabbe SG, Mestman JH, Freeman RK, et al: Management and outcome of class A diabetes mellitus. Am J Obstet Gynecol 127:465, 1977.

Gabbe SG, Mestman JH, Freeman RK, et al: Management and outcome of diabetes mellitus, Classes B–R. Am J Obstet Gynecol 129:723, 1977.

Gabbe SG, Mestman, JH, Hibbard LT: Maternal mortality in diabetes mellitus. Obstet Gynecol 48:549, 1976.

Gillmer MD, Beard RW, Brooke FM, et al: Carbohydrate metabolism in pregnancy. I. Diurnal plasma glucose profile in normal and diabetic women. Br Med J 3:399, 1975.

Goldberg JD, Franklin B, Lasser D, et al: Gestational diabetes: impact of home glucose monitoring on neonatal birth weight. Am J Obstet Gynecol 154:546–550, 1986.

Golde SH, Good-Anderson B, Montoro M, Artal R: Insulin requirements during labor: a reappraisal. Am J Obstet Gynecol 144:556–559, 1982.

Golde SH, Montoro M, Good-Anderson B, et al: The role of nonstress tests, fetal biophysical profile, and contraction stress tests in the outpatient management of insulin-requiring diabetic pregnancies. Am J Obstet Gynecol 148:269–273, 1984.

Gosden C, Ross A, Steel J, et al: Intrauterine contraceptive devices in diabetic women. Lancet 1:530, 1982.

Graber AL, Christman B, Boehm FH: Planning for sex, marriage, contraception, and pregnancy. Diabetes Care 1:202, 1978.

Greene MF, Hare JW, Cloherty JP, Benacerraf BR, Soeldner JS: First-trimester hemoglobin $A_1$ and risk for major malformation and spontaneous abortion in diabetic pregnancy. Teratology 39:225–231, 1989.

Hare JW, White P: Gestational diabetes and the White classification. Diabetes Care 3:394, 1980.

Jovanovic L, Peterson CM: Optimal insulin delivery for the pregnant diabetic patient. Diabetes Care 5(Suppl 1):24, 1982.

Jovanovic L, Peterson CM: Management of the pregnant, insulin-dependent diabetic woman. Diabetes Care 3:63, 1980.

Jovanovic L, Druzin M, Peterson CM: Effect of euglycemia on the outcome of pregnancy in insulin-dependent diabetic women as compared with normal control subjects. Am J Med 71:921, 1981.

Kalkhoff RJ: Effects of oral contraceptive agents on carbohydrate metabolism. J Steroid Biochem 6:949, 1975.

Kalkhoff RK, Kissebah AH, Kim HJ: Carbohydrate and lipid metabolism during normal pregnancy: relationship to gestational hormone action. Semin Perinatol 2:291, 1978.

Karlsson K, Kjellmer I: The outcome of diabetic pregnancies in relation the mother's blood sugar level. Am J Obstet Gynecol 112:213, 1972.

Kenepp NB, Shelley WC, Gabbe SG, et al: Fetal and neonatal hazards of maternal hydration with 5% dextrose before cesarean section. Lancet 1:1150, 1982.

Kennel JH, Trause MA: Helping parents cope with perinatal death. Contemp. Ob/Gyn 12:53, 1978.

Kitzmiller JL, Brown ER, Phillippe M, et al: Diabetic nephropathy and perinatal outcome. Am J Obstet Gynecol 141:741, 1981.

Kitzmiller JL, Cloherty JP, Younger MD, et al: Diabetic pregnancy and perinatal morbidity. Am J Obstet Gynecol 131:560, 1978.

Kobberling J, Bruggeboes B: Prevalence of diabetes among children of insulin-dependent diabetic mothers. Diabetologia 18:459, 1980.

Kowalski K: Helping mothers of stillborn infants to grieve. MCH, January 1977, pp 29–32.

Landon MB, Gabbe SG: Antepartum fetal surveillance in gestational diabetes mellitus. Diabetes 34 (Suppl 2):50–54, 1985.

Langer O, Mazze R: The relationship between large-for-gestational age infants and glycemic control in women with gestational diabetes. Am J Obstet Gynecol 159:1478–1483, 1988.

Lenke RR, Nemes JM: Use of nipple stimulation to obtain contraction stress test. Obstet Gynecol 63:345–348, 1984.

Lev-Ran A: Sharp temporary drop in insulin requirement after cesarean section in diabetic patients. Am J Obstet Gynecol 120:905, 1974.

Lewis SB, Murray WK, Wallin JD, et al: Improved glucose control in nonhospitalized pregnant diabetic patients. Obstet Gynecol 48:260–267, 1976a.

Lewis SB, Wallin JD, Kuzuya H, et al: Circadian variation of serum glucose C-peptide immunoreactivity and free insulin in normal and insulin-treated diabetic pregnant subjects. Diabetologia 12:343–350, 1976b.

Liston RM, Cohen AW, Mennuti MT, et al: Antepartum fetal evaluation by maternal perception of fetal movement. Obstet Gynecol 60:424, 1982.

Manning F, Platt LD, Sipos L: Antepartum fetal evaluation: development of a fetal biophysical profile. Am J Obstet Gynecol 136:787–795, 1980.

Menon RK, Cohen RM, Sperling MA, et al: Transplacental passage of insulin in pregnant women with insulin-dependent diabetes mellitus: its role in fetal macrosomia. N Engl J Med 323:309–315, 1990.

Metzger BE, Freinkel N: Effects of diabetes mellitus on endocrinologic and metabolic adaptations of gestation. Semin Perinatol 2:309, 1978.

Metzger BE, Vileisis RA, Ravnikar V, et al: "Accelerated starvation" and the skipped breakfast in late normal pregnancy. Lancet 1:588, 1982.

Miller E, Hare JW, Cloherty JP, et al: Elevated maternal hemoglobin $A_{1c}$ in early pregnancy and major congenital anomalies in infants of diabetic mothers. N Engl J Med 304:1331, 1981.

Mills JL: Malformations in infants of diabetic mothers. Teratology 25:385, 1982.

Mills JL, Baker L, Goldman AS: Malformations in infants of diabetic mothers occur before the seventh gestational week: implications for treatment. Diabetes 28:292, 1979.

Mills JL, Knopp RH, Simpson JL, et al: Lack of relation of increased malformation rates in infants of diabetic mothers to glycemic control during organogenesis. N Engl J Med 318:671–676, 1988.

Milunsky A, Alpert E, Kitzmiller JL, et al: Prenatal diagnosis of neural tube defects. VIII. The importance of serum alpha-fetoprotein screening in diabetic pregnant women. Am J Obstet Gynecol 142:1030, 1982.

Modanlou MD, Komatsu G, Dorchester W, Freeman RK, Bosu SK: Large-for-gestational-age neonates: anthropometric reasons for shoulder dystocia. Obstet Gynecol 60:417–423, 1982.

National Diabetes Data Group: Classification and diagnosis of diabetes mellitus and other categories of glucose intolerance. Diabetes 28:1039–1057, 1979.

Ney D, Hollingsworth DR: Nutritional management of pregnancy complicated by diabetes: historical perspective. Diabetes Care 4:647, 1981.

Ojomo EO, Coustan DR: Absence of evidence of pulmonary maturity at amniocentesis in term infants of diabetic mothers. Am J Obstet Gynecol 163:954–957, 1990.

Olds SB, London ML, Ladewig PA, et al: Obstetric Nursing. Menlo Park, CA, Addison-Wesley, 1980.

O'Sullivan JB: Body weight and subsequent diabetes mellitus. JAMA 248:949, 1982.

O'Sullivan JB: Prospective study of gestational diabetes and its treatment. In Sutherland HW, Stowers JM (eds): Carbohydrate Metabolism in Pregnancy and the Newborn. Edinburgh, Churchill Livingstone, 1975, p 195.

O'Sullivan JB, Mahan CM, Charles D, et al: Screening criteria for high-risk gestational diabetic patients. Am J Obstet Gynecol 116:895, 1973.

Pedersen J, Pedersen LM, Anderson B: Assessors of fetal perinatal mortality in diabetic pregnancy. Diabetes 23:302, 1974.

Penticuff JH: Psychologic implications in high-risk pregnancy. Nurs Clin North Am 17(1):69–78, 1982.

Peppers L, Knapp RJ: Motherhood and Mourning. New York, Praeger Publishers, 1980.

Perez RH: Protocols for Perinatal Nursing Practice. CV Mosby Co, 1981, St Louis, pp 70–88.

Platt LD, Walla CA, Paul RH, et al: A prospective trial of the fetal biophysical profile versus the nonstress test in the management of high-risk pregnancies. Am J Obstet Gynecol 153:624–633, 1985.

Rancilio N: When a pregnant woman is diabetic: postpartal care. Am J Nurs 79:453, 1979.

Ray M, Freeman R, Pine S, Hesselgesser R: Clinical experience with the oxytocin challenge test. Am J Obstet Gynecol 114:1–9, 1972.

Robert MF, Neff RK, Hubbell JP, et al: Maternal Diabetes and the Respiratory Distress Syndrome. N Engl J Med 294:357, 1976.

Rochard F, Schifrin BS, Goupuil F, et al: Non-stressed

fetal heart rate monitoring in the antepartum period. Am J Obstet Gynecol 126:699–706, 1976.

Roversi GD, Gargiulo M, Nicolini U, et al: A new approach to the treatment of diabetic pregnant women. Am J Obstet Gynecol 135:567, 1979.

Rudolf MCJ, Coustan DR, Sherwin RS, et al: Efficacy of the insulin pump in the home treatment of pregnant diabetics. Diabetes 30:891, 1981.

Sadler TW, Hunter ES III: Hypoglycemia: how little is too much for the embryo? Am J Obstet Gynecol 157:190–193, 1987.

Saylor DE: Nursing response to mothers of stillborn infants. JOGN Nurs 6:39, 1977.

Schiff HS: The Bereaved Parent. New York, Penguin Books, 1977.

Schilthuis MS, Aarnoudse JG: Fetal death associated with severe ritodrine induced ketoacidosis. Lancet 1:1145, 1980.

Schneider JM, Huddleston JF, Curet LB, et al: Pregnancy complicating ambulatory patient management of diabetes. Diabetes Care 3:77, 1980.

Schuler K: When a pregnant woman is diabetic: antepartal care. Am J Nurs 79:448, 1979.

Schulman PK: Diabetes in pregnancy: nutritional aspects of care. J Am Dietetic Assoc 76:585–588, 1980.

Schwartz HC, King KC, Schwartz AL, et al: Effects of pregnancy on hemoglobin $A_{1c}$ in normal, gestational diabetic, and diabetic women. Diabetes 25:1118, 1976.

Second International Workshop-Conference on Gestational Diabetes Mellitus: summary and recommendations. Diabetes 34(Suppl 2):123–126, 1985.

Silfen SL, Wapner RJ, Gabbe SG: Maternal outcome in Class H diabetes mellitus. Obstet Gynecol 55:749, 1980.

Simmons MA, Battaglia FC, Meschia G: Placental transfer of glucose. J Dev Physiol 1:227, 1979.

Skouby SO, Molsted-Pedersen L, Kuhl C: Low dosage oral contraception in women with previous gestational diabetes. Obstet Gynecol 59:325, 1982.

Soler NG, Soler SM, Malins JM: Neonatal morbidity among infants of diabetic mothers. Diabetes Care 1:340, 1978.

Sosenko IR, Kitzmiller JL, Loo SW, et al: The infant of the diabetic mother. Correlation of increased cord C-peptide levels with macrosomia and hypoglycemia. N Engl J Med 301:859, 1979.

Steel JM, Duncan LJP: Contraception for the insulin-dependent diabetic woman: the view from one clinic. Diabetes Care 3:557, 1980.

Steel JM, Johnstone FD, Smith AF, et al: Five years' experience of a pregnancy clinic for insulin-dependent diabetics. Br Med J 285:353, 1982.

Susa JB, Gruppuso PA, Widness JA, et al: Chronic hyperinsulinemia in the fetal Rhesus monkey: effects of physiologic hyperinsulinemia on fetal substrates, hormones and hepatic enzymes. Am J Obstet Gynecol 150:415–422, 1984.

Susa JB, McCormick KL, Widness JA, et al: Chronic hyperinsulinemia in the fetal Rhesus monkey: effects on fetal growth and composition. Diabetes 28:1058, 1979.

Tattersall R, Gale E: Patient self-monitoring of blood glucose and refinements of conventional insulin treatment. Am J Med 70:177, 1981.

Van Assche FA: The fetal endocrine pancreas. In Sutherland HW, Stowers JM (eds): Carbohydrate Metabolism in Pregnancy and the Newborn. Edinburgh, Churchill Livingstone, 1975, pp 68–82.

West TET, Lowy C: Control of blood glucose during labour in diabetic women with combined glucose and low-dose insulin infusion. Br Med J 1:1252–1254, 1977.

White P: Pregnancy complicating diabetes. Am J Med 7:609, 1949.

Wimberley D: When a pregnant woman is diabetic: intrapartal care. Am J Nurs 79(3):451, 1979.

. . . . . . . . . . . . . . . . . . . . . . . . . . . . . . . . . . .

# CHAPTER 27

# Bleeding in Pregnancy

Robert H. Hayashi and Maria S. Castillo

Bleeding or hemorrhage in pregnancy is one of the most frequent contributors to maternal mortality, along with toxemia and infection. Significant blood loss poses a threat to the well-being of both the mother and her fetus. In this chapter, we discuss the clinical entities in pregnancy associated with vaginal bleeding. The entities are grouped according to their occurrence in either early or late pregnancy, during labor, or in the postpartum period. The discussion includes the description, pathophysiology, and management principles of each clinical entity.

## Bleeding in Early Pregnancy
(See Table 27–8)

Vaginal bleeding in the first two trimesters is seen in 16 to 21 percent of pregnancies. In most of these instances, the bleeding occurs from the 9th to the 12th week of pregnancy. Most of the time, the cause of the bleeding remains undetermined; about 10 to 15 percent of pregnancies in which there is bleeding at this time terminate in a spontaneous abortion. The frequency of occurrence of abortion increases as maternal age increases and as the number of previous abortions increases.

The etiology of spontaneous abortion is still not well understood. The role of exogenous factors, such as viral, bacterial, chemical, and trauma, is small. Most often, spontaneous abortion is attributed to chromosomal or embryonic defects that are incompatible with life. Clinical signs and symptoms of all types of abortion are outlined in Table 27–1.

## THREATENED ABORTION

Threatened abortion may occur at any time during the first half of pregnancy. It is diagnosed when vaginal bleeding ensues with or without cramping in the presence of a live fetus. The bleeding is usually slight and may last a few days or even weeks. It may be fresh, bright red bleeding or vary according to the amount of mucus mixed with the blood, or it may be dark brown when it is old blood. The presence of a live fetus can be documented by real-time ultrasonography. After 5 weeks of gestation, a fetus can be seen, and fetal movement as well as fetal cardiac activity can be documented. Also, the diameter of the gestational sac can be measured serially to document an intact growing fetus. In threatened abortion, the cervical os remains closed, although the bleeding may continue, and there will be no evidence of the passage of tissue into the vagina.

Some bleeding about the time of the expected menses is physiologic. Implantation of the blastocyst may cause bleeding about a week prior to the expected menses, resulting in vaginal spotting. The luteoplacental shift of the hormonal support of pregnancy occurs at about 8 weeks and is thought by some to cause vaginal bleeding. Cervical polyps or cervical erosion can also cause bleeding. These lesions could easily be ascertained by a vaginal speculum examination of the cervix.

The usual treatment for threatened abortion is bed rest for 48 hours following each incident of vaginal bleeding. The patient is instructed to count the number of perineal pads used, to note the quantity and color of the blood on the pads, and to look for evi-

Table 27–1
CLINICAL SIGNS AND SYMPTOMS OF ABORTIONS

| Type of Abortion | Fever | Abdominal Cramps | Bleeding | Passage of Tissue | Internal Os Dilatation |
|---|---|---|---|---|---|
| Threatened | No | Slight cramps (may or may not be present) | Slight | No | None |
| Inevitable | No | Moderate | Moderate | No | Open |
| Complete | No | None | Small | Complete placenta with fetus | Partially open with tissue in vagina |
| Incomplete | No | Severe | Severe | Fetal or placental tissue | Open with tissue in cervix |
| Missed | No | None No FHT with Doppler or heart motion on sonar | None to severe if coagulopathy is present | None | None |
| Septic | Yes | Severe | Mild to severe | Possibly; foul smelling discharge | Closed or open with or without tissue |

dence of passage of tissues. She should also abstain from coitus, because increased uterine contractions occur during orgasm. This treatment program is instituted because the exact etiology of the vaginal bleeding is not known. The patient should call her physician if excessive bleeding or pain occurs or if there is rupture of the membranes. At this point, a threatened abortion has progressed to an inevitable abortion.

## INEVITABLE ABORTION

Inevitable abortion is the presence of cervical dilatation, spontaneous rupture of membranes, or both, in addition to vaginal bleeding. Given these conditions, abortion is almost certain to occur. The fetus is generally not viable at this time. The uterine contractility is manifested by painful low abdominal cramps and continues until expulsion of the products of conception occurs. The treatment of this condition is initially expectant, to allow a natural evacuation of the uterine contents. If bleeding is excessive or the process appears to be prolonged or incomplete, a dilatation and curettage under anesthesia is carried out by the physician.

## COMPLETE ABORTION

An abortion occurring before the 10th week of pregnancy usually results in the complete expulsion of the products of conception. This is because the gestational sac has a sufficient amount of decidual tissue surrounding it (decidua capsularis) and the placenta is not too firmly attached to the uterine wall. A careful examination of the tissues passed vaginally confirms a complete abortion. If the uterus is firmly contracted and there is no further active bleeding, the patient may be discharged. She should rest and be cautioned to watch for further bleeding, pain, or fever; a follow-up visit with her doctor should be scheduled.

## INCOMPLETE ABORTION

An abortion occurring after the 10th week of pregnancy usually results in the incomplete expulsion of the products of conception. After the 10th week, there is less decidua between the fetal membranes and the endometrium and they are, therefore, more adherent; the placenta is also more adherent, and the basal plate of the placenta is incompletely formed. Once this basal layer (Nitabuch's layer) is formed, the placenta tends to separate cleanly. Incomplete evacuation of the uterine contents results in continued bleeding, which is the main sign of an incomplete abortion. The retained tissue interferes with myometrial contractility, thereby preventing sufficient constriction around the spiral arteries of the placental site to control bleeding. The amount of bleeding can reach alarming proportions over a period of time. A dilatation and curettage is now necessary for complete removal of all placental tissues, to allow normal control of placental site bleeding.

In any situation in which an abortion has occurred, the practitioners should be cognizant of the patient's emotions and her ability to cope with grief. During the bleeding episodes preceding the abortion, the expectant couple may feel vulnerable and helpless. The thought of hospitalization may be frightening to them. For the woman, the fear of more pain may be predominant in her mind, and heavy vaginal bleeding compounds her fear. A simple and brief explanation of what has occurred and what is being or will be done to help them should be provided. Answering questions for the patient also provides support.

The couple should be permitted to remain together as much as possible. By sharing in the experience, they may provide emotional support to each other immediately and later on. The husband may feel awkward and unsure. He should be reassured that these feelings are normal and that his presence and support to his wife are essential and very important (Pizer and Palinski, 1980).

Anger, disappointment, and guilt are some of the normal emotions a woman may feel after a pregnancy loss. Of these, guilt is usually the strongest. For this reason, it is imperative that she be informed early in the bleeding episode that she may abort in spite of bed rest and all other precautions. Once the abortion has occurred, it should be re-emphasized that the abortion occurred as a result of some abnormality in the developing embryo. Perhaps an illustration of an embryo will help to allay her guilt. If the couple desires and if possible, allow them to see the products of conception, but prepare them for the experience beforehand. Encourage the couple to communicate openly, because they may each experience the loss differently. Another source of emotional support may be for them to talk with another woman or couple who has had a previous pregnancy loss. If there are children in the family, help provide the parents with an explanation that is appropriate for the children's ages. Sharing the experience with the entire family can add additional support to the grieving parents (Pizer and Palinski, 1980).

## MISSED ABORTION

Prolonged retention of the products of conception after embryonic or fetal demise is known as missed abortion. The usual clinical picture is that of a patient who ceases to experience the physiologic changes of pregnancy (such as morning sickness, fatigue, and breast enlargement) following an episode of vaginal bleeding or even without a bleeding history. After fetal death, the hormonal production by the placenta gradually diminishes. The uterus and breasts regress in size. Some patients may present with persistent amenorrhea. Patients with a missed abortion may be amenorrheic for prolonged periods of time. They may eventually resume menses after almost total resorption of the products of conception or they may eventually bleed and pass the tissues spontaneously.

Sonography, urinalysis, and serum pregnancy tests are helpful in making the diagnosis. Real-time sonography demonstrates the absence of fetal life signs (heart action or fetal movements). This sign is very reliable by the sixth week of gestation. Serial pregnancy tests should indicate a decline in placental hormone production. Once the diagnosis of a missed abortion is made or confirmed, a dilatation and curettage can be performed at once or after a waiting period, because 93 percent spontaneously abort within 3 weeks of fetal death (Tricomi and Kohl, 1957). Because of the slow absorption of thromboplastin material in the amniotic fluid into the maternal circulation, about 20 percent of women carrying a dead fetus for longer than 5 weeks may have the manifestations of a consumptive coagulopathy. These patients may have bleeding from the gums and nose and from slight trauma. Patients who are at risk for coagulopathy (over 5 weeks after fetal death) should be followed by weekly serum fibrinogen levels. Evacuation of the uterine contents is indicated if the fibrinogen level begins to decrease. If the level is at or below 100 mg/dl, the patient should be anticoagulated with heparin until the fibrinogen level rises to normal (usually 48 hours) before evacuation of the uterine contents is performed. Occasionally, a patient develops an infection of the dead products of conception. This is manifested by crampy abdominal pain, foul vaginal discharge, and spiking fevers. Cervical and blood cultures should be taken, and systemic broad-spectrum antibiotics should be started and the uterus evacuated.

The usual management of a missed abortion, once the diagnosis is confirmed, is to wait for spontaneous resolution over 3 to 5 weeks, if the patient is emotionally stable, or to induce labor to evacuate the uterine contents using oxytocic agents. Currently the use of prostaglandin $E_2$ vaginal suppositories (20 mg) given repetitively (every 3 hours) has met with good results. The process may take from 6 to 18 hours, and the patient may suffer side effects from the prostaglandin such as nausea, vomiting, diarrhea, and fever, which can be treated palliatively.

## SEPTIC ABORTION

When an illegal abortion is performed, it is often a dilatation and curettage performed under unsterile conditions and it is often an incomplete evacuation of the uterine contents. This results in a serious intrauterine infection that, if left untreated, causes serious sequelae or even the death of the patient. (In fact, before abortions were legalized in the United States, the death rate attributable to illegal abortions contributed significantly to maternal mortality statistics.) The patient usually presents to the hospital emergency room in a septic condition (high fever, tachycardia, and shocky), complaining of abdominal pain and vaginal bleeding. A history of an illegal abortion can usually be elicited.

The patient's condition should be rapidly stabilized with intravenous fluids and blood transfusions. Blood, cervical, and uterine cultures for both aerobic and anaerobic organisms should be obtained. A Gram stain of the uterine discharge should be examined for *Clostridia* and high-dose, multiple-regimen parenteral antibiotics begun. When the patient is stable, a dilatation and curettage with preparations for a possible total hysterectomy should be carried out.

A supportive rather than interrogative atmosphere should be provided for the patient. She may have guilt feelings as well as a fear of persecution because of the illegal abortion. She has already suffered psychologic and physical trauma. She needs a sympathetic ear and emotional support through her recovery.

## HABITUAL ABORTION

Habitual abortion is defined as three or more consecutive spontaneous abortions. Various studies indicate that women who have had a spontaneous abortion are at greater risk for another; thus, the greater the number of previous abortions, the higher the risk (Goldzieher and Benigno, 1958; Warburton and Fraser, 1961).

A specific cause can be found in about two thirds of habitual aborters, usually based on genetic, hormonal, anatomic, immunologic, or infectious factors, or on a chronic systemic illness (Tho et al, 1979).

Genetic factors are the cause of about 25 percent of recurrent abortions, with 13 percent of the cases being due to multifactorial gene abnormalities and 12 percent due to chromosomal abnormalities. The most common chromosomal abnormality is trisomy, with X monosomy with polyploidy being next in frequency. Chromosomal translocations account for 5 to 10 percent of habitual abortions. Paternal factors implicated in recurrent abortion include balanced translocation and polyspermia secondary to hyperspermia (MacLeod and Gold, 1957).

Hormonal causes of recurrent abortion include luteal phase (or progesterone) deficiency. Insufficient corpus luteum function can be related to hyperprolactinemia or a hyperandrogen state, but for the most part, its pathophysiology is poorly understood.

Anatomic abnormalities of the reproductive tract associated with habitual abortion include developmental anomalies of the müllerian duct, such as bicornuate, unicornuate, or subseptate uterus; uterine cavity distortion secondary to myomas; and incompetent cervix.

Chronic systemic illnesses associated with recurrent abortion include lupus erythematosus, advanced diabetes mellitus, and renal and cardiac diseases.

Immunologic factors include maternal levels of sperm-agglutinating or immobilizing antibodies and, possibly human leukocyte antigen (HLA)–related suppression of maternal immunologic response to paternal antigens (Moghissi, 1982).

Finally, chronic reproductive tract infections have been implicated in recurrent abortions. These pathogens are *Toxoplasma gondii, Listeria monocytogenes, Chlamydia trachomatis, Ureaplasma urealyticum* (T-mycoplasma), and herpesvirus (Moghissi, 1982).

When a patient has a recurrent abortion, the medical personnel should make every effort to determine the cause. Carefully collected samples of the products of conception should be sent for genetic analysis. Appropriately collected samples for culture of pathogens should be sent. A thorough pelvic examination, including an intrauterine cavity exploration, should be performed. Finally, a detailed history of the events and factors surrounding the abortion should be recorded. Only by following the above-mentioned protocol can the physician arrive at an etiology and counsel the couple regarding future pregnancy.

## ECTOPIC PREGNANCY
(See Table 27–8)

Ectopic pregnancy is defined as the implantation of the blastocyst at any site other than the endometrium. The vast majority (95 percent) of ectopic pregnancies are located in the fallopian tubes, within which the four most common sites are (in order of frequency) the ampullary, isthmic, fimbrial, and interstitial portions of the tube (Cavanagh and Woods, 1982) (Fig. 27–1). Besides the fallopian tubes, other, less frequent sites include the cervix, ovary, and peritoneal cavity. The incidence of ectopic pregnancy varies widely across the United States, with reports of its occurrence from 1 in 90 to 1 in 200 pregnancies (Cavanagh and Woods, 1982). Etiologic factors that predispose to ectopic pregnancy are any conditions that prevent or retard the passage of the fertilized ovum into the uterus, such as chronic salpingitis, congenital tubal abnormalities, tubal endometriosis, and pelvic adhesions.

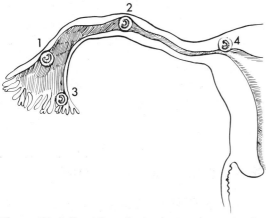

**Figure 27–1.** Location of ectopic pregnancy in the fallopian tube. *1*, Ampullar. *2*, Isthmic. *3*, Fimbrial. *4*, Interstitial. (Locations listed in order of frequency of occurrence.)

Patients wearing an intrauterine device appear to have a higher incidence of ectopic pregnancy. In an ectopic implantation, the trophoblastic cells of the blastocyst proliferate and penetrate the tubal wall and arterial vessels, resulting in internal hemorrhage. The insufficient hormonal production by this faulty placenta stimulates the endometrium to grow; then, as the hormone level fluctuates, the hormonal support for the endometrium fails and vaginal bleeding ensues. There is a wide variation of signs and symptoms, depending on the location of the ectopic pregnancy. Signs and symptoms associated with tubal pregnancy begin with a missed or delayed menses followed by an episode of vaginal bleeding. As the tubal pregnancy begins to rupture, the patient experiences unilateral lower abdominal pain progressing to diffuse lower abdominal pain and vasomotor disturbances (e.g., fainting). The abdomen becomes tender on palpation, and a pelvic mass develops as the blood collects in the cul-de-sac. There is unilateral pain elicited during pelvic examination. In about 50 percent of cases, referred right shoulder pain occurs, resulting from blood irritating the subdiaphragmatic phrenic nerve when the patient is supine. (See Table 27–2 for clinical signs and symptoms of ectopic pregnancy.) Culdocentesis is a most helpful diagnostic tool in establishing a high enough index of suspicion to operate. If a positive tap (free-flowing blood without clots) is obtained, prompt surgical intervention is mandatory.

The patient should be advised about her condition and impending surgical procedures, one of which may be hysterectomy. If possible, she should be queried regarding her desire for future fertility or any history of infertility. This information may influence the type of surgery chosen. Blood (crossmatched) and intravenous fluids are started, but if the patient is in shock, no time should be wasted in stabilizing her, because prompt surgical intervention is required to control the bleeding. Complete excision of the affected tube is the treatment of choice, to prevent a recurrence of an ectopic pregnancy. However, if the patient has another previously damaged tube besides the tube containing the ectopic pregnancy and she desires fertility, one may elect to perform conservative tubal surgery. A linear salpingostomy is performed to evacuate the ectopic pregnancy tissues; the bleeding is carefully controlled, and that tube is conserved. On the other hand, a hysterectomy may be per-

**Table 27–2**
CLINICAL SIGNS AND SYMPTOMS OF ECTOPIC PREGNANCY

| History | Abdomen | Temperature | Pelvic Exam | Uterus |
|---------|---------|-------------|-------------|--------|
| Missed or delayed period; irregular bleeding; unilateral lower abdominal pain progressing to diffuse lower abdomen pain; shoulder pain; fainting | Abdominal distention; lower abdominal pain; rebound tenderness | Subnormal (98.4°F) or mild elevation (99.4°F) | Adnexal mass or mass in cul-de-sac; culdocentesis yields unclotted blood | Normal or slightly enlarged |

formed if the ectopic pregnancy is in the portion of the tube within the uterine wall (interstitial), or if the only remaining tube contains the ectopic pregnancy, provided the patient desires sterility and her condition permits more extensive surgery.

In cases of ectopic pregnancy or abortion, an Rh-negative, unsensitized patient (negative indirect Coombs' test) should receive a hyperimmune gamma globulin (RhoGAM) injection before discharge.

## HYDATIDIFORM MOLE
(See Table 27–8)

Hydatidiform mole is an abnormal development of the placenta resulting in the formation of grapelike vesicles as the fetal part of the pregnancy fails to develop. Unlike the usual abortion that occurs with an abnormal fetus, a mole placenta continues to grow at a very rapid pace to eventually outgrow its own blood supply and degenerate into grapelike vesicles. The incidence in the United States is 1 in 2000 pregnancies. In Asians, the incidence may be as high as 1 in 200 pregnancies. The patient usually experiences exaggerated nausea and vomiting, and she may have intermittent to continuous brownish vaginal discharge associated with frank bleeding by the 12th week. Many times, the patient is more anemic than her bleeding history might indicate. There is a disporportionate rapid growth of the uterus in 50 percent of the cases. There is absence of fetal movement or fetal heart sounds. The uterus is usually tender and boggy because of overstretching of the lower uterine segment. Signs of preeclampsia appear before the 24th week of gestation in some of these patients. Finally, the passage of grapelike vesicles is diagnostic of the condition. The

diagnosis is corroborated by persistently higher than normal titers of human chorionic gonadotropin (hCG) (> 20,000 IU/24 h). Ultrasonography is the most efficacious and reliable test to identify a molar pregnancy. A sonogram demonstrating a large uterus filled with multiple small echoes (vesicles) with the absence of any fetal parts is pathognomonic of a mole pregnancy.

Evacuation of the mole by suction curettage is the treatment of choice. Occasionally, a hysterectomy is required if the molar pregnancy is far advanced (> 20-week uterine size) or if the patient is older, because these two factors increase the risk of malignant degeneration. After the uterine evacuation, continuous follow-up of the patient is needed to detect any malignant changes of the remaining trophoblastic tissues, because choriocarcinoma is reported to occur in 0.5 to 9.5 percent of all patients with hydatidiform mole. Apparently, small groups of the trophoblastic tissues are disseminated in the bloodstream at evacuation and may degenerate into choriocarcinoma. To detect this, serum hCG titers are measured weekly for 6 months and then every 6 months for the next year. The patient should avoid conception during this follow-up period of a year to 24 months, because an increase in titer suggests the development of choriocarcinoma.

Table 27–3 summarizes the clinical signs and symptoms of hydatidiform mole.

# Bleeding in Late Pregnancy

## ANTEPARTUM BLEEDING

The incidence of significant vaginal bleeding in the last half of pregnancy is approximately 3 percent. Several of the conditions

**Table 27-3**
CLINICAL SIGNS AND SYMPTOMS OF HYDATIDIFORM MOLE

| History | Diagnostic Signs | Conclusive Diagnostic Signs | Uterus |
|---------|------------------|------------------------------|--------|
| Hyperemesis; brownish discharge and bleeding by 12th week | Signs of preeclampsia before the 24th week<br>Passage of grapelike vesicles | Persistent hCG > 20,000 U/24 h<br>Ultrasonogram reveals large uterus filled with multiple small echoes (vesicles) and absence of fetal parts | Large for dates; tender and boggy |

that produce vaginal bleeding carry significant risk for the mother and fetus. Over half of these instances are associated with abnormal conditions of the placenta, i.e., placenta praevia and abruptio placentae.

Significant vaginal bleeding is bright red blood not mixed with mucus, as in a "bloody show," and equivalent in amount to that which occurs with menstrual bleeding or more. Hemorrhage that is severe enough to lower maternal cardiac output can impair placental blood flow and place the fetus in jeopardy. A patient in this condition should have her circulating volume expanded quickly by intravenous fluids and blood. Once stable, the patient should have a careful and limited vaginal speculum examination to determine the cause of the bleeding, for example cervical or vaginal trauma, cervicitis, cervical cancer or polyps, or bleeding from cervical, vaginal, or labial venous varicosities. A digital examination should *not* be performed at this time. If the uterine bleeding is not associated with pain, the presumptive diagnosis is placenta praevia. The diagnosis can be confirmed by sonography.

## PLACENTA PRAEVIA
(See Table 27-8)

Placenta praevia is the implantation of the placenta low in the uterus, either overlying or reaching the vicinity of the cervical os. The placenta's position near or over the cervix predisposes to hemorrhage as the placenta separates on cervical dilatation or during the development of the lower uterine segment in late pregnancy. This serious obstetric complication occurs in 0.5 percent of cases (1 in 200 pregnancies). The incidence increases with increasing maternal age (3 times more common in women over 35) and parity of the patient. If the patient has a past history of low-segment cesarean delivery, or placenta praevia, there is a 12 times higher rate of recurrence. Defective vascularization of the decidua appears to be a major contributing factor to the development of placenta praevia. Patients with a history of puerperal endometritis, lower uterine scar, or myomectomy and well-worn uterus (high parity) are at risk. Large low-lying placentas occurring in twin gestation or erythroblastosis also may encroach on the internal cervical os (Hellman and Pritchard, 1971).

The classification of placenta praevia (Fig. 27-2) is as follows (Cavanagh and Woods, 1982):

*Type I*—Low placental implantation, but the lower edge does not reach the internal cervical os.

*Type II*—The lower placental edge reaches the internal cervical os but does not cover it.

*Type III*—The placenta completely covers the internal os when the cervix is closed but only partially covers the internal os when the cervix is dilated.

*Type IV*—The placenta covers the internal cervical os when the cervix is either closed or dilated.

The classic symptom of placenta praevia is painless vaginal bleeding that usually occurs after the 28th week of gestation. This symptom is reported by 80 percent of patients. Ten percent report bleeding and uterine contractions, and the remaining 10 percent are diagnosed incidentally before symptoms appear. This has become more common with the increased use of ultrasound (Huff, 1982). However, the majority of unsymptomatic ultrasound-diagnosed placenta praevia in the midtrimester moves up and away from the internal cervical os as the lower uterine segment develops from cer-

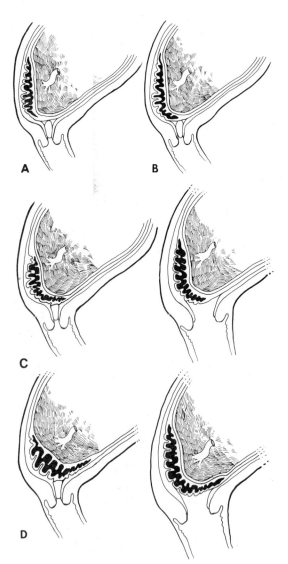

**Figure 27–2.** The classification of placenta previa. *A*, Class I. *B*, Class II. *C*, Class III with closed and partially open cervix. *D*, Class IV with closed and partially open cervix.

vical tissue late in the third trimester (Korducki, 1979). Joupilla (1979) points out that this is especially true if the ultrasound diagnosis of placenta praevia is made in early pregnancy.

The first bleeding episode is generally characterized as occurring while the patient is asleep and is rarely fatal. The bleeding generally ceases only to recur without warning. The earlier in pregnancy the bleeding episodes occur, the more serious the type of placenta praevia (type IV). Fifty percent of patients with type IV placenta praevia have episodic bleeding before the 30th week of

gestation (Cavanagh and Woods, 1982). A type I or type II placenta praevia may not bleed until the onset of labor. Approximately 90 percent of patients with placenta praevia experience at least one episode of bleeding, and 10 to 25 percent develop hypovolemic shock during the course of their pregnancies (Cavanagh and Woods, 1982).

A presumptive diagnosis of placenta praevia should be made with any episode of painless third trimester vaginal bleeding. The diagnosis can be confirmed by the use of ultrasound, which has over 95 percent accuracy in cases of placenta praevia.

Several studies have indicated that placenta praevia can account for intrauterine fetal growth retardation. Bjerre and Bjerre (1976) reported that the most common cause of low-birth-weight infants is placenta praevia. Neri and coworkers (1980) demonstrated fetal growth retardation in 129 cases of placenta praevia. Varma (1973) reported a study indicating that placental insufficiency and fetal growth retardation may be a common problem in patients with placenta praevia who experience recurrent bleeding episodes.

Any patient suspected of having a placenta praevia should be initially hospitalized at bed rest. Initial management should be directed at ascertaining how much bleeding (per hour) the patient had and is having, that is, light (50 ml), moderate (100 ml), or profuse (500 ml). On admission, blood should be drawn for blood count and type and crossmatch for blood and Rh factor. If the bleeding is continuous and significant in amount, an intravenous infusion should be started. The amount of bleeding after the patient is placed in bed should be noted by frequently changing and counting (weighing) the pads under the patient. Periodically, the maternal abdomen should be palpated for uterine activity or rigidity. Expectant management is usually carried out in the hospital. While at bed rest, the patient should be instructed to notify the nurses immediately if she feels fluid escaping from the vagina. External fetal monitoring (nonstress and biophysical profile) should be performed weekly and in conjunction with any bleeding episode, to assess fetal well-being. A hematocrit above 30 is maintained by hematinics or blood transfusions, if necessary. Until the patient is stabilized, vital signs should be taken every 15 minutes including external fetal monitoring, and hourly intake and output assessments. Once the patient is stable, the taking of vital signs can be reduced to once an hour. Once the patient is on the antepartum floor, vital signs with fetal heart tones can be taken every 4 hours, and intake and output determinations and pad counts can be made every shift unless bleeding resumes. Once the bleeding has subsided, an occasional patient may be managed at home, provided that the following criteria are met:

1. The patient fully understands the nature of her condition and that she must remain at bed rest and avoid coitus (see Chapter 14).
2. The patient should have around-the-clock transportation, communication available, and live within 20 to 30 minutes' driving distance from the hospital.
3. The patient must have a hematocrit above 30, to allow some reserve in the face of significant bleeding.
4. The patient must be followed closely (i.e., sonography repeated at 3-week intervals and weekly antepartum fetal testing [nonstress and biophysical profiles]) for fetal growth and fetal well-being.

The expectant management program requires that the patient remain at bed rest until one of the following occurs to terminate the program:

1. The patient goes into labor.
2. The fetus is mature (most reliable indicator is the L/S ratio) or the gestational age reaches 37 weeks.
3. The fetus expires.
4. An intrauterine infection develops.
5. The membranes rupture.
6. The amount of bleeding is excessive or life threatening.

Usually, about one third of patients with placenta praevia can be managed expectantly, as discussed earlier, because over half of the patients are at term when they bleed for the first time. The remainder go into labor or have excessive bleeding.

### Determining the Route of Delivery

The diagnosis of placenta praevia usually indicates delivery by cesarean birth. However, under certain circumstances, such as when there is only partial placental covering of the cervical os or a low-lying placenta, a vaginal delivery may be allowed. Although the placenta can be localized in the lower uterus accurately by ultrasound, the exact relationship of the lower placental edge to the cervical os is less accurate. Also, during the interval of expectant management, the lower uterine segment develops progressively from cervical tissue. Thus, an accurate assessment of the relationship of the lower edge of the placenta to the cervical os must be made to determine the route of delivery. The most definitive method by which to perform this is digital palpation. This method should be performed only after termination of the expectant management program (see earlier) and under double set-up conditions— that is, perform the examination in the operating room with blood ready, intravenous lines in place, anesthesia standing by, and all preparations completed for an immediate cesarean delivery. The palpation of placental tissue covering the cervical os, or part of it, mandates proceeding to cesarean delivery. Occasionally, this palpation of the placenta can evoke profuse bleeding. It should be performed with caution and care, yet firmly enough to make a diagnosis. If no placental tissue is palpated over the cervical os, the examining finger is inserted through the cervical os; if several centimeters of the lower uterine segment can be palpated, diagnosis of a low-lying or marginal placenta praevia is made. A posterior low-lying or marginal placenta usually warrants a cesarean delivery, because this situation is often associated with a significant incidence of intrapartum fetal asphyxia due to cord or placental compression against the sacrum by the presenting part; it is also associated with soft tissue dystocia. On the other hand, a trial of labor may be allowed with an anterior low-lying placenta. The goal of the double set-up examination is to determine the route of delivery only. If a trial of vaginal delivery is to be allowed, induction of labor (amniotomy) should be dictated by the ripeness of the cervix.

Recently, a transvaginal ultrasound probe has been used to carefully delineate the relationship of the placenta implanted in the lower uterus to the internal os of the cervix. As examiners gain experience with ultrasound examination, the double set-up examination may be obviated.

The type of cesarean delivery performed depends largely on the conditions at hand. A low cervical transverse incision is preferred; however, in the case of an anterior placenta praevia, a vertical incision may be required to avoid incising the placenta, which may increase maternal and fetal blood loss. An occasional placenta praevia is complicated by varying degrees of placenta accreta—placental tissue growing right into the myometrial layer of the placental attachment site. This condition usually occurs when there is a previous low cervical cesarean delivery scar. When the separation of the placenta is difficult and it is hard to control bleeding by conservative measures, a hysterectomy is usually required for control of hemorrhage.

## Other Management Concerns

Maternal death from placenta praevia is rare, but the perinatal mortality is still over 5 percent. A pediatrician must attend the delivery, and if a trial of labor is allowed, internal fetal monitoring is recommended. Extreme care must be exercised when placing the intrauterine catheter and scalp electrode. While the patient is undergoing the expectant management program, it is advisable to assign the same nursing personnel to this patient, to alleviate anxiety generated in having to relate to different nurses. During labor and delivery, a 1:1 nurse-to-patient ratio is recommended because of the possibility of bleeding and emergency surgery. Also, vital signs with fetal heart tones should be obtained every 15 minutes and hourly intake and output determinations should be initiated. Throughout hospitalization, the patient should be encouraged to verbalize her concerns and questions. By the time the second bleeding episode occurs, the patient should know and understand the medical and surgical intervention that may be required (Kilker and Wilkerson, 1973). She should understand the principle of expectant management and the reason for the double set-up examination. She should understand that she is at risk for postpartum hemorrhage, because the lower uterine segment does not have the same contractile strength as the upper uterine segment, and that hysterectomy may be necessary because of the placenta's attachment to the thin lower uterine segment.

If the baby is born prematurely, the parents should be encouraged to visit their baby in the neonatal intensive care unit and partake in his or her care as often as possible (Klaus and Kennell, 1976). If the mother wants to breastfeed her baby she should be encouraged to do so. Prematurity is not a deterrent to breastfeeding. She can use a breast pump to supply milk for the baby until the baby is able to feed at her breasts. Breastfeeding also encourages uterine contractility.

## ABRUPTIO PLACENTAE
(See Table 27–8)

Abruptio placentae is premature separation of a normally implanted placenta that results in retroplacental bleeding after the 20th week of gestation and before the fetus is delivered.

Two main types of abruptio placentae occur: (1) that in which the hemorrhage is concealed (20 percent) and, (2) that with external hemorrhage (80 percent). The concealed type of hemorrhage is the more dangerous, because bleeding is not evident and is confined to the uterine cavity and the complications may be severe. In the external type of abruptio placentae, there is vaginal bleeding and complications are fewer and less severe. The most common classification of abruptio placentae is as follows (see also Fig. 27–3 for illustration of types of abruptio placentae):

*Grade 0*—Asymptomatic. Diagnosed after delivery when a small retroplacental clot is discovered. Rupture of a marginal sinus is also included in this category.

*Grade 1*—Vaginal bleeding. Uterine tetany and tenderness may be present. There are no signs of maternal shock or fetal distress.

*Grade 2*—External vaginal bleeding may or may not be present. Uterine tenderness and tetany are present. There are no signs of maternal shock. Signs of fetal distress are present.

*Grade 3*—External bleeding may or may not be present. There is marked uterine tetany, yielding a boardlike consistency on palpation. Persistent abdominal pain, maternal shock, and fetal demise are present. Coagulopathy may become evident in 30 percent of the cases. (Other classification systems would designate this grade as severe abruption.)

Abruptio placentae, in general, is reported to occur in 1 in 250 to 1 in 155 pregnancies.

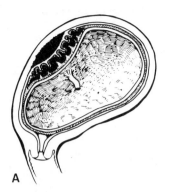 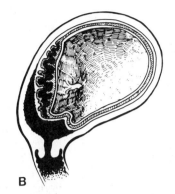 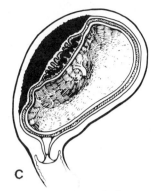

**Figure 27–3.** Types of abruptio placentae. *A*, Mild abruption with some concealed hemorrhage. *B*, Severe abruption with external hemorrhage. *C*, Severe abruption with concealed hemorrhage.

The incidence of severe or grade 3 abruptio placentae is 1 in 500 pregnancies. In about half of the cases, abruptio placentae occurs after the 36th week of gestation. Maternal mortality is about 2 percent if grade 0 is excluded. In the more severe cases associated with fetal demise, maternal mortality increases to 10 percent. The incidence of abruptio placentae is increased with higher parity and previous abruption but not with advanced maternal age.

The exact cause of abruptio placentae is unknown; however, the following conditions seem to be predisposing factors: trauma to the abdomen, short umbilical cord, polyhydramnios, sudden decompression of the uterus, leiomyomas, uterine anomalies, compression or occlusion of the inferior vena cava, circumvallate placenta, and hypertensive disorders. Hypertensive disease in pregnancy is by far the most common predisposing condition. The severity of abruptio placentae increases with parity; furthermore, the woman with a history of abruptio placentae has a risk of recurrence of about 1 in 12 (Pritchard and Brekken, 1967). Some have contended that folic acid deficiency has an etiologic role; however, further studies have failed to substantiate this theory. Naeye and associates (1977) demonstrated a correlation between placental abruption and cigarette smoking and poor maternal weight gain. They suggested that poor maternal nutrition during pregnancy may contribute to the development of abruptio placentae. It is believed that placental abruption is caused by degenerative changes in the small arteries that supply the intervillous space, resulting in thrombosis, decidual degeneration, and rupture of vessels, causing a

retroplacental hematoma (Page et al, 1981). The continued arterial pumping causes further separation of the placenta from its decidual attachment; thus, in the most severe cases, complete separation can occur. If half or more of the placental surface is separated, fetal death is inevitable (Page et al, 1981). A Couvelaire's uterus (retroplacental apoplexy) results in cases of concealed hemorrhage with blood infiltration into the myometrium. The condition was once believed to decrease uterine contractility sufficiently to produce postpartum hemorrhage by disrupting the myometrial bundles; however, the Couvelaire's uterus is not an indication for hysterectomy (Hellman and Pritchard, 1971).

The clinical picture of a severe abruptio placentae usually includes some vaginal bleeding, uterine tetany, uterine tenderness, absence of fetal heart tones, and hypovolemic shock (Table 27–4). With severe abruption, the patient can lose up to one half of her blood volume (2500 ml). The thromboplastin material in the amniotic fluid can find its way into the maternal bloodstream to initiate an acute disseminated intravascular coagulopathy.

Signs of shock may be out of proportion to the amount of hemorrhage evident in concealed hemorrhage; however, uterine rigidity and tenderness is marked. Oliguria due to inadequate renal perfusion before treatment of hypovolemia also may be observed.

In the less severe grades of abruptio placentae (less than half placental separation), fetal distress may be manifested by fetal heart rate patterns of late decelerations, decreased short- and long-term variability, and tachycardia. Internal uterine pressure moni-

**Table 27–4**

CLINICAL SIGNS AND SYMPTOMS OF
ABRUPTIO PLACENTAE

1. Vaginal bleeding may or may not be present
2. Port-wine-colored amniotic fluid
3. ↓ BP, ↑ pulse, dyspnea, pallor, oliguria
4. Symptoms of shock may be out of proportion to the amount of bleeding seen
5. Severe or sudden pain (retroplacental separation) or painless (marginal separation)
6. Uterus with boardlike tone; rigidity or tenderness

toring usually demonstrates an increased resting pressure (> 16 mm Hg) and polysystole (Fig. 27–4).

Although the more severe cases of abruptio placentae are usually heralded by the classic signs and symptoms, the mildest form (grade 0) usually goes unrecognized until after delivery. Thus, in the presence of vaginal bleeding in the third trimester, it is necessary to rule out placenta praevia and other causes of vaginal bleeding by clinical inspection and ultrasound evaluation.

Management of a patient with abruptio placentae requires adherence to the following tenets:

1. Rule of 30's. Maintenance of a minimum urine output of 30 ml/h and a hematocrit of 30 volume percent at all times by intravenous infusion of crystalloid solutions or blood as required.
2. Delivery should be performed as quickly as possible. The goal is a vaginal delivery if the fetus is healthy or dead. A cesarean delivery may be required if fetal distress is present. The use of oxytocin is not

contraindicated, although it is rarely necessary.
3. Early amniotomy to decrease the amnioinfusion into the maternal bloodstream.
4. Intensive maternal and fetal monitoring of vital signs every 15 minutes including circulating volume status (intake and output) every hour. The nurse-to-patient ratio should be 1:1 because of hemorrhage, assessment of nonreassuring fetal heart rate, possible emergency surgery, and the need to provide emotional support for this emergency situation.

Any patient diagnosed as having an abruption (even if it is of a lower grade, because it may progress) should have a reliable, large-bore intravenous line established (two or more in cases of severe abruption), 6 or more units of crossmatched blood, bladder drainage by an indwelling catheter, an amniotomy, internal fetal monitoring with a live fetus, and blood coagulation studies performed. A central venous pressure line or a Swan-Ganz balloon flotation catheter may be necessary in the fluid management of a patient in shock. A peripheral venous blood sample placed in a red-top tube taped to the wall and checked in 7 to 10 minutes indicates the coagulation status of the patient. If the clot is not formed or is fragile, the patient has a coagulopathy. If vaginal delivery is anticipated, correction of the coagulopathy is not necessary and will not alter the outcome (Hellman and Pritchard, 1971). However, careful hemostasis for an episiotomy is required. The coagulopathy usually is present when the patient first enters the hospital, but will be restored to normal 12 to 24 hours

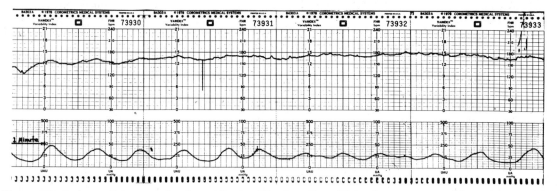

**Figure 27–4.** A cardiotocograph of a patient with abruption. Note the presence of frequent uterine contractions and elevated baseline tone in the bottom panel. Note the presence of "late decelerations" in the upper panel. (From Paul RH, et al: Fetal Intensive Care, Wallingford, CT, Corometrics Medical Systems, Inc, 1979.)

postpartum by a normally functioning liver. If the patient requires an abdominal delivery for obstetric indications (e.g., transverse lie, no progress in labor), the coagulopathy must be corrected with fresh frozen plasma and cryoprecipitate (15 to 20 bags increases fibrinogen 100 mg/dl). At the time of laparotomy, one may encounter a bruised-appearing uterus (Couvelair's uterus). This appearance of the uterus should not belie its ability to contract sufficiently to control bleeding after delivery. A coagulopathy developing with a live fetus would be unusual, but a blood sample should be checked for clotting ability before surgery as a precaution.

By maintaining an adequate circulating volume (rule of 30's) during labor in a patient with an abruption, the incidence of the uncommon sequelae of renal damage, adult pulmonary distress syndrome, and Sheehan's syndrome can be minimized.

The perinatal mortality rate of abruptio placentae is over 50 percent, and the maternal mortality is 1 percent or less.

Continuous fetal and maternal monitoring is *imperative* for the woman who is allowed to labor with a live fetus. Obtaining vital signs at least every 15 minutes, accurate hourly intake and output, central venous pressure readings, and continuous electronic fetal monitoring keep the perinatal team abreast of the maternal and fetal conditions. Observe for signs of shock, hypofibrinogenemia, and acute renal failure (Table 27–5).

At all times, be prepared for emergency or precipitous delivery. To encourage the best placental perfusion, instruct the mother to labor in the lateral position.

---

**Table 27–5**
CLINICAL SIGNS AND SYMPTOMS
OF THE COMPLICATIONS OF
ABRUPTIO PLACENTAE

---

1. Clinical signs of shock
   a. Hypothermia
   b. Tachycardia with weak and thready pulse
   c. Rapid shallow respirations; hypotension with reduced pulse pressure; pale mottled or cyanotic skin; cold, clammy skin
   d. Cerebral manifestation of inadequate perfusion: patient complains of thirst, anxiety, confusion, restlessness
2. Increased bleeding with signs of hypovolemia
3. Decreased urine output (< 30 ml/h)
4. CVP readings ( ↓ *hypovolemia* < 2 cm; ↑ *hypervolemia;* cardiac failure; or fluid overload > 10 cm)
5. Bleeding from puncture sites (coagulopathy)

---

# Intrapartum Bleeding

Significant bleeding during the intrapartum period not associated with placental abruption is rare. Cervical trauma can cause bleeding but is usually not enough to cause problems. There are two causes of intrapartum bleeding that pose a threat to the well-being of the fetus and mother: vasa praevia and uterine rupture.

## VASA PRAEVIA
(See Table 27–8)

Vasa praevia may occur when there is a velamentous insertion of the umbilical cord into a low-lying placenta. In this condition, the cord vessels begin to separate as the cord nears the placental surface, like fingers spreading apart. These single vessels no longer have the gelatinous rubbery protective surrounding as they do in the intact cord, and they often traverse across part of the amniotic membrane to the placental surface. A vasa praevia occurs when the vessel in the amniotic membranes is draped across the cervix in front of the presenting part. When amniotomy is performed, the fetal vessels are torn and fetal bleeding commences. The incidence of this condition is low. Recognition of it requires a high index of suspicion when bleeding follows amniotomy. The determination of a fetal bleed requires the ability to quickly differentiate between fetal and maternal blood (which can result from cervical trauma during the amniotomy procedure), because the baby can die within 1 to 2 minutes if a vessel in the umbilical cord is ruptured. An Apt test can differentiate between maternal and fetal blood (Apt and Downey, 1955). This test is based on the physiologic principle that fetal hemoglobin is alkaline stable, whereas adult hemoglobin is not. (See methodology for Apt test in Table 27–6.) If fetal blood is documented, the baby should be rapidly delivered. Usually, a cesarean delivery is required. During the assessment and diagnosis of this emergency situation, a 2 : 1 nurse-to-patient ratio should be maintained.

## UTERINE RUPTURE
(See Table 27–8)

The major cause of uterine rupture is previous cesarean delivery, and the second most

**Table 27–6**
THE APT TEST METHOD

1. Collect bloody specimen in a lavender-top tube.
2. Concurrently, obtain two controls:
   a. Maternal blood sample
   b. Fetal blood sample—e.g., use cord blood from recent delivery (nursery lab always has a control available)
   c. Sample in question
3. Place 0.2 ml of each sample in a separate test tube (use pipette or tuberculin syringe).
4. Add 2 ml of tap water or distilled water to each test tube (10 : 1 dilution). This lyses the red cells and produces a pink supernatant in all tubes.
5. Centrifuge the tubes for approximately 2 minutes. This step intensifies the color of the supernatant as the sediment falls to the bottom of the tube.
6. Add 1 ml of 0.25 normal (1 percent) NaOH solution to each tube.
7. Read the color change in 2 minutes. If the test solution is adult hemoglobin, its color will change from pink to yellow-brown. If the solution is fetal hemoglobin, its color will remain predominantly pink. It is essential to compare the color change of the test solution with that of the control specimens.
8. If there is any question about the interpretation of the test, and time permits, request the laboratory to perform a Kleihauer-Betke test or hemoglobin electrophoresis.

common cause is overstimulation with oxytocin (Cunningham et al, 1989). Spontaneous rupture of the uterus is a devastating complication of labor, carrying a very high maternal and perinatal mortality. It tends to occur in older, multiparous women, and cephalopelvic disproportion is a significant factor. It occurs once in 1000 to 1500 births and is responsible for at least 5 percent of all maternal deaths. At the height of a uterine contraction, the patient complains of sudden, sharp, shooting abdominal pain. She frequently states that "something has given way" inside her. Uterine contractions cease to bother the patient, and vaginal bleeding is noted. Abdominal palpation reveals tenderness; the presenting part has receded, and two large round objects (one the contracted empty uterus and the other the fetus) can be palpated in the lower abdomen. Shortly thereafter, the patient becomes shocky. A vaginal examination sometimes reveals a rent in the lower uterine segment. The treatment is immediate laparotomy and, frequently, hysterectomy after rapid stabilization of the patient's hypovolemic state. Perinatal mortality is virtually 100 percent. During this obstetric emergency, at least a 1 : 1 nurse-to-patient ratio is recommended. With both vasa praevia and uterine rupture,

maternal vital signs should be taken at least every 15 minutes along with continuous fetal heart rate monitoring.

# Postpartum Hemorrhage
(See Table 27–8)

Postpartum hemorrhage is a significant contributor to maternal mortality today. Most textbooks define it as the occurrence of more than 500 ml of blood loss during and after delivery. However, Pritchard and associates and others have demonstrated that actual blood loss from a normal vaginal delivery exceeds 500 ml (Newton, 1966; Pritchard et al, 1962). Nonetheless, in most large clinical obstetric services, estimates of more than the usual amount of blood loss at delivery and immediately postpartum have been noted in approximately 4 percent of deliveries. Postpartum hemorrhage severe enough to cause signs and symptoms of hypovolemic shock has an incidence of less than 0.5 percent.

The majority of cases of postpartum hemorrhage are due to uterine atony (75 to 80 percent). Other causes include genital tract trauma during delivery, and rarely, placenta accreta, uterine inversion, and coagulopathies.

## UTERINE ATONY

Predisposing factors for uterine atony in the order of their frequency include the following: (1) precipitous labor, (2) $MgSO_4$ treatment in preeclamptic patients, (3) chorioamnionitis, (4) macrosomia (> 4000 g) or multiple gestations, and (5) prolonged labor (Hayashi et al, 1984). Also, patients with a previous history of a postpartum hemorrhage due to uterine atony are likely to repeat that performance. We have found that the majority of patients who experienced a serious postpartum hemorrhage were delivered by cesarean delivery.

When excessive uterine bleeding occurs and the uterus is atonic, the physician usually manually explores the uterus and removes any retained placental fragments or membranes, administers dilute oxytocin intravenously (40 to 60 U added to 1000 ml of intravenous fluid), and gives methyl ergonovine, 0.2 mg intramuscularly (if the patient is not hypertensive). The uterus is manually massaged to increase uterine muscle tone. If bleeding continues despite these standard therapies, the physician must perform an emergency laparotomy to control the hemorrhage by surgical intervention. The use of prostaglandin has been reported to successfully increase uterine tone and abate hemorrhage. Prostaglandin $F_2\alpha$ administered by the intramyometrial route (Jacobs and Arias, 1980; Takagi et al, 1977), prostaglandin $E_2$ that is administered by vaginal suppository (Hertz et al, 1980), and a 15 methyl analogue of prostaglandin $F_2\alpha$ that is 10 times as potent, has a longer duration of action, and is administered by the intramuscular route, have been reported to be very successful (Hayashi et al, 1981; Toppozada et al, 1981). Side effects of prostaglandin treatments have been reported to be mild fever, diarrhea, and vomiting (Hayashi et al, 1981). However, prostaglandins do not affect breastfeeding. Especially with cesarean birth patients, prophylactic antinausea and antidiarrhea medications should be initiated with the prostaglandins. The use of prostaglandins would follow failure of the standard therapies mentioned earlier. Failing all else, the physician may have to ligate the uterine arteries or the hypogastric arteries or even perform a hysterectomy to control the hemorrhage. The perinatal team must recognize when there is a need for rapid volume expansion, to type and crossmatch for many units of blood, and to anticipate the pharmacologic therapy required and have the appropriate agents at hand for immediate use. Notification of the nursing supervisor is important so that an operating room can be made available when necessary. It must be remembered to never inject a bolus of undiluted oxytocin directly intravenously or into the intravenous line, because this practice has been associated with acute hypotension and cardiac arrest. See Table 27–7 for a summary of the aforementioned therapies for postpartum hemorrhage. During these therapies, the nurse-to-patient ratio should be 1:1. Vital signs should be taken at a minimum of every 15 minutes, and an accurate hourly intake and output should be completed.

## GENITAL TRACT TRAUMA

Lacerations of the cervix and vagina occur with spontaneous as well as with instrumented vaginal deliveries. Any patient with excessive postpartum bleeding should be carefully inspected for cervical and vaginal lacerations, even in the presence of atony, to rule out a combined source of bleeding. Genital tract trauma can cause significant blood loss through continuous nonalarming bleeding or bleeding into a dead space to form a large retroperitoneal hematoma over hours.

A careful exploration of the vaginal vault, looking for vaginal and cervical lacerations, should follow every delivery, particularly operative deliveries. Vaginal lacerations are likely to occur over the perineal body and the periurethral area and over the ischial spines in the posterolateral aspects of the vaginal vault. Repair of vaginal lacerations requires good exposure, lighting, and use of the principle of tissue approximation without leaving any dead space. Most important is placing the first suture well above the apex of the laceration. Cervical lacerations are likely to occur at 9 or 3 o'clock and do not need suturing unless they are bleeding. Vaginal and labial hematomas are usually carefully observed, unless they are large or rapidly enlarging, in which case the hematoma should be excised. If no bleeding vessel is identified (as is common), the area should be packed with pressure gauze and observed carefully. Astute observation of the perineal area is mandatory during the postpartum period, especially with any of these lacerations or hematomas. Initially, ice can help to decrease swelling and reduce pain. Later, warm compresses, heat lamps, and analgesic spray can help to decrease discomfort.

*Text continued on page 559*

---

**Table 27–7**

MANAGEMENT OF POSTPARTUM
HEMORRHAGE DUE TO UTERINE ATONY
(IN ORDER OF PROCESSION)

---

1. Standard therapies
   a. Uterine exploration and massage
   b. Intravenous oxytocin (dilute)
   c. Intramuscular methylergonovine (*never intravenous*)
2. Prostaglandin therapy
   a. Prostin 15M, 250 $\mu$g intramuscular or intramyometrial injection
   b. Prostin $F_2\alpha$, 1.0 mg by intramyometrial injection
   c. Prostin $E_2$, 20-mg vaginal suppository
3. Surgical therapies
   a. Uterine artery ligation
   b. Hypogastric artery ligation
   c. Hysterectomy

**Table 27–8**

## PATIENT CARE SUMMARY FOR BLEEDING MANAGEMENT*

| | Antepartum | | | |
| | Outpatient | Inpatient | Intrapartum | Postabortion |
|---|---|---|---|---|
| **ABORTIONS (Nurse-to-Patient Ratio = 1:2)** | | | | |
| BP | — | On admission; then q 1 h & PRN | | q 15 min × 4; then q 30 min × 2; then q 1 h until stable; then on discharge from RR |
| P, R | — | On admission; then q 1 h & PRN | — | q 15 min × 4; then q 30 min × 2; then q 1 h until stable; then on discharge from RR |
| T | — | On admission; then q 4 h | | On admission; then q 4 h; then on discharge from RR |
| Observe for bleeding and tissue passage | Frequently | On admission; then q 30 min | | On admission; then q 1 h until stable; then q 4 h; then on discharge from RR |
| Ultrasound | Gestational dating | — | — | — |
| Sexual limitations | Two weeks' abstention, or until vaginal discharge ceases | | — | Resume activity as tolerated |
| Bed rest | With bathroom privileges | With bathroom privileges | | Resume normal activity as tolerated |

| | Antepartum | | | |
| | Outpatient | Inpatient | Intrapartum | Postsurgery |
|---|---|---|---|---|
| **ECTOPIC PREGNANCY (Nurse-to-Patient Ratio = 2:1)** | | | | |
| BP | — | On admission; then q 1 h | q 15 min during surgery | q 15 min × 4; then q 30 min × 2; then q 1 h until stable; then on discharge from RR |
| P, R | — | On admission; then q 1 h | As above | q 15 min × 4; then q 30 min × 2; then q 1 h until stable; then on discharge from RR |
| T | — | On admission; then q 4 h | — | q 4 h |
| Fetal heart rate | q 1 h | | — | — |
| Check for: | | | | |
| Vaginal bleeding | q 1 h | | — | q 15 min × 4; then 30 min × 2; then q 1 h until stable; then on discharge from RR |
| Tender abdomen | | On admission | — | |
| Right shoulder pain | | On admission | | — |
| Culdocentesis | — | On admission | — | — |
| **HYDATIDIFORM MOLE (Nurse-to-Patient Ratio = 2:1)** | | | | |
| Ultrasound to confirm diagnosis | Performed on all patients suspected of having hydatidiform mole | | — | — |
| BP | — | On admission; then q 1 h | q 15 min during surgery | On admission; then q 15 min × 4; then q 30 min × 2; then q 1 h until stable; then on discharge from RR |
| R, P | — | On admission; then q 1 h | q 15 min during surgery | On admission; then q 15 min × 4; then q 30 min × 2; then q 1 h until stable; then on discharge from RR |

* This table lists *minimal* requirements for taking BP, P, R, and T; presence of excessive bleeding or infection may require more frequent readings.

**Table 27–8**
PATIENT CARE SUMMARY FOR BLEEDING MANAGEMENT* Continued

| | Antepartum | | Intrapartum | Postsurgery |
|---|---|---|---|---|
| | *Outpatient* | *Inpatient* | | |
| T | — | On admission; then q 4 h | — | On admission to RR; then q 4 h |
| Check for bleeding | — | On admission; then q 30 min | — | On admission to RR; then q 15 min × 4; then q 30 min × 2; then q 1 h until stable; then q 4 h |
| Fetal heart rate | — | On admission | — | — |
| hCG titers | — | Follow up for 6–12 months and instruct patient to avoid conception during this time | | |

| | Antepartum | | Intrapartum | Postpartum |
|---|---|---|---|---|
| | *Outpatient* | *Inpatient* | | |
| PLACENTA PRAEVIA—NO BLEEDING (Nurse-to-Patient Ratio = 1 : 6–8 antepartum, 1 : 2 intrapartum) | | | | |
| Ultrasound for placental location and to rule out IUGR | — | q 2–3 weeks | On admission | — |
| BP | — | On admission; then q 4 h | Per cesarean delivery routine if allowed to labor q 15 | On admission; then q 15 min × 4; then q 30 min × 2; then on discharge to PP floor |
| R, P | — | On admission; then q 4 h | Per cesarean delivery routine if allowed to labor q 15 | On admission; then q 15 min × 4; then q 30 min × 2; then on discharge to PP floor |
| T | — | On admission; then q 4 h | q 4 h | On admission; then q 4 h; then on discharge to PP floor |
| Check bleeding (pad count) | Count pads at home | q 8 h and prn | q 1 h and prn | — |
| I & O | | q 8 h | q 8 h (q 1 h with active bleeding) | q shift in RR |
| Bed rest | With bathroom privileges | With bathroom privileges | Yes | Resume activity as tolerated |
| Fetal heart rate monitoring | At office/clinic visit | On admission; then q 8 h | Record q 1 h with continuous monitoring, preferably internal. Without monitor, q 15 min continuously through 2–3 contractions | — |
| Contractions Frequency Duration Quality Resting tone | At office/clinic visit | q shift | Continuous | — |
| Lochia | — | — | — | On admission; then q 15 min × 4; then q 30 min × 2; if stable, then q 4 h |
| NST biophysical profile | Weekly, unless significant bleeding—then repeat immediately | On admission; then weekly unless significant bleeding—then continuous external monitoring | — | — |

*Table continued on following page*

**Table 27–8**
PATIENT CARE SUMMARY FOR BLEEDING MANAGEMENT* Continued

| | Antepartum | | Intrapartum | Postpartum |
|---|---|---|---|---|
| | *Outpatient* | *Inpatient* | | |
| H & H | Weekly | On admission; then weekly | Admission | Morning after delivery |
| Type & crossmatch | — | Keep current | Keep current | — |
| Sexual activity | None | None | — | Resume activity as tolerated |

PLACENTA PRAEVIA WITH BLEEDING (Nurse-to-Patient Ratio = 2:1)

| | *Outpatient* | *Inpatient* | Intrapartum | Postpartum |
|---|---|---|---|---|
| Fetal heart rate | — | Continuous external monitoring PRN while preparing for C/S when indicated | | — |
| BP, P, R | — | On admission; then q 15 min | | q 15 min × 4; then q 30 min × 2; then q 1 h until stable; then q 4 h |
| T | — | On admission; then q 4 h | | On admission to RR; then q 4 h; then on discharge to PP floor |
| I & O | — | Initiate on admission q 1 h while bleeding | — | Hourly while in RR; then q 8 h until stable |
| Check vaginal bleeding | — | Constantly | Constantly until C/S when indicated | q 15 min × 4; then q 30 min × 2; then q 1 h until stable; then q 4 h |
| H & H | — | On admission | On admission to OR | On admission to RR; morning after delivery |
| Clotting studies | — | On admission and PRN | — | — |
| Type & crossmatch | — | On admission Keep current | Keep current | — |
| Bed rest | | Yes | Yes | Yes |
| Prepare for C/S if unable to stop bleeding | | | | |

ABRUPTIO PLACENTAE—SEVERE (Nurse-to-Patient Ratio = 2:1)

| | *Outpatient* | *Inpatient* | Intrapartum | Postpartum |
|---|---|---|---|---|
| BP, P, R | — | — | q 15 min | On admission; then q 15 min × 4; then q 30 min × 2; then q 1 h until stable; then on discharge to PP floor; then q 4–8 hr |
| T | | | On admission | On admission to RR; then q 4 h; then on discharge to PP floor; then q shift |
| Fetal heart rate monitoring | — | — | Continuously during labor, preferably internal Without monitor, q 15 min listening through 2–3 contractions | — |

**Table 27–8**
## PATIENT CARE SUMMARY FOR BLEEDING MANAGEMENT* Continued

| | Antepartum | | | |
| | Outpatient | Inpatient | Intrapartum | Postpartum |
| --- | --- | --- | --- | --- |
| Contractions<br>Frequency<br>Duration<br>Quality<br>Resting tone | — | — | Continuously during labor, preferably internal<br>Without monitor, q 15 min | — |
| I & O | — | — | q 1 h | q shift |
| H & H | — | — | Stat | On admission to RR |
| Type & crossmatch | — | — | On admission keep current | On admissionto RR |

ABRUPTIO PLACENTAE—MILD (Nurse-to-Patient Ratio = 1 : 6–8 antepartum, 1 : 2 intrapartum)

| | Antepartum | | | |
| | Outpatient | Inpatient | Intrapartum | Postpartum |
| --- | --- | --- | --- | --- |
| BP, P, R | — | q 4 h | q 15 min | On admission; then q 15 min × 4; then q 30 min × 2; then q 1 h until stable; then on discharge to PP floor; then q 4–8 hr |
| T | — | On admission; then q 4 h | q 4 h | On admission to RR; then q 4 h; then on discharge to PP floor; then q shift |
| Fetal heart rate monitoring | — | NST biophysical profile weekly FHR q shift | Continuously during labor, preferably internal<br>Without monitor, q 15 min listening through 2–3 contractions | — |
| Contractions<br>Frequency<br>Duration<br>Quality<br>Resting tone | — | FHR q shift | Continuously during labor, preferably internal<br>Without monitor, q 15 min | — |
| I & O | — | q shift | q shift | q shift |
| H & H | — | Daily | — | Morning after delivery |
| Type & crossmatch | — | Keep current | Keep current | |
| Bleeding | — | q shift & PRN | q 1 | On admission; then q 15 min × 4; then q 30 min × 2; then q 1 hr until stable; then on discharge to PP floor; the q 4–8 hrs |

VASA PRAEVIA (Nurse-to-Patient Ratio = 2 : 1)

| | Antepartum | | | |
| | Outpatient | Inpatient | Intrapartum | Postpartum |
| --- | --- | --- | --- | --- |
| Immediate emergency | | | | |
| Prepare for cesarean delivery | | | | |
| Fetal heart rate monitoring | | | Continue until start of cesarean delivery, if possible with internal monitor<br>Without monitor, q 5 min | |

*Table continued on following page*

**Table 27–8**

PATIENT CARE SUMMARY FOR BLEEDING MANAGEMENT* Continued

| | Antepartum | | | |
| | Outpatient | Inpatient | Intrapartum | Postpartum |
|---|---|---|---|---|
| Contractions | | | Continuously during labor, preferably internal / Without monitor, q 30 min | |
| BP, R, P | | | q 15 min before cesarean delivery; routine per surgery | |
| I & O | | | q 1 h | |
| Bleeding | | | Continuously until delivery | On admission; then q 15 min × 4; then q 30 min × 2; then q 1 h until stable; then on discharge to PP floor; q 4–8 h |

UTERINE RUPTURE (Nurse-to-Patient Ratio = 2 : 1)

| | Antepartum | | | |
| | Outpatient | Inpatient | Intrapartum | Postpartum |
|---|---|---|---|---|
| Immediate emergency | | | — | — |
| Prepare for cesarean delivery | | | — | — |
| Fetal heart rate monitoring | | | Continuously until start of cesarean delivery, preferably internal / Without monitor, q 5 min | — |
| Contractions | | | Continuously until start of cesarean delivery, preferably internal / Without monitor, q 15 min | On admission to RR |
| Bleeding | | | Continuously until start of c/s | q 15 min × 4; then q 30–60 min until stable; then q 4–8 h |
| BP, R, P | | | Per cesarean delivery routine q 15 min until surgery | q 15 min × 4; then q 30 min × 2; then q 1 h until stable; then on discharge to PP floor |
| T | | | q 4 h | On admission; then q 4 h; then on discharge to PP floor |
| I & O | | | q 1 h | q 1 h in RR; then q 8 h until stable |

POSTPARTUM HEMORRHAGE (Nurse-to-Patient Ratio = 1 : 1)

| | Antepartum | | | |
| | Outpatient | Inpatient | Intrapartum | Postpartum |
|---|---|---|---|---|
| BP, P, R | | | | q 15 min until stable; then normal routine |
| T | | | | q 1 h if receiving blood / q 4 h if not receiving blood |
| I & O | | | | q 1 h until stable |
| H & H | | | | Yes |

**Table 27–8**
PATIENT CARE SUMMARY FOR BLEEDING MANAGEMENT* *Continued*

| | Antepartum | | Intrapartum | Postpartum |
| | Outpatient | Inpatient | | |
|---|---|---|---|---|
| Type & crossmatch | | | | Yes |
| Lochia assessment | | | | q 15 min minimum until stable; then q 1 hr; then q 4–8 hrs |
| Administer prostaglandins | | | | As needed |
| Perineal assessment | | | | q 15 min |
| Ice compresses | | | | Continuously with trauma |
| **UTERINE INVERSION** (Nurse-to-Patient Ratio = 1:2) | | | | |
| BP, P, R | | | | q 15 min during emergency; then q 15 min × 4; then q 30 min × 2; then q 1 h until stable; then on discharge to PP floor |
| I & O | | | | Continuously until stable |
| Laboratory values | | | | Serial H & H after acute phase |

## UTERINE INVERSION

Uterine inversion is the turning inside out of the uterus in the third stage of labor. The uterus is usually atonic, the cervix open, and the placenta attached. As the fundus of the uterus moves through the vagina, the tugging on the peritoneal structures elicits a strong vasovagal response, leading to hypotension. If the placenta is completely or partially separated, bleeding is excessive. Thus, this condition, unless quickly corrected, is life threatening. Its spontaneous occurrence is rare (1 in 20,000 pregnancies). Improper management of the third stage of labor may increase the risk of its occurrence, particularly when there is fundal placentation, incomplete separation, or an atonic uterus, and a health care provider who exerts fundal pressure with his or her fingers, producing traction on the cord (Watson et al, 1980).

Management of a uterine inversion requires quick thinking and action. The diagnosis is readily apparent when one recognizes a shaggy ball with the placenta attached to it protruding from the vaginal opening. The patient shows signs of hypovolemic shock, so that rapidly infusing intravenous fluids should be instituted and help obtained from other personnel, especially anesthesia standby. (The increased intravenous fluids should *not* contain oxytocin.) The placenta should be manually removed. The physician then institutes a gradual but continuous replacement of the inverted uterus, using the palm of the hand to elevate the uterine fundus through the vagina and into the peritoneal cavity. Once the uterus is replaced, oxytocin or other agents are given to increase uterine tone and to control the bleeding at the placental site.

## PLACENTA ACCRETA

Placenta accreta is an abnormal condition in which the placenta villi grow into the myometrium owing to defective formation of decidua. The placenta is adherent to the myometrium and usually is removed in pieces manually. The result is postpartum hemorrhage. Its occurrence is rare; however it is more likely to occur in a patient with a placenta praevia over a previous low cervical transverse cesarean delivery scar. The usual treatment may require immediate hysterectomy.

## COAGULOPATHIES

These entities are well covered in Chapter 28.

When bleeding occurs in pregnancy, the outcome is potentially disastrous. In early pregnancy, the loss of the fetus requires the perinatal team to be supportive and aware of the grieving process. An understanding of the pathophysiologic processes of abortions, ectopic pregnancy, and hydatidiform mole results in more effective team intervention. In late pregnancy, quick thinking and action, as well as the organizational ability of the team, are essential in dealing with the life-threatening hemorrhage seen with placenta praevia, abruptio placentae, and postpartum conditions such as uterine inversion. The subtleties of the diagnosis of bleeding during labor are important and must not be overlooked. Once recognized, these emergency conditions demand continuous vigilance from the perinatal team, which usually dictates a 1 : 1 nurse-to-patient ratio. Table 27–8 summarizes patient care procedures in the management of various forms of pregnancy-associated bleeding.

## References

Apt L, Downey WS: Melena neonatorum, the swallowed blood syndrome. J Pediatr 47:6, 1955.

Bjerre B, Bjerre I: Significance of obstetrical factors in prognosis of low birth weight children. Acta Paediatr Scand 65:577, 1976.

Cavanagh D, Woods R: Hemorrhage in early pregnancy. *In* Cavannagh D, et al (ed): Obstetric Emergencies. Philadelphia, Harper & Row, 1982, p 133.

Cunningham FG, MacDonald PC, Gant NF: Williams Obstetrics. East Norwalk, CT, Appleton & Lange 1989.

Goldzieher JW, Benigno BB: The treatment of threatened and recurrent abortion: a critical review. Am J Obstet Gynecol 75:1202, 1958.

Hayashi R, Castillo MS, Noah ML: Management of severe postpartum hemorrhage due to uterine atony using an analogue of prostaglandin $F_2\alpha$. Obstet Gynecol 58:426, 1981.

Hayashi R, Castillo MS, Noah ML: Three year experience using Prostin 15M in the management of severe postpartum hemorrhage. Obstet Gynecol 63:806, 1984.

Hellman LM, Pritchard JA (eds): Williams Obstetrics, 14th ed. New York, Appleton-Century-Crofts, 1971.

Hertz RH, Sokol RJ, Dierker LJ: Treatment of postpartum uterine atony with prostaglandin $E_2$ vaginal suppositories. Obstet Gynecol 56:129, 1980.

Huff RW: Third trimester bleeding. Contemp Obstet Gynecol 20:40, 1982.

Jacobs MM, Arias F: Intramyometrial prostaglandin $F_2\alpha$ in the treatment of severe postpartum hemorrhage. Obstet Gynecol 55:665, 1980.

Jensen M, Bobak T: Handbook of Maternity Care. St Louis, CV Mosby Co, 1980, p 189.

Joupilla P: The evaluation of prognosis in threatened early pregnancy. J Perinat Med 8:3, 1980.

Joupilla P: Vaginal bleeding in the last two trimesters of pregnancy: a clinical and ultrasonic study. Acta Obstet Gynecol Scand 58:461, 1979.

Kilker R, Wilkerson B: Nursing care in placenta praevia and abruptio placentae. Nurs Clin North Am 8:479, 1973.

Klaus M, Kennell J: Maternal-Infant Bonding. St Louis, CV Mosby Co, 1976, p 122.

Korducki S: Bleeding late in pregnancy. Wis Med J 78:35, 1979.

MacLeod J, Gold RZ: The male factor in fertility and sterility. Fertil Steril 8:36, 1957.

Moghissi KS: What causes habitual abortion. Contemp Obstet Gynecol 20:45, 1982.

Naeye RL, Harkness WL, Utts J: Abruptio placentae and perinatal death: a prospective study. Am J Obstet Gynecol 128:740, 1977.

Neri A, Goradesky I, Bahary C, et al: Impact of placenta praevia on intrauterine fetal growth. Isr J Med Sci 16:6, 1980.

Newton M: Postpartum hemorrhage. Am J Obstet Gynecol 94:711, 1966.

Page E, Villee C, Villee D: Human Reproduction: Essentials of Reproductive Medicine, 3rd ed. Philadelphia, WB Saunders Co, 1981, p 408.

Pizer H, Palinski O: Coping with a Miscarriage. New York, Plume Books, 1980, p 106.

Pritchard J, Brekken A: Clinical and laboratory studies on severe abruptio placentae. Am J Obstet Gynecol 97:681, 1967.

Pritchard JA, MacDonald PC: Williams' Obstetrics. New York, Appleton-Century-Crofts, 1985.

Pritchard JA, Baldwin RM, Dickey JC, et al: Blood volume changes in pregnancy and the puerperium. II. Red blood cell loss and changes in apparent blood volume during and following vaginal delivery, cesarean section and cesarean section plus total hysterectomy. Am J Obstet Gynecol 84:1271, 1962.

Takagi S, Yoshida T, Togo Y, et al: The effects of intramyometrial injection of prostaglandin $F_2\alpha$ on severe postpartum hemorrhage. Prostaglandins 12:565, 1977.

Tho TP, Byrd JR, McDonough PG: Etiologies and subsequent reproductive performance of 100 couples with recurrent abortion. Fertil Steril 32:389, 1979.

Toppozada M, El Bassaty M, El Rahmin HA, et al: Control of intractable atonic postpartum hemorrhage by 15 methyl prostaglandin $F_2\alpha$. Obstet Gynecol 58:327, 1981.

Tricomi V, Kohl SC: Fetal death in utero. Am J Obstet Gynecol 4:1092. 1957.

Varma T: Fetal growth and placental function in patients with placenta praevia. J Obstet Gynaecol Br Commonw 80:311, 1973.

Warburton D, Fraser FC: On the probability that a woman who has had a spontaneous abortion will abort with subsequent pregnancies. J Obstet Gynaecol Br Commonw 68:784, 1961.

Watson P, Besch N, Bowes W: Management of acute and subacute puerperal inversion of the uterus. Obstet Gynecol 55:12, 1980.

# CHAPTER 28

# Disseminated Intravascular Coagulation, Autoimmune Thrombocytopenic Purpura, and Hemoglobinopathies

Pamela G. Blake, James N. Martin, Jr., and Kenneth G. Perry, Jr.

## Disseminated Intravascular Coagulation

Disseminated intravascular coagulation (DIC) is a pathologic syndrome resulting from an inappropriate activation of the clotting process. DIC is characterized by a disruption of hemostatic mechanisms due to an underlying disease process that causes intravascular consumption of plasma clotting factors and platelets (Fig. 28–1).

DIC is not a primary disease but occurs instead as a consequence of other disease processes. As clotting occurs throughout the microcirculation, fibrin is deposited in small vessels, producing mechanical injury to red blood cells and activating the fibrinolytic process, which attempts to dissolve the fibrin clots. Secondary to clot lysis, an anticoagulant effect results in erythrocyte fragmentation, hemorrhage, tissue ischemia, and anemia. A paradoxic positive feedback system ensues in which clotting is the primary problem, although hemorrhage is the predominant physical finding. DIC is referred to as *consumptive coagulopathy* or *defibrination syndrome* owing to the acute consumption of large amounts of fibrinogen, platelets, and clotting factors (especially factors II, V, and VIII) as the body attempts to regain its hemostatic mechanisms. (Abildgaard, 1968; Perez, 1981).

## INCIDENCE

The incidence of DIC in obstetric patients is difficult to ascertain owing to the wide variation of precipitating events and the exceedingly complex range of clinical manifestations. DIC may range from a mild chronic disease state to a fulminating syndrome with some fatal results. This syndrome of imbalance between the coagulation and fibrinolytic systems may occur in association with a wide variety of obstetric complications including pregnancy-induced hypertension, abruptio placentae, intrauterine fetal death, retained placenta, amniotic fluid embolism, intra-amniotic injection of saline, hemorrhagic shock, and sepsis. Secondary to such a precipitating event or stress, paradoxic coagulation and fibrinolysis occur. To further complicate the situation, the incidence of underlying precipitating events varies according to the population under study. Obstetric-related DIC is encountered in 1 in 500 deliveries for the severe type of DIC and more commonly for milder forms.

## PATHOPHYSIOLOGY

In order to understand the pathophysiology of DIC, one must consider three background components: (1) changes in hemosta-

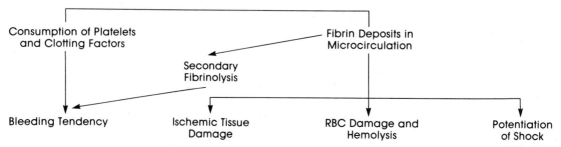

**Figure 28–1.** The disease process of DIC. (From Perez RH: Protocols for Perinatal Nursing Practice. St Louis, CV Mosby Co, 1981, p 356. Adapted from original in Williams WJ: Hematology. New York, McGraw-Hill, 1972.)

sis related to pregnancy; (2) normal blood coagulation; and (3) the fibrinolytic system.

## Hemostasis in Pregnancy

In a normal pregnancy, the components of coagulation and blood volume are altered to facilitate hemostasis. Blood volume of the normal woman late in pregnancy expands approximately 1500 ml. Factors I (fibrinogen), VII, VIII, IX, and X are elevated, but changes in the platelet count are negligible. Throughout the antepartum period, plasminogen levels are elevated, although plasmin activity is relatively normal. When stress such as hemorrhage occurs, plasminogen-to-plasmin conversion is stimulated; thus, coagulation and fibrinolysis are initiated. The greater amounts of available clotting factors may be initiated whenever physiologic insult occurs (Lavery, 1982; Pritchard and MacDonald, 1980).

## Normal Blood Coagulation

The most widely accepted theory of blood coagulation is the Bennett and Ratnoff (1972) cascade theory, which divides the blood coagulation system into two components: (1) the intrinsic system and (2) the extrinsic system (Bennett and Ratnoff, 1972). Common regulatory mechanisms work through the clotting system, and a common convergent pathway brings the intrinsic and extrinsic systems together for the final stages of clot formation.

The intrinsic pathway is so named because its activation is dependent on a substance found in the plasma. When stimulated by pathologic events, factor XII converts factor XI (plasma thromboplastin antecedent) to its activated form. This disruption involves the release of collagen or subendothelial substances, which trigger the intrinsic system. Activated factor XI in the presence of $Ca^{2+}$ causes activation of factor IX (Christmas factor); in turn, activated factor IX in the presence of $Ca^{2+}$, phospholipid, and thrombin-modified factor VIII causes activation of factor X (Stuart-Prower factor) (Bennett and Ratnoff, 1972; Davie and Ratnoff, 1964) (Fig. 28–2).

Tissue thromboplastin released with tissue injury activates the extrinsic pathway. In this system, factor VII and $Ca^{2+}$ activate factor X, a necessary step in association with calcium to convert prothrombin to thrombin (Fig. 28–3). At this point in the clotting mechanism, the extrinsic and intrinsic systems merge into a common pathway for completion of clot formation.

Thrombin from the extrinsic pathway acts on fibrinogen A and B chains to split off fibrinopeptides A and B, resulting in fibrin monomers. Fibrin monomer formation is the initiating event of the formation of a fibrin clot. By linking end to end and side to side, fibrin monomers form an insoluble network, which, when stabilized by thrombin-activated factor XIII, is the basis for clot formation (Perez, 1981; Stefanini, 1974; Talbert and Blatt, 1979).

To a large extent, the coagulation cascade is controlled by the regulatory activities of the serine antiproteinases. Antithrombin III is one of the most important of these proteins. By neutralizing the enzymatic reaction sites of serine proteinases, antithrombin III effectively and progressively acts as an important regulatory mechanism for the control of normal clotting by actively

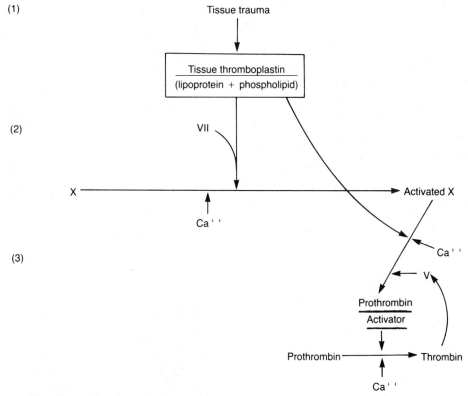

**Figure 28–2.** Clotting mechanism–intrinsic pathway. (From Guyton AC: Physiology of the Human Body. Philadelphia, WB Saunders Co, 1979, p 72.)

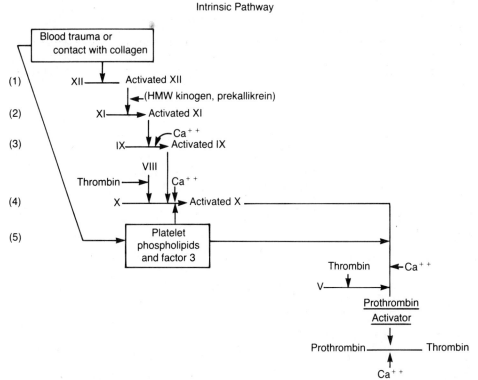

**Figure 28–3.** Clotting mechanism–extrinsic pathway. (From Guyton AC: Physiology of the Human Body. Philadelphia, WB Saunders Co, 1979, p 72.)

neutralizing thrombin, plastin, and activated forms of factors XII, XI, IV, and VII (Gambino and Altman, 1979; Ogston, 1977; Talbert and Blatt, 1979).

Guyton (1976) simplifies the basic pathways of the overall clotting mechanism by pointing out that the extrinsic pathway is explosive in nature. It is initiated within moments following an inciting event. The rapidity of its activation and the magnitude of its effects are limited only by the quantity of tissue factors and tissue phospholipids released from the trauma site and by the amount of factors X, VII, and V available in the blood for consumption. In contrast, the intrinsic pathway by its very nature is much slower and more susceptible to the proteolytic action of plasmin against fibrin, fibrinogen, and factors V and VIII (Guyton, 1976).

### Fibrinolytic System

The fibrinolytic system, or the plasminogen-plasmin system, is the system that is activated in DIC to effect the breakdown of fibrin into soluble fibrin split products (Fig. 28–4). Activation of the fibrinolytic system occurs when plasminogen is converted into circulating plasmin (Guyton, 1976). Plasmin is a potent proteolytic enzyme that not only acts on fibrin but also effectively lyses fibrinogen and factors V and VIII. As fibrinogen and fibrin are lysed, fibrin degradation products are created. The degradation products are known as X, Y, D, and E fragments and have a profoundly negative effect on he-

mostatic mechanisms (Wiman and Collen, 1978). Fibrin degradation products act to inhibit the action of thrombin and render platelets dysfunctional by coating their surfaces. As DIC progresses, fibrin polymerization becomes incomplete and leads to the presence of nonpolymerized fibrin monomers in the peripheral circulation. Fibrin degradation fragments X, Y, D, and E bind with these nonpolymerized fibrin monomers to create the soluble fibrin monomers, which are characteristic of DIC and which can be measured by the protamine sulfate test (Gambino and Altman, 1979; Kaplan et al, 1978; Lavery, 1982; McNichol and Davis, 1973).

## DIAGNOSIS

In its most acute, fulminating form, DIC is a disease process that usually is not difficult to diagnose. In its chronic or milder forms, however, it may pose significant challenges to the practicing physician. Diagnosis of DIC generally is dependent on a sound understanding of predisposing factors, clinical manifestations, and laboratory findings.

### Predisposing Factors

DIC should be suspected in obstetric patients with abruptio placentae; a retained dead fetus for longer than 4 weeks; amniotic fluid embolism; saline-induced abortion; sep-

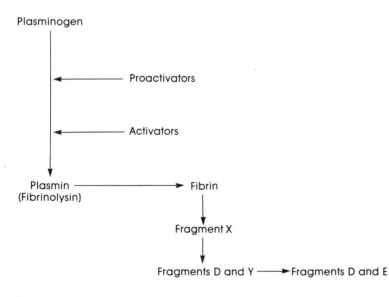

**Figure 28–4.** Fibrinolytic system.

sis; hydatidiform mole; preeclampsia and eclampsia, hemorrhagic shock, and acute fatty liver disease; and less commonly, in a single intrauterine pregnancy, fetal death in a multiple gestation (Finley, 1989; Pritchard, 1959; Pritchard and Brekken, 1967; Roberts and May, 1976; Talbert and Blatt, 1979).

## Clinical Manifestations

The clinical manifestations of DIC relate primarily to hemorrhage, anemia, and ischemia (Ziegel, 1979). Patients generally have frank bleeding or a tendency to bleed from mucous membranes, intravenous line sites, injection sites, and surgical incisions. Abnormal bruising, purpura, petechiae, and ecchymoses frequently are noted. Occult blood usually is present in stool, with frank hematemesis, hematuria, and vaginal bleeding noted often in severe cases. The quantity and character of bleeding are directly related to the severity and explosiveness of the disease process (McGillick, 1982; O'Brian and Woods, 1978). Certainly, in an acute, uncontrolled episode of DIC, a patient can suffer irreparable damage secondary to hypovolemia or intracranial or intraperitoneal bleeding. Ischemia secondary to hemorrhage and anemia is also a life-threatening event in any patient with acute fulminating DIC. The milder cases may have no overt signs of clotting disruption (Lavery 1982; McGillick, 1982).

Al-Gailani and associates (1987) reported that potential thrombogenic state was induced in some gravid patients who underwent chorionic villi sampling (CVS) in early gestation as documented by elevated levels of fibrinopeptide A (Al-Gailani et al, 1987).

## Laboratory Studies

If approached systematically, laboratory findings provide a logical system for differential diagnosis. Because DIC occurs secondary to a disruption of multiple hemostatic mechanisms, laboratory assessment should reflect an alteration in clotting physiology. If DIC is present, laboratory studies reflect the disruption of hemostasis in two or more of its essential components. Initial clotting studies should include hemoglobin, hematocrit, phase platelet count, thrombin time, fibrinogen level, prothrombin time (PT), and par-

tial thromboplastin time (PTT). The prothrombin time tests the extrinsic pathway of coagulation, the partial thromboplastin time assesses the intrinsic pathway of coagulation, and the thrombin time quantitates fibrinogen to fibrin conversion (Bick et al, 1974; Lavery, 1982).

In patients with clinically significant DIC, all studies will be abnormal, supporting a presumptive diagnosis of DIC. To verify the diagnosis, a test for early soluble fibrin monomers should be performed to differentiate between DIC and a primary hyperfibrinolytic syndrome (Bick and Adams, 1974; Gambino and Altman, 1979). For this purpose, a positive protamine sulfate test is used and, if positive, is highly diagnostic of DIC (Table 28–1).

Other laboratory tests are useful for the patient in whom DIC is suspected; however, testing time prohibits or limits their usefulness. They are, however, useful in the long-term management of a patient. Essential information regarding fibrinolysis may be derived from the euglobin lysis time, the fibrin plate assay for plasminogen and plasmin, and assays for demonstrating fibrin degradation products. The tanned red cell hemagglutination inhibition immunoassay is probably most suitable for quantitative evaluation of fibrin degradation resulting from antigen-antibody reaction. These tests do not distinguish between primary fibrinolysis and fibrinolysis secondary to DIC. Hence, they must be considered useful only in reinforcing a presumptive diagnosis. Also useful for the presumptive but not definitive diagnosis of DIC are assays to document decreased factor V or VIII levels (Bick et al, 1974; Gambino and Altman, 1979; Lavery, 1982). In recent years, more sensitive and specific assays of fibrin degradation prod-

**Table 28–1**
LABORATORY FINDINGS IN DIC

| Test | Result |
|------|--------|
| Partial thromboplastin time | prolonged |
| Prothrombin time | prolonged |
| Platelet count | decreased |
| Thrombin generation time | prolonged |
| Fibrinogen | decreased |
| Fibrin and fibrinogen degradation products | increased |
| Protamine paracoagulant test | positive |
| Blood smear | microangiopathic changes |

ucts, such as D-dimer and fibrinopeptide A, have been devised (Boisclair et al, 1990).

All laboratory studies must be used in conjunction with clinical symptomatology to determine the appropriate management of a patient. Laboratory values should be used primarily to confirm clinical impressions and, secondarily, to collect data for ongoing and retrospective understanding of the disease process (Bick et al, 1974) (Table 28–2).

## MANAGEMENT
(Tables 28–3 and 28–4)

The management of DIC should be approached in a systematic and timely fashion, prioritizing and addressing problems one at a time. Foremost is the elimination of the underlying disease process that precipitated the DIC. In obstetrics, this generally indicates termination of the pregnancy. Once this goal is achieved, the DIC may be elimi-

nated by facilitating a return to control of the coagulation mechanism by intact hemostatic pathways. On the other hand, if the underlying process cannot be eliminated or if the DIC has progressed beyond the point of a possible spontaneous, compensatory response, additional therapy is essential (Bick and Adams, 1974; Pritchard and Brekken, 1967).

The perinatal team approach is essential for the diagnosis and optimal treatment of DIC. Outcome for the patient and her neonate may be greatly improved by early identification and assessment of clinical manifestations of DIC. The most subtle sign of bleeding or vascular occlusion may be observed by the care provider and followed by a laboratory assessment to form the basis for diagnosis. Sophisticated laboratory capability is useful only if skilled personnel recognize the need for its use. Open communication and coordination with the blood bank are essential for a consistent, systematic approach to patient care. The initial goal of management should be to stabilize the pa-

**Table 28–2**
A SYSTEMATIC APPROACH TO THE DIAGNOSIS OF DIC

| Responsive Pathology | Screening Tests | Presumptive Tests | Definitive Tests | Adjunctive Tests | Clinical Hints |
|---|---|---|---|---|---|
| Fibrin deposition Thrombocytopenia Platelet function defects | (Combinations of abnormalities are highly significant) Smear for platelets and RBC fragments Platelet count Bleeding time should drop | Progressive thrombocytopenia D-dimer | | Platelet adhesion Platelet aggregation Complement levels Endotoxin | Bruising Petechiae Purpura Ecchymoses Epistaxis |
| Hypofibrinogenemia Factor V decreased Factor VIII decreased Circulating anticoagulants (fibrinolytic degradation) | Thrombin time Fibrinogen screen (Fibrindex) Prothrombin time Partial thromboplastin time | Factor V assay Factor VIII assay Quantitative Fibrinogen FDP | Protamine sulfate test or ethanol gelation test | | Gastrointestinal, genitourinary, intracranial, or interperitoneal bleeding |
| Secondary fibrinolysis Circulating plasma | Clot retraction | Fibrin plate for plasminogen depletion and circulating plasmin Clot lysis | | | Associated clinical conditions |

Adapted from Bick RL, et al: Disseminated Intravascular Coagulation. Etiology, Pathophysiology, Diagnosis, and Treatment. Medical Counterpoint, 1974, p 41.
RBC = red blood cell.

## Table 28–3
### MANAGEMENT OF DIC

**Basic Principles**
Understanding pathophysiology
Prioritize clinical problems
Eliminate underlying cause
Use perinatal team approach for support of patient
  and family
**Procedures**
Stabilize vital signs
Maintain adequate urinary output
Institute and maintain appropraite blood component
  therapy to replace consumable blood clotting factors
  and platelets
Conduct prudent fluid replacement
Perform constant central venous pressure or Swan-
  Ganz monitoring
Use anticoagulant therapy only in critical, individual
  situations

tient's vital signs and maintain adequate urinary output while plans are being made to terminate the pregnancy as soon as possible. A urinary catheter system is helpful to assess urinary output.

The secondary goal should be to institute and maintain appropriate blood component therapy to replace consumable blood clotting factors and platelets. AT III concentrate for replacement therapy is commercially available. If AT III is unavailable, fresh frozen plasma or cryoprecipitate may be administered to replace consumed factors. General guidelines include administration of 2 to 3 U of fresh frozen plasma with subsequent re-evaluation for further replacement. Cryoprecipitate should be administered as needed to attain a fibrinogen level greater than 100 mg/100 ml. This replaces not only fibrinogen but factor VIII as well. Generally, each unit of cryoprecipitate raises the fibrinogen level by 2 to 5 mg/100 ml. Cryoprecipitate is the therapy of choice, because fi-

## Table 28–4
### PATIENT CARE SUMMARY FOR DIC

| | Antepartum | | Intrapartum | Postpartum |
|---|---|---|---|---|
| | **Outpatient** | **Inpatient** | | |
| BP, P, R | — | q 15 min | q 15 min | q 15 min until stable |
| T | — | q 4 h | q 4 h | On admission to RR; then q 4 h |
| Central venous pressure line/ Swan-Ganz | — | Yes | Yes | Yes |
| FHR | — | Continuous fetal monitoring | Continuous fetal monitoring, internal if possible | — |
| Contractions | — | Continuous fetal monitoring | Continuous fetal monitoring, internal if possible | Fundal checks q 15 min until stable; then q 30 min × 2; then q 1 h |
| Laboratory assessment | — | Clot observation Fibrinogen Platelets Fibrinogen-fibrin degradation products Thrombin time Prothrombin time Partial thromboplastin time | Clot observation Fibrinogen Platelets Fibrinogen-fibrin degradation products Thrombin time Prothrombin time Partial thromboplastin time | Clot observation Fibrinogen Platelets Fibrinogen-fibrin degradation products Thrombin time Prothrombin time Partial thromboplastin time |
| I & O | — | q 1 h | q 1 h | q 1 h |
| Observation for signs of shock | — | Continuously | Continuously | Continuously |
| Observation for level of consciousness | — | Continuously | Continuously | Continuously |

Note: Nurse-to-patient ratio, 1 : 1.
BP = Blood pressure; FHR = fetal heart rate; P = pulse; R = respirations; RR = recovery room; T = temperature.

brinogen, once commercially available, has been removed from the market in the United States owing to the significant risk of hepatitis associated with its use (Talbert and Blatt, 1979) (Table 28–5).

Prudent fluid replacement along with component therapy is necessary with constant central venous pressure or Swan-Ganz monitoring of intravascular volume. Infrequently, there is a need for whole blood in the treatment of DIC because component therapy including AT III concentrate, fresh frozen plasma, cryoprecipitate, and platelets usually can be used effectively. When available, blood component therapy can be used with greater effectiveness and versatility, less cost, and a smaller total volume of fluid than fresh whole blood (Lavery, 1982).

One of the longstanding controversies about the management of DIC in obstetrics is related to the appropriate use of anticoagulant therapy. Heparin generally is not used because, following factor replacement therapy and removal of the cause of DIC, it is not needed. The major risk of heparin therapy is hemorrhage due to the enhanced interaction of the serine proteinases and AT III (Corrigan and Jordan, 1970). There is general agreement that heparin is not needed in the treatment of DIC *unless* total defibrination has occurred or the patient has minimal disruption of the vascular system. The hallmarks of decision-making regarding the use of heparin are caution and careful evaluation of risk-to-benefit ratio (Saltzman et al, 1975).

Patients with a retained dead fetus *in utero* may require heparin. Normalization of fibrinogen levels and control of chronic consumption of clotting factors are attempted until vaginal delivery can be performed (Pritchard, 1973). Heparin also is used in cases of fulminating disease in which almost total defibrination has occurred and patient stabilization is necessary to facilitate delivery. When heparin is administered in the treatment of DIC, component replacement must be given—either platelets or cryoprecipitate. Heparin can be administered by constant infusion pump at approximately 500 to 2000 U/h, the approximate dose being 1000 U/h, with adjustments in dosage based on clinical and laboratory response.

Emotional support for the patient and her family is extremely important, because DIC can be life threatening to the woman and her fetus. The nurse should stay with the patient for constant physical assessment as well as emotional support. If the partner can remain with the patient, this is good for his understanding and support as well as emotional support for his mate. If the woman is bleeding, it may be very frightening, and the patient and her significant other should be kept apprised of her and the fetus' condition at all times. In an emergency such as this, it is sometimes difficult to take the time for these explanations, but it will save time in the long run if the patient and her family are informed so they can fully cooperate with treatment modalities.

## OBSTETRIC CONDITIONS ASSOCIATED WITH DIC

There are several well-known events in obstetrics that can precipitate DIC. Abruptio placentae, dead fetus syndrome, amniotic fluid embolism, saline-induced abortion, hemorrhagic shock, pregnancy-induced hypertension, and sepsis have been studied specifically in relation to DIC. Each condition

**Table 28–5**
BLOOD COMPONENT REPLACEMENT THERAPY

| Factor | Volume (ml)* | Supplies |
|---|---|---|
| Platelet concentrate | 40–60 | Increased count of viable platelets by 25,000–35,000 |
| Cryoprecipitate | 30–50 | Fibrinogen |
| | | Factors VIII, XIII (3 to 10 times the equivalent volume of plasma) |
| Fresh frozen plasma | 200 | All factors except platelets; 1 g fibrinogen |
| Packed RBC | 200 | Hematocrit 60% to 65% |
| Fibrinogen† | 300 | Increased fibrinogen (1–2 g) |

Reprinted with permission from Lavery P: When coagulopathy threatens the pregnant patient. Contemporary OB/GYN 20:198, 1982.

* Depends on local blood bank service.

† Not available in the United States.

poses specific challenges for the perinatal care team. Therefore, it is important to understand and manage the underlying problem as well as the DIC.

## Abruptio Placentae

Depending on the criteria used for diagnosis, premature separation of the placenta has been reported to range in incidence from 1 in 75 to 1 in 225 deliveries (Abdella et al, 1984; Karegaard and Gennser, 1986). Patients with abruptio placentae whose babies do not survive have a 38 percent incidence of severe hypofibrinogenemia; thus, any patient with a placental abruption should be considered at risk for the development of DIC (Pritchard and Brekken, 1967). At the time of placental separation, retroplacental hemorrhage occurs. Thromboplastin is released from the traumatized placenta and decidua, activating the extrinsic clotting pathway. Simultaneously, the fibrinolytic mechanisms are activated by thromboplastin and activated procoagulants entering the maternal circulation from the implantation site (Sutton et al, 1971). Pritchard and Brekken recommend prompt vaginal delivery, if possible, with judicious use of oxytocin and amniotomy. In the event of fetal demise, 20 mg prostaglandin $E_2$ (PGE$_2$) suppositories can be used to encourage delivery without cesarean delivery. Cesarean delivery should be used to deliver the patient, with a viable fetus, with abruptio placentae if severe DIC is present and in those who do not progress in labor (Pritchard and Brekken, 1967; Pritchard, 1973). Specific management of DIC is carried out as outlined previously with blood component therapy and fluid replacement based on clinical manifestations and laboratory studies.

## Retained Dead Fetus

Historically, it has been consistently recognized since the early to mid 20th century that the in utero retention of a dead fetus can precipitate abnormal maternal bleeding (Delee, 1901). Significant clotting defects have been linked particularly to the fetus retained for more than 4 weeks after demise. The triggering mechanism for DIC seems to be the release of thromboplastin from the dead fetus. Hence, the ensuing coagulation is slow and chronic in nature with resultant gradual depletion of clotting factors (Pritch-

ard, 1959, 1973). In this situation, in which depletion of clotting factors is chronic rather than acute, heparin occasionally is useful in normalizing fibrinogen levels so that vaginal delivery can be facilitated (Pritchard, 1973). Prostaglandins as well as oxytocin may be used to induce labor (Bailey et al, 1975; Gordon and Pipe, 1975). Component therapy is used to stabilize the patient for delivery or at any time when the chronic DIC process becomes more severe or acute in nature.

## Amniotic Fluid Embolism

Amniotic fluid embolism is a rare complication of pregnancy that is often fatal and always extremely serious. Characterized by respiratory distress, circulatory collapse, and shock, this maternal condition is fatal in 25 percent of patients in the first hour after onset. The secondary complication of hemorrhage is often seen if the patient survives the initial pathophysiologic insult (Pritchard, 1973).

In a recent case report by Dodgson and associates (1987), a gravida undergoing amniocentesis for relief of hydramnios experienced an amniotic fluid embolism. Within minutes, objective symptomatology was present, further documented by laboratory confirmation of DIC. The patient underwent several exchange transfusions with packed red cells and fresh frozen plasma, thus removing the cell debris and appropriately replacing clotting factors. Recognition and expeditious treatment of this antepartal complication resulted in a successful outcome (Dodgson et al, 1987).

Consumptive coagulopathy with hypofibrinogenemia has been the most consistent finding in the surviving parturient secondary to the clot-promoting properties of the amniotic fluid and gestational debris that entered the maternal circulation (Phillips and Davidson, 1972). Management of this acute emergency is immediate recognition and support for the intensive cardiorespiratory distress and shock with constant clinical and laboratory surveillance for DIC. Life-sustaining therapy, including fluid and blood replacement, oxygen therapy, ventilatory support, and digitalization, may be necessary (Halmagyi et al, 1962; Peterson and Taylor, 1970). When diagnosed, DIC should be treated as outlined previously with blood component therapy, fluid replacement, and prompt delivery of the infant.

## Saline-Induced Abortion

Saline-induced abortion has been shown to produce coagulation and fibrinolytic changes frequently. It is hypothesized that DIC is due to thromboplastin release from the uterus or its contents secondary to hypertonic saline injection (Laros and Penner, 1976; Stander et al, 1971; Weiss et al, 1972). Following the intra-amniotic instillation of hypertonic (20 percent) saline to patients desiring second trimester pregnancy termination, Cohen and Ballard (1974) found a 0.01 to 0.25 percent incidence of DIC severe enough to require therapeutic intervention. Medical management is based on the severity of clinical manifestations and laboratory findings.

## Pregnancy-Induced Hypertension

Pregnancy-induced hypertension appears to be a predisposing factor to DIC. The two disease processes are separate entities but occasionally coexist. In the patient with pregnancy-induced hypertension, the triggering mechanism for the development of DIC seems to be vascular endothelial damage secondary to the underlying disease state rather than thromboplastin release from the placenta into the maternal circulation (Roberts and May, 1976).

Hemolysis, elevated liver enzymes, and low platelets (HELLP) syndrome, a variant form of severe preeclampsia, differs from true DIC in that coagulation aberration results from platelet adherence to disrupted endothelial surfaces rather than from an insult activating either the intrinsic or extrinsic coagulation pathways (Naumann and Weinstein, 1985). Although some authors would disagree that HELLP is a DIC variant, recent reports indicate that all HELLP parturients exhibit some degree of DIC if laboratory availability of sensitive tests such as AT III, fibrinopeptide A, fibrin monomer, D-dimer, plasminogen, or fibronectin are readily available (Sibai, 1990; Van Dam et al, 1990).

The complexity of both pregnancy-induced hypertension and DIC poses an extraordinary challenge for the perinatal care team. Management should include expeditious delivery and blood component therapy in conjunction with treatment for the underlying pregnancy-induced hypertension disease process.

## Sepsis

Sepsis commonly incites some level of DIC. It has been speculated that bacterial toxins cause release of platelet phospholipids, which result in platelet clumping (Yoshiwa et al, 1971). Antenatal or postnatal bacterial infections of the respiratory tract, especially group A $\beta$-hemolytic streptococcal, have been reported to result in fulminant DIC and maternal death (Acharya et al, 1988; Kavi and Wise, 1988). Exposure of collagen in the capillary walls very likely also plays a role in the DIC process by activating factor XIII (Colman et al, 1972). Management should reflect a primary concern for treatment of the underlying cause by appropriate antibiotic administration or surgical drainage, if necessary. Once the sepsis itself has been treated, DIC is managed as previously outlined with blood component therapy and supportive therapy as needed.

# Idiopathic (Autoimmune) Thrombocytopenic Purpura

## INCIDENCE

Idiopathic, or autoimmune, thrombocytopenic purpura (aITP) is an acquired immunologic disorder caused by the abnormal development of IgG immunoglobulin, which attaches to platelets and results in their removal by the reticuloendothelial system (Karpatkin, 1980; Kelton and Gibbons, 1982; McMillan, 1977; 1981). It occurs most frequently in young women and is the most common autoimmune disease occurring in the childbearing years. This disease probably affects more pregnant women than had been recognized previously. Both the gravida and the fetus are exposed to significant risks.

## PATHOPHYSIOLOGY

*Thrombocytopenia is defined as a platelet or thrombocyte count less than* 150,000/mm³. The normal adult platelet count in pregnancy is 150,000 to 350,000/mm³ (Romero and Duffy, 1980). As indicated in Table 28–6, thrombocytopenia may complicate several obstetric syndromes (Perkins, 1979), and several types of thrombocytopenia may

**Table 28-6**

CLASSIFICATION OF THROMBOCYTOPENIA

I. Nonfunctional Platelet Disorders
  A. Disorders of decreased platelet survival
    1. Immunologic mechanisms
      a. Autoimmune disease–associated
        (i) aITP (acute/chronic)
        (ii) Alloantibodies (posttransfusion, neonatal)
        (iii) Collagen disorders
        (iv) Lymphoproliferative disorders
      b. Drug-induced
      c. Infection (viral, bacterial, parasitic, HIV)
      d. Localized consumption
    2. Dilution with platelet-poor blood
      a. Massive blood transfusion
      b. Extracorporeal
    3. Disseminated intravascular coagulation
  B. Disorders of decreased platelet production
    1. Aplasia or hypoplasia of bone marrow
      a. Toxic
      b. Idiopathic
    2. Bone marrow malignancy
    3. Megaloblastic anemias
II. Functional Platelet Disorders
  A. Congenital
    1. Storage pool disease and defective release
    2. Glanzmann's thrombasthenia
  B. Acquired
    Drug-induced platelet dysfunction (see above)
III. Combined Platelet and Plasma Abnormalities
  von Willebrandt's disease
IV. Others (TTP, etc)

complicate pregnancy. Actually, the disease of aITP is often referred to as a syndrome, because there is a wide spectrum of possible clinical presentations (Baldini, 1966; 1972). Most parturients with aITP have a primary form of aITP, whereas others develop the condition secondary to a drug reaction or in association with other diseases such as systemic lupus erythematosus, lymphoma, or lymphocytic leukemia. The acute form of aITP typically is found in very young children. In contrast, most young adults with aITP are afflicted with a chronic variety that may last for many years with multiple episodes of relapse and remission. In milder cases, the chronic disease form may be unsuspected unless a screening maternal platelet count taken at the initial visit or at the time of delivery is found to be low or a thrombocytopenic neonate is delivered.

Thrombocytopenia is not always associated with clinical manifestations. The severity of bleeding in this disorder can range from minimal to life threatening, beginning with easy bruising or small petechiae, then minor cutaneous and subcutaneous hemor-

rhages that progress to form purpuric lesions of the skin. More serious mucosal membrane bleeding from the gastrointestinal, genitourinary, or respiratory tract can occur with increasingly severe disease (Table 28–7). In pregnancy, the most frequent manifestations of aITP are epistaxis, gingival bleeding, and ecchymosis. Even with severe thrombocytopenia, maternal intracranial hemorrhage and hemarthroses are uncommon in pregnant patients with aITP.

## DIAGNOSIS

*The diagnosis of aITP is generally one of exclusion* (Wintrobe, 1971). Nonimmune causes of thrombocytopenia, such as preeclampsia and eclampsia (HELLP), infection, intravascular coagulation, and immune etiologies secondary to other diseases, such as systemic lupus erythematosus, usually are evident from their clinical presentation and can be confirmed by appropriate testing. A thorough medical and obstetric history is very important (Table 28–8). Once thrombocytopenia is detected in a parturient patient, the finding should be verified by a phase manual platelet count, because automated counts can be falsely low. If thrombocytopenia is confirmed, further testing should include a complete blood count and a sternal bone marrow aspiration. If the megakaryocytes appear normal and are present in normal or increased numbers, the thrombo-

**Table 28–7**

CLINICAL FEATURES OF aITP

**Mild to Moderate Disease**
None if platelets > 50,000/mm³
Ecchymoses (scattered purplish patches, especially in areas exposed to trauma)
Petechiae (generalized pinpoint hemorrhagic lesions that do not disappear with applied pressure)
Areas of purpura (hemorrhage into the skin or mucous membranes)
Oozing from puncture wound (venipuncture)
**Severe Disease**
Epistaxis
Hematemesis
Hematuria
Melena
Generalized purpura
Hemorrhagic vesicles or bullae (blood blisters) in the oral mucosa
CNS symptoms
Prolonged bleeding time (especially if platelets ≤ or equal to 20,000)

**Table 28–8**

CRITICALLY IMPORTANT COMPONENTS OF MATERNAL HISTORY AND EXAMINATION

Previous operations (especially splenectomy)
History of easy bruising or bleeding
Family history (especially maternal) of bleeding complications
Previous obstetric history
Recent or current infections
Medications taken during or immediately before pregnancy
Collagen vascular diseases
Maternal physical examination (look for splenomegaly)
Laboratory assessment

---

cytopenia is probably secondary to platelet destruction. Hematocrit, hemoglobin, and white blood cell count are usually within normal limits unless there has been a recent hemorrhage. Abnormal megakaryocytes and platelets may be seen on a peripheral blood smear. Coagulation tests (coagulation time, prothrombin time, and partial thromboplastin time) are usually within normal limits. Likelihood of a prolonged bleeding time increases as the platelet count decreases less than 50,000 U/liter. Unless aITP is secondary to another disease, the spleen usually is not enlarged. A demonstration of free or bound platelet-associated antibodies serves to support the diagnosis of an autoimmune thrombocytopenia. Criteria for the diagnosis of aITP are summarized in Table 28–9.

*The maternal antiplatelet factor responsible for aITP is a circulating 7S gamma*

**Table 28–9**

aITP DIAGNOSTIC FINDINGS

Isolated thrombocytopenia ($< 150,000/mm^3$) in the complete blood count
Normal coagulation screens (PT, PTT, thrombin clotting time)
Increased mean platelet volume
Elevated antiplatelet antibody and platelet-associated IgG
Negative antinuclear antibody
Normal to increased megakaryocyte mass in bone marrow aspirate
Absence of splenomegaly
Other causes excluded such as:
  Recent transfusion
  Identified sources of platelet destruction
  Drug ingestion
  Exposure to noxious substances
  Recent infections
  Family history of bleeding
  Preeclampsia and eclampsia (HELLP)

---

*globulin–blocking ("incomplete") antibody,* which attaches to target cell surface antigens on the maternal platelet (Dixon et al, 1975; Harrington et al, 1951; McMillan et al, 1975; Schulman et al, 1965; Sprague et al, 1952). Because the human placenta has receptors for the Fc portion of the IgG molecule and actively transports IgG antibodies of all types from the maternal circulation into the fetal circulation (Kohler and Farr, 1966; Schlamoritz, 1976), these antiplatelet antibodies can cross the placenta to cause fetal and neonatal thrombocytopenia and do so in over half the cases of maternal illness (Goodhue and Evans, 1963; Kelton et al, 1980; Kernoff et al, 1979; McMillan et al, 1975; Minchinton et al, 1980; Territo et al, 1973; Van Leeuwen et al, 1980). Until recently, attempts to detect the presence of platelet antibody have been difficult, inaccurate, and unreliable (McMillan, 1977; Schreiber, 1982).

Severity of the thrombocytopenia depends on the balance between platelet production and destruction (Ahn and Harrington, 1977). This, in turn, varies with the type and quantity of antibody coating the platelet. The usual number of IgG molecules adsorbed on the normal platelet's surface (6000 to 12,000) can be increased from 2 to 20 times in patients with aITP (Dixon et al, 1975). Greater amounts of attached (adsorbed) antibody are related to faster rates of clearance by the spleen and liver. Whereas the spleen preferentially seems to clear lightly coated platelets, the liver can remove from circulation more heavily coated platelets as well as those carrying attached complement.

In the absence of the spleen, the liver acts similarly but less efficiently as an alternative site for platelet sequestration and destruction.

## RISKS OF aITP

The overall course and severity of primary aITP do not seem to be affected by pregnancy in any significant way (Heys, 1966; Tancer, 1960). In contrast, it has been well demonstrated that aITP may have an adverse effect on the mother and baby (Kitzmiller, 1978). The principal maternal risk is hemorrhage associated with either genital tract injury or abdominoperineal incisions employed for operative delivery. Since 1954, only a single maternal death has been attributed to aITP in the literature (Noriega-Guerra et al, 1979; O'Reilly and Taber, 1978). Corticosteroid administration and platelet transfusion, along with the expertise of specialists in medical centers, are significant factors in the virtual elimination of maternal mortality with this disease process, in contrast to the rates as high as 5 to 10 percent reported as recently as the mid 1950s (Heys, 1966; Murray and Harris, 1976; Robson and Davidson, 1950; Rogers, 1959).

Intrapartum and postpartum hemorrhages occur with greater frequency in this disease because bleeding tends to occur during the expulsive efforts of the second stage. Postpartum hemorrhage from trauma to the genital tract still must be anticipated and carefully managed with meticulous surgical technique. Uterine bleeding is not increased markedly, apparently a reflection of the efficient manner in which the uterus contracts to promote postpartum hemostasis. The principle of gentle delivery encouraged primarily out of neonatal concern is also advantageous for the mother to minimize the possibility of cerebral hemorrhage provoked by expulsive efforts in the second stage of labor (Scott, 1976).

There also are sobering concerns for the fetus in the aITP pregnancy. The risk of spontaneous abortion in parturient patients with aITP has been reported to range from 5 to 33 percent as compared with 10 to 15 percent in normal women (O'Reilly and Taber, 1978; Schenker and Polishuk, 1968). Adverse effects on the fetus and neonate are more frequent and more serious, overall perinatal mortality rates having been reported in association with aITP pregnancies to range upward as high as 15 to 25 percent (Laros and Sweet, 1975; Scott, 1976). Since the late 1970s, reported perinatal mortality rates in carefully managed series have been at or less than 5 percent (Horger and Keane, 1979; Jones, 1979; Romero and Duffy, 1980). Reasons for perinatal demise most commonly have been linked to fetal prematurity, intracerebral hemorrhage, and fetal death resulting from maternal hemorrhage and shock (Flessa, 1974; Laros and Sweet, 1975; O'Reilly and Taber, 1978; Territo et al, 1973).

Traditionally, perinatal deaths have been ascribed to intracerebral hemorrhage occurring in thrombocytopenic infants delivered vaginally. Morbidity and mortality, however, may occur more commonly and much earlier in gestation than during labor and delivery. In O'Reilly and Taber's (1978) review of 133 pregnancies in women with aITP, 24 gestations were unsuccessful for a failure rate of 18 percent. Six were lost by first trimester spontaneous abortion, 13 were stillborn, and 5 infants died in the neonatal period. Six of the stillborn infants had evidence of hemorrhage preceding labor and delivery, and three of the neonatal losses were considered due to hemorrhage. Thus, only 9 deaths altogether in the 133 gestations (7 percent) were directly attributable to thrombocytopenia (O'Reilly and Taber, 1978).

Late in gestation, pregnant patients may develop a form of thrombocytopenia identified recently as pseudo ITP (Hart et al, 1986) or incidentally detected mild thrombocytopenia (IDMT) (Burrows and Kelton, 1988). An increased rate of platelet turnover is thought to cause the disorder. Clinical diagnosis is based on (1) a platelet count between 80,000 and 150,000 U/liter; (2) a normal platelet count before or earlier in gestation; (3) presence of an intact spleen; (4) no history of significant signs or symptoms of bleeding either before or during pregnancy; (5) the presence or absence of platelet antibodies; and (6) the absence of other disease processes, such as preeclampsia. The prefix "pseudo" reflects the absence of maternal or perinatal consequences normally associated with ITP. Therefore, neither extensive testing nor operative delivery appears to be indicated for these patients after the platelet count is rechecked, the peripheral blood film is reviewed for abnormality, and a careful history is negative for prior bleeding disorder. Nevertheless, a cord blood sample is obtained following delivery, the neonate is followed closely, and the mother is observed to determine that her platelet count returns to normal postpartum.

A variant of the aITP syndrome may occur in some parturient patients within 4 to 6 weeks after delivery, miscarriage, or spontaneous abortion. Ahn and Harrington (1977) have managed 17 such episodes in 8 postpartum women, describing a pattern of recurring puerperal thrombocytopenia in these parturient patients that follows successive pregnancies. No other recognizable instigating factor or relationship to medication was discovered (Harrington, 1977a; 1977b).

## MANAGEMENT

### Antepartum Period

Once a diagnosis of aITP is made, therapy can be instituted (Table 28–10). *The primary goal of management should be to prevent maternal-fetal hemorrhage.* The overall management of aITP in pregnancy is based on the same general principles as those used in the nonpregnant state. Although it is true in nonpregnant patients that the platelet count alone should not be treated because some nonpregnant individuals tolerate marked thrombocytopenia without complications, marked thrombocytopenia during pregnancy, even without hemorrhage, may be harmful to fetal well-being. A safe platelet count for pregnant women with aITP has never been determined. Not unlike any other individual with aITP, the pregnant woman should be under the careful medical supervision of a well-trained hematologist as well as a competent perinatal team. Obstetric and neonatal care for optimal perinatal outcome probably are best delivered at medical centers where the expertise and resources to respond appropriately to any eventuality are continuously available. Hospitalization should occur whenever there is a platelet count of 20,000 or less or if there is an episode of hemorrhage.

General measures of aITP pregnancy management include the avoidance of not only agents such as aspirin and aspirin-like drugs that impair platelet function but also factors such as trauma (intramuscular injections), fever, infection, azotemia, and increased

**Table 28–10**
ANTEPARTUM MANAGEMENT
CONSIDERATIONS FOR aITP

Frequent outpatient clinic evaluations
Collaboration among obstetrician, hematologist, and
  neonatologist
Periodic platelet counts
Oral iron and folate supplementation
Avoidance of salicylates and related prostaglandin
  synthetase inhibitor medications
Avoidance of trauma
Rapid treatment of fever and infections
Careful clinical, ultrasound, and biophysical
  surveillance of the fetus
Possible use of corticosteroids:
  intravenous immunoglobulins
  other immunosuppressant drugs
  second trimester splenectomy
  platelet transfusion
  plasma exchange

metabolic rate. These complications must be avoided or remedied promptly because they can enhance an aITP patient's tendency to bleed by slowing platelet production, increasing platelet consumption, or impairing platelet function (Ahn and Harrington, 1977; Higby et al, 1974). Adequate vitamin and iron intake must be encouraged to maintain accelerated hematopoietic thrombopoiesis (Karpatkin et al, 1974; Smith et al, 1962).

Specific therapeutic modalities include corticosteroids, splenectomy, immunosuppressive drugs, plasma exchange procedures, platelet transfusions, and high-dose immunoglobulin therapy.

**Corticosteroids.** *Corticosteroids represent the cornerstone of aITP therapy* and are used in the absence of any contraindications. Prednisone appears to improve platelet counts primarily by increasing platelet production (Gernsheimer et al, 1989). Secondarily, its use is associated with decreased antiplatelet antibody production and binding, decreased antibody-coated platelet destruction, and improved capillary stability (Ahn and Harrington, 1977; Cines and Schreiber, 1979; Doan et al, 1960; Fallon et al, 1952; Handin and Stossel, 1975; McMillan et al, 1976; McMillan et al, 1974; Robson and Duttie, 1950; Stefanini and Martino, 1956; Suhrland et al, 1958). Soon after aITP is initially diagnosed or a decision is made to initiate treatment, large doses of prednisone 60 to 100 mg or 1.0 to 1.5 mg/kg/day are employed initially for 2 to 4 weeks or until the platelet count climbs substantially, above $100,000/mm^3$ to $250,000/mm^3$ or more. Higher starting doses may be appropriate if the initial platelet count is less than $10,000/mm^3$. A favorable response to corticosteroid therapy is evidenced by a rise in the platelet count within 7 to 21 days and a lessening in new purpura and hemorrhagic tendencies. Daily therapy by divided dosage has been found to be more effective than single dose or alternate-day therapy (Lacey and Penner, 1977). After remission is achieved, the drug is tapered gradually at 2-week intervals, usually by decreasing the dose 10 to 20 percent. Tapering is continued until the lowest possible dosage compatible with hemostasis is reached (platelet count $> 50,000/mm^3$) and maintained at this level. Relapse following discontinuation of corticosteroid therapy is common. Some patients with aITP will not respond to steroids. *If a significant rise in the platelet count has not* *been observed after 21 days of corticosteroid treatment, another mode of therapy must be considered.*

The majority of gravid patients treated initially with corticosteroids for aITP respond to them, but the quantity and quality of individual responses are highly variable and depend on the duration of disease and level of antibody production (Ahn and Harrington, 1977; Brennan et al, 1975; Heys, 1966; O'Reilly and Taber, 1978). Unfortunately, a sustained remission has been reported in only 14 to 38 percent of treated patients (Thompson et al, 1972). If the platelet count has not reached 50,000/mm$^3$ after 21 days of therapy, splenectomy (Ahn and Harrington, 1977) or immunosuppressive drugs other than corticosteroids can be considered. In the absence of complications secondary to the drug itself or when indications for splenectomy are not met, it has been recommended that corticosteroids be continued throughout pregnancy on at least a daily maintenance level of 5 to 20 mg prednisone, especially in those patients with severe or chronically relapsing disease (Flessa, 1974; Laros and Sweet, 1975; O'Reilly and Taber, 1978). It may be particularly important to administer corticosteroid therapy during the first trimester. Further study is required to accept or refute the alleged beneficial effects on fetal morbidity and mortality during the various stages of gestation.

During the early 1980s, it was recommended that pregnant aITP patients not only have platelets maintained at greater than 50,000 U/liter but also that a bleeding time be evaluated regularly and additional therapy introduced if bleeding exceeded 20 minutes (Hoffman, 1985; Kelton, 1983). Subsequently, the Canadian group of Ballem and associates (1989) recommended that the bleeding time (> 20 min) along with evidence of significantly impaired hemostasis be the primary indicators for therapeutic intervention without regard to maintenance of an absolute platelet value. The routine use of corticosteroids or other agents to maintain an arbitrarily preset platelet count was discouraged. Thus, only seven of 24 patients in their series required treatment, and therapy-related toxicity and expense were spared.

Following a suggestion of Laros and Sweet (1975) that the near-term maternal administration of corticosteroids might prevent or ameliorate fetal thrombocytopenia and

Horger and Keane's (1979) suggestion that the antenatal administration of betamethasone to mothers with aITP might reduce fetal platelet destruction and peripartum hemorrhage, Karpatkin and coworkers (1981) recommended that all women with aITP be treated with a short course of corticosteroids prior to delivery. Although Karpatkin and coworkers' clinical results were suggestive of a positive effect from such a treatment plan, most other investigators were not as successful (Flessa, 1974; Heys, 1966; Robson and Davidson, 1950). Indeed, *the administration of corticosteroids in such a fashion may be contraindicated.* Corticosteroids are known to alter the interaction between IgG antiplatelet antibodies and platelet surface antigens in patients with aITP (Rosse, 1971). Recently, Cines and colleagues (Cines and Schreiber, 1979; Cines et al, 1981; 1982) recorded that high doses of prednisone were associated with a fall in the level of platelet-associated IgG and a positive clinical response in the treated mothers. However, the level of circulating antiplatelet antibody simultaneously increased in the mothers and was associated with the delivery of severely thrombocytopenic infants (Donner et al, 1987).

Corticosteroid administration can be detrimental to the mother and fetus in one of several ways. Although the increased incidence of cleft palate in animal studies has not been substantiated in human investigations and first trimester steroid therapy is not thought to be of great risk in the human, an adverse impact on several human body systems early or later in pregnancy may be possible. Maternal and fetal adrenocortical insufficiency, steroid-induced diabetes mellitus, pregnancy psychosis, and an increased incidence of preeclampsia and eclampsia may occur secondary to prolonged corticosteroid therapy (Flessa, 1974; Gowda et al, 1977; Heys, 1966). Machover-Remisch and associates (1978) reported an increased incidence of intrauterine fetal growth retardation in the offspring of pregnant patients taking more than 10 mg of prednisone per day.

**High-Dose Intravenous Immunoglobulin.** During the last decade, the intravenous infusion of high-dose monomeric polyvalent human immunoglobulin (IgG) has gained acceptance as a therapeutic option for aITP, particularly in patients refractory to corticosteroids and in those in need of acute therapy prior to surgery (Besa et al, 1985; Burke et al, 1989; Davidson et al, 1987; Fabris et al, 1987; Gounder et al, 1986; Imbach et al, 1981; Rose and Gordon, 1985; Schmidt et al, 1981; Tomiyama et al, 1987). Conventional therapy (400 mg/kg/day for 5 days) is associated with response rates (> 100,000 U/liter platelets) in up to 70 percent of patients without significant side effects. Recently, very high-dose intravenous IgG therapy (1000 mg/kg/day) has been shown to be effective in patients previously unresponsive to conventional doses (Bussel et al, 1986; Gibson et al, 1989). The mechanism of action for this mode of therapy is considered to be blockade of immunoglobulin Fc receptors on cells of the reticuloendothelial system. Currently, intravenous IgG is recommended to be first-line treatment for patients with clinical bleeding, because its response rate is superior to prednisone and side effects are minimal (Nydegger, 1988).

**Splenectomy.** Chronic autoimmune thrombocytopenic purpura is a relapsing disease process requiring lifelong therapy beyond the conclusion of pregnancy. Because corticosteroids usually do not effect a permanent remission and long-term medical therapy can be somewhat hazardous, splenectomy usually becomes necessary at some time in most adults with chronic aITP. Removal of the spleen is associated with a permanent remission in 70 to 80 percent of these patients because it eliminates the primary site of platelet destruction (Ahn and Harrington, 1977; Karpatkin et al, 1972) and platelet survival is prolonged (Gernsheimer et al, 1989). Ideally, splenectomy should be performed prior to pregnancy in women with aITP who are planning a family. *Indications for performance of splenectomy during pregnancy* include the failure to respond initially to high-dose corticosteroids (platelet count < 50,000 after 21 days of therapy), a continuing need for intensive medical therapy to remain in remission, and life-threatening hemorrhage (Ahn and Harrington, 1977; Caplan and Berkman, 1976). After splenectomy, a rise in platelet count may be detected within a few hours. Maximum benefit is achieved within 1 to 3 weeks (O'Reilly and Taber, 1978). For cases in which the platelet count rises above 500,000/mm³, anticoagulation has been recommended but not tested rigorously to reduce an alleged increased risk of thromboembolism (Zwaan et al, 1974).

*Benefit of splenectomy to the patient must be weighed carefully against potential risk to the fetus.* In one earlier series, performance of splenectomy was noted to be associated with a 30 percent fetal mortality rate (Peterson and Larson, 1954). In a gravida whose fetus is preterm (ideally midtrimester) and whose aITP is medically unmanageable, splenectomy may be the optimal therapeutic choice. Late in pregnancy, prior to fetal maturity, splenectomy can be carried out through a transthoracic approach (Ahn and Harrington, 1977) or the more standard transabdominal approach. Removal of all accessory splenic tissue, if present, is important. In selected cases in which the mother has poorly controlled severe aITP and a fetus that is term, has mature lungs, or both, splenectomy can be combined with cesarean delivery. The mother's disease may thus be controlled and an atraumatic delivery advantageously performed for the potentially thrombocytopenic infant.

Although there is not a consensus regarding therapeutic merit or degree of use, platelet transfusions often are used preoperatively and intraoperatively in association with splenectomy procedures. Use of platelet transfusions, corticosteroids, better anesthesia, and improved surgical techniques for pregnant splenectomies is responsible for today's much lower operative maternal and perinatal mortality rates than those recorded in the earlier obstetric literature. Formerly, approximately one in ten mothers and one in every four fetuses were lost (Heys, 1966; Laros and Sweet, 1975; Tancer, 1960; O'Reilly and Taber, 1978).

*Splenectomy prior to pregnancy usually decreases the frequency and severity of maternal complications during pregnancy* (Heys, 1966). However, the impression of maternal well-being may lead to a false sense of security on the part of the patient and her obstetrician that the *fetus* is not in danger. *Previous splenectomy has not been shown to effect any improvement in either perinatal mortality or neonatal thrombocytopenia* (Robson and Davidson, 1950; O'Reilly and Taber, 1978; Tancer, 1960; Territo et al, 1973). Splenectomy often results in remission of the aITP disease process, but it does not necessarily cure it (Cines and Schreiber, 1979; Jones, 1979; Karpatkin and Lackner, 1975; Veenhoven et al, 1980). After removal of the spleen, platelet-associated antibody can be produced by the liver, bone marrow, and other reticuloendothelial tissue. Absence of the spleen permits longer survival of antibody-coated platelets and more normal maternal platelet counts but would not be expected to decrease the transplacental passage of free antibody targeted for the fetal platelets (McMillan, 1977).

**Immunosuppressive Drugs.** If severe thrombocytopenia persists despite splenectomy and corticosteroid administration, the administration of other immunosuppressive agents must be considered. Although a number of drugs, including azathioprine, cyclophosphamide, and the vinca alkaloids, have been shown to be beneficial in the treatment of a small number of pregnant patients with severe aITP, controlled clinical trials are sorely needed to investigate the benefit-versus-risk ratio of this therapy as well as its role in treatment (Ahn and Harrington, 1977; Caplan and Berkman, 1976; Gowda et al, 1977). Understandably, immunosuppressive therapy during gestation has been avoided owing to fears of fetal and maternal toxicity, teratogenicity, oncogenicity, fetal growth retardation, and prematurity. Experience with immunosuppressant-treated patients who had undergone organ transplants revealed only an increased frequency of premature growth-retarded infants (Scott, 1977). There is at least one report in which a patient with aITP was treated successfully during the third trimester with cyclophosphamide, and there were no obvious fetal side effects (Horger and Keane, 1979). Much work needs to be done to clarify the uncertainty surrounding the therapeutic indications and to elucidate recommendations for this type of intervention in the pregnant aITP patient. It is especially here that expert hematologic consultation is most valued.

**Plasma Exchange.** An alternative approach to therapy for some gravidas with severe aITP is the removal of antiplatelet antibodies by automated plasma exchange with fresh plasma or purified IgG preparations as part of the replacement medium (Imbach et al, 1981; Marder et al, 1981; Taft, 1982). Published results are mixed, with the best outcome in some patients with acute aITP who respond after only one or two exchanges and the worst outcome in patients with long-standing chronic disease (Branda et al, 1975; 1978; Imbach et al, 1981; Novak and Williams, 1978; Weir et al, 1980). Patient selection criteria must be refined and more investigations performed to study how

plasma exchange can effect a cure. At present, *plasmapheresis should be considered only as an emergency or secondary adjunct* (Taft et al, 1981) *to the primary therapeutic tools* already discussed (Table 28–11).

**Platelet Transfusion.** Platelet transfusion in gravid patients with severe aITP is a temporary measure useful therapeutically for the arrest of life-threatening hemorrhage and useful prophylactically as part of the preparation prior to operative procedures such as splenectomy and cesarean delivery (Baldini, 1972). Although fresh whole blood, platelet-rich plasma, and platelet concentrate are considered vehicles for platelet administration, in general, only platelet concentrates are used therapeutically for patients with aITP. In terms of platelet function, platelet-rich plasma and platelet concentrates begin to lose efficacy with time, with exposure to the 4°C temperature of blood refrigerators, with treatment by the anticoagulant solution acid citrate dextrose and with placement in plastic storage containers (Abbott Laboratories, 1971; Murray and Gardner, 1969).

Optimal practice is to minimize turn-around time from donor to recipient, storing platelets in containers at 4°C for as little as possible of the deadline time of 72 hours. Ideally, platelets should be obtained by single-donor plateletpheresis to reduce the hazards of hepatitis or HIV transmission, increases in numbers of transfused platelet antigens, and febrile reactions. Also, ideally, platelets should be matched not only for ABO and RH blood groups but also for histocompatibility (HLA) and platelet (PL) antigens (Horger and Keane, 1979).

Depending on how much circulating antiplatelet antibody is present and how well the donor platelets have been matched with the patient and her antibody, transfusion of a single unit of platelet concentrate from a carefully collected unit of ABO-compatible

---

**Table 28–11**
POTENTIAL APPLICATIONS FOR PLASMA IN aITP

As preoperative treatment for the adult patient following failed intravenous immunoglobulin, corticosteroid therapy, or both

As emergency treatment for life-threatening hemorrhage

As alternative treatment when other modes of therapy are absolutely or relatively contraindicated

very fresh blood will raise the aITP patient's platelet count significantly less than the 7000 to 11,000/mm³/M² increase observed in normal individuals (Harker and Finch, 1969). There is much variation from one patient to another, and more exact individual needs can be calculated by inserting into the formula depicted in Figure 28–5 the results of blood sampling taken 1 hour after transfusion (American Association of Blood Banks, 1975; Laningham, 1975). For instance, Anguilo and coworkers (1977) demonstrated an increment of 3200 platelets/mm³ per unit of platelet concentrate infused into their patient with aITP. Survival of platelets transfused into an individual with aITP is shortened to 48 to 230 minutes (Harker and Finch, 1969).

Because platelets of patients with aITP are younger and larger and function more efficiently as cofactors of coagulation, it may not be necessary to transfuse enough platelet concentrates to achieve the preoperative platelet count of 60,000 to 70,000/mm³ recommended by Anguilo and colleagues (1977). A maternal count of 50,000/mm³ or less may be adequate (Cavanagh, 1982, particularly in the presence of a bleeding time less than 12 minutes. In our experience, the bleeding time of aITP patients may not be prolonged with only 10,000 to 20,000 platelets. As a reflection of the uncertainty of critical requirements for coagulation, some protocols for aITP management of gravid patients recommend preset transfusion amounts (Cruickshank, 1982). However, the least amount necessary for hemostasis is recommended because platelet transfusion is expensive and carries with it the risk of transmission of infections and development of platelet isoantibodies and alloantibodies. Aisner (1977) recommends that corticosteroids always be administered prior to platelet transfusion to enhance longevity of the transfused platelets.

**Combined and Emergent Treatment.** Infrequently, emergent surgery such as cesarean delivery may become necessary in the symptomatic parturient patient with aITP. The administration of conventional single-agent therapy to correct thrombocytopenia may be impossible owing to inadequate time. In this instance, combination therapy with intravenous corticosteroids, isovolemic plasma exchange, intravenous gammaglobulin (400 mg/kg), and platelet transfusion has been used successfully for a mother in labor with a stressed fetus (Wood and Jacobs, 1989).

### Intrapartum Period

*The most critical and controversial aspect of aITP pregnancy management is the optimal planning of labor and delivery.* Because of the transplacental passage of antiplatelet antibody, infants of women with aITP may be born with thrombocytopenia. Samuels and associates' (1989) data suggest an incidence of 25 percent fetuses with platelet counts less than 100,000 U/liter and 11 percent fetuses with severe thrombocytopenia less than 50,000 U/liter. The most feared perinatal complication is intracranial hemorrhage. Because birth trauma is a major cause of perinatal morbidity and mortality, efforts have been directed toward identification of the fetus at risk and delivery by atraumatic cesarean delivery. Optimal outcome might be achieved by early identification of the thrombocytopenic fetus and its abdominal delivery prior to the onset of labor. Any attempts to select for cesarean delivery only the compromised fetus are advantageous also for the aITP mother's welfare so that she is not subjected to any unnecessary operative intervention and risk.

The maternal platelet count has been ob-

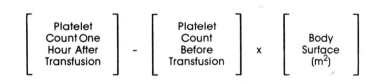

$$\text{Increment in Platelet Count per Unit of Platelets Transfused} = \frac{\left[\begin{array}{c}\text{Platelet Count One Hour After Transfusion}\end{array}\right] - \left[\begin{array}{c}\text{Platelet Count Before Transfusion}\end{array}\right] \times \left[\begin{array}{c}\text{Body Surface (m}^2\text{)}\end{array}\right]}{\text{Number of Units of Platelets Given}}$$

**Figure 28–5.** Calculation of platelet response after transfusion.

served by many to be an unreliable predictor of the fetal or neonatal platelet count (Baele and Thiery, 1978; Carlos et al, 1980; Cines et al, 1982; Kornstein et al, 1980; Laros and Sweet, 1975; Murray and Harris, 1976; Noriega-Guerra et al, 1979; O'Reilly and Taber, 1978; Tancer, 1960; Territo et al, 1973). The discrepancy between maternal and fetal platelet counts may be particularly evident in the splenectomized parturient patient in whom a normal platelet count can be detected despite the presence of considerable amounts of antiplatelet antibodies (Cines and Schreiber, 1979; Jones, 1979; Karpatkin and Lackner, 1975; Veenhoven et al, 1980). In large numbers, the unbound IgG antibodies can traverse the placenta, attach themselves to fetal platelets, and render the antibody-coated platelets subject to destruction by the intact fetal spleen. Clinically, these fetuses have proved to be at greater risk for purpura and death than their counterparts in aITP mothers who have not yet undergone splenectomy.

Samuels and associates (1989) suggest that maternal performance of an indirect platelet antiglobulin test is a useful screen to determine whether or not any fetus is at risk for thrombocytopenia. If the test is positive (predictive value of only 24 percent), determination of fetal platelet count prior to vaginal delivery must be performed by cordocentesis or fetal scalp sampling. If the test is negative, it is 98 percent likely that the fetal platelet count is not less than 50,000 U/liter and, thus, additional testing is unlikely to identify further at-risk fetuses. Other investigators, using different methods, have been unable to demonstrate a similar reliable correlation between the amount of platelet-binding IgG in maternal plasma and neonatal platelet counts (Aster, 1989; Hart et al, 1986).

Because there are no reliable predictors of fetal thrombocytopenia in the patient with aITP, decisions about mode of delivery should be based on actual measurements of the fetal platelet count. Two options exist: fetal scalp sampling and percutaneous umbilical venous blood sampling (PUBS or cordocentesis). Decisions regarding either of these approaches depends on operator expertise, the maternal bleeding time, past obstetric history, placental location, maternal anatomy, technical difficulty, and fetal location.

The measurement of venous platelet counts in fetal scalp blood by direct sampling during early labor was first reported by Ayromlooi (1978). Because this determination should accurately reflect the venous platelet count and reliably predict the risk of fetal hemorrhage, Scott and coworkers (1980) used this novel approach in a small series of parturient patients and found it to be reliable. Sampling was done either during labor or immediately after amniotomy to induce labor at term when the cervix became favorable. If the platelet count was below 50,000/mm$^3$, these investigators delivered the fetus abdominally, but usually, it was higher and a vaginal delivery was supported unless traditional obstetric concerns interfered. Three of 12 parturients with aITP underwent cesarean delivery for fetal counts less than 50,000/mm$^3$, and in all three infants, neonatal platelet counts were less than 20,000/mm$^3$. In fetuses delivered vaginally, the lowest count was 76,000/mm$^3$. Scott and coworkers (1980) recommended sampling for all parturient patients with aITP, whether they are in remission, are taking steroids, or have had a splenectomy.

Fetal scalp sampling (Table 28–12) is not without some risk, and it cannot be accomplished in all patients. Membranes must be ruptured, the head must be the descending part, and the cervix must be partially dilated and effaced. Intracranial hemorrhage already may have occurred at the point in pelvic descent when sampling can be performed. Significant bleeding may occur secondary to the scalp laceration itself. In the hands of Scott and colleagues (1980), there were no untoward fetal bleeding episodes in those fetuses with platelet counts as low as 3000/mm$^3$ so long as pressure was kept on the scalp puncture site through two subsequent uterine contractions.

Cordocentesis permits direct access to the fetal circulation and the determination of the fetal platelet count in cases of suspected fetal thrombocytopenia (Hobbins et al, 1985; Ludomirski and Weiner, 1988; Ludomirski et al, 1987; Moise and Cotton, 1987; Moise et al, 1988; Nicolaides, 1988; Nicolaides et al, 1986). Fetal platelet counts less than 50,000 U/liter are associated with a 6 percent incidence of perinatal death and the potential for intracerebral hemorrhage, especially during parturition. A fetal blood sample is obtained through ultrasound-directed puncture of an umbilical vessel by a 20- to 25-gauge needle. Procedure-related fe-

**Table 28–12**
FETAL SCALP SAMPLING TECHNIQUE

1. Place the patient comfortably on her side in a curled up position with the vaginal introitus near one side of the labor bed; this usually ensures maternal comfort, maximizes uteroplacental blood flow to the fetus, and facilitates a careful performance of the procedure by the obstetrician.*
2. Introduce a plastic cone from a fetal scalp pH set into the vagina and place it against the fetal scalp.
3. Cleanse the designated area on the scalp and make a small incision in the area chosen for sampling.
4. Hold the plastic pipette (from a set such as the Becton-Dickinson Unopipette Test 5855 system, which is used in hospital labs for manual platelet determinations) against the bleeding point and allow it to fill by capillary action; obtain at least two samples.
5. With the Unopipette System, the pipette is then quickly inserted into a reservoir containing diluent and the blood sample is rapidly evacuated into this solution.
6. The platelets then are counted using a standard hemocytometer method.
7. After sampling is completed, maintain steady pressure against the scalp incision with a long-stem cotton swab until oozing has ceased and through at least two uterine contractions.

* Some birthing beds provide a leg support by reversing the stirrup to hold the upper leg during pH blood sampling.

tal mortality is estimated to be 1 to 2 percent. Generally, aITP cordocentesis is performed at 37 to 38 weeks' gestation for fetal platelet count determination. If this is less than 50,000 U/liter, cesarean delivery is performed; otherwise, an attempt at vaginal delivery can be undertaken. The technique appears safe, even when the fetal platelets are as low as 2000 U/liter (Ludomirski and Wiener, 1988). Preparation for prompt cesarean delivery, if needed, is recommended in addition to platelets for possible transfusion. A 4- to 6-hour period is recommended (Scioscia, 1988). The procedure must be repeated if an interval greater than 21 days occurs between sampling and delivery.

If vaginal delivery is elected, a prolonged and difficult labor should be avoided. Electronic fetal monitoring and vigilant attention to basic obstetric principles are critical. For instance, the supine position and overstimulation with oxytocin should be avoided to prevent fetal hypoxia. Platelet counts in term infants are significantly lower in those who have suffered hypoxic episodes (Chadd et al, 1971). Obstetric analgesia is influenced by the patient's hematologic status as well as the skills and preferences of the

obstetric anesthesiologist. General endotracheal anesthesia is used for preplanned cesarean delivery, avoiding potential coagulation problems associated with the placement of an epidural catheter. A maternal platelet count less than 50,000 U/liter has been suggested as minimal requirement prior to vaginal or abdominal surgery, but platelet counts lower than this, particularly in the presence of a normal bleeding time, are satisfactory and safe. Ballem and associates (1989) recommend that the patient's bleeding time should be less than 15 minutes before delivery and less than 12 minutes before any surgical procedure. Anesthesiologists usually are unwilling to perform any type of conduction anesthesia with a platelet count less than 100,000 U/liter.

If the parturient received corticosteroids at any time during gestation, 200 mg of hydrocortisone should be given intravenously as a bolus early in labor or preoperatively. A continuous infusion of 100 mg hydrocortisone every 6 hours should be administered through delivery and the immediate puerperium. Difficult forceps manipulations should be avoided. Episiotomies and any lacerations must be repaired meticulously. Likewise, cesarean delivery technique must be meticulous, the operator making extra efforts to minimize tissue trauma and maximize hemostasis in the surgical field. Intrapartum management considerations for aITP are listed in Table 28–13.

**Table 28–13**
INTRAPARTUM MANAGEMENT
CONSIDERATIONS FOR aITP

Periodic manual platelet counts, bleeding times
Avoidance of intramuscular injections
Avoidance of fetal hypoxia and neonatal asphyxia
Avoidance of difficult or prolonged labor
Avoidance of difficult forceps deliveries
Preferred midline episiotomy
Continuous external electronic fetal monitoring
Internal scalp electrode can be placed after normal scalp sampling for platelet count
Readiness for cesarean delivery immediately after scalp sampling
Appropriate maternal platelet transfusion
Ready availability of blood products for potential maternal and neonatal use
Appropriate corticosteroid use
Potential use of intravenous immunoglobulin therapy
Optimal analgesia and anesthesia
Meticulous operative technique
Selective cesarean delivery
Excellent neonatal care accessibility
Use of intravenous IgG for emergencies

## Postpartum Period

Intensive fetal and maternal surveillance during parturition must be maintained, especially in the immediate postpartum period. Neonatal thrombocytopenia occurs in as many as 70 percent of infants born to women with aITP (Goldswerg and Chediat, 1977; Laros and Sweet, 1975; Noriega-Guerra et al, 1979). It may be severe enough to cause hemorrhagic complications prior to, during, or immediately after the birth process. A review of 98 infants born to women with aITP by Scott and coworkers (1980) revealed no serious bleeding recorded in any infant with a platelet count greater than or equal to 50,000/mm$^3$. Because the passive acquisition of antibody from the mother ceases after the umbilical cord is severed, neonatal thrombocytopenia usually is mild and a self-limited process that peaks 4 to 6 days after delivery and then disappears over a course of weeks to, at the most, 3 months (Pearson and McIntosh, 1978; Scott, 1976). Regardless of the postdelivery platelet count, each neonate of an aITP mother should be monitored for at least 1 week or longer until improvement is noted.

Most often, the neonate requires no special therapy. If neonatal thrombocytopenia is identified, a radiologic study such as a computed tomographic scan can be performed to determine whether or not the newborn has had an intracranial hemorrhage. In the absence of hemorrhage, a number of therapeutic approaches have been advocated, including monitoring only, exchange transfusion with fresh whole blood (Nelson et al, 1979), corticosteroid therapy for 3 weeks pending disappearance of maternal antibody (Laros and Sweet, 1975), platelet transfusion alone, and intravenous gammaglobulin therapy with or without concomitant prednisone therapy (Bussel, 1988). In the presence of ongoing hemorrhage, combined treatment with corticosteroids, intravenous immune gamma globulin (IVIGG), and platelet transfusion is likely to impact immediately.

Early in the puerperium, breastfeeding may induce thrombocytopenia owing to the passage of platelet antibodies in the colostrum (Kelman et al, 1978). In view of this as well as the possible passage of corticosteroids across to the fetus via breast milk, lactation usually is discouraged in these patients (Katz and Duncan, 1975).

For the mother, concerns about future fertility must be addressed prior to hospital discharge (Table 28–14). Because intrauterine devices have an increased failure rate in mothers taking corticosteroids and are associated with increased risks of menorrhagia and uterine perforation in aITP women, low-dose combination birth control pills may be the optimal mode of contraception. If sterilization is desired, we prefer an inpatient procedure via minilaparotomy incision for optimal visualization and handling of tissue for hemostasis.

A summary of patient care procedures in the management of aITP is presented in Table 28–15.

**Table 28–14**
POSTPARTUM MANAGEMENT OF aITP

Continued intensive fetal and maternal surveillance
Reproductive counseling
Contraception by birth control pills or barrier method; avoidance of IUDs
Consider later splenectomy if future childbearing desired
Inpatient sterilization by minilaparotomy if desired; avoidance of laparoscopy
Avoidance of breastfeeding

# Hemoglobinopathies

## ETIOLOGY

Maternal anemia is the *most common* maternal complication noted during gestation and occurs in more than 50 percent of all pregnancies (Morrison, 1981). These anemias can be categorized as acquired and inherited disorders. Of the congenital disorders, there are over 1000 possible genetic abnormalities and most involve the structure of the globin chains of the hemoglobin molecule. By 1990, more than 325 specific abnormalities of the globin molecule have been reported (Perry, 1990). Examples of these defects include hemoglobin S (HbS) and hemoglobin C (HbC), which differ from the normal adult hemoglobin (HbA and HbA$_2$) or fetal hemoglobin (HbF) only by the substitution of one amino acid in the globin chain (Morrison, 1979). Other types of abnormalities involve the diminished production of either the alpha or beta globin chain of the hemoglobin molecule, such as thalassemia

**Table 28–15**
PATIENT CARE SUMMARY FOR aITP

| | Antepartum | | Intrapartum | Postpartum |
| | Outpatient* | Inpatient | | |
|---|---|---|---|---|
| BP, P, R, T | With each clinic visit | Minimum q 4 h, depending on patient's condition | Minimum q 1 h | On admission to RR; then q 15 min × 4; then q 30 min × 2; then q 1 h until stable |
| FHR | With each clinic visit | Weakly NST and CST ≥ 34 weeks | After normal scalp sampling, continuously with fetal monitor, preferably internal; if monitor not available, q 15–30 min in first stage, and q 5 min in second stage | — |
| Scalp sampling | — | — | ×1 in labor room to establish fetal aITP | — |
| Contractions | — | — | Same as FHR | Fundal checks on admission q 15 min × 4; then q 30 min × 2; then q 1 h until stable |
| Lochia | — | — | — | Lochia checks q 15 min until stable; then q 30 min × 2; then q 1 h until stable; then q 4–8 h |
| Sonograms | q 4 wk after 26 weeks | Possible cordocentesis at 37–38 weeks | | |
| Possible plasma exchange Possible platelet transfusions Laboratory values Platelet count Bleeding time | See discussion of management schemes in text; maintain individualized care | | | |
| Observations for signs of shock | — | — | Continuously | Continuously |
| I & O | — | q 8 h | q 1 h | q 1 h until stable |

* Frequent clinic visits (frequency depends on patient's condition).
Note: Nurse-to-patient ratio, 1:6 to 8 antepartum; 2:3 intrapartum; 1:6 to 8 postpartum.
BP = blood pressure; R = respiration; FHR = fetal heart rate; P = pulse; T = temperature; NST = nonstress test; CST = contraction stress test; RR = recovery room.

(HbThal). Fortunately, most of these abnormalities are rare and are inherited in an autosomal codominant or recessive manner. Sickle hemoglobin is one of the most common structural variants and is also clinically important because of the increased maternal mortality and morbidity as well as fetal and neonatal wastage encountered during pregnancy in parturient patients with severe disease.

## INCIDENCE

Inherited abnormal hemoglobins may be classified as mild or severe, depending on their clinical appearance (Table 28–16). The *most common type of hemoglobinopathy* is sickle cell trait (HbS) (Foster, 1980), which occurs in 1 per 12 African Americans or those of Mediterranean descent. Fortunately, this is usually a benign syndrome during preg-

**Table 28–16**
CLASSIFICATION OF HEMOGLOBINOPATHIES

Mild (Benign Forms)
    Sickle cell trait (Hb A-S)
    Hemoglobin S-E disease (Hb S-E)
    Hemoglobin S-D disease (Hb S-D)
    Hemoglobin S-Memphis (Hb S-Memphis)
    Hemoglobin C disease (Hb C-C)
Sickel Cell Disease
    Sickle cell anemia (Hb S-S)
    Hemoglobin S-C disease (Hb S-C)
    Hemoglobin S-thalassemia (Hb-S-Thal)
    Hemoglobin B-thalassemia

nancy, and sickle cell patients usually are not treated differently than patients with normal hemoglobin with the exception that HbA-S patients receive intensive antepartum scrutiny for infections, specifically those related to the urinary tract. Other variants, such as hemoglobin S-E, S-D, and S-Memphis, are usually benign during pregnancy and are exceedingly rare (Morrison, 1979). Finally, hemoglobin C disease (HbC-C and HbA-C) is the sixth most common hemoglobinopathy and affects 1 per 4400 African Americans. It also does not have a significant adverse effect on either the mother or the fetus.

As shown in Table 28–16, patients with severe hemoglobinopathies include those with clinically significant forms of thalassemia and those with sickle cell disease. Sickle-cell disease is composed of sickle-cell anemia (HbS-S), hemoglobin S-C (HbS-C), and hemoglobin S-thalassemia (HbS-Thal), which occur in 1 per 600, 1 per 850, and 1 per 1600 patients, respectively (Foster, 1980). In pregnant patients, these hemoglobinopathies are usually thought to increase the risk for the mother and the fetus. Those with homozygous beta thalassemia or Cooley's anemia usually do not live to conceive, and those with homozygous alpha thalassemia are rarely born alive (Perry, 1990). Therefore, the disorders that constitute sickle-cell disease are the ones most clinically applicable to the perinatologist.

## PATHOPHYSIOLOGY

The molecular alteration that distinguishes HbS from normal hemoglobin A (HbA) is a minor structural change that involves only 2 of the 574 amino acids in normal hemoglobin. The single base replacement at the sixth position in the beta chain where the neutral amino acid valine is substituted for negatively charged glutamic acid drastically diminishes the oxygen-carrying capacity and survival time of the red blood cell in those patients who have sickle hemoglobin. As shown in Figure 28–6, this amino acid replacement allows the beta chains of various hemoglobin molecules within the red cells to interlock by hydrophobic bonding with other HbS molecules. Long microfilaments form, which then coalesce into large microcables. Once these helical structures polymerize in the deoxygenated state, they distort the membrane of the erythrocyte in the classic sickled shape. Once the cell loses water, the cell membrane may be hardened by calcium deposits and, thus, the cell becomes irreversibly sickled and is destroyed.

If a sickle cell patient is exposed to acidosis or hypoxia, the sickling of the HbS–containing cells occurs more often, which causes sludging of the cells in the microcirculation (Fig. 28–7). With subsequent capillary obstruction there is increased blood viscosity within the capillaries and more sickling occurs, which leads to further deoxygenation. This completes the vicious circle of increased intravascular sickling, and thus, a painful vaso-occlusive crisis is clinically set in motion (Martin and Morrison, 1982). Clinically, these crises produce sudden pain involving the abdomen, chest, vertebrae, and extremities. The manifestations usually follow a repetitive pattern from one crisis to the next, but during pregnancy, such findings may be intensified. Although vaso-occlusive crises are more common during pregnancy, hematologic crises can occur and are characterized by reticulocytopenia and a rapid decline in the hematocrit (Hct). These patients are usually more pale but less icteric than patients having a vaso-occlusive crisis. Splenic sequestration is another example of a hematologic crisis but occurs more commonly during childhood.

## EFFECTS ON PREGNANCY

Older reports regarding pregnant patients with sickle-cell disease (HbS-S, HbS-C, HbS-Thal) revealed maternal mortality figures between 10 and 20 percent, maternal morbidity between 50 and 80 percent, and perinatal wastage rates of 40 to 60 percent (Table

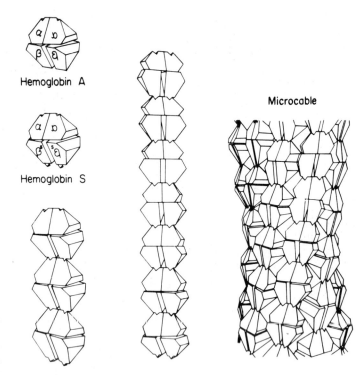

**Figure 28–6.** Sickle cell microcables. Hemoglobin filaments coalesce into a semisolid gel to form microcables. These microcables further polymerize to form helical structures that distort the cell into its characteristic sickle shape.

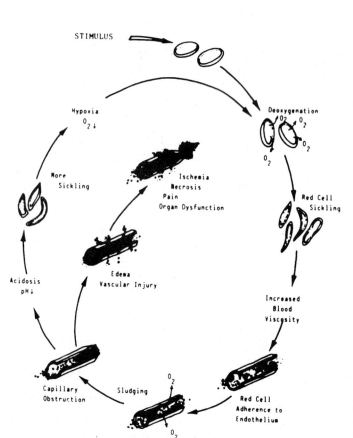

**Figure 28–7.** The sickle cell crisis cycle. A dangerous sequence is set in motion when HbS-containing red cells become deoxygenated, sickled, and obstructive of blood flow in the microvasculature. (From Martin JN Jr, Morrison JC: Managing the parturient with sickle cell crisis. Clin Obstet Gynecol 27:39, 1984.)

28–17) (Fort et al, 1971; Freeman and Ruth, 1969). Through meticulous care and intensive medical therapy, these percentages have been reduced to the point that it is no longer rare to expect a normal pregnancy outcome for mother and infant (Morrison and Wiser, 1976; Perkins, 1971; Powars, 1986). Nevertheless, patients with sickle cell disease are considered at high risk and are a continuing problem for the physician (Koshy et al, 1988; Morrison et al, 1980a).

## DIAGNOSIS AND COUNSELING

It is prudent that each African American patient be assessed for sickle hemoglobin. If the screening test is positive, she should have a hemoglobin electrophoresis to differentiate the type of abnormal hemoglobin present (Table 28–18). It is unlikely that sickle-cell anemia patients without prior symptoms would be discovered, but some subjects with HbS-C or HbS-Thal have been found, and even if milder disorders such as HbA-S are diagnosed, proper education and counseling can be offered. For those with mild disorders, the avoidance of stress, high altitudes, infection, and hypoxia should be mentioned, but reassurance of their normalcy is underscored. Avoidance and early recognition of infection and crises are very important in those with major hemoglobinopathies. Educating the public as to the extent of the disease and its cause is also important. Therefore, antepartum screening is recommended for African Americans to detect sickle hemoglobinopathies. It is also essential to test the cord blood to determine the presence of HbS in the newborn so that the family can be counseled, if necessary (Kramer et al, 1979). Infants rarely have crises before 3 to 6 months of age because there is ample fetal hemoglobin to protect the cells from sickling.

### Laboratory Findings

As shown in Table 28–18, the most common laboratory finding in patients with hemoglobinopathies is anemia (Morrison, 1981). In general, those with Hct less than 20 or Hb less than 6 g/dl usually have HbS-S or Cooley's beta thalassemia. Patients with HbS-C or HbS-Thal may have a hematocrit value of 20 to 25 percent and even 30 percent on some occasions. Patients with heterozygous beta or alpha thalassemia as well as the mild sickle hemoglobinopathies, including sickle cell trait, have hematocrit values of 30 to 35 percent. The reticulocyte count is usually elevated in the range of 10 to 20 percent, and thrombocytosis is common in patients with sickle hemoglobinopathies. The serum

**Table 28–17**
PREGNANCY OUTCOME WITH SEVERE SICKLE HEMOGLOBINOPATHIES

| Reference | Number of Gestations | Maternal Values (%) | | Neonatal Values (%) | |
|---|---|---|---|---|---|
| | | *Morbidity* | *Mortality* | *Morbidity* | *Mortality* |
| Statistics prior to 1970 | | | | | |
| Adams (1953) | 25 | 65 | 35 | 17 | 22 |
| Curtis (1959) | 64 | 35 | 8 | 46 | 42 |
| Anderson (1960) | 28 | 0 | 48 | — | 80 |
| Rimer (1961) | 25 | 0 | — | — | 42 |
| McCurdy (1964) | 34 | 75 | 3 | 17 | 29 |
| Laros (1967) | 67 | 15 | — | — | 19 |
| Freeman (1969) | 67 | — | — | 21 | 42 |
| Statistics after 1970 | | | | | |
| Perkins (1971) | 109 | 13 | 0 | 12 | 12 |
| Hendricks (1972) | 61 | 13 | 0 | 12 | 12 |
| Horger (1972) | 54 | 96 | 8 | 51 | 24 |
| Pritchard (1973) | 128 | — | 1.5 | 29 | 33 |
| Morrison (1976) | 36 | 4 | 0 | 16 | 3 |
| Charache (1979) | 74 | 45 | 1.4 | 33 | 28 |
| Milner (1980) | 181 | — | — | — | 5.3 |
| Morrison (1980) | 75 | 14 | 0 | 9 | 2.6 |
| Miller (1981) | 63 | — | 0 | — | — |
| Powars (1986) | 56 | 28.6 | 1.2 | — | 0 |
| Tuck (1987) | 51 | — | 0 | — | 1.9 |
| Koshy (1988) | 189 | — | 0 | — | 2.1 |

**Table 28–18**
DIAGNOSIS OF HEMOGLOBINOPATHIES

A. Screening Tests (Sickledex—Ortho, etc.)
  1. Based on solubility and color change
  2. High false-positive rate, rare false-negative result
  3. Confirm with sodium metabisulfate slide test
  4. Definitive diagnosis—hemoglobin electrophoresis
B. Genetic Diagnosis
  1. Chorionic villous sampling by DNA analysis
  2. Amniotic fluid uncultured cells by DNA analysis
  3. Fetal blood sampling
  4. Family pedigree
C. Hemoglobin Electrophoresis
  1. Hb A-S: 25 to 35%-S, 60%-$A_1$, normal $A_2$, F
  2. Hb S-S: 90 to 95%-S, normal $A_2$, normal to increased F, no $A_1$
  3. Hb S-C: normal $A_2$ and F, 45 to 48 percent of both S and C, no $A_1$
  4. Hb S-Thal: 35 to 50%-S, 40 to 60 percent $A_1$, normal to increased $A_2$ and F
  5. B-Thal heterozygous: 90%-$A_1$, increased $A_2$ and F
  6. A-Thal heterozygous: 95%-$A_1$, normal $A_2$ and F
D. Hemoglobin and Hematocrit Values
  1. Hb A-S: Hb 11 to 12 g%, Hct 32 to 37 percent
  2. Hb S-S: Hb 5 to 8 g%, Hct 15 to 22 percent
  3. Hb S-C: Hb 8 to 10 g%, Hct 25 to 30 percent
  4. Hb S-Thal: Hb 9 to 10 g%, Hct 28 to 32 percent
  5. B or A-Thal: Hb 9 to 12 g%, Hct 28 to 36 percent
E. Other Indices
  1. Blood films of sickling (Hb S), target cells—thalassemia
  2. Indices—normochromic, normocytic unless associated iron deficiency
  3. Reticulocyte count increased 3 to 20 percent
  4. Serum iron—variable
  5. Bilirubin elevated in Hb S-S and SC even when not in crisis

bilirubin is normally elevated (1 to 7 mg/dl) and can reach 15 to 20 mg/dl during crisis. The prothrombin, partial thromboplastin, and clotting times are normal in patients with hemoglobinopathies, but platelet counts, fibrinogen, and fibrin split products may be abnormal, particularly during crisis (Martin and Morrison, 1982).

## MANAGEMENT

### Antepartum Period

**Conservative Versus Transfusion Therapy.** *All authorities recommend careful and frequent antepartum visits* beginning early during gestation. The severity of anemia, reticulocyte counts, bilirubin levels, degree of

sickling, and presence of infection and crisis should be intensively assessed at each visit (Table 28–19). Many authors recommend continued observation during gestation if the patient with a severe sickle hemoglobinopathy has a benign prior history, elevated HbF, or ho hint of infection or crisis (Charache et al, 1980; Desforgres and Warth, 1974; Koshy et al, 1988; Perkins, 1971; Tuck et al, 1987). On the other hand, others who have noted deterioration in such patients during pregnancy recommend prophylactic treatment with partial exchange or simple transfusions to remove HbS-containing cells, replacing them with normal donor cells containing HbA (Cunningham et al, 1979; Morrison et al, 1980b). Therefore, one group advocates conservative management of pregnant patients with severe sickle hemoglobinopathies, whereas another recommends intensive therapy with prophylactic transfusions. Each group has good statistics to warrant the use of its approach (see Table

**Table 28–19**
ANTEPARTUM ASSESSMENT OF PREGNANT PATIENTS WITH HEMOGLOBINOPATHIES

A. Hemoglobin Testing
  1. Sickle screen to black patients with unknown hemoglobin
  2. Hemoglobin electrophoresis with unexplained or unresponsive anemia
  3. Husband, family members of known hemoglobinopathy patients
  4. Consider genetic amniocentesis if both parents have hemoglobinopathy
B. Education and Counseling After Identification
C. Prenatal Visits
  1. Encourage early entry into prenatal clinic
  2. If asymptomatic, visits every 2 weeks until 20 weeks, then weekly
  3. Close scrutiny for signs of infection, crisis, or labor
D. Laboratory Tests
  1. Routine prenatal assessment
  2. Baseline fibrinogen, platelet count, and CP
  3. Reticulocyte count, bilirubin, hematocrit, hemoglobin, urinalysis twice monthly
  4. Hemoglobin electrophoresis twice monthly if patient has received transfusions
E. Fetal Assessments
  1. NST and CST weekly beginning at 32 weeks
  2. USG 16 to 18 weeks, repeat at 28 to 30 weeks
  3. Fetal movement—30 minutes, three times daily beginning at 32 weeks
  4. Umbilical artery velocimetry if suspect IUGR.

CP = Chemistry profile; CST = contraction stress test; NST = nonstress test.

28–17). During infection or crisis, most authors recommend the use of blood products as a major therapeutic modality.

For those recommending prophylactic transfusions, several techniques are available. Prior to 1978, most persons used the manual method, but this type of therapy is expensive and cumbersome (Cunningham et al, 1979; Morrison and Wiser, 1976). Continuous automated erythrocytopheresis has been recommended by several authors as a method that can lead to a more accurate estimation of the amount of blood infused and withdrawn as well as allow the clinician to perform these transfusions on an ambulatory basis (Keeling et al, 1980; Key et al, 1980; Morrison et al, 1982). The IBM 2997 Cell Separator and the Haemonetics Model 30 have both been useful in this maneuver. If the newer methods are not available, the manual method can be used (Table 28–20). The method of manual transfusion as well as critical levels for follow-up are listed in Table 28–20. The benefits and risks of this technique are listed in Table 28–21.

**Table 28–20**
PROTOCOL FOR MANUAL PARTIAL
EXCHANGE TRANSFUSION

1. Obtain hematocrit (Hct) and Hb A%; match, type, and crossmatch.
2. Infuse 200 to 500 ml of normal saline (60 min).
3. Phlebotomize 500 ml (30 min).
4. Give 2 units (150 to 200 ml/unit) buffy coat–poor, washed RBC (90 min).
5. Repeat entire procedure.
6. Allow 12 hours for equilibration.
7. Obtain Hct and Hb A%.
8. If Hct > 30% and Hb A > 40%, discharge patient; if not, repeat procedure.
9. Assess Hct and Hb A every 2 weeks.
10. Repeat entire procedure:
    a. At 36 to 38 weeks.
    b. When Hct < 25% and Hb A < 20%.
    c. If crisis occurs.
    d. If labor ensues.
Comments:
    a. Infuse buffy coat–washed RBC warmed and under pressure.
    b. If Hct falls rapidly (1–2 weeks) post-transfusion, check hemolysis:
       (1) reticulocyte count
       (2) bilirubin
       (3) antibody screen
       (4) plasma hemoglobin
    c. In Hb S-C patients, it may be difficult to raise Hb A > 35%.
    d. Interval between exchanges usually 4 to 8 weeks.

**Table 28–21**
BENEFITS AND RISKS OF
TRANSFUSION THERAPY

| Benefits | Risks |
| --- | --- |
| Decreases number of HB S cells | Hepatitis |
| Increases number of Hb A cells | Transfusion reaction |
| | Isosensitization |
| Decreases erythropoiesis of HB S cells | HIV infection |
| | Febrile reactions |
| Can abort a crisis | Premature labor |
| Increased sense of well-being | Temporary measure only |
| Can be used in congestive heart failure or renal disease | |

**Crisis Management.** If a vaso-occlusive crisis occurs during pregnancy, one must consider medical and surgical or obstetric disorders in the differential diagnosis, because pain does not always mean crisis in a sickle-cell patient. Up to one third of crises during adulthood are associated with apparent or occult infections, and most crises commonly include the lung and urinary and intestinal tracts. To differentiate bacterial infection from simple vaso-occlusive crisis without infection, the total number of segmented leukocytes (rarely above 1000 bands/$\mu$ in crisis), leukocyte alkaline phosphatase activity (normal in vaso-occlusive crisis alone), and isoenzymes (1 and 2) of serum lactate dehydrogenase (higher during crisis) are helpful assessments (Martin and Morrison, 1982).

The treatment of the crisis itself should be directed toward relieving the pain, preventing dehydration, and treating concurrent infections as well as other complications. Acetaminophen is the antipyretic and mild analgesic of choice, although during crisis, meperidine is usually required for alleviating severe pain. Morphine is avoided because of its potential smooth muscle constrictive properties. It is important to use these drugs only for severe pain because of the possibility of drug abuse or addiction. If infection is thought to be a problem, then antibiotics should be begun as soon as appropriate cultures are taken. Fluid and electrolyte replacement are essential because of the increased insensible fluid loss and hyposthenuria that occur during sickle cell crisis. Many compounds used to alkalize the maternal serum (and prevent further sickling) have been assessed as therapeutic agents but have not been effective. The efficacy of oxygen administration is also questionable unless the patient has evidence of a respiratory infection or other problems that would cause the $Pa_{O_2}$ level to be less than 70 mm.

The administration of blood components with HbA-containing cells is the cornerstone of crisis therapy. Many prefer the exchange transfusion method using the IBM 2997 for erythrocytopheresis. Only if the Hct is less than 15 is it necessary to give packed red cells prior to initiating an exchange transfusion. Buffy coat–poor washed erythrocytes are returned to the patient with her own plasma and leukocytes by erythrocytopheresis. Usually, this method aborts the crisis within 30 minutes after beginning the infusion. It is critically important to make certain that properly matched and administered red blood cells are used. Impeccable blood banking technique is important in ensuring the patient the maximal benefits and minimal risks of transfusion therapy. Table 28–22 outlines a step-wise fashion for antepartum management of these patients with suggested nursing actions.

## Intrapartum Period

**General Principles.** During the intrapartum period, spontaneous labor is managed with intensive maternal and fetal surveillance. Determination of Hct, Hb, and percentage of HbA are useful during the intrapartum period. Similarly, blood smears for potential crisis (assessment of the percentage of sickle cells), coagulation studies, and serial maternal blood gases also may be helpful. Frequent vital signs assessments in the mother as well as adequate fluid administration to avoid dehydration are recommended. Central venous lines and Foley and uterine catheters should be avoided, unless necessary, to reduce infectious morbidity. Although oxygen is not generally recommended, it may be used in labor, particularly if there are signs of fetal compromise. Intensive electronic monitoring of the fetal heart rate and maternal contractions is helpful to assess the fetal response to the contractions. Likewise, fetal scalp sampling can be helpful when alarming patterns are seen on the fetal heart rate monitor.

**Table 28–22**
ANTEPARTUM MANAGEMENT OF HEMOGLOBINOPATHY CRISIS

A. General
  1. Environment—quiet, comfortable, supportive
  2. Prevent dehydration—Ringer's lactate, NS
  3. Monitor I & O
  4. Monitor vital signs during labor
B. Analgesia
  1. Acetaminophen
  2. Meperidine
  3. Sedatives
C. Blood Component Replacement (most important)
  1. Method—simple, manual partial exchange transfusion, antenatal erythrocytopheresis
  2. Meticulous blood banking, volunteer donor, fresh as possible
  3. Buffy coat—poor washed donor RBCs, VDRL, and hepatitis B
D. Antibiotics
  1. 25 percent of crisis associated with infection
  2. Use broad-spectrum coverage until culture return
E. Others
  1. Oxygen—may or may not be of benefit (3 liters/min nasal and biprong)
  2. Alkalinization—not useful
  3. Catheters (bladder, uterine, central venous—avoid if possible
  4. Laboratory test—CP, blood film, hemoglobin studies
F. Special Cases
  1. Labor—continuous FHR monitoring and scalp sampling, maternal ABG
  2. Hemolytic crisis—plasma hemoglobin, but no increased bilirubin
  3. Infection—urinary tract, pulmonary, bone, gallbladder—unusual organisms

ABG = Arterial blood gases; CP = chemistry profile; FHR = fetal heart rate; NS = normal saline; RBCs = red blood cells; VDRL = Venereal Disease Research Laboratory.

**Blood Component Therapy.** It is best if the HbA level is greater than 20 percent and the Hct is greater than 25 percent. If transfusions are needed because the patient is in crisis during labor or there is a low Hct and HbA, labor is not a contraindication to the infusion or exchange transfusion of blood. Adequate pain relief with meperidine can be used during early labor, and this treatment can be combined with pudendal, local, or nitrous oxide anesthesia at delivery. If an obstetric anesthesiologist is present, conduction anesthesia with a light segmental epidural block may be used, but spinal, caudal, and paracervical blocks are best avoided. For cesarean birth, balanced endotracheal general anesthesia has provided best results.

## Postpartum Period

During the postpartum period, the patient should be assessed for signs of crisis due to the stress of labor. These patients are also prone to infection, and early recognition of signs of fever or foul-smelling lochia with prompt treatment is essential.

Sterilization is often recommended to these patients because of the risk not only to the fetus but also to the patient. If the patient desires future pregnancies, an effective means of birth control is imperative so that future pregnancies can be planned. Estrogen-progestin combination oral contraceptives are probably contraindicated in women with sickle cell anemias, because erythrocyte sequestration and vascular occlusion may be intensified. Contraception is a difficult issue, but is probably best handled by barrier techniques. It is possible that the use of the progestin-only pill (mini-pill) as well as the extremely low-dose estrogen pill (< 35 mg) may prove safe in the future. Nevertheless, the association of coagulation changes with sickle cell anemia and estrogens makes the use of the oral contraceptives undesirable at this time. Similarly, use of the intrauterine device, because it is associated with infectious problems, cannot be recommended. Surgical sterilization is considered only in those who choose to limit their family.

Counseling for these patients is important. If the patient is newly diagnosed, emotional support as well as education regarding her disease is needed. Information on the effects of chronic illness on the mother and her family is necessary to help these families cope. If the patient has had the disease for some time, the effect of pregnancy on her disease should be discussed, including the maternal and fetal morbidity and mortality.

Genetic counseling is important in helping the couple decide on sterilization. If both parents have the trait form of the disease, there is a 25 percent chance with each pregnancy that the child will be affected. If one parent has the trait and the other has the hemoglobinopathy, there is a 50 percent chance with each pregnancy that the child will develop the hemoglobinopathy; in such cases, a child born without the hemoglobinopathy will have the trait form. If both parents have a hemoglobinopathy, then all of their children will be affected. Despite aggressive genetic counseling, many young couples have children regardless of risk assessment (Neal-Cooper, 1988).

## Hemoglobinopathy in the Newborn

Because most of the hemoglobin in the red blood cells is fetal hemoglobin, hemolytic anemia characteristics of these hemoglobinopathies are not operational in utero or at birth. As more red blood cells that contain more abnormal hemoglobin are synthesized, the disease becomes clinically apparent. Even so, neonatal screening for hemoglobinopathies has been recommended in order to initiate ongoing care and appropriate intervention for those at high risk of early morbidity and mortality (Pearson, 1986).

## NEW DEVELOPMENTS

### Therapeutics

The prospects for new and successful therapy for sickle cell hemoglobinopathies have never looked brighter. Most of these new therapeutic regimens are aimed at the atomic interaction that actually triggers a sickle cell crisis (Klotz et al, 1981). The new agents are divided into three major categories: (1) those that inhibit the actual polymerization of sickle hemoglobin by disrupting the hydrophobic bonding (see Fig. 28–6); (2) those that inhibit the polymerization by decreasing the concentration of deoxygenated HbS; and (3) those that interact with the erythrocyte membrane. Of the agents that effect molecular bonding, several drugs, such as urea, organic solvents, and detergents, have been used but have proved too toxic for use in humans. New agents in this category that are most promising are the small peptides that can bind to the surface of the HbS molecule and prevent the intramolecular contacts necessary for polymerization. The major advantage of the use of these peptides is that they contain only amino acids, which, because they are naturally occurring compounds, have very low toxicities.

The second approach to this problem (decrease in the concentration of deoxy HbS) simply involves an increase in the oxygen affinity so that HbS binds to oxygen more tightly. The drug cyanate has been used in humans but produced toxic effects such as neuropathy and has been withdrawn. One possible solution would be to use this drug only with some type of extracorporeal procedure. Another way of attacking the deoxyhemoglobin is to increase the volume in the erythrocyte itself, as in creating hyponatremia. In one clinical trial, chronic hyponatremia has reduced (in nonpregnant patients) the frequency of painful crises. Unfortunately, this is an extreme form of therapy, with the potential for water intoxication, and probably would not be applicable except for the most severely affected patients. The most exciting modality in this group, however, is the induction of fetal HbF or hemoglobin A in patients with hemoglobinopathies.

It was first demonstrated, in 1982, that chemotherapeutic agents could stimulate the production of HbF (Ley et al, 1982). Since then, numerous cytotoxic drugs as well as erythropoietin have been under investigation. Most recently, hydroxynurea has been shown to augment HbF production with minimal toxicity (Charache et al, 1987). Another exciting possibility is induction of HbA synthesis from DNA inserted into the patient's bone marrow. Unfortunately, it is dif-

**Table 28–23**
PATIENT CARE SUMMARY FOR HEMOGLOBINPATHIES

| | Antepartum | | Intrapartum | Postpartum |
|---|---|---|---|---|
| | *Outpatient* | *Inpatient* | | |
| BP, P, R | q visit | Minimum q 4 h | q 1 h | On admission q 15 min × 4; then q 30 min × 2; then q 1 h until stable |
| T | q visit | Minimum q 4 h | q 4 h | On admission; then q 4 h |
| FHR | Weekly NST and CST | Weekly NST and CST | Continuous electronic fetal monitoring, preferably internal; if no monitor available, q 15 to 30 min in first stage, and q 5 min in second stage | — |
| Contractions | — | — | Continuous electronic monitoring; if no monitor available, q 1 h | Fundal checks on admission; then q 15 min × 4; then q 30 min × 2; then q 10 min until stable; then q 4 h |
| Lochia assessment | | | | Lochia checks with fundal checks |
| Laboratory values | | | | |
| Hemoglobin and hematocrit | q visit | Weekly | At onset of labor | On admission to RR; qid until discharge |
| Screening | First visit of all black and Mediterranean patients | — | — | — |
| Observation for signs of: Pulmonary complications Congestive heart failure Sickle cell crisis | q visit | q shift | q 1 h | q 1 h until stable; then q 4 h |
| Sonogram | As appropriate to rule out IUGR | | | |

Note: Nurse-to-patient ratio, 1 : 6 to 8 antepartum, 2 : 3 intrapartum, 1 : 6 to 8 postpartum.

BP = Blood pressure; CST = contraction stress test; FHR = fetal heart rate; IUGR = intrauterine growth retardation; NST = nonstress test; P = pulse; R = respiration; RR = recovery room; T = temperature.

ficult to extrapolate this technology to the gravid patient, because clinical trials continue in the nonpregnant patient with sickle cell disease. Genetic engineering to induce normal hemoglobin in persons with structurally deficient hemoglobin such as S and C could also be applied to those who produce less hemoglobin A than they should, such as patients with major thalassemia. Inherited disorders that were previously thought to be incurable may at last be eliminated.

In the category of agents that would act on the erythrocyte membrane, there are several drugs that inhibit the cell membrane from stiffening so that the cell becomes permanently sickled. Among these, cetiedil, a local anesthetic; zinc acetate; and thioridazine, a tranquilizer, have all been used with good results. Human studies are beginning in this area. Therefore, it is apparent that the near future may hold exciting potential treatment agents for those with sickle hemoglobinopathies.

## Diagnosis

An exciting development in the prenatal diagnosis of hemoglobinopathies is the analysis of fetal DNA. Techniques most recently applied to this analysis include restriction endonuclease mapping, linkage analysis of restriction fragment length polymorphisms, oligonucleotide probes, and polymerase chain reaction. DNA for these studies may be secured from (1) chorionic villus cells obtained by chorionic villus sampling, (2) amniotic fluid cells obtained by amniocentesis, and (3) leukocytes obtained by cordocentesis. In addition, prenatal diagnosis can be undertaken using ion exchange high pressure liquid chromatography (HPLC) and electrophoresis of fetal blood. Each of these techniques has advantages and disadvantages. However, techniques such as chorionic villous sampling and amniocentesis that offer earlier diagnosis obviously are advantageous for a couple with the propensity to produce a severely affected offspring. Clearly, then, the choice of continuation of the pregnancy or abortion would be open to the parents. Here again, education and diagnostic testing of the mother and father play very important roles.

The hemoglobinopathies can drastically affect the mother and fetus during gestation. Through aggressive prenatal care and cur-

rent as well as future therapeutic interventions, the risk of sickle cell and other major hemoglobinopathies has been reduced to a much lower level than in the past. Continued progress in this area is expected in the future.

A summary of patient care procedures in the management of hemoglobinopathies is presented in Table 28–23.

### Acknowledgment

Acknowledgment is given to Marcella L. McKay, RN, MSN, MEd, for her contribution to the first edition.

## References

*Disseminated Intravascular Coagulation*

Abdella TN, Sibai BM, Hays JM Jr, et al: Perinatal outcome in abruptio placentae. Obstet Gynecol 63:365, 1984.

Abildgaard CF: Recognition and treatment of intravascular coagulation. J Pediatr 74:163, 1968.

Acharya U, Lamont CAR, Cooper K: Group A beta-haemolytic streptococcus causing disseminated intravascular coagulation and maternal death. Lancet 1:595, 1988.

Al-Gailani F, Elias S, Simpson JL, et al: Fibrinopeptide A increases after chorionic villus sampling. Prenatal Diagnosis 7:557, 1987.

Bailey CDH, Newman C, Elinas SP, et al: Use of prostaglandin $E_2$ vaginal suppositories in intrauterine fetal death and missed abortion. Obstet Gynecol 45:110, 1975.

Bennett B, Ratnoff OD: The normal coagulation mechanism. Med Clin North Am 56:95, 1972.

Bick RL, et al: Disseminated Intravascular Coagulation: Etiology, Pathophysiology, Diagnosis, and Treatment. Medical Counterpoint, October, 1974, p 38–43.

Boisclair MD, Ireland H, Lane DA: Assessment of hypercoagulable states by measurement of activation fragments and peptides. Blood Rev 4:25, 1990.

Cohen E, Ballard CA: Consumptive coagulopathy associated with intra-amniotic saline instillation and the effect of intravenous oxytocin. Obstet Gynecol 43:300, 1974.

Colman RW, Robboy SJ, Minna JD: Disseminated intravascular coagulation: an approach. Am J Med 52:679, 1972.

Colman RW, Minna, JD, Robboy SJ: Disseminated intravascular coagulation: a problem in critical-care medicine. Heart Lung 3:789, 1974.

Corrigan JJ, Jordan CM: Heparin therapy in septicemia with disseminated intravascular coagulation. N Engl J Med 283:778, 1970.

Davie EW, Ratnoff OD: Waterfall sequence for intrinsic blood clotting. Science 145:1310, 1964.

Delee JB: A case of fatal hemorrhagic diathesis with premature detachment of the placenta. Am J Obstet 44:45, 1901.

Deykin D: The clinical challenge of disseminated intravascular coagulation. N Engl J Med 283:636, 1970.

Dodgson J, Martin J, Boswell J, et al: Probable amniotic fluid embolism precipitated by amniocentesis and treated by exchange transfusion. Br Med J 294:1322, 1987.

Finley BE: Acute coagulopathy in pregnancy. Med Clin North Am 73:723, 1989.

Gambino SR, Altman P: The FDP test. Lab 79, Jan/Feb, 1979, pp 34–36.

Gordon H, Pipe NGH: Induction of labor after intrauterine fetal death. A comparison between prostaglandin $E_2$ and oxytocin. Obstet Gynecol 45:44, 1975.

Guyton AC: Disseminated intravascular clotting. *In* Textbook of Medical Physiology, 5th ed. Philadelphia, WB Saunders Co, 1976, p 109.

Halmagyi DFJ, Starzecki B, Shearman RP: Experimental amniotic fluid embolism: mechanism and treatment. Am J Obstet Gynecol 84:251, 1962.

Kaplan AP, Castellino FJ, Collen D, et al: Molecular mechanisms of fibrinolysis in man. Thromb Hemostasis 39:263, 1978.

Karegaard M, Gennser G: Incidence and recurrence rate of abruptio placentae in Sweden. Obstet Gynecol 67:523, 1966.

Kavi J, Wise R: Group A beta-haemolytic streptococcus causing disseminated intravascular coagulation and maternal death. Lancet 1:993, 1988.

Larus RK, Penner A: Pathophysiology of disseminated intravascular coagulation in saline-induced abortion. Obstet Gynecol 48:353, 1976.

Lavery JP: When coagulopathy threatens the pregnant patient. Contemp Obstet Gynecol 20:191, 1982.

McGillick K: DIC: the deadly paradox. RN 42:41, 1982.

McNichol GP, Davis JA: Fibrinolytic enzymes system. Clin Haematol 2:23, 1973.

Naumann RO, Weinstein L: Disseminated intravascular coagulation—the clinician's dilemma. Obstet Gynecol Surv 40:487, 1985.

O'Brian BS, Woods S: The paradox of DIC. Am J Nurs 78:1878, 1978.

Ogston D: The protease inhibitors of blood coagulation, fibrinolysis and the complement system. Rec Adv Hematol 2:375, 1977.

Perez RH: Protocols for Perinatal Nursing Practice. St Louis, CV Mosby Co, 1981.

Phillips LL, Davidson EC: Procoagulant properties of amniotic fluid. Am J Obstet Gynecol 113:911, 1972.

Pritchard JA: Hematologic problems associated with delivery, placental abruption, retained dead fetus and amniotic fluid embolism. Clin Haematol 2:563, 1973.

Pritchard JA: Fetal death in utero. Obstet Gynecol 14:573, 1959.

Pritchard JA, Brekken AL: Clinical and laboratory studies on severe abruptio placentae. Am J Obstet Gynecol 97:681, 1967.

Pritchard JA, MacDonald PC: Williams Obstetrics, 16th ed. New York, Appleton-Century-Crofts, 1980.

Roberts JM, May JW: Consumptive coagulopathy in severe pre-eclampsia. Obstet Gynecol 48:163, 1976.

Salzman FW, Deykin D, Shapiro RM, et al: Management of heparin therapy. N Engl J Med 292:1046, 1975.

Sibai BM: The HELLP syndrome (hemolysis, elevated liver enzymes, and low platelets): much ado about nothing? Am J Obstet Gynecol 162:311, 1990.

Stander RW, Flessa HC, Gleuck HI, et al: Changes in maternal coagulation factors after intraamniotic injection of hypertonic saline. Obstet Gynecol 27:660, 1971.

Stefanini M: Disseminated intravascular coagulation: how to recognize an insidious culprit. Mod Med Feb 1974, pp 31–39.

Sutton DMC, Houser R, Kulapongs P, et al: Intravascular coagulation in abruptio placentae. Am J Obstet Gynecol 109:604, 1971.

Talbert LM, Blatt PM: Disseminated intravascular coagulation in obstetrics. Clin Obstet Gynecol 22:889, 1979.

Van Dam PA, Renier M, Baekelandt M, et al: Disseminated intravascular coagulation and the syndrome of hemolysis, elevated liver enzymes, and low platelets in severe preeclampsia. Obstet Gynecol 73:97, 1989.

Weiner CP: The obstetric patient and disseminated intravascular coagulation. Clin Perinatol 13:705, 1986.

Weiss AE, Esterling, WE, Odom MH, et al; Defibrination syndrome after intra-amniotic infusion of hypertonic saline. Am J Obstet Gynecol 113:868, 1972.

Wilde JT, Kitchen S, Kinsey S, et al: Plasma D-dimer levels and their relationship to serum fibrinogen/fibrin degradation products in hypercoagulable states. Br J Haematol 71:65, 1989.

Ziegel EE: Disseminated intravascular coagulation. *In* Ziegel EE, Van Blarcom CC: Obstetric Nursing, 7th ed. New York, Macmillan, 1979, p 638.

### Idiopathic (Autoimmune) Thrombocytopenic Purpura

Ahn YS, Harrington WJ: Treatment of idiopathic thrombocytopenic purpura. Ann Rev Med 28:299, 1977.

Abbott Laboratories: The Use of Blood. Chicago, 1971.

Aisner J: Platelet transfusion therapy. Med Clin North Am 61:1133, 1977.

American Association of Blood Banks: Blood Component Therapy, 2nd ed. 1975.

Angiulo J, Temple JT, Corrigan JJ, et al: Management of cesarean section in a patient with idiopathic thrombocytopenic purpura. Anesthesiology 46:145, 1977.

Aster RH: The immunologic thrombocytopenia. *In* Kunicki TJ, George E (eds): Platelet immunology. Philadelphia, JB Lippincott Co, 1989, p 387.

Ayromlooi J: A new approach to the management of idiopathic thrombocytopenic purpura in pregnancy. Am J Obstet Gynecol 130:235, 1978.

Baele G, Thiery M: Management of gravidas with idiopathic thrombocytopenic purpura. Am J Obstet Gynecol 130:248, 1978.

Baldini MG: Idiopathic thrombocytopenic purpura. N Engl J Med 274:1245, 1302, 1360, 1966.

Baldini MG: Idiopathic thrombocytopenic purpura and the ITP syndrome. Med Clin North Am 56:47, 1972.

Ballem PJ, Buskard N, Wittmann BK, et al: ITP in pregnancy: use of the bleeding time as an indicator for the treatment. Blut 59:132, 1989.

Besa EC, MacNab MW, Solan AJ, et al: High-dose intravenous IgG in the management of pregnancy in women with idiopathic thrombocytopenic purpura. Am J Hematol 18:373, 1985.

Branda RF, McCullough JJ, Tate DY, et al: Plasma exchange in the treatment of fulminant idiopathic (autoimmune) thrombocytopenic purpura. Lancet 1:688, 1978.

Branda RF, Moldow CF, McCullough JJ, et al: Plasma exchange in the treatment of immune disease. Transfusion 15:570, 1975.

Brennan MF, Rappeport JM, Maloney WC, et al: Correlation between response to corticosteroids and splenectomy for adult idiopathic thrombocytopenic purpura. Am J Surg 129:490, 1975.

Burke G, Casey C, Chamberlain P, et al: Refractory immune thrombocytopenic purpura in pregnancy managed with multiple courses of high dose immunoglobulin. Ir J Med Sci 158:69, 1989.

Burrows RF, Kelton JG: Incidentally detected thrombocytopenia in healthy mothers and their infants. N Engl J Med 319:142, 1988.

Bussel JB: Management of infants of mothers with immune thrombocytopenic purpura. J Pediatr 113:497, 1988.

Bussel JB: Intravenous immunoglobulin therapy for the treatment of idiopathic thrombocytopenic purpura. Prog Hemostasis Thrombosis 8:103, 1986.

Bussel JB, Cunningham-Rundles C, Abraham C: Intravenous treatment of autoimmune hemolytic anemia with very high dose gammaglobulin. Vox Sang 51:264, 1986.

Caplan SN, Berkman EM: Immunosuppressive therapy of idiopathic thrombocytopenic purpura. Med Clin North Am 60:971, 1976.

Carloss HW, McMillan R, Crosby WH: Management of women with immune thrombocytopenic purpura. JAMA 244:2756, 1980.

Cavanagh D: Clotting disorders in pregnancy. In Cavanagh D, Woods RF (eds): Obstetric Emergencies, 3rd ed. Philadelphia, JB Lippincott, 1982, p 7.

Chadd NA, Elwood PP, Gray OP: Coagulation defects in hypoxic full term newborn infants. Br Med J 4:516, 1971.

Cines DB, Schreiber AD: Immune thrombocytopenia use of Coombs' anti-globulin to detect platelet IgG and $C_3$. N Engl J Med 300:106, 1979.

Cines DB, Dusak B, Tomaski A, et al: Immune thrombocytopenic purpura and pregnancy. N Engl J Med 306:826, 1982.

Cines DB, Dusak B, Tomaski A, et al: Immune thrombocytopenia in pregnancy. Clin J Res 29:516A, 1981.

Cruickshank DP: Idiopathic thrombocytopenic purpura. In Quennan JT, Hobbins JC (eds): Protocols for High Risk Pregnancies. A contemporary Ob/Gyn book. Oradell, NJ, Medical Economics Co, 1982, p 89.

Davidson BN, Rayburn WF, Bishop RC, et al: Immunoglobulin therapy for autoimmune thrombocytopenia purpura during pregnancy. A report of two cases. J Reprod Med 32:107, 1987.

Dixon R, Rosse W, Ebbert L: Quantitative determination of antibody in idiopathic thrombocytopenic purpura. N Engl J Med 292:230, 1975.

Doan CA, Bouroucle BA, Wiseman BK: Idiopathic and secondary thrombocytopenic purpura. Clinical study and evaluation of 381 cases over a period of 28 years. Ann Intern Med 53:861, 1960.

Donner M, Aronsson S, Holmberg L, et al: Corticosteroid treatment of maternal ITP and risk of neonatal thrombocytopenia. Acta Paediatr Scand 76:369, 1987.

Fabris P, Quaini R, Coser P, et al: Successful treatment of a steroid-resistant form of idiopathic thrombocytopenic purpura in pregnancy with high doses of intravenous immunoglobulins. Acta Haematol 77:107, 1987.

Fainstat T: Cortisone-induced congenital cleft palate in rabbits. Endocrinol 55:502, 1954.

Fallon WW, Greene RW, Losner EL: the hemostatic defect in thrombocytopenia as studied by the use of ACTH and cortisone. Am J Med 13:12, 1952.

Flessa HC: Hemorrhagic disorders and pregnancy. Clin Obstet Gynecol 17:236, 1974.

Gernsheimer T, Stratton J, Ballem PJ, et al: Mechanisms of response to treatment in autoimmune thrombocytopenic purpura. N Engl J Med 320:974, 1989.

Gibson J, Laird PP, Joshua DE, et al: Very high dose intravenous gammaglobulin in thrombocytopenia of pregnancy. Aust N Z J Med 19:151, 1989.

Goldswerg H, Chediak J: Quantitative and qualitative platelet disorders that complicate pregnancy. J Reprod Med 19:205, 1977.

Goodhue PA, Evans T: Idiopathic thrombocytopenic purpura in pregnancy. Obstet Gynecol Surv 18:671, 1963.

Gounder MP, Baker D, Saletan S, et al: Intravenous gammaglobulin therapy in the management of a patient with idiopathic thrombocytopenic purpura and a warm autoimmune erythrocyte panagglutinin during pregnancy. Obstet Gynecol 67:741, 1986.

Gowda VJ, Appuzio J, Langer A, et al: Pregnancy complicated by refractory idiopathic thrombocytopenic purpura and diabetes mellitus. J Reprod Med 19:147, 1977.

Handin RI, Stossel TP: Effect of corticosteroid therapy on the phagocytosis of antibody-coated platelets. Blood 46:1016, 1975.

Harker LA, Finch CA: Thrombokinetics in man. J Clin Lab Invest 48:963, 1969.

Harrington WJ: Chronic idiopathic thrombocytopenic purpura. In The Blood Platelets, 1971, p 264.

Harrington WJ: Differential diagnosis and management of thrombocytopenia. Med Times 99:53, 1971b.

Harrington WJ, Sprague CC, Minnich V, et al: Demonstration of a thrombocytopenic factor in the blood of patients with thrombocytopenic purpura. J Lab Clin Med 38:1, 1951.

Hart D, Dunetz C, Nardi M, et al: An epidemic of maternal thrombocytopenia associated with elevated antiplatelet antibody. Am J Obstet Gynecol 154:878, 1986.

Heys RF: Childbearing and idiopathic thrombocytopenic purpura. J Obstet Gynecol Br Commonw 73:205, 1966.

Heys RF: Steroid therapy for idiopathic thrombocytopenic purpura during pregnancy. Obstet Gynecol 23:532, 1966.

Higby DJ, Cohen E, Holland JF, et al: The prophylactic treatment of a thrombocytopenic leukemic patients with platelets: a double blind study. Transfusion 14:440, 1974.

Hobbins JC, Grannun PA, Romero R, et al: Percutaneous umbilical blood sampling. Am J Obstet Gynecol 152:1, 1985.

Hoffman PC: Idiopathic thrombocytopenic purpura in pregnancy. Clin Perinatol 12:599, 1985.

Horger EO, Keane MWD: Platelet disorders in pregnancy. Clin Obstet Gynecol 22:843, 1979.

Imbach P, Barandum S, d'Apuzzo V: High dose intravenous gamma globulin for idiopathic thrombocytopenic purpura in childhood. Lancet 1:1228, 1981.

Imbach P, d'Appuzzo V, Hirt A, et al: High dose intravenous gamma globulin for idiopathic thrombocytopenic purpura in childhood. Lancet 1:1228, 1981.

Jones WR: Tissue-specific autoimmune diseases in pregnancy. Clin Obstet Gynecol 6:473, 1979.

Karpatkin M, Porges RF, Karpatkin S: Platelet counts in infants of women with autoimmune thrombocytopenia: effect of steroid administration to the mother. N Engl J Med 305:936, 1981.

Karpatkin S: Autoimmune thrombocytopenic purpura. Blood 56:329, 1980.

Karpatkin S, Gang SK, Freedman ML: Role of iron as a regulator of thrombopoiesis. Am J Med 57:521, 1974.

Karpatkin S, Lackner HL: Association of antiplatelet antibody with functional platelet disorders: autoimmune thrombocytopenic purpura, systemic lupus erythematosus and thrombopathia. Am J Med 59:599, 1975.

Karpatkin S, Strick N, Suskind GW: Detection of splenic anti-platelet antibody synthesis in idiopathic autoimmune thrombocytopenic purpura. Br J Med 23:167, 1972.

Katz FH, Duncan BR: Entry of prednisone into human breast milk. N Engl J Med 293:1154, 1975.

Kelemen E, Szalay F, Petefy M: Autoimmune (idiopathic) thrombocytopenic purpura in pregnancy and the newborn. Br J Obstet Gynaecol 85:239, 1978.

Kelton JG: Management of the pregnant patient with idiopathic thrombocytopenic purpura. Ann Int Med 99:796, 1983.

Kelton JG, Blanchette VS, Wilson WE, et al: Neonatal thrombocytopenia due to passive immunization: prenatal diagnosis and distinction between maternal platelet alloantibodies and autoantibodies. N Engl J Med 302:1401, 1980.

Kelton JG, Gibbons S: Autoimmune platelet destruction: idiopathic thrombocytopenia purpura. Semin Thromb Hemostas 8:83, 1982.

Kelton JG, Inwood MJ, Barr RM, et al: The prenatal prediction of thrombocytopenia in infants of mothers with clinically diagnosed immune thrombocytopenia. Am J Obstet Gynecol 144:449, 1982.

Kelton JG, Moore J, Gaudie J, et al: The development and evaluation of a serum assay for platelet bindable IgG (S-PBI IgG). J Lab Clin Med 98:272, 1981.

Kernoff LM, Malan E, Gunston R: Neonatal thrombocytopenia complicating autoimmune thrombocytopenia in pregnancy: evidence for transplacental passage of anti-platelet antibody. Ann Intern Med 90:55, 1979.

Kitzmiller JL: Autoimmune disorders: maternal, fetal and neonatal risks. Clin Obstet Gynecol 21:385, 1978.

Kohler PF, Farr RS: Elevation of cord over maternal IgG immunoglobulin: evidence for an active placental IgG transport. Nature 210:1070, 1966.

Kornstein M, Smith JR, Stockman JA III: Idiopathic thrombocytopenic purpura: mother and neonate. Ann Intern Med 92:128, 1980.

Lacey JV, Penner JA: Management of idiopathic thrombocytopenic purpura in the adult. Semin Thromb Hemostas 3:160, 1977.

Laningham JET: Platelet transfusion. Bull Lab Med Univ N Carolina, 1975, p 3.

Laros RK, Sweet RL: Management of idiopathic thrombocytopenic purpura during pregnancy. Am J Obstet Gynecol 122:182, 1975.

Ludomirski A, Weiner S: Percutaneous fetal umbilical blood sampling. Clin Obstet Gynecol 31:19, 1988.

Ludomirski A, Nemiroff R, Johnson A, et al: Percutaneous umbilical blood sampling: A new technique for prenatal diagnosis. J Reprod Med 32:276, 1987.

Machover-Reinisch J, Simon NG, Karow WG, et al: Prenatal exposure to prednisone in human and animal retards intrauterine growth. Science 202:436, 1978.

Marder VJ, Nusbacher J, Anderson FW: One-year follow-up of plasma exchange therapy in 14 patients with idiopathic thrombocytopenic purpura. Transfusion 21:291, 1981.

McMillan R: Chronic idiopathic thrombocytopenic purpura. N Engl J Med 304:1134, 1981.

McMillan R: The pathogenesis of immune thrombocytopenic purpura. CRC Crit Rev Clin Lab Sci 8:303, 1977.

McMillan R: Platelet-associated IgG: an assay of anti-platelet antibodies in immune thrombocytopenic purpura. Blood 46:1039, 1975.

McMillan R, Longmire RL, Tavassoli M, et al: In vitro platelet phagocytosis by splenic leukocytes in idiopathic thrombocytopenic purpura. N Engl J Med 290:249, 1974.

McMillan R, Longmire R, Yelenosky R: The effect of corticosteroids on human IgG synthesis. J Immunol 116:1592, 1976.

Minchinton RM, Dodd NJ, O'Brien H, et al: Autoimmune thrombocytopenia in pregnancy. Br J Haematol 44:451, 1980.

Moise KJ Jr, Carpenter RJ Jr, Cotton DB, et al: Percutaneous umbilical cord blood sampling in the evaluation of fetal platelet counts in pregnant patients with autoimmune thrombocytopenia purpura. Obstet Gynecol 72:346, 1988.

Moise KJ Jr, Cotton DB: Discordant fetal platelet counts in a twin gestation complicated by idiopathic thrombocytopenic purpura. Am J Obstet Gynecol 156:1141, 1987.

Morgan AD: An update on the clinical application of blood components. JSC Med Assoc 74:532, 1978.

Murray JM, Harris RE: The management of the pregnant patient with idiopathic thrombocytopenic purpura. Am J Obstet Gynecol 126:449, 1976.

Murray S, Gardner FH: Effect of storage temperature on maintenance of platelet viability—deleterious effect of refrigerated storage. N Engl J Med 280:1094, 1969.

Nelson W, Vaughan V, McKay R (eds): Textbook of Pediatrics, 11th ed. Philadelphia, WB Saunders Co, 1979, p 1416.

Nicolaides KH: Cordocentesis. Clin Obstet Gynecol 31:123, 1988.

Nicolaides KH, Rodect CH, Soothill PW, et al: Ultrasound guided sampling of umbilical cord and placental bleed to assess fetal well-being. Lancet 1:1065, 1986.

Noriega-Guerra L, Aviles-Miranda A, de la Cadena OA, et al: Pregnancy in patients with autoimmune thrombocytopenic purpura. Am J Obstet Gynecol 133:439, 1979.

Novak R, Williams J: Plasmapheresis in catastrophic complication of idiopathic thrombocytopenic purpura. J Pediatr 92:434, 1978.

Nydegger UE: New aspects of immunoglobulin treatment for idiopathic thrombocytopenic purpura. Plasma Ther Transfus Technol 9:83, 1988.

O'Reilly R, Taber B: Immunologic thrombocytopenic purpura and pregnancy. Obstet Gynecol 51:590, 1978.

Pearson HA, McIntosh S: Neonatal thrombocytopenia. Clin Haematol 7:111, 1978.

Perkins RP: Thrombocytopenia in obstetric syndromes: a review. Obstet Gynecol Surv 34:101, 1979.

Peterson O, Larson P: Thrombocytopenic purpura in pregnancy. Obstet Gynecol 4:454, 1954.

Pitkin RM: Autoimmune diseases in pregnancy. Semin Perinatol 1:161, 1977.

Robson HN, Davidson LSP: Purpura in pregnancy, with special reference to idiopathic thrombocytopenic purpura. Lancet 2:164, 1950.

Robson HN, Duttie JJR: Capillary resistance and adrenocortical activity. Br J Med 2:971, 1950.

Rogers TE: Thrombocytopenia in pregnancy following splenectomy. Am J Obstet Gynecol 78:806, 1959.

Rolbin SH, Abbott D, Musclow E, et al: Epidural anesthesia in pregnant patients with low platelet counts. Obstet Gynecol 71:918, 1988.

Romero R, Duffy TP: Platelet disorder in pregnancy. Clin Perinatol 7:327, 1980.

Rose VL, Gordon LI: Idiopathic thrombocytopenic purpura in pregnancy. Successful management with immunoglobulin infusion. JAMA 254:2626, 1985.

Rosse WF: Quantitative immunology of immune hemolytic anemia. II. The relationship of cell-bound antibody to hemolysis and the effect of treatment. J Clin Invest 50:734, 1971.

Sacher RA, King JC: Perinatal diagnosis of passive ITP;

use of percutaneous umbilical blood sampling (PUBS). Blut 59:128, 1989.

Samuels P, Bussel JB, Braitman LE, et al: Estimation of the risk of thrombocytopenia in the offspring of pregnant women with presumed immune thrombocytopenic purpura. N Engl J Med 323:229, 1990.

Samuels P, Tomaski A, Bussel J et al: The natural history of immune thrombocytopenic purpura in pregnancy. Proceedings of Ninth Annual Meeting of the Society of Perinatal Obstetricians, 1989, Abstract #11.

Schatz M, Patterson R, Zeitz S, et al: Corticosteroid therapy for the pregnant asthmatic patient. JAMA 233:804, 1975.

Schenker JG, Polishuk WZ: Idiopathic thrombocytopenia in pregnancy. Gynecologia 165:271, 1968.

Schlamoritz M: Membrane receptors in the specific transfer of immunoglobulins from mother to young. Immunol Communications 5:481, 1976.

Schmidt RE, Bodde V, Schafer G, et al: High-dose intravenous gammaglobulin for idiopathic thrombocytopenic purpura. Lancet 2:475, 1981.

Schreiber AD: Immunohematology. JAMA 248:1380, 1982.

Schulman NR, Marder VJ, Weinrack RS: Similarities between known antiplatelet antibodies and the factors responsible for thrombocytopenia in idiopathic purpura: physiologic, serologic and isotopic studies. Ann NY Acad Sci 124:499, 1965.

Scioscia AL, Grannum PAT, Copel JA, et al: The use of percutaneous umbilical blood sampling in immune thrombocytopenic purpura. Am J Obstet Gynecol 159:1066, 1988.

Scott JR: Fetal growth retardation associated with maternal administration of immunosuppressive drugs. Am J Obstet Gynecol 128:668, 1977.

Scott JR, Cruikshank DP, Kochenour NK, et al: Fetal platelet counts in the obstetric management of immunologic thrombocytopenic purpura. Am J Obstet Gynecol 136:495, 1980.

Scott JS: Immunological diseases in pregnancy. In Scott JS, Jones WJ (eds): Immunology of Human Reproduction. London, Academic Press, 1976, p 229.

Sitarz AL, Driscoll JM Jr, Wolff SA: Management of isoimmune neonatal thrombocytopenia. Am J Obstet Gynecol 124:39, 1976.

Smith MD, Smith DA, Fletcher M: Hemorrhage associated with thrombocytopenia in megaloblastic anemia. Br Med J 1:982, 1962.

Sprague CC, Harrington WJ, Lange RD et al: Platelet transfusions and the pathogenesis of ITP. JAMA 150:1193, 1952.

Stefanini M, Martino NB: Use of prednisone in the management of some hemorrhagic states. N Engl J Med 254:313, 1956.

Strother SV, Wagner AM: Prednisone in pregnant women with idiopathic thrombocytopenic purpura. N Engl J Med 319:178, 1988.

Suhrland LG, Anguilla ER, Weisberger AS: The effect of prednisone on circulating antibody formulation in animals immunized with human platelet antigen. J Lab Clin Med 51:724, 1958.

Taft EG: Apheresis in platelet disorders. Plasma Ther 2:181, 1982.

Taft E, et al: Apheresis in platelet disease states. In Kasprisin DO, Vaithianathan T: Proceedings of the Second Annual Apheresis Symposium. Chicago, 1981, p 138.

Tancer ML: Idiopathic thrombocytopenic purpura and pregnancy. Am J Obstet Gynecol 79:148, 1960.

Territo M, Finklestein J, Oh W, et al: Management of autoimmune thrombocytopenia in pregnancy and in the neonate. Obstet Gynecol 41:579, 1973.

Thompson RL, Moore RA, Hess CE et al: Idiopathic thrombocytopenic purpura: long-term results of treatment and the prognostic significance of response to corticosteroids. Arch Intern Med 13:730, 1972.

Tomiyama Y, Mizutani H, Tsubakio T, et al: High-dose intravenous IgG before delivery for idiopathic thrombocytopenic purpura: transplacental treatment of the fetus. Acta Haematol Jpn 50:890, 1987.

Van Leeuwen EF, von dem Borne AE, Oudesluijs-Murphy AM, Ras-Zeijlmans GJ: Neonatal alloimmune thrombocytopenia complicated by maternal autoimmune thrombocytopenia. Br Med J 281:27, 1980.

Veenhoven WA, van der Schans GS, Nieweg HO: Platelet antibodies in idiopathic thrombocytopenic purpura. Clin Exp Immunol 39:645, 1980.

Weir AB III, Poon M, McGowan EI: Plasma exchange in idiopathic thrombocytopenic purpura. Arch Intern Med 140:1101, 1980.

Wintrobe MM: Clinical Hematology, 7th ed. Philadelphia, Lea & Febiger, 1974, p 1071.

Wood L, Jacobs P: Emergency caesarian section and symptomatic immune thrombocytopenic purpura. Am J Hematol 31:67, 1989.

Zwaan FE, deKoning J, Eernisse JG: Idiopathic thrombocytopenic purpura. Neth J Med 17:140, 1974.

*Hemoglobinopathies*

Anyaegbunam A, Langer O, Brustman L, et al: The application of uterine and umbilical artery velocimetry to the antenatal supervision of pregnancies complicated by maternal sickle hemoglobinopathies. Am J Obstet Gynecol 159:544, 1988.

Baum KF, Dunn DT, Maude GH, et al: The painful crisis of homozygous sickle cell disease. A study of risk factors. Arch Intern Med 147:1231, 1987.

Boehm CD: Use of polymerase chain reaction for diagnosis of inherited disorders. Clin Chem 35:1843, 1989.

Charache S, Dover GJ, Moyer MA, et al: Hydroxyurea-induced augmentation of fetal hemoglobin production in patients with sickle cell anemia. Blood 69:109, 1987.

Charache S, Scott J, Niebyl J, et al: Management of sickle cell disease in pregnant patients. Am J Obstet Gynecol 55:407, 1980.

Cunningham FG, Pritchard JA, Mason R, et al: Prophylactic transfusion of normal red blood cells during pregnancy complicated by sickle cell hemoglobinopathy. Am J Obstet Gynecol 135:994, 1979.

Desforges JE, Warth J: The management of sickle cell disease in pregnancy. Clin Perinatol 1:385, 1974.

Fort AT, Morrison JC, Berreras L, et al: Counseling the patient with sickle cell disease about reproduction: pregnancy outcome does not justify the maternal risk. Am J Obstet Gynecol 11:324, 1971.

Foster HW: Managing sickle cell anemia in pregnant patients. Contemp Obstet Gynecol 16:21, 1980.

Freeman MG, Ruth GJ: SS disease and CC disease: obstetric considerations and treatment. Clin Obstet Gynecol 12:134, 1969.

Kan YW, Dozy AM: Antenatal diagnosis of sickle cell anemia by DNA analysis of amniotic fluid cells. Lancet 2:910, 1978.

Kazazian HH Jr, Phillips DG, Dowling CE, et al: Prenatal diagnosis of sickle cell anemia—1988. Ann New York Acad Sci 565:44, 1989.

Keeling MM, Lavery JP, Clemons AU et al: Red cell exchange in the pregnancy complicated by a major hemoglobinopathy. Am J Obstet Gynecol 138:185, 1980.

Key TC, Horger EO, Walker EM, et al: Automated erythrocytopheresis for sickle cell anemia during pregnancy. Am J Obstet Gynecol 138:731, 1980.

Klotz IM, Haney DN, King LC: Rational approaches to chemotherapy: antisickling agents. Science 213:724, 1981.

Koshy M, Burd L, Wallace D, et al: Prophylactic red-cell transfusions in pregnant patients with sickle cell disease. N Engl J Med 319:1447, 1988.

Kramer MS, Rooks Y, Johnston D, et al: Accuracy of cord blood screening for sickle hemoglobinopathies. JAMA 241:139, 1979.

Ley TJ, DeSimone J, Anagnou NP, et al: 5-Azacytidine selectively increases $\beta$-globin synthesis in a patient with $\beta$ thalassemia. N Engl J Med 307:1469, 1982.

Martin JN Jr, Morrison JC: Sickle cell crisis: recognizing it and treating it. Contemp Obstet Gynecol 20:171, 1982.

Martin JN Jr, Martin RW, Morrison JC: Acute management of sickle cell crisis in pregnancy. Clin Perinatol 13:853, 1986.

Maugh TH: Sickle cell (II): many agents near trials. Science 211:468, 1981.

Miller JM, Horger ED, Key TC, et al: Management of sickle cell hemoglobinopathies in pregnant patients. Am J Obstet Gynecol 141:37, 1981.

Moore ML: Realities in Childbearing, 2nd ed. Philadelphia, WB Saunders Co, 1983.

Morrison JC: Anemia associated with pregnancy. In Sciarra JJ (eds): Gynecology and Obstetrics, Vol. 3. New York, Harper & Row, 1981, pp 1–38.

Morrison JC: Hemoglobinopathies and pregnancy. Clin Obstet Gynecol 22:819, 1979.

Morrison JC, Propst MG, Blake PG: Sickle hemoglobin and the gravid patient: a management controversy. Clin Perinatol 7:273, 1980a.

Morrison JC, Douvas SG, Martin JN, et al: Erythrocytopheresis in pregnant patients with sickle hemoglobinopathies. Obstet Gynecol 149:912, 1984.

Morrison JC, Schneider JM, Whybrew WD, et al: Prophylactic transfusions in pregnant patients with sickle hemoglobinopathies: benefit versus risk. Obstet Gynecol 56:274, 1980b.

Morrison JC, Wiser WL: The use of prophylactic partial exchange transfusion in pregnancies associated with sickle cell hemoglobinopathies. Obstet Gynecol 48:516, 1976.

Neal-Cooper F, Scott RB: Genetic counseling in sickle cell anemia: experiences with couples at risk. Public Health Rep 103:174, 1988.

Pearson HA: A neonatal program for sickle cell anemia. Adv Pediatr 33:381, 1986.

Pearson HA: Neonatal testing for sickle cell diseases—a historical and personal review. Pediatrics 83:815, 1989.

Perkins RP: Inherited disorders of hemoglobin synthesis and pregnancy. Am J Obstet Gynecol 111:120, 1971.

Perry KG Jr, Morrison JC: Red blood cell disorders. In Gleicher N (ed): Principles of Medical Therapy in Pregnancy, 2nd ed. New York, Plenum, 1990.

Perry KG Jr, Morrison JC: The diagnosis and management of hemoglobinopathies during pregnancy. Semin Perinatol 14:90, 1990.

Posey YF, Shah D, Ulm JE, et al: Prenatal diagnosis of sickle cell anemia. Hemoglobin electrophoresis versus DNA analysis. Am J Clin Pathol 92:347, 1989.

Powars DR, Sandhu M, Niland-Weiss J, et al: Pregnancy in sickle cell disease. Obstet Gynecol 67:217, 1986.

Rouyer-Fessard P, Plassa F, Blouquit Y, et al: Prenatal diagnosis of haemoglobinopathies by ion exchange HPLC of haemoglobins. Prenatal Diagnosis 9:19, 1989.

Tuck SM, James CE, Brewster EM, et al: Prophylactic blood transfusion in maternal sickle cell syndromes. Br J Obstet Gynaecol 94:121, 1987.

# CHAPTER 29

# Additional Medical Complications in Pregnancy

Charles J. Ingardia and Elizabeth Frances Pitcher

Pregnancy causes or aggravates many medical conditions in addition to those presented in the preceding chapters. Some of its effects can be minor; others may cause major difficulties for parturient patients. Some of the more frequently observed medical complications are presented in this chapter.

## Rh Isoimmunization

### Rh ANTIGEN AND SENSITIZATION

Although the actual structure of the Rh antigen is still unclear, unlike the A and B antigens, its presence is confined to the surface of red blood cells (RBCs). The genetic locus for the Rh antigen is on the short arm of chromosome number 1, but the actual number of genes controlling Rh expressivity as well as the number of Rh antigens is unclear. There have been several systems proposed for their nomenclature, the Fischer-Race concept being the most popular. In this model, there are three closely linked genes and their alleles controlling antigenic variation (Dd, Cc, Ee) (Race, 1948).

In this concept, all alleles (except for "d") have a corresponding distinct cell surface antigen. The frequency of distribution of these antigens varies, with geographic and racial differences noted. CeDe, CDe, and cde are the most common antigenic arrangements and are present in 35, 20, and 16 percent of the population, respectively. The presence

of D determines Rh positivity, whether in a homozygous or heterozygous individual. Each of the other Rh antigens is capable of engendering a specific antibody reaction (i.e., anti-e), but multiple antibody reactions can be observed, particularly if anti-D is present.

An Rh-negative individual is at risk when exposed to Rh-positive RBCs. Two major determinants affect the risk of sensitization: the volume of Rh-positive cells transfused (i.e., transplacental hemorrhage) and the ABO compatibility status of mother and infant. As little as 0.1 to 0.25 ml of Rh-positive blood can engender an immune response.

Following exposure to Rh-positive antigen, an initial response of primarily gamma M immunoglobulin (IgM) (saline reacting) is followed by a gamma G immunoglobulin (IgG) antibody (albumin reacting) response. The IgG antibody produced is of the $IgG_1$ and $IgG_3$ subclasses. Immune suppression appears to be effective until the appearance of the IgG response. A secondary immune response can be elicited with a very small transplacental hemorrhage (0.1 ml) (Bowman, 1978).

By 6 months, up to 8 percent of exposed Rh-negative individuals will have a detectable antibody response. In another 8 to 10 percent of exposed Rh-negative individuals, however, the antibody response may only be detectable in a subsequent pregnancy when the fetus is Rh-positive. The overall risk then of an ABO-compatible pregnancy of Rh immunization following delivery is approximately 16 to 17 percent.

## Tests to Detect
## Transplacental Hemorrhage

**Acid Elution (Kleihauer-Betke) Test.** Fetal RBCs are detected by adding an acid buffer, which causes adult hemoglobin (HbA) to leave the RBC membrane, leaving ghost cells. Fetal hemoglobin (hemoglobin F, or HbF), however, is resistant to this acid elution and remains intact. Fetal RBCs then can be distinguished from maternal RBCs on smear (Fig. 29–1).

Although fetal hemoglobin can almost always be assumed to be from RBCs, persistent HbF exists in about 2 percent of the population and has been associated with a false-positive acid elution test in a patient transfused with blood from such an individual.

The fetomaternal bleed can be calculated using the following formula:

$$\frac{\dfrac{\text{number of fetal RBCs}}{\text{number of maternal RBCs}} \times (\text{ml FMH})}{\text{estimated maternal blood volume (ml)}} =$$

**Other Tests.** Other tests that can be used to detect fetomaternal hemorrhage (FMH) are the Fetaldex test, alpha fetoprotein test, microscopic Du test, Rho-gam cross match test, and enzyme-linked antiglobulin test (ELAT).

## ABO Incompatibility

The presence of ABO-incompatible blood decreases the risks of sensitization, probably owing to removal of fetal RBCs from maternal circulation at a faster rate or to sequestration of fetal RBCs at a site in the maternal reticuloendothelial system (e.g., liver) where recognition lymphocytes are scarce. Both anti-A and anti-B are complement fixing; therefore, intravascular hemolysis of fetal RBCs occurs with destruction of the Rh antigen.

It has been demonstrated by Bowman (1978) that the risk of Rh sensitization with ABO incompatibility between mother and infant is about 2 percent. In ABO-compatible pregnancies, the risk is 16 to 17 percent. Other influences of sensitization are paternal genotype (homozygous or heterozygous) and fetal genotype (Rh antigenic position affects antigenicity).

## ERYTHROBLASTOSIS FETALIS

### Pathogenesis

The basic pathogenetic process in erythroblastosis fetalis is the destruction of fetal Rh-positive erythrocytes by maternal anti-D (IgG) antibody. The mechanism of hemolysis is not completely understood. It is known that anti-D (mostly $IgG_1$ and $IgG_3$) can activate the complement cascade but cannot fix complement; therefore, direct erythrolytic activity is unlikely. Most IgG-tagged red blood cells are hemolyzed through the extravascular phagocytic system in the spleen.

The resultant fetal anemia leads to an increased production of erythropoietin and eventual extramedullary erythropoiesis in the liver and spleen, resulting in enlargement

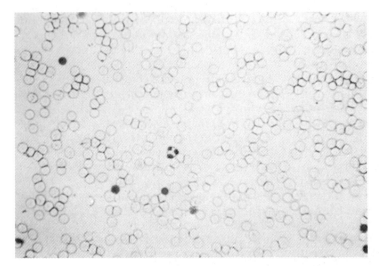

**Figure 29–1.** Acid elution smear depicting fetal RBCs and maternal "ghost" RBCs. (From Scott JR, and Warenski, JC: Tests to detect and quantitate fetomaternal bleeding. Clin Obstet Gynecol 25:279, 1982.)

of these organs. Immature RBC erythroblasts are released into the circulation. Further progression leads to extensive erythropoiesis with enlargement and distortion of liver parenchyma. Although it was once believed that myocardial failure was primarily related to the anasarca and ascites associated with erythroblastosis fetalis, it is more likely the result of increased portal hypertension due to hepatosplenomegaly. Fetal edema is further complicated by fetal hypoproteinemia due to decreased hepatic protein synthetic function. Some authors have found that hydropic fetuses have a total protein concentration of less than 3 g/dl and albumin levels less than 2 g/dl (Grannum and Copel, 1988). This increased portal hypertension is probably also related to the increase in placental edema and hypertrophy (placentomegaly) characteristic of the disease. The placental enlargement probably alters the flow of oxygen and nutrients across the placental bed and, along with the significant anemia, places the fetus at risk for hypoxia and fetal demise.

### Ultrasound Detection

Sonographic analysis of sensitized pregnancies, although not as sensitive as either direct HbF analysis or spectrophotometric analysis of amniotic fluid bilirubin, can be a helpful adjunct in the management of erythroblastosis. Ultrasonographic changes consistent with hydrops fetalis include polyhydramnios, placental enlargement, and fetal hepatosplenomegaly. Also observed is the presence of fetal ascites, pleural effusion, and pericardial effusion. Unfortunately, abdominal circumference and umbilical vein diameter do not appear to be useful in predicting the degree of anemia (Nicolaides et al, 1988).

### Antibody Detection

Antibodies can be detected in several ways.

**Saline Agglutination.** If Rh-positive RBCs are suspended in isotonic saline, they will not agglutinate if anti-D is added to the solution. The RBC membranes lie relatively too far to be bridged by the IgG antibody (160,000 mw). IgM, however, can bridge this gap owing to its larger molecular size (900,000 mw). The absence of agglutination

in saline, then, cannot rule out significant anti-D (IgG) production.

**Albumin Agglutination.** With the addition of a 22 percent bovine albumin solution, the RBC membranes are aligned closer and, subsequently, agglutinate and hemolyze when anti-D (IgG) or anti-D (IgM) is added. The presence of a negative saline agglutination and a positive albumin agglutination indicates an anti-D (IgG) response.

**Antiglobulin Testing (Indirect Coombs' Test).** The introduction of anti-human globulin (produced by rabbits, goats, and so on) to a suspension of known washed Rh-positive RBCs mixed with the patient's serum, which has anti-D antibody, agglutinates those RBCs (positive indirect Coombs'). This indirect method for testing for RBC antibody is very sensitive. Other techniques include enzyme-treated RBCs and autoanalyzer analysis.

## NURSING CONSIDERATIONS

Perinatal nurses collaborate with the physician in explaining disease process, therapy, and need for frequent monitoring of fetus. Communicate parameters to be measured and normal values (see Table 29–1). Explain indications for administration of RhoGAM including implication for subsequent pregnancies.

### Evaluation and Management

**Use of Titers.** The Rh-negative patient who is identified by initial prenatal laboratory analysis should have an associated antibody screen test performed to rule out the presence of anti-D antibody. Even if the antibody screen is initially negative, it must be repeated at 20, 24, 28, 32, and 36 weeks, because in one half of sensitized women, the antibody cannot be detected until the subsequent pregnancy. Negative titers at these weeks warrant no further investigation.

Once a positive anti-D titer is obtained, the paternal blood type should be obtained. If he is Rh positive, an attempt to determine zygosity should be made. If he has fathered Rh-negative children, he is clearly a heterozygote (Dd+), and there is a 50 percent chance of the fetus being Rh positive. If he is homozygous (DD), it can be assumed the fetus is Rh positive, and a series of spectro-

**Table 29–1**

PATIENT CARE SUMMARY FOR Rh ISOIMMUNIZATION*

| | Antepartum | | Intrapartum | Postpartum |
|---|---|---|---|---|
| | *Outpatient* | *Inpatient* | | |
| BP, P, R | Each visit | q 8 h (if normal, BP may be deleted during the night) | q 1h | On admission to RR: q 15 min × 4; then q 30 min × 2; then q 1 h until stable On postpartum floor: q 4 h |
| T | Same as above | Same as above | q 4 h | Same as above |
| FHR | Weekly NST and CST starting at 32 weeks | Weekly NST and CST starting at 32 weeks | Continuous electronic fetal monitoring, preferably internal; if no monitor available, q 15 min in first stage and q 5 min in 2nd stage | — |
| Contractions | Each visit | q shift | Continuous electronic fetal monitoring, preferably internal; if no monitor available, q 1 h by palpation | Fundal checks and lochia assessment same as BP, P, R |
| Laboratory studies Rh titers | 20, 24, 28, 32, and 36 weeks | 20, 24, 28, 32, and 36 weeks | Collect cord and maternal blood at time of delivery to assess need for RhoGAM | — |
| Amniocentesis | Performed at any maternal titer or critical titer as established by your laboratory | | — | — |
| Sonograms | At 24 weeks (dating ultrasound plus R/O hydropic changes); then q 3–4 weeks to detect early hydropic changes | | | |
| RhoGAM administration | At 28 weeks and postamnio for nonsensitized women | — | — | Given within 72 h after delivery to Rh-negative mothers with Rh-positive babies |

*Nurse-to-patient ratio: *Antepartum,* 1:6 to 8; *intrapartum with fetal distress,* 1:1; *intrapartum without fetal distress,* 2:3; *postpartum,* 1:6 to 8.

BP = Blood pressure; CST = contraction stress test; FHR = fetal heart rate; NST = nonstress test; P = pulse; R = respiration; T = temperature.

photometric amniotic fluid evaluations should be instituted. The Rh-paternal genotype may be helpful in determining zygosity in fetuses in which the father is known to be heterozygous for the D-antigen (Bowman, 1980). Percutaneous umbilical fetal blood analysis of Rh type can help evaluate which fetuses need serial spectrophotometric analysis.

Queenan (1977) and Bowman (1981), in reviewing the relationship between antibody titers and perinatal outcome, found a relationship between titers and outcome only if pregnancy represented the "first immunized pregnancy," i.e., one characterized by a negative antibody titer at the initial visit with subsequent detection of anti-D antibody. Previous history should be negative for stillbirths or previous infants that required ex-change transfusion. In Bowman's experience with titers of less than 1:8 (Queenan: < 1:32), no intrauterine death has occurred. These patients are not followed by serial amniocentesis but, rather, have serial antibody titers performed every 3 to 4 weeks. If a rise over this critical titer occurs, spectrophotometric analysis of amniotic fluid bilirubin is performed.

If the patient has anti-D antibody on initial screen or has a previously affected infant, titers alone are not predictive of outcome. An important point to remember is that each laboratory must determine its own critical titer. With the general decline in Rh immunization, some authors conclude it is impossible for most laboratories to develop their own critical titer. Even in the first Rh-isoimmunized pregnancy, the presence of an

Rh-positive fetus can be associated with severe involvement in up to 20 percent of cases.

At the present time, then, it is clear that spectrophotometric analysis of amniotic fluid for bilirubin pigment remains the most important index of severity of fetal hemolytic involvement.

**Spectrophotometric Analysis.** This technique was pioneered by Liley and is based on the measurement of the deviation, or peak, produced by bilirubin pigment in amniotic fluid at 450 mU on the spectra absorption curve. The values are plotted on semilogarithmic paper, with wave length as the linear horizontal coordinate and optical density as the vertical coordinate (see Fig. 29–2).

Timing of the initial analysis can be based on both previous pregnancy history and serial antibody titers. With previous severely affected neonates or stillbirths, the initial analysis may be performed as early as 22 to 24 weeks. A sudden increase in titer level over previous values also may indicate an earlier analysis. With the typical presentation of a patient with no previously affected children but with a significant but stable anti-D titer, the initial amniocentesis is performed at 24 to 28 weeks. Subsequent analyses are gauged by the result of spectrophotometric examination and usually range from 1 to 3 weeks but may be repeated as early as 5 days following the previous amniocentesis. Declining trends allow for spacing every 3 weeks. This spacing allows for the bilirubin trend to be clearly revealed and removes the likelihood that spectrophotometric distortion has occurred because of an amniotic fluid blood contamination from the previous tap. Sources of error in interpretation include:

- Blood (peak 415 mU)
- Meconium (peak at 410 to 415 mU)
- Polyhydramnios (fall in Δ OD 450 values)
- Light (reduction in Δ OD 450 values)
- Congenital anomalies (evaluation of values)

*Liley's Zone Method.* In 1961, Liley (1961) reported on a method of amniotic fluid spectrophotometric analysis that offered ongoing evaluation of fetal hemolysis using bilirubin absorption curves plotted against gestational age. Liley demonstrated in over 100 cases that the trend in normal pregnancy is declining levels toward term. He subdivided these trends into three prediction zones (Fig. 29–2). Declining levels into zone 1 heralded no *in utero* mortality and, generally, little fetal involvement. Increasing trends into zone III indicated an ominous prognosis with severe hydrops fetalis or fetal death, occurring in 7 to 10 days. Zone II values needed to be followed closely to determine whether they would move into zones I or III. The zone boundaries decline as the gestation advances. The significance of a normal trend is that values that are initially in high zone II but plateau on serial examination move into zone III with advancing gestational age. With regard to singular values, extremely high (> 0.28 to 0.30) or extremely low (< 0.02) values may be helpful in predicting outcome, but only after sequential sampling do trends emerge that more adequately anticipate fetal and neonatal status.

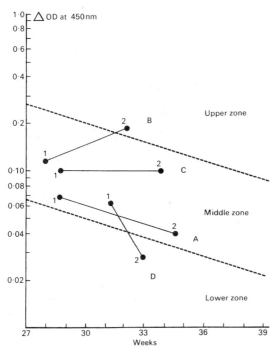

**Figure 29–2.** Liley's prediction zones. *A*, Usual reduction in Δ OD 450 results with advancing gestational age. *B*, Upward trend indicating severe hemolytic involvement. *C*, Plateauing of Δ OD 450 results, indicating need to intervene because the normal fall with gestational age is not seen—indicates moderate to severe involvement. *D*, Steeply falling values indicate unaffected or mildly affected neonate. (From Whitfield CR: Amniotic fluid analysis. *In* Beard RW, and Nathanielsz PW [eds]: Fetal Physiology and Medicine. London, WB Saunders Co Ltd, 1976, p 333.)

Three basic trends emerge in serial evaluation. Rising values into zone III or the upper 20 percent of zone II indicate significant fetal involvement and the need for intervention. With significant prematurity (< 30 weeks), this intervention should be intrauterine transfusion. Once evidence of pulmonary lung maturity is obtained, delivery should be accomplished. Plateauing values can be watched without intervention with serial analysis unless they enter zone III or upper zone II; treatment is similar to that used for rising values. Declining values can be watched until term with serial analysis. A recent review suggests that all patients with evidence of anti-D production be delivered by 38 weeks, because some morbidity can occur even with very low Δ OD 450 values.

***Whitfield's Action Line Method.*** Whitfield and coworkers (1968), in their analysis of 641 spectrophotometric values during a 3-year period, proposed a curve action line, which delineated at any one point in gestation when intervention is mandatory (Fig. 29–3). In general, the action line follows Liley's zone III and zone II border until about 34 weeks, when it drops into zone II range. If the Δ OD 450 remains less than 0.035, the pregnancy is allowed to continue until term.

In Whitfield's original series, intrauterine transfusion was performed if the action line was crossed (or extrapolated to be crossed) at less than 33 weeks' gestational age. Beyond 33 weeks, delivery was accomplished when the action line was crossed.

More recent advances in the care of the premature infant and the availability of more sophisticated methods of diagnosis and therapy (i.e., percutaneous blood sampling and ultravascular transfusions) have allowed intervention at an earlier gestational age. Some have questioned, however, the validity of extrapolation of Liley's curves to lengths of gestation between 16 and 25 weeks. The limitation of spectrophotometric analysis has led one author to suggest that direct fetal hemoglobin analysis is the only accurate method of determining fetal anemia in the second trimester. (Nicolaides et al, 1986)

**Intrauterine Transfusion.** Since Liley introduced the technique of intrauterine transfusion in 1963, many refinements have been proposed to reduce the risks involved. The goal of intrauterine transfusion is the deposition of unsensitized (Rh-negative) packed RBCs into the fetal peritoneal cavity. There, they are taken up by the subdiaphragmatic lymphatics and eventually deposited into the intravascular compartment. These unsensitized RBCs help correct severe fetal anemia and help to postpone the onset of hydropic changes associated with poor prognosis.

***Intrauterine Intravascular Transfusion.*** The introduction of high-resolution ultrasound in the early 1980s has allowed for more direct access to fetal circulation for both diagnosis and therapeutic purposes. Rodeck and Nicolaides (1983) introduced fetoscopically directed intravascular transfusion. The percutaneous technique has been described by several authors (deCrespigny et al, 1985; Grannum et al, 1986).

Two basic techniques have been described: (1) simple and (2) exchange transfusion. Although exchange transfusions may have an advantage in the terminally ill hydropic fetus, most centers use simple transfusion.

The site of transfusion may be cord insertion to the placenta, cord insertion to the fetus, mid cord loop, hepatic vein portion of umbilical cord, and rarely, cardiac puncture. Most centers use the placental cord insertion

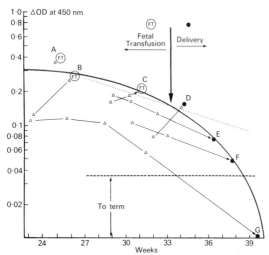

**Figure 29–3.** Whitfield's "action line." When Δ OD 450 results cross or are extrapolated to be crossed, intervention is mandatory. If this crossing occurs at less than 33 weeks, fetal intrauterine transfusion (FIT) is performed. If over 34 weeks, delivery is indicated. The horizontal broken line indicates initial Δ OD 450 value of 0.035 mu (no serial amniocentesis is performed). (From Whitfield CR: Amniotic fluid analysis. *In* Beard RW and Nathanielsz PW [eds]: Fetal Physiology and Medicine. London, WB Saunders Co Ltd 1976, p 334.)

site, the fetal cord insertion site, or both. The mother is medicated with a tocolytic agent and, occasionally, a mild tranquilizer. A 22-g or 20-g needle is introduced under direct ultrasound guidance, and the umbilical vein is entered. A medication to induce fetal paralysis is given (0.1 mg/kg EFW of pancuronium bromide). A fetal hematocrit is obtained. Washed, irradiated, 0-negative packed RBCs, with high hematocrit (85 to 90 percent) and screened for human immunodeficiency virus (HIV) and cytomegalovirus (CMV) contamination, are prepared. The quantity of blood to be transfused can be calculated by the following formula:

V = Estimated normal blood volume (160 ml/kg EFW)
Hct 1 = Pretransfusion Hct
Hct 2 = Hct of transfused blood
Hct 3 = Desired Hct (usually 35 to 45 percent)

$$\frac{V \, (Hct \, 3 - Hct \, 1)}{Hct \, 2} = \text{ml blood to be transfused}$$

It is important to check the hematocrit approximately half to two thirds of the way through the procedure. Nonstress testing (NST), biophysical assessment, or both should be performed both prior to and after the transfusion.

In most series, repeat transfusions are performed at 2-to-3 week intervals. Knowledge of the previous intervals is helpful in planning the next appropriate interval between transfusions. A 1 percent daily drop in fetal Hct has been shown in one center (Grannum and Copel, 1988) and may be helpful in guiding repeat timing of transfusion and timing of delivery.

*Complications.* Complications observed in association with intravascular transfusion include chorioamnionitis (Grannum and Copel, 1988), fetal distress and death (Seeds, 1989), cord puncture and hematoma (Keckstein et al, 1990; Moise et al, 1987), fetomaternal hemorrhage, and failed procedure.

## NURSING CONSIDERATIONS

In collaboration with the physician, supply information regarding intrauterine transfusion, if required. Explain use of ultrasound during procedure and assessment of fetus with NST following.

## SUPPLEMENTAL ANTEPARTUM TESTING IN Rh ISOIMMUNIZATION

### NST and OCT

Routine antepartum fetal heart rate monitoring should be performed from 32 weeks until delivery in the Rh-sensitized pregnant patient. The frequency of testing should be based, in part, on the degree of fetal involvement suspected by Δ OD 450 analysis. An NST should be performed twice a week when values place the fetus in upper zone II or zone III or if there is a rising trend in values. With declining levels, the NST may be performed weekly. All nonreactive NSTs should be followed by an oxytocin challenge test (OCT), a biophysical assessment, or both.

The presence of a sawtooth or sinusoidal fetal heart rate pattern (Fig. 29–4) has been described in the fetus with erythroblastosis (Baskett and Koh, 1974; Freeman et al, 1991). It also has been reported with fetal acidosis, alphaprodine administration, and acute fetal anemias (Gray et al, 1978; Modanlou et al, 1977). The presence of a persistent sinusoidal fetal heart rate pattern in an Rh-sensitized pregnancy indicates significant anemia and mandatory intervention.

### Biophysical Assessment

This modality of assessing fetal well-being by determining the presence of fetal breathing, fetal tone, amniotic fluid volume, and gross body movement along with the NST has proved to be helpful in predicting fetal hypoxemia. It has not been studied extensively in isoimmunized pregnancies, although fetal movement has been observed in the presence of fetal anemia (Parer, 1988).

### Doppler Velocimetry

Doppler flow-velocity waveform appears to be helpful in predicting fetal Hct in Rh-sensitized pregnancies. Kirkinen and associates (1983) studied 18 fetuses and demonstrated that an inverse relationship exists between cord hematocrit and umbilical blood flow. This increase in flow in fetal anemia is probably due to increase flow velocity. Other authors (Copel et al, 1988; Rightmire et al, 1986) also have demonstrated the accuracy of this modality in predicting fetal anemia.

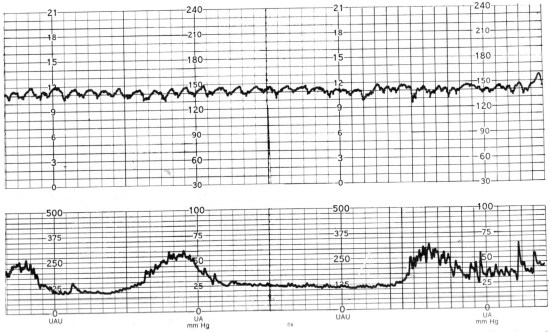

**Figure 29–4.** Sinusoidal heart rate pattern. (From Veren D, Boehm FH, and Killam AP: The clinical significance of sinusoidal fetal heart rate pattern associated with alphaprodine administration. J Reprod Med 27:412, 1982.)

There is no consensus, however, on the value of following fetuses post-transfusion and whether or not Doppler velocimetry can be useful in determining transfusion interval.

# Rh-IMMUNE GLOBULIN (RhIg) IN TREATMENT OF Rh ISOIMMUNIZATION

## The Remaining Problems

It has become clear that although RhIg has reduced sensitization, certain problems remain that have prevented its total elimination. The major problems of underuse and inadequate dosage still need to be corrected. Another unproven theory, the grandmother theory, asserts that the Rh-negative female infant is sensitized by Rh-positive blood from her mother at birth (Taylor, 1967). More important is the issue of antenatal sensitization that occurs during the course of normal pregnancy owing to accidental breaks in the feto-maternal circulation, allowing Rh-positive fetal RBCs to enter the maternal circulation. The majority (> 95 percent) of these breaks occur in the last trimester (Bowman, 1978). This transplacental leak prior to delivery is,

for the most part, silent and goes undetected by the usual means of acid elution testing.

## Routine Antenatal Use

If accidental breaks in placental circulation occur regularly, with the antenatal transfusion of fetal RBCs accounting for up to 2 percent of cases of Rh sensitization, then routine antenatal administration of RhIg prior to the third trimester can eliminate this problem. A clinical triad of antenatal RhIg prophylaxis in Canada (300 μg at 28 and 34 weeks' gestation) (Bowman, 1978) was followed by a trial of only one dose (300 μg at 28 weeks' gestation), with equal efficacy (Bowman, 1978). If, at delivery, the infant is found to be Rh positive, another injection is given. It is apparent that RhIg reduces the incidence of antenatal sensitization by 93 percent.

## Du Variant

About 3 to 5 percent of Rh-negative mothers are Du-positive (variant). Because the Du factor represents an incomplete D antigen, its antigenicity and ability to produce anti-D are also variable. Hemolytic disease of the newborn has been reported in a Du variant infant born to an Rh-sensitized, Rh-negative mother (Lacey, 1978). Conversely, an Rh-negative, Du-positive, Coombs-negative mother who delivers an Rh-positive fetus runs the risk, albeit small, for full anti-D sensitization and antibody production (Hill et al, 1974).

Another problem that may arise is the detection of the Du factor. In the postpartum period, enough fetal blood from an Rh-positive fetus may enter maternal circulation to modify the interpretation of her Rh status. In these circumstances, the Rh-negative woman with a large fetomaternal hemorrhage from an Rh-positive fetus is inaccurately classified as Du-positive. If these mothers are then mistakenly assumed to be genetically Du-positive, RhIg is often withheld. Unfortunately, it is these mothers with the large transplacental hemorrhage who are at even higher risk of being sensitized. These problems could be eliminated by routine administration of RhIg to all Rh-negative, Du-positive mothers or those mothers found to be only Du-positive in the postpartum period. In mothers found to be Du-positive after delivery, the volume of fetomaternal bleeding should be determined.

## Atypical Antibodies

With the development of prophylactic immune globulin, the incidence of hemolytic disease of the newborn has declined dramatically. Although 98 percent of all hemolytic disease of the newborn is related to the Rh antigen, approximately 2 percent is due to antibody produced by other blood group antigens, the so-called irregular or atypical antibodies. Sources of sensitization are similar to those of the Rh antigen (i.e., fetal blood, transfused blood, or both). It is clear that not all atypical antibodies are capable of producing hemolytic disease of the newborn, either because of the nature of the immunoglobulins (IgM versus IgG) that may prevent transplacental transfer or because the antibodies have no effect on RBC integrity, sequestration, or clearance. Other antibodies can produce hemolytic disease of the newborn similar in appearance to Rh hemolytic disease, and amniotic fluid studies need to be performed (Weinstein, 1976).

The finding of an atypical antibody indicates the need for analysis of paternal blood. If the father is antigen-negative, no further analysis is performed. If he is positive for the antigen in question, the management scheme proposed by Weinstein (1976) should be followed. A partial list of common atypical antibodies that can lead to hemolytic disease of the newborn is seen in Table 29-2.

## Clinical Use

To be effective in preventing Rh isoimmunization, RhIg must be given in sufficient amounts to compensate for the extent of antigen (Rh-positive fetal RBCs) exposure. Presently, RhIg is available in 300 $\mu$g (RhoGAM) and 50-$\mu$g doses (Mic-RhoGAM). Greater than expected fetomaternal hemorrhage can be associated with abruption, cesarean delivery, manual exploration, and so on, and these situations warrant an acid elution (Kleihauer-Betke) or ELAT test to determine the amount of fetomaternal hemorrhage. No delay in the administration of RhIg should be tolerated after delivery of an Rh-positive infant to an Rh-negative Coombs' mother. General dosage guidelines for the usual obstetric conditions are listed in Table 29-3.

## OTHER MODALITIES OF TREATMENT

Other methods in the treatment of Rh isoimmunization include plasmapheresis, oral desensitization, and the use of immunosuppressive drugs such as steroids and promethazine hydrochloride.

**Table 29-2**
ATYPICAL ANTIBODIES ASSOCIATED WITH MODERATE TO SEVERE HEMOLYTIC DISEASE OF THE NEWBORN

| | |
|---|---|
| Kelly (k) | Public Antigens |
| Duffy (Fy[a]) | Yt[a] |
| Kidd (Jk[a], Jk[b]) | EN[a] |
| MNS$_s$ | Co[a] |
| Diego (Di[a], Di[b]) | Private Antigens |
| P | Biles |
| | Good |
| | Heibel |
| | Radin |
| | Wright[a] |
| | Zd |

**Table 29–3**
GENERAL RhIg DOSAGE GUIDELINES FOR
OBSTETRIC CONDITIONS

| Condition | Dosage (µg) |
|---|---|
| Spontaneous vaginal delivery | 300 |
| Cesarean delivery | 300 |
| Cesarean delivery with hemorrhage* | |
| Abortion | |
| < 13 weeks | 50 |
| > 13 weeks | 300 |
| Ectopic pregnancy | |
| < 13 weeks | 50 |
| > 13 weeks | 300 |
| Amniocentesis+ | 300 |
| Chorionic villus sampling | 50 |
| Percutaneous umbilical blood sampling | 300 |
| Fetal surgery | 300 |
| Transfusion mix | 20 (per ml packed RBCs) |
| match+ | 10 (per ml whole blood) |

* Need Kleihauer-Betke test to determine dosage.
+ RhIg may be delayed in late amniocentesis if delivery is anticipated within 48 hours.

## DELIVERY CONSIDERATIONS

Once the decision is made to deliver the isoimmunized patient, the choice of delivery method and labor conduction should be based on the usual obstetric indications with very few modifications. Vaginal delivery should be conducted with direct fetal heart rate monitoring and use of fetal scalp sampling when worrisome fetal heart rate patterns exist. The association of polyhydramnios with isoimmunization can lead to uterine overdistention, abruption, and occasional desultory labor patterns. With an unfavorable cervix, in which case internal monitoring is not possible from the onset, or with significant fetal distress, fetal malpresentation, or both, primary cesarean delivery is indicated. Care of the isoimmunized patient is summarized in Table 29–1.

# Cardiopulmonary Complications

## ASTHMA

Bronchial asthma complicates approximately 0.5 to 1 percent of all pregnancies. The disease may occur as episodic attacks of various degrees of severity or may be more chronic in nature with persistent dyspnea. Bronchoconstriction is the basic pathophysiologic mechanism, although this hyperactivity may be triggered by a number of antigenic stimuli that lead to release of chemical mediators (histamine, kinins, slow reactivity substance, and 5-hydroxy tryptamine). Prostaglandins and $\beta$-adrenergic receptors also play a role in mediating bronchospasm.

Arterial hypoxemia, occasionally severe, results from ventilation perfusion inequity. This is due to varying degrees of airway obstruction produced by bronchoconstriction, bronchial edema, and bronchial mucus plugging. Decreased $CO_2$ is a major reflection of the disease severity and an important management guideline. Although decreased arterial $P_{CO_2}$ is most commonly observed, $P_{CO_2}$ may be elevated because of hypoventilation. Retention of $CO_2$ (increased $P_{CO_2}$) occurs in approximately 15 to 20 percent of patients with severe disease, and when renal bicarbonate concentration is not adequate, respiratory acidosis ensues. Death due to asthma is a result of asphyxiation. Pathologically, widespread mucous impactions and distentions of bronchioles, which are approximately 5 ml wide, are found throughout the lungs. The importance of mucous stagnation must be remembered, particularly in the context of management.

## Effect of Pregnancy on the Course of Asthma

One might expect that, owing to the increase in plasma cortisol, prednisone, and histaminase in normal pregnancy, some predictable clinical improvement in most asthmatic patients should occur, particularly during the first trimester. However, clinical observations of pregnant asthmatic patients have not demonstrated any consistent ameliorative effect. Unfortunately, certain obstetric medications may exacerbate asthma. These include prostaglandins and ergonovine. Also, certain physiologic changes associated with pregnancy (i.e., gastroesophageal reflux and reduction of pulmonary residual capacity) also may make asthmatic attacks more common. Asthma in pregnant patients may remain stable, may worsen, or may improve. In a study by Gluck and Gluck (1976), the authors followed 47 pregnant asthmatic patients through delivery. Compared with their prepregnant asthmatic state, 20 patients became worse (43 percent), 20 patients were the same (43 percent), and 7 patients improved (14 percent). These changes were examined in relation to severity of their preconceptual asthma. In the group with mild disease, 12 percent improved, 72 percent were unchanged, and 16 percent became worse. In the group that was moderately affected, 40 percent improved, 60 percent became worse, and there were three admissions for asthma conditions. Finally, in the group with severe disease no patients improved, 17 percent were unchanged, and 83 percent became worse, with nine hospitalizations for asthma. The authors felt that the severity of asthma before pregnancy definitely correlated with the response of asthma in pregnancy; patients with mild asthma generally were unchanged, whereas those with severe asthma were usually worse (Gluck and Gluck, 1976).

A common problem in evaluating the response of asthma in pregnancy is the fact that in normal nonasthmatic pregnancies there can be breathing difficulties and orthopnea. Hence, the appearance of these symptoms during pregnancy, particularly in the last trimester, does not necessarily indicate the presence of asthma or its worsening.

It has been shown by most authorities that worsening of the asthmatic condition during pregnancy never occurs before the fourth month of gestation and that the majority occur in the sixth or seventh month. It was also noted by Gluck and Gluck (1976) that rising or stable IgE levels (normally decreased in pregnancy) in pregnant asthmatic patients prognosticated worsening of the disease during the pregnancy. The severe asthmatic patient is at the highest degree of deterioration during the second half of her pregnancy, and one can anticipate improvement after delivery. Likewise, patients who had improvement of their asthma during pregnancy noted it primarily during the first trimester. In a large study by Schaffer and Silverman (1961), there was no improvement in asthmatic patients after the 16th week of pregnancy.

## Effect of Asthma on the Pregnant Woman, the Fetus, and the Neonate

Severe asthma may severely affect pregnancy. A study by Gordon and colleagues (1970) reviewed 277 patients under active treatment for asthma in which 16 were classified as severe asthmatics. Those 16 women with severe asthma had the highest perinatal mortality and morbidity, with an incidence of 35 percent low-birth-weight infants and 12.5 percent neurologically abnormal infants at 1 year of age. There were also four deaths among the women with severe asthma. However, with mild-to-moderate disease, asthma had little effect on pregnancy outcome. In a review of 293 pregnant patients with asthma by Schaffer and Silverman (1961), the spontaneous abortion rate and prematurity rate did not exceed those of their normal controls. In a large prospective study (Gluck JC and Bluck PA, 1976) in which asthma was medically managed, perinatal mortality rates were not elevated in asthmatic mothers. Pregnancy-induced hypertension was more common in asthmatic gravidas, although this was observed primarily with severe asthma. There was no difference in gestational age, birth weight, or incidence of congenital malformations.

The issue of desensitization during pregnancy has been raised. In a review by Schaffer and Silverman (1961), desensitization was performed in 44 of their patients; they noted no deleterious effects from desensitization. In a survey of the literature of 212 pregnant patients who were desensitized during gestation, 11 percent showed constitutional reactions, including mild cramping and bleeding, but none had abortions.

## Management
(Table 29–4)

**History and Physical Examination.** Inquiries into the duration of the attack, precipitating events, present medications, and presence of associated cough, fever, upper respiratory infection, and so on should be made. Physical examination should be conducted with vital signs (rectal temperature) recorded. Findings specifically concerned with pulmonary status, such as associated rales, wheezing, bronchi, decreased breath sounds, and so on, should alert the perinatal team to bronchospasm as well as a contributing factor (e.g., pneumonia, bronchitis).

**Laboratory Studies.** Management of the pregnant woman with asthma should include the following laboratory studies:

- Blood gases

Table 29–4
PATIENT CARE SUMMARY FOR ASTHMA*

| | Antepartum | | Intrapartum | Postpartum |
|---|---|---|---|---|
| | *Outpatient* | *Inpatient* | | |
| BP | Each visit | q 8 h | q 1 h | On admission; then q 15 min × 4; then q 30 min × 2; then q 1 h until stable; then q 4–8 h |
| P, R | Same as above | q 2 h | q 30 min | Same as above |
| T | Same as above | Same as above with acute attack NST/CST then, q 2 h | q 1 h | On admission; then q 4 h |
| FHR/contractions | | | Continuous electronic fetal monitoring, preferably internal | Fundal checks and lochia assessment same as BP above |
| Laboratory values Blood gases CBC with differential Theophylline levels (goal 10–20 μ/g/dl) Electrolytes Sputum with gram stain and culture Chest x-ray with study abdominal shielding Steroids (if patient is on therapy) | q 1 month until 28 weeks, then q 2 weeks (or after each adjustment) | On admission and repeated as needed | 100 mg Solu-Cortef q 8 h × 3 doses | |

\* Nurse-to-patient ratio: *Antepartum,* 1:6 to 8; *intrapartum,* 2:3; *postpartum,* 1:6 to 8.
BP = Blood pressure; CST = contraction stress test; FHR = fetal heart rate; NST = nonstress test; P = pulse; R = respiration; T = temperature.

- CBC with differential
- Electrolytes
- Sputum with Gram's stain and culture
- Chest x-ray study with abdominal shielding if there is no immediate improvement or if fever, rales, and so on are present

## Medications
### *Aqueous Epinephrine*

Dose—0.3 to 0.5 ml (1/1000 solution) every 15 to 20 minutes subcutaneously in the absence of severe hypertension or cardiac arrhythmias).

### *Theophylline*

Loading dose—250 mg in anhydrous theophylline (6 mg/kg) in 50 to 100 ml $D_5W$ over 20 minutes.
Maintenance dose—0.9 mg/kg/h intravenously (50 to 70 mg/h in $D_5W$ solution).
Long-term maintenance—Theodur 100 to 300 mg bid; Staphylline 125 to 250 mg q 8 h; Quibron t/SR 200 to 300 mg bid.

Theophylline level should be 10 to 20 μg/ml.
*Side Effects.* If persistent nausea and vomiting, tachycardia, hypotension, cardiac arrhythmias, or convulsions occur, the dosage should be reduced or discontinued.
*Use in Pregnancy.* At the present time, theophylline is considered safe in pregnancy without evidence of teratogenic effect. Theophylline toxicity (jitteriness, tachycardia, and so on) has been reported, however, in neonates who received the drug transplacentally near delivery as well as those who were breastfed. Owing to decreased clearance of theophylline in the third trimester, theophylline levels need to be monitored more frequently. Theophylline concentration in breast milk peaks 1 to 3 hours after oral dosage.

### β Agonist
### *Terbutaline (Brethine)*

Loading Dose—0.25 mg subcutaneously q 30 min.
Maintenance Dose—0.25 mg q 5 h.
Long-Term Maintenance—5 mg tid.

*Side Effects.* The use of β agonists has been associated with a number of metabolic and clinical side effects. The most common side effects include tachycardia, widening of pulse pressure, anxiety and restlessness, and increased water retention. Hyperglycemia, hyperlipemia, and increased renin production also occur.

*Use in Pregnancy.* Betamimetics should be used with caution because of the frequency of at least minor side effects. All betamimetics have been shown to reduce uterine activity. Pulmonary edema has been reported, particularly with intravenous administration for preterm labor. Experience with patients in preterm labor demonstrates few neonatal problems, but if they occur, they center on cardiac stimulation effects (i.e., tachycardias) as well as hypoglycemia due to hyperinsulinism. No serious neonatal adverse reactions have been reported in medicated mothers breastfeeding their infants.

*Inhalant Therapy.* Intermittent positive-pressure breathing can be given with isoproterenol via nebulizer, 20 to 30 breaths every 45 minutes. Aerosols, 2 to 3 breaths every 2 to 3 hours, can also be used with bronchodilators such as terbutaline (Brethine), 2.5 to 5 mg, and metaproterenol (Alupent), 10 to 20 mg.

### Glucocorticoids

**Loading Dose—hydrocortisone (Solu-Cortef) 100 to 200 mg intravenously, then 100 mg q 8 h in D₅W.**

**Maintenance Dose—Prednisone 60 to 100 mg/ day with gradual tapering to lowest effective dose.**

*Side Effects.* The side effects of glucocorticoids include hypertension, hypokalemia, hypernatremia with water retention, hyperglycemia, susceptibility to infections, peptic ulcers, and cushingoid features. Osteoporosis and ecchymosis have been associated with long-term use.

*Use in Pregnancy.* Glucocorticoids should be used with caution in pregnancy. Long-term studies are incomplete; however, animal data indicating a potential problem with neurologic development suggest they be used only in cases of asthma that are resistant to other therapy (theophylline, betamimetics). Their use as a therapy to enhance fetal pulmonary lung maturity is still controversial. Patients should seek advice from their pediatrician as to whether they may breastfeed while taking these drugs.

### Antibiotics (Ampicillin)

**Initial Dose—1 g IV, then 500 mg q 6 h.**
**Maintenance Dose—500 mg p.o. qid × 10 to 14 days.**
Use with evidence of bronchitis, pneumonia, and so on.

## NURSING CONSIDERATIONS

Assess for level of impairment and effect of medications (see Table 29–4).

Assess present level of knowledge regarding use of medications. Supply information as needed. Mother may need to know about fetal effects sooner than maternal effects.

Supply clear, concise explanations regarding status of the fetus and mother. Any information regarding medications' effect on the fetus and condition of the mother relieves anxiety. May help interrupt anxiety and dyspnea cycle.

## PULMONARY EDEMA

Acute pulmonary edema is a medical emergency that demands prompt diagnosis and early therapy. The most common causes of pulmonary edema in the pregnant and nonpregnant state are cardiac disease (atherosclerosis, hypertension, cardiomyopathy) and excessive positive fluid balance. Excessive positive fluid balance is especially true in pregnant patients treated for preterm labor with β sympathomimetics with or without associated glucocorticoid use for acceleration of fetal pulmonary lung maturity. Pregnancy-induced hypertension also may lead to a noncardiogenic cause of pulmonary edema. This is thought to be due to damage at the pulmonary capillary bed leading to an egress of fluid into the pulmonary interstitium.

Acute myocardial failure occurs in all instances in which left ventricular function can no longer effectively eject normal (or increased) stroke volume. This failure of complete left ventricular ejection during systole causes a rise in left ventricular diastolic pressure, which leads to a rise in left atrial and pulmonary venous pressures. Under normal circumstances, the plasma oncotic pressure prevents a substantial diffusion of intravascular fluid into interstitial tissues. However, with the increased hydrostatic pressure of the elevated pulmonary venous system, movement of the fluid into the lung, interstitium, and alveoli occurs. This movement of fluid into interstitium and alveoli interferes with alveolar and capillary bed oxygen exchange, which results in hypoxia. The various etiologies of pulmonary edema are listed in Table 29–5.

## Diagnosis

Diagnosis of acute pulmonary edema should be considered when any patient complains of acute shortness of breath, whether at night (paroxysmal nocturnal dyspnea) or any other time the patient assumes a sitting or upright position (orthopnea). The condition may be accompanied by cough and occasional hemoptysis. Chest pain (substernal) can accompany other symptoms.

Confirmatory signs include presence of rales at lung bases, engorged hepatojugular veins, and a protodiastolic gallop ($S_3$) on cardiac auscultation. With progressive disease, patients may become cyanotic and semicomatose or may display confusion.

## Management
(Table 29–6)

Initial management should involve seeking the mechanism of left ventricular failure. Adjuvant testing that should proceed while therapy is initiated includes:

- Electrocardiogram (ECG)
- Chest x-ray study
- Serial blood gas analysis
- Electrolytes
- Hemodynamic monitoring—central venous pressure (CVP) or pulmonary arterial balloon catheter

Once the initial management is under way, secondary management steps can be taken. Betamimetic therapy and steroids should be discontinued if they are being used. Steps to improve ventilation and oxygenation should be initiated. The goals are $P_{CO_2}$, 35 to 45 mm Hg; $P_{O_2}$, 80 mm Hg; and normal pH. The patient can be placed in a sitting position, or oxygen can be administered via nasal prongs. If the $P_{CO_2}$ is greater than 50 mm Hg or the $P_{O_2}$ is less than 60 mm Hg despite therapy, intubation and mechanical ventilation are indicated. *Caution:* High $F_{IO_2}$ (greater than 50 to 60 percent) observed with assisted ventilation can lead to oxygen toxicity and adult respiratory distress syndrome.

### Diuretic Therapy

**Dose—Furosemide 40 mg intravenously.**

Diuretic therapy causes a prompt diuresis, which reduces the hydrostatic pressure as well as directly affects the venous vasculature, causing vasodilatation. These two effects cause a reduction in the pulmonary wedge pressure and improved cardiac output. Ethacrynic acid has been associated with fetal and maternal totoxicity and, therefore, should not be used, if possible.

*Side Effects.* Commonly reported complications include hypovolemia, nausea, vomiting, abdominal pain, and diarrhea. Furosemide decreases uric acid excretion, and hyperuricemia may develop. Tinnitis also

---

**Table 29–5**
ETIOLOGIES OF ACUTE PULMONARY EDEMA IN PREGNANCY

| Cardiac Etiology | Noncardiac Etiology |
|---|---|
| A. Left ventricular failure<br>  Acute decompensation of chronic left<br>   Ventricular disease (i.e., hypertensive<br>   heart disease)<br>  Myocardial infarction<br>  Cardiomyopathy<br>B. Mitral valve disease<br>  Congenital (i.e., mitral stenosis)<br>  Acquired (i.e., rheumatic valvular disease)<br>C. Volume overload—particularly with risk factors<br>  Preeclampsia and eclampsia with or without<br>   renal impairment<br>  Betamimetic use with or without associated<br>   glucocorticoid use<br>  Transfusion therapy<br>  Underlying cardiac disease | A. Altered capillary membrane permeability<br>  Bacteremia<br>  DIC<br>  Uremia<br>  Toxic agent inhalation<br>B. Decreased plasma oncotic pressure—hypoalbuminemia<br>C. Pulmonary embolism |

Table 29–6
## PATIENT CARE SUMMARY FOR PULMONARY EDEMA*

| | Antepartum | Intrapartum | Postpartum |
|---|---|---|---|
| BP, P, R | q 15 min until stable | q 15 min | q 15 min until stable; then q 30 min × 2; then q 1 h |
| T | q 4 h | q 4 h | q 4 h |
| FHR | NST/CST | Continuous electronic monitoring, preferably internal; if no monitor available, then q 15 min in first stage and q 5 min in second stage | — |
| Contractions | q 1 h | Continuous electronic monitoring, preferably internal; if no monitor available, then q 30 min | Fundal checks on admission to RR; then q 15 min × 4; then q 30 min × 2; then q 1 h until stable; then q 4 h Lochia: Same as above |
| ECG<br>Chest x-ray study<br>Blood gases<br>Electrolytes } | On admission and as needed | As needed | As needed |
| CVP and Pulmonary arterial balloon catheter | If necessary | If necessary | If necessary |
| I & O | q 1 h | q 1 h | q 1 h until stable; then q 8 h |

* Nurse-to-patient ratio: *Antepartum,* 1:6 to 8; *intrapartum,* 1:1; *postpartum,* 1:6 to 8.

BP = Blood pressure; CST = contraction stress test; FHR = fetal heart rate; I & O = intake and output; NST = nonstress test; P = pulse; R = respiration; RR = recovery room; T = temperature.

has been reported. Significant other complications from diuretic therapy include hypokalemia, hyponatremia, and occasionally, metabolic alkalosis. Severe hypokalemia is a contraindication to diuretic therapy, although potassium supplementation may help correct depletion so that it may subsequently be used.

*Use in Pregnancy.* The use of furosemide during pregnancy has been associated with increased maternal and fetal uric acid. Fetal urinary output does increase following maternal administration. Severe volume depletion, which can occur following its use, can lead to decreased uterine blood flow. No serious neonatal reactions have been reported in breastfed infants of medicated mothers.

### Morphine

#### Dose—Morphine sulfate 3 to 4 mg intravenously, repeated as needed.

Morphine helps to improve the status of acute pulmonary edema via a reduction in the work of breathing by reducing hyperventilation (central effect). It also can act directly as an agent to cause vasodilatation, which leads to reduced volume return to the decompensated ventricles. Small intravenous doses of morphine are the method

of choice, because intramuscular or subcutaneous depositions are erratically absorbed.

*Side Effects.* Morphine's side effects include nausea and vomiting and, occasionally, profound hypotension and decreased respirations. Therefore, it should be used with great caution in patients with preexisting hypotension (systolic pressure < 100 mm Hg), chronic obstruction pulmonary disease, or atrioventricular (AV) block. Respiratory acidosis is a contraindication to its use.

*Use in Pregnancy.* Morphine can depress the fetal central nervous system if given close to delivery. Breast milk excretion has been observed. Morphine also has been associated with vasoconstriction of placental vessels (impairing $O_2$ and $CO_2$ transfer); however, human documentation of deleterious effects is lacking. Narcotic antagonists should be available at the time of delivery.

### Digitalis

#### Dose—(Complete digitalization) Digoxin 0.50 mg; then 0.25 mg q 6 h × 3 doses. Follow with digoxin levels (< 3 ng/ml).

Although probably not necessary in many patients, digitalis should be used in patients who exhibit cardiac disease, particularly those with cardiomegaly. Digitalis, however, should not be used when there has been a recent myocardial infarction (increased cardiac oxygen requirement). When used for pulmonary edema, it should be given as an intravenous dose. Ionotropic effect can be seen prior to full digitalization.

*Side Effects.* Common side effects with digitalis include nausea, vomiting, skin rashes, eosinophilia, and occasionally, AV block and arrhythmias due to digitalis intoxication. As previously mentioned, digitalis increases myocardial contractility while increasing cardiac oxygen requirement, and recent myocardial infarction militates against its use. It must not be used in patients with pre-existing heart block (second or third degree), bradycardia, obstructive cardiomyopathies, and digitalis toxicity (toxic effects may be seen in patients with digoxin levels > 3 ng/ml). Hypokalemia potentiates the cardiotoxic effects and should be corrected prior to its use.

*Use in Pregnancy.* Digoxin crosses the placenta and can concentrate in the fetal heart. It may even be used to treat fetal tachyarrhythmias with congestive changes. Fetal toxic effects have not been reported.

### Vasodilatory Therapy (Afterload Reduction)

**Dose—Nitroprusside 20 μg/kg/min (hemodynamic monitoring is essential).**

Newer agents have been proposed that reduce peripheral vascular resistance and dilate venous capillary beds in the patient with acute pulmonary edema. This reduced resistance causes a lowering of the impedance to left ventricular ejection, thereby allowing improved ventricular emptying. These drugs, although helpful in refractory cases, should not be used in initial therapy. Nitroprusside is the drug of choice, because the ganglionic blockers phentolamine, trimethaphan, and hexamethonium primarily lead to arterial vasodilatation, whereas nitroprusside affects both arterial and venous vascular tone. Nitroprusside should be given intravenously as a continuous drip.

*Side Effects.* Nitroprusside's side effects center on its hypotensive effects, and therefore, patients in shock should not receive the drug. Cyanide toxicity has been reported because this is a byproduct of its metabolism.

*Use in Pregnancy.* Although increased fetal serum cyanide levels are reported with maternal administration, the risk to the fetus is unclear.

**Phlebotomy and Rotating Tourniquets.** Once considered a mainstay of therapy, phlebotomy and rotating tourniquets should only be used to temporize prior to initiating other therapy. Removal of 500 ml initially helps to reduce plasma volume and, thereby, decreases an end-diastolic ventricular volume. Patients may, if necessary, be reinfused with their own blood (packed cells) after plasmapheresis. Rotating tourniquets can be used to help reduce venous return, but care must be taken not to impede arterial flow to the extremities in the process.

### Hemodynamic Monitoring in Pulmonary Edema

Hemodynamic monitoring with the use of a pulmonary arterial balloon catheter can prove to be an invaluable aid both in diagnosis of the etiology (cardiogenic versus noncardiogenic) and in guiding therapy. Although central venous pressure monitoring historically has been used in the management of this complication, it is clear that there can be a discrepancy between CVP and pulmonary capillary wedge pressure (PCWP) measurements. In one recent series, the CVP value correlated with PCWP in only one third of patients (Benedetti, 1982).

### NURSING CONSIDERATIONS

Administer oxygen and monitor ABGs as indicated. The patient should maintain a sitting position, with uterus displaced to the left. Administer medications as ordered and monitor for effectiveness (see Table 29–6).

Concern over infant may be a mother's primary concern. Keeping parents informed of fetal status helps to reduce anxiety.

## Thromboembolic Complications

### DEEP VEIN THROMBOSIS (THROMBOPHLEBITIS)

The true incidence of superficial and deep thrombophlebitis in pregnancy is unknown, but in a review by Aaro and Juergens (1971), it has been estimated to complicate approximately 1 in 70 pregnancies. Friend and

Kakkar (1970) estimated that deep vein thrombosis is less common than thrombosis in the superficial veins, and that thrombosis occurs in 1.6 to 4.7 per 1000 deliveries. The onset of thrombophlebitis is three times more likely to occur in the postpartum period than antenatally. Factors associated with increased pregnancy risk include maternal age greater than 35 years, obesity, immobilization, cardiopulmonary disease, diabetes mellitus, and previous history of thromboembolism. Mode of delivery also seems to be a risk factor, with cesarean delivery three times more likely to engender thromboembolic problems than vaginal delivery. Thrombi are often bilateral, although only one calf appears affected. The most common sites include the venous sinuses within the soleus muscle, the pocket of valve cups, and the left ileofemoral venous segment.

## Pathophysiology

Virchow (1846) described a classic triad of venous stasis, hypercoagulable blood, and venous intimal injury as the prerequisite for thromboembolism.

Pregnancy is characterized by an increase in venous stasis in the lower extremities and groin area owing to the enlarging gravid uterus. Compression of the inferior vena cava causing this stasis is most pronounced when the pregnant patient is in the supine or sitting position. Pregnancy is also characterized by some marked changes in the coagulation and fibrinolytic systems. There is a moderate rise in all coagulation factors except factors XI and XIII. A dramatic rise in fibrinogen and factors III, X, and VIII can be seen. In addition to this rise in coagulation factors, there is also a suppression of the fibrinolytic system, specifically a depression of plasminogen activator and anti-thrombin III, both of which play crucial roles in clot lysis. Intimal vessel injury probably plays no role in initiation of thrombosis in pregnancy except for the possibility of injury during cesarean delivery, which could conceivably trigger a pelvic vein thrombophlebitis.

## Diagnosis

The clinical signs of calf tenderness, swelling, erythema, and pain elicited with dorsal flexion of the foot (Homans' sign) are the most common manifestations. The pain may be particularly noticeable with ambulation. The swelling may not be discernible to the naked eye, and calf measurements should be taken. A difference of 2 cm in circumference (measured equidistant from the patella) is significant. An area of warmth or distinct erythema may be noted over the involved area.

Confirmatory testing of the presence of thrombosis can be accomplished by the noninvasive techniques of Doppler ultrasound or plethysmography or the invasive techniques of venography or [125]I-fibrinogen scanning.

### Noninvasive Testing

*Doppler Ultrasound.* Doppler testing is based on ultrasonic velocity detection. The flow pattern after Valsalva's maneuver, respirations, or alternating compression is noted. Distortions in the flow pattern indicate thrombosis. Small nonocclusive thrombi can be missed, but major emboli can be detected. It is less effective in detecting emboli above the groin area.

*Plethysmography.* This testing is based on electrical impedance of the calf and its alteration when thrombosis is present. The plethysmographic tracing is a measurement of the rate of emptying after venous occlusion induced by inflating and rapidly releasing a thigh cuff. Respirations also cause a fluctuation in the impedance tracings. Deviation from normal patterns is diagnostic of thrombosis.

Problems in interpretation arise when both the Doppler ultrasound and plethysmographic techniques are used in assessing the gravid patient. Approximately 10 to 15 percent of normal pregnant patients have abnormal tests if they are supine. It is imperative, then, that all abnormal tests be confirmed while the patient is in the lateral recumbent position.

### Invasive Testing

*Venography.* The injection of radioopaque dye into a vein in the foot with follow-up x-ray studies has remained a mainstay of diagnosis for many years. Because it is difficult to adequately shield the fetus from radiation, particularly while examining the inguinal area, this technique has become less popular during pregnancy. If used, a pronounced collateral venous system can be observed in the afffected calf owing to thrombosis. False-positive results can result from hematomas, local edema, or popliteal cysts. Subiliac lesions can be missed occasionally. The contrast medium also can induce phlebitis in and of itself.

$^{125}$**I-fibrinogen Scan.** The incorporation of radioactive tracer compound into the thrombus leads to a hot spot that can be detected. The use of radioactive iodine, however, is contraindicated in pregnancy because of fetal thyroid concentration, although the radiation risk is probably small.

## Management
(Table 29–7)

**Initial Management.** The initial management of thrombophlebitis consists of the following elements:

1. Bed rest with elevation of affected leg for 5 to 7 days or until symptoms clear.
2. Analgesia.
3. Support hose—thigh-high lightweight elastic.
4. Laboratory studies:
   a. Prothrombin time (PT), partial thromboplastin time (PTT)
   b. Fibrinogen
   c. Complete blood count with platelets
5. Anticoagulation—heparin 40,000 U/day as continuous drip infusion (1500 to 1700 U/h) until PTT is 2.5 to 3 times control and plasma heparin is 0.3 U/ml.

Initial therapy continues to 10 to 14 days.

## Table 29–7
### PATIENT CARE SUMMARY FOR DEEP VEIN THROMBOSIS*

| | Antepartum | | Intrapartum | Postpartum |
|---|---|---|---|---|
| | *Outpatient* | *Inpatient* | | |
| BP, P, R | Each visit | q 4 h | q 1 h | On admission to RR; then q 15 min × 4; then q 30 min × 2; then q 1 h until stable; then q 4 h PP |
| T | Each visit | q 4 h | q 4 h | On admission to RR; then q 4 h |
| FHR | Each visit | NST and CST, then q shift | Continuous electronic monitoring, preferably internal; if no monitor available, q 15 min in first stage and q 5 min in second stage | — |
| Contractions | Each visit | q shift | Continuous electronic monitoring; if no monitor available, q 1 h by palpation | Fundal checks on admission to RR; then q 15 min × 4; then q 30 min × 2; then q 1 h until stable; then q 4 h Lochia: Same as above |
| Bed rest | Yes | Yes | Yes | Yes |
| Support hose | Yes | Yes | Yes | Yes |
| Laboratory studies PT PTT Fibrinogen CBC with platelets | At initial visit; then q month | Yes | Yes | q 1 month until therapy discontinued |
| Assessment of thrombosis site including Homans' sign | Each visit | q 4 h | q 1 h | q 1 h in RR q 4 h on PP floor |

* Nurse-to-patient ratio: *Antepartum*, 1:6 to 8; *intrapartum*, 2:3; *postpartum*, 1:6–8.
BP = Blood pressure; CBC = complete blood count; CST = contraction stress test; FHR = fetal heart rate; NST = nonstress test; P = pulse; PP = postpartum; PT = prothrombin time; PTT = partial thromboplastin time; R = respiration; RR = recovery room; T = temperature.

### Subsequent Anticoagulation

*Maintenance Dose.* Heparin, 20,000 U/ day (or 10,000 U bid) subcutaneously, may be given throughout pregnancy. Warfarin, 5 mg tid (15 mg/day) until PT is 1.5 to 2 times controlled values, may be given to postpartum patients *only.*

*Intrapartum Management.* Heparin can be stopped when labor commences without risk of excessive intrapartum or postpartum bleeding. Rarely is there a need to reverse heparin therapy, but if excessive bleeding exists, protamine sulfate (1 mg intravenous push inactivates approximately 100 U of heparin) can be used. Heparin is again initiated postpartum, and a switch to warfarin can be made over the next few days. Anticoagulation should be continued for 4 to 6 weeks.

Anticoagulation in pregnancy is discussed more fully elsewhere in this chapter.

## NURSING CONSIDERATIONS

Supply parents with information concerning the disease process and the effect of heparin. Aim of therapy is to provide for rest and to prevent stasis by the use of elevation and support hose. Monitor as indicated (see Table 29–7).

Explanation of need to thin the blood to reduce risk of embolism. Heparin is the drug with the least effect on the fetus and can be discontinued at time of delivery. Explain side effects and need to report them to care givers.

Institute instruction as soon as heparin therapy is started. Allow patient to handle equipment before need for actual self-administration.

## PULMONARY EMBOLISM

Pulmonary embolism occurs once in every 2500 to 3000 pregnancies. If the condition is left untreated, the condition can result in a mortality rate of 50 percent. It is believed that the underlying pathophysiology is similar to that of deep vein thrombosis. Approximately 35 percent of patients who develop pulmonary embolism give an antecedent history of deep vein thrombosis. The remaining pulmonary embolism patients may develop silent deep vein thrombosis with migration to the pulmonary arterial branches or thrombi that arise *de novo* as cardiopulmonary emboli without deep vein origin.

## Diagnosis

Dyspnea remains the most common symptom of pulmonary embolism and is present in over 80 percent of cases. Pleuritic chest pain (72 percent) and apprehension (60 percent) are also commonly present. Other signs and symptoms may include hemoptysis (34 percent), rales, tachypnea (90 percent), a loud pulmonic closure, and pleuritic friction rub. Confirmatory findings include a $P_{O_2}$ less than 80 mmHg and an abnormal ventilation-perfusion lung scan or angiography. A chest x-ray study may reveal an infiltrate indicating an elevated hemidiaphragm or pleural fluid. ECG often reveals a right axis shift or right bundle-branch block. Lactic dehydrogenase and bilirubin levels are often elevated.

The mainstays of diagnosis are arterial blood gas analysis and lung scanning. If $P_{O_2}$ is greater than 85 mm Hg, pulmonary embolism is unlikely, although up to 14 percent of patients with pulmonary embolism have $P_{O_2}$ greater than 85 mm Hg. Values less than 90 mm Hg can represent smaller emboli. Ventilation perfusion lung scans using $^{99}Tc$ and xenon gas can be helpful particularly when a mismatch pattern is observed. This mismatch pattern indicates normal ventilation with decreased perfusion. Fetal irradiation risks from these agents are probably minimal, and the importance of establishing the diagnosis is so great that the physician should not hesitate to use this technique. The specificity of the lung scan can be reduced if the patient has congestive heart failure or chronic obstructive lung disease. In equivocal cases, pulmonary angiography with abdominal shielding can be helpful, although smaller emboli can be missed.

## Management
(Table 29–8)

The management of pulmonary embolism consists of the following elements:

1. Laboratory studies
   a. Serial blood gas analysis
   b. PT
   c. PTT
   d. CBC with differential
2. ECG
3. Chest x-ray study
4. $O_2$ therapy—1 to 2 liters/min via nasal prongs

5. Sedation—10 mg morphine sulfate subcutaneously or 4 mg intravenously
6. Aqueous theophylline—250 mg in 50 ml $D_5W$ over 15 to 20 minutes
7. Digitalization (with massive pulmonary embolus) 0.50 mg intravenously, then 0.25 mg q 8 h × 3
8. Anticoagulation therapy, fibrinolytic therapy, or surgical intervention

### Anticoagulation Therapy

#### Heparin

**Initial Dose—10,000 U intravenous bolus, then 1000 to 2000 U/h as continuous intravenous infusion until PTT is 2.5 to 3 times controlled (plasma heparin 0.3 U/ml).**

**Maintenance Dose—1000 U/h continuous intravenous for 10 days, then 10,000 U bid as subcutaneous injection. This lower dose rarely affects PTT.**

*Side Effects.* Hemorrhage is the most frequent side effect associated with heparin. Other side effects include anaphylactoid reactions, alopecia, thrombocytopenia, and with long-term use, osteoporosis. The use of salicylates, phenylbutazone, indomethacin, clofibrate, and dipyridamole may increase the risk of excessive bleeding. Quinine drugs and d-tubocurarine may decrease the anticoagulant effect.

*Use in Pregnancy.* The use of heparin appears to be safe during the course of pregnancy without added risks to mother or fetus. Because heparin does not cross the placenta, it does not lead to fetal anticoagulation and perinatal hemorrhage. It remains the drug of choice for anticoagulation during pregnancy.

#### Warfarin

**Maintenance Dose (in postpartum patients *only*)—5 mg tid (15 mg/day) until PT is 1.5 to 2 times controlled.**

*Side Effects.* The major side effect of warfarin is hemorrhage. This hemorrhage may be so brisk that administration of fresh frozen plasma and blood may be required. Less frequently encountered side effects include nausea, vomiting, diarrhea, alopecia, and dermatitis. Overdosage may be managed by intravenous or subcutaneous vitamin K administration. Certain drugs, including phenylbutazone, anabolic steroids, broad spectrum antibiotics, salicylates, and chloramphenicol, enhance the anticoagulant response to warfarin. Barbiturates, griseofulvin, and glutethimide may diminish anticoagulant response.

*Use in Pregnancy.* The fetus and neonate appear to be extremely sensitive to warfarin and warfarin drugs because of their lower concentration of vitamin K–dependent coagulation factors. Risk of perinatal hemorrhage in up to 5 to 10 percent of cases has been reported. Warfarin drugs also may induce fetal malformation (warfarin embryopathy), which is reported to occur in approximately 15 to 25 percent of prenatal exposures (Hall et al, 1980). This syndrome includes nasal hypoplasia, stippling of bones, ophthalmologic abnormalities, intrauterine growth retardation, and mental delay. Because of these concerns, warfarin should be considered contraindicated in pregnancy.

Warfarin is excreted in breast milk, but whether or not neonatal effects can be observed is controversial.

**Intrapartum Management.** Heparin dosage can be lowered to 20,000 U the day of delivery and increased to previous levels after delivery. Warfarin can be added postpartum. Anticoagulation therapy at maintenance levels should be continued for 6 to 8 months following pulmonary embolism.

**Fibrinolytic Therapy.** The thrombolytic agents streptokinase and urokinase are available for clot dissolution. Both act to increase active plasmin, which then hydrolyzes the fibrin in clots. Lytic therapy has been demonstrated to result in quicker lysis of clots than has heparin therapy; however, whether this translates into reduced recurrence risks or overall improvement in long-term status is unclear. These agents need to be used with great caution, because frank hemorrhage may occur with biopsies, arterial punctures, and so on. Patients need to be at strict bed rest, and blood products (packed RBCs, fresh frozen plasma) should be available. Allergic and pyrogenic side effects have also been reported. The experience with these agents in pregnancy is limited, and they should be used only in very selective cases, if ever.

**Surgical Intervention.** Emergency surgical removal of a pulmonary embolus has limited applicability, because most patients respond to anticoagulation therapy and over 90 percent of the fatalities associated with pulmonary embolism occur within 1 hour, usually before surgical intervention could be initiated. At the present time, embolectomies

**Table 29–8**
PATIENT CARE SUMMARY FOR PULMONARY EMBOLISM*

| | Antepartum | Intrapartum | Postpartum |
|---|---|---|---|
| BP, P, R | q 15 min | q 15 min | q 15 min until stable; then q 30 min × 2; then q 1 h; then q 4 h on PP floor |
| T | q 4 h | q 4 h | On admission; then q 4 h |
| FHR | Weekly NST/CST | Continuous electronic monitoring, preferably internal; if no monitor available, q 15 min in first stage and q 5 min in second stage | — |
| Contractions | q 8 h | Continuous electronic monitoring, preferably internal; if no monitor available, q 1 h by palpation | Fundal checks on admission; then q 15 min × 4; then q 30 min × 2; then q 1 h until stable; then q 4 h on PP floor<br>Lochia: Same as above |
| I & O | q 1 h until stable; then q 8 h | q 1 h | q 1 h until stable; then q 8 h |
| CVP | Yes | Yes | Yes |
| ECG | Yes | Yes | Yes |
| Laboratory studies<br>  Serial blood gases<br>  PT<br>  PTT<br>  CBC with differential | At initial evaluation; then as needed during anti-coagulation therapy | — | — |
| Chest x-ray study | At initial evaluation; then as needed | — | — |
| O₂ therapy | 1 to 2 liters/min nasal prong (depending on ABGs or pulse meter) | 1 to 2 liters/min face mask | 1 to 2 liters/min nasal prong |

* Nurse-to-patient ratio = 1:1.
  BP = Blood pressure; CST = contraction stress test; CVP = central venous pressure; ECG = electrocardiogram; FHR = fetal heart rate; I & O = intake and output; NST = nonstress test; P = pulse; PP = postpartum; PT = prothrombin time; PTT = partial thromboplastin time; R = respiration; T = temperature.

are reserved for those few patients who do not respond to anticoagulation therapy yet demonstrate persistent hypotension, hypoxemia, or both. When performed in a timely manner, the survival rate approaches 50 percent (Sasahara and Barsamian, 1973).

Vena cava interruption is another surgical technique used in patients with pulmonary embolism in whom deep vein origin is demonstrated and in whom anticoagulation is contraindicated or deep vein thrombosis failed to resolve after anticoagulation. Other candidates include patients with septic pulmonary emboli from pelvic vein thrombophlebitis.

A variety of procedures (clip, ligation, filters) of vena cava interruption have been proposed. Recurrence risks, however, are approximately 10 percent owing to emboli arising from areas above the ligation or from ovarian vein thromboembolism or even em-

boli arising from the ligation site itself (Bernstein, 1973).

Side effects include venous stasis of the legs and perineum. Clearly, this is a procedure to be used selectively.

## NURSING CONSIDERATIONS

Administer medications and oxygen as ordered. Monitor for changing condition of mother and fetus (see Table 29–8).

Patients may be extremely anxious, related to sudden onset of pain and dyspnea. Offer firm emotional support and reassurance regarding therapy. The nurse should give care efficiently without displaying fear.

Supply information to patient and significant other as condition allows. Clear, concise sentences help reduce the stress of the situation. Explain effect of medications as condition allows.

# References

Aaro LA, Juergens JL: Thrombophlebitis associated with pregnancy. Am J Obstet Gynecol 109:1128, 1971.

Baskett TF, Koh KS: Sinusoidal fetal heart rate pattern—a sign of fetal hypoxia. Obstet Gynecol 44:379, 1974.

Benedetti TJ, Cotton DB, Read JC, Miller FC: Hemodynamic observations in severe preeclampsia with a flow-directed pulmonary artery catheter. Am J Obstet Gynecol 136:465, 1980.

Bernstein EF: The place of venous interruption in the management of pulmonary embolism. In Moser KM, Stein M (eds): Pulmonary Thromboembolism. Chicago, Year Book Medical Publishers, 1973.

Bowman JM: Blood-group incompatibilities. In Iffy L, Kaminetzky HA (eds): Principles and Practice of Obstetrics and Perinatology. New York, John Wiley & Sons, 1981, p 1193.

Bowman JM: Hemolytic Disease of the Newborn. In Conn HF, Conn RB Jr (eds): Current Diagnosis, 6. Philadelphia, WB Saunders Co, 1980.

Bowman JM: The management of Rh-isoimmunization. Obstet Gynecol 52:1, 1978.

Bowman JM, Manning FA: Intrauterine fetal transfusions: Winnepeg, 1982. Obstet Gynecol 61:203, 1983.

Bowman JM, Pollack JM: Antenatal Rh prophylaxis: 28 weeks gestation service program. Can Med Assoc J 118:627, 1978.

Bowman JM, Chown B, Lewis M, et al: Rh-isoimmunization during pregnancy: antenatal prophylaxis. Can Med Assoc J 118:623, 1978.

Copel JA, Grannum PA, Belanger K, et al: Pulsed Doppler flow velocity waveforms before and after intrauterine intravascular transfusion for severe erythroblastosis fetalis. Am J Obstet Gynecol 158(4):768–74, 1988.

deCrespigny LC, Robinson HP, Quinn M, et al: Ultrasound-guided fetal blood transfusion for severe rhesus isoimmunization. Obstet Gynecol 66:529–532, 1985.

Freeman RK, Garite TJ, Nageolte MP: Fetal Heart Rate Monitoring, 2nd ed. Baltimore, Williams & Wilkens, 1991.

Friend JR, Kakkar VV: The diagnosis of deep vein thrombosis in the puerperium. J Obstet Gynaecol Br Commonw 77:820, 1970.

Gluck JC, Bluck PA: The effects of pregnancy on asthma: a prospective study. Ann Allergy 37:164, 1976.

Gordon M, Niswander KR, Barendes H, et al: Fetal morbidity following potentially anoxigenic obstetric conditions. VII. Bronchial asthma. Am J Obstet Gynecol 106:421, 1970.

Grannum PA, Copel JA: Prevention of Rh isoimmunization and treatment of the compromised fetus. Semin Perinatol 12(4):324–35, 1988.

Grannum PA, Copel JA, Plaxe SC, et al: In utero exchange transfusion by direct intravascular injection in severe erythroblastosis fetalis. N Engl J Med 314(22):1431–34, 1986.

Gray JH, Cudmore DW, Luther ER, et al: Sinusoidal fetal heart rate pattern associated with alphaprodine administration. Obstet Gynecol 52:678, 1978.

Hall JG, Pauli RM, Wilson K: Maternal and fetal sequelae of anticoagulation during pregnancy. Am J Med 68:122, 1980.

Hill Z, Vacl-Kalasova E, Clabkova M, et al: Hemolytic disease of the newborn due to anti-D antibodies in Du positive mothers. Vox Sang 27:92, 1974.

Keckstein G, Tschurtz S, Schneider V, et al: Umbilical cord hematoma as a complication of intrauterine intravascular blood transfusion. Prenat Diagn 10(1): 59–65, 1990.

Kirkinen P, Jouppila P, Elk-nes S: Umbilical vein blood flow in Rhesus isoimmunization Br J Obstet Gynaecol 90:640–3, 1983.

Lacey P: An unexpected case of severe hemolytic disease of the newborn due to anti-D (Abstract). Transfusion 18:642, 1978.

Liley AW: Liquor amnii analysis in management of pregnancy complicated by rhesus sensitization. Am J Obstet Gynecol 82:1359, 1961.

Liley AW: Intrauterine transfusion in the foetus in haemolytic disease. Br Med J 2:1107, 1963.

Modanlou HT, Freeman RK, Ortiz O, et al: Sinusoidal fetal heart rate pattern and severe fetal anemia. Am J Obstet Gynecol 49:537, 1977.

Moise KJ, Carpenter RJ, Huhta JC, et al: Umbilical cord hematoma secondary to in-utero intravascular transfusion for Rh isoimmunization. Fetal Ther 2(2):65–70, 1987.

Nicolaides KH, Fontanarosa M, Gabbe SA, et al: Failure of ultrasonographic parameters to predict the severity of fetal anemia in Rhesus isoimmunization. Am J Obstet Gynecol 158:920–26, 1988.

Nicolaides KH, Rodeck CH, Mibashan RS, et al: Have Liley charts outlived their usefulness? Am J Obstet Gynecol 155:90–4, 1986.

Parer JT: Severe Rh isoimmunization—current methods of in utero diagnosis and therapy. Am J Obstet Gynecol 158:1323–9, 1988.

Queenan JT: Intrauterine transfusion—a cooperative study. Am J Obstet Gynecol 104:397, 1969.

Queenan JT: Modern Management of the Rh Problem, 2nd ed. Hagerstown, MD, Harper & Row, 1977.

Race RR: The Rh genotype and Fisher's theory. Blood 3:27, 1948.

Rightmire DA, Nicolaides KH, Rodeck CH, et al: Fetal blood velocities in Rh isoimmunization: relationship to gestational age and to fetal hematocrit. Obstet Gynecol 68:233–6, 1986.

Rodeck CH, Nicolaides KH: Fetoscopy and fetal tissue sampling. Br Med Bull 39:332–7, 1983.

Sasahara AA, Barsamian EM: Another look at pulmonary embolectomy. Ann Thorac Surg 16:317, 1973.

Schaffer G, Silverman F: Pregnancy complicated by asthma. Am J Obstet Gynecol 82:182, 1961.

Seeds J, Chescheir N, Bowes W, et al: Fetal death as a complication of intrauterine intravascular transfusion. Obstet Gynecol 74:461–463, 1989.

Taylor JF: Sensitization of Rh negative daughters by their Rh positive mothers. N Engl J Med 276:547, 1967.

Weinstein L: Irregular antibodies causing hemolytic disease of the newborn. Obstet Gynecol Surv 31:581, 1976.

White CA, Goplerud CP, Kissker CT, et al: Intrauterine fetal transfusion, 1965–1976, with an assessment of surviving children. Am J Obstet Gynecol 130:933, 1978.

Whitfield CR, Neely RA, Telford ME: Amniotic fluid analysis in rhesus iso-immunization. J Obstet Gynecol Br Commonw 75:121, 1968.

# CHAPTER 30

# Critical Care of the Pregnant Patient*

Gary D.V. Hankins and Carol J. Harvey

An explosion of information and technology over the past 20 years, which is expected to continue into the foreseeable future, has resulted in the subspecialty of critical care obstetrics. Numerous medical and nursing textbooks are devoted to addressing the subject of this chapter (Baldwin and Hanson, 1984; Berkowitz, 1983; Clark et al, 1990; Harvey, 1991).

The spectrum of pathophysiologic conditions and treatment of various disease states, which would have previously precluded pregnancy, includes women with structural cardiac lesions; prosthetic heart valves; history of deep venous thrombosis and pulmonary embolus; and microangiopathic anemias, including thrombotic thrombocytopenic purpura and hemolytic uremic syndromes in pregnancy. The challenge in providing care for women with these conditions resulted in the recognition by the American Board of Obstetrics and Gynecology in 1978 of the subspecialty of maternal and fetal medicine. Similar significant advances in the fields of internal medicine, surgery, and anesthesia resulted in the formation of the Society of Critical Care Medicine in 1980. The American Association of Critical Care Nurses and the Society of Critical Care Medicine have been instrumental in establishing guidelines for the care of patients in the intensive care unit, spanning the gamut from physical plant design to staffing to patient care protocols (Frigoletto and Little, 1988;

Society of Critical Care Medicine, 1988; Shuman, 1989).

The most practical, efficient, and economical means of caring for the critically ill obstetric patient who requires invasive monitoring, ventilatory support, or both, depends on the number of pregnant women cared for at the facility and the referral patterns to that facility. Although some obstetric services have a sufficient volume of patients with this acuity, the majority of obstetric services see fewer then 20 such patients per year. Accordingly, arrangements need to be in place either to care for these women in existing surgical or medical intensive care units or to have specialized rooms designated in the labor and delivery suite where the necessary equipment can be quickly assembled to provide the needed care for these patients. For the woman whose pregnancy is ongoing, the ideal care would be provided by specially trained obstetricians and obstetric nurses. In the absence of a specially trained obstetric team, it is necessary to assemble a team of physicians and nurses, each with special areas of expertise sufficient to manage all problem areas that a patient may present to the health care team. The members of the team should include an obstetrician and be augmented by a combination of other health care providers, including anesthesiologists, pulmonologists, cardiologists, and intensivists. An obstetric and an intensive care nurse are required in the care of a patient with a viable pregnancy. Although the obstetric team may be intimidated by ventilators, pulmonary artery catheters, pressure transducers, and alarms, the intensive care team may be just as intimi-

---

* The opinions expressed in this chapter are those of the authors and not necessarily those of the United States Air Force or the Department of Defense.

dated by the gravid uterus, fetus, and fetal monitors. Even in those circumstances in which a dedicated obstetric intensive care unit exists, liberal consultation is still encouraged.

Regardless of the location where care is provided, the use of flow sheets, such as those used in intensive care units (Perinatal Innovations, Salt Lake City, UT), is encouraged (Fig. 30-1). These documents facilitate quick assessment of the patient's condition by all members of the health care team. Key components of flow charts include assessment of hemodynamic parameters; ventilator settings and blood gas analyses; temperature; intake and output, including the specific fluids infused; medications; and daily weights. The severity of the illness necessitating such intensive care frequently requires daily assessment by a 12-lead echocardiogram as well as frequent radiologic studies, particularly a chest radiograph. In the event that the patient remains pregnant, shielding of the abdomen for any nonabdominal radiologic procedures should be carried out. In caring for these women, it is incumbent that patient care standards established for both the obstetric patient as well as the intensive care unit patient be met and that achievement of such standards be documented in the patient's chart. This is especially important because patients requiring such care frequently have (1) severe complications from their disease processes, (2) multiple organ system failure, and (3) the possibility of long-term residual effects from their illness or death. These factors make it highly likely that the care we have delivered to these women, and the documentation of that care, will be subject to review.

Proper equipment for care of the pregnant woman with a life-threatening complication is a prerequisite. All equipment required in a labor and delivery setting is also mandatory for any obstetric intensive care unit or surgical unit during that interval that the pregnant woman is present for care. Multiple oxygen and suction outlets should be available for both the mother and her neonate. In addition to the obstetric supplies, standard critical care equipment also is needed. The minimal equipment often required is listed in Table 30-1. When purchasing equipment, a primary consideration should be whether the information generated by the equipment will be used entirely for patient care or whether information collected will be stored

for future analysis and research. Obstetric services involved in multiple research projects require more data storage and retrieval options from the technology than the service that provides patient care alone. Consideration should be given to a system composed of modular units that can be interchanged to make the system fit the needs of the patient.

# Application of Invasive Technologies

The flow-directed pulmonary artery catheter transformed a tool used exclusively by the cardiac catheterization and research laboratories into a clinical instrument available at the woman's bedside for ongoing monitoring of cardiovascular status and function (Swan et al, 1970). Information obtained from its use can facilitate diagnosis, management, and evaluation of therapeutic decisions. Often, clinical impressions can be reinforced or refuted with accurate hemodynamic measurements in critically ill women. The indications for the use of invasive hemodynamic monitoring are much the same in obstetrics as in any other area of medicine (Hankins, 1988), and it is reasonable to expect that similar results can be gained from its use in pregnant women (Clark et al, 1985b). Moreover, understanding of the pathophysiology of many conditions unique to obstetrics, such as pulmonary edema associated with the use of $\beta$ agonists and the hemodynamics of preeclampsia and eclampsia, has been advanced significantly by invasive cardiovascular monitoring (Benedetti et al, 1982; Clark and Cotton, 1988; Hankins et al, 1984; Hauth et al, 1983; Lee et al, 1988).

## VENOUS ACCESS

Venous access for invasive monitoring usually is obtained via the internal or external jugular vein or the subclavian vein. The femoral and antecubital veins are used less frequently because of greater difficulty in positioning the catheter. Additionally, use of the inguinal area in obstetrics may limit access to and manipulation of the catheter at critical times, such as during delivery. Un-

*Text continued on page 628*

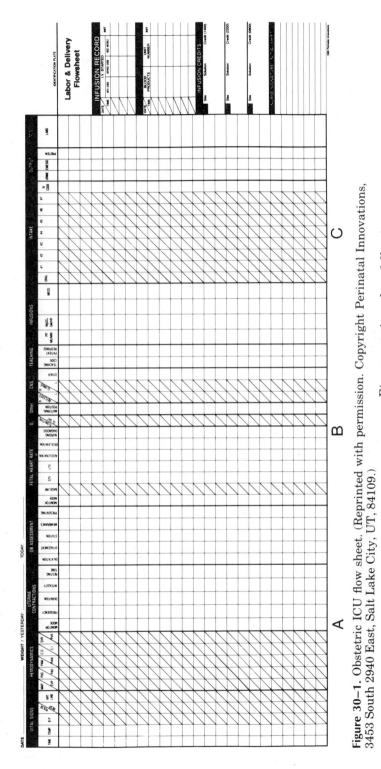

**Figure 30–1.** Obstetric ICU flow sheet. (Reprinted with permission. Copyright Perinatal Innovations, 3453 South 2940 East, Salt Lake City, UT, 84109.)

*Figure continued on following page*

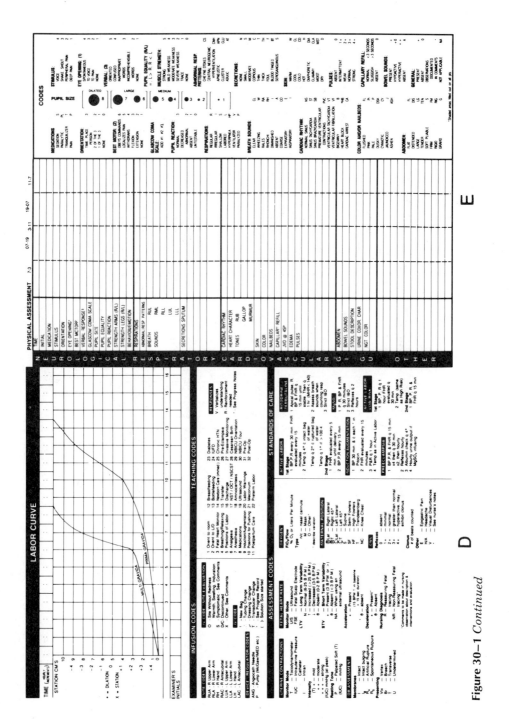

Figure 30–1 Continued

622

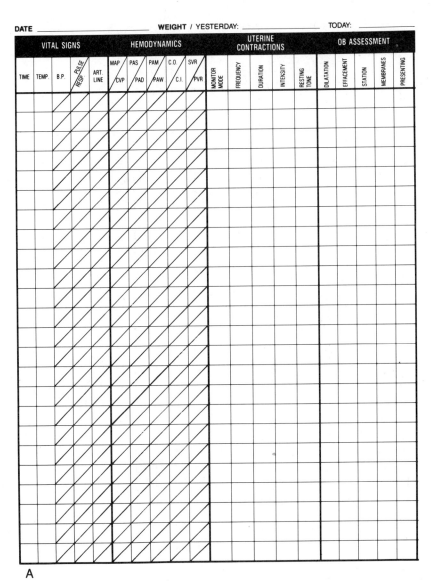

**Figure 30–1A.**

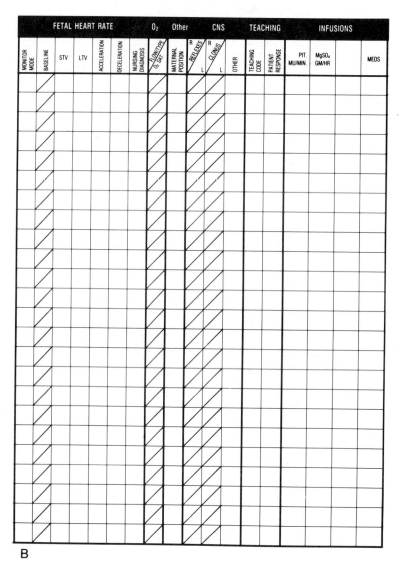

B

**Figure 30–1B.**

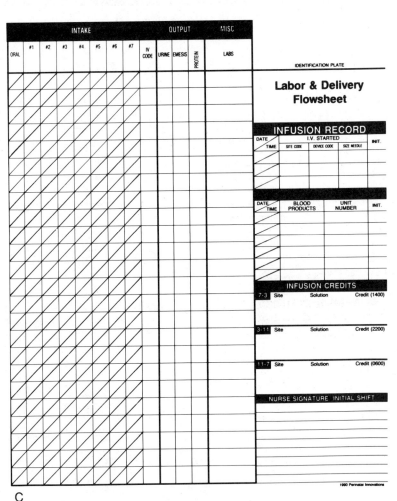

C

**Figure 30–1C.**

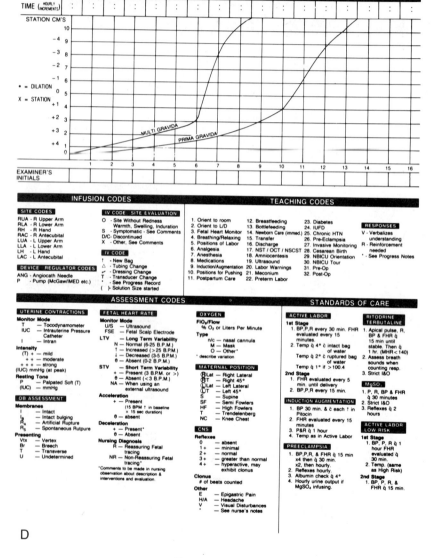

D

Figure 30–1D.

**PHYSICAL ASSESSMENT** 7-3   07-19   3-11   19-07   11-7

**NEUROLOGICAL**

| | |
|---|---|
| TIME | |
| INITIAL | |
| MEDICATION | |
| STIMULUS | |
| ORIENTATION | |
| EYE OPENING[1] | |
| BEST MOTOR[2] | |
| VERBAL RESPONSE[3] | |
| GLASCOW COMA SCALE | |
| PUPIL SIZE | |
| PUPIL EQUALITY | |
| PUPIL REACTION | |
| STRENGTH ARMS (R/L) | |
| STRENGTH LEGS (R/L) | |
| BEHAVIOR/EMOTION | |

**RESPIRATORY**

| | |
|---|---|
| RESPIRATIONS | |
| ABNORMAL RESP. PATTERNS | |
| BREATH SOUNDS RUL | |
| RML | |
| RLL | |
| LUL | |
| LLL | |
| SECRETIONS SPUTUM | |

**CARDIOVASCULAR**

| | |
|---|---|
| CARDIAC RHYTHM | |
| HEART CHARACTER | |
| TONES RUB | |
| GALLOP | |
| MURMUR | |
| SKIN | |
| COLOR | |
| NAILBEDS | |
| CAPILLARY REFILL | |
| JVD @ 45° | |
| EDEMA | |
| PULSES | |

**GI-GU**

| | |
|---|---|
| ABDOMEN | |
| BOWEL SOUNDS | |
| STOOL DESCRIPTION | |
| URINE: COLOR, CHAR. | |
| NGT: COLOR | |

**OTHER**

---

**CODES**

**MEDICATIONS:**
| | |
|---|---|
| SEDATION | S |
| PARALYTIC | PL |
| TRANQUILIZER | T |
| PAIN | P |

**ORIENTATION:**
| | |
|---|---|
| TIME, PLACE, PERSON | 3 |
| 2 OF THE 3 | 2 |
| 1 OF THE 3 | 1 |
| NONE | 0 |

**BEST MOTOR: (2)**
| | |
|---|---|
| OBEYS COMMANDS | 6 |
| LOCALIZES PAIN | 5 |
| WITHDRAWS | 4 |
| FLEXION | 3 |
| EXTENSION | 2 |
| NONE | 1 |

**GLASGOW COMA SCALE:** ADD #1, #2, #3.

**PUPIL REACTION:**
| | |
|---|---|
| NORMAL | 3 |
| DECREASED, ABNORMAL | 2 |
| ABSENT | 1 |
| UNTESTABLE | 0 |

**RESPIRATIONS:**
| | |
|---|---|
| REGULAR | R |
| IRREGULAR | I |
| SHALLOW | S |
| LABORED | L |
| HYPERPNEA | HP |
| VENTILATOR | V |
| PARALYZED | P |

**BREATH SOUNDS:**
| | |
|---|---|
| CLEAR | CL |
| WHEEZING | W |
| RALES | RA |
| RHONCHI | RH |
| DIMINISHED | i |
| ABSENT | A |
| COARSE | CO |
| EXPIRATORY | E |
| INSPIRATORY | I |

**CARDIAC RHYTHM:**
| | |
|---|---|
| NORMAL SINUS | NS |
| SINUS TACHYCARDIA | ST |
| SINUS BRADYCARDIA | SB |
| PREMATURE VENTRICULAR CONTRACTIONS | PVC |
| VENTRICULAR TACHYCARDIA | VT |
| VENTRICULAR FIBRILLATION | VF |
| BIGEMINY | B |
| HEART BLOCK | *HB |
| CARDIAC ARREST | CA |

**COLOR AND/OR NAILBEDS:**
| | |
|---|---|
| FLUSHED | FL |
| PINK | Pi |
| PALE | P |
| DUSKY | DSK |
| CYANOTIC | CY |
| JAUNDICED | J |
| ASHEN | ASH |

**ABDOMEN:**
| | |
|---|---|
| FLAT | FL |
| DISTENDED | DIS |
| LARGE | LG |
| TENDER | TEN |
| SOFT, PLIABLE | S |
| FIRM | FM |
| RIGID | RIG |
| GRAVID | G |

**STIMULUS:**
| | |
|---|---|
| VOICE | 4 |
| SHAKE, SHOUT | 3 |
| PERIPHERAL PAIN | 2 |
| DEEP PAIN | 1 |

**EYE OPENING: (1)**
| | |
|---|---|
| SPONTANEOUS | 4 |
| TO VOICE | 3 |
| TO PAIN | 2 |
| NONE | 1 |

**VERBAL: (3)**
| | |
|---|---|
| ORIENTED | 5 |
| CONFUSED | 4 |
| INAPPROPRIATE WORDS | 3 |
| INCOMPREHENSIBLE WORDS | 2 |
| NONE | 1 |

**PUPIL EQUALITY (R/L)**
=; L> R; R < L

**MUSCLE STRENGTH:**
| | |
|---|---|
| STRONG | 5 |
| MILD WEAKNESS | 4 |
| MODERATE WEAKNESS | 3 |
| SEVERE WEAKNESS | 2 |
| TRACE | 1 |
| NONE | 0 |

**ABNORMAL RESP. PATTERNS:**
| | |
|---|---|
| CHEYNE-STOKES | CS |
| CENTRAL NEUROGENIC HYPERVENTILATION | CNH |
| APNEUSTIC | APN |
| CLUSTER | CLU |
| ATAXIC | AT |

**SECRETIONS:**
| | |
|---|---|
| NONE | N |
| SMALL | S |
| MODERATE | M |
| COPIOUS | C |
| THIN | T |
| THICK | TH |
| FOUL | F |
| BLOOD TINGED | BT |
| SEROSANGUINOUS | S |

**SKIN:**
| | |
|---|---|
| WARM | W |
| COOL | CL |
| COLD | CD |
| HOT | H |
| DIAPHORETIC | DIA |
| CLAMMY | CLA |
| MOIST | MST |
| DRY | D |

**PULSES:**
| | |
|---|---|
| ABSENT | 0 |
| INTERMITTENT | 1+ |
| WEAK | 2+ |
| NORMAL | 3+ |
| STRONG | 4+ |

**CAPILLARY REFILL:**
| | |
|---|---|
| NORMAL | <3 SECONDS |
| SLUGGISH | >3 SECONDS |
| ABSENT | 0 |

**BOWEL SOUNDS:**
| | |
|---|---|
| PRESENT | + |
| HYPOACTIVE | +0 |
| HYPERACTIVE | ++ |
| ABSENT | A |

**GENERAL:**
| | |
|---|---|
| PRESENT | + |
| ABSENT | 0 |
| OBSERVATIONS DOCUMENTED | |
| IN COMMENTS | • |
| NOT APPLICABLE | NA |

**PUPIL SIZE** DILATED 8 / LARGE 7 6 / MEDIUM 5 4 3 2 1

*Shaded areas filled out on all pts.

E

**Figure 30–1E.**

**Table 30–1**

MINIMAL EQUIPMENT FOR AN OBSTETRIC
INTENSIVE CARE PATIENT

Fetal monitor

Continuous electrocardiogram monitor—with high
and low alarms and printer

Temperature monitor

Continuous arterial pressure monitor—invasive and
noninvasive

Central venous pressure monitor

Pulmonary artery pressure monitor

Cardiac output monitor

Equipment to maintain the airway: laryngoscopes,
endotracheal tubes

Equipment to ventilate, including ambu bags,
ventilators, $O_2$, and compressed air

Emergency resuscitation equipment (including
defibrillators and cardioverters and emergency
drugs)

Equipment to support hemodynamics: infusion pumps,
blood warmer, pressure bags, blood filters

Birthing beds with removable headboard and
adjustable position to deep Trendelenburg's position

Adequate lighting for bedside procedures

Suction

Hypo-hyperthermia blanket

Scale

Temporary pacemaker

Continuous inspired $O_2$ monitoring capability for
ventilators

Capnography for ventilators

Transcutaneous $O_2$ monitor or pulse oximeter for
patients receiving $O_2$

Transport monitor

der certain conditions, such as the patient with a coagulopathy, the antecubital approach may be prudent to avoid the possibility of an intrathoracic bleed. In such cases, venous access may be easier to achieve by venous cutdown as opposed to percutaneous cannulation of the vessel. Additionally, sonography can assist in locating the catheter tip and altering the position of the woman's arm to facilitate its final positioning in the pulmonary artery. The nurse's role during the procedure is to instruct the patient on the procedure, position the patient in a slight Trendelenburg's position with a hip wedge to produce venous distention, and assist the operator in the procedure.

The majority of the complications of invasive hemodynamic monitoring relate to two factors: (1) gaining venous access, and (2) the experience and skill of the operator. In gaining venous access, Seldinger's technique or a modification of this technique is recommended. After inquiring as to whether or not the patient has any allergies, the site selected is sterilized, prepared, and draped, usually with a povidone-iodine solution. The operator puts on his or her gown and gloves for gaining venous access and for positioning the pulmonary artery catheter. If the internal jugular approach is selected, the patient is positioned, and her head is tilted below the horizontal position and turned to the side opposite the vessel selected for cannulation. Using 1 percent Xylocaine and a 21- or 22-gauge 2-inch needle, the skin is injected, and a wheal is made over the carotid artery. The needle is then directed into the patient's neck and toward the ipsilateral nipple at a 45 degree angle, aspirating for blood as a tract toward the vessel is anesthetized (Fig. 30-2). Often, the vein walls collapse by the pressure of the needle, and the vessel is completely penetrated without blood returning. Accordingly, if a tract the entire length of the needle has been anesthetized and no blood has returned, the operator should slowly withdraw the needle while maintaining a small amount of negative pressure on the syringe. If free-flowing blood returns, the needle should be disconnected from the syringe and

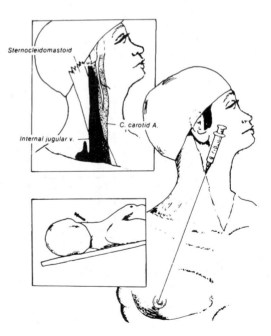

**Figure 30–2.** Use of the modified Seldinger technique for vessel cannulation. The technique uses sequentially larger caliber needles for vessel localization; the vessel is wired and, finally, a vein dilator and catheter port is passed over the wire. Emphasis is on avoidance of trauma to the patient or her vessel.

left free in the the patient's neck to serve as a guide for cannulation of the vessel with a larger bore catheter. Failure to achieve blood return merits repositioning the patient and further attempts, each time redirecting the angle of approach of the 21-gauge needle by approximately 5 degrees medial or lateral to the prior attempt. Once the vessel is located, an 18-gauge needle can be used to recannulate it, following which, a vascular wire is passed into the vessel. The wire should pass freely and without resistance and should *never* be withdrawn through the cutting edge of the needle because the wire may be severed. After the wire is passed into the vessel, the needle is withdrawn over the wire. A scalpel is used to make a 3- to 4-mm cut about the wire, following which, the larger 7.5 or 8 Fr. vascular access catheter is passed, with the assistance of a vein dilator, over the wire. The wire and dilator are then withdrawn, and one should be able to extract blood readily through the catheter introducer. If doubt exists as to whether the blood is arterial or venous, blood gas analysis can be performed. Self-contained kits for acquisition of vascular access are available from a variety of companies.

## CATHETER ANATOMY

The standard flow-directed thermodilution pulmonary artery catheter (Fig. 30–3) includes a distal lumen at the catheter tip, a proximal lumen 30 cm from the catheter tip, a balloon lumen, and a thermistor. The distal lumen provides continuous pulmonary artery pressure measurements when the balloon is deflated, and pulmonary capillary wedge pressures (PCWP) when the balloon is inflated. The proximal port can be used to monitor venous pressure or administer fluids or drugs. Both the proximal and distal lumina of the catheter may be used to withdraw samples or venous blood for laboratory studies. Cardiac output and central core temperature can be measured when the pulmonary artery catheter is used in conjunction with a thermodilution cardiac output computer. Catheters are available with additional ports through which medications can be administered. The small size of these ports renders them ineffective for rapid acute infusion of large volumes of fluid or blood; however, they are appropriate for the administration of vasopressors, antibiotics, and other slower controlled infusions. Fiberoptic pulmonary artery catheters also are gaining popularity in the treatment of critically ill patients that, in conjunction with a bedside microprocessor and strip chart recorder, can provide a continuous reading of the patient's mixed venous oxygen saturation. The standard adult pulmonary artery catheter is 7 Fr. and requires a 7.5 Fr. venous introducer, whereas the fiberoptic catheters are 7.5 Fr. and require an 8.0 Fr. introducer.

The pulmonary artery catheter is directed into position by venous return to the heart. Its passage is reflected indirectly by pressure waveforms viewed on an oscilloscope that are characteristic of the specific heart chambers (Fig. 30-4). Continuous electrocardiographic monitoring is necessary during catheter positioning to observe for ventricular ectopia and arrhythmias. Prior to catheter insertion, the proximal and distal lumens should be flushed and purged of air and the balloon checked for symmetric inflation, absence of an air leak, and ease of spontaneous deflation. The catheter is then advanced through

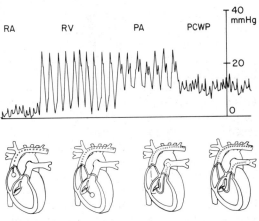

**Figure 30–4.** Pressure waveforms observed on an oscilloscope as the pulmonary artery catheter passes through the right atrium (RA), right ventricle (RV), and pulmonary artery (PA), to the pulmonary capillary wedge position (PCWP).

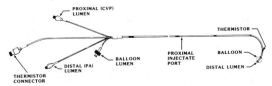

**Figure 30–3.** Diagram of a flow-directed pulmonary artery catheter.

an introducer at the venous access site. The balloon is inflated after insertion of approximately 15 cm of the catheter. If resistance to balloon inflation is encountered, the catheter should be advanced further into the vessel, and a repeat attempt should be made at inflation. This usually is successful, because the caliber of the vessel increases when the catheter is centrally advanced. If undue resistance is met, the balloon should not be inflated, because this could result in rupture of a blood vessel with catastrophic hemorrhage. As the balloon-tipped catheter is carried along by venous blood flow, the chest cavity is entered and a low-amplitude pressure tracing is obtained, which demonstrates respiratory variation (i.e., in the woman who is spontaneously breathing, the pressure falls with inspiration and rises with expiration). Continued advancement of the catheter tip into the right ventricle results in a spiking waveform with a baseline pressure of 0 mm Hg. Subsequently, as the pulmonary artery is entered, another spiking waveform of lower amplitude is identifiable that measures diastolic pressures above 0 mm Hg. The next waveform obtained, a dampened tracing with respiratory variation, is the PCWP. When the balloon is deflated, a pulmonary artery tracing reappears. A true PCWP is verified by (1) conversion of a pulmonary artery pressure tracing to a PCWP tracing when the balloon is inflated, (2) the presence of a respiratory variation in the pressure tracing, and (3) a calculated mean pulmonary artery pressure higher than the PCWP.

The ability to obtain accurate tracings over prolonged periods can be enhanced with two devices that are particularly useful in situations that mandate catheter repositioning. A catheter introducer system (Cordis Corporation, Miami, FL; Arrow Corporation, Reading, PA) containing a one-way valve allows a malfunctioning catheter to be advanced, withdrawn, or changed without loss of the venous access. Additionally, sheaths are available that fit over the catheter itself and attach to the introducer port. The sheaths maintain sterility of a segment of the pulmonary artery catheter, allowing its advancement or withdrawal, as necessary, to obtain accurate pressure tracings. Routine chest radiography to verify catheter positioning is not necessary when catheter insertion is uncomplicated and one is certain the chest cavity was not entered. Verification of proper positioning of the pulmonary artery catheter depends on obtaining a high-quality and appropriate pressure tracing and not by chest radiograph. Most women with pulmonary problems have complications that require sequential chest radiographs, however, and on every film the position of the catheter should be checked and the patient should be observed for the development of pneumothorax, hemothorax, and hydrothorax.

## DATA COLLECTION

Continuous central venous and pulmonary artery pressures and intermittent PCWP measurements are afforded directly by use of the pulmonary artery catheter. Cardiac output can be measured, as necessary, by the thermodilution technique. Both the heart rate and rhythm are observed through the use of continuous electrocardiographic monitoring. Systemic arterial pressure can be measured by manual or automatic sphygmomanometer or percutaneous arterial catheterization. Percutaneous arterial catheterization also readily provides access for arterial blood sampling and analysis but risks damage to the vessel and to the extremity supplied by the vessel. The radial, axillary, and pedal vessels are the most commonly used vessels, in that order. Prior to cannulation of the radial artery, Allen's test should be performed to assess collateral circulation into the hand. This is accomplished by compressing both the radial and ulnar arteries simultaneously while having the patient repetitively open and close her hand. After approximately 30 seconds, open the hand and release pressure from the ulnar artery. The hand should resume a normal pink color promptly if collateral circulation is adequate.

Mean pressure values are of clinical significance and can be determined for both the pulmonary arterial and systemic circulations by electronic dampening of the respective tracing, or they can be calculated with the following equation

$$\text{mean pressure} = \frac{\text{systolic pressure} + 2(\text{diastolic pressure})}{3}.$$

The PCWP, a dampened pressure tracing, has a mean value that is the average of its maximum and minimum deflections on the oscilloscope. Although oscilloscopic readings are usually adequate for clinical management, strip chart recordings are recommended when dealing with complex waveforms, such as those that may be encountered with mitral valvular disease or with data collection for clinical research. If marked respiratory variations exist, these pressures should be read directly from the oscilloscope or the strip chart recorder because reliance on the digital display underestimates the wedge pressure when the patient is spontaneously breathing and overestimates it when positive pressure ventilation is being used.

Various other hemodynamic values that reflect cardiac function and vascular resistance can be calculated or derived from a particular formula (Table 30-2). Stroke volume is a measure of the amount of blood pumped per contraction by the heart. Both the cardiac output and the stroke volume may be corrected for body size by division of the values by body surface area to obtain cardiac index and stroke index. Because body surface area nomograms have not been developed for pregnant women nor keyed to gestational age, adult nomograms must be used to derive body surface area. Resistance to flow can be calculated from right and left ventricles through determinations of the pulmonary vascular resistance and systemic vascular resistance, respectively. Pulmonary shunts and arterial-venous content differences are calculated by analyses of simultaneously obtained samples of mixed venous

blood (drawn from the distal port of the pulmonary artery catheter) and arterial blood. Blood from the central venous pressure line should not be used. It yields, on average, a 20 percent error of shunt calculation because it does not contain the venous drainage from the heart and often is not fully mixed, depending on where the central venous pressure catheter port (the right atrial port) is positioned.

Recently derived normal values for healthy nonpregnant and pregnant subjects are given in Table 30-3 (Clark et al, 1989). These values are obtained from middle-class Caucasian women late in their third trimester, and again, several weeks postpartum. In each instance, their pregnancies had been without complications.

## INTERPRETATION OF DATA

In an assessment of cardiac function, four areas are addressed: preload, afterload, contractile or inotropic state of the myocardium, and heart rate (Braunwald, 1971; Braunwald, 1974a; Braunwald, 1974b; Herman and Gorlin, 1969; Mason et al, 1970; Soonenblick et al, 1970).

**Preload.** Preload is determined by intraventricular pressure and volume, thus setting the initial myocardial muscle fiber length. Clinically, the right and left ventricular end-diastolic filling pressures are assessed by central venous pressure and PCWP, respectively. A plotting of cardiac output against central venous pressure or PCWP gives a cardiac function curve for the right or left ventricle (Fig. 30–5). The ventricular function curve demonstrates that a failing heart requires a higher preload or filling pressure to achieve the same cardiac output as a normally functioning heart (Fig. 30–6). Therapeutic manipulation of the ventricular filling pressures and simultaneous measurement of cardiac output allows calculation of the optimal preload (i.e., the construction of a Starling's ventricular function curve at the patient's bedside). The preload can be increased by the administration of crystalloid, colloid, or blood and can be decreased by the use of diuretic, a vasodilator, or phlebotomy.

**Afterload.** Afterload is defined as the ventricular wall tension during systole and is dependent on the end-diastolic radius of

**Table 30–2**
FORMULAS FOR DERIVING VARIOUS
HEMODYNAMIC PARAMETERS

Stroke Volume (SV) (mL/beat)
$SV = CO/HR$
Stroke Index (SI) (ml/beat/m$^2$)
$SI = SV/BSA$
Cardiac Index (CI) (ml/min/m$^2$)
$CI = CO/BSA$
Systemic Vascular Resistance (SVR) (dyne
  $\times$ sec $\times$ cm$^{-5}$)
$SVR = [(MAP - CVP)/CO] \times 80*$
Pulmonary Vascular Resistance (PVR)
  (dyne $\times$ sec $\times$ cm$^{-5}$)
$PVR = [(MPAP - PCWP)/CO] \times 80*$
* Conversion factor: 1 mm Hg/l/min − 80 dyne
  $\times$ sec $\times$ cm$^{-5}$

* BSA, body surface area (m$^2$); CO, cardiac output (l/min);
CVP, central venous pressure (mm Hg); HR, heart rate
(beats/min); MAP, mean systemic arterial pressure (mm Hg);
MPAP, mean pulmonary artery pressure (mm Hg);
PCWP, mean pulmonary capillary wedge pressure (mm Hg).

**Table 30–3**
CENTRAL HEMODYNAMIC NORMAL VALUES

|  | Nonpregnant | Pregnant |
| --- | --- | --- |
| Cardiac output (l/min) | 4.3 ± 0.9 | 6.2 ± 1.0 |
| Heart rate (beats/min) | 71 ± 10.0 | 83 ± 10.0 |
| Systemic vascular resistance (dyne · cm · sec⁻⁵) | 1530 ± 520 | 1210 ± 266 |
| Pulmonary vascular resistance (dyne · cm · sec⁻⁵) | 119 ± 47.0 | 78 ± 22 |
| Colloid oncotic pressure (mm Hg) | 20.8 ± 1.0 | 18.0 ± 1.5 |
| Colloid oncotic pressure—pulmonary capillary wedge pressure (mm Hg) | 14.5 ± 2.5 | 10.5 ± 2.7 |
| Mean arterial pressure (mm Hg) | 86.4 ± 7.5 | 90.3 ± 5.8 |
| Pulmonary capillary wedge pressure (mm Hg) | 6.3 ± 2.1 | 7.5 ± 1.8 |
| Central venous pressure (mm Hg) | 3.7 ± 2.6 | 3.6 ± 2.5 |
| Left ventricular stroke work index (g · m · m⁻²) | 41 ± 8 | 48 ± 6 |

the ventricle, the aortic diastolic pressure, and the ventricular wall thickness (Lappas et al, 1977). The extent to which the right or left intraventricular pressure rises during systole depends primarily on the pulmonary or systemic vascular resistance (Fig. 30–7). In the presence of heart failure, increases in afterload worsen the degree of failure by decreasing both the stroke volume and the cardiac output (Cohn and Fanciosa, 1977).

Afterload, like preload, can be increased or decreased therapeutically as mandated by the clinical setting. Increases in afterload are mediated through modulation of the α-adrenergic system; phenylephrine is an agent with almost pure α-agonist effects. Decreases in afterload or systemic vascular resistance can be achieved with numerous agents. Sodium nitroprusside by continuous intravenous infusion is used most commonly to decrease afterload in the intensive care

setting, whereas hydralazine is the agent most commonly used in obstetrics. The intermittent intravenous administration of small, incremental doses of hydralazine, without continuous arterial pressure monitoring, has been proved safe for both mother and fetus. Sodium nitroprusside and nitroglycerine infusions should not be used unless continuous intra-arterial blood pressure monitoring has been instituted. Additionally, the potential for fetal cyanide toxicity exists when nitroprusside is used (Naulty et al, 1976; Strauss et al, 1980). It has been recommended arbitrarily that antepartum use be limited to 30 minutes.

**Contractile or Inotropic State of Heart.** Contractile or inotropic state of the heart is defined as the force and velocity of ventricular contractions when preload and afterload are held constant. Although cardiac output can be measured directly, its adequacy must

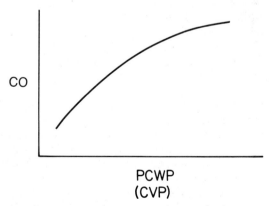

**Figure 30–5.** Ventricular function (Starling) curve for the normal heart. Pulmonary capillary wedge pressure (PCWP) or central venous pressure (CVP) represents fiber length, and cardiac output (CO) represents fiber shortening.

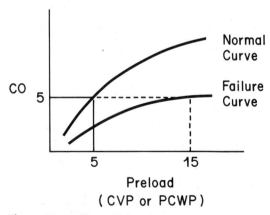

**Figure 30–6.** Ventricular function curve for the heart in failure. To maintain cardiac output (CO), the failing heart is required to function at higher preloads (PCWP or CVP).

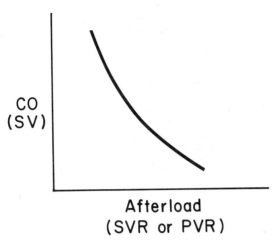

**Figure 30–7.** Relationship of afterload (SVR or PVR) to cardiac output (CO) or stroke volume (SV) at a constant preload.

be assessed indirectly from acid-base status, arterial-venous oxygen content differences, mixed venous oxygen content or saturation, and urinary output. In low-output cardiac failure, both preload and afterload should be optimized through therapeutic manipulation. If this method fails to restore the cardiac output to an acceptable level, attention should be directed to improving myocardial contractility. β-sympathomimetics, such as dopamine and isoproterenol, are effective in improving cardiac output acutely. Depending on the cause of myocardial failure, either short-term or long-term therapy with digitalis may be necessary.

**Heart Rate.** Heart block is rare in pregnant women, but cardiac output can be compromised when the heart rate is too slow. In this circumstance, either treatment with atropine or cardiac pacing is indicated. Conversely, sustained tachycardia can lead to congestive heart failure because of shortened systolic ejection and diastolic filling times or myocardial ischemia, especially in the clinical setting of valvular heart disease. The pathophysiologic basis of tachycardia should be determined (fever, hypovolemia, pain, hyperthyroidism) and corrected. Treatment with propranolol, digoxin, or a calcium channel blocker such as verapamil is seldom required in obstetric patients; however, when indicated, all can prove effective in limiting heart rate.

## MIXED VENOUS BLOOD ANALYSIS

Fiberoptic pulmonary artery catheters and bedside microprocessors now make it possible to continuously plot the mixed venous blood oxygen saturation. In nonpregnant subjects, the mixed venous oxygen content may fall before any other evidence of hemodynamic instability appears, making it potentially useful as an early warning system (Divertie and McMichan, 1984; Schmidt et al, 1983).

Traditionally, mixed venous blood samples have been analyzed in the same manner used for arterial blood samples; intermittently and often paired with an arterial specimen. As with arterial blood, mixed venous blood can be analyzed for oxygen tension ($PvO_2$ in mm Hg) and for saturation ($SvO_2$ as a percent). Mixed venous blood saturation reflects the balance between oxygen delivery and oxygen use. It reflects tissue perfusion, the variation in oxygen requirements for different organs, and the affinity of hemoglobin to accept and subsequently to release oxygen. The normal value for $PvO_2$ is 40 mm Hg with an average saturation of 73 percent; saturations below 60 percent are interpreted as abnormally low (Schmidt et al, 1983). Pericapillary interstitial fluid $PO_2$ is 10–20 mm Hg and intracellular $PO_2$ is estimated to be 6 mm Hg. To maintain an adequate intravascular-to-interstitium-to-cellular gradient, a minimal capillary $PO_2$ of 30 mm Hg is required. Values below this result in impaired oxygen delivery and anaerobic metabolism. In women, unconsciousness accompanies a $PvO_2$ of less then 20 mm Hg, and irreversible brain damage occurs below 12 mm Hg (Gibbs et al, 1940; Thews, 1960).

The advantages of continuous monitoring of mixed venous blood saturation ($SvO_2$), as opposed to arterial blood saturation, are numerous. First, arterial blood samples usually have a saturation of 90 percent or greater, corresponding to $PO_2$ of 60 to 100 mm Hg or greater. Because of the shape of the hemoglobin dissociation curve (Fig. 30–8), fluctuations at these higher levels of oxygen tension are reflected by very small corresponding changes in saturation. Conversely, at the lower levels of oxygen present in venous blood a linear relationship exists between saturation and tension, making $SvO_2$ a sensitive marker for detection of physiologic instability. Secondly, although an arterial blood analysis provides useful information

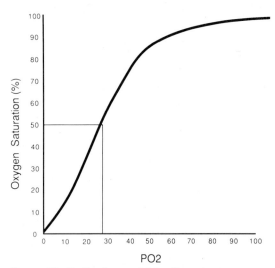

**Figure 30–8.** Oxyhemoglobin dissociation curve. Note that the mixed venous oxygen saturations operate on the "dissociation" or linear phase of the curve and are very sensitive to physiologic instability.

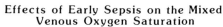

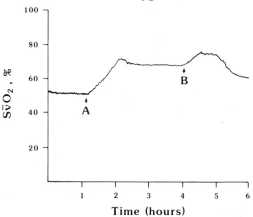

**Figure 30–9.** The effects of sepsis on $SvO_2$. At point A, the cardiac output has already increased disproportionate to oxygen utilization even before the patient has clinically apparent infection, resulting in an increase in $SvO_2$. At point B, the patient develops rigors with a further increase in both cardiac output and $SvO_2$.

concerning pulmonary oxygen exchange, ventilation, and shunt, it provides little information regarding the overall adequacy of oxygen delivery to peripheral tissues. Because the mixed venous gas reflects the end product of supply and demand, it is superior in this respect. Finally, the addition of a thermodilution cardiac output measurement, in conjunction with a mixed venous gas, can support or refute clinical assumptions made on the basis of the mixed venous oxygen saturation. For example, improvement of mixed venous oxygen saturation with stable cardiac output is a good prognostic sign and heralds clinical improvement. If, however, the same change in the mixed venous oxygen saturation is accompanied by a 100 percent increase in cardiac output, it may simply be the first sign of sepsis.

Continuous monitoring of $SvO_2$ is advocated for titration of vasoactive and inotropic drugs, adjustment of positive end-expiratory pressure (PEEP), evaluation of fluid therapy, routine patient care, and as an early warning system for changes in cardiorespiratory status. In Figure 30–9, the effect of sepsis on $SvO_2$ is demonstrated. Because the rise in cardiac output exceeds the increase in tissue oxygen demands, $SvO_2$ increases even before clinical sepsis is apparent (point A). Shortly

before and during rigors (point B), a further increase is noted. In another patient care scenario, the titration of optimal or best PEEP using $SvO_2$ is demonstrated in Figure 30–10. Incremental increases in PEEP at points A and B resulted in airway recruitment, decreased shunt, and improved oxygen delivery. At point C, however, increased PEEP resulted in a fall in venous return and a fall in cardiac output, with a proportional fall in oxygen delivery, reflected in a declining

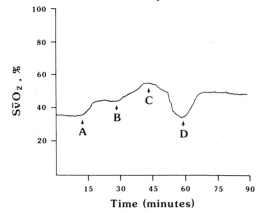

**Figure 30–10.** Use of $SvO_2$ to select the best PEEP.

$SvO_2$. At point D, the amount of PEEP is reduced, venous return increases, and both cardiac output and $SvO_2$ improve. Thus, the $SvO_2$ can be a very simple and efficient method to define PEEP.

Pregnancy produces physiologic alterations of the mixed venous blood gas. Because the increase in cardiac output exceeds the increase in oxygen use, the $PvO_2$ and $SvO_2$ both normally increase (Kerr, 1976). During labor, both are abnormally low when measured during contractions because of the return of desaturated venous blood from the uterus, placenta, and lower extremities. Between contractions, however, $PvO_2$ and $SvO_2$ are again abnormally high relative to nonpregnant levels (Ueland and Hansen, 1969).

Little data is available on the use of this relatively new technology in pregnant women. We anticipate, however, that continuous monitoring of mixed venous oxygen saturation may be particularly useful in women who develop the adult respiratory distress syndrome (ARDS) or who have very prolonged illnesses and intensive care unit stays.

# Etiology and Treatment of Pulmonary Edema

The greatest use of invasive hemodynamic monitoring in obstetrics may lie in the differentiation of the pulmonary edema of heart failure (hydrostatic pulmonary edema) from that of lung failure (permeability pulmonary edema) (Rinaldo and Rogers, 1982), because only after the correct diagnosis has been made can therapy be optimized (Fig. 30–11).

McHugh and colleagues (1972) correlated radiographic findings of pulmonary edema with absolute PCWP in patients with myocardial infarction. Pulmonary congestion is apparent, first, at a pressure of 18 mm Hg, is mild to moderate at 18 to 25 mm Hg, and is moderate to severe at 20 to 30 mm Hg. Development of frank pulmonary edema at a PCWP above 30 mm Hg was noted. This model represents pure hydrostatic pulmonary edema secondary to left ventricular failure or acute volume overload. In pulmonary edema of this origin, therapy should be directed at improving myocardial contrac-

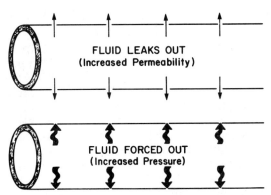

**Figure 30–11.** Mechanisms that would reduce intravascular volume even though extravascular extracellular fluid is increased.

tility and reducing the preload to a high-normal range.

Pulmonary edema also can result from damage to the pulmonary alveolar capillary membrane by any of a host of insults, ranging from sepsis (most common) to hypersensitivity reactions mediated by non-human leukocyte antigen leukoagglutinins at the time of blood transfusion (Anderson et al; 1979; Petty, 1982; Thompson et al, 1971; Trambaugh et al; 1980). In this model, there is a disturbance of membrane permeability resulting in the flux of both protein and water into the pulmonary interstitium and the alveolus despite normal cardiac function and filling pressures. Unlike the situation in hydrostatic or pressure-induced pulmonary edema, which resolves within a few hours after normal PCWP is restored, alveolar membrane lesions require days to heal. This process may eventuate into ARDS if the source of the injury is not eradicated, such as a focus of infection leading to septic emboli. The therapeutic goals in pulmonary edema due to permeability defects are (1) to maintain filling pressures in the low-normal range to minimize transudation of protein and fluid into the lungs, and (2) to eradicate the source of injury.

To illustrate these concepts, let us consider the hypothetical case of a pregnant woman with premature labor who is being treated with intravenous magnesium sulfate. On initial presentation, she was treated with bed rest and hydrated with 2 liters of normal saline but had continued contractions. Despite 4 g/h of intravenous magnesium sulfate, her contractions are increasing in intensity and frequency, and her cervix is progressively dilating. Eighteen hours after beginning tocolytic therapy, acute dyspnea develops and physical findings are consistent with pulmonary edema. Concomitantly, the patient's temperature is 39°C (102.2°F) and, for the first time, uterine tenderness is elicited. A number of factors could account for this edema, including (1) sepsis with alveolar membrane injury, (2) heart failure secondary to tocolytic therapy (i.e., hydrostatic pulmonary edema), and (3) iatrogenic volume overload causing hydrostatic pulmonary edema. The diagnosis and management of this patient may be enhanced by invasive hemodynamic monitoring with precise knowledge of myocardial function and ventricular filling pressures.

# Cardiovascular Monitoring and Obstetrics

Currently, the flow-directed pulmonary artery catheter is used in obstetrics in (1) the management of critically ill patients or those at risk for sudden cardiovascular decompensation and (2) clinical investigations that attempt to define the pathophysiology of various disease processes or evaluate therapy of a specific condition.

Obstetric patients with cardiac or pulmonary complications who are critically ill or whose condition is subject to rapid deterioration (Clark et al, 1985; Hankins, 1988; Lee et al, 1988) are essentially the same patients who would receive invasive cardiovascular monitoring in medical or surgical intensive care units. Management of patients with severe sepsis complicated by hypotension or oliguria (Lee et al, 1988) and of patients with heart failure or pulmonary edema of unclear etiology might be aided by placement of a pulmonary artery catheter (Cunningham et al, 1987). Women with sudden intraoperative cardiovascular decompensation are also candidates for hemodynamic monitoring. For example, the diagnosis of amniotic fluid embolism is facilitated by the demonstration of pulmonary hypertension and a high degree of pulmonary shunting. Additionally, fetal squamous cells or amniotic fluid debris might be obtained in smears of blood aspirated from the pulmonary artery (Clark

et al, 1985a). Similarly, patients with massive blood loss and large transfusion requirements (e.g., with placental abruption or uterine rupture) may benefit from invasive monitoring, particularly when oliguria or pulmonary edema is present.

Another group of high-risk obstetric patients for whom invasive hemodynamic monitoring of labor and delivery affords a margin of safety are those with chronic cardiovascular disease. Patients with significant structural lesions or physiologic disturbances of the heart or great vessels, in addition to those with symptoms due to compromised cardiac status, are at risk for peripartum decompensation. Included in this group at high risk for cardiac decompensation are all patients who are categorized as New York Heart Association functional class III and IV. Particularly dangerous structural or physiologic disturbances include primary pulmonary hypertension, Eisenmenger's physiology, aortic coarctation, and mitral stenosis (Clark et al, 1985a; Clark et al, 1985c; Hankins et al, 1985a). More precise assessment of their baseline condition, both early in pregnancy, to assess the risk of continuing the pregnancy, and during labor and delivery, as well as prompt evaluation of complications and subsequent therapeutic decisions, should affect favorably both management and outcome.

Patients with coronary artery disease exhibited by angina or a history of myocardial infarction also should be monitored invasively during labor, delivery, and the early postpartum period (Hankins et al, 1985b). Similarly, women with a cardiomyopathy should be monitored irrespective of the cause of the cardiac lesion (Cunningham et al, 1986). Additional high-risk patients include those with uncontrolled hyperthyroidism or pheochromocytomas in the predelivery or perioperative period. Although a number of indications have been listed, this list is by no means inclusive nor will all women with the conditions listed earlier require invasive monitoring.

## THE NURSE'S ROLE IN INVASIVE MONITORING IN OBSTETRICS

The nurse's role in caring for the patient with a pulmonary artery catheter, an arterial catheter, or both, is to (1) collect and interpret the data from the technology; (2) communicate critical data points to the team members; (3) alter nursing actions and plan of care based on the hemodynamic findings; and (4) prevent, recognize, and treat complications of invasive hemodynamic monitoring. The periodic acquisition and recording of hemodynamic data or profiles typically includes the patient's mean arterial pressure (MAP), central venous pressure, pulmonary artery pressure (PAP), PCWP, cardiac output, and the derived parameters of stroke volume, systemic vascular resistance, and pulmonary vascular resistance (PVR). If the patient has a continuous $SvO_2$ pulmonary artery catheter, the additional data points of oxygen delivery and consumption including the hemoglobin level, $SaO_2$, $SvO_2$, $CaO_2$ (arterial oxygen content), $CvO_2$ (venous oxygen content), arteriovenous oxygen difference ($AVDo_2$), oxygen availability ($O_2AV$), oxygen consumption ($VO_2$), and oxygen extraction ratio ($O_2ER$) are collected. The patient's condition dictates the frequency of acquiring complete hemodynamic profiles and calculations.

The nurse must interpret the hemodynamic profile and alter the patient's plan of care based on the data. For example, Ms. Dobbs is a 31-year-old gravida 2, para 1, at 35 weeks' gestation diagnosed with chronic hypertension and superimposed pre-eclampsia. A pulmonary artery catheter is inserted owing to hypertensive crisis unresponsive to hydralazine. Oliguria and shortness of breath are also present. Hemodynamic data on insertion is a MAP of 158, central venous pressure is 7 mm Hg, PAP is 42/30, PCWP is 28, and cardiac output is 3.3 liters/min. The derived systemic vascular resistance and PVR are 3660 and 34 respectively. The plan of care prior to catheter insertion was the administration of a $\beta$ blocker to lower the patient's blood pressure. Because the hemodynamic data show a depressed cardiac output and a profoundly elevated systemic vascular resistance, the altered plan of care includes the administration of an arterial dilating agent to decrease the systemic vascular resistance instead of a $\beta$ blocker that will further decrease the cardiac output. The nursing assessment includes the evaluation of altered cardiac output on the mother's tissue perfusion, the pulmonary system, and the neurologic system, and the adaptation of the fetus to the stress-influenced environment and subsequent treatment modalities.

Inherent in the nurse's role in critical care obstetrics is the component of team communication and collaboration. Also important is the psychophysiologic support of the patient and her family. Open visitation policies should be encouraged, and family members should be allowed to remain at the patient's bedside. If the patient has delivered and the neonate's condition allows, frequent mother-baby visitation and interaction should be a priority of the team. Breastfeeding or at least initiation of breast-pumping should be initiated as early as the maternal and newborn conditions allow.

It is impossible to cover in one chapter what others have devoted entire textbooks to. Our purpose in this chapter is to briefly review the evolution of the field of critical care obstetrics, a subspecialty of maternal-fetal medicine. Additionally, we hope to offer guidance to those physicians and nurses charged with the care of these critically ill women regarding the selection of the most appropriate location and team of providers who care for these women. It is our belief that the pregnant woman and her fetus rank as one of our highest medical priorities. We are dealing with two lives with an expected cumulative longevity in excess of 100 years when the acute processes in the mother can be reversed and both her and the fetus' health are preserved. Those accepting the challenge of providing care to the woman and her fetus must be aware that they will be held to applicable standards, not only in the field of obstetrics but also of critical care medicine. The technology available to us for the care of pregnant women has exploded over the past 20 years, and a continuing evolution of this technology and its applications is anticipated. Similarly, the data base concerning the woman, the physiology of pregnancy and the fetus, and our understanding of the pathophysiology of many diseases has burgeoned. The challenge is great, as are the demands. Notwithstanding, the rewards of critical care medicine are far greater than perhaps in any other area of medicine. Frequently, our patients are healthy prior to some acute event that precipitated their need for admission to a critical care setting. Accordingly, our outcome for these patients should exceed that of our colleagues in other specialties whose patients often suffer from chronic and debilitating disease processes.

## References

Anderson RR, Holliday RL, Driedger AA, et al: Documentation of pulmonary capillary permeability in the adult respiratory distress syndrome accompanying human sepsis. Am Rev Respir Dis 119:869–877, 1979.

Baldwin RWM, Hanson GC (Eds): The Critically Ill Obstetric Patient. London, Farrand Press, 1984.

Benedetti TJ, Hargrove JC, Rosene KA: Maternal pulmonary edema during premature labor inhibition. Obstet Gynecol 59:335, 1982.

Berkowitz RL: Critical Care of the Obstetric Patient. New York, Churchill Livingston, 1983.

Braunwald E: On the difference between the heart's output and its contractile state. Circulation 43:171–174, 1971.

Braunwald E: Regulation of the circulation (Part I). N Engl J Med 290:1124, 1974a.

Braunwald E: Regulation of the circulation (Part II). N Engl J Med 290:1420, 1794b.

Clark SL, Cotton DB, Lee W, et al: Central hemodynamic assessment of normal term pregnancy. Am J Obstet Gynecol 161:1439–1442, 1989.

Clark SL, Cotton DB, Hankins GDV, Phelan JP: Critical Care Obstetrics, 2nd ed. Oradell, NJ, Medical Economics Books, 1990.

Clark SL, Cotton DB: Clinical opinion: clinical indications for pulmonary artery catheterization in the patient with severe pregnancy-induced hypertension. Am J Obstet Gynecol 158:453, 1988.

Clark SL, Horenstein JM, Phelan JP, et al: Experience with the pulmonary artery catheter in obstetrics and gynecology. Am J Obstet Gynecol 152:374–378, 1985b.

Clark SL, Montz FJ, Phelan JP: Hemodynamic alterations associated with amniotic fluid embolism: a reappraisal. Am J Obstet Gynecol 151:617–621, 1985a.

Clark SL, Phelan JP, Greenspoon J, et al: Labor and delivery in the presence of mitral stenosis: central hemodynamic observations. Am J Obstet Gynecol 152:984–988, 1985c.

Cohn JN, Franciosa JA: Vasodilator therapy of cardiac failure. N Engl J Med 297:247, 1977.

Cunningham FG, Lucas MJ, Hankins GD: Pulmonary injury complicating antepartum pyelonephritis. Am J Obstet Gynecol 156:797–807, 1987.

Cunningham FG, Pritchard JA, Hankins GD, et al: Peripartum heart failure: idiopathic cardiomyopathy or compounding cardiovascular events? Obstet Gynecol 67:157–168, 1986.

Divertie MG, McMichan JC: Continuous monitoring of mixed venous oxygen saturation. Chest 85:423, 1984.

Frigoletto FD, Little GA (eds): Guidelines for Perinatal Care, 2nd ed. Washington, DC, American Academy of Pediatrics and American College of Obstetricians and Gynecologists, 1988.

Gibbs FA, Williams D, Gibbs EL: Modification of the cortical frequency spectrum by changes in $CO_2$, blood sugar, and $O_2$. J Neurophysiol 3:49, 1940.

Hankins GD, Brekken AL, Davis LM: Maternal death secondary to a dissecting aneurysm of the pulmonary artery. Obstet Gynecol 65:45S–48S, 1985a.

Hankins GDV, Wendel GD Jr, Cunningham FG, Leveno KJ: Longitudinal evaluation of hemodynamic changes in eclampsia. Am J Obstet Gynecol 150:506–512, 1984.

Hankins GD, Wendel GD Jr, Leveno KJ, Stoneham J: Myocardial infarction during pregnancy: a review. Obstet Gynecol 65:139–146, 1985b.

Hankins GDV: Techniques and principles of invasive hemodynamic monitoring in obstetrics and gynecology. ACOG Technical Bulletin #121, Oct 1988.

Harvey CJ (ed): Critical Care Obstetric Nursing. Gaithersburg, Maryland, Aspen Publishers, 1991.

Hauth JC, Hankins GD, Kuehl TJ, Pierson WP: Ritodrine hydrochloride infusion in pregnant baboons. I. Biophysical effects. Am J Obstet Gynecol 146:916–924, 1983.

Herman MV, Gorlin RV: Implications of left ventricular asynergy. Am J Cardiol 23:538, 1969.

Kerr MG: Maternal cardiovascular adjustments in pregnancy and labor. In Goodwin JW, Gooden JO, Chance GW (eds): Perinatal Medicine: The Basic Science Underlying Clinical Practice. Baltimore, MD, Williams & Wilkins Co, 1976, pp 395–408.

Lappas DG, Powell WM, Daggett WM: Cardiac dysfunction in the perioperative period. Pathophysiology, diagnosis and treatment. Anesthesiology 47:117, 1977.

Lee W, Clark SL, Cotton DB, et al: Septic shock during pregnancy. Am J Obstet Gynecol 159:410–416, 1988.

Mason DT, Spann JF Jr, Selis R, et al: Alterations of hemodynamics and myocardial mechanics in patients with congestive heart failure. Pathophysiologic mechanisms and assessment of cardiac function and ventricular contractility. Prog Cardiovasc Dis 12:507, 1970.

McHugh TJ, Forrester JS, Alder L, et al: Pulmonary vascular congestion in acute myocardial infarction: hemodynamic and radiologic correlations. Ann Intern Med 76:29, 1972.

Naulty JS, Cefalo R, Rodkey FL: Placental transfer and fetal toxicity of sodium nitroprusside. Presented at the Annual Meeting of the American Society of Anesthesiology, San Francisco 1976 (Abstract 543).

Petty TL: Adult respiratory distress syndrome. Semin Respir Med 3:219, 1982.

Rinaldo JE, Rogers RM: Adult respiratory distress syndrome. Changing concepts of lung injury and repair. N Engl J Med 206:900, 1982.

Schmidt CR, Frank LP, Estafanous FG: Utility of continuous pulmonary artery oximetry as an early warning monitor in cardiac surgery patients. Presented at the 5th Annual Meeting, Society of Cardiovascular Anesthesiologists, San Diego, CA, April 1983.

Shuman DJ: Standards for Obstetric-Gynecologic Services, 7th Ed. Committee on Professional Standards of the American College of Obstetricians and Gynecologists, Washington, DC, 1989.

Society of Critical Care Medicine: Recommendations for Critical Care Unit Design. Task Force on Guidelines, Society of Critical Care Medicine. Crit Care Med 16:796–806, 1988.

Soonenblick EH, Parmley WW, Ursch ICS, et al: Ventricular function: evaluation of myocardial contractility in health and disease. Prog Cardiovasc Dis 12:449, 1970.

Strauss RG, Keefer JR, Burke T, Civetta JM: Hemodynamic monitoring of cardiogenic pulmonary edema complicating toxemia of pregnancy. Obstet Gynecol 55:170–174, 1980.

Swan HJC, Ganz W, Forrester J, et al: Catheterization of the heart in man with use of a flow-directed balloon-tipped catheter. N Engl J Med 283:447, 1970.

Thews G: Die sauerstoff diffusion im gehirn. Ein beitrag zur frage sauerstoff diffusion der organe. Pflugers Arch 271:197, 1960.

Thompson JS, Severson CD, Parmely MF: Pulmonary hypersensitivity reactions induced by transfusion of non-HLA leukoagglutinins. N Engl J Med 284:1120, 1971.

Trambaugh RF, Lewis FR, Christensen JM, et al: Lung water changes after thermal injury—the effects of crystalloid resuscitation and sepsis. Ann Surg 192: 479, 1980.

Ueland K, Hansen JM: Maternal cardiovascular dynamics. II. Posture and uterine contractions. Am J Obstet Gynecol 103:1–7, 1969.

**PART III**

Follow Up

# CHAPTER 31

# Newborn Care in the Delivery Room

Kathryn E. TePas and M. Douglas Cunningham

The birth of an infant is a moment of uncertainty. Modern obstetrics and neonatology attempt to maximize the options for effective therapy of complications befalling the fetus or infant of a woman with a high-risk pregnancy. It is essential for newborn care in the delivery room of high-risk pregnancies to declare the presence of fetal-neonatal compromise, document severity, and immediately treat the adverse physiologic states. Delivery room care for sick newborn infants begins with a high state of preparedness for the rapid implementation of resuscitation measures.

Perinatal asphyxia presents the neonatologist-pediatrician with the pathophysiologic effects of impaired respiration. Hypoxia and acidosis are the overriding events to be relieved by ventilation of the newborn lungs. The transformation from dependence on maternal respiration to independent respiration requires a great deal of energy and vitality on the part of normal newborn infants but it may be an impossible task for compromised neonates. Prior to delivery, the lungs are filled with fluid and largely bypassed from the standpoint of cardiac output. At the moment of birth, they must be rapidly relieved of the fluid and instantly inflated and perfused. Impediments to this transformation preclude the infant's only immediate means for reversing the metabolic acidosis of perinatal asphyxia and the deterioration of vital signs. Successful newborn resuscitation depends on effective restoration of respiratory function.

## Antepartum Considerations

### PREGNANCY RISK FACTORS

Numerous maternal conditions can be related to an increased risk for fetal well-being and birth asphyxia. Table 31–1 lists most conditions that allow time to prepare for a high-risk delivery and prompt resuscitation of the sick newborn.

Pregnancy-risk scoring systems have been advocated for nearly 25 years, but their acceptance has varied and is generally limited to larger medical centers. Indexing high-risk pregnancies affords the opportunity to weigh various risk factors and distinguish the more ominous situations. Numerous scoring systems have been proposed. The Maternal-Child Health Care Index, offered by Nesbitt and Aubry (1969), relies on maternal history and physical examination and subtracts positive risk data from a perfect score of 100. A simple 1 +, 2 +, 3 + system, initiated at the University of Colorado and adapted for the University of California, San Diego, (Resnick, 1976), weighs breech delivery at 1 +; drug abuse, 2 +; and premature rupture of membranes, 3 +. More recent publications have emphasized problem-oriented algorithms (Friedman et al, 1987). Irrespective of form, some manner of high-risk assignment sets the stage for anticipatory measures to be taken should an asphyxiated or otherwise handicapped infant be delivered.

A retrospective analysis of 96 cases of ce-

**Table 31–1**
PREGNANCY RISK FACTORS

**Antepartum Conditions Suggesting Advanced
  Preparations for Delivery and Resuscitation**
Rh isoimmunization
Toxemia
Diabetes mellitus
Prolonged rupture of fetal membranes
Premature delivery
Prolonged labor (especially prolonged second stage)
Post-term delivery
Breech presentation
Chorioamnionitis
Thyroid disease
Acute pyelonephritis or other urinary tract infection
Severe anemia (such as sickle cell or thalassemia)
Severe maternal respiratory distress
Myasthenia gravis
Multiple gestation
Oligo- and polyhydramnios
Maternal drug therapy or usage:
  Propylthiouracil
  Propranolol
  Lithium
  Magnesium
  Alcohol
  Amphetamine
  Cocaine
  Heroin
  Methadone
  Ritodrine
  Terbutaline
Intrauterine growth disturbance
  Very low birth weight
  Intrauterine growth retardation
  Small- or large-for-gestational-age fetuses
Meconium staining of amniotic fluid
Apparent anomalies
  Myelomeningocele
  Omphalocele
  Gastroschisis
**Intrapartum Events that Occur with Little Notice
  and Require a Constant State of Preparedness**
Abruptio placentae
Placenta praevia
Precipitous labor
Mid-forceps rotation
Prolapsed umbilical cord
Maternal hypotension
Cord tightly around neck (nuchal cord)
Shoulder dystocia
Ruptured uterus

rebral palsy revealed that many high-risk pregnancies did not receive special care and that potentially avoidable problems, of either obstetric or neonatal care, could have been identified in the antepartum period (McManus et al, 1977). More recent data have reaffirmed these observations by identifying a multiplicity of conditions leading to cerebral palsy, of which 53 percent are attributable to congenital disorders and only 14 percent to birth asphyxia (Naeye et al,

1989). Whether the stress is pre-existing or acute, identifiable high-risk factors (as in Table 31–1) may have similar neurologic sequelae.

## ASSESSMENT OF FETAL WELL-BEING

Fetal assessment for growth and development attempts to establish normal growth and allows for the assumption that the fetus can withstand the stresses of labor, birth, and the adaptation to an extrauterine existence. Various methods are now available for assessing fetal condition and intrauterine environment.

Ultrasonography affords detection and monitoring of intrauterine growth and the presence of anomalies. Decreased biparietal diameters for fetal head growth suggest intrauterine growth retardation. Anomalies such as hydrocephalus, omphalocele, and myelomeningocele can be documented as well as estimates of uterine size and amniotic fluid volume. Ultrasound examinations revealing disproportionate twin growth and the presence of hydramnios can lead to the diagnosis of twin-to-twin transfusion. Ultrasonographic and electrophysical studies of fetal reactivity, muscle tone, breathing movements, and amniotic fluid volume comprise a biophysical profile of the fetus (Vintzileos et al, 1989). Additionally, percutaneous umbilical blood sampling and chorionic villus biopsy are two new techniques for assessing fetal well-being.

Amniotic fluid studies obtained by amniocentesis are a major aid to fetal assessment. Resuscitation preparations are mandatory for those Rh-sensitized pregnancies with rising amniotic fluid $\Delta$ OD 450 levels. Phospholipid analysis of amniotic fluid for lung maturation has led to improved awareness and preparation for prematurity. Low lecithin-sphingomyelin (L/S) ratios and absence of phosphatidylglycerol are associated with increased risk for birth asphyxia (Gluck, 1978).

Antepartum nonstress testing, contraction stress testing, and biophysical profile are used to assess fetal well-being prior to the onset of labor. During labor, awareness by the resuscitation team of nonreassuring fetal heart rate tracings alerts the team to possible fetal compromise.

Fetal heart rate monitoring can be complemented by sampling of capillary blood to determine intrapartum fetal acid-base status. Scalp blood pH values of 7.25 or less signal a diminishing capability of the fetoplacental unit to maintain acid-base balance. Fetal blood pH values of 7.15 or less are associated with at least a 90 percent incidence of the clinical diagnosis of birth asphyxia. Alternatively, immediate postpartum cord blood arterial and venous samples enable the resuscitation team to establish the presence or absence of significant fetal-neonatal hypoxemia and acidosis. Normative umbilical cord blood gas values are being determined. Institutional normal values are important to establish for appropriate care in the newborn period.

## COMMUNICATION

Introduction of the parents to the neonatal physician and nurses by the obstetric team before delivery confirms continuity of care and prepares them for future interaction. A myriad of strangers under difficult circumstances is an unnecessary burden for the parents. If a patient has been identified as high risk before the intrapartum period, a tour of the neonatal intensive care nursery also may help to alleviate stress. A recent study demonstrated that an antepartum tour or information presented to the mother at the bedside reduced the maternal stress more than when no intervention was given (Chappel, 1988). If labor has already begun, pictures of the unit may be helpful to the parents.

Interdisciplinary communication among anesthesiology, obstetric, and neonatology personnel eliminates confusion and enhances sharing of information and coordination of efforts to resuscitate and stabilize a sick newborn. The use and effects of analgesic and anesthetic agents must be made known to the resuscitation team. Resuscitation of an infant must follow the established Standard for Neonatal Resuscitation of the American Heart Association and the American Academy of Pediatrics (Cropley and Bloom, 1989).

Once a high-risk delivery has been defined and plans for infant resuscitation established, notification of the neonatal intensive care unit should be made. Advance notice allows for preparation of an acute care bed and the placement of additional nursing personnel on standby status. Sick infant transport to the nearest neonatal intensive care facility also may be required. Advance notice to the transporting agency allows time to assemble equipment and alert personnel.

# Anticipation of Resuscitation

During final preparations for delivery, the obstetric staff need only update the neonatal resuscitation team. The physical environment, equipment, and medications required for resuscitation of an infant must be organized in the delivery area at all times. Last-minute scrambling by the neonatal team in preparation for the arrival of a sick infant is inexcusable. Daily inventories and rechecking before and after each delivery are necessary to ensure smooth and orderly resuscitations.

## DESIGNATION AND PREPARATION OF PERSONNEL

If the infant is known beforehand to be at risk for asphyxia, a neonatal resuscitation team is requested. All deliveries should be attended by a nurse who is qualified to perform initial newborn assessments and is capable of initiating resuscitation measures. The nurse should be free to deal with the infant and devoid of responsibilities for the mother.

The neonatal resuscitation team should consist of at least one neonatal physician and two nurses or one neonatal nurse practitioner and one special care nurse. One team member must be experienced in endotracheal intubation of infants, especially low-birth-weight premature newborns. One member must assume the role of team leader to determine and delegate specific tasks and responsibilities before the actual delivery. Three team members facilitate resuscitation at a high-risk delivery. One assumes responsibility for airway management, the second monitors cardiovascular function, and the third prepares and administers medication and records the sequence of events.

The objective of the team is to function together smoothly, quickly reverse the effects of asphyxia, and stabilize the infant. To achieve these goals, physicians and nurses who maintain certification in neonatal resuscitation are able to work comfortably as a team.

## THE PHYSICAL ENVIRONMENT

In many cases, delivery room management of the sick newborn is just the beginning of many days of intensive care. In others, it constitutes an intensive period of care for the infant, albeit for an hour or less. Bearing in mind the nature of care, the physical space allocated for newborn resuscitation should meet the recommendations of the American Academy of Pediatrics and the American College of Obstetricians and Gynecologists (1992) for a neonatal intensive care station. One hundred and fifty square feet of floor space meets minimal requirements for a resuscitation bed, two to three team members, and usable space for monitoring equipment and supplies. It also must provide space for the set-up of sterile trays for umbilical catheterization or thoracostomy trays when needed.

The resuscitation area can be either within the delivery room or in an immediately adjacent room. The latter is often preferred by neonatologists. A large delivery room may adequately accommodate the 40-square-foot space requirement (Guidelines for Perinatal Care, 1992). Properly equipped, a resuscitation area in the delivery room should suffice for all low-risk and most high-risk deliveries.

The advantages of a resuscitation room include having an isolated environment dedicated entirely to the needs of a neonate requiring vigorous resuscitation. It provides space for mounted equipment and storage of supplies (Fig. 31–1). If emergency x-ray studies are required, portable equipment can be brought in without disturbing the obstetric team. If mechanical ventilation is required, respiratory care practitioners can enter without violating the sterile field. Lastly, a resuscitation room buffers parents and others from the sights, sounds, and dialogue of full scale resuscitation, and the resuscitation team can work without being distracted by frightened and distraught parents.

Conversely, others may choose to use an area within a family-centered birthing facility. Adequate space and equipment can be

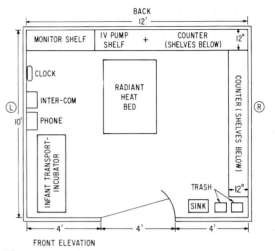

**Figure 31–1.** Overhead schematic for distribution and arrangement of resuscitation room facilities. Note counter space and shelving for monitoring and support equipment.

provided in the labor, delivery, recovery, and postpartum (LDRP) care concept. Other personnel need to be ready to assist the resuscitation team by redirecting family members and support persons in the event of extreme circumstances.

Temperature and air flow in the delivery room are traditionally regulated for the comfort of the mother and obstetric staff. A complicating feature of birth asphyxia is hypothermia (Sheldon, 1977), and the advent of effective radiant heat warmers in the delivery room often is accompanied by a false sense of security that thermal stability is no longer a problem. The high-risk infant quickly loses heat following delivery by evaporation, conduction, radiation, and convection. The design of the resuscitation area must take into account all four routes of heat loss. Evaporative, conductive, and radiant heat loss can be minimized by placing the infant in warm blankets or towels under a radiant warming bed and rapidly drying the skin. As soon as the skin is dry, towels and blankets should be removed and a servo-control probe attached to allow for temperature stabilization. However, convective heat loss (dependent on ambient temperature and the velocity of air flow over the infant) must be considered separately. Air conditioning ducts are a major source of convective losses in many delivery rooms. It is important to ensure that the resuscitation area is not within the cross draft of ducts. Keeping the delivery room temperature at or above 24.4°C (76°F) (usual nursery or neonatal intensive care room temperature) helps minimize convective losses.

The resuscitation station must include adequate utilities to supply technical support systems. Good ceiling lighting is essential for accurate assessment of the neonate. A surgical spotlight is helpful for umbilical vessel catheterizations. If attached to the bed, the spotlight is available without taking up additional floor space.

Sufficient numbers of electrical outlets for the operation of support equipment is critical to any intensive care (resuscitation) setting. Ten outlets with emergency generator backup are usually adequate to power the radiant warmer, infusion pumps, spotlight, cardiac monitor, and blood pressure monitor. The electrical outlets should be immediately adjacent to the neonatal station (Fig. 31–2) and should not in any way be required by the obstetric staff for care of the mother.

Two vacuum outlets are required: one for airway suction and the other for use with thoracostomy drainage systems. The station should have two oxygen outlets and one air outlet. One oxygen outlet attaches to the respirator Flowmeter and supports hand bag ventilation. An air outlet and the second oxygen outlet are made available for a ventilator, should one be needed. Air, oxygen, and vacuum outlets also should be separate from the maternal supply.

Although seldom considered, waste materials are a fact of resuscitative efforts. A large amount of trash accumulates (syringe packages, sterile wrappings, empty vials and ampules, expended syringes, and used linens). A waste receptacle and sharps container within arm's reach decreases the clutter associated with rapid intervention. These materials should be collected in accordance with universal precautions and OSHA guidelines.

## EQUIPMENT

It is imperative that equipment be organized and immediately accessible to the infant resuscitation team: this means within arm's reach of the infant's bed. Supplies should be checked periodically throughout the day and kept restocked at all times. Responsibility for this should be delegated to each nursing shift.

The items required for delivery room management of the high-risk infant are listed in Table 31–2. The radiant warmer should be turned on prior to delivery to eliminate warm-up time. Stethoscope, facemasks, anesthesia bag, and laryngoscope blade should be on the bed to be kept warm and in plain view. The infant servo-control temperature probe for the radiant warmer should be ready for attachment to the infant.

Mounting the cardiac monitor on a wall shelf conserves floor space. Blood pressure monitoring is made easier by the use of pneumatic monitors or Doppler pulse sensors. Several small arm cuff sizes are necessary. Blood pressure monitoring is essential for evaluating the recovery of an infant from asphyxia. Universal precautions for avoidance of contact with blood or body fluids should be observed by persons caring for the newborn. The amniotic fluid, vernix, blood, and oral-tracheal secretions are possible sources of contact and contamination. Equipment for observing universal precautions by newborn care-givers should include gowns, gloves, masks, and disposable eye protection.

## PHARMACEUTICALS

The most essential drugs for use in resuscitation efforts are listed in Table 31–3. Displaying both medications and supplies on a

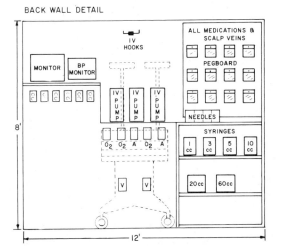

BACK WALL DETAIL

**Figure 31–2.** View of wall behind resuscitation bed. Easy access to supplies and visibility of monitors is stressed. Note number of oxygen (O$_2$), air (A), and vacuum (V) outlets behind the bed.

Table 31–2
EQUIPMENT FOR RESUSCITATION

Large surface radiant warmer with:
  Servo-control mechanism and probe
  Observation lights
  Spotlight
  Thermometer
Infant resuscitation bag (for delivery of 90 to 100
  percent oxygen)
  Pressure manometer
  Pressure release valve
  Masks; premature and newborn
Flowmeters for oxygen and air with tubing
Wall suction with extension tubing and negative
  pressure gauge
Stethoscope with infant dome and diaphragm
Laryngoscope: Miller 0 blade (8 cm) and extra
  batteries and light bulbs
Endotracheal tubes—2.5 mm to 4.5 mm inner
  diameter
Soft wire stylet
DeLee suction trap #10 with suction adapter to wall
  suction
Meconium suction adapter
Hand suction bulb
Cord clamps
Suction catheters, sizes 5, 6, 8 and 10 Fr
Umbilical catheterization trays with umbilical
  catheters, sizes 3.5 and 5 Fr
Betadine solution
Cardiac monitor with leads and electrodes
Blood pressure device with infant cuffs, sizes 2.5, 3.5,
  and 4.0 cm
Needles, 27 to 18 gauge
Scalp vein needles, 21 to 25 gauge
Syringes, size 1 to 60/ml
Sterile gloves
Benzoin solution
Adhesive tape, ½″ and 1″
Three-way stopcocks
Scissors
Thoracostomy tray
Thoracostomy catheters, sizes 10, 12 and 16 Fr
Chest drainage system with underwater seal
Intravenous fluids: dextrose 5 percent in water and
  dextrose 10 percent in water in 250-ml or 500-ml
  containers

pegboard seems to be the most practical storage system (Fig. 31–3). It provides immediate visualization of the presence or absence of items, takes up no counter space, and allows for the individual labeling of items. Color-coded and easy-to-read labels facilitate quick retrieval of appropriate items.

Figures 31–1, 31–2, and 31–3 are examples of a resuscitation station with equipment and supplies that meet American Academy of Pediatrics and American College of Obstetrics and Gynecology (1992) criteria for space, organization, and use for resuscitation.

# Need for Resuscitation

## PATHOPHYSIOLOGY OF ASPHYXIA

Asphyxia is the failure to exchange carbon dioxide and oxygen and maintain body acid-base balance. Survival of the fetus is dependent on the continued respiratory function of the placenta. Intermittent intrauterine asphyxia may occur for periods lasting several days if marginal respiratory compensation can be achieved by the fetoplacental circulation. Progressive fetal asphyxia and intrauterine death may result, or the fetus may survive until the onset of labor only to suffer increasing asphyxia with the stress of advancing labor. Fetal asphyxia also may occur acutely as in maternal shock following abruptio placentae, uterine rupture, or compromise of the umbilical vessels by prolapse of the cord. In the fetus, a loss of heart rate beat-to-beat variability and fetal heart rate decelerations may be signs of limited myocardial ability to withstand the stress of uterine contractions because of acute or chronic intrauterine asphyxia.

In contrast to the fetus, asphyxia in the newborn is always acute and related to intrapartum events or failure of the newborn airway to become established with sustained spontaneous ventilation. Frequently, in the asphyxiated newborn, the lungs fail to become adequately aerated or perfused owing to central nervous system depression and absence of respiratory drive or airway obstruction by secretions. Failure to establish spontaneous ventilation immediately leads to continuing hypoxia and greatly aggravates the existing consequences of intrauterine asphyxia.

Oxygen deprivation leads to the deteriorating pathophysiologic events listed in Table 31–4. Hypoxia, especially of the larger muscle masses and organs, causes tissue metabolism to revert to an anaerobic state with an accumulation of blood lactic acid. Failure of respiration leads to carbon dioxide accumulation, increasing production of carbonic acid. The end result is uncompensated metabolic and respiratory acidosis. The increased hydrogen ion concentration leads to a failure of bicarbonate buffering of the blood. Other blood-buffering mechanisms, principally phosphates and hemoglobin, are overwhelmed, and whole blood buf-

**Table 31–3**
MEDICATIONS FOR USE IN NEONATAL RESUSCITATION

| Drug | Indication | Route | Dose |
|---|---|---|---|
| Epinephrine (1:10,000 dilution) | Bradycardia | intratracheal intravenous | 0.1–0.3 ml/kg |
| Volume expander 5 percent albumin whole blood normal saline | Hypovolemia | intravenous | 10 ml/kg |
| Sodium bicarbonate | Metabolic acidosis | intravenous | 2 mEq/kg |
| Naloxone | Opiate narcosis | intravenous intratracheal | 0.1 mg/kg |
| Dopamine | Hypotension | Continuous intravenous infusion | 5 $\mu$g/kg/minute |

Data from Cropley C, Bloom RS (eds): Textbook of Neonatal Resuscitation. Dallas, TX; American Heart Association/American Academy of Pediatrics, 1989; and Kaufmann RE, Banner W, Blumer J, et al: Naloxone dosage and route of administration for infants and children: addendum to emergency drug doses for infants and children. Pediatrics 86:484, 1990.

fering capability fails, a base deficit rapidly accrues, and blood pH falls rapidly.

Worsening hypoxia and hypercapnia, at first, cause a maximal ventilatory effort in either the fetus or the newborn, but with advancing asphyxia, ventilatory efforts fail and primary apnea ensues (see Table 31–4). A second effort at ventilation occurs at approximately 5 minutes as irregular gasping. Dawes (1968) described the second effort to breathe and noted that it gives way to a final period of apnea after 10 minutes of asphyxia.

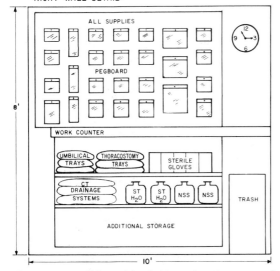

**Figure 31–3.** Schematic for supply storage and pegboard storage of frequently used supplies requiring easy and quick retrieval.

Secondary apnea may last up to 20 minutes with occasional agonal gasping movements, usually associated with fixed blood pH values of 6.8 or less.

Concomitant to these metabolic derangements of respiratory failure are changes in cardiac rhythm. Heart rate increases initially, causing increased cerebral vascular flow, myocardial perfusion, and slightly increased cardiac output.

Like the fetal heart rate, the asphyxiated newborn heart is tachycardic, initially, followed by progressive bradycardia (see Table 31–4). After 5 minutes of asphyxia, a plateau of bradycardia at 50 beats/min usually is noted. If resuscitation is not effective, the heart rate declines further to a slow dysfunctional rhythm with idioventricular contractions and, finally, asystole.

Following the initial increased cardiac output, progressive asphyxia and bradycardia result in an ever diminishing cerebral blood flow. Cerebral ischemia and brain damage are most likely between 5 and 10 minutes of severe asphyxia in both the fetus and newborn. Similar perfusion losses occur in the gut and kidneys.

In the fetus, pulmonary vascular flow is unchanged, but the newborn experiences a rapid decrease in pulmonary blood flow. In addition to the severe acid-base derangements brought on by asphyxia, glucose and calcium metabolism are also disturbed. Because of poor cardiac output and decreased peripheral perfusion, large muscle groups and abdominal organs are deprived of oxygen and revert to anaerobic metabolism.

Table 31–4
PATHOPHYSIOLOGIC EVENTS AND CONSEQUENCES OF BIRTH ASPHYXIA

| Physiologic Factor | Time from Birth | | | |
|---|---|---|---|---|
| | *1 min* | *3 min* | *5 min* | *10 min* |
| Respiratory effort | Rapid | Primary apnea | Returns briefly as irregular gasping | Fails again and becomes secondary apnea followed by agonal breathing |
| Approximate blood pH | 7.25 | 7.15 | 7.00 | 6.75 |
| Heart rate | Increased | Falls | Plateau about 50 beats/min | < 50 beats/min becomes idioventricular |
| Cardiac output | Slightly increased | Decreasing | Falling | Minimal |
| Pulmonary blood flow | Decreases rapidly | Decreasing | Minimal | Negligible |
| Cerebral blood flow | Slightly increased | Decreasing | Rapidly falling | Ischemia resulting in brain damage |
| Renal perfusion | Unchanged | Decreasing | Rapidly declining | Ischemia, cortical necrosis |

Glucose use becomes inefficient, and energy demands of the brain and myocardium are met by an increased glucose consumption and depletion of glycogen stores.

## IMMEDIATE ASSESSMENT OF THE NEONATE

The need for resuscitation is dictated by the pathophysiologic events of asphyxia, but clinical indicators for initiating vigorous resuscitative procedures must be recognized immediately at birth from the infant's appearance. Virginia Apgar (1953) proposed a scheme for rapid clinical assessment that has become known as the Apgar Scoring System (Table 31–5). The severely compromised infant with a heart rate of 50 or less is hardly overlooked (Apgar score = 1), but varying degrees of birth asphyxia, with scores be-

tween 1 and 7, require immediate attention and extended periods of close observation.

Any distressed infant (asphyxiated or suffering from other forms of shock) provides evidence for the Apgar scoring parameters. Gluck (1978) described variations of the basic Apgar observations for initial asphyxia for which prompt corrective measures ensure a return to normal. Like the fetus, the newborn signals early distress (shock, asphyxia, or both) with tachycardia (heart rate 140 to 160) with periods up to 200. With deepening but still reversible distress, heart rate begins to decline to rates of 120 to 100.

Other signs of early but reversible neonatal asphyxia and distress noted by Gluck (1978) include heightened respirations, overreaction to stimuli, excessive body movements, and exaggerated reflexes. Skin color and the general appearance of a distressed infant include a duskiness of forehead, lips, hands, and feet overlaying a deeper pinkish

Table 31–5
APGAR SCORING SYSTEM

| Criteria | Scores | | |
|---|---|---|---|
| | *2* | *1* | *0* |
| *Heart Rate* | > 100 | < 100 | Asystole |
| *Respiratory Effort* | Crying with regular breath sounds easily heard | No crying, irregular efforts, gasping, weak breath sounds | Apnea |
| *Reflex Irritability* | Crying, grimacing, and withdrawal from painful stimuli | No crying, grimacing only, apathetic, minimal to no withdrawal from painful stimuli | Areflexia |
| *Muscle Tone* | Limb flexion, fetal positioning, voluntary activity | Minimal movement, weak response to stimulation | Atonia |
| *Color* | Completely pink | Central pinkness with blue hands and feet | Ashen |

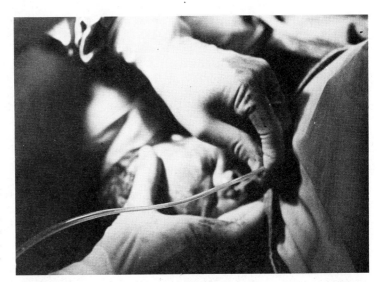

**Figure 31–4.** Fetus's head presenting on the perineum, and obstetrician using DeLee trap suctioning of nasopharynx. This procedure is of special importance before the first breath in the presence of meconium-stained amniotic fluid.

color that has been described by Gluck as "pink-on-blue" or "blue-on-pink." This unusual color calls attention to an early sign of neonatal distress. It is distinct from poor peripheral perfusion or vasoconstriction with mottling and an underlying gray cyanosis.

## Steps for Resuscitation

### AIRWAY AND VENTILATION

Recognition of respiratory failure requires immediate attention and the establishment of a patent airway in any resuscitation attempt. In the neonate, clearing of the airways should have taken place with delivery of the head on the perineum and prior to the infant taking its first breath. As the head and neck of the fetus present, bulb suctioning of the mouth and nose are necessary. If excessive secretions appear in the pharynx, a DeLee suction catheter with trap connected to wall suction can be used to clear the upper airway and then advanced to empty the stomach (Fig. 31–4). OSHA regulations prohibit the practitioner from sucking on the DeLee tubing. If delivery is by cesarean section, a similar approach to clearing the airway can be taken. A 10 or 12 Fr suction catheter is more effective if thick or tenacious secretions are encountered. Immediately on delivery of the infant, the head should be held slightly downward in a Trendelenburg position to avoid aspiration of any retained secretions.

As soon as the cord has been clamped and cut, the high-risk infant should be transferred to a radiant warmer in either the delivery room or an adjacent resuscitation room. The infant must be thoroughly dried and the wet towels discarded. The infant should be positioned under the radiant warmer with its head slightly lower than its feet. Suctioning of the mouth, first, and nose with bulb syringe follows.

During this period, deep suctioning of the upper airway should be avoided. Care must be taken not to overly stimulate the posterior pharynx and produce vagal stimulation with reflex bradycardia. Tactile stimulation can take the form of brisk rubbing with a warm towel to dry the infant. Drying the infant reduces heat loss by evaporation while providing safe stimulation. Stimulating the birth-depressed infant by gentle rubbing may be helpful for initiating respiratory efforts. Slapping the soles of the feet is acceptable but no more than twice. Tactile stimulation can be used only for a short period of time. If the infant does not respond, resuscitation efforts must quickly advance to bag-and-mask ventilatory support (Cropley and Bloom, 1989). Other forms of tactile stimulation, such as slapping the buttocks or rasping the infant's back with one's knuckles, are condemned.

If apnea persists and the heart rate falls below 100 (within 1 to 3 minutes of life), asphyxia is worsening. Suctioning to provide a clear upper airway permits the next step: bag-and-mask ventilation in accordance with American Heart Association and American Academy of Pediatrics Standards for Neonatal Resuscitation (Cropley and Bloom, 1989). Monitoring of the heart rate should begin with the first minute, by stethoscope, and later, electronically, when time permits lead attachment. Heart rate greater than 100 by 1 minute of age allows for continued attempts to give tactile stimulation and observe for spontaneous respirations.

Adequate lung inflation can be judged by the rise of the chest with each mechanical breath and by the equality of breath sounds heard by stethoscope. Adequate ventilation is noted by a surge in heart rate from below 100 to a rate of 120 or higher. Mucous membrane color changing to pink, increased skin perfusion, and spontaneous breathing movements are additional signs of the infant's improving condition and the abatement of asphyxia.

The majority of term infants with prolonged apnea and early bradycardia in the first 2 minutes of life respond satisfactorily to airway management and recover from mild-to-moderate asphyxia at birth, but low-birth-weight infants, premature infants, and infants who have prolonged and chronic intrauterine hypoxia are less likely to do so.

With a persistent heart rate of less than 100 with no return of respiratory effort, endotracheal intubation becomes mandatory for reversal of the worsening effects of persistent hypoxia.

Establishment of an adequate airway and initiation of effective ventilation and respiration are the keys to successful infant resuscitation. All other measures become secondary to placing an adequate airway (Fig. 31–5).

Endotracheal intubation should be undertaken only by persons certified by completion of the course for Standards of Neonatal Resuscitation by the American Heart Association and the American Academy of Pediatrics (Cropley and Bloom, 1989). In addition, the procedure should be carried out with an assistant familiar with all phases of infant resuscitation and the equipment (Table 31–6).

As soon as possible after resuscitation, a chest roentgenogram should be taken for lung appearance and endotracheal tube placement. Blood gas determinations should also be made as soon as possible to verify the effectiveness of the neonate's ventilation (i.e., restoration of oxygenation and compensation of acidosis).

After endotracheal intubation, placement of arterial and venous umbilical catheters should be considered. Umbilical artery catheters afford blood gas sampling and central arterial blood pressure monitoring. An umbilical vein catheter allows for venous blood gas monitoring and central venous pressure monitoring if it can be documented by roentgenography to be above the diaphragm. Umbilical vein catheters can be quickly placed and secured and can serve as routes for drug, intravenous fluid, or colloid solution administration.

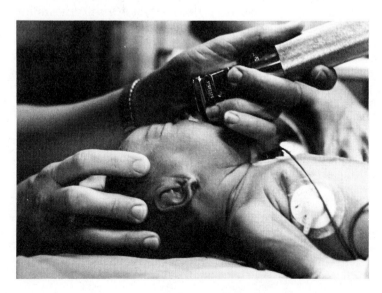

Figure 31–5. Left-handed laryngoscopy, leaving right hand free to pass endotracheal tube. Note only slight neck extension with insertion of blade.

Table 31–6
ENDOTRACHEAL TUBE SIZE

| Birth Weight (g) | Endotracheal Tube Internal Diameter (mm) | Comments |
|---|---|---|
| > 3000 | 4.0 | Needed for passage of 10 Fr suction catheter to clear larger volume of secretions |
| 2000–3000 | 3.5 | Usually passes easily into trachea; easy to pass 8 Fr suction catheter |
| 1000–2000 | 3.0 | Most likely size to pass |
| < 1000 | 2.5 | Larger endotracheal tube not likely to fit |

## CIRCULATION

Support of circulation of the asphyxiated infant begins with effective ventilation and restoration of respiration. However, if the heart rate should fail to rise above 100, external cardiac massage must be considered. If heart rate is documented at 80 beats/min or less, external cardiac massage is mandatory (Cropley and Bloom, 1987). During the first minute of life, only estimates of the heart rate can be made. The stethoscope usually is used to count heart rate, but palpation of cord pulse also may be useful. Attachment of electronic monitor leads may be difficult or impossible, and time should not be lost attempting technological finesse. Stethoscope monitoring in the first 1 to 2 minutes by use of the 6-second method (heart rate = beats/ 6 seconds × 10) informs the resuscitation team of cardiac status and responses to airway placement and management.

Cardiac compression for the newborn infant, and especially the low-birth-weight infant, is specifically different from that described in most basic life support courses and guidebooks. First noted by Todres and Rogers (1975) and included in standards of the American Heart Association and American Academy of Pediatrics for neonatal resuscitation (Cropley and Bloom, 1989), it calls for open-handed encirclement of the newborn chest with thumb over sternum for cardiac compression (Fig. 31–6). The fingers of both hands interlace to form posterior support of the spine and ribs. The palms sta-

bilize the lateral walls of the chest, localizing the mediastinum medially. The thumbs (side-by-side on larger infants, or overlapped on smaller infants) are pressed downward (posteriorly) 1 to 2 cm. The chest should be compressed approximately 100 times per minute with maximum thumb pressure over the lower third of the sternum. In the author's experience, the two-finger method (also included in the standards for neonatal resuscitation) is an effective alternative but less so for low-birth-weight infants. Adequate cardiac compression can be documented if an umbilical artery line is in place, and a pulse wave form can be observed. Occasionally, palpation of the femoral artery by an assistant can be used to confirm adequate external cardiac compression. If continued mechanical ventilation and cardiac compression do not bring about improved heart rate (> 100 beats/min) and improved color of the infant, drug therapy must then be considered.

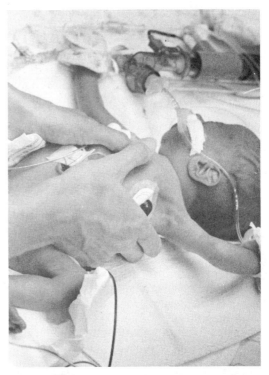

**Figure 31–6.** Simulated two-handed chest-encircling midsternal method of external cardiac massage. Note that in this very small infant the thumbs override, but in a larger infant, the thumbs would be side-by-side.

## PHARMACOLOGIC ADJUNCTS

Severe birth asphyxia may not respond to the previously mentioned measures, and drug support may be needed. It must be emphasized that only severe asphyxiating circumstances should be expected to include drugs for support of continued resuscitative efforts.

Certain medications have become recognized as the principal choices for infant resuscitation. Extensive lists of drugs for inclusion in resuscitation preparations lead to confusion. Table 31–3 lists those drugs most frequently noted for use in standardized resuscitation of neonates (Cropley and Bloom, 1989).

Epinephrine (0.1–0.3 ml/kg; 1:10,000 dilution) increases the rate and strength of cardiac contractions. It should be administered via the intratracheal or intravenous route if the heart rate is 0 or remains below 80 beats/min, despite a minimum of 30 seconds of adequate ventilation with 100 percent oxygen and chest compressions. Epinephrine may be repeated every 5 minutes. The complications of excessive use include tachycardia, hypertension, and ventricular fibrillation.

Persistent bradycardia with severe metabolic acidosis may not be readily relieved by ventilation within the first 3 to 5 minutes. Alkali use may have to be considered. Sodium bicarbonate given intravenously should improve the pH and support improved cardiac responsiveness to ventilation. It is important to continue ventilation during the administration of sodium bicarbonate. Moreover, the use of alkalizing agents can improve cardiac response to both endogenous and exogenous catecholamines with a concomitant chronotropic effect.

Volume expansion is indicated if there is evidence of acute bleeding or other signs of hypovolemia. Those signs would include pallor despite oxygenation, weak pulse with rapid heart rate, poor response to resuscitative effort, and low blood pressure. Current recommendations call for the use of 5 percent albumin solution (Table 31–3) in the delivery room. Alternative volume expanders include whole blood, normal saline, fresh frozen plasma, plasma protein fraction, and Ringer's lactate. Albumin is preferred, however, because of its availability and demonstrated effectiveness in a number of newborn conditions.

Central nervous system hemorrhage following sodium bicarbonate use in low-birth-weight infants has been associated with resuscitation and the need to give large volumes of hypertonic solutions. Studies to date raise concerns about rapid expansion of blood volume in the absence of autoregulation of cerebral blood flow. Infusions of alkali and colloid substances in volumes of 5 to 10 ml must be given slowly in asphyxiated newborns, especially those of low birth weight with a propensity to central nervous system hemorrhage.

Hypoglycemia complicates birth asphyxia, and initiating a continuous infusion to keep intravenous and intra-arterial lines open also allows maintenance of body glucose. Excessive glucose administration and hyperglycemia is to be avoided. Monitoring capillary glucose by test strips through the first hour of life is essential to maintaining euglycemia.

If, following the use of epinephrine, sodium bicarbonate, and a volume expander, the infant continues to have poor peripheral perfusion, a weak pulse, and signs of shock, a vasopressor is needed to further support an infant's resuscitation. A continuous infusion of dopamine is recommended, beginning with 5 $\mu$g/kg/min (Cropley and Bloom, 1989).

Occasionally, antepartum analgesia with morphine or other opiates results in respiratory depression of the newborn. Usually, respiratory depression is observed as primary apnea with heart rate remaining stable and tactile stimulation transiently improving heart rate and respirations. If the immediate antepartum history is positive for opiate analgesia, naloxone (Narcan) is a rapidly acting antagonist.

Administration of drugs during resuscitation carries considerable risk because of the uncertainty of the route of administration. Umbilical vessels are used because of availability and the need for expediency. Hypertonic and sclerosing solutions are dangerous to hepatic portal vessels, and if administered through unbilical arteries, renal, intestinal, and lower limb arteries are threatened. Intravenous routes are recommended. Umbilical vessels must be used cautiously. The endotracheal route for epinephrine and naloxone is effective and approved.

Throughout the process of resuscitation following a high-risk pregnancy, attention must be paid to the environment. Thermoregulation to avoid hypothermia in the infant is paramount. Hypothermia alone causes hypoglycemia, acidosis, dysrhythmia, and shock. If allowed to occur, no amount of resuscitative effort can successfully reverse both asphyxia and profound hypothermia. No data exist to support the notion that hypothermia is protective or helpful to the asphyxiated infant. Availability and use of servo-control mechanisms for conserving infant body heat are mandatory for all resuscitation settings.

Accidents can occur if care in handling electrical outlets and high pressure lines is not exercised. Unnoticed suction lines have found their way to the skin of infants and produced suction-induced blisters.

# After Resuscitation

At some point in the management of a sick infant, it is necessary to reassess the infant's condition with regard to moving him or her from the resuscitation area to either the neonatal intensive care unit or a tertiary care facility. This depends largely on the infant's response to intervention. The resuscitation team leader decides when and where the infant should be moved. Following a brief physical examination, the infant's destination is confirmed and the receiving facility notified of the mode of transport, expected time of arrival, and current condition of the infant. The parents should be apprised as soon as possible of the plans for transfer, their infant's condition, and the immediate expectations for the infant.

## PHYSICAL EXAMINATION

A brief physical examination of the infant should be completed before the infant leaves the delivery and resuscitation area, with special consideration being given to cardiovascular and respiratory function (Table 31–7). Inspection for bruising, lacerations, paralysis, and fractures is necessary. An attempt to establish gestational age should be made, especially looking for age and size discrepancies. An evaluation of pulmonary and cardiovascular adjustment to extrauterine life includes

1. Color (in and out of oxygen)
2. Ease of respirations
3. Presence of excessive secretions

4. Quality of breath sounds
5. Peripheral perfusion
6. Blood pressure
7. Presence of murmurs

A general assessment of the infant's overall condition should note tone, activity, and alertness with a final determination of body temperature, heart rate, respiratory rate, and blood pressure.

## DISPOSITION AND OBSERVATION

All infants in high-risk delivery situations should be observed closely for at least 4 to 6 hours whether mother and child are bonding in a recovery room or the infant has been removed to an observation nursery. Constant observation by skilled personnel include 15-minute reassessment of temperature, respirations, heart rate, color, tone, and behavior. Generally, this should continue until all vital signs have been continuously normal for 1 hour.

Thermal control is a major concern, even for seemingly normal infants, but it should not be a problem if the naked infant is placed against the mother's skin with warm blankets covering both. Overhead radiant warmers may provide supplemental heat if needed, but Freeman (1979) found that infant temperatures were warmer with skin-to-skin contact and blankets than with the use of a radiant warmer. If, for reasons of maternal health, a bonding period is not feasible with this attention to thermal control, then admission of the infant to the observation nursery is strongly recommended rather than a protracted period of observation in the delivery suite.

Special care facilities are required for any infant who has not made a smooth transition to extrauterine life. A preterm infant requiring oxygen and ventilation should be admitted to an intensive or special care nursery. Infants who require immediate special care include those with suspected pneumothorax, asphyxia, poor peripheral perfusion, poor muscle tone, hypertonia, or seizure-like activity. Any infant for whom vigorous resuscitation was required should be monitored in the intensive care unit for the sequelae of birth asphyxia. If the delivering institution does not have facilities for intermediate or critical intensive care, consultation with a neonatal referral center should be considered.

**Table 31-7**
GUIDE FOR GENERAL ASSESSMENT IN THE DELIVERY ROOM

| Feature | General Condition | Trauma | Maturity ≥ 36 weeks |
|---|---|---|---|
| General | Color and peripheral perfusion | | Pink skin<br>Flexion all limbs<br>Diminishing vernix |
| Head | Appropriate size<br>Dysmorphologic features | Large cephalohematoma or caput<br>Bruising<br>Petechiae<br>Lacerations<br>Depressed skull fracture | Quick ear pinnae recoil<br>Incurving 2/3 pinnae<br>Head circumference > 31 cm |
| Face | Alertness<br>Obvious defects of palate and lip<br>Copious secretions | Bruising<br>Lacerations<br>Paralysis (7th cranial nerve) | Absent facial lanugo |
| Thorax | Ease of respirations<br>Quality of breath sounds<br>Peripheral perfusion<br>Blood pressure<br>Murmur | Pneumothorax<br>Diaphragmatic paralysis | 1–2 mm breast tissue |
| Abdomen | Distended or scaphoid<br>Number of cord vessels<br>Masses<br>Liver size<br>Patent anus | | Few visible vessels |
| Back | Deformities | Bruising<br>Petechiae<br>Lacerations | Patchiness of absence of lanugo |
| Limbs | Color<br>Deformities<br>Range of motion<br>Muscle tone | Bruising<br>Lacerations<br>Fractures | Sole creases, anterior 2/3;<br>100 degree popliteal angle<br>20 degree ankle angle<br>45 degree wrist angle |
| Genitals | Sex distinction | | Testes in scrotum<br>Anterior scrotal rugae and rubor<br>Labia majora cover labia minora<br>Mons pubis present |
| Neuromuscular condition | Alertness<br>Spontaneous activity<br>Muscle tone | Upper extremity paralysis (Erb's or Klumpke's) | Recoil arms and legs<br>Strong grasp reflex<br>Strong rooting reflex<br>Complete Moro's reflex |

## PARENT CONTACT

The only circumstance under which an infant should leave the delivery area without parental contact is if the father is not present and the mother is under general anesthesia. If appropriately transported, a few moments can be made available for the parents to have face-to-face contact with the infant and time to touch a hand or foot. It is unlikely that this will jeopardize the infant's condition. Failure to have even this brief contact may interfere with the parental attachment process later. Marut (1978) describes the earliest phase of the postpartum attachment process as the time in the delivery room when the mother identifies the child as her own. A few seconds of contact establishes reality and assists the woman in assuming her new role as a mother.

During this brief contact, the parents should be informed of the general condition of the infant and the immediate plans for its care. Although it is important to be honest with the parents when they ask the inevitable, "Will the baby be all right?", it is also important to be as supportive as possible. Parents may have difficulty dealing with the reality of having an infant in crisis. Benfield and coworkers (1976) describe grief reaction in parents as often being out of proportion to the level of illness in the infant. The resuscitation team members should accept the parents' behavior and allow them to use their coping mechanisms to deal with their grief. The many technical details of the infant's condition or predicted hospital course can be relayed to them as their awareness of reality develops. The prime objectives of the resuscitation team at the time of transport are to allow parent-infant contact, establish the reality of having an ill neonate, and build rapport with the parents.

## TRANSPORT

During transport of the infant from the resuscitation area to an observation nursery or special care unit, three things should be provided for: (1) thermal control, (2) maintenance of required ventilatory support, and (3) visibility of the infant. Much ground is lost if, after extensive resuscitation efforts, a sick infant becomes cold or disconnected from life support equipment while en route to a special care nursery. Radiant heat warming with skin temperature control allows personnel attending the infant and the parents to touch the infant without interruption of thermal control. New disposable thermal pads can be placed under the infant and can maintain temperature for up to 4 hours. A transport incubator equipped with a ventilator and cardiopulmonary monitors is required for referral to special care centers. Good visibility of the infant is of special importance to prevent life support mechanisms from becoming dislodged.

# Special Considerations

Some high-risk infants require special attention in addition to resuscitation because of certain problems.

## MECONIUM STAINING

The passage of meconium *in utero* is a presumed fetal response to asphyxia, but it is uncommon before 34 weeks' gestation despite other signs of fetal distress. Amniotic fluid that is stained dark green and appears thickened poses a greater risk to the newborn than does yellowish fluid. The mere presence of meconium-stained fluid increases the risk of perinatal morbidity and mortality. Preventing the neonate from aspirating meconium present in the hypopharynx before delivery of the chest is the most

effective means of minimizing pulmonary complications (Perez, 1981). As soon as the head and neck are delivered on the perineum or through an abdominal incision, the obstetrician should suction the nasopharynx (Fig. 31–4). The amniotic fluid must be observed, and the meconium staining confirmed. If it is meconium stained, a determination as to its character is important to the neonatal resuscitation team. The meconium staining may be yellow in color and thin in consistency, or it may be dark green, thick, and contain particulate material. Immediately after delivery, the infant should be examined with a laryngoscope to observe the vocal cords. If meconium is seen on or below the vocal cords, the infant should have endotracheal intubation and suction using an adapter and wall suction. Mechanical suction only is recommended in keeping with Centers for Disease Control universal precautions for communicable diseases (Holtzman et al, 1989). If thick meconium is found in the endotracheal tube, the procedure should be quickly repeated. Positive pressure ventilation should not be administered until after direct laryngoscopy and suction have been performed. The infant should receive free oxygen during the procedure via a catheter held close to the nose or mouth. Many of these infants will be depressed at birth, but some may be vigorous and crying. Nevertheless, it is recommended that after suctioning on the perineum by the obstetrician these infants be considered for laryngoscopy to clear any aspirated meconium in the upper airway. The morbidity and mortality of infants with meconium aspiration may be significantly decreased if they are thoroughly suctioned on the perineum and undergo direct tracheal suction immediately following birth (Bascik, 1977). Conversely, if the meconium is thin and the fetal heart rate was normal, and the newborn heart rate and respiratory rates are normal, endotracheal intubation and suction do not need to be performed. These infants can be managed like otherwise normal newborn infants with the same expectations for an uncomplicated outcome (Holtzman et al, 1989).

## IMMATURITY

Birth asphyxia is a major hazard for the premature infant. Primarily owing to the immature respiratory system, it is often complicated by such perinatal conditions as antepartum hemorrhage, intrauterine infection, breech presentation, and protracted labor.

During aggressive delivery room management to reverse asphyxia, it is especially difficult to keep premature infants warm. Their absence of subcutaneous fat (as an insulator) and large surface-to-volume ratio leads to exaggerated heat losses. Quick, gentle drying, removing wet linen, and servo-operated radiant warmers helps to maintain normal body heat.

Bruising as a result of delivery trauma and excessive stimulation after delivery are common, because these infants have poor capillary integrity. Bruising may lead to excessive red blood cell breakdown and neonatal hyperbilirubinemia. Gentle handling is a must.

Intraventricular hemorrhage, a common complication of asphyxia associated with prematurity, may be precipitated or exacerbated by a sudden rise in arterial pressure and a concomitant rise in cerebral blood flow.

Rapid administration of bolus medications is to be avoided during resuscitation efforts because of the potential loss of cerebral blood flow autoregulation. Arterial pressure also can be elevated following infusion of hyperosmolar solutions and colloids. Infusion of all solutions and volume expanders should be performed *slowly* to minimize the risk of intracranial hemorrhage (Volpe and Koenigsberger, 1981).

The use of exogenous surfactant for the treatment of expected respiratory distress syndrome has been established and approved. Two approaches are currently in use: (1) early prophylactic administration in the delivery room to very low-birth-weight infants and (2) rescue administration between 2 and 24 hours of age. Recent information suggests that prophylactic treatment in the delivery room may not be more effective than rescue therapy, which follows stabilization and evaluation in the neonatal intensive care unit. Further studies and evaluation of clinical experience are in progress (Fujiwara et al, 1990).

Table 31–8
SOME BIRTH ANOMALIES WHOSE PRESENCE ALTERS DELIVERY ROOM MANAGEMENT

| Anomaly | Recognition | Problems | Intervention |
|---------|-------------|----------|--------------|
| Encephalocele myelomeningocele | | Contamination leading to infection<br>Respiratory impairment<br>Increased heat loss through defect | Sterile gloves<br>Warm sterile saline dressings and sterile plastic-bowel bag<br>May require continued assisted ventilation |
| Choanal atresia | Cyanotic and distressed at rest<br>Pink when cries | Hypoxia<br>Acidosis | Tape oral airway in place<br>Position on back or abdomen |
| Diaphragmatic hernia | Scaphoid abdomen<br>Absent breath sounds<br>Cyanosis | Severe respiratory distress secondary to abdominal contents in chest | Nasogastric tube to suction<br>If ventilation required, intubate trachea |
| Esophageal atresia with tracheo-esophageal fistula | Hoarse cry<br>Excess oral secretions<br>Respiratory distress | Aspiration of saliva<br>Aspiration of stomach contents | Elevate head<br>Prevent aspiration<br>Continuous upper airway suction |
| Gastroschisis/ omphalocele | External abdominal contents with or without protective membrane | Increased heat loss through exposed viscera<br>Risk of infection<br>Risk of bleeding if traumatized | Maintain thermal control<br>Sterile gloves<br>Warm sterile saline dressings |
| Ambiguous genitalia | | | Make parents aware of problem early<br>Do not assign sex role |
| Epidermolysis bullosa | Large fluid-filled bullae<br>Excoriated skin | Increased risk of infection<br>Increased fluid loss<br>Increased heat loss<br>Exfoliated skin obstructing airway or gastrointestinal tract | Sterile linen, gloves<br>Mask<br>Minimal handling<br>No tape<br>Do not apply identification bands |

Although representing less than 1 percent of all live births, the extremely immature infant of less than 30 weeks' gestation accounts for most neonatal deaths and neurologically handicapped infants born without congenital malformations. At the present time, many infants of 25 to 30 weeks' gestation (600 to 1500 g) respond well to intensive care (Sachs et al, 1989). If at all possible, these infants should be delivered in a setting with tertiary obstetric and neonatal services.

## MULTIPLE BIRTHS

Twin and other multiple births require provisions for additional resuscitation teams. Advance preparations for extra supplies and equipment should be made to ensure readiness at the time of delivery. Although the second fetus (or additional fetuses) is at greater risk for intrapartum asphyxia, the teams should be prepared to treat asphyxia in either infant. Premature onset of labor, premature rupture of membranes and the need for cesarean delivery due to malpresentation are common complications of preterm deliveries. Birth weight discrepancies between the fetuses can be a sign of twin-to-twin transfusion and the resulting polycythemia of one infant and anemia of the other. (See Chapter 24.)

## BIRTH ANOMALIES

Although approximately 4 percent of children are born with some major birth defect, few require alteration in delivery room management of the infant. However, some conditions can be identified as requiring special attention in the delivery room (Table 31–8).

Myelomeningocele and encephalocele are examples of neural tube defects that are obvious in the delivery room. Care must be taken to prevent infection due to contamination of the exposed meninges. Use sterile technique, wet-to-dry sterile dressings. Position the infant on his abdomen to avoid pressure on the lesion.

Infants are obligate nasal breathers. Choanal atresia must be suspected if the newborn is distressed and cyanotic at rest yet pink when crying (mouth breathes). The diagnosis is strongly suggested if a soft rubber catheter cannot be easily passed through each nostril. Position the infant on his or her side or abdomen and tape an oral airway in place to provide adequate intake of air.

Diaphragmatic hernia occurs once in every 3000 live births and should be suspected in the infant who has a scaphoid abdomen and is greatly distressed at birth. These infants should be intubated but ventilated with caution, because hypoplastic lungs and pneumothoraces are common complications. A nasogastric tube is required to keep the stomach decompressed and reduce thoracic pressure caused by the displacement of dilated bowel. These infants require transport to a tertiary center for emergency surgery, and possible extracorporeal membrane oxygenation (ECMO).

Infants who have esophageal atresia with tracheoesophageal fistula may present in the delivery room with excess oral secretions, a hoarse cry, and respiratory distress. Aspiration pneumonia is the immediate danger. These infants should be positioned with the head elevated to reduce gastric acid aspiration through the fistula; with a nasogastric tube placed in the pouch, intermittent suction helps the infant avoid aspiration of saliva.

Gastroschisis and omphalocele present with bowel external to the abdominal wall. Omphaloceles are covered with a translucent membrane that may or may not remain intact through delivery. In either instance, risk of trauma to the bowel and infection are of prime concern. Delivery room management should include gentle handling with sterile gloves and wrapping the sac, bowel, or both, with warm saline dressings. The infant will have increased heat loss via the exposed bowel, and added thermal control is needed.

The use of sterile plastic bowel bags with drawstrings have proved to be an excellent means of maintaining body temperature while minimizing evaporative fluid loss and infection.

Ambiguous genitalia are mentioned because all parents are anxious to know whether their infant is a boy or a girl. Hurried sex assignment without understanding the infant's anatomy, endocrine physiology, and chromosome constitution can have serious social and emotional consequences for the family in later years. If the genitalia appear indeterminate, the problem of sex assignment should be discussed with the parents in the delivery room.

**Table 31–9**
DRUGS THAT MAY AFFECT THE NEWBORN IN
THE DELIVERY ROOM

| Antepartum Drugs | Immediate Effects on Neonate |
|---|---|
| Propylthiouracil | Fetal goiter with airway obstruction |
| Propranolol | Hypoglycemia |
| | Respiratory depression |
| | Bradycardia |
| Lithium | Hypotonia |
| | Respiratory distress |
| Magnesium | Respiratory depression |
| | Hypotonia |
| | Hypotension |
| | Hypocalcemia |
| Alcohol | Hypoglycemia |
| | Hypotonia |
| Heroin | Respiratory depression (reversed with naloxone) |
| Ritodrine or Terbutaline | Hypoglycemia |
| | Hypotension (may be unresponsive to volume expansion) |
| | Hypocalcemia |

## DRUGS

There are many medications that affect the growth and development of the fetus if taken by the mother during pregnancy. Certain drugs, regardless of their long-term effect on the fetus, alter or compromise the fetus and newborn's ability to adapt to extrauterine life. Drugs that may affect the newborn in the delivery room are listed in Table 31–9 (narcotic agents have been mentioned with birth depression).

## INFANTS OF DIABETIC MOTHERS

Despite careful obstetric and anesthetic management, infants of diabetic mothers remain at greater risk for birth asphyxia. The incidence of hyaline membrane disease is 5 to 6 times greater for premature and near-term infants of diabetic mothers. Maternal hyperglycemia predisposes the infant to hypoglycemia, and continuous serum glucose monitoring is mandatory until values remain within normal limits and regular feedings are established (See also Chapter 26.)

## Rh ISOIMMUNIZATION AND HYDROPS FETALIS

Erythroblastosis fetalis following Rh isoimmunization of the mother may be mild and may require only minimal attention at delivery. However, hydrops fetalis is a severe manifestation of Rh disease, and delivery room preparations for resuscitation must be maximal. In addition to airway management, circulatory assessment is especially important. Most Rh-affected hydropic infants have low hematocrit and hemoglobin values. The resuscitation team must plan for an early packed red blood cell exchange transfusion. O-negative, low-titer, anti-A and anti-B blood should be immediately available. A packed red blood cell isovolumetric exchange transfusion to increase the hematocrit to 32 to 40 percent within the first hour of life may be life saving in cases of severe hydrops fetalis and cardiopulmonary failure. (See also Chapter 29.)

## Routine Care

When the newly delivered infant requires vigorous resuscitation for survival, some of the routine newborn procedures may be forgotten. Identification procedures, gonococcal eye prophylaxis, and vitamin K administration remain important aspects of the newborn infant's delivery room care.

The infant should be identified before leaving the delivery room even if he or she is in crisis at the time. Identification bands (prepared before delivery and including mother's name, hospital number, infant's sex, and date and time of delivery) can be attached to the infant's arm and leg without interrupting resuscitation efforts. Footprinting can be omitted. Individual institutional protocols differ, but arm and leg banding is the *minimal* recommendation for identification before the infant leaves the delivery room. If properly banded, the infant's footprint impressions may be obtained after he or she is admitted to a nursery.

Documentation of gonococcal eye prophylaxis ensures that, if the procedure has not been completed in the delivery room (commonly owing to the poor condition of the infant), the nursery staff will be aware of the need to complete it.

The neonate is deficient in vitamin K–dependent coagulation factors and may develop significant bleeding. The administration of 0.5 to 1.0 mg of intramuscular vitamin K corrects prolonged prothrombin time. Stressed and premature infants are at a great risk for developing these bleeding problems and should receive vitamin K in the delivery room or on admission to the nursery.

## Long-Term Outcome

Low Apgar scores and ultimate infant outcome are difficult to correlate. Information originating from the Collaborative Project on Cerebral Palsy, Mental Retardation, and Other Neurological and Sensory Disorders of Infancy and Childhood (Drage and Berendes, 1966) reported poor neurologic outcome with low 1- and 5-minute Apgar scores. Later studies of very low-birth-weight infants have revealed more encouraging results. Nelson and Ellenberg (1981) found that for children who had Apgar scores of 0 to 3 at 10 minutes or later and survived with intensive resuscitation, 80 percent were free of major handicaps at an early school age. Similarly, Westgren and colleagues (1982) reported that intensive obstetric and neonatal management of 72 infants weighing less than 1500 g resulted in 88 percent of all surviving infants being neurologically normal at 2 years of age. One third of these infants had prolonged asphyxia with Apgar scores of less than 7 at 10 minutes.

Current studies indicate that associated risk factors of the prenatal and postnatal period are more predictive of neurologic outcome for full-term and preterm infants. A prospective 6 year study of high-risk infants, with 39 percent occurrence of Apgar scores of 0 to 3 at 1 and 5 minutes, failed to reveal the score as a single long-term indicator of cerebral palsy. It was concluded that a more predictable factor was the association of low Apgar scores *and* abnormal neurologic signs and symptoms. The combination of these observations were better predictors of poor lifetime outcome.

Apgar scoring should not be looked on as a predictor of outcome but as a scheme to call forth appropriate resuscitative measures. Attempts to correlate scores with fetal and newborn scalp serum pH values have shown wide discrepancies (Sykes et al, 1982). Apgar scores of 0 at 1 to 5 minutes should not preclude a maximal first response by the resuscitation team.

## Parent Information and Education

Often, parents are given only a brief view of their high-risk infant before he or she is transferred to the intensive care area. To understand the impact this may have on the parent-infant unit, it is necessary to briefly look at the development of parent-infant attachment and how the imperfect child may interfere with that process.

Although a common worry for all pregnant couples is that their infant will not be normal, they may become anxious with the onset of labor. Prospective mothers and fathers carry set expectations with them to the delivery suite, and if all has gone well up to the time of admission, they expect a healthy infant. Delivery of the healthy infant tends to reinforce their previous expectations of their baby. Contact with the infant facilitates the bonding process. Bonding at this stage (in the first hours after delivery) is primarily unidirectional (parent-to-infant), rapid, and facilitated by physical contact (Taylor, 1980).

High-risk parents have different perceptions of their pregnancies. Johnson (1979) has identified several feelings that are associated with parents during high-risk pregnancies, including denial, guilt, feelings of failure, and anticipatory grief. Denial may be used as a defense against prenatal attachment to an infant who may die. Pregnancy is thought of as a normal physiologic process, and parents (especially the mother) may feel guilty, blaming themselves for being unable to have a normal pregnancy. If the parents associate success as a man or woman with successful childbearing, they may have feelings of failure. Anticipatory grief is used by these parents to prepare themselves for loss of the child they envision. These feelings develop with their increasing knowledge of the high-risk pregnancy and accompany the parents to the delivery room.

During the activity of preparation in the delivery room, it is important for the parents to receive ongoing support from the staff. Honesty is crucial. Johnson (1979) reports that although information regarding the status of the fetus may be stressful, lack of information is more stressful. Relating positive as well as negative information is important. A positive statement about fetal heart tones sounding good, when spoken in an encouraging manner, helps parents to cope with their fears.

If the high-risk mother has required prolonged hospitalization in the obstetric area, it is helpful if the obstetrician introduces the parents to members of the neonatology team. Parents are reassured to see familiar persons whose only concern is the welfare of their baby. Because most people have a great fear of the unknown, it is helpful if the neonatology team has briefly described to the parents what immediate steps will be taken for their infant.

After delivery, both parents focus immediately on the infant. During the resuscitation, it is vital that someone provide them with information about the baby. Unfortunately, the parents' need for information comes at a time when the resuscitation team is most preoccupied. The leader of the neonatal team should decide what is to be said and how, so that the parents do not receive conflicting reports.

If the infant is immature or ill, the parents must be told the reality of the situation. The mother's condition may not permit her to visit the nursery for hours or days, and the initial delivery room contact will help her to begin to know her infant. Pictures may be provided to help her identify with her infant until she is able to visit. Unless healthy, the infant will differ from the infant the parents have anticipated during the pregnancy. Delivery room personnel must be prepared for the anxiety and grief displayed by parents when faced with the appearance of their infant (Affonso, 1976). Generally, the specifics of long-term outcome are not dealt with in the delivery room for the simple reason that they are usually not known at the time.

Before leaving the delivery room, the neonatal team should assure the parents that they will return with specific information regarding the child's status as soon as possible. At this time, the neonatology team can begin to explain the infant's condition and what interventions are to be undertaken once the infant reaches the special care nursery.

For the parents, delivery of an immature, sick, or deformed infant is just the beginning of a period of attachment and adjustment to the fact that the infant is not healthy. The maternal-infant dyad is most fragile when the infant is imperfect. Although the delivery room time is brief, supportive behavior by the obstetric and neonatal staff can have a positive influence in reducing stress for the parents by providing honest information, understanding their grief, supporting their coping mechanisms, and promoting contact with their infant.

## References

Affonso D: The newborn's potential for interaction. J Obstet Gynecol Nurs 5:9, 1976.

Allen MC, Capute AJ: Neonatal neurodevelopment examinations as a predictor of neuromotor outcome in premature infants. Pediatrics 83:498, 1989.

Apgar V: A proposal for a new method of evaluation of the newborn infant. Anesth Analg 32:260, 1953.

Avery ME, Fletcher BD, Williams RG: The lung and its disorders. *In* The Newborn Infant. Philadelphia, WB Saunders Co, 1981, p 338.

Bascik RT: Meconium aspiration syndrome. Pediatr Clin North Am 24:463, 1977.

Benfield D, Leib S, Reuter J: Grief response of parents after referral of the critically ill newborn to a regional center. N Engl J Med 294:975, 1976.

Chappel J: Antepartum Orientation of High Risk Mothers to Neonatal Intensive Care Units: Effect on Maternal Anxiety Following Premature Birth. Gainesville, FL, University of Florida, 1988. Thesis.

Cropley C, Bloom RS (eds): Textbook of Neonatal Resuscitation. Dallas, TX, American Heart Association/American Academy of Pediatrics, 1989.

Dawes G: Foetal and Neonatal Physiology. Chicago, Year Book Publishers, 1968, p 149.

Drage JS, Berendes H: Apgar scores and outcome of the newborn. Pediatr Clin North Am 13:635, 1966.

Freeman M: Giving family life a good start in the delivery room. Am J Maternal Child Nurs 4:51, 1979.

Friedman EA, Acker DB, Sachs BP (eds): Obstetrical Decision Making. Philadelphia, BC Decker Inc, 1987.

Fujiwara T, Konishi M, Chida S, et al: Surfactant replacement therapy with a single post-ventilatory dose of a reconstituted bovine surfactant in preterm neonates with respiratory distress syndrome: final analysis of a multi-center, double-blind, randomized trial and comparison with similar trials. Pediatrics 86:753, 1990.

Gluck L: Special problems of the newborn. Hosp Pract 13:75, 1978.

Gluck L: Fetal lung maturity. *In* Proceedings of the Seventy-Eighth Ross Conference on Pediatric Research. Columbus, 1979, p 256.

Gregory GA: Resuscitation of the newborn. Anesthesiology 43:225, 1975.

Guidlines of Perinatal Care, 2nd ed. American Academy of Pediatrics and the American College of Obstetricians and Gynecologists, 1992.

Holtzman RB, Banzhaf WC, Silver RK, et al: Perinatal management of meconium staining of the amniotic fluid. Clin Perinatol 16:835, 1989.

Johnson SH: High Risk Parenting. Philadelphia, JB Lippincott Co, 1979, p 10.

Kaufmann RE, Banner W, Blumer J, et al: Naloxone dosage and route of administration for infants and children: addendum to emergency drug doses for infants and children. Pediatrics 86:484, 1990.

Korones SB: High Risk Newborn Infants: The Basis for Intensive Nursing Care. St Lous, CV Mosby Co, 1981, p 68.

Marut JS: Special needs of cesarian mothers. Am J Maternal Child Nurs 3:202, 1978.

McManus F, Rang M, Chance G, et al: Is cerebral palsy a preventable disease? Obstet Gynecol 50:71, 1977.

Naeye RL, Peters EC, Bartholomew M, et al: Origins of cerebral palsy. Am J Dis Child 143:1154, 1989.

Nelson KB, Ellenberg JH: Apgar scores as predictors of chronic neurologic disability. Pediatrics 68:36, 1981.

Nesbitt REL, Aubry RH: High-risk obstetrics II. Value of semi-objective grading system in identifying the vulnerable group. Am J Obstet Gynecol 103:972, 1969.

Perez R: Protocols for Perinatal Nursing Practice. St Louis, CV Mosby Co, 1981, p 224.

Resnick R: Principles of organization of an obstetrical unit from scratch. Clin Perinatol 3:323, 1976.

Sachs BP, Ringer SA: Intrapartum and delivery room management of the very low birthweight infant. Clin Perinatol 16:809, 1989.

Sheldon, R: Management of perinatal asphyxia and shock. Pediatr Ann 6:15, 1977.

Standards and Recommendations for Hospital Care of Newborn Infants. Evanston, IL, American Academy of Pediatrics, 1977, p 25.

Sykes GS, Johnson P, Ashworth F, et al: Do Apgar scores indicate asphyxia? Lancet 1:494, 1982.

Taylor PM: Parent-Infant Relationships. New York, Grune & Stratton, 1980, p 81.

Todres ID, Rogers MC: Methods of external cardiac massage in the newborn infant. J Pediatr 86:781, 1975.

Vintzileos AM, Campbell WA, Rodis JF: Fetal biophysical profile scoring: current status. Clin Perinatol 16:661, 1989.

Volpe JJ, Koenigsberger R: Neurologic disorders. *In* Avery GB (ed): Neonatology: Pathophysiology and Management of the Newborn. Philadelphia, JB Lippincott Co, 1981, p 943.

Westgren M, Ingemarsson I, Ahlström H, et al: Delivery and long-term outcome of very low birth weight infants. Acta Obstet Gynecol Scand 61:25, 1982.

# CHAPTER 32

· · · · · · · · · · · · · · · · · · · · · · · · · · · · · · · · · · · ·

# Genetic Counseling

Anne L. Matthews and Ann C. M. Smith

Genetic counseling is "a communication process which deals with the human problems associated with the occurrence or the risk of occurrence of a genetic disorder in a family" (Ad Hoc Committee on Genetic Counseling, 1975). The multifaceted process of genetic counseling involves a team approach to assist families or individuals in dealing with genetic disorders and their implications for the family. In general, the process includes five major areas of concentration:

1. Providing information concerning the disorder or problem and all its ramifications, including diagnosis, prognosis, and future risk.
2. Helping the family comprehend the information provided.
3. Discussing client management options and referring to appropriate health care resources.
4. Presenting alternatives with respect to future family planning.
5. Supporting the family in its decisions and assisting them in making the best possible adjustment to the problem.

By its very nature, genetic counseling demands the expertise, effort, and time of many health care professionals in order to be an effective avenue of health care maintenance and prevention. This chapter discusses the overall impact of genetic disease, basic patterns of inheritance, environmental influences, appropriate indications for genetic counseling, and the genetic counseling process. Emphasis has been placed on the family's most common questions and concerns regarding pregnancy and reproduction.

## Incidence of Genetic Disease

Health professionals have become increasingly aware of a need for genetic services in virtually every aspect of health care. Since the time of Gregor Mendel in the 1800s, the knowledge base in the arena of human genetics has dramatically increased, with huge strides having been made since the 1950s. McKusick's (1990) catalog presently lists over 4000 disorders with known inheritance patterns. Additionally, many common disorders, such as cancer, mental illness, diabetes, coronary heart disease, and gout, are now known to have a genetic component. For the woman who is pregnant or considering pregnancy, a normal healthy infant is the desired outcome; yet, 0.5 to 1 percent of all liveborn infants have a chromosome abnormality, 4 to 7 percent of perinatal deaths are due to chromosome aberration, and it is estimated that at least half of all first trimester miscarriages have abnormal chromosome complements (Hassold, 1986). Among the newborn population, 3 to 5 percent will have a major congenital malformation, most of which are found to have a genetic component. In the United States alone, this accounts for more than a quarter of a million affected children each year. If one then examines the impact (social, financial, emotional, and so on) of these children on their families, birth defects affect more than 15 million Americans.

Another area of importance is mental retardation. Approximately 3 percent of the general population is mentally retarded (Opitz, 1980). In the severe form of mental retardation, the risk of illness and death early in life is high. Further, it is estimated that 70 percent of mental retardation in the general population can be attributed to genetic causes (Opitz, 1980). Clearly, then, the effect of genetic disorders is not isolated to a few affected individuals but extends to thousands of individuals and their families. Pregnancy initiates a heightened awareness of particular risks and concerns. The future of genetic counseling services in the detection, treatment, and prevention of genetic disorders is promising. Through increased awareness by health care providers and collaborative efforts, genetic counseling services offer a reasonable and important avenue of preventive health care.

# Development of Cytogenetic Techniques

Tjio and Levan (1956) opened a new era in the field of human cytogenetics by developing an effective technique for analyzing human chromosomes. Based on their technique, it was documented that humans have 46 chromosomes in each somatic cell, instead of 48 as previously reported. Lejeune and colleagues (1959) described the chromosomal basis of Down syndrome, thereby opening the way for rapid advances in clinical genetics. Over the past 30 years, cytogenetic techniques have continued to become more precise, and many syndromes have been found to have a chromosomal etiology. Recent advances in molecular genetic techniques, coupled with these newer cytogenetic techniques, have allowed for the identification of submicroscopic chromosomal changes and further delineation of some syndrome etiologies.

## THE HUMAN GENOME

In each human somatic cell, there are 46 chromosomes (*diploid* number). The germ cells, such as the sperm and egg, contain the *haploid* number of chromosomes, 23. Chromosomes are the structural elements in the cell nucleus composed of DNA (deoxyribonucleic acid) and proteins that contain genes, the smallest inherited unit of the genome. For each somatic cell there are 23 pairs of *homologous* chromosomes, with one member of each pair being inherited from each parent. Of the 23 homologous pairs, 22 are known as autosomes (non–sex chromosomes), and one pair is known as the sex chromosomes, X and Y. In the normal female, the sex chromosomes are represented by two X chromosomes, and in the normal male, they are represented by an X and a Y chromosome (Figs. 32–1 and 32–2).

During the metaphase stage of cell division, human chromosomes can be seen under the microscope as distinct entities with identifiable landmarks. Chromosomes are described as having two arms joined at a central region, the *centromere* (Fig. 32–3). Chromosomes are then arranged according to a standardized format based on size known as a *karyotype*. This pictorial display of chromosomes can be obtained by doing a chromosome analysis. Although any tissue in the body can be used (e.g., skin, bone marrow, amniotic fluid), the analysis is usually performed on peripheral blood lymphocytes. The obtained cells are first stimulated to undergo mitosis and are then arrested during metaphase by the use of colchicine. The preparation is then placed in a hypotonic solution so that the cell membrane swells and bursts, allowing the chromosomes to spread. The preparation is stained and placed under a microscope. The chromosomes are then photographed, enlarged during the printing process, and arranged (by hand or computer) so that a complete karyotype is provided.

With the advent of new banding techniques (G, R, C, and high-resolution banding), it is possible to identify not only abnormalities of chromosome number but small additions or deletions of chromosome material as well as rearrangements of chromosome material (Caspersson et al, 1968). The new banding techniques have identified many individuals who were diagnosed as having normal chromosomes as actually having abnormal chromosome constitutions. This becomes an important finding, because even small aberrations in chromosomes can cause clinical abnormalities such as slow growth and development and mental retardation. What is important for the clinician to note is that a child need not have gross major malformations to be affected by a chromosome abnormality. Thus, chromosome analysis may be appropriate even when clinical manifestations are subtle (Table 32–1). In either case, it would appear that too much or

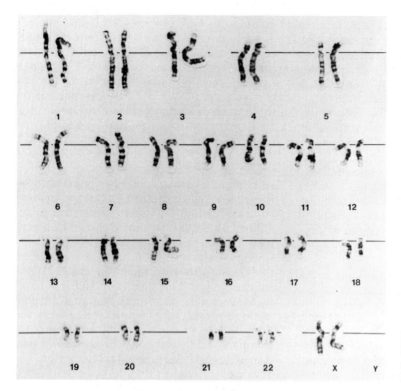

**Figure 32–1.** Normal female karyotype: 46,XX. (Courtesy of The Children's Hospital, Denver, CO.)

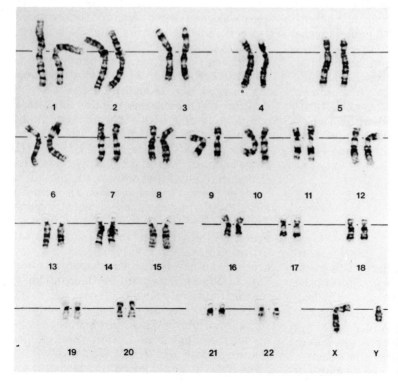

**Figure 32–2.** Normal male karyotype: 46,XY. (Courtesy of The Children's Hospital, Denver, CO.)

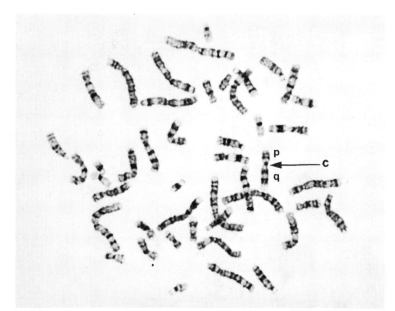

**Figure 32–3.** Metaphase spread. Note: p = short arm of chromosome; q = long arm of chromosome; c = centromere. (Courtesy of The Children's Hospital, Denver, CO.)

too little chromosome material produces adverse effects on normal physical and mental development.

## CLASSIFICATION OF CHROMOSOME ABNORMALITIES

Abnormalities of chromosomes occur in both the autosomes and sex chromosomes. Two major categories of abnormalities can occur: (1) those of chromosome number and (2) those of chromosome structure. Following the discussion of these categories, specific clinical aspects of chromosome abnormalities are presented.

**Table 32–1**
INDICATIONS FOR
CHROMOSOME ANALYSIS

Suspected chromosome syndrome
Multiple malformations with or without associated mental retardation
Positive family history of X-linked mental retardation (fragile-X syndrome)
Ambiguous genitalia
Abnormal sexual development (primary amenorrhea, lack of secondary sexual characteristics)
Multiple miscarriages
Possible balanced translocation carrier
Acquired chromosomal abnormality (leukemias, environmental hazards)

## Numeric Abnormalities (Aneuploidy)

Cells with abnormalities of chromosome number (aneuploidy) have an unbalanced set of chromosomes due to either an excess or deficiency of an entire chromosome. Aneuploidy can arise through a variety of mechanisms. The most common cause is *nondisjunction,* which is the failure of two homologous chromosomes to separate during meiosis. The resulting gamete may then contain one too many or one too few chromosomes. Union of this aneuploid gamete with a normal gamete then leads to aneuploidy in the zygote. For example, if the gamete containing the extra chromosome unites with a normal gamete, then the individual will have 47 chromosomes. That individual is considered *trisomic* for whatever chromosome is extra.

The most common trisomy noted is trisomy 21, known as Down syndrome (Fig. 32–4). Other common autosomal trisomies seen in live-born infants are trisomy 13 and trisomy 18 (Thompson et al, 1991). Trisomy 16 is the most common autosomal trisomy observed in spontaneous abortuses; it has never been observed in live-born infants (Hassold and Jacobs, 1984).

A *monosomy* occurs when a gamete is missing a chromosome and is united with a normal gamete, resulting in a zygote that has 45 chromosomes. Monosomy of an entire chromosome appears to be incompatible with

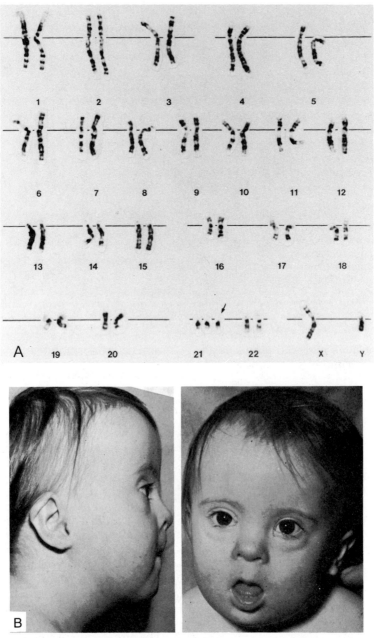

**Figure 32–4.** *A*, Karyotype of a patient with trisomy 21, Down syndrome: 47,X + 21. *Arrow* denotes extra chromosome 21. *B*, Infant with Down syndrome. (*A* courtesy of The Children's Hospital, Denver, CO. *B* from Smith DW: Recognizable Patterns of Human Malformation, 3rd ed. Philadelphia, WB Saunders Co, 1982, p 13.)

fetal survival with the exception of the sex chromosomes. A female fetus can survive and be born with only one X chromosome, a condition called Turner syndrome, 45,X.

If nondisjunction occurs after fertilization (i.e., mitotic nondisjunction), then the resulting zygote has a mixture of normal and aneuploid cells. This produces two or more cell lines with different chromosome numbers within the individual. This specific type of nondisjunction is known as *mosaicism*. Mitotic nondisjunction may occur any time after fertilization. For example, in Down syndrome mosaicism, one tissue may contain cells with 47 chromosomes (trisomy 21), whereas another contains the normal number of chromosomes. The concept of mosaicism becomes particularly important in diagnosis and prognosis for the individual. In the situation of an infant with Down syndrome mosaicism, the clinical findings may be classic, minimal, or nonapparent, depending on the degree and location of the mosaicism. Thus, an individual with Down syndrome who has normal or near-normal intelligence should be investigated for the possibility of mosaicism. Additionally, it may be necessary to examine more than one tissue system (e.g., blood and skin) to define the location and degree of mosaicism present.

## Structural Abnormalities

Thus far, we have discussed abnormalities of chromosome number only. Abnormalities of chromosome structure involve a loss, gain, or repositioning of the chromosome material. Structural abnormalities are deletions, additions, duplications, inversions, and translocations. By definition, partial trisomies and monosomies result from structural rearrangements. Structural abnormalities have been observed in every chromosome (deGrouchy and Turleau, 1984). A deletion is a loss of chromosome material. In humans, the most common deletion observed involves a loss of chromosome material at the end of the chromosome (terminal deletion). Occasionally, loss of an intervening segment (interstitial deletion) occurs. Deletions may be associated with phenotypes that range from mild to severe. One of the more common deletion syndromes is the cri du chat syndrome (cat cry syndrome) caused by the deletion of the short arm of chromosome 5 (5p-).

Structural abnormalities involving the presence of additional chromosome material are classified as duplications or additions. Duplications arise through errors in chromosome replication or errors in crossing over during cell division. The term *partial trisomy* is used to describe the presence of segments of additional or duplicated chromosome material.

When two breaks occur in a single chromosome and the intervening segment becomes inverted (turned upside down), the resulting abnormality is known as an *inversion*. If the inverted segment includes the centromere, the inversion is known as a *pericentric inversion*. If the inverted material does not involve the centromere, the inversion is known as a *paracentric inversion*. Prior to the availability of new banding techniques, inversions were difficult to detect.

A translocation involves the exchange of chromosome material between two or more chromosomes. There are two categories of translocations: (1) robertsonian (centric fusion) and (2) reciprocal. If all the essential genetic material is present, although rearranged, the individual is a *balanced translocation carrier* and, generally, is phenotypically normal. When the translocation results in the loss or addition of chromosome material, the individual has an *unbalanced translocation* and may have an associated abnormal phenotype.

One of the most common unbalanced robertsonian translocations occurs between chromosomes 21 and 14, resulting in translocation Down syndrome. These individuals are phenotypically indistinguishable from individuals who have the classic trisomy 21. In this case, the karyotype reveals 46 individual chromosomes with a structurally abnormal number 14 chromosome. On further analysis, there is an extra number 21 chromosome fused to the number 14 chromosome (Fig. 32–5). Unlike the karyotypically normal parents of children with trisomy 21 Down syndrome, some cases of translocation Down syndrome have been inherited from one of the parents. The parental karyotype reveals 45 chromosomes, with one of the number 21 chromosomes fused to a number 14 chromosome (Fig. 32–6). Figure 32–7 illustrates the possible zygotes resulting from the mating of a balanced translocation carrier and his or her spouse.

Couples in which one of the partners is a carrier of a balanced translocation are at an increased risk of having a child with an unbalanced chromosomal rearrangement. The specific recurrence risk figures given in genetic counseling depend on the type and amount of chromosomal material involved in the translocation.

## ETIOLOGIES OF CHROMOSOME ABNORMALITIES

With the continuing refinement of techniques for chromosome analysis, medical genetics has been able to illuminate some of the possible etiologies of chromosome abnormal-

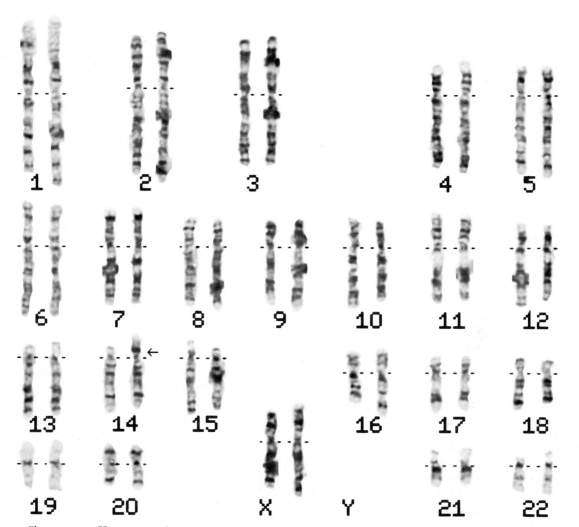

**Figure 32–5.** Karyotype of a patient with Down syndrome as a result of an unbalanced 14/21 translocation. *Arrow* denotes an extra 21 chromosome fused to a 14 chromosome. (Courtesy of Dr. Loris McGavran, The Children's Hospital, Denver, CO.)

ities. Three major areas have been identified that are important for the primary health care provider to be aware of: (1) advanced parental age; (2) radiation absorbed by the individual; and (3) gene regulation.

Advanced parental age traditionally has focused on the age of the mother at conception. It has been documented that women 35 years and older are at an increased risk for a fetal chromosome abnormality (Goad et al, 1976). It is hypothesized that the maternal age of the ovum in combination with environmental factors interferes with normal spindle function during meiosis and results in nondisjunction. Paternal age has tradi-

tionally been associated with an increase of mutations at the gene level and has been investigated as a possible cause for chromosome abnormalities (Stene et al, 1977). Studies of data from live births and amniocentesis registries have indicated no evidence for a consistent paternal age effect independent of maternal age (Cross and Hook, 1982).

X-ray and other sources of radiation have been documented to cause chromosomal breakage and possible rearrangements, thereby increasing the risk for a chromosome abnormality (Uchida, 1977). Routine preventive measures to minimize the amount of radiation exposure should be taken when-

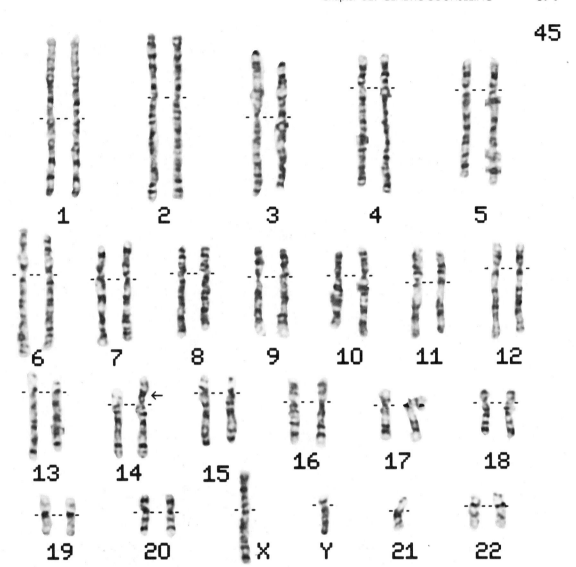

45

**Figure 32-6.** Karyotype of a clinically normal parent who is a balanced 14/21 translocation carrier. (Courtesy of Dr. Loris McGavran, The Children's Hospital, Denver, CO.)

ever possible (i.e., shielding and not scheduling elective x-ray studies within 10 days of the onset of the last menstrual period).

Genes regulating nondisjunction have been documented in other species, and thus, similar hypotheses have been raised in human beings (Thompson et al, 1991). Empiric data have demonstrated that in some families that have a family member with a trisomy there is an increased risk for future offspring to also have a trisomy. This genetic predisposition does not include families in which there is a familial translocation (Pelz et al, 1988; Rudd et al, 1984).

## CLINICAL ASPECTS OF AUTOSOMAL ABNORMALITIES

A few common chromosome disorders are discussed in this section. The following sections are intended as an outline or guide and are not an exhaustive discussion of any of the disorders.

### Down Syndrome

Down syndrome is the most common chromosome abnormality, with an incidence of

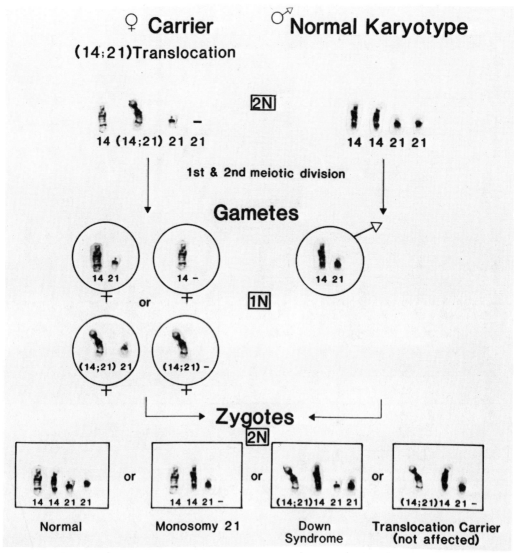

**Figure 32–7.** Possible zygotes resulting from a mating between a balanced (14/21) translocation carrier female and a karyotypically normal spouse. Note that the zygote giving rise to a fetus with Down syndrome results from the maternal gamete, which contains both the translocated chromosome and a normal chromosome 21. Monosomy 21 is lethal, and this pregnancy would result in early spontaneous abortion. (Courtesy of The Children's Hospital, Denver, CO.)

approximately 1 in 600 live births. In the absence of major complications such as severe cardiac abnormalities, individuals with Down syndrome live fairly long lives and are usually moderately to severely mentally retarded (Gayton and Walker, 1974; Penrose and Smith, 1966). Because the disorder has significant sequelae, it is important to diagnose it as soon after birth as possible. When the diagnosis is suspected, a chromosome analysis should be performed to delineate the specific etiology of the disorder (trisomy versus translocation). This information be-

comes paramount in providing the family with accurate genetic counseling. For families who have a child with trisomy 21, the risk of recurrence for future pregnancies is approximately 1 percent (Thompson et al, 1991). The risk of Down syndrome, if the mother is a carrier of the balanced translocation, is approximately 10 percent. If the father carries the translocation, then the risk is lower, approximately 2 to 5 percent (Thompson et al, 1991).

The phenotypic features of individuals with Down syndrome are often obvious at birth. The major clinical features are (see Fig. 32–4B):

Central nervous system: Mental retardation
Hyptonia at birth; improving with age
Head: Depressed nasal bridge
Mongoloid slant of eyes
Epicanthic folds
Brushfield's spots (white speckling of the iris)
Protruding tongue
High-arched palate
Low-set ears
Flattened occiput
Broad short neck
Extremities: Shortened metacarpals
Abnormal dermatoglyphics:
Transverse palmar crease (simian line)
Increased number of ulnar loops
Arch tibial on hallucal area

Congenital heart disease is present in approximately one half of individuals affected with Down syndrome; gastrointestinal and urinary tract abnormalities are also reported. There are no reported cases in the literature of affected males reproducing (unless mosaicism was present), but affected females have been known to reproduce (Riccardi, 1977).

## Trisomy 18

Trisomy 18 (Edwards syndrome) is a severe chromosome abnormality occurring in approximately 1 in 6000 live births. Major features include (Fig. 32–8):

Central nervous system: Mental retardation
Severe hypertonia
Microcephaly
Head: Prominent occiput
Low-set and malformed ears
Corneal opacity
Ptosis (drooping of the eyelids)
Micrognathia
Extremities: Overriding clenched fingers
Abnormal dermatoglyphics
Rocker bottom feet
Other: Congenital heart disease
Single umbilical artery

Renal abnormalities
Cryptorchidism
Gastrointestinal tract abnormalities

The diagnosis of trisomy 18 should be confirmed because the prognosis is grim; 30 percent of affected infants die within the first month of life, 90 percent by 1 year, and 99 percent by age 10. Those infants who have survived the first year of life have been found to be profoundly retarded (Taylor, 1968).

## Trisomy 13

Trisomy 13 (Patau syndrome) is noted in about 1 in 5000 live births. The major clinical findings include (Fig. 32–9):

Central nervous system: Mental retardation
Brain abnormalities
Head: Microcephaly
Microphthalmia
Malformed ears
Micrognathia
Cleft lip and palate
Extremities: Polydactyly
Abnormal posturing of fingers
Abnormal dermatoglyphics
Other: Congenital heart defects
Gastrointestinal tract defects
Reproductive system defects
Hemangiomas
Scalp defects

As in trisomy 18, the prognosis for infants born with trisomy 13 is extremely poor. Over one half of the affected individuals die within the first month of life, and 95 percent succumb by 3 years of age. All affected individuals have been profoundly retarded, and no individuals are known to have survived to adulthood with the exception of those with documented mosaicism (Taylor, 1968).

## Deletion 5p-

The cri du chat syndrome results from a loss of the short arm of chromosome number 5. The diagnosis is often suspected on the basis of the characteristic catlike cry. Other features include:

Central nervous system: Mental retardation
Microcephaly

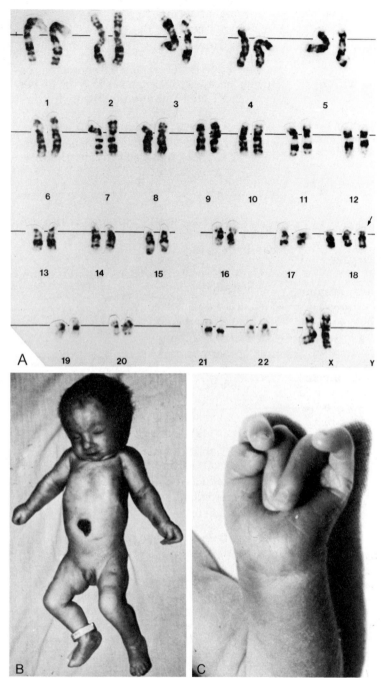

**Figure 32–8.** *A*, Karyotype of a patient with trisomy 18: 47,XX + 18. Arrow denotes extra chromosome 18. *B*, Newborn with trisomy 18. *C*, Characteristic posturing of the fingers of a newborn with trisomy 18. (Courtesy of The Children's Hospital, Denver, CO.)

Head: Hypertelorism
  Epicanthic folds
  Downward slanting palpebral fissures
  Low set ears
  Micrognathia

In addition to the deletion 5p- syndrome, there are a number of other chromosomal deletion syndromes that have been recog-

nized with the development of high-resolution cytogenetic techniques (deGrouchy and Turleau, 1984). Moreover, disorders previously not thought to be associated with chromosomal aberrations are now found to have a chromosomal abnormality. For example, Prader-Willi syndrome, which is characterized by initial failure to thrive, obesity, mental retardation, hypogonadism,

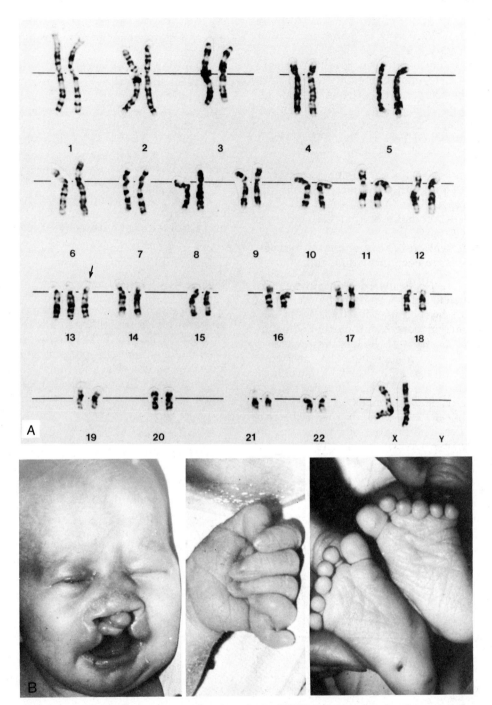

**Figure 32–9.** *A*, Karyotype of a patient with trisomy 13: 47,XX, + 13. *Arrow* denotes extra chromosome 13. *B*, Newborn with trisomy 13. Note bilateral cleft lip and palate and polydactyly of hands and feet. (Courtesy of The Children's Hospital, Denver, CO.)

and small hands and feet, has been found to be associated with an interstitial deletion of chromosome 15 (q11-q12) in approximately 50 percent of cases with that diagnosis (Butler, 1990).

## Sex Chromosome Abnormalities

Abnormalities of the sex chromosomes are relatively common, occurring in approximately 1 in 400 to 700 live births (Linden et al, 1990). In addition, they account for approximately 25 percent of spontaneous abortions (Riccardi, 1977).

A discussion of the abnormalities involving the sex chromosomes requires an understanding of the Lyon hypothesis. In response to questions concerning sex chromatin and gene dosage compensation, Mary Lyon (1961) published her *inactive X hypothesis,* which proposes the following:

1. Females at an early embryonic stage inactivate one of the two normal X chromosomes present.
2. All descendants of that cell have the same inactivated X.
3. Inactivation is a random and independent process in each individual cell.

The inactive X forms a dark-staining mass in the nucleus known as the *Barr body,* or X chromatin body (Fig. 32–10A). Cells containing one or more X chromatic bodies are chromatin positive; those lacking these bodies are chromatin-negative. The most common procedure used to observe X chromatin is the buccal smear. Cells, which are scraped from the inside of the cheek, are stained and microscopically examined for the presence of Barr bodies. The number of Barr bodies observed is always one less than the number of X chromosomes present. In normal females, there is one Barr body, representing the inactive X chromosome. A normal male is Barr body–negative because he has only one X chromosome. Because a buccal smear is only a screening technique, a chromosome analysis should be performed to confirm the diagnosis of the suspected sex chromosome abnormality.

A similar technique is used to screen for the presence of the Y chromosome. After staining buccal mucosal cells with a fluorescent dye, the Y chromosome appears as a very bright body within the cell nucleus. The number of Y bodies in a cell is equal to the number of Y chromosomes present. Normal males have one Y body and normal females have no Y bodies (Fig. 32–10B).

Two of the most common sex chromosome abnormalities are Turner syndrome (45,X) and Klinefelter syndrome (47,XXY).

## Turner Syndrome

Turner syndrome has a frequency of approximately 1 in 5000 female live births. However, the 45,X karyotype represents the most common chromosome abnormality found in spontaneous abortions (Hassold and Jacobs, 1984). Major clinical findings in females with Turner syndrome include:

Short stature
Webbed neck
Low posterior hairline
Shieldlike chest
Widely spaced nipples
Cubitus valgus
Primary amenorrhea
Streaked ovaries
Underdeveloped secondary sex characteristics
Congenital heart disease (30 percent with coarctation of the aorta)
Renal abnormalities

Intellectually, females with Turner syndrome are usually within the normal range, although some learning disabilities, particularly perceptual difficulties, have been noted (Linden et al, 1990).

The diagnosis of Turner syndrome often is not made until puberty, when the absence of menses and short stature become concerns. Occasionally, the diagnosis can be suspected in female infants at birth by the presence of redundant skin on the back of the neck and marked lymphedema of the dorsum of the hands and feet (Fig. 32–11).

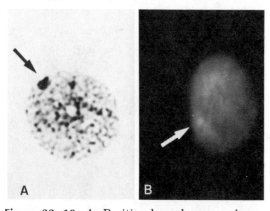

**Figure 32–10.** *A,* Positive buccal smear. *Arrow* denotes Barr body within the cell nucleus. *B,* Nucleus of lymphocyte noting fluorescent Y body. (Courtesy of The Children's Hospital, Denver, CO.)

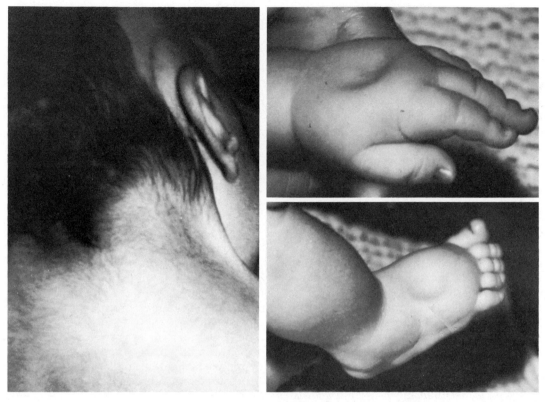

**Figure 32–11.** Newborn with Turner syndrome. Note webbed neck, low posterior hairline, and marked lymphedema of hand and foot. (Courtesy of The Children's Hospital, Denver, CO.)

## Klinefelter Syndrome

The incidence of 47,XXY karyotype in newborn males is approximately 1 per 800 (Linden et al, 1990). In general, the term Klinefelter syndrome refers to those males with a 47,XXY chromosome constitution and the following phenotypes:

Normal appearance

Tall stature

Normal onset of puberty with subsequent decrease in testicular size

Azoospermia

Gynecomastia and eunuchoid body shape observed in approximately 30 percent

Intellectual development ranging from normal intelligence to mild mental retardation has been reported in males with Klinefelter syndrome (Robinson et al, 1979). A 25-year longitudinal study of males with 47,XXY karyotypes has shown that cognitively delayed language development, articulation problems, and poor reading skills are areas of great deficiency. Additionally, there may be some deficit of gross motor skills (Linden et al, 1990).

A number of other sex chromosome abnormalities have been described. It would appear that in most cases, an increasing number of X and Y chromosomes leads to an increasing number of physical and mental abnormalities.

Given the number of different chromosome abnormalities and the variability of clinical findings, any infant or child with multiple anomalies should be considered for banded chromosome analysis regardless of whether or not the infant fits any known chromosomal syndrome. This analysis becomes extremely important in delineating the etiology, treatment, and prognosis of such an affected child.

## MENDELIAN INHERITANCE

Single gene disorders that follow the classic mendelian patterns of inheritance are classified as autosomal dominant, autosomal recessive, X-linked dominant, or X-linked recessive. In these disorders, the abnormality occurs at the gene level and is the result of either a single gene or pair of abnormal genes. For any given trait an individual possesses, there is a pair of genes working in concert with one another. The paired genes are located on homologous chromosomes and occupy a specific place on the chromosome, known as the *locus*. An individual is *homozygous* for a particular trait when two genes at a given locus are identical. The individual is *heterozygous* for a particular trait when two different genes are present at a given locus. Alternate forms of genes occurring at a given locus are known as *alleles*. For many traits, there may be only one form of a particular gene; for others, multiple alleles may exist. For example, an individual may be homozygous for blood type A (AA), in which both genes at the ABO locus are identical, or the individual may be heterozygous for blood type A, such as AB. In this case, one gene is the A allele and the other gene is the B allele. Any change in a gene's form is known as a *mutation*. Although the majority of mutations are inconsequential to normal growth and development, on occasion, a gene mutation results in a disease process or malformation. A discussion of the major types of mendelian inheritance patterns follows.

## Autosomal Dominant Inheritance

A condition is inherited in an autosomal dominant fashion when the disorder manifests itself in the heterozygous state. That is, the abnormal or mutant gene overshadows the normal gene. Autosomal dominant disorders are characterized by the following (Fig. 32–12):

1. Multiple generations of affected individuals. An affected individual usually has one affected parent.

2. Both males and females are affected, and both sexes can transmit the gene.

3. There is male-to-male transmission. This concept is important, as it rules out X-linked inheritance.

4. Offspring of affected individuals have a 50 percent risk of inheriting the gene.

5. Individuals who do not have the abnormal gene cannot transmit the disorder to their offspring.

6. New mutations may occur. Given a negative family history and normal parents, a child with an autosomal dominant disorder is presumed to represent a new mutation. Parents in this case would not be at increased risk in future pregnancies.

7. Variable expressivity may exist with respect to phenotype. That is, clinical findings may differ among affected individuals.

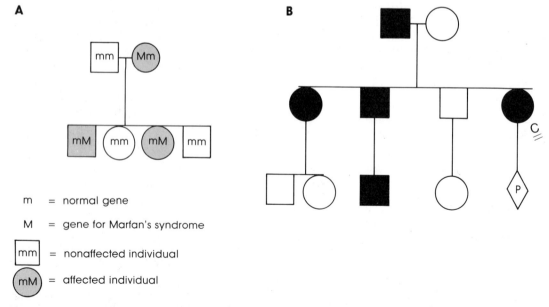

m = normal gene

M = gene for Marfan's syndrome

mm = nonaffected individual

mM = affected individual

**Figure 32–12.** *A,* Potential genotypes of a mating between an affected female and an unaffected spouse. *B,* Autosomal dominant pedigree.

This becomes important to the clinician when making a diagnosis, because there may be only mild symptoms in affected individuals.

McKusick's (1990) catalog currently lists over 2000 autosomal, dominantly inherited disorders. Some of the more common are Huntington's chorea, neurofibromatosis (von Recklinghausen's disease), and polycystic kidney disease. Dominant disorders with particular importance for the pregnant woman are achondroplasia; connective tissue disorders, such as Marfan's syndrome; bleeding disorders, particularly von Willebrand's disease; and acute intermittent porphyria.

### Autosomal Recessive Inheritance

A condition is inherited in an autosomal recessive fashion when the disorder manifests itself in the homozygous state. To be affected, the individual must have two abnormal genes. The individual is considered to be a carrier in the heterozygote state with the normal gene overshadowing the abnormal gene. Carriers are usually phenotypically normal. Autosomal recessive disorders are characterized by the following (Fig. 32–13):

1. Most affected individuals have phenotypically normal parents. Pedigrees show affected individuals within sibships.

2. Both males and females are affected, and both sexes can transmit the gene.

3. Parents who are carriers of the same abnormal gene have a 25 percent risk with each pregnancy of having an affected child.

4. Unaffected offspring of two carrier parents have a two-thirds chance of being a carrier.

5. A consanguineous mating is often present. There is a higher probability that two related individuals will have the same gene in common than that two unrelated individuals will.

6. The affected individual's clinical picture is often relatively severe.

7. In instances in which affected individuals reproduce, all of the offspring must be carriers for the disorder.

The majority of biochemical disorders are inherited in an autosomal recessive manner. For a number of these disorders, biochemical assays are available to detect the heterozygote carrier state. For example, carriers of Tay-Sachs disease have approximately half the normal enzyme activity for hexosaminidase A. Thus, the phenotypically normal carrier is biochemically abnormal.

Common autosomal recessive disorders observed are cystic fibrosis, galactosemia, and phenylketonuria (PKU). Recessive disorders that should have special consideration during pregnancy are PKU and the hemoglobinopathies, such as sickle cell anemia and SC disease (Thompson et al, 1991).

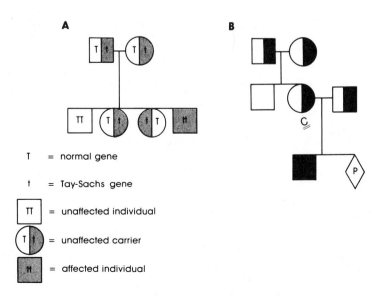

**A**

**B**

T = normal gene

t = Tay-Sachs gene

TT = unaffected individual

(T t) = unaffected carrier

tt = affected individual

**Figure 32–13.** *A*, Potential genotypes of a mating between two carrier parents. *B*, Autosomal recessive pedigree.

## X-Linked Recessive Inheritance

X-linked (sex-linked) disorders are those for which the abnormal gene is located on the X chromosome. Females, who have two X chromosomes, are considered to be heterozygote carriers; that is, the normal gene on the chromosome overshadows the abnormal gene on the other X chromosome. In general, carrier females are clinically normal. Males who have a gene for an X-linked recessive disorder are affected because they have only one X chromosome. Genes located on the Y chromosome have not been shown to be paired with those on the X chromosome. The most distinguishing characteristic delineating X-linked disorders from autosomal disorders is the absence of male-to-male transmission. As males pass on their Y chromosomes to sons, a son cannot receive an X-linked disorder from this father. Only females are able to pass on an X-linked disorder to male offspring. Other major characteristics of X-linked recessive disorders are (Fig. 32–14):

1. Usually, only males are affected. On rare occasions, carrier females exhibit some clinical signs and symptoms of the disorder.
2. Affected males are related through carrier females.

3. There is a 50 percent risk that a female carrier will have an affected son.
4. There is a 50 percent risk that a female carrier will have a daughter who is a carrier.
5. Males affected with an X-linked disorder cannot pass the disorder on to their sons; conversely, all of their daughters are *obligate* carriers.
6. If only one affected male is observed in a pedigree, the possibility of a new mutation should be considered. Approximately one third of lethal disorders affecting males are caused by new mutations. (Thompson et al, 1991).

There are approximately 200 X-linked disorders now described (McKusick, 1990). Common X-linked disorders include glucose-6-phosphate dehydrogenase deficiency (G-6-PD), Duchenne muscular dystrophy, color blindness, hemophilia, and Lesch-Nyhan syndrome. X-linked disorders that need to be followed closely during pregnancy are hemophilia A and B.

## Fragile-X Syndrome

Fragile-X syndrome is now recognized as the most common familial form of mental retardation, with an incidence of 1 in 1000

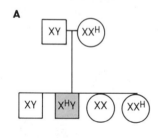

X = X chromosome with normal gene

X$^H$ = X chromosome with hemophilia gene

XY = unaffected male

XX = unaffected female

X$^H$Y = affected male

XX$^H$ = carrier female

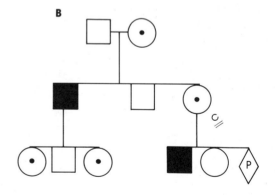

**Figure 32–14.** *A,* Potential genotypes of a mating between a carrier female and an unaffected spouse. *B,* X-linked recessive pedigree.

(Hagerman, 1987). The Marker X, or fragile X, was first described by Lubs (1969) in a family with X-linked mental retardation. However, it was not until the 1980s that cytogenetic analysis for the fragile-X chromosome (fragile site at Xq27.3) was routinely used for the diagnosis of fragile-X syndrome.

In 1991, the gene for fragile-X syndrome (FMR-1) was localized and shown to contain a variable repetitive sequence of DNA (Rousseau et al, 1991). This paved the way for the use of DNA mutation analysis, which is more sensitive than cytogenic analysis in distinguishing fragile-X carrier females and transmitting males from normal individuals.

The fragile-X syndrome is characterized by mental retardation in association with a recognized constellation of physical and behavioral characteristics (Hagerman and Silverman, 1991). Inherited in X-linked fashion, fragile-X syndrome occurs predominantly in males. Females can be affected but usually to a lesser extent. Among the affected males studied, mental retardation varies from mild to severe, with the majority of adolescent adult males being moderately to severely retarded, whereas prepubescent males often are only mildly retarded. Only rarely do males with the fragile-X gene have normal IQs, and even then, they frequently have learning disabilities. Approximately, one third of carrier females have some degree of mental impairment, ranging from mild learning disabilities to mental retardation. Characteristics of fragile-X syndrome include

Mental impairment: Mental retardation (mild to severe)
  Learning disabilities (especially among females)
Physical findings:
  Macro-orchidism
  Large or prominent ears
  Long, narrow face
  Connective tissue problems (e.g., double-jointed fingers, mitral valve prolapse, and flat feet)
Behavioral abnormalities:
  Hyperactivity
  Autisticlike behavior (e.g., repetitive behavior, poor eye contact, and violent outburst)
Sensory integration deficits
Tactile defensiveness

In general, recurrence risks for genetic counseling in fragile-X syndrome are similar to those given for X-linked mental retardation. However, the inheritance of fragile-X syndrome differs from the classic X-linked model by the incidence of transmitting or nonpenetrant males (20 percent of males with fragile-X gene) and the increased frequency of affected females (33 percent).

Prenatal diagnosis is available for fragile-X syndrome, but it, too, has its limitations. Although amniocentesis and chorionic villus sampling have been used with fragile-X syndrome, both techniques have experienced false-positive and false-negative results. It is important that prenatal diagnosis for fragile-X syndrome be performed by an experienced laboratory. Consequently, all couples considering prenatal diagnosis for fragile-X syndrome should be referred for genetic counseling to discuss the benefits as well as the limitations of prenatal diagnosis (Hagerman, 1987).

## X-Linked Dominant Inheritance

Relatively few genetic disorders exhibit X-linked dominant inheritance. The most common is the Xg blood group system. In this particular pattern, the abnormal gene located on the X chromosome overshadows the normal gene; therefore, heterozygous females as well as males are affected. The major characteristics include the following:

1. No male-to-male transmission.
2. All daughters of an affected male will be affected.
3. Affected females have a 50 percent risk of having affected offspring regardless of sex.

## MULTIFACTORIAL INHERITANCE

In contrast to mendelian disorders in which a single gene pair is involved, multifactorial disorders are believed to result from an additive effect of *many genes* interacting with environmental factors. In the majority of cases, the environmental factors cannot be identified. Usually, this pattern of inheritance is more complex and less straightforward than mendelian inheritance and is associated with smaller risk figures. The frequency of multifactorial disorders may vary with respect to ethnic background. For example, neural tube defects have an increased incidence among English and Irish populations. Some of the most common and familiar isolated malformations are inherited in a multifactorial fashion, such as cleft lip and palate, neural tube defects (anencephaly and meningomyelocele), clubfoot, dislocated hips, hypospadias, and pyloric stenosis. Additionally, there are many other common disorders considered to have a multifactorial etiology, including diabetes, allergies, cancers, cardiac disorders, affective disorders, and some forms of mental retardation. Major characteristics of multifactorial inheritance include

1. Risk figures based on empiric data. In general, there is a 2 to 5 percent risk of recurrence among first-degree relatives of an affected individual.
2. There is often a sex bias; for instance, pyloric stenosis is more common in males; congenital dislocated hips are more common in females.
3. The risk of recurrence is greater if the affected individual is of the less commonly affected sex.
4. The risk of recurrence increases with the severity of the disorder. For example, parents of a newborn with congenital aganglionic megacolon (Hirschsprung's disease) involving a long segment of bowel have a greater risk of recurrence in future offspring than if only a small segment of bowel is affected.
5. The more family members affected, the greater the risk of recurrence. This is in contrast to mendelian disorders, in which risk remains constant.

## THE ENVIRONMENTAL ETIOLOGY OF MALFORMATIONS

In the newborn population, 2 to 4 percent of infants have a recognizable malformation. If the period of ascertainment is extended beyond the first year of life, this figure increases to 4 to 6 percent because those previously unrecognized malformations present themselves. Earlier in this chapter, congenital malformation of a known genetic etiology is discussed. This section concentrates on the environmental causes of malformations.

Congenital malformations are structural defects present at birth resulting from abnormal tissue differentiation, abnormal tissue and organ interaction during fetal development, or both (Warkany, 1971). Approximately 10 percent of congenital anomalies are known to have an environmental etiology (Wilson, 1973). Since Gregg (1941) first demonstrated a relationship between maternal rubella during pregnancy and fetal malformations, it has become increasingly evident that a variety of environmental agents can have a deleterious effect on the developing fetus. Those agents capable of causing malformation are classified as teratogens and include drugs and chemicals, radiation, congenital infection, and maternal environment.

### Prerequisites for a Teratogenic Effect

When considering the teratogenic effect of agents on the developing embryo, four major factors must be considered:

1. genetic susceptibility of the fetus;
2. time of exposure to the agent;
3. pharmacologic properties of the agent; and
4. dosage.

The *genetic susceptibility (or predisposition) of the fetus* is an important factor in determining whether or not a specific agent is teratogenic. Although the majority of research regarding the teratogenicity of agents has been generalized from animal models, caution must be taken when extrapolating these data to humans. Agents shown to be teratogenic in certain animals may have no association with birth defects in humans and vice versa. For example, evidence implicating the drug thalidomide as a teratogen in the human embryo was overwhelming, whereas early animal data demonstrated little or no evidence of a teratogenic effect. Additionally, susceptibility within species may vary according to individual genetic makeup. Thus, the risk to the fetus may vary even in the presence of a documented teratogenic agent.

The *time of exposure* to a teratogenic agent is an important determinant of the effect on the developing fetus. The *period of embryogenesis from 2 to 8 weeks after conception appears to be the most vulnerable time for the fetus.* Exposure to a teratogenic agent during this time may result in multiple malformations. Exposure prior to this time (conception through implantation) results in either early fetal wastage or no apparent effect. During the second and third trimesters, exposure to these agents does not result in gross malformations but may produce functional pathology.

The *nature and pharmacologic properties of an agent* determine its interaction with developing fetal tissues. Prior to the early 1960s, it was a common belief that the placental barrier offered effective protection to the fetus. However, current data have shown that most agents and their breakdown products readily cross the placental barrier in both animals and humans. Thus, a single agent may not prove to be teratogenic, but its breakdown products represent a significant risk to the developing embryo.

The *dose of an agent* represents another important determinant in producing a teratogenic effect. In many animal models, a dose-response relationship has been demonstrated (McClearn, 1979). This hypothesis has now been extrapolated to humans and appears to be appropriate, at least in some instances. For example, a dose-response curve has been demonstrated in fetal alcohol syndrome, with a higher blood alcohol level being associated with a more severe clinical outcome (Smith, 1980).

### Teratogenic Agents

**Radiation.** Ionizing radiation was the first environmental agent shown to be teratogenic in humans (Warkany, 1971). During the 1920s, pregnant women who were treated with therapeutic doses of radiation for pelvic malignancy gave birth to children with severe birth defects including microcephaly, skeletal defects, and mental retardation (Heinonen et al, 1977). An increased incidence of congenital malformations was also noted in children born to women who were pregnant at the time of the Hiroshima and Nagasaki atomic bomb explosions (Satow and West, 1955; Wood, 1969).

From a genetic standpoint, radiation exposure is cumulative and may result in a variety of outcomes. Radiation may produce a change at the gene level (mutagenic), at the chromosome level (clastogenic), at the cell level (oncogenic), or at the tissue and organ level (teratogenic). The effects of radiation depend on the dosage and time of exposure. Fetal tissues are most susceptible to radiation damage during the first trimester, when the cells are rapidly dividing and differentiating. Exposure to high doses of radiation ($> 10$ rads) during the first 3 weeks following conception is more likely to result in spontaneous abortion, whereas weeks 4 through 12 place the fetus at increased risk for major malformations (Swartz and Reichling, 1978). Radiation exposure after the first trimester is not likely to cause either miscarriage or anomalies; however, it has been associated with an increased incidence of childhood leukemias (Stewart and Kneale, 1970).

For couples who wish to minimize their risks, the following precautions are appropriate: shielding of the pelvis and abdomen whenever possible; for females, scheduling of elective x-ray studies during menses or within 10 days of onset; and, for males, delaying conception for 6 to 8 weeks following exposure.

**Drugs and Chemicals.** It is important to understand the effects of drugs during pregnancy, because they represent an area over which there is some control. In general, the time during gestation when the drug is taken determines whether or not and what type of embryotoxicity will result. A variety of mechanisms by which drugs produce abnormalities have been hypothesized. Drugs may (1) disturb a critical phase in embryologic development by causing cell death, altering cell migration, or both; (2) alter the hormonal environment; or (3) interfere with physiologic functions. Relatively few drugs have been positively implicated as being teratogenic in humans. A variety of drugs are suspected of having a teratogenic potential, although they have yet to be clearly established as known teratogens. On the other hand, certain drugs have been used widely enough in controlled situations to warrant exclusion from the list of potential teratogens. Table 32–2 lists some of the drugs that have been documented to represent a definite or suspected hazard to the fetus.

Thalidomide demonstrates the classic example of a teratogen. Introduced as a remedy against influenza in the mid 1950s, thalidomide also was recommended as a sedative and tranquilizer. Five years later, after the birth of over 8000 infants with similar limb malformations, the drug was withdrawn. Thalidomide proved to be extremely teratogenic when taken 6 to 8 weeks after the last menstrual period (Goldman, 1980).

**Alcohol.** In 1973, Jones and colleagues described a group of children with a character-

**Table 32–2**
DEFINITE, SUSPECTED, AND NONTERATOGENIC DRUGS

| Drug | Clinical Findings |
|---|---|
| **Definite Hazards** | |
| Alcohol | Fetal alcohol syndrome |
| Accutane (isotretinoin) | CNS, cardiac and ear abnormalities |
| Hormones | |
| Androgens | |
| Folic acid antagonists (aminopterin, methotrexate) | Labial fusion and clitoral hypertrophy |
| Anticoagulants (Coumadin) | Cranial and skeletal abnormalities; microcephaly |
| | Nasal hypoplasia; fetal hemorrhage; stippled epiphyses; psychomotor delay |
| Cocaine | IUGR; vascular disruptions |
| Anticonvulsants | |
| Dilantin | Fetal hydantoin syndrome |
| Tridione | Craniofacial abnormalities |
| Valproic | Neural tube defects; craniofacial abnormalities |
| Thalidomide | Craniofacial, skeletal (limbs), and cardiac abnormalities |
| **Suspected Hazards** | |
| Estrogens/progestins | VACTERL syndrome |
| Amphetamines | Cardiac malformations |
| Lithium | Cardiac malformations |
| **No Evidence of Teratogenic Effect** | |
| Salicylates | |
| Antihistamines | |
| Heparin | |
| Antibiotics (penicillins, sulfonamides) | |
| Narcotics | |

istic phenotype born to mothers who had been chronic alcoholics during their pregnancies. This phenotype, known as the fetal alcohol syndrome, includes the following clinical findings (Fig. 32–15):

Prenatal, postnatal growth retardation, or both

Mental retardation

Microcephaly

Microphthalmia, short palpebral fissures, or both

Underdeveloped philtrum

Carp-shaped mouth

Thin upper lip, flattened maxillary area, or both

Although fetal alcohol syndrome can be diagnosed in the neonate, the syndrome may not be recognized until postnatal growth retardation and developmental delay become more apparent at 1 to 2 years of age. Although no one clinical finding is pathognomonic for the syndrome, the diagnosis should be considered in light of the previously mentioned phenotype and a positive history of maternal alcohol use.

In general, infants diagnosed as having the fetal alcohol syndrome have been born to mothers who were chronic alcoholics and drank heavily during pregnancy. It is known that alcohol freely crosses the placenta, reaching the same concentration in the fetus as that in the mother's blood. The critical factor appears to be the blood alcohol level; there is a direct relationship between the amount of alcohol consumed and the severity of the syndrome (Hanson et al, 1978). The fetal alcohol syndrome is believed to be a consequence of disharmonic growth, that is, a diminished cell number, which is more profound in some tissues than in others (Smith, 1980).

Fetal alcohol syndrome represents the extreme end of the spectrum of problems related to the effects of alcohol during pregnancy. A second term, the fetal alcoholic effect, is now being used to describe those infants who exhibit only mild or partial manifestations of the syndrome (Rossett et al, 1981). There continues to be controversy regarding the minimum amount of alcohol intake necessary to produce an effect. Partial features of the fetal alcohol syndrome were seen in 11 percent of offspring whose mothers consumed two to four drinks (hard liquor) per day as opposed to 19 percent of offspring whose mothers consumed four or more drinks per day (Hanson et al, 1978). Additionally, it has been reported that the con-

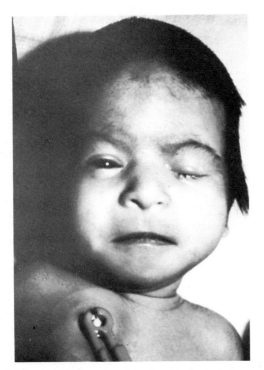

**Figure 32–15.** Infant with the fetal alcohol syndrome. (Courtesy of The Children's Hospital, Denver, CO.)

sumption of two drinks per day is associated with infants whose only clinical finding is decreased birth weight (Little, 1977). Although it is still unclear "how much alcohol is too much alcohol," it has been documented that a reduction of alcohol consumption as late as 24 to 26 weeks' gestation is associated with an improved neonatal outcome (Rossett et al, 1981).

**Anticonvulsants.** Women with documented seizure disorders taking anticonvulsants during pregnancy have been found to have an increased incidence of offspring with characteristic abnormalities. One of the more well-known teratogenic anticonvulsants is phenytoin (Dilantin) which is associated with the fetal hydantoin syndrome. This syndrome is characterized by the following:

Prenatal and postnatal growth deficiency
Motor and mental retardation
Microcephaly
Short upturned nose
Broad and depressed nasal bridge
Epicanthic folds
Nail and distal phalangeal hypoplasia

Other associated malformations are cleft lip (6 percent) and cardiac defects (9 percent) (Hanson et al, 1976). Hanson (1986) reviewed the clinical effects of phenytoin during pregnancy and found that approximately 5 to 10 percent of exposed infants have the fetal hydantoin syndrome; subtle changes, such as the hydantoin effect, can be found in 30 percent of exposed offspring.

Other anticonvulsants also have been documented to be teratogenic, such as trimethadione, carbamazepine (Tegretol), and valproic acid. Because the known teratogenicity of trimethadione is substantial, it is now contraindicated in pregnancy.

Valproic acid has been implicated as a human teratogen with a phenotype similar to the fetal hydantoin syndrome, namely, craniofacial findings and nail and distal digital hypoplasia (Ardinger et al, 1988). Moreover, the greatest risk that has emerged is a 1 to 2 percent increased risk for spina bifida in pregnancies in which the mother is taking valproic acid. This risk is similar to that for women who have already had a child with a neural tube defect (Oakeshott and Gillian, 1989). Thus, it is suggested that women taking valproic acid during pregnancy have the pregnancy monitored with alpha-fetoprotein (AFP) measurements and careful ultrasound examinations of the fetal spine (Serville et al, 1989).

There continues to be considerable discussion regarding the teratogenicity of anticonvulsants versus the maternal disease state. Whether it is the seizures or the *in utero* exposure to the anticonvulsants that acts as a teratogen remains unclear. New research being conducted by Buehler and colleagues (1990) has found an association between the fetal hydantoin syndrome phenotype and inherited levels of activity of the oxidative enzyme, epoxide hydrolase, with low activity corresponding to occurrence of the syndrome. Whether or not infants at risk for malformations can be indentified prenatally by the measurement of epoxide hydrolase activity awaits further research; however, preliminary results are encouraging.

**Vitamin A.** Although vitamin A is well known as an essential nutrient for maintaining normal growth and regulating the proliferation and differentiation of epithelial tissues, it also is now recognized to be a human teratogen when taken during pregnancy. The vitamin A analogues retinoids are used in the clinical management of dermatologic diseases such as acne and psoriasis. The major drugs that have been implicated to be teratogenic are isotretinoin (Accutane) and etretinate (Tigason), an aromatic retinoid (Lammer et al, 1985). Lammer and colleagues found that isotretinoin-exposed infants were 26 times more likely to have brain, cardiac, or ear malformations than were unexposed infants. These malformations include:

Hydrocephalus
Microcephaly
Cardiac septal defects
Malformed ears
Stenotic and atretic external ear canals
Micrognathia
Facial asymmetry
Cleft palate

Because of the known teratogenicity of these drugs, the Teratology Society has issued a position paper recommending that all women of childbearing age be informed that the use of these drugs during pregnancy may put the fetus at increased risk for major congenital malformations (Teratology Society Position Paper, 1987).

**Cocaine.** With the dramatically increased use of cocaine in the United States, studies have documented an increased risk for severe sequelae in infants exposed to cocaine *in utero* (MacGregor et al, 1987) (see Chapter 10).

Because most drugs have not been thoroughly investigated regarding their teratogenic potential, it is best to avoid all unnecessary drugs during pregnancy. If a drug is indicated, the potential benefits for that drug must be weighed against the potential hazzards to the fetus.

**Congenital Infections.** As previously stated, Gregg (1941) was one of the first to recognize an association between maternal rubella infection and abnormal fetal development. Other infectious diseases that have been documented to produce deleterious effects in the fetus are cytomegalovirus, toxoplasmosis, herpes simplex, syphilis, and human immunodeficiency virus (HIV).

Congenital infections may result in a wide spectrum of clinical pathology, ranging from major malformations to fetal and newborn infection. Fig 32–16 illustrates the major consequences of an intrauterine infection. After the mother is exposed and infected, she develops an acute viremia. The infection itself may or may not produce any maternal

symptoms. The virus then reaches the fetus via the placenta, where it may persist for the remainder of the pregnancy and early neonatal life. The type and severity of pathology observed is dependent on the nature of the virus and the time of fetal infection. Table 32–3 lists the major types of problems observed with several of the more well-defined congenital infectious agents.

It is now appropriate to add to the list of potential teratogens HIV, because women are at increasing risk for infection with HIV and the resulting diseases of aquired immunodeficiency syndrome (AIDS). The virus crosses the placenta, and the fetus is at risk for infection. Blanche and colleagues (1989) report that approximately one third of infants born to seropositive women were found to have AIDS by 18 months of age. Of this group, about 20 percent died of complications of the disease by 2 years of age. There has been less information available regarding the risk for malformations to fetuses exposed to the HIV virus *in utero*. To date, no specific syndrome has been identified (Qazi, 1988). However, there are many questions that remain unanswered, such as whether or not a fetus is at greater risk if the mother is nonsymptomatic or symptomatic and whether or not the infection initially occurs during pregnancy. Until more research is available, it is difficult to counsel women regarding the risks associated with HIV and AIDS (see Chapter 8).

The diagnosis of a congenital infection is important for genetic counseling to help establish the correct recurrence risk in future pregnancies. Thus, when a congenital infection is suspected, appropriate diagnostic tests should be obtained, such as viral cultures, antibody titers on both mother and infant, and radiologic examination for intercranial calcifications.

**Maternal Environment.** The previous discussion centered on fetal exposure to external agents such as drugs, radiation, and congenital infections. We now briefly discuss the effects of the maternal environment from both physical and metabolic standpoints.

Constraints placed on the fetus because of the mother's uterine cavity may on occasion result in certain types of malformations known as *deformations*. Uterine constraints may affect different parts of the forming embryo, mimicking other malformation syndromes. For example, the Pierre Robin sequence can result from a single gene

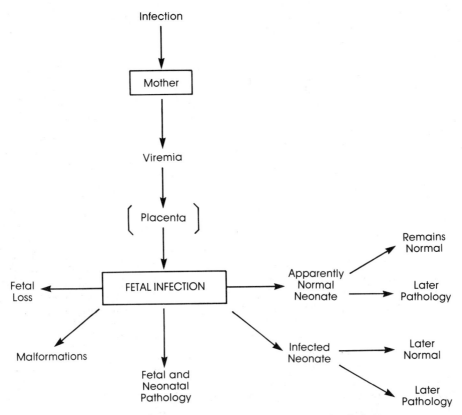

**Figure 32–16.** Major consequences of an intrauterine infection.

disorder, can be associated with other major anomalies and be indicative of a chromosome abnormality, or may be the result of the infant's being positioned against the wall of the uterus, thereby inhibiting growth of the lower mandible. In the latter case, the Pierre Robin sequence would be considered a deformation secondary to uterine constraint.

The metabolic environment of the mother also may have a profound effect on the developing fetus. An entire chapter has been devoted to treating the diabetic mother, but

**Table 32–3**
INTRAUTERINE INFECTIONS

| Disease | Time of Susceptibility | Infant Findings* |
|---|---|---|
| Rubella (virus) | First trimester | Microcephaly; cataracts; deafness, congenital heart disease, MR |
| | Second and third trimesters | Hearing loss, congenital or progressive |
| Cytomegalic Inclusion disease (virus) | All trimesters | Severe form: Micro- or hydrocephaly; MR; cerebral calcifications; seizures; chorioretinitis; deafness. Some infants excrete virus but are asymptomatic. |
| Toxoplasmosis (parasite) | All trimesters | Severe form: Micro- or hydrocephaly; seizures; choioretinitis |
| Herpes (virus) | First trimester | One half end in miscarriage |
| | Third trimester | Encephalitis; chorioretinitis; pneumonitis |
| Syphilis (bacteria) | All trimesters (100 percent cure if treated by 16 weeks of age) | None at birth 2 to 4 weeks: Lacrimation; snuffles, osteochondritis Later sequelae: Saddle nose; Hutchinson's teeth; deafness |

* Systemic findings may be seen in all the above infections except syphilis. These include hepatosplenomegaly, jaundice, apnea, tachypnea, cyanosis, hypothermia, fever, lethargy, and poor feeding.

from the genetic standpoint, it is important to be aware that infants born to diabetic mothers are at an increased risk for congenital malformations.

In a large study of 4929 live-born and still-born infants with congenital malformations (Becerra et al, 1990), the relative risk (compared with nondiabetic mothers) for major malformations among infants of mothers with insulin-dependent diabetes mellitus was 7.9 percent. The absolute risk (per 100 live births) was 18.4 percent. For major cardiovascular defects and central nervous system abnormalities among offspring of diabetic mothers as compared with nondiabetic mothers, the risks were 18.0 percent and 15.5 percent, respectively. Moreover, infants born to mothers with gestational diabetes mellitus who required insulin during the pregnancy were 20 times more likely to have major cardiac defects than infants born to nondiabetic mothers (Becerra et al, 1990). These figures are indicative of a stronger association of congenital malformations and insulin-dependent diabetes than has routinely been reported. The study also implicates gestational diabetes mellitus as a major risk factor for congenital cardiovascular abnormalities.

PKU is an autosomal recessive disorder involving an abnormality in the metabolism of the amino acid phenylalanine. Lacking the enzyme phenylalanine hydroxylase, women with PKU have high levels of serum phenylalanine. During pregnancy, these high levels represent a serious threat to the developing fetus. Infants born to women with PKU have been documented to have a high incidence of mental retardation and microcephaly. The risk for mental retardation may be as high as 90 to 100 percent (Richards, 1975). Although current literature suggests that placing a woman with PKU on a low phenylalanine diet prior to and during pregnancy decreases the risk for mental retardation, there is no documentation that this method completely eliminates the risk. Clearly, this problem represents a significant risk, because an increasing number of women diagnosed to have PKU during the newborn period have been treated and are currently of reproductive age.

Smoking has been associated with increased perinatal mortality and small-for-gestational-age infants. After adjusting for multiple variables, Meyer and Tonascia (1977) documented an increased risk of approximately 20 percent to infants whose mother smoked one pack a day as opposed to a 35 percent risk of perinatal mortality in women who smoked more than one pack a day. In addition, an increased incidence of placenta praevia as well as spontaneous abortions has been reported (Fielding, 1978). Although smoking has not been documented to cause malformations, it must be recognized as a potential hazard to the developing fetus.

The maternal environment also may pose problems when that environment is the result of a single gene disorder, such as myotonic dystrophy, a dominantly inherited condition. Although the mother may be mildly affected, the pregnancy and fetus are at risk for a number of different complications. Maternal myotonic dystrophy has been associated with recurrent miscarriage, stillbirth, polyhydramnios, poor fetal movement, and neonatal death (Bell and Smith, 1972). The infants are extremely hypotonic at birth; however, this condition improves over time. Intellectual development usually is impaired (Dubowitz, 1969). In a recent study by Rutherford and colleagues (1989), of 14 infants born to mothers with myotonic dystrophy, all had ventricular dilatation, 13 had asphyxia at delivery, 11 were premature, 4 had intrauterine growth retardation, 9 were found to have rib anomalies, and 5 had raised right hemidiaphragms. Most of the infants had major respiratory complications and had to be ventilated as a result of pulmonary hypoplasia. All four infants who needed to be ventilated longer than 4 months died. Obviously, the fetus of a mother with myotonic dystrophy is at considerable risk for a number of complications both before and after delivery.

In terms of genetic counseling, the documentation of a teratogenic etiology is important, because the risk of recurrence in the absence of a teratogen is low for the majority of families, and they can be reassured during future pregnancies. The importance of a detailed pregnancy history including exposure to any possible teratogenic agents cannot be overemphasized. With continued careful documentation of exposure to environmental agents during pregnancy, we will gain a better understanding of the potential relationship between these agents and fetal malformations.

# Preconception Counseling

In the past, genetic counseling has been primarily provided retrospectively, that is, after the birth of a child with birth defects or a genetic disorder. With technologic advances and an increasing public awareness, it has become imperative that health care practitioners provide information on a prospective basis. There are three major areas to be considered when counseling a couple who are planning a pregnancy: (1) reproductive history; (2) family history and screening pedigree; and (3) consanguinity.

## MATERNAL REPRODUCTIVE HISTORY

From the genetic standpoint, the reproductive history should include any type of pregnancy loss, spontaneous abortion, stillbirth, and perinatal death. For those couples with three or more miscarriages for which no maternal anatomic or physiologic explanation can be found, cytogenetic analysis should be considered. In studies of couples with a history of repeated reproductive failure, 5 to 10 percent have been documented to have a chromosome rearrangement or sex chromosome mosaicism (Ward et al, 1980; Watson et al, 1981).

Stillbirths and perinatal deaths should be investigated whether or not obvious malformations are present. As previously mentioned, a very small chromosomal deletion or unbalanced rearrangement can produce increased morbidity and mortality without the identification of major structural malformations. Additionally, congenital infections and genetic disorders can go undetected and result in the family not knowing the specific cause of death. Other areas included are infertility, duration and types of contraception, how pregnancy was confirmed, environmental exposures, and potential health histories of the couple.

## FAMILY HISTORY

The family history and screening pedigree can be extremely helpful in determining the family at risk. The screening pedigree can identify inherited conditions that may or may not have immediate implications for obstetric management. However, the family should be advised that other conditions may occur that were predictable from this pedigree.

The pedigree itself is a fairly simple but often productive method for ascertaining high-risk families. The health professional can obtain the necessary information and draw a screening pedigree in approximately 15 to 20 minutes. Information that should be obtained from the family when drawing the pedigree includes the following: full names and maiden names, if appropriate; birth dates of the immediate family members; names and ages of the rest of the family with a description of their health status; causes of death and age at death; and any other information that the family believes is pertinent. The screening pedigree usually includes the affected individual or the individual for whom the family is concerned and his or her siblings, parents, aunts, uncles, and grandparents (Fig. 32–17).

Ethnicity is another important aspect of the screening pedigree. A couple's ethnic background may be useful in determining the applicability of screening tests. For example, couples of Ashkenazi Jewish descent are at an increased risk for being carriers of the gene for Tay-Sachs disease. The carrier rate is approximately 1 in 30 (Greenberg and Kaback, 1982). African Americans are at an increased risk for sickle cell anemia, and the Mediteranean populations have been shown to be at risk for thalassemias.

## CONSANGUINITY

The screening pedigree also may identify those families in which consanguinity is an issue; that is, the partners are related to one another. For example, first cousins have one sixteenth of their genes in common. Because all individuals are carriers of five to seven lethal recessive genes, related couples may be at an increased risk for having a child with an autosomal recessive condition. For consanguineous couples with a known inherited disorder in the family, more specific risk figures can be provided.

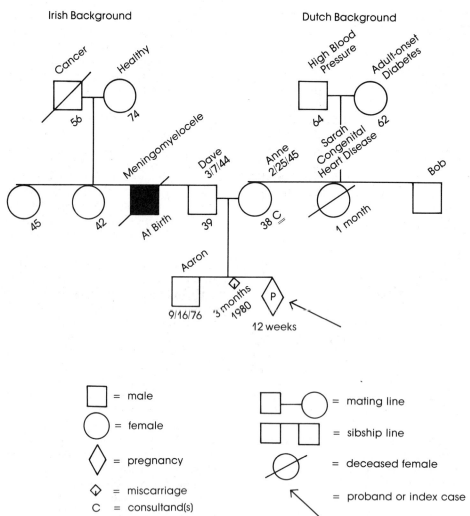

**Figure 32–17.** Screening pedigree obtained from a couple seeking prenatal diagnosis. Note positive family history for a neural tube defect (■ = affected).

# Postconception Counseling

Although preconception counseling is extremely helpful in identifying at-risk couples, the majority of couples receiving genetic counseling are at the postconception stage. These families, generally, can be grouped into two major categories: (1) those couples who are pregnant and have an appropriate indication for prenatal diagnosis and (2) those couples who have given birth to a child with birth defects or a genetic disorder.

## PRENATAL DIAGNOSIS

Prenatal diagnosis, the *in utero* determination of fetal disease, is an important part of genetic counseling. Rapid advances in prenatal diagnostic techniques represent a significant breakthrough in clinical genetics. These techniques have made it increasingly possible for a couple to make more informed reproductive decisions.

A number of different prenatal diagnostic techniques are now available (Table 32–4). The most widely known and used techniques

Table 32–4
TECHNIQUES FOR PRENATAL DIAGNOSIS

| Technique | Abnormalities Detectable |
|---|---|
| **Noninvasive** | |
| Maternal serum alpha-fetoprotein | Neural tube defects; problems with fetal well-being; Down syndrome (low maternal serum alpha-fetoprotein) |
| Ultrasonography | Skeletal malformations; major organ malformations; polyhydramnios; oligohydramnios; hydrops |
| **Invasive** | |
| Genetic amniocentesis | Chromosomal abnormalities; inborn errors of metabolism; hemoglobinopathies and other biochemcial disorders; alpha-fetoprotein detection for neural tube defects |
| Chorionic villus sampling | As above for genetic amniocentesis except does *not* include alpha-fetoprotein analysis |
| Fetal blood sampling (PUBS) | Hemoglobinopathies, biochemical disorders, inborn errors, rapid karyotype |
| Fetoscopy | Fetal skin or liver biopsy; external malformations |
| X-ray | Skeletal malformations |
| Amniography | External malformations; GI and GU malformations |

are genetic amniocentesis, ultrasonography, and chorionic villus sampling. Other techniques used are percutaneous umbilical blood sampling (PUBS), fetoscopy (amnioscopy), amniography, and x-ray study. Additionally, screening of maternal serum for such products as AFP, unconjugated estriol, and human chorionic gonadotropin are commonly performed to screen for the presence of a number of different disorders such as neural tube defects and chromosomal abnormalities.

Genetic amniocentesis presently allows for the detection of chromosome abnormalities, hundreds of biochemical disorders, neural tube defects, some ventral wall defects, as well as for DNA analysis for the diagnosis of a number of single gene disorders. The procedure involves the transabdominal withdrawal of fluid from the amniotic sac at approximately 15 to 16 weeks of pregnancy. Early amniocentesis, performed between 12 and 14 weeks' gestation, also is offered in some centers. Data regarding fetal loss following early amniocentesis is still being collected (Thayer et al, 1990).

Regardless of when the procedure is performed, prior to it, couples should receive adequate counseling to discuss the indications for the amniocentesis, the procedure itself, and any risks that may be involved. Ultrasound is performed to localize the placenta and fetus, determine approximate fetal gestation, and rule out the presence of twins. Under sterile conditions, approximately 30 ml of amniotic fluid is removed via a 22-gauge needle. Amniotic cells that originate from fetal skin, amnion, and fetal mucous

membranes are then grown in culture and may be analyzed for fetal chromosomes, fetal DNA fragments, or fetal enzyme activity (Huisjes, 1978).

Prenatal diagnosis should be considered for couples presenting with the following indications:

1. Maternal age (35 years or older).
2. Previous child with a chromosome abnormality or positive family history.
3. Parental balanced translocation carrier.
4. Mother a known or at-risk carrier for an X-linked disorder.
5. Parents carriers of an autosomal recessive disorder diagnosable *in utero.*
6. A parent affected with an autosomal dominant disorder diagnosable *in utero.*
7. Positive family history for neural tube defects.

Advanced maternal age has been associated with an increased risk for fetal chromosome abnormalities (Epstein and Golbus, 1977). The actual risk figures given to couples depend on whether figures are quoted from the newborn population or amniocentesis data (Fig. 32–18). Nationwide, genetic amniocentesis is usually offered at maternal age 35, because the risk tends to rise at this time. In general, the risk increases from approximately 1 percent at age 37 to 10 to 12 percent at age 45 or older.

Couples who have had a previous child with trisomy 21 have a 1 to 2 percent recurrence risk in future pregnancies (Epstein and Golbus, 1977). Additionally, there is some evidence that families with children affected with other chromosome aberrations also may

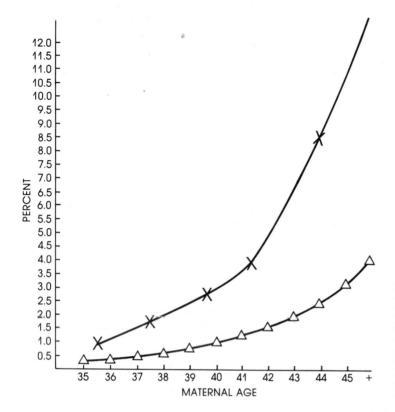

**Figure 32–18.** Incidence of chromosome abnormalities at midtrimester amniocentesis (X) and Down syndrome at term (△) as a function of maternal age. (Redrawn from Antenatal Diagnosis. US Department of Health, Education, and Welfare, NIH Publication #79-173, April 1979, p I-51.)

be at increased risk in future pregnancies (Hecht, 1979). Prenatal diagnosis should be made available to any couple who have had a child with a chromosome abnormality. Further, if a positive family history for a chromosome abnormality is ascertained, prenatal diagnosis should be considered. As stated previously, a parent who is a carrier of a balanced translocation is at an increased risk for having offspring with an unbalanced rearrangement. Genetic amniocentesis is appropriate for these couples and can delineate the specific chromosome constitution of the fetus.

Mothers who are documented carriers or at risk for being a carrier of an X-linked disorder may find genetic amniocentesis an appropriate option. With the rapid technologic advances in cytogenetics and molecular genetics, a number of X-linked disorders are now diagnosable with DNA analysis. If, however, the disorder itself cannot be diagnosed, the sex of the fetus can be determined and the pregnancy electively terminated in the presence of a male fetus. The decision to terminate a pregnancy in light of this knowledge must be discussed at length and the family's decision supported. Once again,

DNA analysis and gene localization have negated the necessity of this option in many disorders such as classic hemophilia and Duchenne muscular dystrophy.

Prenatal diagnosis has been accomplished for a variety of biochemical disorders, some of which are listed in Table 32–5. A diagnosis of specific inborn errors of metabolism is made by analysis of amniotic fluid or cultured fibroblasts. The majority of these disorders are inherited in an autosomal recessive fashion, putting couples at a 25 percent risk with each pregnancy.

The diagnosis of neural tube defects is a common indication for prenatal diagnosis. The spectrum of neural tube defects ranges from anencephaly and myelomeningocele to spina bifida occulta. Neural tube defects are seen in approximately 1 in 1000 live births and are inherited as multifactorial disorders. Regardless of the numerical risk given, families with a positive history of neural tube defects should be offered prenatal diagnosis. The specific risk can be reduced by as much as 90 percent through AFP determination.

AFP is a glycoprotein and a major component of fetal blood. Small amounts of AFP are found in the amniotic fluid of normal

Table 32–5

SOME INHERITED BIOCHEMICAL DISORDERS THAT CAN BE DIAGNOSED PRENATALLY
IN CULTURED FETAL CELLS

| Error in the Metabolism of | Disorder | Metabolic Defect | Brief Description of Phenotype |
|---|---|---|---|
| **Amino Acids** | Maple sugar urine disease (AR)* | Deficiency of enzymes needed in breakdown of some amino acids (leading to large excesses of leucine, isoleucine, and valine) | Poor development, convulsions, and early death. Urine has maple sugar odor. Diet therapy seems promising. |
| | Cystinosis (AR) | Primary defect unknown (but leading to accumulation of cystine in cells) | Several forms. In severe form, kidney function is impaired, leading to poor development, rickets, and childhood death. |
| **Sugars** | Galactosemia (AR) | Deficiency of enzyme needed in the metabolism of galactose (derived primarily from milk) | Liver and eye defects, mental retardation, and early death if untreated. Restrictive diet can control adverse symptoms. |
| **Lipids** | Tay-Sachs disease (AR) | Deficiency of enzyme needed in the breakdown of a complex lipid (allowing its accumulation in nervous tissue) | Progressive physical and mental degeneration, paralysis, blindness, and death in infancy. |
| | Adrenogenital syndromes (AR) | Deficiency of enzymes needed in the synthesis of sex hormones and of steroids controlling salt and water balance. | Mild and severe forms. In the most common form, dehydration and early death. In females, virilization is often seen. |
| **Purines** | Lesch-Nyhan syndrome (XR) | Deficiency of enzyme involved in the metabolism of purines (resulting in excessive production of uric acid) | Mental retardation, muscular spasms, compulsive self-mutilation. Patients may survive into adulthood. |
| **Complex Polysaccharides** | Hurler syndrome (AR) Hunter syndrome (XR) | Defects of connective tissue (allowing accumulation of mucopolysaccharides in cells) | Dwarfism, grotesque facial features, mental retardation. Hunter's syndrome less severe. |
| **Heme** | Porphyria (AD) | Deficiency of enzyme needed in the synthesis of heme | Attacks of abdominal pain accompanied sometimes by impairment of mental functions. |

* AR = autosomal recessive, AD = autosomal dominant, XR = X-linked recessive. Altogether, about 100 diseases can be detected prenatally.

Table from Genetics. Human Aspects by Arthur and Elaine Mange, copyright © 1980 by Saunders College Publishing, reprinted by permission of the publisher.

fetuses as well as in maternal serum. In the presence of an open neural tube defect, concentrations of AFP in amniotic fluid are greatly increased (Brock, 1977). Elevated levels also may be associated with a number of other malformations (Campbell et al, 1978; Seppala, 1975; Seppala and Unnerus, 1974).

More recently, AFP determination of maternal serum has become a valuable screening method not only for determining neural tube defects but for predicting fetal well-being and outcome at delivery. It has been demonstrated that when elevations in ma-

ternal serum alpha-fetoprotein (MSAFP) are present and the appropriate adjustments for such factors as gestational age, maternal weight, race, and maternal disease (e.g., diabetes) have been made, an elevation of MSAFP may be indicative of poor fetal outcome including prematurity, low birth weight, impending or actual fetal demise, and a number of other malformations, such as omphalocele, gastroshisis, and renal malformations (Thomas and Blakemore, 1990).

A new approach to noninvasive screening for trisomy 21 (Down syndrome) recently has been advocated by a number of researchers. It has been demonstrated that low levels of MSAFP have been associated with fetal trisomies, in particular, trisomy 21 (Palomaki and Haddow, 1987). This measurement has allowed clinicians to calculate specific risk figures in women under the age of 35. The best timing to administer this screening test is between 16 and 18 weeks' gestation (Albright et al, 1988). These figures must be carefully calculated and adjusted for a number of factors (maternal weight, race, gestational age, maternal diabetes), as is the case with elevated levels of MSAFP. At the present time, a new investigative laboratory method is being tested that combines data from MSAFP, unconjugated estriol, and human chorionic gonadotropin. This triple test or MSAFP plus is also performed at 16 to 18 weeks of gestation and is combined with maternal age to calculate a new, patient-specific risk. In the presence of a fetus with Down syndrome, it has been found that not only may the MSAFP level be low but also the unconjugated estriol. The human chorionic gonadotropin has been found to be elevated. With these two additional screening tests, it is estimated 60 percent of cases with Down syndrome can be identified (Wald et al, 1988). However, it must be clear to both patients and practitioners that these tests are screening procedures only and are *not* diagnostic. A normal cytogenetic evaluation following amniocentesis rules out the presence of Down syndrome and other chromosomal abnormalities, whereas a negative screening test can only reduce the risk, not rule it out.

Most prenatal diagnostic centers follow specific protocols to evaluate increases or decreases of MSAFP and other screening tests that allow for the identification of normal fetal etiologies such as those found with twins or advanced gestation and abnormal fetal etiologies that are associated with malformations and poor fetal outcome.

The most recent technique currently being used for the prenatal diagnosis of genetic disorders is chorionic villus sampling (Brambati et al, 1985). Chorionic villus sampling (CVS) procedures can be accomplished in either one of two methods: (1) transcervically or (2) transabdominally. If performd transcervically, a sterile catheter is introduced into the cervix under continuous ultrasonographic guidance and a small portion of chorionic villi (placenta) is aspirated with syringe suction. If performed transab-

dominally, an 18-gauge spinal needle with stylet is inserted under sterile conditions percutaneously through the abdominal wall into the chorion frondosum under continuous ultrasonographic guidance. The stylet is then withdrawn, and a syringe aspirates out the chorionic tissue (Elias et al, 1989). In either method, the villi are then selected out from the obtained sample for direct harvest and culturing for chromosomal analysis, and when indicated, processed for DNA or enzymatic analysis. The advantages of these methods of prenatal diagnosis are that they can be performed between the 9th and 12th weeks of pregnancy, results are available within a few days, and if a fetal abnormality is detected and termination of the pregnancy is decided, a first-trimester abortion, which carries a lower morbidity and mortality risk than a midtrimester termination (Castadot, 1986), can be performed.

At the present time, a number of large studies are being conducted to assess the efficacy and risks of transcervical and transabdominal chorionic villus sampling (Brambati et al, 1990; Canadian Collaborative study, 1989; Rhoads et al, 1989). Spotting or bleeding (approximately 10 percent) and uterine cramping (2.5 percent) are stated to be the most common complications. Risk for fetal loss following the procedure has been demonstrated to be between 2 percent and 5 percent with those centers having the most experience being at the 2 percent level (Brambati et al, 1990). The other major disadvantage is that amniotic fluid is not obtainable using this method. Thus, families at risk for neural tube defects would need to employ other techniques, such as amniocentesis and ultrasound, for that specific diagnosis.

PUBS is offered when fetal blood is needed for diagnosis. The procedure is usually performed between 16 and 18 weeks' gestation; however, it is most commonly performed following the detection of an abnormality on ultrasonography and there is need for a rapid karyotype (Golbus, 1990). This procedure also is commonly used to monitor fetal hematocrits in Rh-immunized patients before and after transfusion procedures.

As ultrasonography techniques and equipment have become more refined, fetal observation has become more detailed. Gestational age, twinning, placental localization, and the presence of poly- or oligohydramnios often are screened for by this technique routinely in many centers. The number of structural abnormalities being detected has continued to grow. Craniospinal defects (hydrocephalus, anencephaly, and microcephaly), renal malformations (obstruction or dysplasias), gastrointestinal malformation (obstructions, gastroschisis, omphalocele, and skeletal dyplasias are only a few of the disorders that have been diagnosed *in utero* by ultrasound (Sabbagha et al, 1981). At the present time, there is no evidence of problems to either the fetus or the mother from exposure to ultrasound.

Fetal observation also can be achieved by x-ray study. The fetal skeleton is sufficiently ossified by approximately 16 weeks of gestation to allow observation of bony abnormalities and gross limb malformations. An x-ray study of the fetus taken on an oblique axis at 20 weeks of pregnancy has been used to rule out such disorders as hypophosphatasia and metatrophic dwarfism. The need for x-ray study has steadily declined as other techniques for the prenatal diagnosis of skeletal malformations have been perfected. However, in a few instances, such as when hypophosphatasia is suspected, x-ray study is the most appropriate method of evaluation and should be considered.

Fetoscopy (amnioscopy) via a fiberoptic endoscope allows for the direct visualization of the fetus. Initially, the procedure was used predominantly for fetal blood sampling to diagnose beta thalassemia and sickle-cell anemia (Alter and Nathan, 1976; Jensen et al, 1979). These disorders are now diagnosable via DNA analysis of amniocytes. Additionally, owing to rapid advances in the other prenatal techniques that carry lower risks to the fetus, fetoscopy is seldom employed.

Recent advances in molecular genetics have provided an entirely new arena for the prenatal diagnosis of many genetic disorders. This field of molecular biology and the resulting knowledge of the content and structure of the human genome has dominated most of the advances in clinical genetics in the past few years. Gene defects and their chromosomal locations are being identified daily. Advances in recombinant DNA technologies have allowed carrier testing, prenatal diagnosis, paternity testing, forensic diagnosis, and presymptomatic detection to become realities for a large number of genetic conditions.

DNA testing, and thus prenatal diagnosis, is now available for a number of more well-known genetic disorders, including cystic fibrosis, neurofibromatosis, sickle cell anemia, beta- and alpha-thalassemias, hemophilia A and B, Huntington's disease, phenylketonuria, alpha-1 antitrypsin deficiency, and Duchenne and Becker muscular dystrophies. Couples with a family history of these disorders and those couples at increased risk because of being members of a high-risk population for a genetic disorder, such as African Americans for sickle cell anemia, may consider having DNA testing carried out either for postconception diagnosis or for prenatal diagnosis.

In general, there are two ways to approach DNA analysis. First, there are several laboratory methods to directly detect the specific mutation of a genetic disorder. Second, if the specific mutation is not yet known, indirect methods, such as linkage with DNA polymorphisms, may be available. Many disorders, which were initially only detectable by the indirect linkage method, have moved over to the direct methods as the specific mutation has been identified, such as sickle cell anemia and Duchenne muscular dystropy.

Restriction endonuclease analysis to detect point mutations that alter restriction sites is a major direct method used when a single base change is responsible for the disorder. For example, sickle cell anemia is caused by a single nucleotide substitution in the sixth codon of the beta-globin gene. The DNA from amniotic fluid or any nucleated cell is subjected to the action of restriction endonucleases, which cleave to the DNA at specific locations. Separated by electrophoresis, the DNA fragments are hybridized with complementary DNA (Abelson, 1977). The diagnosis of sickle cell anemia or alpha-thalassemia is based on the absence of normal hybridized patterns (Panny et al, 1979; Phillips et al, 1979).

The new technology known as polymerase chain reaction (PCR) became available in 1987 and made the prenatal diagnosis of sickle cell anemia and other disorders much easier and faster. This technology is used to amplify specific regions of DNA up to about 10-million–fold in approximately 3 hours (White et al, 1989). In the case of sickle cell anemia, primers are used to amplify the specific region in the beta-globin gene. After amplification and electrophoresis of the DNA, a single strong band of the particular specifically amplified DNA is detected. Because the amplified DNA is observed by chemical staining techniques and does not need radioactive probes to be detected, it is more rapid and less expensive (Gelehrter and Collins, 1990).

Another frequently used technique is that of Southern blot analysis, used to detect major deletions or rearrangements of DNA. At the present time, this method is used to diagnose Duchenne muscular dystrophy, which has been shown to be the result of deletions in the gene for Duchenne muscular dystrophy in more than 60 percent of cases (Gelehrter and Collins, 1990). This technique also has demonstrated that 70 percent of all individuals with cystic fibrosis share the same mutation, namely the deletion of a phenylalanine residue at position 508, known as a deletion of delta F508. The cystic fibrosis gene has been localized to chromosome 7q31 (Rommens et al, 1989).

As mentioned previously, not all disorders are amenable to direct detection and, thus, linkage analysis is still appropriate for diagnosis. Linkage analysis first came into widespread use in 1978, when Kan and Dozy (1978) identified a restriction fragment length polymorphism at the beta-globin locus. Strategies were devised such that it became possible, using genetic linkage analysis, to identify DNA markers close to human disease loci (Beaudet et al, 1990). Hemophilia A requires this technique, because the specific mutation is still unknown. In this instance, the analysis is one of looking at specific markers that are known to be very closely linked to the hemophilia A gene. Usually, it is necessary to analyze the DNA from several family members to decide what markers are associated with the disorder. Presymptomatic and prenatal diagnosis of Huntington's disease is also accomplished in this manner (Kazazian, 1990).

As one can note, prenatal diagnosis does not guarantee the birth of a normal infant but can only provide information regarding those malformations or disorders that are specifically looked for. With the enormous strides being made in the area of molecular genetics, the number of diagnosable disorders grows daily. However, many genetic diseases are not amenable to prenatal diagnosis and practitioners as well as families must understand the limits of our technologies. The family must be apprised of what prenatal diagnosis can and cannot provide.

Thus, it becomes imperative that adequate genetic counseling precede any diagnostic procedure.

For some couples, the detection of an abnormal fetus and termination of pregnancy offer an alternative to having affected offspring. For other couples, the abnormalities detected prenatally may be amenable to surgical correction (e.g., omphalocele) or medical management at birth. For those couples who elect to continue the pregnancy after the prenatal detection of a fetal abnormality, counseling and ongoing support should be made available. Resources such as mental health counseling, social services, and spiritual guidance should be sought to help families to begin the grief process as they mourn the loss of the expected "perfect baby" and begin to deal with the anticipated problems or possible death of the malformed infant (Matthews, 1990). In any case, it is appropriate to discuss all the available options with the family. By far, the majority of those couples undergoing prenatal diagnosis are given reassuring results and thus find peace of mind throughout the remainder of the pregnancy.

## POSTNATAL DIAGNOSIS

Infants with birth defects and genetic disorders usually can be grouped into three major categories: (1) those presenting with obvious malformations at birth, (2) those who have a "stormy" neonatal period, and (3) those who appear normal at birth but subsequently develop an abnormal clinical course. As previously stated, the majority of these infants are detected during the early neonatal period.

It is the general expectation of couples and their primary health care team that pregnancy outcome will result in the birth of a normal healthy infant. Consequently, when an infant with an obvious malformation is born, both the parents and the health care professionals involved are faced with an emotional crisis and, often, a medical emergency. The first major step in determining the course of action for the infant is to make an accurate diagnosis. Often, a genetic evaluation is warranted to assist in this process. In making an accurate diagnosis, data from a number of sources need to be obtained and evaluated. These sources include but are not limited to

1. Pregnancy history
2. Family history and pedigree
3. Detailed physical examination
4. Growth and developmental history
5. Laboratory procedures
6. Photographs

Each of these areas is discussed in the section dealing with the principles and practices of genetic counseling.

When evaluating the infant with a malformation, the clinical geneticist tries to identify specific patterns of abnormalities. Two major questions are considered: (1) Is the malformation restricted to one organ system or does it involve multiple systems, and (2) does the malformation have a genetic or nongenetic etiology? If multiple major and minor malformations are present, the geneticist must consider chromosomal, single gene, and nongenetic etiologies. These etiologies frequently have a recognizable pattern of malformations, thus making it imperative that the clinician have expertise in syndrome recognition (Riccardi, 1977). It is the specific combination and frequency of a constellation of clinical findings that are significant for syndrome identification. For example, in Down syndrome any one of the specific clinical findings can be found in normal infants, such as a single flexion crease (simian line), clinodactyly, or mongoloid slant. However, when these findings are found in combination, the diagnosis of Down syndrome is considered. In the presence of a single malformation or malformations affecting only one organ system, multifactorial, single-gene, and developmental etiologies are considered. For example, isolated congenital heart disease is inherited in a multifactorial fashion. Skeletal dysplasias (including achondroplasia and other dwarfisms) usually affect only the skeletal system but may be inherited as autosomal dominant or recessive disorders. These conditions often can only be distinguished on the basis of skeletal x-ray study. Some malformations are considered to be developmental in nature and represent an abnormality of embryonic development that is not explained by known or possible genetic mechanisms or by known teratogens (Riccardi, 1977). For example, the presence of an isolated limb anomaly in the absence of a positive family history would make one consider a developmental etiology.

In the case of a stillborn infant, a careful examination (including an autopsy) for any major or minor abnormalities is indicated. Photographs can be of assistance to the geneticist in establishing the correct diagnosis. As previously mentioned, tissue for cytogenetic analysis should be obtained in the presence of minor malformations with or without major malformations.

Many genetic disorders are not associated with congenital malformations but may be identified during the neonatal period by a stormy clinical course. Such findings as nausea and vomiting, organomegaly, abnormal central nervous system function (seizures, hypo- or hypertonia), and metabolic electrolyte imbalances may warrant investigation for a possible genetic cause. Because many inborn errors of metabolism are associated with these findings, laboratory screening, such as that for amino and organic acids, is indicated. Documentation of a metabolic condition as early as possible is imperative given the availability of treatment protocols for some of these disorders (e.g., PKU, galactosemia, thyroid abnormalities). If the etiology of the problem is of an infectious nature, a toxoplasmosis, rubella, cytomegalovirus, and herpes simplex (TORCH) screen should be requested.

In some instances, infants with inborn errors of metabolism or other genetic disorders have a normal neonatal course and do not present with clinical findings until several months of age. Unfortunately, many of these disorders are not diagnosed until clinical symptoms become more severe. The classic example of a metabolic disorder presenting in this manner is Tay-Sachs disease. The affected infant appears normal and reaches developmental milestones until approximately 4 to 6 months of age. At this time, further development ceases and signs of neurologic degeneration are noted.

Since the early 1960s, most states have mandated programs to screen the entire newborn population for PKU. Newborns in many centers are now screened for additional genetic disorders (Table 32–6). The major purpose of these programs is the early identification and initiation of appropriate treatment modalities for affected newborns. With this approach, devastating irreversible damage is usually avoided and the affected

**Table 32–6**
NEWBORN SCREENING*

Phenylketonuria
Hypothyroidism
Sickle cell anemia
Galactosemia
Maple syrup urine disease
Homocystinuria

\* Some centers may screen for other disorders.

infant can be expected to have a normal developmental course.

# The Practice of Genetic Counseling

Genetic counseling is appropriate for any family that asks the question "Will it happen again?" Referrals to the genetic counseling team may be made by the family itself or any health care professional. Major indications for referral are summarized in Table 32–7.

## INFORMATION GATHERING

The multifaceted process of genetic counseling begins at the time of referral. As previously outlined, information is gathered from a variety of sources. The principles involved include establishing an accurate diagnosis, discussing prognosis and treatment

**Table 32–7**
MAJOR INDICATIONS FOR REFERRAL FOR GENETIC COUNSELING

Genetic counseling is appropriate for any family concerned about the diagnosis, etiology, recurrence risk, prognosis, and treatment of a specific disorder.
A. Positive family history with:
  1. Congenital malformations
  2. Mental retardation with or without malformations
  3. Chromosome abnormality
  4. Single gene disorders
  5. Family disorders (multifactorial)
  6. Sensory defects
  7. Neurologic, neuromuscular disorders, or both
B. Consanguinity
C. High-risk ethnic group
D. Recurrent miscarriages
E. Potential teratogenic effect
F. Prenatal diagnosis

when appropriate, providing risks of recurrence, and presenting reproductive alternatives. Two clinical cases are presented to illustrate the genetic counseling process and to outline what families can expect.

> Case # 1: A gravida III, para 0, AB II 26-year-old mother delivered a male infant with bilateral cleft lip and palate, congenital heart disease, hypotonia, and multiple minor anomalies including abnormal dermatoglyphics.
>
> Case # 2: A 38-year-old woman, who is pregnant, was referred for prenatal diagnosis for maternal age. The family history indicated that her husband's sibling died at birth with a large meningomyelocele.

## PHYSICAL EXAMINATION

The primary purpose of the initial counseling session is to establish an accurate diagnosis. In Case # 1, the physical examination is paramount in helping to establish the diagnosis. Beyond the obvious major malformations, special attention should be given to the presence or absence of minor anomalies, which are frequently overlooked. Facial features should be described, such as positioning of eyes (hypertelorism, hypotelorism, mongoloid slant), configuration of the nose and mouth (depressed nasal bridge, anteverted nostrils, downturned mouth), development of the jaw (micrognathia), positioning and shape of the ears, overall skull shape, sutures, and hair patterns. Neck and trunk features should include such descriptions as webbed neck, low posterior hairline, and chest configuration. Hyperpigmented or depigmented areas of the skin should be described with attention to size, shape, location, and number.

Dermatoglyphic analysis can be helpful in delineating the etiology of some genetic disorders. Dermatoglyphics is the study of the dermal ridge configurations on the digits, palms, and soles (Preus and Fraser, 1972). The ridges begin development at approximately the 13th week of gestation and are complete by the 19th week. Thus, many genetic disorders that affect multiple systems also affect the dermatoglyphics. Some of the more well-known aberrations of dermatogly-

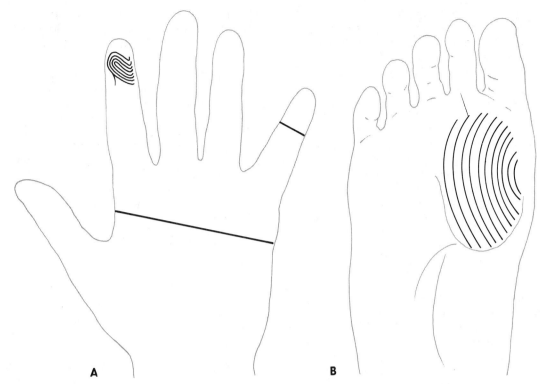

**Figure 32–19.** Dermatoglyphic findings common in Down syndrome. *A,* Note single palmar crease (simian line), single flexion crease on 5th digit, ulnar loop pattern on index finger, and *B,* open field pattern (arch tibial) on hallucal area of foot.

phics are found in Down syndrome. A single flexion crease (simian line) on the palms is a common finding as well as an increased number of ulnar loops on the fingertips (Fig. 32–19*A*). In addition to changes of the hand print patterns, a characteristic pattern known as an arch tibial may be found on the hallucal region of the feet (Fig. 32–19*B*).

## LABORATORY ANALYSES

The next step in evaluating an infant is to collect data from laboratory analyses. Beyond the routine laboratory analyses performed (electrolytes, blood count, x-ray study), there are a number of specific studies that may be appropriate in evaluating Case # 1. In light of multiple malformations, blood for chromosome analysis should be obtained. If the infant's status is critical and management plans are in question, then cytogenetic analysis of a direct bone marrow preparation may be warranted. Results from bone marrow preparations usually can be obtained within a day. As a precautionary mea-

sure, a blood specimen should also be obtained simultaneously to ensure satisfactory results. If one suspects an infectious etiology, viral cultures and a TORCH screen are appropriate. In the presence of hypotonia and failure to thrive, a detailed neurologic examination and possibly a computed axial tomography (CAT) scan should be obtained. An ophthalmologic examination is often beneficial because many disorders, including congenital infections, metabolic abnormalities, and chromosome aberrations, are associated with specific eye findings.

## FAMILY HISTORY AND PEDIGREE

An extensive family history and a pedigree are essential elements of establishing any diagnosis. The family pedigree serves three additional purposes: (1) establishes the mode of inheritance, (2) identifies other areas of concern, and (3) identifies additional family members at risk.

The detailed history should include information concerning conception, pregnancy, and labor and delivery as well as neonatal and developmental data. The history may be extremely helpful in determining whether the problem is prenatal (congenital) or postnatal in onset and whether the disorder is familiar or nongenetic.

As illustrated by Case # 2, the family history identified an additional risk for the couple, that is, an increased risk for neural tube defects. Had this been overlooked, appropriate testing may not have been offered. When conducted correctly, the family history and pedigree becomes a powerful tool in the process of genetic counseling.

## TIMING OF GENETIC COUNSELING

Another issue of importance is the timing of genetic counseling. Although, ideally, counseling should be prospective, that is, before the birth of an affected child, it usually occurs retrospectively. In retrospective counseling, timing is a crucial factor. One needs to appreciate the parameter of the grief process that confronts couples who have just given birth to an abnormal infant and be cognizant of family differences. It may be appropriate for the genetic counselor to approach the family in the newborn nursery, obtain some preliminary information to assist with the immediate evaluation, and suggest counseling at a future date. This allows the family time to recover from the initial stages of shock and be more receptive to accepting any information given.

The period of time between the initial referral for genetic evaluation and the final genetic counseling session may include a single consultation or many sessions over a period of months. The final counseling is based on all the available information, published literature, and collaborative expertise of the genetics team. The session includes a discussion of the diagnosis and medical facts, prognosis and management, risk of recurrence, and reproductive alternatives.

## DISCUSSION OF REPRODUCTIVE ALTERNATIVES

An important aspect of genetic counseling is a discussion of reproductive alternatives. Options that may be discussed include continuing previous reproductive plans (having another child), sterilization, adoption, artificial insemination, delayed childbearing, prenatal diagnosis, and early detection and treatment. For many families, the risk of recurrence and burden of the disorder in question is low or is perceived as low, and the couple elects to have more children. For those couples who view their risk as being too high or the burden too great and for whom prenatal diagnosis is not available, sterilization may represent the only acceptable alternative.

Artificial insemination by donor may be an appropriate option in specific situations: (1) when the husband has an autosomal dominant disorder, artificial insemination by donor decreases the recurrence risk to that of the general population; (2) when the husband has an X-linked disorder, artificial insemination by donor prevents the continuation of the disorder through obligate carrier daughters; (3) when both parents are carriers for an autosomal recessive disorder, artificial insemination by donor decreases the risk of recurrence to considerably less than 25 percent, and if donor carrier testing is available, to 0 percent; and (4) for those couples with a high risk of recurrence for a multifactorial disorder. It is imperative when artificial insemination by donor is used for genetic reasons that a careful family history and appropriate carrier tests be obtained on the sperm donor. Patients also should be informed that the risk of AIDS is rare with properly screened semen.

Because technology in medical genetics and health care continues to make rapid advances, many couples may decide to delay childbearing until methods of early detection and treatment are available. For example, hydrocephalus has been successfully treated surgically via *in utero* shunting (Clewell et al, 1982).

## THE PRINCIPLES OF GENETIC COUNSELING

Geneticists and health care professionals must adhere to certain principles of practice in order for genetic counseling to be an effective avenue of health care. These principles include *establishing an accurate diagnosis, offering nondirective counseling, maintaining confidentiality, providing referral and follow-up,* and *using a team approach.* The importance of an accurate diagnosis cannot be stressed enough. With the establishment of the diagnosis, genetic counseling should proceed in a nondirective manner. A major component of nondirective counseling is the ability to present information in a truthful yet sensitive manner. The counselor must strive to create a nonthreatening and non-coercive atmosphere and refrain from inter-jecting his or her own biases and opinions. In addition to providing information, the coun-selor provides assistance and support. The counselor may find that some families need assistance in defining personal priorities and making decisions appropriate to their partic-ular situation. Once a family has decided on a particular course of action, the decision should be supported, regardless of what that course of action is.

As with any patient-professional relation-ship, confidentiality and trust are para-mount features. Occasionally, confidentia-lity becomes an issue. For example, what is the moral obligation of the counselor if an autosomal dominant disorder is diagnosed and the patient refuses to share this informa-tion with at-risk relatives? Although this sit-uation is rare, the counselor should encour-age the family to share this information with relatives, stressing the reason for doing so.

Families receiving genetic counseling should be provided with a written summary of the discussion. Additionally, the counselor should be in contact with the primary health care provider so that continued follow-up may be coordinated. For some families, refer-rals to other health services may be appro-priate, such as infant stimulation programs, social services, physical therapy, family counseling, special clinics, and parent groups. As an outgrowth of the counseling process, other family members identified to be at increased risk also may benefit from genetic counseling and should be referred.

Genetic counseling is a complex and multi-faceted process and therefore *cannot* be per-formed efficiently or effectively in isolation. The genetics team consists of health care professionals and scientists representing a variety of backgrounds and expertise. The genetics team is usually composed of a medi-cal geneticist, genetic counselor (genetic as-sociate, nurse geneticist, or both), social worker, and laboratory specialists (cyto-geneticist, biochemical geneticist, immuno-geneticist). The expertise of many other health professionals is drawn on, including other medical and nursing specialists, popu-lation geneticists, and the clergy.

The genetics team continually strives to inform and assist the primary physician or nurse clinician before, during, and after counseling. It is hoped that these primary health care providers use the genetics team as a resource group for consultation and as-sistance in the care of their patients.

## References

Abelson J: Recombinant DNA: examples of present-day research. Science 196:159, 1977.

Ad Hoc Committee of Genetic Counseling: Genetic coun-seling. Am J Hum Genet 27:240, 1975.

Albright SG, Lingley LH, Seeds JW: Pitfalls of gesta-tional age reassignment in evaluation of low mater-nal serum alpha-fetoprotein levels. Am J Obstet Gynecol 159:369, 1988.

Alter BP, Nathan DG: Antenatal diagnosis of haemato-logical disorders—"1978." Clin Haematol 7:195, 1976.

Ardinger HH, Atkin JF, Blackston RD, et al: Verifica-tion of the fetal valproate syndrome phenotype. Am J Med Genet 29:171, 1988.

Beaudet AL, Scriver CR, Sly WS, et al: Introduction to Human Biochemical and Molecular Genetics. McGraw-Hill, 1990.

Becerra JE, Khoury MJ, Cordero JF, Erickson JD: Dia-betes mellitus during pregnancy and the risks for spe-cific birth defects: a population based case control study. Pediatrics 85(1):1, 1990.

Bell DB, Smith DW: Myotonic dystropy in the neonate. J Pediatr 81:83, 1972.

Blanche S, Rouzioux C, Moscato ML, et al: A prospective study of infants born to women seropositive for human immunodeficiency virus type 1. N Engl J Med 320: 1643, 1989.

Brambati B, Lanzani A, Tului L: Transabdominal and transcervical chorionic villus sampling: efficiency and risk evaluation of 2,411 cases. Am J Med Genet 35:160, 1990.

Brambati B, Simoni G, Danesino C, et al: First trimester fetal diagnosis of genetic disorders: clinical evalu-ation of 250 cases. J Med Genet 22(2):92, 1985.

Brock DJ: Biochemical and cytological methods in the diagnosis of neural tube defects. Prog Med Genet New Series 2:1, 1977.

Buehler BA, Delimont D, Van Waes M, Finnell RH: Prenatal prediction of risk of the fetal hydantoin syn-drome. New Engl J Med 322(22):1567, 1990.

Butler MG: Prader-Willi syndrome: current under-standing of cause and diagnosis. Am J Med Genet 35:319, 1990.

Campbell S, Rodeck C, Thomas A, et al: Early diagnosis of exomphalos. Lancet 1:1098, 1978.

Canadian Collaborative CVS-Amniocentesis Clinical Trail Group: Multicentre randomised clinical trail of chorionic villus sampling and amniocentesis. Lancet. 1:1, 1989.

Carr DH, Gedeon M: Population cytogenetics of human abortuses. *In* Hook EB, Porter IH (eds): Population Cytogenetics: Studies in Humans. New York, Aca-demic Press, 1977.

Caspersson T, Farber S, Foley GE, et al: Chemical dif-ferentiation among metaphase chromosomes. Exper Cell Res 49:219, 1968.

Castadot RG: Pregnancy termination: techniques, risks,

and complications and their management. Fertil Steril 45:5–17, 1986

Chasnoff IJ, Griffith DR: Cocaine: clinical studies of pregnancy and the newborn. Ann NY Acad Sci 562:260–266, 1989.

Clewell WH, Johnson ML, Neier RP, et al: A surgical approach to the treatment of fetal hydrocephalus. N Engl J Med 306:1320, 1982.

Cross PK, Hook EB: Paternal age and Down syndrome—a continuing dilemma: data from prenatal cytogenetic studies from the New York State chromosome registry and implications for genetic counseling. Am J Hum Genet 34:121A, 1982.

deGrouchy J, Turleau C: Clinical Atlas of Human Chromosomes, 2nd ed. New York, John Wiley & Sons, 1984.

Dubowitz V: The floppy infant. London, Heinemann, 1969.

Elias S, Simpson JL, Shulman LP, et al: Transabdominal chorionic villus sampling for first-trimester prenatal diagnosis. Am J Obstet Gynecol 160:879–886, 1989.

Epstein CJ, Golbus MS: Prenatal diagnosis of genetic diseases. Am Sci 65:703, 1977.

Fielding JE: Smoking and pregnancy. N Engl J Med 298:337, 1978.

Firshein SI, Joyer LW, Lazarchick J, et al: Prenatal diagnosis of classic hemophilia. N Engl J Med 300: 937, 1979.

Gayton WF, Walker L: Down syndrome: informing the parents. Am J Dis Child 127:510, 1974.

Gelehrter TD, Collins FS: Principles of Medical Genetics. Baltimore, Williams & Wilkins, 1990.

Goad WB, Robinson A, Puck T: Incidence of aneuploidy in a human population. Am J Hum Genet 28:62, 1976.

Golbus MS: Fetal diagnosis and therapy: an update. In Fine BA, Gettig E, Greendale K, et al (eds): Strategies in genetic counseling: reproductive genetics and new technologies. The National Foundation—March of Dimes, Birth Defects Original Article Series, 26:19, 1990.

Golbus MS, Stephens JD, Mahoney MJ, et al: Failure of fetal creatine phosphokinase as a diagnostic indicator of Duchenne muscular dystrophy. N Engl J Med 300: 860, 1979.

Goldman AS:Critical periods of prenatal toxic insults. In Schwartz RH, Yaffe SJ (eds): Drug and Chemical Risks to the Fetus and Newborn. New York, Alan R Liss, 1980.

Greenberg DA, Kaback MM: Estimation of the frequency of hexosaminidase A variant alleles in the American Jewish population. Am J Hum Genet 34:444, 1982.

Gregg NM: Congenital cataract following German measles in the mother. Trans Ophthal Soc Aust 3:35, 1941.

Hagerman RJ: Fragile X syndrome. Curr Prob Pediatr 17:623–674, 1987.

Hagerman RJ, Silverman AC: Fragile X Syndrome: Diagnosis, Treatment and Research. Johns Hopkins University Press, 1991.

Hanson JW: Teratogen update: fetal hydantoin effects. Teratology 33:349–353, 1986.

Hanson JW, Streissguth AP, Smith DW: The effects of moderate alcohol consumption during pregnancy on fetal growth and morphogenesis. J Ped 92:457, 1978.

Hanson JW, Myrianthopoulos NC, Sedwick H, et al: Risks to the offspring of women treated with hydantoin anticonvulsants, with emphasis on the fetal hydantoin syndrome. J Ped 89:662, 1976.

Hassold T: Chromosome abnormalities in human reproductive wastage. Trends Genet 2:105–110, 1986.

Hassold T, Jacobs P: Trisomy in man. Annu Rev Genet 18:69–97, 1984.

Hecht T: Chromosome 18 Trisomy syndrome. In Bergsma D (ed): Birth Defects Compendium. New York, Alan R Liss, 1979.

Heinonen OP, Slone D, Shapiro S: Birth Defects and Drugs in Pregnancy. Littleton, MA, PSG Publishing, 1977.

Herbest D, Miller J: Nonspecific X-linked mental retardation: the frequency in British Columbia. Am J Med Genet 7:461, 1980.

Hook EB, Hamerton JL: The frequency of chromosome abnormalities detected in consecutive newborn studies—differences between studies—results by sex and severity of phenotypic involvement. In Hook EB, Porter IH (eds): Population Cytogenetics, Studies in Humans. New York, Academic Press, 1977.

Huisjes HS: Cytology of the amniotic fluid and its clinical applications. In Fairweather D, Eskes J (eds): Amniotic Fluid: Research and Clinical Application, 2nd ed. Amsterdam, Excerpta Medica, 1978.

Jensen M, Zahn V, Rauch A, et al: Prenatal diagnosis of beta thalassemia. Klin Wochenschr 57:37, 1979.

Jones KL, Smith DW, Ulleland N: Pattern of malformation in offspring of chronic alcoholic mothers. Lancet 1:1267, 1973.

Kan YW, Dozy AM: Polymorphism of DNA sequence adjacent to human beta-globin structural gene: relationship to sickle mutation. Proc Natl Acad Sci USA 75:5631, 1978.

Kazazian HH: Current status of prenatal diagnosis by DNA analysis. In Fine BA, Gettig E, Greendale K, et al (eds): Strategies in genetic counseling: reproductive genetics and new technologies. The National Foundation March of Dimes, Birth Defects Original Article Series, 26:210–216, 1990.

Lammer EJ, Chen DT, Hoar RM, et al: Retinoic acid embryopathy. N Engl J Med 313(14):837–841, 1985.

Lejeune J, Gautier M, Turpin R: Etude des chromosomes somatiques de neuf infants mongoliens. CR Acad Sci 248:1721, 1959.

Linden MG, Bender BG, Robinson A: Conspectus: clinical manifestations of sex chromosome anomalies. Compr Ther 16(5):3–10, 1990.

Little R: Alcohol consumption during pregnancy and decreased birth weight. Am J Pub Health 67:1154, 1977.

Lubs HA: A marker X chromosome. Am J Hum Genet 21:231, 1969.

Lyon MF: Gene action in the X-chromosome of the mouse (mus musenlus L). Nature 190:372, 1961.

MacGregor SN, Keith LG, Chasnoff IJ, et al: Cocaine use during pregnancy: adverse perinatal outcome. Am J Obstet Gynecol 157:686–690, 1987.

Matthews AL: Known fetal malformations during pregnancy: a human experience of loss. In Fine BA, Gettig E, Greendale K, et al (eds): Strategies in genetic counseling: reproductive genetics and new technologies. The National Foundation March of Dimes, Birth Defects Original Article Series, 26:168–175, 1990.

McClearn GE: Genetics and drug-related behaviors (invited theme symposium). Am J Hum Genet 31:4A, 1979.

McKusick VM: Mendelian Inheritance in Man, 9th ed. Baltimore, The Johns Hopkins University Press, 1990.

Meyer MB, Tonascia JA: Maternal smoking, pregnancy complications, and perinatal mortality. Am J Obstet Gynecol 128:494, 1977.

Moore TR, Sorg J, Miller L, et al: Hemodynamic effects

of intravenous cocaine on the pregnant ewe and fetus. Am J Obstet Gynecol 155:883–888, 1986

Nora AH, Nora JJ: A syndrome of multiple congenital anomalies associated with teratogenic exposure. Arch Environ Health 30:17, 1975.

Oakeshott P, Gillian MH: Valproate and spina bifida. BMJ 298:1300–1301, 1989.

Opitz J: Mental retardation: biologic aspects of concern to pediatricians. Ped Rev 2:41, 1980.

Palomaki GE, Haddow JE: Maternal serum AFP, age, and Down syndrome risk. Am J Obstet Gynecol 156:460, 1987.

Panny SR, Scott AF, Phillips JA: Prenatal diagnosis of sickle cell disease by restriction endonuclease analysis. Limitations and advantages. Am J Hum Genet 31:58A, 1979.

Pelz L, Götz J, Krüger G, Witt G: Increased methotrexate-induced chromosome breakage in patients with free trisomy 21 and their parents. Hum Genet 81:38, 1988.

Penrose LS, Smith GF: Down's Anomaly. Boston, Little, Brown & Co, 1966.

Phillips JA, Scott AF, Kazazian HH, et al: Prenatal diagnosis of hemoglobinopathies by restriction endonuclease analysis: pregnancies at risk for sickle cell anemia and S-OArab. Johns Hopkins Med J 145:57, 1979.

Preus M, Fraser F: Dermatoglyphics and syndromes. Am J Dis Child 124:933, 1972.

Qazi AH: Lack of evidence for craniofacial dysmorphism in perinatal human immunodeficiency virus infection. J Pediatrics 112:7–11, 1988.

Rhoads GG, Jackson LG, Schlesselman SE. The safety and efficacy of chorionic villus sampling for early prenatal diagnosis of cytogenetic abnormalities. N Engl J Med 320:609–617, 1989.

Riccardi V: The Genetic Approach to Human Disease. New York, Oxford University Press, 1977.

Richards BW: Observations on the familial appearance of diseases associated with metabolic disorders of the mother. Ann Hum Genet 39:189, 1975.

Robinson A, Puck M, Pennington B, et al: Abnormalities of the sex chromosomes: a prospective study on randomly identified newborns. In Robinson A, Lubs HA, Bergsma D (eds): Sex Chromosome Aneuploidy: Prospective Studies in Children. The National Foundation—March of Dimes, Birth Defects Original Article Series, Vol XV:203, 1979.

Rommens JM, Iannuzzi MC, Kerem BS, et al: Identification of the cystic fibrosis gene: chromosome walking and jumping. Science 245:1059–1065, 1989.

Rossett HL, Weiner L, Edelin KC: Strategies for prevention of fetal alcohol effects. Obstet Gynecol 57:1, 1981.

Rousseau F, Heitz H, Biancalana V, et al: Direct diagnosis by DNA analysis of the fragile X syndrome of mental retardation. N Engl J Med 325(24):1673–1681, 1991.

Rudd NL, Hoar DI, Martin RH, et al: Factors distinguishing couples at risk for nondisjunction. Can J Genet Cytol 26:595, 1984.

Rutherford MA, Heckmatt JZ, Dubowitz V: Congenital myotonic dystrophy: respiratory function at birth determines survival. Arch Dis Child 64(2):191–195, 1989.

Sabbagha R (NMI), Tamura RK, DalCompo S (NMI): Antenatal ultrasonic diagnosis of genetic defects: present status. Clin Obstet Gynecol 24:1103, 1981.

Satow WU, West E: Studies on Nagasaki (Japan) children exposed in utero to atomic bomb. Roentgenographic survey of skeletal system. Am J Roentgenol 74:493, 1955.

Seppala M: Fetal pathophysiology of human alpha fetoprotein. Ann NY Acad Sci 259:59, 1975.

Seppala M, Unnerus H: Elevated amniotic fluid alpha fetoprotein in fetal hydrocephalus. Am J Obstet Gynecol 119:270, 1974.

Serville F, Carles D, Guibaud S, Dally D: Fetal valproate phenotype is recognizable by mid pregnancy. Letter to the J Med Genet 26:348, 1989.

Smith DW: Alcohol effects on the fetus. In Schwarz RH, Yaffe SJ (eds): Drug and Chemical Risks to the Fetus and Newborn. New York, Alan R Liss, 1980, p 73.

Smith DW: Teratogenicity of anticonvulsive medications. Am J Dis Child 131:1337, 1977.

Stene J, Fischer G, Stene E, et al: Paternal age effect in Down's syndrome. Ann Hum Genet 40:299, 1977.

Stewart A, Kneale GW: Radiation dose effects in relation to obstetric X-rays and childhood cancers. Lancet 1:1185, 1970.

Swartz HM, Reichling BA: Hazards of radiation exposure for pregnant women. JAMA 239:1907, 1978.

Taylor GI: Autosomal trisomy syndrome: a detailed study of 27 cases of Edwards' syndrome and 27 cases of Patau's syndrome. J Med Genet 5:227, 1968.

Teratology Society Position Paper: Recommendations for vitamin A use during pregnancy. Teratology 35:269–275, 1987.

Thayer B, Braddock B, Spitzer K, Miller W: Clinical and laboratory experience with early amniocentesis. In Fine BA, Gettig E, Greendale K, et al (eds): Strategies in genetic counseling: reproductive genetics and new technologies. The National Foundation—March of Dimes, Birth Defects Original Article Series, 26:58, 1990.

Thomas RL, Blakemore KJ: Evaluation of elevations in maternal serum alpha fetoprotein: a review. Obstet Gynecol Survey, 45(5):269–283, 1990.

Thompson ML, McInnes RP, Willard HF: Thompson and Thompson's Genetics in Medicine, 5th ed. Philadelphia, WB Saunders Co, 1991.

Tjio J, Levan A: The chromosome number in man. Hereditas 42:1, 1956.

Uchida JA: Maternal radiation and trisomy 21. In Hook EB, Porter IA (eds): Population Genetics: Studies in Humans. New York, Academic Press, 1977.

Van Allen MI: Fetal vascular disruption: mechanisms and some resulting birth defects. Pediatr Annals 10(6):31–50, 1981.

Wald NJ, Cuckle HS, Densem JW, et al: Maternal serum screening for Down's syndrome in early pregnancy. Br Med J 297:883–887, 1988.

Ward BE, Henry GP, Robinson A: Cytogenetic studies in 100 couples with recurrent spontaneous abortions. Am J Hum Genet 32:549, 1980.

Warkany J: Congenital Malformations. Chicago, Year Book Medical Publishers, Inc, 1971.

Watson JD, Ward BE, Mosher G, et al: Evaluation of 175 couples with reproductive failure. Am J Hum Genet 33:39A, 1981.

White TJ, Arnheim N, Erlich HA: The polymerase chain reaction. Trends Genet 5:185–189, 1989.

Wilson JG: Environment and Birth Defects. New York, Academic Press, 1973.

Wood RW: Delayed radiation effects in atomic bomb survivors. Science 166:569, 1969.

# CHAPTER 33

• • • • • • • • • • • • • • • • • • • • • • • • • • • • •

# Parent Counseling

John H. Kennell and Marshall H. Klaus

More than two decades ago, a study of the mother-infant bond began, when nurses and physicians in intensive care nurseries observed that sometimes, after extraordinary efforts had been taken to save small premature infants, the infants would return to emergency rooms injured by their parents even though they had been sent home intact and thriving. This chapter reviews recent human attachment studies and applies their findings to the care of the parents of a premature infant, a malformed infant, a stillborn child, or a neonate who has died.

A mother's and father's actions and responses toward their infant are derived from a complex combination of their own genetic endowment; the way the baby responds to them; a long history of interpersonal relations with their own families and each other; past experiences with previous pregnancies; the absorption of the practices and values of their cultures; and, probably most important, how each was raised by his or her own parents. The mothering or fathering behavior of each woman and man, their ability to tolerate stresses, and their need for special attention differ greatly and depend on a mixture of these factors.

The actual process of parent-to-infant attachment, or bond formation, is not yet completely understood, but a diversity of observations are beginning to make it possible to piece together some of the various phases. The time periods that are apparently crucial for this process are shown in Table 33–1.

Many mothers are initially disturbed by feelings of grief and anger when they become pregnant because of factors ranging from economic and housing hardships to intraper-

sonal difficulties. However, by the end of the first trimester, the majority of women who initially rejected pregnancy have accepted it. This initial stage, as outlined by Bibring and associates (1959, 1961), is the mother's identification of the growing fetus as an integral part of herself.

The second stage is a growing perception of the fetus as a separate individual, usually occurring with the awareness of fetal movement. After quickening, a woman generally begins to have some fantasies about what the baby may be like, attributes to the infant some human personality characteristics, and develops a sense of attachment and value toward the baby. At this time, further acceptance of the pregnancy and marked changes in attitude toward the fetus may be observed. Unplanned, unwanted infants may now seem more acceptable. With the frequent use of ultrasound for high-risk patients, it is apparent that visualization of a moving fetus has an accelerating effect on the attachment process for both father and mother. Objectively, the health care worker usually finds some outward evidence of the mother's prep-

**Table 33–1**
STEPS IN ATTACHMENT

Planning the pregnancy
Confirming the pregnancy
Accepting the pregnancy
Fetal movement
(Observation by ultrasound)
Accepting the fetus as an individual
Birth
Touching and smelling the baby
Hearing and seeing the baby
Caretaking

aration by such actions as the purchase of clothes or a crib, the selection of a name, and the arrangement of space for the baby.

# Parenting Considerations in High-Risk Antepartum Care

## ASSESSMENT AND COUNSELING

We have found it useful to pick out in advance the mother who is most likely to have special difficulties in relating to her infant. Blau and colleagues (1963) noted that mothers who deliver premature infants have more negative attitudes toward their pregnancies, greater emotional immaturity, and more body narcissism. Cohen (1966) emphasizes that after the first trimester, behaviors that suggest rejection of pregnancy include (1) a preoccupation with physical appearance, (2) excessive emotional withdrawal or mood swings, (3) excessive physical complaints, (4) absence of any response to quickening, and (5) lack of any preparation for the baby during the last trimester. In our experience, mothers who have a high incidence of severe mothering difficulties often have one of the following characteristics:

1. The previous loss of a newborn infant, including miscarriage and induced abortion;
2. A fertility problem, with no living children;
3. A previous seriously ill newborn infant;
4. Primiparity, if younger than 17 or older than 38 years;
5. A medical problem with which the infant may be affected, such as Rh disease, toxemia, or diabetes; and
6. The unmarried mother and the mother without social support.

Certain management principles for obstetric and pediatric health care professionals apply to all these situations.

1. In almost all high-risk situations, the odds are heavily in favor of the birth of a live baby who will ultimately be healthy and normal, so it is reasonable to stress the positive and be optimistic. This is essential for the mother's later relationship with her baby, which is, in turn, extremely important for the infant's development. After a physician reads the literature or a physician's report about a woman's new or rare condition, it is tempting to tell her about the problems and pitfalls that may develop. But this may only make the course of the pregnancy more turbulent for the mother and the obstetrician. Mentioning the possibility of a symptom or complication is comparable to telling the young boy just starting to ride a bicycle that there is one big tree in the middle of the playground.

2. The obstetric team should include the pediatric team early and continue to involve them in decisions and plans for the management of the mother and baby. "After the fact" recriminations are almost eliminated when everyone is involved in the ongoing decision-making.

3. Prepare the mother for the anticipated aspects of care for her newborn.

4. Cohen (1966) suggests that the following questions be asked to learn the special needs of each mother:

   a. How long have you lived in this immediate area, and where does most of your family live?
   b. How often do you see your mother or other close relatives?
   c. Has anything happened to you in the past (or do you currently have any condition) that causes you to worry about the pregnancy or the baby?
   d. What was your husband's (partner's) reaction to your pregnancy?
   e. What other responsibilities do you have outside the family?

It is wise to inquire about how the pregnant woman was mothered. Did she have a neglected and deprived infancy and childhood, or did she grow up with a warm and intact family life? There is evidence that the loss of a parent in the first 11 years of life is a major psychologic risk factor for new fathers and mothers; therefore, information about the health of the parents' parents can be valuable (Brown and Harris, 1978).

## PRENATAL HOSPITALIZATION

With the advances in high-risk perinatal care, the benefits of prenatal hospitalization for selected patients are established. The fetus can gain significant medical advantages from this sophisticated hospital care. The nurses and physicians working in high-risk prenatal units are aware of the upsetting emotional effects on pregnant women when they are hospitalized for periods of a month or more for the management of medical problems such as hypertension, diabetes, premature labor, or a slow-growing fetus. Investigations by Merkatz (1978) disclosed that mothers who had prolonged antenatal hospitalization were principally concerned about the baby they were carrying and only secondarily concerned about their own medical condition. She reported the great loneliness of these women, their fears about the baby, and their reactions to separation from home and family. Merkatz stressed the need for unlimited visits for the hospitalized woman by her husband or boyfriend, children, and parents. She noted that families need privacy and unrestricted time together so that family members can assist each other to cope with fear, uncertainty, and anxiety. To encourage strong family support requires changes in visiting policies for young siblings-to-be, extra beds for fathers-to-be so that they can stay overnight with their wives, special dining rooms for the family to eat together, and other alterations to make the hospital more like a home. On a number of occasions, women who had prolonged prenatal hospitalization mentioned how everybody seemed interested in the high-risk pregnancy but not in them as a person or the baby as an individual. Individualized care plans worked out with the women are necessary because of their highly individualized response to the high-risk pregnancy and hospitalization.

## CONTINUITY OF PERINATAL CARE

It is only during this century that the change was made from a system in which there was one continuous caretaker, the family doctor or midwife, who was available to the mother during her pregnancy, labor, and birth and who provided the care for both the mother and baby during the postpartum period. Observations by Larson (1980) reveal a significant change in the mother's ability to parent if a home health caretaker, such as a visiting nurse, made contact with the mother before birth and 48 hours after the birth rather than starting 6 weeks after delivery. This suggests that interventions in the perinatal period should begin during the pregnancy rather than after the mother has

taken her baby home. The study gives added impetus for family physicians; pediatric, obstetric, and public health nurses; and pediatricians to arrange visits to meet and talk with the mother during the pregnancy.

## FAMILY-CENTERED CESAREAN CHILDBIRTH

The National Institutes of Health Consensus Development Conference on Cesarean Childbirth (1980) emphasized the importance of the father's presence at a cesarean birth. There has been no evidence of harm to mother, neonate, or father when family-centered maternity care has been extended to the cesarean birth family. The presence of fathers in the operating room and closer contact between mother and neonate appeared to improve all postcesarean behavioral responses of the families. Greater involvement of fathers with their infants has been a consistent finding in studies of postcesarean birth families.

The mother who has had a cesarean birth may be somewhat passive and dependent in her early postpartum period. Most of her focus is on her own needs. Therefore, the nurse should be respectful and understanding of this and bring the baby to the mother when she is comfortable. Rooming-in beginning as soon after delivery as possible should be encouraged. There is an important role for the father or other family member, that is, to be present during the day and evening to bring the baby from the bedside crib to the mother for feedings or holding. Frequent, early breastfeedings enhance the milk output and the chances of success. If the baby cannot come out of the nursery to visit with the mother, pictures should be provided to the mother. As soon as the mother becomes more comfortable, she should be assisted to the nursery (sometimes this may necessitate a wheelchair). Some mothers have even been taken on a stretcher if space permits and the condition of the fetus is critical. As the mother is more able to care for herself and her baby, rooming-in can then be made available to her.

During this time of separation, the father may become fatigued and frustrated as he tries to divide his time between the mother and the infant. He, too, needs support from the nursing staff during this difficult period.

# Parenting Considerations in Normal and High-Risk Intrapartum Care

1. The less anxiety the mother experiences during labor and delivery, the better will be her immediate relationship with her baby. Therefore, she and her husband should visit the maternity unit to see where labor and delivery will take place. She should also learn about the anesthetic (if she is to receive one), delivery routines, and all the procedures and medication she will receive before, during, and after delivery. By reducing the possibility of surprise, such advance preparation will increase confidence during labor and delivery. The better the father is prepared, the more supportive he can be. As for a child entering the hospital for surgery, the more meticulously every step and event are detailed in advance for an adult, the less the subsequent anxiety.

2. The mother must have continuous support during her labor and delivery. Three randomized trials involving nearly 1200 women have demonstrated the clinical importance of continuous emotional support by a woman (doula) companion during labor and delivery (Kennell et al, 1991; Klaus et al, 1986; Sosa et al, 1980). In a recent study in the United States, primiparous women supported continuously by a doula had fewer cesarean deliveries (18 percent versus 8 percent), shorter labors, and less use of pitocin (17 percent versus 44 percent) and epidural anesthesia (18 percent versus 55 percent) compared with mothers who did not have continuous support (Kennell et al, 1991). In another study, mothers with a supportive companion were more likely to remain awake and had more affectionate interactions, talking to, smiling at, and stroking their newborn infants more often than in a control group of mothers in the first 25 minutes after leaving the delivery room (Sosa et al, 1980). A recently reported study from South Africa showed that mothers supported by a doula were less anxious and reported less postpartum depression, and were more likely to be breastfeeding exclusively at 6 weeks (51 percent versus 29 percent), to believe they had coped well during labor, and to have more confidence in adapting to parenthood (Hofmeyr et al, 1991). Fathers are present with mothers during labor for about 80 percent of deliveries in the United States. When questioned, both fathers and mothers say it is important for the father to be present and report the support provided to a couple by a doula through labor and delivery to be extremely valuable (Bertsch et al, 1990). Doulas are present during an increasing number of labors, to support mothers, couples, and sometimes family members.

3. The mother also must be satisfied with the arrangements that have been made to maintain her home during her hospitalization. This gives her freedom to concentrate on the needs of the baby and to enjoy her family in the process. It relieves the pressure on the father so that he can reserve his energies for the family.

4. In an effort to reduce the amount of tension on the mother, she should labor and deliver in the same room, preventing the need to rush to a delivery room in the last minutes of labor. In some hospitals, this option is available not only to low-risk mothers but also to high-risk mothers. Once the delivery is completed and the mother has had a quick glance at the infant, it is important for her to have a few seconds to regain her composure before she proceeds to the next task— taking on the infant. It has been our experience that it is best not to give a mother her baby until she indicates that she is ready to take it on. It should be her decision. However, once she makes this decision, the health care team should make every effort to facilitate her decision.

5. In many hospitals, it is customary to put the baby on the mother's chest for 1 or 2 minutes shortly after delivery. This is helpful, but the lack of privacy, the narrow table, and the short time period do not allow sufficient opportunity for the mother to touch and explore the baby. Although it is a reasonable procedure, it is not sufficient to optimize maternal attachment.

6. After delivery, it is extremely helpful for the father, mother, and baby to have a period alone in either the delivery room or an adjacent room (labor or recovery room). Obviously, this is possible only if the infant is normal and the mother is well. The mother should have the infant with her on the bed so she can hold him or her—the infant should not be off in a bassinet where she can only see his or her face (Fig. 33–1). She should be given the baby nude and allowed to examine him or her completely. We have found it valuable to encourage the mother to move

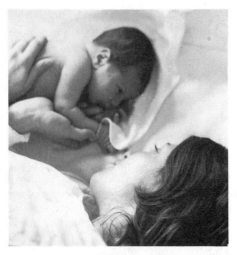

**Figure 33–1.** Mother receiving infant in the first minutes of life. (From Klaus MH and Fanaroff AA: Care of the High Risk Neonate, 2nd ed. Philadelphia, WB Saunders Co, 1979.)

over in her regular hospital bed so that she only takes up about half of it, leaving the other half for her partially dressed or nude infant. A heat panel easily maintains or, if need be, increases the body temperature of the infant. Several mothers have told us of the unforgettable experience of holding their nude baby against their own bare chest. The father may also participate in this skin-to-skin contact with his infant. This allows both parents to become acquainted with their new baby. Because the eyes are so important for both the parents and baby, we withhold the ocular application of silver nitrate ($AgNO_3$) or other ophthalmic prophylaxis until after this rendezvous. (Many hospitals now apply an antibiotic ointment, which is not as irritating to the infant's eyes.)

7. We have found it valuable for the mother, father, and infant to be together for at least 1 hour. After 30 to 45 minutes, the mother and baby often fall asleep. Usually, the mother and father never forget this shared experience. It helps some parents to begin to attach to their infant. We emphasize that this should be a private session. Keep in mind that some parents take days to fall in love with their infant and that this gradual process is entirely normal.

Affectional bonds develop further in the succeeding days and weeks through continued close association of baby and mother, particularly when she cares for him. Close contact with her husband and other children also is obviously important. Based on what parents have told us and our own observations, we believe that every parent has a task to perform during the postpartum period. In particular, the mother must look at and take in her real, live infant and then synchronize or reconcile the fantasized image of the infant she anticipated with the one she actually delivered (Figure 33–2). Many cultures recognize the need for this by providing the mother with a doula, or aunt, who relieves the mother of her other responsibilities so she can devote herself completely to this task.

At the present time, the period in the hospital for most mothers and babies in the United States has been greatly abbreviated to a stay of a few hours to 2 days for mothers who deliver vaginally, and about 3 to 4 days for mothers who have a cesarean delivery. This results in a rushed experience, with little time for the mother to interact with and get to know her new baby. This makes it crucial to stress to the family the importance of providing food, support and protection for the mother and infant in the first days at home so that the mother can have long periods of protected time to observe and fall in love with her baby. This protection and support of the mother-infant dyad in the first days and weeks is a standard cultural practice in 183 of 186 representative nonindustrialized societies, and is provided in most industrialized nations by parental leave and measures such as daily visits by health visitors, home help, and more availability of extended family members. In the United States, the burden of this protection and nurturing often falls on the father. If he can handle the telephone calls, answer the door, manage the household chores, and restrict visiting to a minimum for the first 4 weeks, the mother can then have the protected and relaxed time to interact with her baby, start the attachment process, and establish her breastfeeding schedule. For mothers without this support, the nursing, social service, and medical staffs should mobilize this assistance by calling on other family members or community services, such as the Visiting Nurse Association.

8. If the baby must be moved to a hospital with an intensive care unit, we find it helpful to give the mother a chance to see, touch, and if possible, hold her infant, even if the baby has respiratory distress, is in an oxygen hood, and is being ventilated. The health

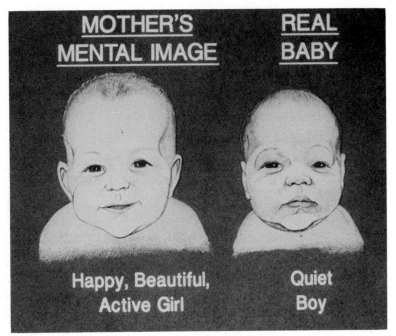

**Figure 33–2.** The mother's mental image of her baby during pregnancy is always different from the baby she delivers. (From Klaus MH and Fanaroff AA: Care of the High Risk Neonate, 3rd ed. Philadelphia, WB Saunders Co, 1986.)

care provider stops in the mother's room with the transport incubator and encourages her to touch her baby and look at him or her at close range. A comment about the baby's strength and healthy features may be long remembered and appreciated. A picture of the infant given to the mother can help her remember her baby until she can see him again.

9. We encourage the father to follow the transport team to our hospital so he can see what is happening with his baby. He uses his own transportation so that he can stay in the premature unit for 3 to 4 hours. This extra time allows him to find out how the infant is being managed, to get to know the nurses and physicians in the unit, and to talk with them about what will happen to the baby in the succeeding days. We allow him to come into the nursery and explain in detail everything that is going on. We ask him to help act as a link between us and his family by carrying information back to his wife and request that he come to our unit before he visits his wife so that he can let her know how the baby is doing. We suggest that he take a Polaroid picture, even if the infant is on a respirator, so that he can show and describe to his wife in detail how the baby is being cared for. Mothers often tell us how valuable the picture is in keeping some contact with their infant, even while physically separated.

## Parenting Considerations in High-Risk Postpartum Care

During the past several years, many changes have been made in the physical arrangements for mothers and obstetricians' approach to them. If the mother has not yet visited her baby, we find it best to describe what the infant looks like and how the infant will appear to her physically. We do not talk about chances or survival rates or percentages but stress that most babies survive in spite of early and often worrisome problems. We do not emphasize problems that may occur in the future. We do try to anticipate common developments (e.g., the need for bilirubin reduction lights for jaundice in small premature infants). The following guidelines may be helpful.

1. A mother's room arrangements should be adjusted to her individual needs. Mothers are often best able to express themselves and work out their problems when they are alone, but some need companionship during this stressful period.

2. If at all possible, mother and infant should be kept near each other in the same hospital, ideally on the same floor.

3. It is useful to talk with the mother and father together whenever possible. When

this is not possible, it is often wise to talk with one parent on the phone in the presence of the other. At least once a day, we discuss with the parents how the child is doing; we talk with them at least twice a day if the child is critically ill. It is necessary to find out what the mother believes is going to happen or what she has read about the problem. We move at her pace during any discussion.

4. It is highly desirable for one professional (primary nurse or physician) to do most of the communicating with the family about the medical problem and the infant's progress. When more than one member of the hospital staff speaks with the parents, the parents often go on a stressful roller-coaster ride from optimism to pessimism as they receive varying information about the baby's problems and possible complications and interventions. Thus, it is best for one individual to collect and synthesize the varied opinions of the members of the health care team and speak with one consistent voice.

5. The health care team should not relieve their own anxieties by adding their worries to those of the parents. If there is a possibility, for example, that the child has Turner's syndrome, it is not necessary to share this with the parents while the infant is still acutely ill with other problems and while affectional bonds are still weak. If the health care professionals are worried about a slightly high bilirubin level, it is not necessary to discuss kernicterus.

6. Before the mother comes to the neonatal unit, the nurse or physician should describe in detail what she will see. When she makes her first visit, it is important to anticipate that she may become distressed when she looks at her infant. We always have a stool nearby so that she can sit down, and a nurse stays at her side during most of the visit, describing in detail the procedures being carried out, such as the monitoring of respiration and heart rate.

7. The nurse should go into some detail in describing all the equipment surrounding the infant and should be nearby to answer questions and give support during the difficult period when the mother is first seeing her infant.

8. It is important to remember that feelings of love for the baby are often elicited through contact. Therefore, we turn off the lights and remove the eye patches from an infant under bilirubin lights so that the mother and infant can see each other. Phototherapy blankets are very helpful. Because they wrap around the infant, the parents can hold the baby while phototherapy is continued. An additional advantage is that eye pads are not necessary and, therefore, eye-to-eye contact is not interrupted.

9. Extended visiting or rooming-in for the mother of a normal full-term infant around the clock or throughout the day and evening, when the mother is able to handle and completely care for her infant, has been found to be a useful practice. This also pertains to the mother of a high-risk infant. In almost all intensive care units, visiting hours for parents and grandparents are unlimited. As soon as possible, we describe to both the father and mother the value of touching the infant in helping them get to know him or her, reducing the number of apneic episodes (if this is a problem), increasing weight gain, and hastening the infant's discharge from the unit. This encourages them to visit the baby frequently for extended periods.

10. An innovative model of care for preterm infants and their parents is provided at the Ramon Sarda Mother and Infant Hospital in Buenos Aires (Kennell and Klaus, 1988). This public hospital for low socioeconomic–level families has a remarkably warm, supportive environment for parents and a dormitory residence for mothers who live-in, breastfeed, and provide the care for their preterm infants throughout their hospital stay. The objectives of this program are to strengthen the emotional ties between mother and infant, enhance breastfeeding, and develop maternal abilities by learning through experience, by sharing ideas, and by imitation within the group of resident mothers. If this model were applied in the United States, it would be expected to be of most benefit to those mothers who visit their premature infants least and who have the greatest need for strong emotional ties to their infants and guidance in mothering. The individualized evaluation and the preparation of an environmental care plan for every low-birth-weight infant has been reported (Als et al, 1986) to improve the outcome and shorten the hospital stay. This approach involves parents in observing their infant closely and then participating in decision-making. This should enhance the parents' involvement and participation with their infant.

11. The nursery should keep a record of all

phone calls and visits by parents. Our data reveal that when there are fewer than three phone calls or visits in a 2-week period, there is a high incidence of subsequent severe mothering disorders, such as failure-to-thrive, battering, or giving up the baby. This may vary with different units. Therefore, if the visiting pattern of the mother is less than that of most mothers, the mother is given extra help in adapting to the hospitalization. In the last decade, when a mother did not visit her infant frequently, this was a warning that the woman was likely to have problems with chemical abuse, usually of crack cocaine. Therefore, even more so than in the past, an irregular, infrequent, or absent visiting pattern is an important indicator that the baby may be abandoned in the hospital or seriously neglected or abused if discharged home. As a consequence, this type of pattern requires careful investigation of the mother's situation as soon as possible.

12. Clinical observations and studies suggest that prolonged antepartum hospitalization may interfere with the mother's bonding to her new baby. Some of these mothers have indicated a need to go home and be with their family and their other children. It is important to respect this need, which arises from a stressful separation and isolation. It is a reminder of the value of open visiting by the family during the mother's hospitalization. Keeping in mind the mother's emotional turmoil during this stressful period, and to provide follow-up care at the home when it might be necessary, health care professionals may find it helpful to encourage these mothers to visit and to go out of their way to call to keep them informed about the baby's progress.

13. To help the family during the infant's hospitalization, there must be a good working relationship among the health care professionals. Meetings with the nursery staff in the intensive care unit should be held every 2 weeks. This provides an opportunity for members of the team to express their concerns about a father's and mother's behavior and to work out a plan to assist them.

14. It may be possible to enhance normal attachment behavior in the mother several days or weeks following birth by permitting a special short nesting period of 3 or more days of close physical contact with privacy and virtual isolation during which the mother provides complete care for her small infant, with help and nursing support

readily available nearby. Early discharge combined with a period of isolated physical contact with caretaking may help to normalize mothering behavior for infants discharged from intensive care nurseries.

15. Communicate with the mother about her condition and the baby's condition. This is important before, during, and after the birth. At times, this communication is brief and incomplete, but it is essential. For example, when there is evidence of fetal distress, the mother can be told, "We have evidence that your baby should be delivered quickly, so we are proceeding with this, and we will need your full cooperation." Or, when a baby shows stress or fails to breathe after birth, the parents can be told, "The baby has a problem. We will be working with the baby and will let you know more about this just as soon as we can."

Clinically, we have been impressed and disturbed by the devastating and lasting untoward effects on the mothering capacity of women who have been frightened by the physician's pessimistic outlook about the chances of survival and normal development of an infant. For example, when a 3-lb premature baby is doing well but the mother is told that there is a reasonable chance that the baby may not survive, the mother will often show evidence of mourning (as if the baby were already dead) and reluctance to become attached to her baby. We have repeatedly observed that such mothers may refuse to visit or will show great hesitation about any physical contact.

When discussing such a situation with a physician who has spoken pessimistically with the mother, we have often been told that it is important to share all worries with a mother so that she will be prepared in case of a bad outcome. If there is a close and firm bond between the mother and infant (which occurs after an infant has been home for several months) there may be no reason for the physician to withhold concern. However, while the ties of affection are still forming, they can be easily retarded, altered, or permanently damaged. It is not easy to keep from sharing all the possible or potential problems with a mother, but with the evidence available at present, it is our conviction that health care personnel should do their best to hold back. This does not mean that they should be untruthful, because parents quickly sense their true feelings. They must base their statements on the present situation (infant mortality rates in low-birth-weight nurseries have decreased steadily year by year), not on yesterday's high mortality figures. Today, many extremely immature babies live and are normal.

# Caring for Parents of Infants with Congenital Malformations

## PARENTAL REACTIONS AND ADAPTATIONS TO THE MALFORMED INFANT

The birth of an infant with a congenital malformation presents complex challenges to the health care providers who will care for the affected child and the family (Johns, 1971). Despite the relatively large number of infants with congenital anomalies, our understanding of how parents develop an attachment to a malformed child remains incomplete. Although previous investigators agree that the child's birth often precipitates major family stress, relatively few have described the process of family adaptation during the infant's first year of life (Hare et al, 1966; Johns, 1971; Roskies, 1972). Solnit and Stark's (1961) conceptualization of parental

reactions emphasized that a significant aspect of adaptation is that parents must mourn the loss of the normal child they had expected. Other observers have noted pathologic aspects of family reactions, including the chronic sorrow that envelops the family of a defective child (Olshansky, 1962; Zuk, 1959). Less attention has been given to the more adaptive aspects of parental attachment to children with malformations.

Parental reactions to the birth of a child with a congenital malformation appear to follow a predictable course. For most parents, initial shock, disbelief, and a period of intense emotional upset (including sadness, anger, and anxiety) are followed by a period of gradual adaptation, which is marked by a lessening of intense anxiety and emotional reaction (Fig. 33–3). This adaptation is characterized by an increased satisfaction with and ability to care for the baby. These stages in parental reactions are similar to those reported in other crisis situations, such as those involving terminally ill children. The shock, disbelief, and denial reported by many parents seem to be an understandable attempt to escape the traumatic news of the baby's malformation, news so at variance with their expectations that it is impossible for it to register except gradually.

The intense emotional turmoil described by parents who have produced a child with a congenital malformation corresponds to a period of crisis (defined as "upset in a state of equilibrium caused by a hazardous event

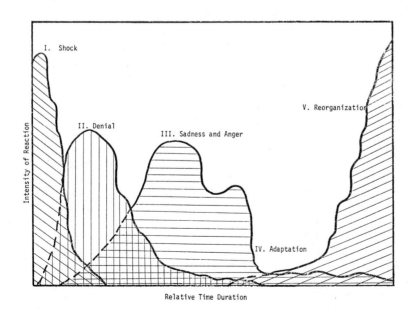

**Figure 33–3.** Hypothetical model of a normal sequence of parental reactions to the birth of a malformed infant. (Adapted from Drotar D, Baskiewicz A, Irwin N, Kennell J, and Klaus M: Pediatrics 56:710–715, 1975. Copyright American Academy of Pediatrics 1975. Reproduced by permission of Pediatrics.)

which creates a threat, a loss, or a challenge for the individual") (Bloom, 1963; Rappoport, 1965). A crisis consists of a period of impact, a rise in tension associated with stress, and finally, a return to equilibrium. During such crisis periods, a person is, at least temporarily, unable to respond with his or her usual problem-solving capabilities. Roskies (1972) noted a similar "birth crisis" in her observations of mothers of children with birth defects caused by thalidomide.

Solnit and Stark (1961) have likened the crisis of the birth of a child with a malformation to the emotional crisis following the death of a child, in that the mother must mourn the loss of her expected normal infant. In addition, she must become attached to her actual living, damaged child (Figure 33–4). However, the sequence of parental reactions to the birth of a baby with a malformation differs from that following the death of a child in another respect. Because of the complex issues raised by the continuation of the child's life and the demands of his or her physical care, the parents' sadness, which is initially important in their relationships with the child, diminishes in most instances once they take over the physical care. Parents reach a point at which they are able to adequately care for their child and effectively cope with disrupting feelings of sadness and anger.

The mother's initiation of the relationship with her child is a major step in reducing the anxiety and emotional upset associated with the trauma of the birth. As with normal children, the parents' caretaking experience with their infant seems to release positive feelings, which aid the mother-child relationship following the stresses associated with the news of the child's anomaly and, in many instances, the separation of mother and child in the hospital (Zuk, 1959). Lampe and coworkers (1977) noted significantly greater hospital visiting by the parents if an infant with an abnormality had been at home for a short while.

## PRACTICAL SUGGESTIONS FOR FACILITATING PARENTAL ATTACHMENTS TO THE MALFORMED INFANT

1. We have come to believe that, if medically feasible, it is better to leave the infant with the mother for the first 2 to 3 days or discharge the baby home. If the child is rushed to the hospital where special surgery will eventually be performed, the mother will not have enough opportunity to become attached to him or her. Even if immediate surgery is necessary, as in the case of bowel obstruction, it is best to bring the baby to the mother first, allow her to touch and handle him, and point out to her how normal he or she is in all other respects.

2. The parents' mental picture of the anomaly often may be far more alarming than the actual problem. Any delay in seeing the child greatly heightens their anxiety and causes their imaginations to run wild. Therefore, we suggest that it is helpful to bring the baby to both parents when they are together as soon after delivery as possible.

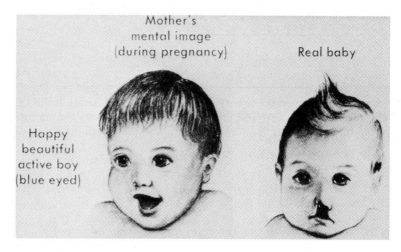

**Figure 33–4.** The major change in mental image that the mother of a malformed baby must make following delivery. The mental portrait of the expected perfect baby must be changed to that of the baby with an abnormality. (From Klaus MH and Fanaroff AA: Care of the High Risk Neonate, 3rd ed. Philadelphia, WB Saunders Co, 1986.)

Mother's mental image (during pregnancy)

Real baby

Happy beautiful active boy (blue eyed)

3. We believe that parents should not be given tranquilizers, which tend to blunt their responses and slow their adaptation to the problem. However, a sedative at night is sometimes helpful.

4. Parents who are adapting reasonably well often ask many questions and, indeed, at times appear to be almost overinvolved in clinical care. We are pleased by this and are more concerned about the parents who ask few questions, who appear stunned or overwhelmed by the problem, or who withdraw and visit infrequently. Parents who become involved in trying to find out what the best procedures are and who ask many questions about care are sometimes annoying but often make the best adaptation in the end.

5. Many anomalies are very frustrating to the physicians and nurses as well. There is a temptation for them to withdraw from the parents who ask many questions and then appear to forget and ask the same questions over and over.

6. We have found it best to move at the parents' pace. If we move too quickly, we run the risk of losing the parents along the way. It is beneficial to ask the parents how they view their infant.

7. Each parent may move through the sequence of shock, denial, anger, guilt, and adaptation at a different pace. If they are unable to talk with each other about the baby, their own relationship may be disrupted. Therefore, we use early crisis intervention and meet several times with the parents. During these discussions, we ask the mother how she is doing, how she feels her husband is doing, and how he feels about the infant. We then reverse the questions and ask the father how he is doing and how he thinks his wife is progressing. The hope is that they not only will think about their own reactions but will begin to consider each other's as well.

## Summary of Care for Parents of Preterm, Sick, or Malformed Infants

1. When an infant weighs between 3 and 5 lb and appears to be doing well without grunting and retractions, we have found it useful and safe for the mother to have the baby placed in her bed for 20 to 30 minutes in the first hours of life with a heat panel above both of them. We do not recommend this unless the physician feels relaxed and sure about the infant's health.

2. When the long-term significance of early mother-infant contact is kept in mind, a modification of restrictions and territorial traditions usually can be arranged so that a mother and her infant can be kept near each other in the same hospital. It is helpful if the mother can have some private sessions with her infant in a separate room close to the unit.

3. Transporting the mother and baby together to the medical center that contains the intensive care nursery, either before or after delivery, should be encouraged for its immediate and long-term benefits.

4. The intensive care nursery should be open for parental visiting 24 hours a day and should have flexible rules about visits from others such as grandparents, supportive relatives and, on certain occasions, siblings. Provided proper precautions are taken, infections will not be a problem.

5. A mother should be permitted to enter the premature nursery as soon as she is able to maneuver easily.

6. We also encourage grandparents, brothers, sisters, and other relatives to view the infant through the glass window of the nursery so that they will begin to feel attached to the infant.

7. If there is any chance that the infant will survive, we are optimistic in our talks with the parents from the beginning. There is no evidence that if a favorable prediction proves to be incorrect and the baby dies, the parents will be harmed by the early optimism. There is almost always time to prepare them before the baby actually dies. If the infant lives and the spokesperson for the health care team has been pessimistic, it is almost impossible for parents to become closely attached after they have figuratively dug a few shovelfuls of earth. We recognize that this recommendation is contrary to many old customs and places a heavy burden on the primary professional. It is our belief that if the infant does die, we must still work with the parents and help them with the mourning period.

8. Once the possibility that a baby has brain damage has been mentioned, the parents will not forget it. Therefore, unless we are 100 percent sure that the baby is dam-

aged, we do not mention the possibility of any brain damage or retardation to the parents. On many occasions we have cared for neonates who have appeared to be brain damaged but who later were perfectly normal.

9. It is important to emphasize that if we have a clear objective finding, such as a cardiac abnormality or a specific congenital malformation, we see no reason to hide this from the parents. We would never lie to a parent.

10. We should continue to study interventions such as rooming-in, nesting, the Sarda dormitory residence (in Argentina), and kangaroo baby carrying (Whitelaw, 1990), as well as transporting a healthy premature infant to be with his or her mother. It is necessary to try out these various interventions in different hospital settings and evaluate their ability to reduce the severe anxiety that many parents presently face during the prolonged hospitalization and the early days following discharge.

11. In all these interventions, it is critical that nurses take mothers under their wings, especially supporting and encouraging them during these early days and weeks. The nurse's guidance in helping a mother with simple caretaking tasks can be extremely valuable in helping to overcome some of her anxiety. In this sense, the nurse assumes the role of the mother's own mother and contributes much more than merely teaching her basic caretaking techniques. Praise for what the mother notes or does for her baby (if appropriate), asking the mother for her ideas and suggestions, and encouraging her to perform caretaking tasks with her baby can enhance the mother's self-esteem and affection for her baby.

12. It is necessary to identify high-risk parents who are having special difficulties in adapting so that interventions can begin early. These parents often visit rarely and for short periods, appear frightened, and usually do not ask the medical staff questions about the infant's problems. Sometimes, these mothers and fathers are hostile or irritable and show inappropriately low levels of anxiety.

13. As we develop a further understanding of the process by which normal mothers and infants interact with each other during the first months and the first year of life, it appears that recommendations for stimulation may be detrimental to normal develop-ment, at least at certain ages. Rather than suggesting stimulation, it may be important for a mother to naturally and unconsciously use imitation to learn about and find her own infant. The timing and appropriateness of this recommendation for different infants and mothers requires further study.

14. Many infants weighing from 4 to 5 lb who were previously separated from their mothers immediately after birth and admitted to neonatal intensive care units can now be kept safely with their mothers on postpartum divisions. This requires special training for the nurses but proves to be popular with nurses and mothers (Whitby et al, 1982).

It is probable that in the future several of these interventions will be combined so that a mother may have early postdelivery contact with her premature infant, if it is healthy, then have the baby stay with her on the postpartum division or, if smaller or sicker, brought to her bedside in the maternity unit from the neonatal intensive care unit on several occasions early in the course of the infant's stay in the hospital and then, before early discharge, live in and nest with the mother for 3 or 4 days.

# References

Als H, Lawhon G, Brown E, et al: Individual behavioral and environmental care of very low birthweight infants at risk for broncho-pulmonary dysplasia: neonatal intensive care and developmental outcome. Pediatrics 78:1123–1132, 1986.

Bertsch T, Nagashima-Whalen L, Dykeman S, et al: Labor support by first-time fathers: direct observations. J Psychosom Obstet Gynecol 11:251, 1990.

Bibring GL: Some considerations of the psychological processes in pregnancy. Psychoanal Study Child 14:113, 1959.

Bibring GL, Dwyer TF, Huntington DS, Valenstein AF: A study of the psychological processes in pregnancy and of the earliest mother-child relationship. I. Some propositions and comments. Psychoanal Study Child 16:9, 1961.

Blau A, Slaff B, Easton K, et al: The psychogenic etiology of premature birth: a preliminary report. Psychosom Med 25:201, 1963.

Bloom B: Definitional concepts of the crisis concept. J Consult Psychol 27:42, 1963.

Brown GW, Harris T: Social Origins of Depression: A Study of Psychiatric Disorder in Women. New York, The Free Press, 1978.

Chappel J: Stresses Encountered by Hospitalized Antepartum Patients and Implications for the NICU Nurse. (Unpublished study report.) University of Florida, 1983.

Cohen R: Some maladaptive syndromes of pregnancy and the puerperium. Obstet Gynecol 27:562, 1966.

Hare E, Lawrence K, Paynes H, et al: Spina bifida cystica and family stress. Br Med J 2:757, 1966.

Hofmeyr CJ, Nikodem VC, Wolman W-L, Chalmers B, Kramer T: Companionship to modify the clinical birth environment: effects on progress and perceptions of labour and breastfeeding. Brit J Obstet Gynecol 98:756, 1991.

Johns N: Family reactions to the birth of a child with a congenital abnormality. Med J Aust 7:277, 1971.

Kennell J, Klaus M: The perinatal paradigm: is it time for a change? Clin Perinatol 15:801–813, 1988.

Kennell JH, Klaus MH, McGrath S, et al: Continuous emotional support during labor in a U.S. hospital: a randomized controlled trial. JAMA 265:2197, 1991.

Klaus MH, Kennell JH, Robertson S, Sosa R: Effects of social support during parturition on maternal and infant morbidity. Br Med J 293:585, 1986.

Lampe J, Trause M, Kennell J: Parental visiting of sick infants: the effects of living at home prior to hospitalization. Pediatrics 59:294, 1977.

Larson C: Efficacy of prenatal and postpartum home visits on child health and development. Pediatrics 66:191, 1980.

Merkatz R: Prolonged hospitalization of pregnant women: the effects on the family. Birth Family J 5:204, 1978.

Moore ML: Potential Alterations in Attachment: Maternal and/or Neonatal Illness. NAACOG Update Series.

Princeton, NJ, Continuing Professional Education Center, Inc, 1983.

National Institutes of Health: Cesarean Childbirth Consensus Development Conference Summary. Bethesda, MD, 1980, Vol 3, No 6.

Olshansky S: Chronic sorrow: a response to having a mentally defective child. Soc Case 43:190, 1962.

Rappoport L: The state of crisis: some theoretical considerations. In Parad H (ed): Crisis Intervention. New York, Family Service Association, 1965.

Roskies E: Abnormality and Normality: The Mothering of Thalidomide Children. New York, Cornell University Press, 1972.

Solnit A, Stark M: Mourning and the birth of a defective child. Psychoanal Study Child 16:523, 1961.

Sosa R, Kennell J, Klaus M, et al: The effect of a supportive companion on perinatal problems, length of labor, and mother-infant interaction. N Engl J Med 303:597, 1980.

Whitby C, DeCates CR, Roberton NRC: Infants weighing 1.8–2.5 kg: Should they be cared for in neonatal units or postnatal wards? Lancet 322, 1982.

Whitelaw A: Kangaroo baby care: just a nice experience or an important advance for preterm infants? Pediatrics 85:604–606, 1990.

Zuk G: Religious factor and the role of guilt in parental acceptance of the retarded child. Am J Ment Defic 64:145, 1959.

# CHAPTER 34

# Grief Counseling

Kenneth R. Kellner and Marian F. Lake

The loss of a baby through stillbirth or neonatal death is a devastating experience for a woman. It precipitates intense emotional turmoil in the woman, her family and friends, and the medical professionals providing care during and after her pregnancy. If this emotional response is unrecognized and unattended, serious sequelae may develop.

The national perinatal death rate is 14.4 per 1000 live births (Vital Statistics, 1988). In most industrialized countries, the neonatal death rate equals the fetal death rate. Nurses, physicians, and other health care providers, although informed of the technologies available to achieve fetal and neonatal survival, are often well intentioned but ill prepared to care for the woman and her family when perinatal death occurs.

Perinatal death causes a grief and mourning response as severe as, and perhaps even more disruptive than, that seen in families in whom adult members have died. Information presented here allows readers to increase their awareness of the characteristics of normal grief and mourning, increase their appreciation of the significance and implications of the loss to the family, and assimilate methods designed to guide their care of the patient and her family.

## Prenatal Maternal Attachment

It is often difficult for family members, friends, and medical professionals to understand the intensity of the woman's emotional response to the death of her fetus or newborn. It may be difficult to understand these emotions that seem to represent a deep, loving attachment to a baby who did not survive intrauterine life or never left the intensive care nursery. Unfortunately, the assumption may be made that because the baby was not, for example, full term or born alive or taken home and cared for by the mother, she has not been able to develop an attachment to the baby and, therefore, should be able to easily cope with the death, carry on with her life, and make a rapid, full recovery. In fact, an intense emotional attachment develops between the woman and her baby long before delivery and, frequently, long before conception.

The process involved in the development of the maternal-infant bond has been described by Klaus and Kennell (1982). The attachment of mother to infant begins long before birth and physical care giving. As a young girl's socialization begins and she perceives a societal role as wife and mother, she may subconsciously begin the process of bonding to her baby through her fantasies of marriage, motherhood, and family, that is, years before a pregnancy is actually conceived.

After conception, the bond between mother and fetus intensifies. Prior to the woman's detection of fetal movement, she may view the fetus as part of herself rather than as a separate individual. The perception of fetal movement allows and encourages her to identify the baby as an individual, now separate from her. Fantasizing about the baby's appearance and sex, the mother ascribes personality characteristics to the fetus, often giving the baby nicknames. The fetus develops an individual identity. Long before delivery, the woman thinks about and plans for the baby's childhood, adolescence, and adult life. The death of a fetus or newborn cannot be viewed as the death of a baby whose identity and personality are unknown to the mother. It is the death of a perfect, idealized baby whose life has been long established for the woman and with whom she has developed an intense, loving relationship.

The existence of prenatal maternal attachment is further supported in the literature. The expression of grief after perinatal death may be viewed as evidence of that attachment (Kirkley-Best, 1981). The emotional expression of grief occurs irrespective of the woman's pleasure with being pregnant and the extent of parent-infant contact after delivery. Kennell and colleagues (1970), using grief scores to evaluate parental response to neonatal death, found that "clearly identifiable mourning" was present in each of the women interviewed, whether or not the pregnancy had been planned and whether or not the mother had touched the baby after death. Similar findings are reported in a study of 50 women experiencing neonatal death (Benfield et al, 1978). Both investigators found a grief response to be evident whether the baby was nonviable by weight or weighed over 4000 g. Thus, a woman, even one whose unplanned or unwanted pregnancy ends in the delivery of a nonviable fetus with whom she has had no physical contact, experiences a reaction demonstrating a pre-existing emotional attachment to the baby.

The health professional must not assume that a woman will make a quick, full recovery from a perinatal death because she has had no opportunity to become attached to the baby. *Intense prenatal maternal attachment exists long before delivery* and is evident, irrespective of circumstances surrounding the pregnancy.

# Grief and Mourning: Definitions

Information in the literature over the past few decades has increased our understanding of and sensitivity to the expression of grief following the loss of a loved one. Research concerning the survivor's grief after the death of an adult or child predominates.

Although little attention has been directed to a systematic evaluation of the emotional implications of a perinatal death, the available information clearly demonstrates that the family's response to this catastrophe parallels the descriptions of what families experience after the death of a child or adult. Experience with families after the delivery of a stillborn or the death of a neonate suggests to the authors that it may in fact be more disruptive.

*Mourning is the process by which an individual reorganizes and adapts following the death of a loved one. The emotion that dominates this process is grief.* Mourning is now recognized as a series of phases through which an individual passes after experiencing a loss (Bowlby, 1961; Lindemann, 1944; Parks, 1972). Although descriptions differ slightly, the process involves the following four phases:

1. Shock and disbelief
2. Yearning, searching, and anxiety
3. Disorganization, despair, and depression
4. Reorganization

The phase of *shock and disbelief* is characterized by a period of denial, which is usually short lived. A sense of apathy, numbness, and unexpected calm typifies this period. Concentration and the ability to make decisions are severely impaired. A typical response is to think a mistake has been made and that the loved one is still alive. The denial and inability to react are useful, self-protective defense mechanisms in that they allow the individual time to mobilize resources to cope with the shock. Patients relate that the emotions apparent in this phase are most intense during the first few weeks after the death. Denial that persists may constitute an abnormal response (Bowlby, 1961).

*Yearning, searching, and anxiety* make up the painful second phase of mourning. Preoccupied by thoughts and images of the deceased, the mourner cries, expresses anger and guilt, and often relates loneliness, sleeplessness, lack of strength and appetite, and a general loss in normal behavior patterns. This disruption in behavior results in confusion and anxiety. The grieving person is angry and needs to affix blame for the death. That blame may be directed at the survivor, the deceased, or, not uncommonly, health care professionals and those attempting to provide comfort. The intense emotional turmoil of this phase often prompts a feeling of profound personality changes and approaching insanity. The characteristics of this phase are most intense between the second week and fourth or fifth month after the death (Davidson, 1979).

*Disorganization, despair, and depression* predominate when the reality of the death becomes apparent and life is viewed without the relationship to the deceased. This phase, usually most intense 4 to 6 months after the death, typically lasts several months. Previous meaningful aspects of life now carry little significance, and activities are carried out only with effort. Work may be accomplished only by "going through the motions." Restlessness and aimless movements are common. Anorexia, insomnia, and malaise often prompt the mourner to make frequent calls to her physician seeking medical remedies.

*Reorganization* begins as time passes and preoccupation with the deceased wanes. The mourner is able to re-enter actitivies of daily life without the oppressive feelings characteristic of the preceding three phases. Memory of the deceased is not gone; rather, it may be recalled but with feelings of sadness that do not disrupt daily functioning. Life is reorganized to allow the survivor to incorporate the severed relationship into her continuing life. The capacity to interact is no longer reduced. The emotional responses of each of the four phases are summarized in Table 34–1.

Health care providers coming in contact with grieving couples who have experienced a perinatal death must keep the following in mind:

1. *The process of mourning is both normal and painful.* The expression of grief is expected, and the pain is inevitable.

2. *The process is not static.* Emotional responses typically intensify and wane over a period of 2 years, with characteristics of each phase overlapping one another.

3. Although the process is presented in an orderly progression, *the individual's response may not be immutable.* The behavioral sequence may be described with the following progression: (1) anxiety, (2) anger, (3) pain, (4) despair, and (5) hope. In reality, anger, for example, may precede anxiety, may not surface at all, or may persist through the whole process.

The length of time that passes before reorganization is reached varies. Full resolution may not be apparent for up to 2 years after the death. The duration of the response is influenced by what has been described as *grief work,* that is, the ability to come to terms with the reality of the first 3 phases (Lindemann, 1944). To complete this difficult, often exhausting work, the bereaved must:

1. Accept the pain of the death,
2. Review their relationship with the deceased and emancipate themselves from it,
3. Readjust to their environment, and
4. Form new relationships.

Psychologic sequelae of bereavement are ameliorated by adequate grief work. Reorganization is delayed if the process is impeded or, in fact, not encouraged.

**Table 34–1**
CHARACTERISTIC RESPONSES DURING THE PHASES OF MOURNING

| **Shock and Disbelief** | **Yearning, Searching, and Anxiety** | **Disorganization** | **Reorganization** |
|---|---|---|---|
| Denial | Tears | Restlessness | Daily functioning not disrupted |
| Unexpected calm | Anger | Aimless movement | Memories recalled with |
| Apathy | Guilt | Insomnia | appropriate sadness |
| Numbness | Insomnia | Anorexia | Oppressive feelings have lifted |
| Impaired concentration | Anorexia | Malaise | Capacity to interact has |
| Impaired decision-making | Need to affix blame | Life seems | returned |
| "There must be a mistake" | Confusion | meaningless | |
| | Preoccupation with deceased | | |
| | Loneliness | | |
| | Disruption in normal patterns of behavior | | |

# Pathologic Grief Reactions

When the normal process of mourning and the expression of grief are blocked or suppressed, pathologic reactions can occur. In this instance, grief work is delayed, inhibited, or absent. The emotional expression of grief after perinatal death, vital to a healthy resolution, is often avoided by the woman and suppressed by those individuals with whom she comes into contact. Discussions of her pregnancy, her delivery, and the baby are avoided. Her need for support remains unmet. The silence and isolation she perceives may be interpreted as a lack of support, and attempts to review her relationship with the baby are thwarted. Often lacking any tangible evidence that the baby in fact ever existed, the woman's attempts to appreciate the reality of her baby's death also are blocked, and she is placed at even further risk of developing a morbid grief response (Bowlby, 1961; Schoenberg, 1980). Such factors added to the unique physical, psychologic, and sociocultural climate in which the death occurs create a setting high in risk for the development of pathologic grief reactions (Condon, 1986).

Pathologic responses may be identified as either prolonged grief or absent, inhibited grief. Both have been described following perinatal death. Jensen and Zahourek (1972) found evidence of chronic depression, an aspect of prolonged grief, in six of ten women 1 year after the death of a newborn. In a study of 56 women evaluated 1 to 2 years after a neonatal death, Cullberg (1971) found that 19 exhibited symptoms of a pathologic reaction. An additional study reports the incidence to be 26 percent of the population evaluated (Rowe et al, 1978).

Two groups of women seem to be at particular risk for an unsatisfactory outcome: women with pregnancies occurring less than 6 months after a stillbirth, and women whose pregnancies involved a surviving twin. The British Stillbirth and Neonatal Death Association suggests that pregnancies occurring less than 6 months after a stillbirth can be associated with catastrophic grief reactions (Lockwood and Lewis, 1980). Additionally, in a group of nine women who either became pregnant within 5 months after a perinatal death or had a surviving twin, five developed morbid responses (Rowe et al, 1978). Although this study group is small, it is apparent that women in these circumstances need psychologic follow-up.

As the phase of resolution is reached and the woman has incorporated the death of her baby as a part of her life, the symptoms of grief and mourning wane. This does not mean the baby's death will ever be perceived as fair or justifiable. Parents never forget the loss. It merely becomes less painful to remember. The dates of delivery, death, and burial, in addition to certain holidays, are anniversaries that may precipitate sadness and tears. This "shadow grief," as described by Peppers and Knapp (1980), may linger for a lifetime and does not constitute a morbid grief reaction. It is not a debilitating grief but rather represents the normal surfacing of memories and concomitant sadness.

# Grief After Abortion

The woman who experiences abortion, whether elective or spontaneous, grieves and mourns in the same manner as the woman whose baby is stillborn or dies as a neonate. Women relate intense feelings of depression, anger, and guilt in the weeks and months after the abortion. The woman's fetus is often referred to as tissue or products of conception rather than as a baby with his or her own identity. No funerals are held, and the woman usually has no opportunity to see or hold her baby. She may hear such responses as "Better that it happened now, before you got to know the baby," or "It's for the best." These circumstances may culminate in what the woman perceives as a clear message from health care providers, family members, or friends that it is inappropriate for her to grieve for the loss of this baby.

The majority of women whose pregnancies end in spontaneous abortion experience grief and mourning but do not experience disabling, pathologic grief reactions (Niswander, 1967; Peck, 1966; Simon et al, 1967). However, there is evidence that suggests the length of gestation at the time of perinatal loss influences the grief response. Blumberg and associates (1975) propose that preoccupation with the loss is prolonged after fetal movement has been perceived, that is, after the fetus may have assumed an identity of its own. This assessment is supported by information that describes a more intense emotional response after stillbirth and neonatal death as compared with that seen after spontaneous abortion (Kirkley-Best, 1981; Toedter et al, 1988). Although this information suggests that the intensity of grief and mourning may be less intense in women experiencing abortion, it is nonetheless evident (Lovell, 1983; Peppers and Knapp, 1980). Supportive counseling should be provided so that individual needs can be assessed and questions can be answered (Leppert and Pahlka, 1984; Seibel and Graves, 1980).

Women who undergo elective termination of pregnancy for potential or realized fetal abnormalities may experience particular difficulty in resolving their loss. When a woman or couple decides to end a pregnancy because of the risk of fetal abnormality, that decision-making process, with its inherent assumption of responsibility, may intensify the feelings of guilt. Doubt and regret may delay resolution and place the woman at risk for an abnormal emotional response (Black, 1990; Donnai et al, 1981; Niswander and Patterson, 1967).

The grief women experience after elective or spontaneous abortion must not be ignored. The same type of attention to the emotional needs of these women that is provided for families experiencing stillbirth or neonatal death promotes a healthy resolution to their grief.

# Grief at the Event of Stillbirth

The concept of prenatal maternal attachment and a body of literature replete with anecdotal descriptions of parental responses allow us to appreciate the emotional impact of fetal and neonatal death (Kirkley-Best and Kellner, 1981). Health care providers caring for women experiencing stillbirth need to consider this tragedy's special characteristics carefully.

The sense of emptiness, typical of any mourning response, may be particularly acute in the case of fetal death. The developing relationship between mother and fetus is abruptly terminated as evidenced by the fact that the growing, moving fetus is now quiet. In addition to losing a part of her body that had been relied on for recognition and gratification, the woman may experience profound disturbances in her body image. A sense of uncleanliness and loss of body integrity may predominate (Grubb, 1976; Kish, 1978).

Clearly, one of the most outstanding characteristics of the grief response at stillbirth is guilt. Both mother and father may experience it, but there is evidence to suggest that guilt is more intense and more prolonged in the woman (Helmrath and Steinitz, 1978). "What did I do that made my baby die?" and "What did I neglect to do?" are questions parents repeatedly ask. A woman often spends extended periods of time reviewing the pregnancy to find where she was at fault. Often, irrational or seemingly insignificant events are perceived as the cause of death; for example, neglecting a prenatal vitamin, missing a prenatal visit, walking up a flight of stairs, or contemplating an abortion early in the pregnancy. A father may assume guilt for leaving his partner home alone during the day, not insisting that she take her vitamins, or continuing sexual activities.

A woman's response to stillbirth has implications beyond her grief for the baby. A situation that has been described as a double crisis occurs (Quirk, 1979). The woman is confronted with not only the crisis of death but also an implied inability to nurture and protect her baby. If the ability to complete a pregnancy and deliver a healthy infant is perceived as proof of femininity and womanhood, the woman whose baby was stillborn may grieve for lack of this proof. Pregnancy has been described as the fulfillment of a wish fantasy (Deutsch, 1944). If this wish is unfulfilled, intense feelings of anger, guilt, and depression can be expected.

# Overcoming Obstacles to Parental Grief Work

Davidson (1977) studied 15 women and their families who had experienced a perinatal death. He identified three occasions when the mother seems most vulnerable to disorientation: (1) when she tries to confirm perceptually who died, (2) when she tries to get emotional support, and (3) when she compares her feelings with those of others. Although the work refers to mothers, fathers have similar problems. Each of these periods of vulnerability can be looked at as an obstacle to parental grief work. From this concept, methods to help families overcome each obstacle can be developed.

## CONFIRMING PERCEPTUALLY WHO DIED

When an adult or older child dies, it is clear who that person was. There are memories, photographs, personal possessions, and mementos. Remembrances can be shared with relatives and friends. In contrast to this concrete, well-defined image of the person who has died, parents may be left with only vague feelings and images when perinatal death occurs. This is most pronounced with stillbirth, because the baby never existed as a separate, living human being outside its mother. Parents are left with hopes and dreams of the future that are unique to each individual and not easily shared. Mothers' memories of fetal movement and fathers' external perceptions of this may be the only physical contact with the baby. Parents who never see their dead baby and who are surrounded by silence from the medical staff know that something is missing but have difficulty conceptualizing what. Women who had stillbirths 20 or 30 years ago have asked, "How do I know my baby was dead? Maybe it was alive and they gave it to someone else." Such an occurrence has been reported in the lay press (LeBlanc, 1982). These women can be trapped in the phase of searching and yearning, never really believing their child is dead. Only when parents can believe and admit that the baby is dead can they progress to a satisfactory resolution of their grief.

These parents are also subject to disorientation because of the loss of control over their lives. All people need to feel that they have some control over their own destinies. When events occur over which we have no control, it can be very frightening. Because parents' plans and efforts are directed toward a healthy, normal baby, when this does not occur, an overwhelming feeling of loss of control can take over that can make any further effort seem useless. To give back control, parents should be encouraged to make their own choices about the care of themselves and their baby. Letting parents make choices helps restore personal integrity (Lippman and Carlson, 1977) and removes

responsibility from the staff, who are usually anxious over their perceived responsibility for the tragedy.

Labor and delivery should be conducted as planned in order to help keep the parents oriented. There is no reason why the father cannot be present. Medical procedures such as episiotomy should be performed when indicated and not avoided to spare the mother the discomfort. Above all, parents' individual wishes and desires must be respected. Davidson (1977) describes a woman with a previable baby who did not want to push at the end of her labor because she saw that as actively participating in the baby's death.

The simplest and probably most important way to help parents confirm who died is to let them *see the baby* (Bourne, 1979; Cohen et al, 1978; Davidson, 1977; Kennell and Trause, 1978; Kowalski and Bowes, 1976; Lewis, 1982; Lewis, 1972; O'Donohue, 1978; Seitz and Warrick, 1974). Davidson (1977) found no adverse reactions in mothers who had viewed their babies, and some seemed to adapt more easily to their loss. Cohen and coworkers (1978) found a higher percentage of nonviewers among mothers requiring psychiatric treatment than among those who resolved their grief satisfactorily. At the University of Florida, 91 percent of 164 parents chose to see their dead baby when offered the choice (Kellner et al, 1984). No correlation was found between the baby's appearance (maceration, malformation) and the desire to view the baby. This choice should be presented before delivery so that parents have time to decide. They should be told what the baby will look like. If they choose not to see the baby at delivery, it should be available at a later time. The normal, positive aspects of the baby's appearance should be pointed out, because this is what parents focus on and remember (Bourne, 1979; Cohen et al, 1978; O'Donohue, 1978). A majority of parents also choose to *hold the baby* (Kellner et al, 1984), and they should be given time alone with it. They should be asked if there are other family or friends whom they would like to have view or hold the baby.

*Naming the baby* helps acknowledge the reality of the death and helps parents and others think and talk about the child. Parents are usually surprised when told that they can name a stillborn baby, and more than three fourths will do so when given the opportunity (Kellner et al, 1984).

Tangible evidence of the baby's existence

is appreciated by parents. They may desire the baby's blanket, identification bracelet, or a lock of hair. A very simple memento is a set of the baby's *footprints* on the standard hospital form. In addition to confirming the actuality of the baby, the footprints reinforce the normality of the baby (normal feet and toes) and provide information about site, time, and staff involved, which can help the parents review events later.

*Photographs* are strongly desired by almost all families. These photographs should be good quality, because they are how parents will remember the child. Although instant photographs taken during labor and delivery may be adequate (Chez, 1982), photographs of the baby carefully wrapped in a blanket better facilitate acceptance (Kellner et al, 1981). Attempts should be made to avoid the harshness of typical pathology pictures and to photograph the baby in a manner that demonstrates compassionate care (Fig. 34–1). Graham and associates (1987) found that women who had received pictures of their infant were less depressed at the

postpartum visit than those who had not. Davidson (1979) found that after being shown photographs of their babies, women who had not seen their babies previously stopped hearing phantom crying.

After delivery, patients should be given the choice of *where to recover*. Depending on the facilities, the value of being away from mothers and babies should be weighed against the expertise of the obstetric staff to handle the physical and emotional problems of the postpartum period. Lamb (1982) suggests using a color code on charts to signify mothers with sick or dead babies. She also presents a checklist form for the chart so that interventions and responses can be noted and not duplicated. Although there has been a traditional tendency to discharge these women as quickly as possible, many mothers, especially those with poor support systems at home, may benefit from longer contact with counseling personnel in the hospital.

*Baptism* may be requested (Kirkley-Best et al, 1982). This may be performed by the

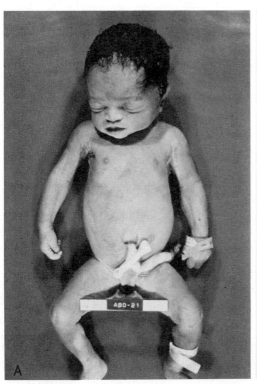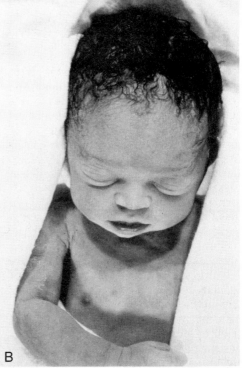

**Figure 34–1.** *A,* The harshness of the typical pathology photograph of a dead infant provides inadequate comfort to the family. *B,* When the baby is photographed in a manner that demonstrates compassionate care, acceptance is facilitated.

appropriate clergy either in the hospital or after discharge or by staff members familiar with the procedure. Religious practices vary (Hollingsworth and Pasnau, 1977) and should be considered when discussing choices.

An *autopsy* can help families in many ways. By providing a detailed description of the baby, it helps parents confirm that this was a real human being. Because almost all stillborns are completely normal, it can help restore feelings of value and self-esteem to the parents. An autopsy also can help answer the two questions that are central to the family's feelings: "Why did my baby die?" and "Will it happen again?" When a definite cause of death is found, parental guilt can be reduced and realistic recurrence risks given to relieve anxiety. Even when no cause of death is found, the normality of the child can be stressed and the low risk of recurrence reassured. Such information can also be a comfort to the health care providers. A copy of the autopsy report should be given to the parents so that they can review it later, when emotions have eased; it also serves as a sign that nothing is being held back or concealed. Several authors have reported that parents are interested in autopsy results and will return to get them (Clyman et al, 1980; Cohen et al, 1978; Kellner et al, 1984). The autopsy request, therefore, should be part of the care given the patient rather than an end in itself. Berger (1978) provides an excellent discussion of the value of the autopsy and how the request should be made. The request should come from the team member most involved with the patient's care, but he or she must be knowledgeable to answer the parents' questions about what will be performed and when, where, and how much it will cost.

Information also must be available about options for disposition of the baby. An explanation of how the hospital disposes of the body should be given if appropriate, because what happens to the body can be a source of long-lasting concern (Cohen et al, 1978). A *funeral* for a stillborn is perfectly appropriate, and the hospital should assist in facilitating this choice. A funeral can facilitate the grieving process in several ways. It formalizes the death as something real and important. It provides family and friends an opportunity to support the bereaved by sharing in this ritual. The grave provides a place where the parents can visit to be with their baby and where sadness can be expressed. Even if cremation is chosen, a small service can be held. Parents remember the funeral as a positive experience and often see it as the time when the past was closed and they started looking toward the future.

Hospital staff members often feel pressure to talk with parents about autopsy and disposition of remains in order to "get the paperwork over with." However, it must be appreciated by the staff, and it is helpful to acknowledge to the parents that they are being asked to make very difficult choices under circumstances in which they would rather not be making any choices. There is rarely a circumstance in which parents cannot have several days to make these critical decisions about the care of their deceased baby.

Seeing, holding, and naming the baby; mementos; and the autopsy and funeral all help the parents confirm that this was indeed a baby, their baby who died, and serve as remembrances of the event. As Stack (1982) says, "The end point of the grieving process is not to help the person forget the lost loved one, but to remember without pain."

## GETTING EMOTIONAL SUPPORT

Society, family, and friends often do not consider fetal loss to be a significant life event. Such solicitudes as "It's better the baby died before you got to know it," "You're young, you can have lots more babies," or "You have other children at home so what's the big deal?" are wrong and tend to isolate the bereaved from these often well-meaning people who do not understand what has happened.

Medicine also has traditionally shared this view and focused on the medical aspects of managing fetal death (ACOG, 1979). Health care providers are also hampered from giving support because the death raises their own anxieties. This is discussed in greater detail later. Cullberg (1972) found that staff responded to the anxiety engendered by perinatal death by avoiding the situation, by projecting their feelings of anger and blame onto the parent, and by denial and "magical repair." These strategies resulted in the staff's avoiding the family as much as possible or not being sensitive to their needs. Parents experiencing neonatal death report concern and many phone calls while the infant was ill, but once the baby died there was a "conspiracy of silence" around the parents as if they had never had a baby (Helmrath and Steinitz, 1978).

Families can be helped to overcome this obstacle by receiving support. First, health care providers must realistically evaluate their own anxieties and feelings so that they can help the family manage theirs. Staff with special training or interest in this field can be very helpful. Second, professionals must *volunteer to help*. Families are quick to pick up both verbal and nonverbal cues that staff are uncomfortable and, thus, tend to be silent and compliant to minimize distress. The staff interpret the parents' behavior as indicating that they do not want to talk, so they stay away, which completes the cycle of silence. Physicians and nurses must break the cycle by taking the initiative and entering the patient's room. It is not necessary to spend a long time. Several 10- to 15-minute contacts during the day may be better than one long one, but this must be individualized. Schreiner and colleagues (1979) found that a simple, caring phone call to parents after the death of their newborn resulted in a decrease in the number and intensity of subsequent emotional problems.

The question that is always asked is "What do I say?" A simple statement that shows your feelings, acknowledges the reality of the event, and offers continuity of support is ideal, such as "I'm sorry your baby died. Is there anything I can do for you?" This also gives the parents permission to express their feelings. Lippman and Carlson (1977) stress the concept of realistic support in this circumstance. This is a time when the staff person can purposely encourage the family to express themselves concerning the death and can listen patiently. As they point out, this may be easier said than done for health care personnel accustomed to providing tangible care. However, the importance of listening as a therapeutic modality cannot be overemphasized. A mother of a stillborn said, "I can understand why they avoided me, because they didn't know what to say . . . but sometimes you really don't have to say anything."

It is also helpful to bring up certain topics that parents may be reticent to raise or have not anticipated because of the acute stress of the situation. Clyman and associates (1980) found that over half the mothers they interviewed had difficulty telling their other children of the death or in dealing with subsequent behavior problems such as nightmares. Discussions with siblings must be tailored to the children's ages and previous experience and discussions about death. In general, though, it is recommended that parents explain that the child was in no way responsible for the death and that he or she is safe from a similar fate. This is discussed in more detail later in this chapter. Couples experiencing a first pregnancy are naturally concerned whether or not they will ever have a healthy baby. Although a definitive answer should not be given until all studies are complete, parents usually can be assured that stillbirth will not recur. Parents should also be warned that other people may not appreciate the magnitude of the tragedy that has occurred. Telling parents the type of things people may say and asking them to think about how they will respond is helpful preparation.

The mother may appreciate being able to discuss with a staff member how best to dispose of nursery items and baby clothes purchased before the loss of her child. It should be stressed, however, that the mother should handle this in a manner comfortable for her and not let others perform these functions while she is in the hospital. As one mother said, "Sometimes other people do your thinking for you and that's bad." There is no right or wrong. The mother may feel more comfortable having things put away before she gets home, doing it herself, or closing the nursery door and not going in for 6 months. It should be up to the parents alone.

It is beneficial to inquire, at a follow-up visit, about the couple's sexual relationship. This topic rarely is raised by parents even when significant problems have developed as a result of the death. As with sexual problems under other circumstances, giving parents permission to talk about it may be beneficial in itself. Showing parents how this problem fits into their overall grieving reactions and explaining that this is an understandable and common problem is helpful.

Religion can be a variable source of support (Kirkley-Best et al, 1982). Depending on ideology, parental participation, and formal support structures, religion may be great comfort or a source of distress. Support should be given so that parents can sort out their feelings and commitments.

In summary, parents have difficulty getting support because of a lack of understanding by society as well as health care professionals of their need for emotional support. The simplest way to help them overcome this obstacle is to volunteer our help and experience. Parents who receive adequate comfort and support are less depressed and have higher levels of self-esteem and psychologic well-being (Murray and Callan, 1988).

## COMPARING THEIR FEELINGS WITH THOSE OF OTHERS

As has been stressed, parents encounter many people who do not understand. These may be people whom the parents have formerly depended on for examples of appropriate behavior. In the case of perinatal death, the clues may be that parental mourning and feelings of grief are inappropriate and abnormal (Helmrath and Steinitz, 1978). The mother who tells her bereaved daughter to "eat to keep up her strength" and asks, "Why all the tears, it's been a month?" can cause very disorienting and uncomfortable feelings in the woman experiencing an acute and normal grief response. Likewise, the father who has just suffered the most devastating tragedy in his life and returns to work to find his friends silent and acting as if nothing has happened can become very confused (Davidson, 1977). He may react in anger and hostility, further alienating potential sources of support, or he may convince himself that his feelings are abnormal and hold them within. The normal intense emotions of grieving are difficult enough to bear without the added burden of feeling that those emotions are abnormal. "I feel like I'm going crazy" is a common complaint of the unprepared.

Problems also arise because of a lack of appreciation of the duration of mourning. Helmrath and Steinitz (1978) point out that the period of acute grief lasts 6 months to 1 year; Davidson (1979) believes that it takes a majority of adults 18 to 24 months to complete the mourning process. Although the overall intensity gradually decreases and most couples may appear to be functioning normally in public at 6 months, it is common for mothers returning for gynecologic examinations 1 or 2 years later to cry when given permission to talk about the death. Unfortunately, this lengthy period can be a strain on family and friends who are not sharing these feelings and grow impatient with the sadness and mourning. This adds to the couple's alienation.

This obstacle can be overcome by discussions of what grieving is like. *Education* should include not only the parents but also their family and friends whenever possible. Perinatal mortality counseling programs should have education as a major objective (Kellner et al, 1981).

It is tempting to describe normal grieving to couples so that it will not be perceived as abnormal and the distress intensified. However, such counseling may merely intellectualize the death and retard resolution. In addition, because each person reacts according to his or her individual personality and emotional experiences, predictions of an individual's feelings and behaviors are highly inaccurate. One woman at the time of an early stillbirth was given a detailed list of the signs and symptoms of grieving and was disturbed later that she had not experienced all of them. One successful approach is to stress the individuality of responses to the death and introduce specific feelings with phrases such as "Some mothers have felt . . . ," "Some fathers have told us . . . ," "You may or may not feel that way. Whatever happens is right for you and O.K."

A discussion of anniversaries, such as due date, confirmation of pregnancy, and the baby's death, as events that bring back painful memories can assuage the discomfort. It is like a deep wound, which, although healed, still hurts when traumatized.

Education and reassurance can do much to help parents understand and express their feelings. This can result in a healthier resolution of their grief. Obstacles to parental grief work and methods to help overcome these obstacles are summarized in Table 34–2.

# Fathers

If the emotion at perinatal death is the forgotten grief, then the father is certainly the forgotten mourner. As one mother said, "After the baby died, all the cards and flowers were addressed to me." Several factors may conspire to make it even more difficult for the father to resolve his feelings in a healthy way than for the mother.

**Table 34–2**
METHODS TO OVERCOME THE OBSTACLES TO
NORMAL PARENTAL GRIEF

| Confirming Perceptually Who Died | Getting Emotional Support | Comparing Feelings with Others' |
|---|---|---|
| See the baby | Volunteer time | Educate parents |
| Hold the baby | Volunteer topics | Educate family |
| Name the baby | Provide follow-up | Educate staff |
| Footprints | | |
| Mementos | | |
| Photographs | | |
| Autopsy | | |
| Funeral | | |

Data from Davidson G: Death of the wished-for child: a case study. Death Educ 1:265, 1977.

There can be no doubt that in almost all cases, prenatal maternal attachment to the baby is stronger than prenatal paternal attachment (Davidson, 1977). The physical intimacy shared by the woman and the baby developing within her can never be matched by the paternal experience. Peppers and Knapp (1980) have labeled this difference between the mother's and father's experience incongruent bonding. Bugen (1977) proposed that the intensity and duration of a grieving response are directly proportional to the closeness of the relationship between the deceased and the bereaved. LaGrua (1979), studying families following perinatal death, found that grieving in this situation fits this model. It would, therefore, be expected that fathers, having a less intimate relationship with the fetus, would grieve less than mothers, and this seems to be the case (Benfield et al, 1978; Helmrath and Steinitz, 1978). Peppers and Knapp (1980) have called this difference between the mother's and the father's experience incongruent grieving.

Another important obstacle to paternal grief work is society's expectations that the man be strong and not show emotion. The father's response to the death tends to be determined by how he believes he should act as a man, rather than how he needs to act to work through his grief (Cordell and Thomas, 1990). The father tries to give strength to his spouse and thereby denies his own feelings. While the mother is in the hospital and sheltered during the initial intense and overwhelming stages of grief, the father must go home and tell the children, tell the friends, arrange for the funeral, and interact with the hospital. The man is more likely consciously not to grieve, and when he does, he may be more upset by his emotions than the mother (Kennell et al, 1970). It is important to recognize, however, that the emotions of a father experiencing a stillbirth are also strong (Kotzwinkle, 1975).

The obstacles to paternal grief work not only increase the chances of a poor resolution of grief for the father but put his relationships with his wife at great risk. One third of the women studied by Cullberg (1972) reported marital difficulties. Feelings of anger and blame may be misdirected at a spouse, and the couple may be unable to accept each other as they did before. The incongruent grieving can easily lead to conflict because the husband quickly tires of his wife's intense emotions, whereas she accuses him of being unfeeling and not having loved the baby. This often affects their sexual relationship (Peppers and Knapp, 1980).

The solution is support and education. The father needs acknowledgment of his role in the pregnancy and his feelings about the death. He should be allowed to show his emotions, and other family members and friends should be encouraged to share the feelings with him and handle whatever personal affairs they can to lighten his burden. The husband and wife should be treated as a couple. The husband should be allowed to be with his wife as much as possible, and ideally they should be allowed to stay together continuously in the hospital. Communication between partners is the cornerstone of a satisfactory resolution of the crisis. The difference in grieving responses should be discussed and tolerance stressed. It can be very helpful to meet with the parents both together and separately to facilitate the expression of their feelings.

# Siblings

In one perinatal mortality counseling program, almost half of the parents experiencing a perinatal death had living children (Kellner et al, 1981). These parents must face the problem of telling siblings about the death and appreciate help in doing so.

*The age of the child is an important consideration.* Grollman (1977) found that from ages 3 to 5, children deny that death is a regular or final process. From ages 5 to 9, they understand death to be final but do not recognize it as universal or something that will eventually happen to themselves. After age 9, the inevitability of death is acknowledged. This provides a general guideline to the type of information the child can process and may prepare parents for the child's responses. For example, young children, because they do not understand the finality of death, repeatedly ask the parents where the baby is and when it is coming home. This can be very upsetting to the parents. At the same time is very important that the child's questions be answered and concerns addressed (Leon, 1990).

*Difficulty also stems from the different feelings that parents and siblings have about the future child.* Furman (1978) points out that whereas parents usually view the coming baby with anticipation as a happy addition to the family, a child may see it as a rival and feel jealousy and envy. It is easy to conceive a child's having destructive fantasies about the baby. When the baby dies, the child may be faced with guilt over his or her wishes coming true coupled with his or her fear of what the parents may do if they find out (Leon, 1986). In addition, parents may interpret a child's short attention span as the child's lack of interest in the death and, therefore, not discuss it. Parents appreciate it when staff make them aware of these issues.

*Parents may also wonder whether or not siblings should attend the funeral.* Schowaiter (1980) believes the decision should be based on the child's level of development and the amount of environmental support available. Children less than 7 years old tend to be disruptive and should attend only if it is important to the parents. Those older than 7 should be allowed to be part of the decision after a discussion between the parents and child. If the child attends, the service should be conducted with his or her presence in mind; he or she should be allowed to leave at any time, and a specific person should be assigned to care for the child (Schreiner et al, 1979).

The impact of the death on surviving or subsequent siblings also must be appreciated. Leon (1990) found significant psychiatric disturbance in patients that could be traced to a sibling's death many years earlier. In some cases, his patient was a replacement child (see next section), but in others, lack of understanding and poor family support were the cause.

# The Next Pregnancy

Almost every woman asks, "When can I get pregnant again?" Becoming pregnant right away may seem to be a good strategy, but it is not.

Cain and Cain (1964), studying disturbed children of families who had experienced a previous child's death, found that one half of the physicians had suggested getting pregnant quickly as a means of forgetting the death or giving the mother something to do. Horowitz (1978) found that 38 of 40 mothers who had suffered a poor outcome in pregnancy either got pregnant again to replace the loss or purposely did not use contraception.

Unfortunately, *immediately replacing the dead child may have serious consequences.* Rowe and associates (1978) found that, in a sample of 26 mothers followed between 12 and 20 months after stillbirth, the only predictor of morbid grief reactions was the presence of a surviving twin or subsequent pregnancy within 5 months of the loss. Forrest and colleagues (1982) found that women who conceived within 6 months of their baby's death had a higher rate of detectable psychiatric disorders than those who conceived later. Jolly (1976) has likewise warned against replacing the dead infant with another child, as has Oglethorpe (1989).

It must be remembered that the child who died was an ideal child. There was never a chance or the need to reconcile a real child with that image. In addition, the dead child represented hopes, dreams, plans, and perhaps an important part of his or her parents' identification and defense systems (Bourne, 1979; Cain and Cain, 1964). The replacement child must bear the burden of that image and those fantasies and a lifelong sense of impossible destinies to fulfill.

Parents must have truly resolved their grief before they can successfully embark on having a new child who must be an individual in his or her own right (Klaus and Kennell, 1982). Parents must come to realize that yes, they can have another child, but no, they can never have the child that died. This should form the basis for counseling on this subject.

Regardless of when the next pregnancy occurs, it must be acknowledged that concerns about the present fetus' safety are normal and to be expected (Theut et al, 1989). Parents should be encouraged to voice their fears at every opportunity. The health care provider can then offer nonpatronizing reassurance.

## Physicians and Nurses

*Health care personnel have feelings, too.* The inability to recognize and deal with those feelings appropriately can interfere with the care of patients. A stillborn or neonatal death arouses strong emotions in physicians and nurses that may mirror those of the parents. The physician may have feelings of helplessness, defeat, guilt, resentment, and failure (Stack, 1982). Queenan (1978a) titled an editorial on fetal death "The Ultimate Defeat."

Peppers and Knapp (1980) believe that because of their training, health care personnel and physicians, in particular, have difficulty dealing with death. "Death becomes something to work against, to avoid if possible, at any cost. It is not to be accepted; it is to be rejected. When death does occur it is considered the result of medical accident or technical error." Obstetricians and pediatricians dealing constantly with the beginning of life and so rarely with death may have particular problems accepting perinatal death. So too may nurses and social workers in areas where life begins.

*Stillbirth arouses anxiety in the staff* that, unless recognized, can be another contributing factor to parents not getting the support they need. Rowe and coworkers (1978) found that 60 percent of families were dissatisfied with the information they received or the way they received it, specifically with contacts with their physician. This is because of the way most physicians and nurses respond to anxiety (Cullberg, 1972; Stack, 1982). Reactions of health care personnel include avoidance of the situation, either by physical separation or dissociation, that is, separating one's feelings from the reality of the situation. They also project their personal feelings of guilt and anger onto the patient in the form of aggressive or accusing behavior and use denial to make believe nothing has happened by not showing the mother her dead baby and discharging her from the hospital early.

Just as these defenses may further isolate the parents and result in a cyclic degeneration of the relationship between them and the staff, the staff's recognition of their own feelings can be a positive factor in helping these families. As Queenan (1978b) says, "Never underestimate the help the obstetrician can offer bereaved parents." Peppers and Knapp (1980) and Kellner (1990) offer practical advice for physicians in this difficult situation. When the time comes to talk with the family about what has happened or what will happen, it should be conducted in a quiet, private place. Appropriate family or friends may be present. It is helpful to plan ahead how the words will be spoken. It is best to keep the information simple and honest. Time should be allocated for understanding and questions. It is important to note that parents may remember only some of what they are told but those words they will remember forever. Physical contact, such as touching a hand or putting an arm around the father, can be very comforting. In one program, staff always sit down when in the room and remove their white coats (Kellner et al, 1981). Handing a box of tissues to the father gives him permission to express his emotions.

A plan for an ongoing relationship of contact and follow-up is needed. A phone call a week after the event (Schreiner et al, 1979) and an office visit for a discussion of autopsy reports should be the minimal contact. Contact with the family must be maintained until the parents feel it is no longer needed. Referral for professional counseling may be appropriate.

Physicians and nurses themselves also need support. They should share their feelings either in group discussion sessions (Scupholme, 1978) or individually, with colleagues or professionals. It is a disservice to themselves and their patients for them to ignore their feelings.

## Counseling and Support Programs

Just as the parents feel disoriented and overwhelmed after a perinatal death, so may individual physicians and nurses. The team approach can be very helpful in this situation. Several hospitals have developed formal programs, and these have been described in the literature (Carr and Knupp, 1985; Davidson and Goldenberg, 1979; Kellner et al, 1981; Kennell and Trause, 1978; Lake et al, 1983; Lippman and Carlson, 1977; O'Donohue, 1978). Formal support and counseling have been shown to shorten the duration of bereavement after perinatal death (Forrest et al, 1982) and to decrease anger and physical symptoms (Lake et al, 1987).

A typical counseling team might be composed of an attending obstetrician, an obstetric resident on rotation, a pathologist, a nurse, and a social worker. It is believed that the interdisciplinary nature of this team is best suited to resolving the many problems these families have. Different family members often relate best to different team members, which facilitates the expression of feelings. In addition, the team allows a sharing of the emotional burden, which would be overwhelming for one person. Each member not only provides emotional support to other team members and hospital staff but also shares his or her particular area of expertise. At the same time, each team member can pursue his or her own interests in this field, which include formal teaching of residents, students, nurses, and hospital staff.

Parents are seen at the time of diagnosis, at prenatal visits, at delivery, during their postpartum stay in the hospital, at the postpartum visit, and at a final follow-up visit. This is the minimum contact, because additional telephone contacts usually are made. A data form is kept that serves two purposes: (1) noting of personal data so that at later interviews a personal relationship can be conveyed (Schreiner et al, 1979) and specific areas followed up, and (2) ensuring that interventions (such as giving footprint mementos) are performed and areas of counseling (such as what to tell siblings) are not unnecessarily repeated by different team members (Lamb, 1982).

These counseling programs were originally developed to aid families experiencing stillbirth, because these families did not fall into any already established program. However, proficiency in this field has grown, and they are now also providing aid to families with a congenital malformation diagnosed *in utero* and to pregnant patients with cancer who must make decisions about termination. Such teams now often function as a resource for hospital and community personnel faced with any poor-outcome pregnancy.

The single most constant source of support for parents is another person who has been through the same experience. This is often a friend or relative who experienced a miscarriage or stillbirth many years ago, unbeknownst to the bereaved. Parents are amazed at the number of people who "come out of the closet" and share feelings that may have been suppressed for years. This can be very beneficial for both sets of parents.

In an effort to capitalize on this source of support, several parent groups have been formed at local, national and international levels. Peppers and Knapp (1980) provide an excellent discussion of the function and organization of these groups as well as addresses for additional information.

Perinatal death strikes the unprepared, the young, and the inexperienced. It is, as Bourne (1979) says, "one of nature's obscenities." How physicians and nurses handle this situation can have lasting consequences for parents and their families.

It is now clear that there is strong prenatal parental attachment to the baby. When that attachment is broken by perinatal death, intense grief is the appropriate, expected response. The resolution of this crisis depends on how health care providers respond to the grieving parents and family.

Learning what is helpful is only the first step. Professionals gladly share in their patients' joy when a healthy baby is born. They have an even stronger obligation to share in their patients' sorrow when the pregnancy ends in tragedy.

## References

ACOG: Diagnosis and management of missed abortion and antepartum fetal death. ACOG Tech Bull No 55, November 1979.

Benfield DG, Leib SA, Vollman JH: Grief response of parents to neonatal death and parent participation in deciding care. Pediatrics 62:171, 1978.

Berger LR: Requesting the autopsy: a pediatric perspective. Clin Pediatr 17:445, 1978.

Black RB: Prenatal diagnosis and fetal loss: psychosocial consequences and professional responsibilities. Am J Med Genet 35:586, 1990.

Blumberg BD, Golbus MS, Hanson KH: The psychological sequelae of abortion performed for a genetic indication. Am J Obstet Gynecol 122:799, 1975.

Bourne S: Coping with perinatal death. Midwife Health Visit. Community Nurse 15:89, 1979.

Bowlby J: Processes of mourning. Int J Psychoanal 42:317, 1961.

Bugen LA: Human grief: a model for prediction and intervention. Am J Orthopsychiatry 47:196, 1977.

Cain AC, Cain BS: On replacing a child. J Am Acad Child Psychiatry 3:443, 1964.

Carr D, Knupp SF: Grief and perinatal loss. A community hospital approach to support. J Obstet Gynecol Neonatal Nurs 14:130, 1985.

Chez RA: Symposium: helping parents and doctors cope with perinatal death. Contemp Ob/Gyn 20:98, 1982.

Clyman RI, Green C, Rowe J, et al: Issues concerning parents after the death of their newborn. Crit Care Med 8:215, 1980.

Cohen L, Zilkha S, Middleton J, et al: Perinatal mortality: assisting in parental affirmation. Am J Orthopsychiatry 48:727, 1978.

Condon J: Management of established pathological grief reaction after stillbirth. Am J Psychiatry 143:8, 1986.

Cordell AS, Thomas N: Fathers and grieving: coping with infant death. J Perinatol 10:75, 1990.

Cullberg J: Mental reactions of women to perinatal death. In Psychosomatic Medicine in Obstetrics and Gynecology: Proceedings of Third International Congress, London, 1971. Basel, Karger, 1972, pp 326–329.

Davidson G: Understanding Death of the Wished-for Child. Springfield, IL, OGR Service Corporation, 1979.

Davidson G: Death of the wished-for child: a case study. Death Educ 1:265, 1977.

Davidson CS, Goldenberg RL: Report on counseling elicited by symposiums on fetal death (equal time). Contemp Ob/Gyn 13:13, 1979.

Deutsch H: The Psychology of Women: A Psychoanalytic Interpretation; Vol 2: Motherhood. New York, Grune & Stratton, 1944.

Donnai P, Charles N, Harris R: Attitudes of patients after "genetic" termination of pregnancy. Br Med J 282:621, 1981.

Forrest GC, Standish E, Baum JD: Support after perinatal deaths: a study of support and counselling after perinatal bereavement. Br Med J 285:1475, 1982.

Furman E: The death of a newborn: care of the parents. Birth Fam J 5:214, 1978.

Graham MA, Thompson SC, Estrada M, et al: Factors affecting psychological adjustment to a fetal death. Am J Obstet Gynecol 157:254, 1987.

Grollman EA: Explaining death to children. J School Health, June 1977, pp 336–339.

Grubb CA: Body image concerns of a multipara in the situation of intrauterine fetal death. Matern Child Nurs 5:93, 1976.

Helmrath TA, Steinitz EM: Death of an infant: parental grieving and the failure of social support. J Fam Pract 6:785, 1978.

Hollingsworth CE, Pasnau RO: The Family in Mourning: A Guide for Health Professionals. New York, Grune & Stratton, 1977.

Horowitz NH: Adolescent mourning reactions to infant and fetal loss. Soc Casework, November 1978, pp 551–559.

Jensen JS, Zahourek R: Depression in mothers who have lost a newborn. Rocky Mountain Med J 71:61, 1972.

Jolly H: Family reactions to stillbirth. Proc R Soc Med 69:835, 1976.

Kellner KR: Helping families who experience stillbirth. OB/GYN Reports 2:435, 1990.

Kellner KR, Donnelly WH, Gould SD: Parental behavior after perinatal death: lack of predictive variables. Obstet Gynecol 63:809, 1984.

Kellner KR, Kirkley-Best E, Chesborough S, et al: Perinatal mortality counseling program for families who experience a stillbirth. Death Educ 5:29, 1981.

Kennell JH, Trause MA: Helping parents cope with perinatal death. Contemp Ob/Gyn 12:53, 1978.

Kennell JH, Sylter H, Klaus MH: The mourning response of parents to the death of a newborn infant. N Engl J Med 283:344, 1970.

Kirkley-Best E: Grief in response to prenatal loss: an argument for the earliest maternal attachment. University of Florida (Gainesville), Doctoral Dissertation, 1981.

Kirkley-Best E, Kellner KR: Grief at stillbirth: an annotated bibliography. Birth Fam J 8:91, 1981.

Kirkley-Best E, Kellner KR: The forgotten grief: a review of the psychology of stillbirth. Am J Orthopsychiatry 52:420, 1982.

Kirkley-Best E, Kellner KR, Gould S, et al: On stillbirth: an open letter to the clergy. J Pastoral Care 36:17, 1982.

Kish G: Notes on C. Grubb's body image concerns of a multipara in the situation of intrauterine fetal death. Matern Child Nurs J 7:111, 1978.

Klaus M, Kennell J: Parent-Infant Bonding, 2nd ed. St Louis, CV Mosby Co, 1982.

Kotzwinkle W: Swimmer in the Secret Sea. New York, Avon Books, 1975.

Kowalski K, Bowes WA: Parents' response to a stillborn baby. Contemp Ob/Gyn 8:53, 1976.

LaGrua PM: Grieving responses of parents to the death of their newborn infant. University of Florida (Gainesville), Master's Thesis, 1979.

Lake MF, Johnson TM, Murphy J, et al: Evaluation of a perinatal grief support team. Am J Obstet Gynecol 157:1203, 1987.

Lake MF, Knuppel RA, Murphy J, et al: The role of a grief support team following stillbirth. Am J Obstet Gynecol 146:877, 1983.

Lamb JM: In Chez, R.: Symposium: Helping parents and doctors cope with perinatal death. Contemp Ob/Gyn 20:98, 1982.

LeBlanc RD: My baby can't be dead. Readers Digest, March 1982, pp 73–77.

Leon I: The invisible loss: the impact of perinatal death on siblings. J Psychosom Obstet Gynaecol 5:1, 1986.

Leon I: When A Baby Dies: Psychotherapy for Pregnancy and Newborn Loss. New Haven, Yale University Press, 1990.

Leppert PC, Pahlka BS: Grieving characteristics after spontaneous abortion: a management approach. Obstet Gynecol 64:119, 1984.

Lewis E: Reactions to stillbirth. In Psychosomatic Medicine in Obstetrics and Gynecology: Proceedings of Third International Congress, London, 1971. Basel, Karger, 1972, pp 323–325.

Lewis E: Comments. In Klaus MH, and Kennell JH: Parent-Infant Bonding, 2nd ed. St Louis, CV Mosby Co, 1982.

Lindemann E: Symptomatology and management of acute grief. Am J Psychiatr 101:141, 1944.

Lippman C, Carlson K: A Model Liaison Program for the Obstetrics Staff: Workshop on the Tragic Birth. In Hollingsworth CE, Pasnau RO (eds): The Family in Mourning: A Guide for Health Professionals. New York, Grune & Stratton, 1977, pp 17–28.

Lockwood S, Lewis IC: Management of grieving after stillbirth. Med J Aust 2:308, 1980.

Lovell A: Some questions of identity: late miscarriage, stillbirth and perinatal loss. Soc Sci Med 17:755, 1983.

Murray J, Callan VJ: Predicting adjustment to perinatal death. J Med Psych 61:237, 1988.

Niswander KR, Patterson RJ: Psychologic reaction to therapeutic abortion. Obstet Gynecol 29:702, 1967.

O'Donohue N: Perinatal bereavement: the role of the health care professional. QRB, 4:30, 1978.

Oglethorpe RJL: Parenting after perinatal bereavement—a review of the literature. J Reprod Infant Psych 7:227, 1989.

Parks CM: Bereavement: Studies of Grief in Adult Life. New York, International University Press, 1972, pp 13–26.

Peck A, Marcus H: Psychiatric sequelae of therapeutic interruption of pregnancy. J Nervous Mental Dis 143:417, 1966.

Peppers L, Knapp R: Motherhood and Mourning, New York, Praeger, 1980.

Queenan J: The ultimate defeat. (Letter from the Editor-in-Chief.) J Contemp Ob/Gyn 11:7, 1978a.

Queenan J: Never underestimate the help you can offer bereaved parents. (Letter from the Editor-in-Chief.) Contemp Ob/Gyn 12:9, 1978b.

Quirk TS: Crisis theory, grief theory and related psychosocial factors: the framework for intervention. J Nurse Midwife 24:13, 1979.

Rowe J, Clyman R, Green C, et al: Follow-up of families who experience a perinatal death. Pediatrics 62:166, 1978.

Schoenberg BM (ed): Bereavement Counseling. Westport, CT, Greenwood Press, 1980, pp 75–76.

Schowaiter J: Children and funerals. Pediatrics Rev 1:337, 1980.

Schreiner RH, Gresham EL, Green M: Physicians' responsibility to parents after death of an infant. Am J Dis Child 133:723, 1979.

Scupholme A: Who helps? Coping with the unexpected outcomes of pregnancy. JOGN Nurs 7:36, 1978.

Seibel M, Graves WL: The psychological implications of spontaneous abortions. J Reprod Med 25:161, 1980.

Seitz P, Warrick L: Perinatal death: the grieving mother. Am J Nurs 74:2028, 1974.

Simon NM, Senturia AG, Rothman D: Psychiatric illness following therapeutic abortion. Am J Psychiatry 124:97, 1967.

Stack J: Reproductive casualties. Perinatal Press 6:29, 1982.

Theut SK, Pedersen FA, Faslow MJ, et al: Perinatal loss and parental bereavement. Am J Psychiatry 146:635, 1989.

Toedter LJ, Lasher JN, Alhadeff JM: The perinatal grief scale: development and initial validation. Am J Orthopsychiatry 58:435, 1988.

Vital Statistics of the United States 1986, Vol II. Part A. DHHS Publ No (PHS) 88-1122. Washington, DC, United States Public Health Service, US Government Printing Office, 1988.

# CHAPTER 35

# The Nature of Lawsuits Related to Obstetric Care

Stuart Z. Grossman

In this chapter, those areas of obstetric care that engender the greatest number of medical negligence cases are reviewed. From my experience in dealing with medicolegal issues, I identify particular actions that physicians, nurses, and other hospital personnel can take to avoid serious legal consequences. Although some of these areas are controversial in regard to medical management, these recommendations are my opinions as to how the obstetric team can avoid lawsuits. It is not my intention to dictate management of the pregnant patient. The obstetric team should be aware of the constantly changing technology in the practice of obstetrics and should keep abreast of these changes because they reflect the national standards of patient care.

## Why Obstetrics Has One of The Highest Malpractice Litigation Rates

The obstetric health care team practices in what is perhaps the most emotionally charged area of medicine. The arrival of the newborn is anticipated as a moment of joy rarely equalled in life. For most mothers, pregnancy is the first period of long-term contact with a physician. The close attention paid to her health and the well-documented physical and emotional changes undergone during pregnancy cause her to feel deserving of a healthy baby. Anticipation builds with the expectation of a healthy baby.

The expectant father also has high hopes. He is relying on the medical profession to guide his wife through this period and feels, at times, awkward and helpless, yet proud and hopeful. The financial obligation that giving birth places on the father cannot be underestimated. In cases in which the mother has been working prior to birth, an interruption in her career is often regarded as a personal sacrifice despite the fact that the child may have been very much wanted. Expectant parents are knowledgeable consumers, expecting that the fees charged them by all of the health care providers involved will purchase appropriate care, often translated by the parents as a healthy baby.

Therefore, when an unhealthy baby arrives and joy turns to despair, an explanation is often asked of a lawyer if the health care team has not provided an explanation. The obstetric health care team is charged with the responsibility of practicing obstetrics within the accepted standard of care; its failure to do so often results in litigation. In an attempt to define these areas of litigation, the health care team should pay particular attention to the following areas of practice.

## Why Obstetricians Get Sued

### THE USE OF OXYTOCIN

The ground for litigation arising out of the use of oxytocin usually is divided into two categories: (1) the injudicious use of the drug and (2) the failure to appropriately monitor the patient during its administration.

Most of the cases involving the alleged negligent use of oxytocin occur when the obstetrician decides that oxytocin is needed to augment labor. However, arrest of labor is often an indication of a complication. Often, this potent medication, joined with the forces of labor, causes some of the worst neonatal injuries observed.

It is hoped that a labor curve indicates to the obstetrician his patient's condition and assists him or her in determining whether or not oxytocin should be used.

Continuous monitoring with electronic fetal monitoring can provide an accurate assessment of the maternal and fetal response to oxytocin. Frequency of assessment and documentation should meet national standards.

### ADVICE TO THE PRACTITIONER

Every labor should be graphed using a Friedman labor curve or an alternative uterine activity graphing method so that the decision to use oxytocin can be shown to be a judicious one.

Once the decision to use oxytocin is made, the nurse and the obstetrician in attendance should be aware of the fact that oxytocin may cause hyperstimulation, which may in turn cause uteroplacental insufficiency. Knowledge of these effects, which can be adverse to the fetus, mandates that appropriate monitoring be ordered and accomplished. The American College of Obstetricians and Gynecologists (ACOG, 1978) recommends that the physician be immediately available when oxytocin is used. This has been interpreted by some to mean that the physician be in the hospital or at least within 10 minutes of the hospital (Braun and Cefalo, 1983). Because it is well known that oxytocin can increase the duration, intensity, and frequency of uterine contractions and also elevate the baseline resting tone, internal electronic monitoring is mandated. External monitors, reliable only for measuring frequency and duration of contractions, are not deemed sufficient under these circumstances. Because oxytocin is used to augment a slow labor or to induce labor in high-risk patients, fetal heart rate changes can occur. Therefore, the internal fetal heart rate electrode should be used to most accurately observe the baseline, any decelerations, and any changes in the variability of the fetal heart rate. ACOG (1991) recommends "fetal heart rate and uterine contraction monitoring similar to that recommended for high risk patients in active labor."

Notwithstanding the revised AAP/ACOG Guidelines for Perinatal Care (1992), which allow the hospital to write its own policy on fetal assessment, the NAACOG Practice Resource (1988a) states "electronic fetal monitoring should be used for continuous recording of fetal heart rate and uterine activity" with oxytocin administration.

### ADVICE TO THE PRACTITIONER

Use of internal fetal monitoring during the administration of oxytocin is mandatory.

## DIFFICULT VAGINAL DELIVERY

Three examples of difficult vaginal deliveries that spawn litigation are midforceps, breech, and multiple births. Years ago, high-forceps deliveries were deleted from obstetric practice. Today, it has been shown that midforceps delivery can increase morbidity and mortality for the infant and cause trauma to the mother. In most cases in which the infant cannot deliver spontaneously or by outlet (low) forceps, cesarean delivery is a safer alternative, especially for the infant.

### ADVICE TO THE PRACTITIONER

(1) Beware of midforceps or difficult forceps deliveries.

(2) After delivery, make a careful, complete record of what was done and why it was done.

Some routine uses of cesarean delivery are being re-evaluated. One such circumstance is some breech presentations. Breech deliveries are associated with an increased risk of perinatal morbidity and mortality, even for skilled obstetricians. When cesarean delivery is used for premature breech deliveries, a low-vertical uterine incision is most practical to ensure safe delivery of the after-coming head.

### ADVICE TO THE PRACTITIONER

(1) Be sure of the presenting part prior to or in early labor. If there is a question, get an ultrasound or x-ray study.

(2) Avoid vaginal breech delivery.

(3) Use a low-vertical uterine incision in cesarean delivery for breech presentations in the premature and term infant in which the lower uterine segment is not well developed.

With multiple births, most commonly twins, litigation concerning damage to the second baby is becoming increasingly common. Usually, the cause is either traumatic vaginal delivery or abruption of the placenta after delivery of the first infant.

ADVICE TO THE PRACTITIONER

Consider cesarean delivery when you are aware of multiple births. Recognize multiple births whenever possible, using ultrasound in pregnancy either routinely or whenever clinical conditions suggest a multiple pregnancy.

Vaginal birth after cesarean delivery (VBAC) is being encouraged under certain circumstances. These include previous low-transverse cesarean deliveries, especially those performed for nonrepeating indications such as fetal distress, malpresentation, or both in the previous pregnancy. Nevertheless, adherence to a strict VBAC protocol can be hazardous legally. Uterine rupture can occur, and hence, the delivery team must be prepared to deal with this anticipated complication. In planning a VBAC, therefore, flexibility is the key.

## CHOICE OF ANESTHESIA

Traditionally, obstetricians took comfort in thinking that the choice of anesthesia and any untoward results would be the responsibility of the anesthesiologist. However, the lines of liability have merged, and an obstetrician can and will be held liable for the choice of anesthesia even though an anesthesiologist administers the drug and approves the decision. Specifically, general anesthesia has a significant risk for the pregnant patient, because the second leading cause of maternal death is aspiration during general anesthesia. This fatal complication can occur even with a skilled anesthesiologist. If general anesthesia is used, intubation of the pregnant patient is mandatory.

ADVICE TO THE PRACTITIONER

(1) Know the propensities of anesthesia, and choose the safest method for cesarean delivery dictated by circumstances.

(2) Avoid general anesthesia whenever regional anesthesia can safely and skillfully be administered.

## ATTENDANCE

Owing to the unpredictable events of birthing, physicians have been known to miss the labor and delivery of patients. Often, and unrealistically, a high level of responsibility is placed on the labor nurse to provide coverage for the absent obstetrician. If a disaster occurs, a lawsuit follows.

ADVICE TO THE PRACTITIONER

The obstetrician has a legal duty to attend to his or her patient. If attendance is impossible, coverage is mandatory. An organized group practice should be seriously considered to provide this coverage. It is best for an obstetrician to be present during labor.

## RESUSCITATION

Every obstetrician has had the experience of delivering a child with an Apgar score of 8 or higher who later turns blue somewhere between the delivery room and the nursery. Although most hospitals do not have a pediatrician in attendance at the time of the delivery, the obstetrician should remain in attendance until the newborn is safely situated in the nursery or until a pediatrician is with the infant. Should a neonatologist be available through the hospital, it is recommended that the obstetrician freely use his or her services.

If a problem is noted before delivery, it is a standard of care to request the presence of a pediatrician or resuscitation team at the delivery. Many salvageable newborns are further damaged by inappropriate resuscitation, especially (1) by not using a DeLee suction when meconium is present, as the the fetal head delivers on the perineum (or through the uterine incision) before the chest is delivered, and (2) bagging the infant before suctioning has occurred.

ADVICE TO THE PRACTITIONER

(1) Stay with the newborn after birth.

(2) If there are any indications that a medical complication will arise with this newborn prior to birth, make arrangements for a neonatologist, pediatrician, or resuscitation team to attend the delivery.

(3) The baby is your patient also and must not be abandoned. Develop a good working relationship with the anesthesiologist or nurse anesthetist and establish a role for each of you when resuscitation is needed.

(4) When meconium is present, use a DeLee suction with delivery of the head.

(5) Always suction the infant before bagging is begun.

## PROLONGED LABOR

The labor graph (discussed previously in conjunction with oxytocin) is a great source of information that protects the obstetrician.

Because labor is a stress test for the baby, the internal monitor used in conjunction with the labor graph is an excellent way to follow the progress of the fetus and the mother.

### ADVICE TO THE PRACTITIONER

Get in the habit of using a labor graph, and become proficient at interpreting internal electronic fetal monitoring tracings. If your hospital has internal fetal monitoring available and you are not using it, you may encounter legal difficulties. The recognition and treatment of labor problems are important ways to prevent unwanted results.

## SHOULDER DYSTOCIA

Cases of shoulder dystocia have emerged as a leading cause of malpractice suits. Obstetricians must avoid predisposing factors such as the injudicious use of oxytocin in patients with arrested labor, due to cephalopelvic disproportion, and difficult forceps deliveries. In addition, obstetricians should have a careful management plan, maneuver by maneuver, to avoid excessive downward traction on the fetal head, which can injure the brachial plexus. One often ignored maneuver that may result in successful delivery of the anterior shoulder is the McRoberts' procedure followed by manual suprapubic pressure. If this method is also unsuccessful, the posterior arm should be delivered first. The nurse should recognize that fundal pressure is inappropriate in this situation and can further impact the anterior shoulder. Nurses should assist with the McRoberts' procedure and suprapubic pressure.

The obstetrician should dictate a detailed summary of how he or she managed the problem, not just that there was shoulder dystocia. This way, if his or her management was proper and the infant still sustained a brachial plexus injury, it can be defended better, because in some cases of severe shoulder dystocia, these brachial plexus injuries cannot be avoided.

### ADVICE TO THE PRACTITIONER

(1) Be mindful of predisposing factors; that is, try not to use oxytocin in patients in whom an arrest in the active phase of labor may be due to cephalopelvic disproportion, and avoid difficult forceps deliveries.

(2) Have a logical plan for management of shoulder dystocia, and perform it system-

atically, keeping in mind the McRoberts' maneuver, if needed.

(3) Avoid excessive downward traction of the fetal head.

(4) After the delivery, chart what you did in careful, well-organized detail.

## FETAL MONITORING

The fetal monitor should be used to assess fetal status during labor. Not only can it alert you to problems but it can reassure you that the fetus is doing well. If an electronic monitor is not used, be certain that auscultation of the fetal heart rate is performed properly and documented every 15 to 30 minutes in the first stage of labor and, more frequently, every 5 to 15 minutes in the second stage. Listening for the fetal heart rate should take place through several contractions. Palpation of contractions through several contractions is necessary to assess uterine activity properly. Palpation is also necessary when using the tocotransducer and should be documented.

### ADVICE TO THE PRACTITIONER

(1) Auscultate appropriately when electronic monitoring is not used.

(2) Use external monitoring when problems are not apparent, and do not rely on variability in this mode.

(3) Use internal monitoring when any problems with the fetal heart rate or contractions are apparent.

(4) Become proficient at interpretation of fetal heart rate tracings.

(5) Continue fetal monitoring in the delivery or operating room.

## CHARTING

The patient's chart is a legal document; just as important, the patient's chart documents the reasoning or rationale for the many obstetric decisions that are made. During labor, the obstetrician must chart his or her own examinations and write progress notes. Likewise, nurses must chart their own observations and actions thoroughly. The patient's chart should be completed at the conclusion of each office visit and reviewed before it is sent to the hospital to be available in the labor and delivery suite prior to the patient's arrival.

## ADVICE TO THE PRACTITIONER

The chart tells you the whole story and either supports you or condemns you if your judgment and care are questioned. It must be understood by nurses who are going to assist you in the labor and delivery process. Never, under any circumstances, change your chart once it has come into issue in a legal forum. Even if there is a basis for making a change, you will appear guilty. If changes need to be made during documentation, draw a single line through the error, and date and initial it. Rewrite the correct information.

## APPROPRIATE PRENATAL TESTING

The obstetrician should be aware of the increased use of maternal serum alpha-fetoprotein testing and amniocentesis and recommend these to all appropriate obstetric patients. Information on its use in screening chromosomal defects and other abnormalities should be available to all prospective parents, regardless of their age, if they elect additional screening.

In regard to the recognition of problems during pregnancy, patients must be observed carefully for any high-risk problems. If the mother becomes high risk, she should be observed more frequently, and appropriate tests, such as ultrasound and nonstress and contraction stress tests, should be performed.

### ADVICE TO THE PRACTITIONER

Although some tests are routine, stay alert to the clinical signs. Attempt to treat each patient individually by taking enough time to listen to her, and follow up on her complaints, which are often subtle. Follow up complications appropriately.

## SHOULD THIS PROCEDURE BE PERFORMED IN THE HOSPITAL?

A recent trend in all medical fields is the increased use of the medical office for many medical procedures previously performed in a hospital. Along with this convenience comes the concomitant responsibility to the patient should an untoward event occur. If a decision has been made not to perform a procedure in the hospital, be certain that your office is equipped with appropriate resuscitation facilities. Personnel must be educated for new procedures, such as the reading of a nonstress test or an ultrasound. Information regarding a contraction stress test or more sophisticated ultrasound could be missed owing to the level of the technician's education. The practitioner should be familiar with the limitations that a hospital has with respect to set-up time, operating room personnel, recovery room facilities, anesthesia service, ultrasound, and all other items that may be needed routinely as well as in an emergency.

### ADVICE TO THE PRACTITIONER

You are responsible for knowing what is available in your medical community. Because you are responsible for ordering tests, be sure that you advise patients where these tests can be completed so that they can make arrangements in advance. Be conscious of the time it takes for your hospital to set up for emergency procedures, and always leave a margin of safety so that patients can receive the treatment they need at the hospital in a timely fashion. Finally, recognize the limitations of your office and your office staff in determining whether or not procedures should be performed there.

## PRETERM LABOR

Recently, litigation surrounding the failure to diagnose preterm labor has increased. Symptoms such as vaginal bleeding, contractions, and low back pain must alert the obstetrician to the possible onset of preterm labor. Having considered this diagnosis, the physician should manage the patient conservatively, including recommending bed rest, and if she is managed as an outpatient, home monitoring should be performed by a reputable home health care agency. The patient should be made aware of the importance of communicating all symptoms to the obstetrician, the home health care attending nurse, or both.

### ADVICE TO THE PRACTITIONER

It is incumbent on the attending obstetrician to be alert to preterm labor and to make available to the patient a treatment plan that may include home monitoring of the uterus. The practitioner must be sure to communicate with the home health care nurse about the patient's ongoing condition.

# Why Obstetric Nurses Get Sued

The law no longer accepts the legal proposition that the nurse is a mere servant to the physician. The nurse, unlike most physicians, is an employee of the hospital and is responsible to the hospital. The hospital assumes responsibility for the actions of the nurse. Thus, if a nurse is negligent, he or she can be sued independently and the hospital can be sued for the actions of its employee (vicarious liability).

Today, the nurse is specialized and must attain the requisite level of knowledge and education for use in daily practice. With so many coexisting levels of nursing, from the technician to the clinical specialist, the level of practice can vary considerably. It should be clear that any patients at risk should be attended by a registered nurse. This is especially true in the labor and delivery areas. At the present time, many hospitals provide exclusively registered nurse coverage for their labor and delivery areas, because these have become intensive care areas where changes in even normal patients can occur quickly and proper assessment is essential. Nevertheless, nurses who should be practicing appropriately in the following areas of knowledge and expertise are frequently being sued for deficiencies.

## CHARTING

If it is true that the chart is the documentation of antepartum management, labor and delivery progress, and postpartum recovery, then it must follow that an incomplete chart is an indication of incomplete nursing care. With unfortunate frequency, charts left incomplete or blank in important areas provide an opportunity for the creation of an unwanted scenario. Items such as frequency of vital signs, labor progress, treatments and medications given, and notations of notifications to physicians are important in terms of satisfying national standards and are uniformly demanded within individual institutions.

A nurse is not faulted for caring for a patient and then completing the chart after the delivery has been accomplished or the complication resolved. Temporary nursing notes, which are later translated into a complete chart, are acceptable when the chart is not readily available.

### ADVICE TO THE OBSTETRIC NURSE

Consider the chart the best evidence of what you did for the patient. Be sure your observations and actions are charted. If you did something for the patient and it is not charted, the assumption in court will probably be that it was not done.

## TAKING VITAL SIGNS

The assumption that nurses are responsible for taking vital signs of patients and correlating these signs with the patient's underlying conditions (or certainly reporting the vital signs to a physician if they are troubling) is a cornerstone of a nurses's duties to the patient and, hence, a cornerstone of that nurse's legal liability. The sources that a patient's attorney uses to determine whether or not the vital signs were taken with appropriate frequency are the hospital's, clinic's, and office's own regulations and national standards. Yet, a surprising number of nurses remain unaware of these requirements concerning vital signs.

### ADVICE TO THE OBSTETRIC NURSE

Be certain that you are aware of your hospital's regulations and national standards concerning the taking (and charting) of vital signs. Do not be lulled into skipping the taking of vital signs because the patient appears to be stable.

## THE IDENTIFICATION OF HIGH-RISK PATIENTS

The identification of high-risk patients is often the responsibility of the nurse *because the high-risk status does not appear until the patient has begun labor.* Frequently, the physician is not in attendance at that time, and it may take him or her a while to arrive at the hospital. Unfortunately, sometimes patients become high risk and have relatively subtle signs. This is, of course, another reason for diligence in monitoring both the mother and the fetus. Knowledge of the predisposing factors and subtle signs of high-risk pregnancy and the appropriate treatment is a standard to which every nurse is held responsible.

## ADVICE TO THE OBSTETRIC NURSE

Know what constitutes a high-risk patient. If in doubt, ask a fellow nurse for assistance in making the diagnosis. Communicate this to the attending obstetrician as soon as possible, and recommend that he or she come to the hospital, clinic, or office if he or she is not there to see the patient. Chart your communication. Do not hesitate to ask the advice of another physician if the patient's own physician is unavailable. Finally, be sure that the person who attends a high-risk patient is a registered nurse and not a licensed practical nurse.

## FETAL MONITORING

The hospital purchases fetal monitoring equipment with the intention that it be used. Its very existence within the labor and delivery suite mandates that it be used properly. This, of course, means that electronic fetal monitoring tracings should be evaluated appropriately by the attending nurse and that this nurse should have the knowledge to undertake treatment, when necessary. A nurse should not hesitate to call on another nurse for consultation if there is any difficulty in interpreting the fetal tracing. Once any type of nonreassuring pattern is recognized, the attending obstetrician should be notified immediately and treatment instituted.

Unfortunately, not all physicians are experienced in electronic fetal monitoring, and some avoid the use of these monitors because of their lack of experience. Most hospitals have policies concerning when electronic fetal monitoring should be used, such as in conjunction with the use of oxytocin. However, it is imperative that the patient's well-being have the highest priority; therefore, the physician should be encouraged to allow the nurse to use the monitor. If the monitor is not used, specific procedures for auscultation should be used (see Chapter 18).

The fetal heart rate tracing is a permanent part of the patient's chart and should be treated as such. It should be retrievable.

The placement of the fetal heart rate electrode and intrauterine catheter by nurses is a subject of some dispute. Some institutions permit this, and some do not. Certainly, this should be attempted only if the nurse has been educated and certified in its placement. NAACOG (1981) recommendations stated

that certified nurses could place the electrode but not the catheter. However, later NAACOG (1986) recommendations state that the qualified nurse can apply any of the fetal monitoring appliances. The 1981 NAACOG standards stated that nurses could not rupture membranes, but this statement has been removed in the 1986 NAACOG standards. However, the NAACOG (1988b) states that nurses should not rupture membranes. The state Nurse Practice Acts regulate their procedures, usually with broad statements that cover certified procedures. However, in some states, Nurse Practice Acts disallow the placement of electrodes and catheters by nurses. In any event, if electronic fetal monitoring is mandatory, then the nurse must aggressively pursue the attending physician if he or she is responsible for attaching this electrode. It is suggested that the tracings be reviewed periodically by the nursing staff together with the physicians and that unique patterns be discussed freely and openly. Quality improvement is also a good way to investigate problem outcomes.

## ADVICE TO THE OBSTETRIC NURSE

(1) Labor nurses should be able to interpret fetal monitor tracings and treat nonreassuring patterns.

(2) Know how the fetal monitor functions and how to interpret tracings and continuously update your knowledge and the knowledge of your colleagues by reviewing these tracings.

(3) Know the limitations of your state Nurse Practice Act and how it affects your practice.

(4) Document tracing interpretation treatments and outcomes.

(5) Use quality improvement to evaluate adverse outcomes.

## THE NURSE AS A PATIENT ADVOCATE—AVOIDING FETAL OR MATERNAL INJURY

This is currently the most sensitive area of litigation. The obstetrician used to be considered the "captain of the ship." It was his or her choice to attend or not attend the patient and his or her exclusive responsibility to make certain diagnoses. The ultimate responsibility for the pregnancy's outcome rested with the physician. This concept is now treated in the law like high-risk forceps are treated in obstetrics: it is obsolete. Specialization among nurses is established and recognized (particularly in the fields of labor and delivery and neonatology nursing), and the level of knowledge that the nurse is required to attain is significantly higher than in the past. Concomitant with this level of knowledge is the fact that the nurse is expected to communicate any untoward findings promptly so that fetal or maternal injury can be prevented. What does the nurse do when the obstetrician is not appropriately handling a situation or, perhaps, not even attending to a situation? There is always the chain-of-command. It should be the hospital's responsibility to provide a clear chain-of-command policy for nurses to follow, when necessary. The hospital should encourage nurses to follow the policy without fear of penalty. If the nurse's assessments are inappropriate, then he or she should be educated appropriately.

In an emergency, however, the nurse may have to go to any source that is available to help the patient. The nurse has a duty, as the patient's advocate, to be certain that the requisite standard of care is carried out.

### ADVICE TO THE OBSTETRIC NURSE

Labor nurses should be assertive when they are in a situation in which fetal or maternal injury could occur. The chain-of-command should be used, but if it is not working in time to help the patient, then it should be abandoned and the patient's interests should receive top priority. The role of the nurse as a patient advocate is the modern trend in law; defense by the "captain of the ship" theory is outmoded.

## INDUCTION OF LABOR

National standards and hospital regulations often differ as to whether or not nurses can begin the induction of labor without the presence of the attending obstetrician. Indeed, questions concerning the management of the intravenous administration of oxytocin are also often left unresolved. Each nurse should be aware of the NAACOG standards and the regulations of the hospital where he or she works before attempting to induce labor, change the intravenous flow of oxytocin, or both. Obviously, along with this, a complete and thorough working knowledge of the propensities of oxytocin must be obtained, including the only appropriate route of administration, which is the intravenous route. (Please see previous discussion with respect to the use of electronic fetal monitoring in conjunction with oxytocin.)

### ADVICE TO THE OBSTETRIC NURSE

Complete knowledge of the use of oxytocin involves not only the propensities of the drug but conjunctive use of monitoring and the treatment of oxytocin-induced complications. Chart the dose of oxytocin in milli-units per minutes and know the appropriate dose and when to increase and stop it.

## RESUSCITATION

Frequently, babies are born in need of resuscitation; with even more frequency, pediatricians are not in attendance. This often can be avoided by notifying the pediatrician or resuscitation team when the first signs of fetal distress appear. Once they have been called, the nurse should be alert to their timely arrival. More than one notification may be necessary if delivery is about to occur and they have not arrived yet. The obstetrician is attending to the mother, and when the need for resuscitation arises, it is the labor and delivery nurse who is left to carry out resuscitation if the pediatrician or resuscitation team has not arrived. Therefore, resuscitation should be learned and practiced with skill by each nurse who may be called on to resuscitate an infant. Resuscitation mandates that an orderly procedure take place and that management be documented on the chart. If a physician's assistance is required or is available, then an orderly system by which resuscitation is carried out that defines the role of each individual involved is necessary. Those not directly involved in resuscitation should assist by notifying a pediatrician and making whatever other arrangements are necessary.

### ADVICE TO THE OBSTETRIC AND NEONATAL NURSE

Learn how to resuscitate an infant and develop a system by which the resuscitation will be carried out in an orderly fashion, including the call for assistance and transfer of the infant, when necessary.

## MULTIPLE RESPONSIBILITIES

With the advent of the LDRP programs that are currently in vogue at hospitals, an obstetric nurse must be qualified in the labor room, delivery room, nursery, and postpartum areas. Because hospitals provide this service that is attractive to the pregnant consumer, more nurses are being cross-trained in all areas. The nurse must be aware of the fact that he or she is going to be legally responsible for practicing adequate and standard nursing in each of these areas. These multiple responsibilities must be met by adequate education and cross-training in these areas.

### ADVICE TO THE OBSTETRIC AND NEWBORN NURSE

Recognize that you have strengths in some areas and weaknesses in others so that when you are called to perform as a nurse in an LDRP, you have taken all necessary steps to be trained in these areas to fully, adequately, and safely perform your duties. Resist the temptation to treat a patient in an area in which you are not fully qualified; let your supervisor or administrator know of your areas of weakness and your willingness to be trained to better serve your patients.

## STAFFING

Hospital nurses and auxiliary staff are sometimes not optimal for the care of patients. This is particularly true in labor and delivery, in which the number of patients can fluctuate greatly even within a 24-hour period. It is often difficult to pull nurses experienced in labor and delivery from another floor. Often, the absence of a ward clerk or an aide can justify the placement of another nurse on the unit. "On call" staffing from within the department can be very helpful in solving this problem. One small hospital in Florida has its entire labor and delivery staff "on call." When labor patients come to the hospital, the nurse is called in and stays with the patient. Therefore, nurses are not in the hospital when there are no laboring patients and adequate staff is available when needed. Trained casual pool staff can also expand staffing when it is necessary.

### ADVICE TO THE OBSTETRIC NURSE

Do not abandon your patients because of lack of staffing. Your help is better than no help. Document the lack of staffing to the hospital supervisor to avoid further problems.

# Liability of Clinicians and Educators

Clinicians and nurse practitioners are expected to have more knowledge and experience than staff nurses, and their practice should reflect this advanced knowledge. Therefore, clinicians and nurse practitioners should take an active part in writing appropriate policies and procedures for the obstetric units to maintain optimal standard patient care. Educators should be active in preparing the staff for new policies and procedures as well as maintaining current policies and procedures. Obstetric educators should be responsible for the orientation of new employees. They should assess these new employees, who should not be allowed to practice independently until they are ready.

Nurse practitioners and clinicians also take on a more independent practice than a staff nurse. However, if there are any questions regarding patient care, they must defer to the physicians or follow the chain-of-command. However, educator, clinician, and nurse practitioner litigation rarely has been observed.

### ADVICE TO EDUCATORS; CLINICIANS, AND NURSE PRACTITIONERS

Keep the staff well informed with educational programs. Provide current policies and procedures. Practice within the nurse's scope.

It is hoped that this discussion is a practical tool for the health care provider to use in the obstetric setting. Our emphasis is the avoidance of malpractice.

**Acknowledgment**

The author is greatly indebted to Charles Kalstone, M.D., of Coral Gables, Florida, for his invaluable assistance in updating the original version of this text and is belatedly thanked for his efforts in the creation of the original chapter that appeared in the first edition of this text. Acknowledgment is given to J. B. Spence, JD, for his contribution to the first edition.

# References

ACOG: Induction-Augmentation of Labor. ACOG Technical Bulletin No 157, July, 1991.

ACOG: Intrapartum Fetal Heart Rate Monitoring. ACOG Technical Bulletin No 132, September, 1989.

ACOG/NAACOG: Electronic Fetal Monitoring. Joint statement by ACOG/NAACOG Task Force Committee, March, 1986.

American Academy of Pediatrics (AAP) and ACOG: Guidelines for Perinatal Care, 3rd edition, 1992.

Braun A Jr, Cefalo R (eds): Guidelines for Perinatal Care. Washington, DC: AAP and ACOG, 1983.

Clark DM: Oxytocin Guidelines (collective letters). International Correspondence Society of Obstetricians/Gynecologists 24(9):66–69, 1983.

Frigoletto F, Little G: Guidelines for Perinatal Care, 2nd ed. Washington, DC: ACOG/AAP, 1988.

Gilfix MG: Electronic fetal monitoring: physician liability and informed consent. Am J Law Med 10(1):31, 1984.

Isil OA: Legal Risks and Perinatal Health Care. NAACOG Update Series, Lesson 13, Vol 1, 1984.

NAACOG: (Practice Resource) Fetal Heart Rate Auscultation, March, 1990.

NAACOG: The nurse's role in the induction/augmentation of labor, January, 1988a.

NAACOG: Standards for the Nursing Care of Women and Newborns, 4th edition, 1991.

NAACOG: Statement on "Nursing responsibilities in implementing intrapartum fetal heart rate monitoring," 1988b.

NAACOG: Practice Competencies and Educational Guidelines for Nurse Providers of Intrapartum Care, 1988c.

NAACOG: Obstetric, Gynecologic, and Neonatal Nursing Functions and Standards, 1986.

NAACOG: Obstetric, Gynecologic, and Neonatal Nursing Functions and Standards, 1981.

NAACOG: The Nurse's Role in Electronic Fetal Monitoring. NAACOG Technical Bulletin No 7, July 1980.

Parke, Davis & Co: "Pitocin." Morris Plains, NJ, 1979.

Shane J: Medical-legal ramifications of difficult labor and delivery. Clin Perinatol 8:3, 1981.

Wiley J: The nurse's legal responsibility in obstetrical monitoring. J Obstet Gynecol Neonatal Nurs 5:5 (Suppl), 1976.

# Index

Note: Page numbers in *italics* refer to illustrations; page numbers followed by t refer to tables.

**743**